THE ILLUSTRATED
ENCYCLOPEDIA OF

Healing
Remedies

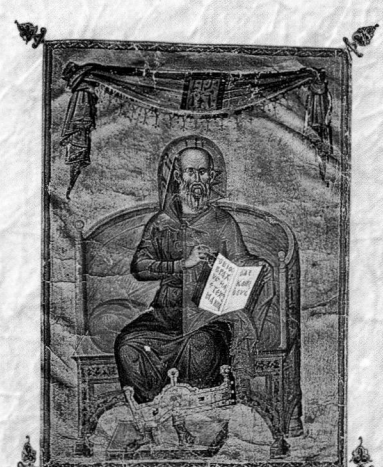

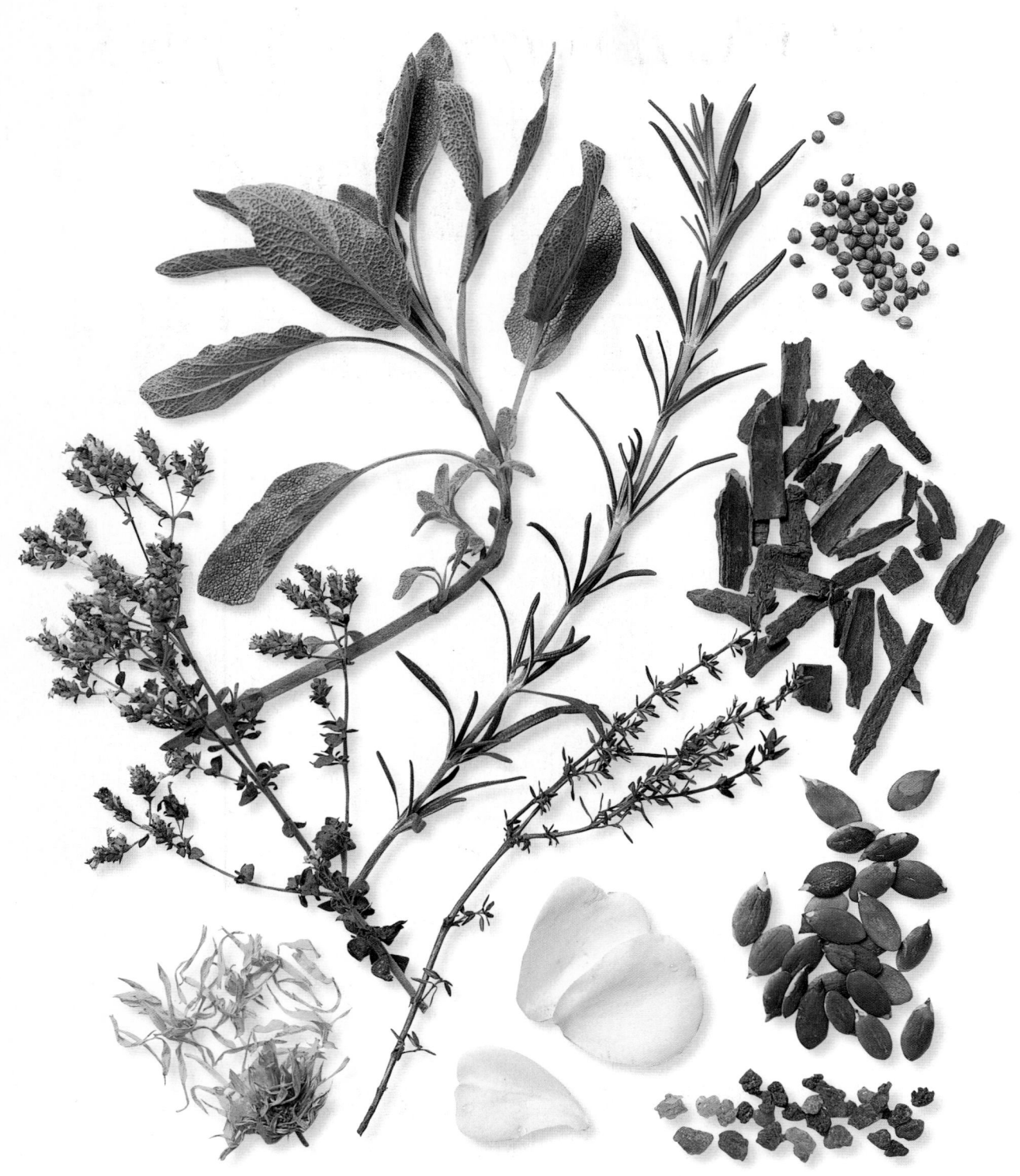

THE ILLUSTRATED
ENCYCLOPEDIA OF
Healing
Remedies

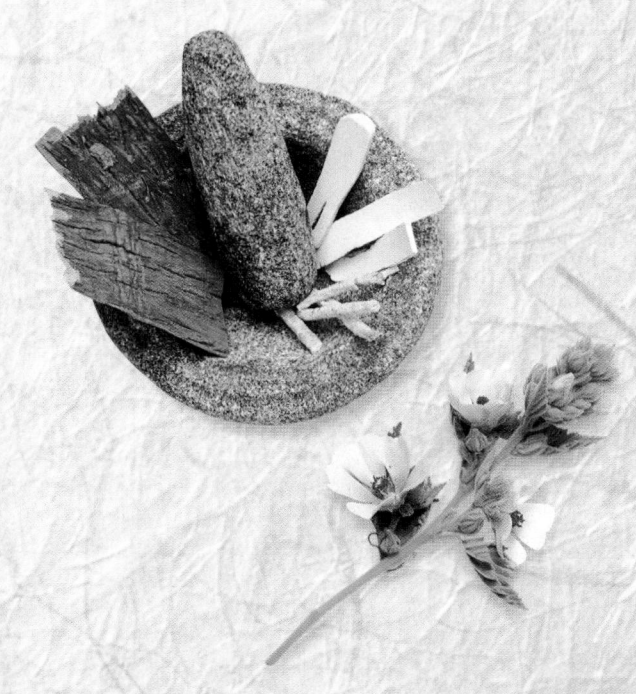

C. NORMAN SHEALY
M.D., Ph.D.

ELEMENT

Shaftesbury, Dorset • Boston, Massachusetts • Melbourne, Victoria

© Element Books Limited 1998

First published in Great Britain in 1998 by
ELEMENT BOOKS LIMITED
Shaftesbury, Dorset, SP7 8BP

Published in the USA in 1998 by
ELEMENT BOOKS INC
160 North Washington Street, Boston, MA 02114

Published in Australia in 1998 by
ELEMENT BOOKS
and distributed by Penguin Australia Ltd
487 Maroondah Highway, Ringwood, Victoria 3134

NOTE FROM THE PUBLISHER
Any information given in this book is not intended
to be taken as a replacement for medical advice.
Any person with a condition requiring medical attention
should consult a qualified practitioner or therapist.

Editor in Chief **C. Norman Shealy** M.D., Ph.D.
General Editor **Karen Sullivan**

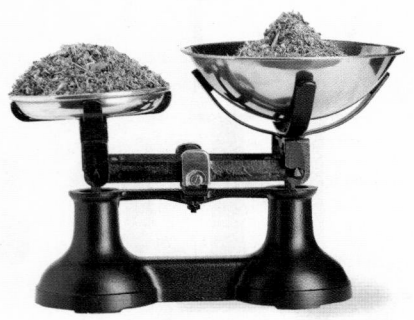

Designed and created with
THE BRIDGEWATER BOOK COMPANY LIMITED

ELEMENT BOOKS LIMITED
Editorial Director Julia McCutchen
Managing Editor Miranda Spicer
Editor Katie Worrall
Production Director Roger Lane
Production Sarah Golden

THE BRIDGEWATER BOOK COMPANY
Art Director Terry Jeavons
Designers Jane Lanaway, Glyn Bridgewater
Page layout John Christopher, Richard Constable,
Chris Lanaway, Andrew Lawes, Angela Neal,
Michael Whitehead, and Ginny Zeal
Managing Editor Anne Townley
Picture research Vanessa Fletcher
Three-dimensional models Mark Jamieson
Studio photography Guy Ryecart, Ian Parsons
Illustrations Michael Courtney, Lorraine Harrison,
Ivan Hissey, Mainline Design

Repro by
Appletone Graphics Ltd., Bournemouth, England

Printed and bound in Italy by
Graphicom

British Library Cataloguing in Publication
data available

Library of Congress Cataloging in Publication
data available

ISBN 1–86204–187–3 HB

ISBN 1–86204–516–X PB

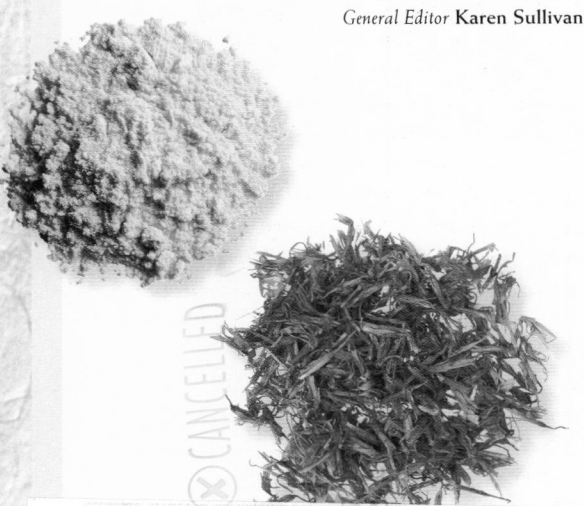

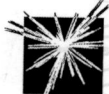

ACKNOWLEDGMENTS

The publishers wish to thank the following for the use of pictures:

A–Z BOTANICAL pp. 28T, 32BR, 33TR, 79TR, 92TL, 97C, 116CL, 132BR, 183TR, 184TR, 203BL, 229TL, 229TR, 230CL, 232TR, 239TL, 239TR, 240TL, 241T

AUSTRALIAN BUSH ESSENCES pp. 230BL, 230TR, 231TR. 238TL. 240BL

C. W. DANIEL PUBLISHERS pp. 141CR, 141BR

BRIDGEMAN ART LIBRARY pp. 2, 78

e.t.archive pp. 18–19

GARDEN PICTURE LIBRARY pp. 41CL, 107TL, 153CR, 16TL, 185CR, 197TR, 213B, 218BL, 222TL, 22BR, 225TR, 233TL

HARRY SMITH pp. 33C, 152CL

HOUSES AND INTERIORS p. 93CR

HUTCHISON PICTURE LIBRARY pp. 68BL, 70B, 105BR, 189B, 190BL

IMAGE BANK pp. 18TL, 18BL, 80BL, 291TR

NATURAL HISTORY PHOTOGRAPHIC AGENCY: pp. 99BR, 199L, 216B

OXFORD SCIENTIFIC FILMS pp. 188TL, 176T

SCIENCE PHOTO LIBRARY pp. 75L, 184B, 196CR, 277BR, 390TL, 341BR, 398TL, 424, 448TR

WELEDA UK LTD, manufacturers of homeopathic remedies pp. 174TL, 174CL, 174BL,

ZEFA pp. 10BL, 10/11, 11TR, 18CL, 34BL, 40TL, 45CB, 47BL, 50T, 51BL, 58TL, 69T, 74C, 75R 77B, 78/79, 88T, 95BL, 105TL, 105BC, 108CL, 141TR, 155TL, 168BR, 174TR, 193TL, 197BL, 201TR, 207C, 210/211, 212BL, 214T, 215CR, 228BR, 237TL, 237TR, 242TR, 242BR, 244/245, 261T, 266CR, 267T, 276TL, 287T, 307, 324L, 330TR, 335BR, 391, 417TR, 427, 439

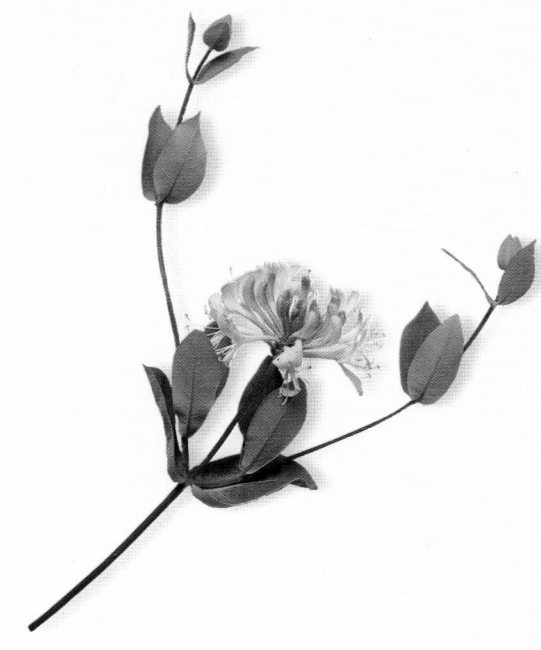

SPECIAL THANKS TO

Maria Anderson, Philip Auchinvole, Tony Bannister, Jan Boyle, Glyn Bridgewater, Stephanie Brotherstone, Deena Bunn, Kimberley Bunn, Adam Carne, Rob Chappell, Judith Cox, Naomi Denny, Juliette Denny, Nina Downey, Rebecca Drury, Cathy Glendinning, Paul Golding, Rachel Gould, Paul Harley, Deborah Heath, Julia Holden, Simon Holden, Natalie Jerome, Carolyn Jikeimi-Roberts, Mette Lauritzen, Jan Lewington, Kay Macmullan, Jack Martin, Jim McClean, Norma McClean, Henry Milne, Helen Omand, Elin Osmond, Wendy Oxberry, Sunny Pitcher, Caron Riley, Vincent Riley, Warren Saunders, Michelle Sawyer, Stephen Sparshatt, Sarah Stanley, Andrew Stemp, Neil Strowger, Jenny Sullivan, Bethany Sword, Lauren Sword, Sheila Sword, Gav Tuffnell, Mary Watson, Derek Watts, Louise Williams, Robert Williams.

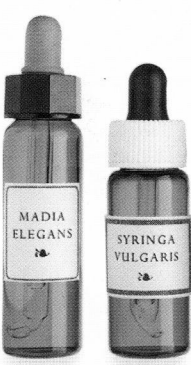

MADIA ELEGANS

SYRINGA VULGARIS

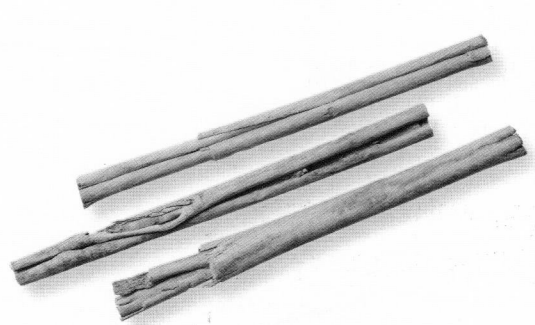

CONTENTS

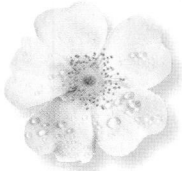

FOREWORD 8
INTRODUCTION 10
HOW TO USE THIS BOOK 14

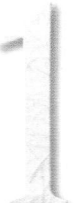

PART ONE

THERAPIES AND HEALING
REMEDY SOURCES

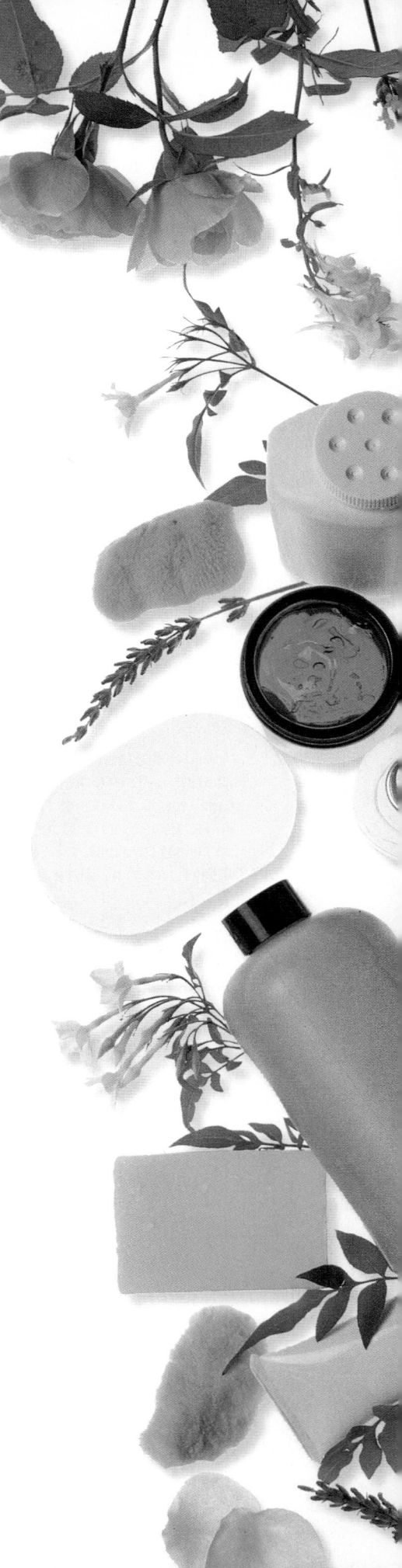

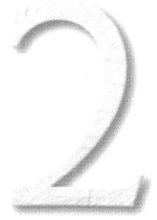

PART TWO

TREATING COMMON AILMENTS

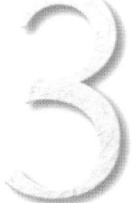

PART THREE

REFERENCE SECTION

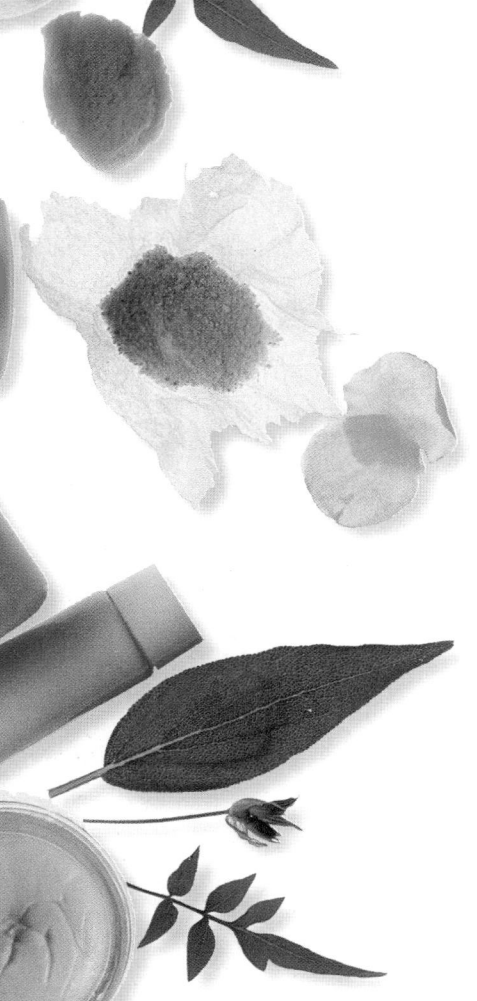

FOREWORD

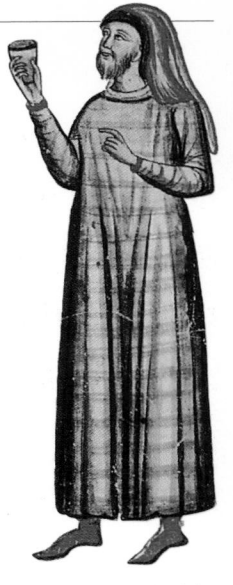

THE "FATHER OF MEDICINE" is generally considered to be Hippocrates, who was born around 460 B.C.E. on the island of Cos, and died around 370 B.C.E. The body of work that is attributed to Hippocrates consists of 79 books and 59 treatises on which modern medicine is said to be founded. It is particularly interesting that a great deal of his writing addresses the role model of the physician — he should look healthy and well-nourished, wear decent clothes, and have a degree of friendliness. Other than that, the most consistent commentary is on attention to anatomical detail, and precautions about the limitations of therapy, especially surgery.

ABOVE *The role of the physician was central to the work of Hippocrates who is considered to be the founder of modern medicine.*

In terms of theory, modern medicine dates from the work of Hippocrates, although the history of natural therapy extends back to long before his time. From those early days in Greece, two major schools of thought have dominated Western medicine — on the one hand rationalism, and on the other empiricism. Essentially the rationalists believe that science can ultimately know all the answers about life, and even create it. The "success" of recent experiments into cloning has certainly appeared to give credence to this view. In contrast, empiricists, or naturalists, believe in the ineffable quality of the universe, the natural order of life, and a concept of the divine, or vital force. Interestingly, empiricism has been embraced to a greater extent by the general public and rationalism by the Western medical society. Individuals seem to feel much more at home with a way of understanding health and disease that relies on sensory input and personal experience.

ABOVE *Eastern philosophy is based on a belief in wholeness which is at odds with much of Western thinking about medicine.*

The dramatic increase in popularity of Ayurveda and Chinese Medicine in the West can be seen as a return to what is in essence a naturalist or empiricist approach, although both these therapies have developed into organized

RIGHT *Holistic therapies address both the spiritual and physical aspects of illness and disease.*

systems. Homeopathy was developed very much later, at a time when Western medicine was in a remarkably non-scientific pit of superstition and useless therapy which was often worse than no therapy at all. It is a very subtle approach to healing, perhaps ultimately dealing at an anatomic level in the "vital force" of the universe, and its popularity is also increasing. These therapies, and the others covered in this book, put the reader back in touch with empirical approaches to health, giving him or her the opportunity to grasp and use insights which Western physicians have largely ignored. The idea is to choose remedies from this book according to intuition, with the introductory chapters as a guide, and judge their results according to your own sensory perception.

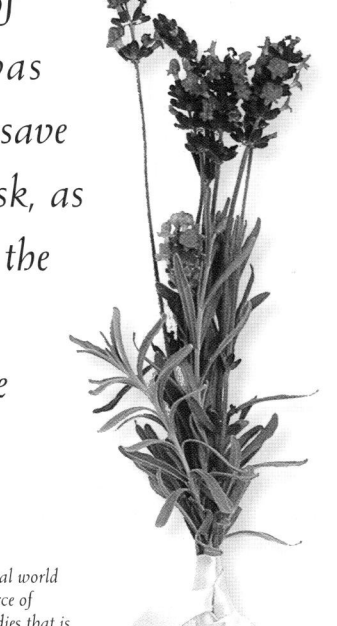

ABOVE *Attention to diet is an important part of almost every natural therapy.*

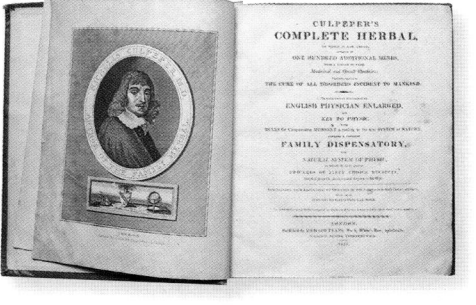

ABOVE *There is a wealth of medical knowledge enshrined in old texts that is now being rediscovered by new generations.*

When I asked my Professor of Medicine, Eugene A. Stead Jr., M.D., in 1978 what he considered to be the role of a physician, he answered that it is to be a triage officer. "Triage" is a term which is often used in connection with battle or disaster victims, and means the allocation of treatment to patients according to the principle of maximizing the number of survivors. A triage officer would stand at the door when a patient was significantly ill and advise when medicine or surgery was truly needed to save life or function. Dr. Stead advised that when life and function are not at risk, as in the vast majority of symptomatic illnesses, the patient should "go into the department stores and choose that which most appeals."

In this wonderful and comprehensive book, you have a remarkable department store of choices. May your browsing be healing.

C. NORMAN SHEALY M.D., PH.D
Missouri

RIGHT *The natural world around us is a source of health-giving remedies that is open to all.*

INTRODUCTION

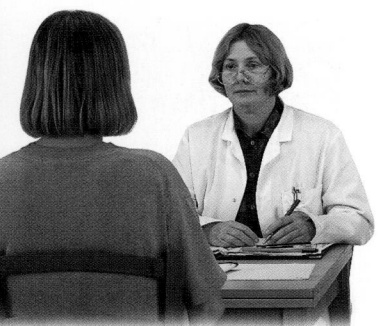

ABOVE. *The claims of conventional medicine are today being questioned by increasing numbers of people.*

T*he increased use of natural medicines and remedies over the past decade has prompted one of the most exciting developments in healthcare in our time. Many of the tenets of modern medicine have been challenged, and the crisis that conventional healthcare is now facing is the result of its own philosophy. The main premise of conventional medicine is that curing disease will lead to good health. This ignores the fundamental concept that pathology is individual to the sufferer, and that prevention is ultimately more important than treatment for the population at large.*

This idea is borne out by the fact that modern medicine is simply not as efficient or effective as we have been led to believe; indeed, evidence suggests that it may cause and create more fatal diseases than it cures, and despite the huge sums of money invested, the populations of the U.K., Australia, the U.S. and most of Europe do not live as long or as healthily as people from other cultures, where healthcare investment is substantially lower.

Adverse drug reactions and side-effects are one of the 10 most common reasons for hospitalization in the U.S., and a 1997 survey indicates that avoidable deaths from unnecessary surgery total nearly 100,000 per year. The information provided to doctors and physicians throughout the course of their careers is largely funded by the pharmaceutical industry, which earns billions each year from sales of prescription and over-the-counter medicines. As a result, we,

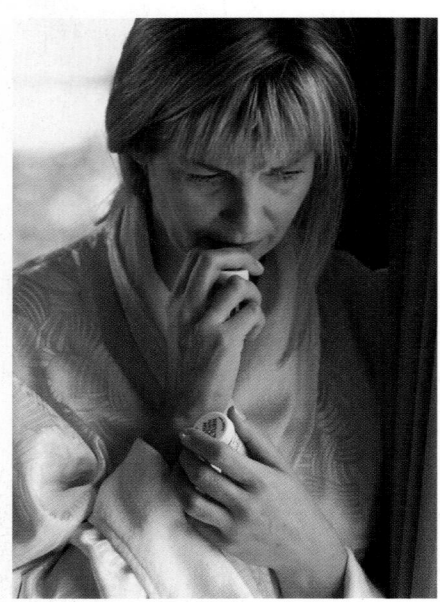

BELOW *The quick fix, pill-dispensing option of much modern medicine neglects underlying causes of ill health.*

in the West, have been encouraged to adopt a "pill-popping" approach to health – taking an average of 26.5 million pills per hour. Sleeping tablets, analgesics (painkillers), antihistamines, sedatives, and antidepressants rank among the top 20 drugs prescribed by physicians, and more than 52 million aspirin or paracetamol tablets are taken each day in the U.S.

Perhaps the most alarming result of this over–dependence upon drugs is the fact that we have stopped taking responsibility for our own health. When we have a headache, we take a painkiller; when we have a

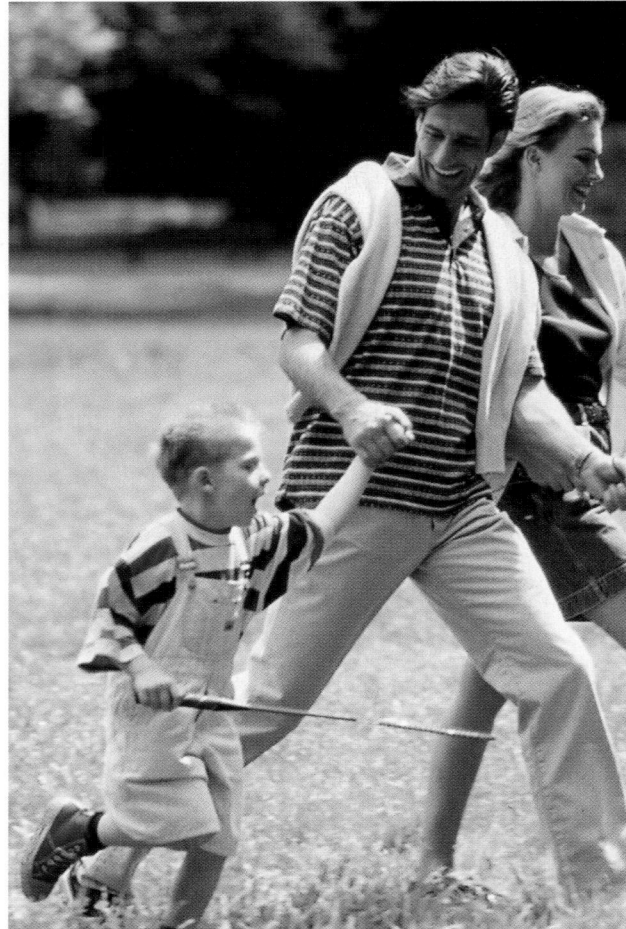

cold, we might take an antihistamine. We suppress the symptoms of health conditions because we want to feel better; we no longer accept the logic that pain or discomfort is a message from our body that something is wrong. We have become used to the idea that someone or something else can deal with our health problems. By taking a pill or conventional medicine in some form, we do experience a relief from symptoms, but what is important to

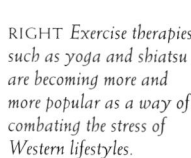

RIGHT *Exercise therapies such as yoga and shiatsu are becoming more and more popular as a way of combating the stress of Western lifestyles.*

BELOW *By ensuring the health of our children, we will be promoting the well-being of future generations.*

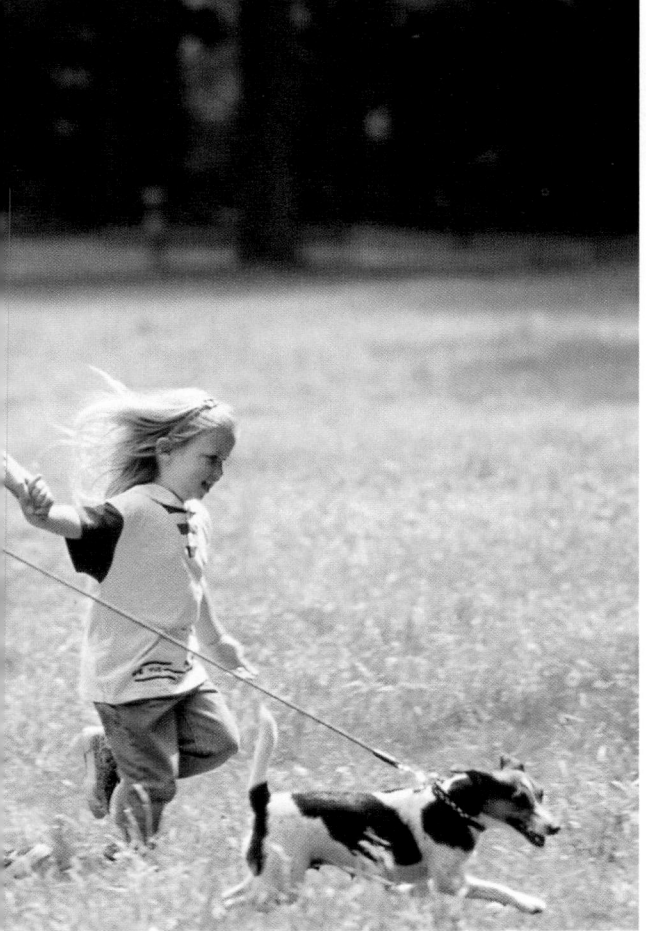

Recently, this trend has begun to change. Scares about the side-effects and long-term effects of immunization, abuse of painkillers, anti-histamines, and antibiotics have proved that conventional medicine, despite its many miracles, has been overused and we have become far too dependent on it. Many of us are no longer happy to accept the risks of prescription drugs, and are realizing that there are natural, healthy alternatives. With the increased interest in diet, emotional health and well-being, and exercise, we are becoming more in tune with our bodies and are choosing to listen to the messages they give. Even more importantly, we are taking steps to prevent illness rather than simply treat it when it does arise, and for this reason we are willing to try natural substances that not only treat health conditions, at cause level, but work with the body to keep it well. Natural remedies are more likely to make you feel better, more vital and more alert; they have fewer side-effects and because they work actively to prevent illness, they are, perhaps, the answer to the healthcare crisis that has been spiraling out of control.

Our understanding of how different cultures approach healthcare is blossoming, and figures show that many of the most common Western illnesses, such as eczema, asthma, cancer, chronic fatigue syndrome, and digestive problems simply do not exist

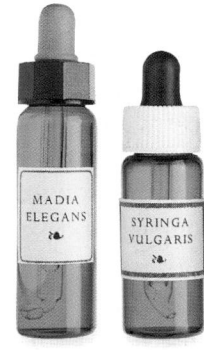

to the same degree in other countries. We have a cornucopia of information at our fingertips, and a greater understanding of how disease can be prevented and cured using herbs, oils, homeopathic remedies, food, vitamins and nutritional supplements, and other substances that encourage our bodies to work at their optimum level.

remember is that the cause of the pain or illness remains. By treating the symptoms, or suppressing them, we are doing nothing to treat the root cause. Eczema sufferers apply ointments and creams to the surface of the skin; they may take anti-inflammatories or antihistamines to ease the itching, but the cause of the eczema is still there and the body's reaction has been masked by drugs. They have not been cured; their illness has merely been controlled.

ABOVE RIGHT *The time may be approaching when remedies derived from natural sources will supplant the synthetic medicines of Western healthcare.*

RIGHT *A wide range of ailments can be alleviated by holistic therapies, from life-threatening diseases like cancer to minor disorders like the common cold.*

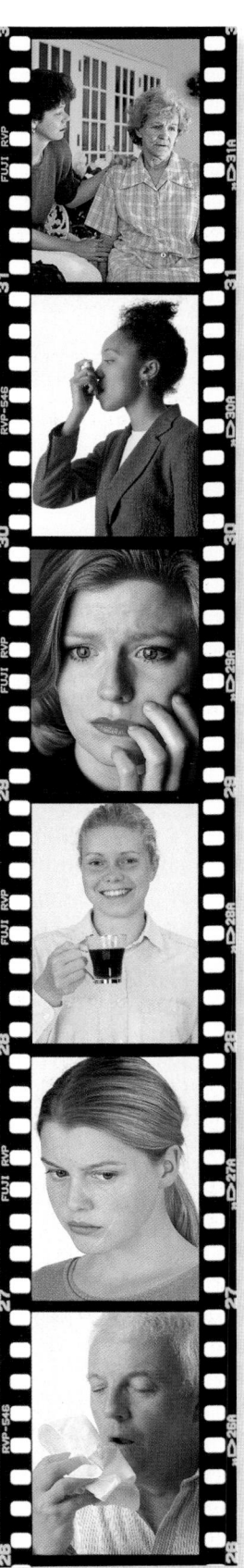

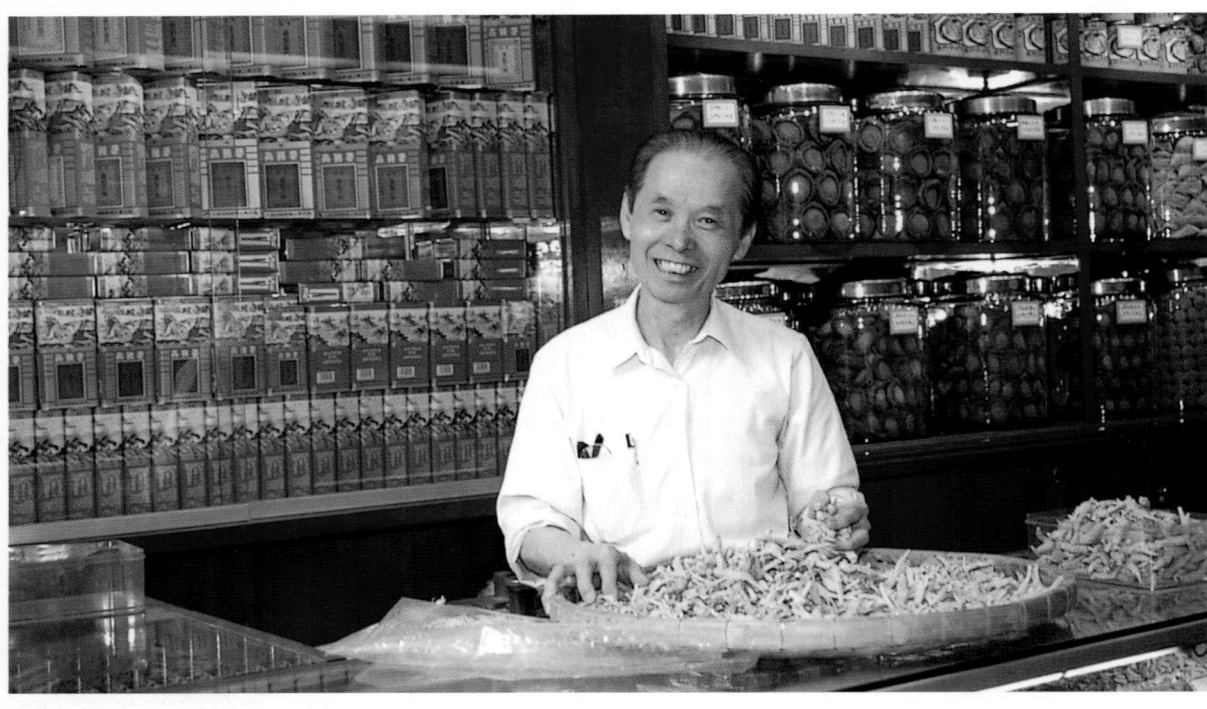

LEFT *Traditional Chinese Medicine is one of the most popular natural therapies.*

A HEALTHY MIND IN A HEALTHY BODY

The modern clinical emphasis on separating different aspects of our physical, mental, and spiritual health has resulted in a dehumanizing of medicine. By treating the whole person, holistic therapies can restore the proper balance and promote a sense of complete well-being, inside and out.

The sale of natural products has increased by over 200 percent over the last five years, and more than 20 percent of the U.S. population has consulted a natural health practitioner over the last year. Our approach to our health is changing dramatically, and this increased interest is being fed by a broad range of products from around the world that are now available in our local shops and stores.

Our growing understanding of holistic treatment has encouraged us to examine the healing practices of cultures from around the world, and from each we can gather invaluable information about diet, lifestyle, illness, health and well-being.

This book concentrates on the remedies that form the basis of eight international therapeutic disciplines: homeopathy, aromatherapy, Chinese herbal medicine, herbalism, Ayurveda, flower essences, folk or traditional medicine (also called home remedies), and nutrition. These remedies can be used to encourage and enhance good health and

ABOVE *Ayurveda, the traditional medicine of India, uses herbal treatments to restore the body's natural balance.*

to treat and prevent illnesses, both chronic and acute. Many of these remedies are derived from plants, which have a wide variety of therapeutic uses; indeed, up to 140 conventional drugs in use today are based on plants and herbs.

A large percentage of these remedies have been in use for thousands of years, and it was the practice of herbalism and other disciplines that made it possible for so many of our conventional drugs to be created. However, in practice, pharmaceutical companies isolate and often synthesize the active ingredient of a plant or herb, and many practitioners believe that this causes side-effects and other problems that do not occur when the substance is taken in its whole, natural form.

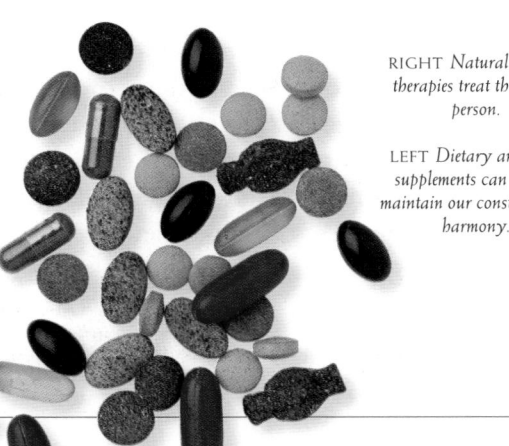

RIGHT *Natural healing therapies treat the whole person.*

LEFT *Dietary and other supplements can help to maintain our constitutional harmony.*

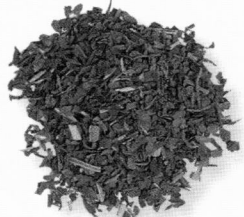

AYURVEDA
Ayurvedic tea is a simple form of healing remedy.

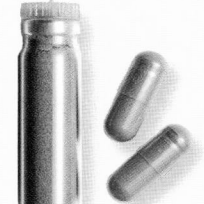

CHINESE HERBS
Chinese herbal remedies come in various forms including lozenges and powders.

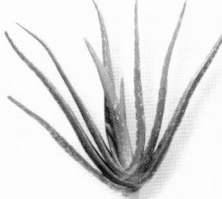

HERBS AND PLANTS
The leaves, shoots, seeds, and even roots of many plants have therapeutic qualities.

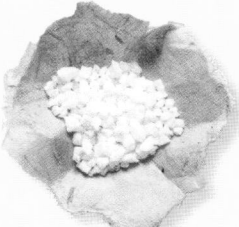

HOMEOPATHY
Homeopathic remedies are most often given in the form of tablets.

Isolating the active ingredients of plants produces powerful and often toxic drugs, while medical herbalism offers a gentler, safer, and less disruptive effect, allowing the body to undertake its own natural healing process.

There are over 1000 remedies outlined in this book, many of which you can grow in your own garden or on the windowsill, or purchase from a reputable health shop. Others will be items from your larder or store cupboard – everyday goods with healing and therapeutic properties that may surprise you. Each of the remedy sources has a data file of features, cautions, and other useful information, and there are often recipes for practical applications. Each of the main eight disciplines is also introduced, which helps you to understand how, for instance, the use of something like cinnamon or ginseng differs between Western and Chinese herbalism, and between folk medicine and Ayurveda. You'll learn how a rose aromatherapy oil is different from a rose flower essence, how vitamin C and healthy bacteria can encourage good health, and how Belladonna, a poisonous substance, can be taken in tiny dilutions to relieve fevers and other problems. You'll discover natural alternatives to caffeine and

BELOW *A well-stocked herb garden, used with care and skill, will be of more therapeutic benefit than any number of proprietary medicines.*

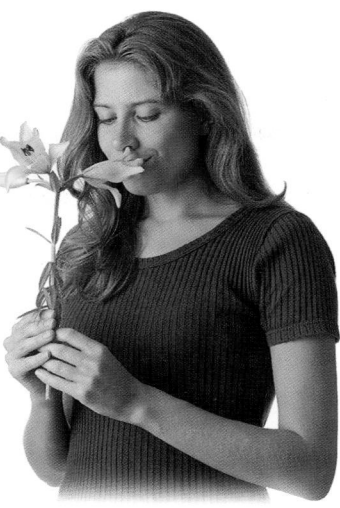

ABOVE *The restoration of the body's natural rhythms is an important aspect of holistic therapy.*

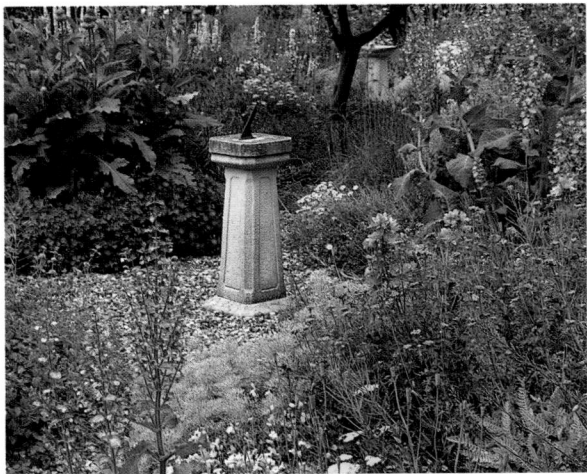

sleeping pills, laxatives, and antacids, in remedies that strengthen your mind and body, lift your mood, calm your nerves, and enhance your resistance to infection and illness.

Over 200 common ailments are also discussed in detail, with practical examples of how you can use the remedies from around the world to cure or prevent them. There are also suggestions for stocking a complete home medicine chest, so you can have on hand all the essential remedies to keep you healthy.

We are on the brink of an exciting new era in healthcare, and with the benefit of these remedies, presented in easy-to-follow files, grouped by the discipline in which they are most often used, you and your family can experiment with safe substitutes to conventional medicines by following the comprehensive instructions. The remedies in this book form the basis of a "stay-well" philosophy, with substances to boost immunity, help prevent cancer and heart disease, encourage emotional well-being and relaxation, enhance your strength, and keep your body's systems functioning the way they should. These remedies are the medicine of the future, and this is the essential guide for anyone who wants to take responsibility for their own health. By using only a few of these remedies, you can live longer and with a better quality of life. These are the secrets of good health from around the world; experiment with care and you'll be amazed at the results.

KAREN SULLIVAN
London, 1998

ABOVE *A simple plant like Meadowsweet is a treasure store of healing properties waiting to be unlocked.*

HOW TO USE THIS BOOK

This exhaustive and gloriously illustrated reference work is dedicated to the whole spectrum of alternative healing remedies. Aimed at the general reader, this comprehensive book covers the origins, methods, principles and remedies of eight alternative therapies – Ayurveda, Aromatherapy, Flower Remedies, Chinese Herbal Medicine, Herbalism, Homeopathy, Vitamins and Minerals, and Traditional Home and Folk Remedies.

PART ONE: **Therapies and Healing Remedy Sources.** Eight chapters cover the different therapies. In each case, the background and history of the therapy are covered together with how it works, information on visiting a practitioner and extensive guidelines for self-help. Following the introduction to the therapy, the major remedies and remedy sources are covered with details on how the substance is obtained or made, what they treat and how they should be taken. "Therapy Connections" highlights the remedy sources which are common to more than one therapy, giving a full picture of the properties and various uses of one particular remedy source.

PART TWO: **Treating Common Ailments.** 185 pages of common ailments and the relevant remedies with which they can be treated. In many cases, information on how the remedies should be prepared will be accompanied by step-by-step photographic sequences. Caution boxes will make clear the situations in which the remedies are not suitable. Cross-referencing directs the reader back to Part One, where the source of the remedy, its properties and uses are outlined in detail. A final chapter is devoted to the best remedies to be kept in your Home Remedy Chest.

PART THREE: **Reference Section.** Consists of a full glossary of terms, a list of useful addresses and books for further reading.

Color coding identifies the particular alternative therapy

Introduction to the history and background of each therapy

The principles behind the therapy and how it works

The background of each therapy is covered in Part One.

Full-color photographs illustrate the tools of each therapy, the sources of the remedies and prominent figures in its history

The remedy source is described and illustrated

"Therapy Connections" refer you to other therapies which use the same remedy source

The remedy sources are listed in Part One.

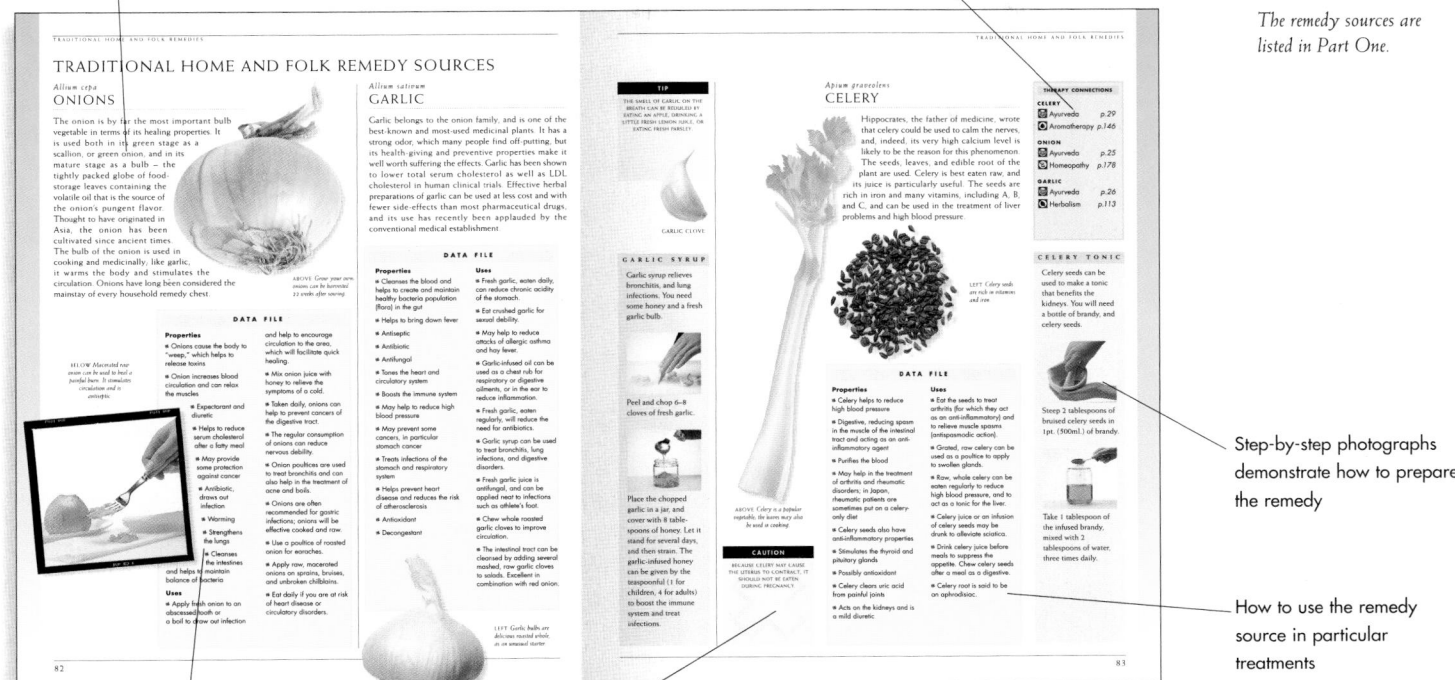

Step-by-step photographs demonstrate how to prepare the remedy

How to use the remedy source in particular treatments

Bullet points highlight the properties of the remedy source

Cautions warn when it is inadvisable to use a particular remedy

Ailments, grouped according to the body system affected, each have a descriptive introduction

The different remedies for the ailment in question are listed with cross-references to its detailed entry in the therapy chapter in Part One

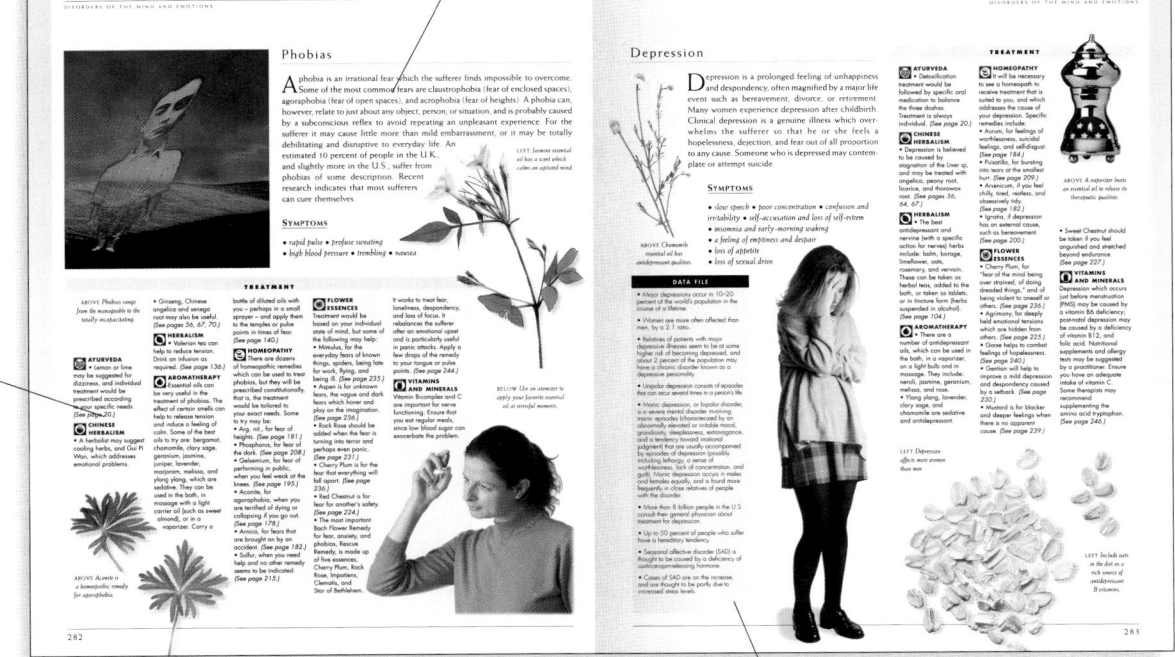

Specific illnesses appear in Part Two, Treating Common Ailments.

A "Data File" gives the latest facts and figures about this ailment

1

THERAPIES AND HEALING REMEDY SOURCES

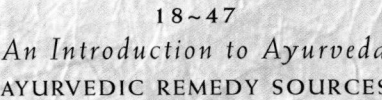

AYURVEDA

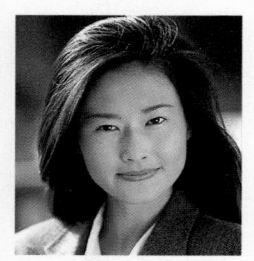

ABOVE *We are all unique. Ayurveda recognizes this and treats us individually.*

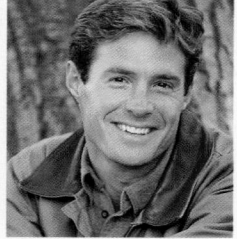

ABOVE *No two people will have the same personality, views, and lifestyle.*

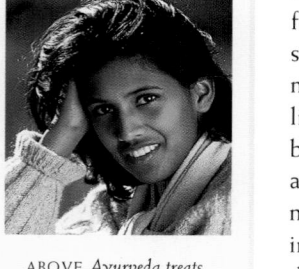

ABOVE *Ayurveda treats all the issues that are integral to health.*

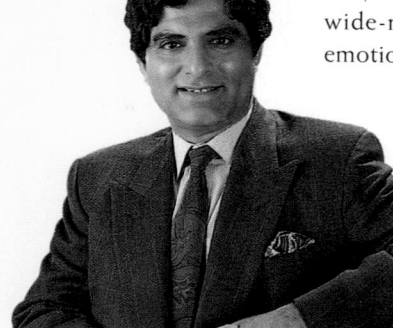

ABOVE *Deepak Chopra has been influential in bringing Ayurveda to mainstream American medicine.*

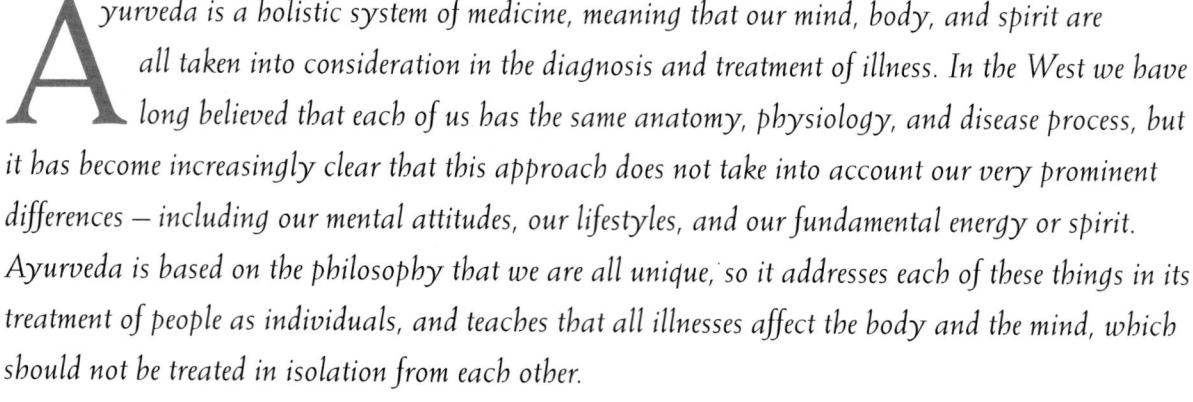

Ayurveda is a holistic system of medicine, meaning that our mind, body, and spirit are all taken into consideration in the diagnosis and treatment of illness. In the West we have long believed that each of us has the same anatomy, physiology, and disease process, but it has become increasingly clear that this approach does not take into account our very prominent differences – including our mental attitudes, our lifestyles, and our fundamental energy or spirit. Ayurveda is based on the philosophy that we are all unique, so it addresses each of these things in its treatment of people as individuals, and teaches that all illnesses affect the body and the mind, which should not be treated in isolation from each other.

WHAT IS AYURVEDA?

Ayurvedic medicine is the traditional system of medicine practised in India and Sri Lanka. Like Traditional Chinese Medicine, Ayurveda is a complete system of healthcare, designed to contribute to a way of life, rather than an occasional treatment.

The word "Ayurveda" means "science" or "wisdom" of life, and it embraces elements as diverse as medicine, philosophy, science, spirituality, astrology, and astronomy. Although Ayurveda has been practised for over 3,000 years, it is a sophisticated and advanced system of living that is as relevant today as it was so many years ago. In fact, as we begin to realize the limitations of our conventional Western approach, it becomes clear that Ayurveda can offer much to treat and prevent many modern diseases that conventional medicine has been unable to treat. Some of these include ME (myalgic encephalomyelitis), stress-related disorders, arthritis, impotence, asthma, eczema, and chronic illness. It offers natural herbal remedies to counter imbalances in the body, and detoxification, diet, exercise, meditation, spiritual guidance, and wide-ranging techniques to improve mental and emotional health.

PRANA – THE ENERGY OF LIFE

The fundamental belief in Ayurveda is that everything within the universe is composed of energy, or "prana." Like everything else, we too are comprised of energy, which changes according to our circumstances, our environment, our diets and lifestyles, and the world around us. Some of these changes can be positive, and others negative, and in order to ensure that most of the changes are positive, we must live in a way that encourages energy balance. Energy controls the functions of every cell, thought, emotion, and action, so every aspect of our lives, including the food we eat and the thoughts we think, affects the quality of our energy, and consequently our health.

Ayurvedic medicine teaches that there is no single prescription for health that is appropriate for everyone. In Ayurveda every person must be treated individually. The skill of the practitioner lies in his ability to correctly identify each individual's constitution, diagnosing the causes of imbalance and then treating the patient accordingly.

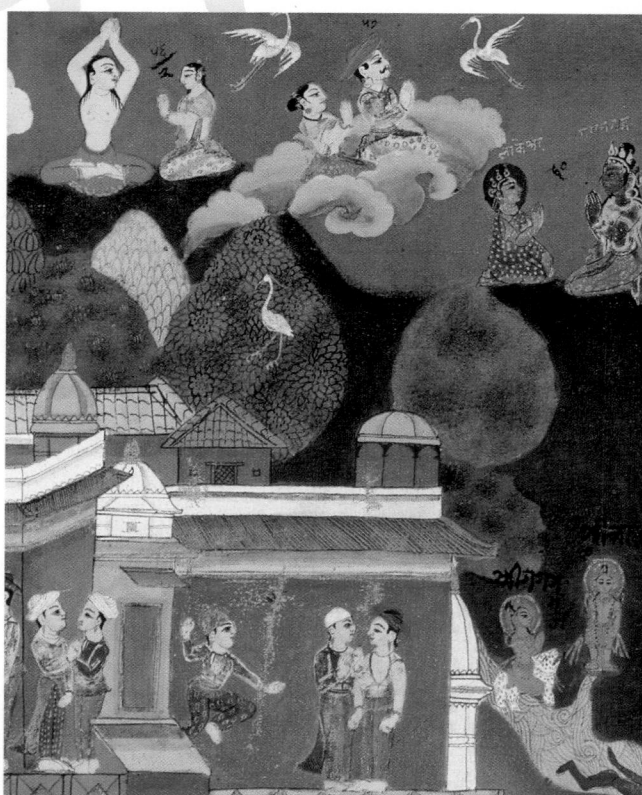

A HISTORY OF AYURVEDA

Over 3,000 years ago, 52 great *Rishis*, or seers, of ancient India discovered through meditation the "Veda," or the knowledge of how our world and everything within it works. Contained within the knowledge of the Veda were the secrets of sickness and health. These secrets were organized into a system called Ayurveda, the sophistication of which is apparent in the most famous of all ancient Ayurvedic texts, the *Charaka Samhita*. The knowledge of the Rishis had three main components: etiology (the science of the cause of illness and disease), symptomatology (the study of symptoms), and finally medication (the process of treating individuals to cure disease or relieve pain).

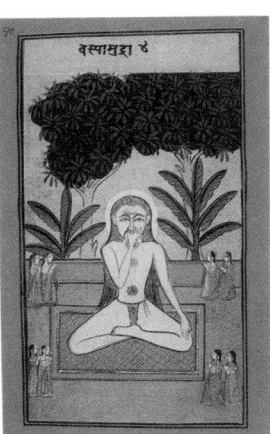

ABOVE *Through meditation the Rishis gained an understanding of the world.*

The beliefs were founded on Hindu philosophy, and were enlarged and enhanced by the teachings of the Lord Buddha (d. 483 B.C.E.), who taught that the mind could be enriched through correct thinking. Today Buddhism is one of the fastest-growing belief systems in the West. The eightfold path of Buddhism encompasses:

- ☸ *right understanding*
- ☸ *right concentration*
- ☸ *right livelihood*
- ☸ *right mindfulness*
- ☸ *right action*
- ☸ *right thought*
- ☸ *right effort*
- ☸ *right speaking*

Another important Ayurvedic text, the *Sushruta Samhita*, offers guidance on surgery, surgical equipment, suturing, and the importance of hygiene during and after an operation. Detailed medical information is teamed with commonsense advice on how to live a healthy and meaningful life.

In Vedic philosophy our lives become meaningful when we strive to fulfill our potential, but that cannot be achieved without basic good health.

CAUSES OF DISEASE

Ayurvedic practitioners believe that disease may be triggered by many external causes, including planetary influences, acts of god, fire and accidents, harmful gases (which we would today call pollution), poisons and toxins, and evil spirits. As well as this, there are two other main causes of illness, an imbalance of the "tri-doshas" (vátha, pitta, and kapha, *see page 20*) and mental imbalance.

The purpose of Ayurveda is to enable people to avoid serious illness by understanding how we become ill. For the most part, it works on a preventive basis, but when we do become ill it offers a wide range of treatments to help the body heal itself. Every Ayurvedic remedy is free of side effects, is made from natural substances, and is nontoxic. In order to benefit from Ayurveda, it is not necessary to understand or believe in the complex spirituality that goes hand-in-hand with the system. All that is necessary is an open mind and a desire to be healed.

LEFT *The word "Ayurveda" means "wisdom of life." Life encompasses body, mind, and soul.*

RIGHT *The teachings of Buddha were integrated into the philosophy of Ayurveda.*

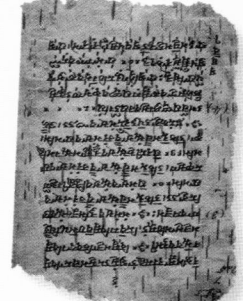

HOW DOES IT WORK?

The universe consists of five elements, Ether (space), Air, Earth, Fire, and Water. Our bodies consist of a combination of these elements. All five elements exist in all things, including ourselves.

❋ **ETHER** corresponds to the spaces in the body: the mouth, nostrils, thorax, abdomen, respiratory tract, and cells.

❋ **AIR** is the element of movement so it represents muscular movement, pulsation, expansion and contraction of the lungs and intestines, even the movement in every cell.

❋ **FIRE** controls enzyme functioning. It shows itself as intelligence, fuels the digestive system, and regulates metabolism.

❋ **WATER** is in plasma, blood, saliva, digestive juices, mucous membranes, and cytoplasm, the liquid inside cells.

❋ **EARTH** manifests in the solid structures of the body: the bones, nails, teeth, muscles, cartilage, tendons, skin, and hair.

The five elements also relate to our senses: sound is transmitted through Ether; Air is related to touch; Fire is related to sight; Water is related to taste; and Earth is connected to smell.

Ayurveda teaches that all organic matter is formed from the Earth element, which "gave birth" to other matter. All five elements may be present in all matter: Water, when it is frozen, becomes solid like Earth; Fire melts it back to Water; Fire can turn Water to steam, which is dispersed within the Air and the Ether.

Our constitutions are very important in Ayurveda, and each of us is individual, according to our specific energies. We inherit many aspects of our constitution, and we can live a healthy and happy life if we strive to attain a good quality of spirit (with no envy, hatred, anger, or ego), and maintain a healthy diet and lifestyle.

Your constitution is determined by the state of your parents' doshas at the time of your conception, and each individual is born in the "prakruthi" state, which means that you are born with levels of the three doshas that are right for you. But, as we go through life, diet, environment, stress, trauma, and injury cause the doshas to become imbalanced, a state known as the "vikruthi" state. When levels of imbalance are excessively high or low it can lead to ill health. Ayurvedic practitioners work to restore individuals to their "prakruthi" state.

THE THREE DOSHAS

There are three further bio-energies, called doshas, which exist in everything in the universe, and which are composed of different combinations of the five elements. The three doshas affect all body functions, on both a mental and a physical level. Good health is achieved when all three doshas work in balance. Each one has its role to play in the body.

☸ VÁTHA is the driving force; it relates mainly to the nervous system and the body's energy.

☸ PITTA is Fire; it relates to the metabolism, digestion, enzymes, acid, and bile.

☸ KAPHA is related to Water in the mucous membranes, phlegm, moisture, fat, and lymphatics.

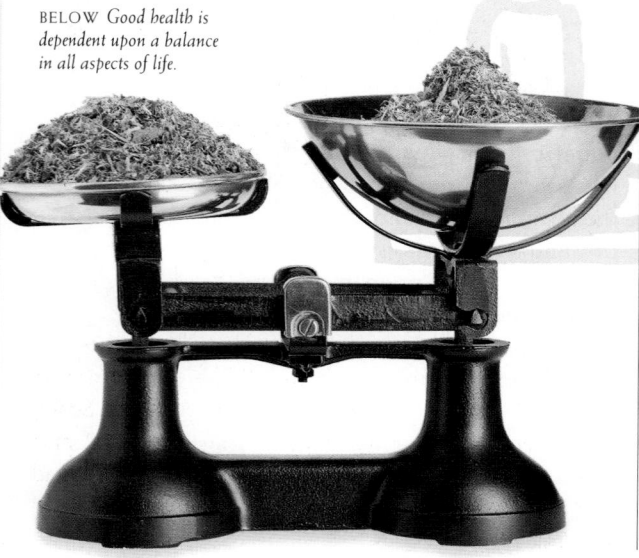

BELOW *Good health is dependent upon a balance in all aspects of life.*

VÁTHA is a combination of the elements Air and Ether, with Air being the most dominant. Its qualities are light, cold, dry, rough, subtle, mobile, clear, dispersing, erratic, and astringent. Váhta is the lightest of the three doshas, portrayed by the color blue. Predominantly váhta people are thin with dry, rough, or dark skin; large, crooked or protruding teeth; a small, thin mouth, and dull, dark eyes.

Characteristics:
❋ Often constipated
❋ Frequent but sparse urine and little perspiration
❋ Highly original and creative mind
❋ Poor long-term memory
❋ Rapid speech
❋ Tendency to anxiety and depression
❋ High sex drive (or none at all)
❋ Love of travel
❋ Dislike of cold weather

RIGHT *Vátha people tend to be thin, with light bones.*

The balance of the three doshas depends on a variety of factors, principally correct diet and exercise, maintaining good digestion, healthy elimination of body wastes, and ensuring balanced emotional and spiritual health.

We will be made up of a combination of two or all three types of dosha, although we may tend to be predominantly one. Some sub-groups include vátha-pitta, vátha–kapha or pitta–kapha.

THE FUNDAMENTAL QUALITIES

The principle of qualities in Ayurveda is similar to the Chinese concept of yin and yang, in that every quality has its opposite, and good health depends on finding a balance between the two extremes of qualities such as slow and fast, wet and dry, cloudy and clear. For example, hot and cold exist together as a pair of qualities, and everything in between is composed of levels of heat and cold. Heat relates to pitta, an imbalance of which can cause problems such as fevers, heartburn, or emotional disturbances such as anger or jealousy. If you have an excess of pitta you need to reduce your heat quality by eating fewer pitta foods, such as onions, garlic, and beef, and introduce more "cooling" foods, such as eggs, cheese, and lentils.

AYURVEDA

PITTA

PITTA is mostly Fire with some Water. Its qualities are light, hot, oily, sharp, liquid, sour, and pungent. Pitta is "medium" and portrayed by the color red. Pitta types seem to conform to a happy medium, and are of medium height and build, with soft, fair, freckled, or bright skin; soft, fair, light brown, or reddish hair that goes prematurely gray; small, yellowish teeth, and an average-sized mouth.

Characteristics:
* Speaks clearly, but often sharply
* Enjoys light but uninterrupted sleep
* Intelligent
* Clear memory
* Jealous
* Ambitious
* Passionately sexual
* Interested in politics
* Dislikes heat
* Loves luxury
* Loose stools and a tendency to diarrhea
* Strong appetite
* Great thirst

RIGHT *Pitta people are of medium build, and fair-skinned.*

KAPHA

KAPHA is a combination of mostly Water and some Earth. Its qualities are heavy, cold, oily, slow, slimy, dense, soft, static, and sweet. Kapha is the heaviest of the doshas, and is portrayed by yellow. Kapha people tend to be large-framed and often overweight, with thick, pale, cool, and oily skin; thick, wavy and oily hair, either very dark or very light; strong white teeth, and a large mouth with full lips.

Characteristics:
* Speaks slowly and monotonously, and needs plenty of deep sleep
* Sluggish or slow but steady appetite
* Heavy sweating
* Large soft stools
* Business-like
* Good memory
* Passive, bordering on lethargic
* Dislikes cold and damp
* Delights in good food and familiar places

RIGHT *Kapha people are often large and overweight.*

THE THREE DOSHAS

The three doshas, or tridoshas, come from the five basic eternal substances, the pancha-mahabhutas. Each is made up of different elements.

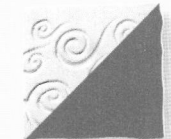

ABOVE *Vátha Sanskrit symbol and icon. Vátha consists of vayu (air) and akasha (ether).*

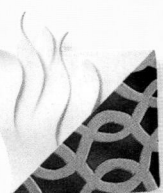

ABOVE *Pitta Sanskrit symbol and icon. Pitta consists of tejas (fire) and jala (water).*

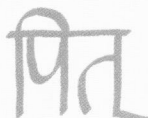

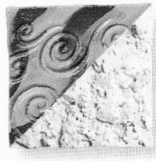

ABOVE *Kapha Sanskrit symbol and icon. Kapha consists of jala (water) and prthvi (earth).*

AGNI AND DIGESTION

In Ayurveda good digestion is the key to good health. Poor digestion produces "ama," a toxic substance that is believed to be the cause of illness. Ama is seen in the body as a white coating on the tongue, but it can also line the colon and clog blood vessels. Ama occurs when the metabolism is impaired as a result of an imbalance of "agni." Agni is the Fire which, when it is working effectively, maintains normality in all the functions of the body. Uneven agni is caused by imbalances in the doshas, and such factors as eating and drinking too much of the wrong foods, smoking, and repressing emotions.

MALAS

Malas represent the effective elimination of waste products and there are three main types:
* *Sharkrit or pureesha (feces)*
* *Mootra (urine)*
* *Sweda (sweat)*

Ama is a fourth type of waste, which cannot be eliminated, and an accumulation of which causes disease. Comprised of toxic materials, a build-up of ama is the result of an unhealthy diet and lifestyle, and the ingestion of toxins.

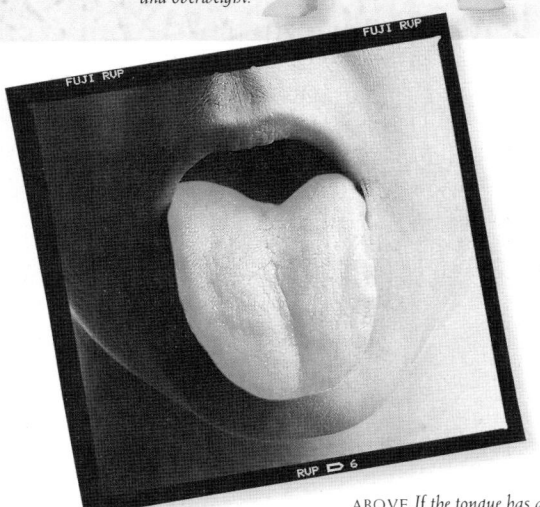

ABOVE *If the tongue has a white coating, it indicates that the body is out of balance.*

THE SEVEN TISSUES

Imbalance in the doshas also causes imbalance in the seven body tissues, or "dhatus." These are: plasma (rasa), blood (raktha), muscle (mamsa), fat (madas), bone (asthi), marrow and nerves (majja), and reproductive tissues (shukra). The dhatus support and derive energy from each other, so when one is affected the others also suffer.

AYURVEDIC TREATMENT

WHAT CAN AYURVEDA TREAT?

- Allergies
- Anxiety
- Arthritis
- Back pain
- Bronchitis
- Circulation problems
- Colds
- Digestive complaints such as irritable bowel syndrome, constipation, indigestion
- Dyslexia
- Eczema
- Headaches
- High blood pressure
- Insomnia
- Irritability and emotional stress
- Obesity
- Skin problems
- Water retention

Ayurveda will keep the immune system strong and capable of fighting off infection, and able to address chronic disorders from within.

SHODANA

In Ayurvedic medicine it is essential to detoxify the body before prescribing restorative treatment. Shodana is used to eliminate disease, blockages in the digestive system, or any causes of imbalance in the doshas. Where shodana is required the practitioner can use "panchakarma" therapy, and sometimes a preparatory therapy called "purwakarma." Purwakarma breaks down into two types of preparatory treatment, known as "snehana" and "swedana":

Snehana involves massaging herbal oils into the skin to encourage elimination of toxins. Blended oils are used to treat specific disorders, such as stress, anxiety, insomnia, arthritis, or circulation problems. Oils can also be massaged into the scalp for depression, insomnia, and memory problems. Snehana can sometimes involve lying in an oil bath, which is thought to be even more effective at allowing you to absorb the properties from herbal oils.

Swedana means sweating. It is sometimes used in conjunction with the oil treatment, but on a separate day. Steam baths are used to encourage the elimination of toxins through the pores, and, together with the oil treatments, they make the detoxification process much more effective.

PANCHAKARMA

This is a profound detoxification. It is traditionally a fivefold therapy, but all five aspects are used only in very rare cases. You may need only two or three of the following treatments:

Nirhua vasti (*oil enema therapy*). The oil is passed through a tube to the rectum, using gravity, rather than pressure, so that it does not cause damage. Oil enemas are often used to eliminate vátha or pitta-oriented problems, such as in the treatment of constipation, irritable bowel syndrome, diarrhea, indigestion, and fungal infections.

Ánuvasana vasti (*herbal enema*). The practitioner makes a herbal decoction and passes it through the tube. The selection of a herbal enema rather than an oil one depends on the patient's problem and the contraindications.

Vireka (*herbal laxative therapy*). Vireka is used as a normal part of any detoxification therapy, and is also used to treat pitta-oriented disease, such as gastrointestinal problems, and vátha problems, such as constipation and irritable bowel syndrome. It also helps with inflammatory skin complaints, fluid retention, liver problems, and energy problems.

Vamana (*therapeutic vomiting*). This is a traditional treatment for respiratory and catarrhal problems such as bronchitis, sinusitis, and asthma, but it is rarely used today.

Nasya (*herbal inhalation therapy*). This treatment involves inhaling the vapor from medicinal herbs infused in boiling water. It is used mostly to eliminate kapha-oriented problems, ear, eyes, nose and throat disorders, headaches, migraine, neuralgia, sinusitis, catarrh, and bronchitis.

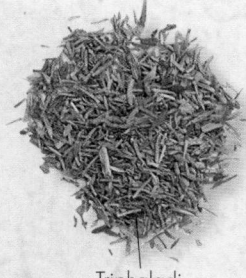
Triphaladi choornum

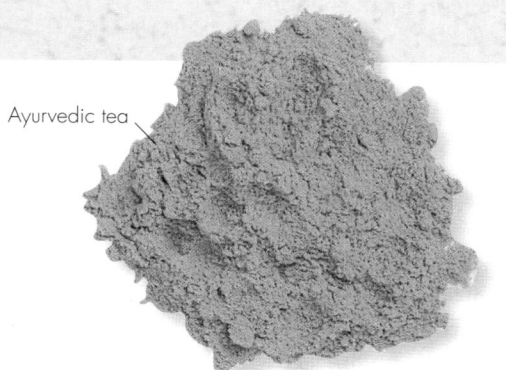
Guggul

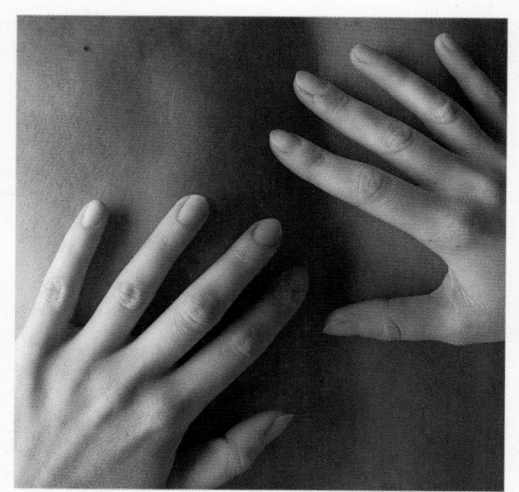
ABOVE *Snehana uses herbal oils to help eliminate toxins from the body.*

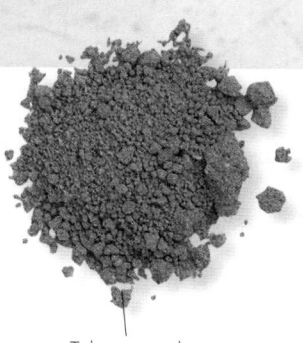
Taleespatradi vatakam

Ayurvedic tea

SAMANA

After the detoxification process the practitioner may prescribe herbal or mineral remedies to correct imbalances in the doshas. These are to stimulate agni and restore balance in the doshas. They are not prescribed to eradicate disease, because the disease is just a symptom of doshic imbalance. Herbal remedies are usually prescribed in liquid form or as dried herbs, although they can also come in powder or tablet form. The ingredients are pre-prepared, but the blends are prescribed for the individual. Each ingredient is classified by the effect it has on lowering or increasing the levels of the doshas.

Prescriptions are usually made up of groups of herbs, to which you add eight cups of water and boil until the liquid is reduced to one cup. You may have to take the remedy two or three times a day.

Your practitioner will also advise on lifestyle, food, and exercise. There is no single healthy diet in Ayurveda – just a diet that is best for you. It is important to eat to suit your constitution, and the practitioner may prepare a diet sheet for you to use.

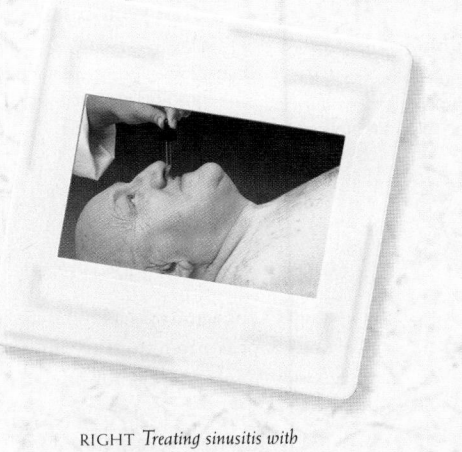

RIGHT *Treating sinusitis with nasya (nasal drops). Nasya is one of the five Ayurvedic purification therapies.*

Ashwagandha

Ayurvedic tea

PLANT POWER

In many cases the whole plant is used in an Ayurvedic treatment; in others, only part. All plants are associated with the following properties and effects:

✪ THE THREE DOSHAS. Plants can be used to increase or decrease an influence as required.

✪ SHAD RASA (the tastes). Every plant contains one or more of the six basic tastes, which are sweet, acidic, salty, pungent, bitter, and astringent.

✪ GUNAS (the properties). The gunas are distinctive characteristics that can be related to matter, thoughts, and ideas. There is a belief that everything in the universe is made up of complementary opposites (*see yin and yang, in Chinese Herbal Medicine, page 48*). There are 20 gunas: hot and cold, hard and soft, oily and dry, light and heavy, dull and sharp, subtle and gross, slimy and rough, unmoving and mobile, turbid and transparent, solid and liquid. The properties of each guna are related to the doshas, and specific substances, which are characterized by specific gunas, can increase or decrease dosha influence throughout the body. The properties of each guna can affect the doshas.

Many herbs are used in Ayurvedic preparations, and are sold as essences, pills, powders, pastes, and potencized remedies. Often they are herbs that are known and used in the West, although they are used differently in Ayurvedic medicine.

Herbs can have many effects on the body, including purifying the blood, binding stools, aiding digestion, expelling worms, improving coagulation, healing fractures, increasing appetite, lowering fever, reducing toxins, balancing the tridoshas (or increasing or decreasing the three doshas), strengthening the heart, among others.

It is usually safe to combine taking Ayurvedic herbal remedies and orthodox medicines. However, you should inform your Ayurvedic practitioner of any medication you are currently taking or have taken in the past.

LEFT *Yoga harmonizes mind and body, and can thus be regarded as an Ayurvedic treatment.*

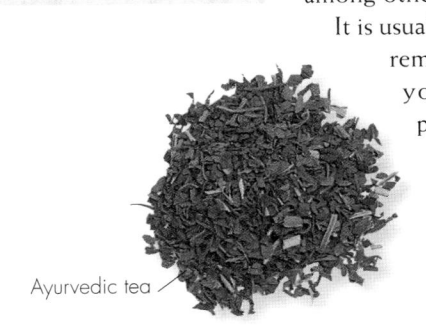

LEFT *Ayurvedic remedies come in many forms, some ready to use: liquid herbal remedies, dried herbs, powders, capsules, and tablets.*

OTHER USEFUL AYURVEDIC TREATMENTS INCLUDE:

❧ Meditation
❧ Breathing exercises
❧ Marma puncture (rather like acupuncture; adjusting energy levels in the body by stimulating energy points in the body, which can stimulate some of its functions and maintain health
❧ Marma therapy, applying pressure or massage to marma points
❧ Yoga
❧ Unblocking chakras, which are centers of energy located along the midline of the body which distribute energy to the 107 marma points on the body
❧ Rejuvenation therapy, or rasayana, which helps to promote and preserve health and longevity in the healthy, and to cure disease in the sick
❧ Psychotherapy or counseling

AYURVEDIC REMEDY SOURCES

Achillea millefolium
YARROW *GANDANA*

Yarrow is a sacred plant to many cultures. In China, yarrow stalks were used to cast the I Ching, to read the future for the emperor. Ayurvedics use the herb as a "heal-all" because it has so many uses – allowing you to keep your head in the heavens and your feet on the ground. Yarrow balances emotional upsets, and is a frequent addition to treatments during the menopause.

LEFT *Yarrow flowers in early summer. Gather it at this time.*

DATA FILE

Properties

Yarrow is bitter, pungent, astringent, cooling, and drying. It acts as a diaphoretic, antispasmodic, anti-inflammatory, antiphlogistic, antiseptic, and tonic. Yarrow is carminative, alterative, sedative, vulnerary, and emmenagogic.

Part of Plant Used

The leaves, stalks, flowers, and fruits.

Conditions Treated

Used for hemorrhages, ulcers, measles, colds, fever, nosebleeds, abscesses, vaginitis, varicose veins, headache, menopause, hemorrhoids, gout, cellulite, acne, sunburn, smallpox, and chicken pox. Yarrow has healing effects on mucous membranes, eases diarrhea, and improves blood clotting.

Form Taken

Skin patches, lotion, bath, compress, massage oil.

Used With Other Herbs?

Angelica, cedarwood, cinnamon, clove, lavender, lemon, licorice, myrrh, myrtle, sarsaparilla, St. John's wort, turmeric.

CAUTION

DO NOT ADMINISTER YARROW TO CHILDREN UNDER TWO YEARS OLD.

THOSE WITH SENSITIVE SKIN MAY BE IRRITATED WHEN EXPOSED TO THE SUN WHILE USING YARROW.

IT SHOULD NOT BE USED IN CASES OF HIGH VÁTHA.

HOW TO USE

🍃 Yarrow reduces pitta and kapha; it increases vátha with its cooling, drying properties.
🍃 **Legend has it that Achilles used yarrow to staunch his soldiers' wounds during the Trojan War.** 🍃 For wound treatment, simply press fresh leaves and flower tops into cuts and scrapes on the way to washing and bandaging them.
🍃 **As an infusion to relieve menstrual cramps or hot flushes,** steep 2 teaspoons of the dried herb in a cup of boiling water for about 10 minutes. Add honey to taste, and drink warm.

RIGHT *Yarrow leaves can be used on a cut until you get the chance to clean it at home.*

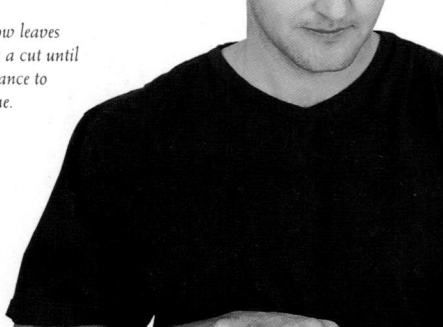

Acorus calamus
CALAMUS ROOT *VACHA*

Also known as sweet flag or myrtle flag, this rhizome is a reddish, hairy root, known throughout Asia for its medicinal properties. The word "vacha" means speech in Sanskrit, and calamus root is traditionally used as a brain tonic and to improve the capacity for speech.

DATA FILE

Properties

This herb is pungent and bitter, with astringent qualities. It is a stimulant, a heating/drying agent which warms vátha and decreases kapha states. It can be used as a decongestant and expectorant. Calamus root is emetic and anticonvulsive; it is a bronchio-dilator, increases circulation to the brain, and so can reduce brain toxins.

Part of Plant Used

The root.

Conditions Treated

Calamus strengthens the adrenals, improves muscle tissue, helps circulation

and is useful in periods of weakness. It has a beneficial effect on gingivitis (gum disease), and a massage with calamus oil will stimulate lymphatic drainage. The herb increases endurance and stamina, and has been used for the treatment of arthritis, shock, coughs, and nagging sinus headaches.

Form Taken

Use the herb externally in a compress or as massage oil.

Used With Other Herbs?

Calamus mixes well with ginger, yarrow, lemon, orange, cinnamon, and also with cedar.

HOW TO USE

🍃 Calamus reduces kapha and vátha, and increases pitta. 🍃 **Calamus root is often used to improve the memory.** 🍃 A simple formula for boosting your brain power: mix ¼ of a teaspoon of the powdered root with a ½ teaspoon of honey. Take internally every morning and evening. Use any time you are experiencing mental stress and overstimulation. A great help at exam time!

LEFT *Calamus leaves and young rhizome (rootstock). Rhizomes are thick horizontal underground stems.*

CAUTION

CALAMUS CAN CAUSE BLEEDING DISORDERS, SUCH AS NOSEBLEEDS AND HEMORRHOIDS, IF USED IN EXCESS.

USE ONLY THE RECOMMENDED DOSE.

CALAMUS CAN HAVE A VERY STRONG AND LONG-LASTING ODOR. IT MAY BE APPROPRIATE TO USE IT IN CONJUNCTION WITH ROSEMARY, LAVENDER, OR A SWEET-SMELLING HERB.

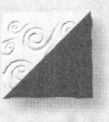

VÁTHA
Reduces Vátha
Calamus, Onion
Increases Vátha
Yarrow

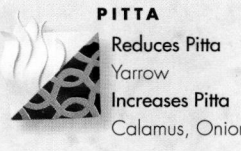

PITTA
Reduces Pitta
Yarrow
Increases Pitta
Calamus, Onion

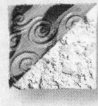

KAPHA
Reduces Kapha
Yarrow, Calamus, Onion

Allium cepa
ONION *DUNGRI*

Onion and its relative garlic are members of the lily family. They are some of the oldest known medicinal plants, rich in trace elements, minerals, and sulfur. Remedies using onion date back to 3000 B.C.E. Ayurvedic practitioners prescribed onion for cancer and leprosy. Onion stimulates the production of saliva and digestive juices, as well as the flow of tears!

RIGHT *Slices of raw onion can be placed directly on a burn to soothe the pain.*

DATA FILE

Properties
Onion is a pungent, sweet bulb with heating and drying qualities. It is an excellent stimulant, carminative, and expectorant. The juice is disinfectant, rejuvenative, and antispasmodic. Onion has a rejuvenating effect on all tissues and body systems: the digestive, respiratory, nervous, reproductive, and circulatory systems.

Part of Plant Used
The bulb.

Conditions Treated
Onion has been used to treat a broad spectrum of ailments, including but not limited to nerve rejuvenation, colds, skin disease, parasites, bronchial disorders, asthma, joint problems and arthritis, cysts and growths, fluid retention. Onion helps eliminate lead and other heavy metals from the body, and is beneficial for diabetics and patients with cancer.

Form Taken
Onion can be peeled and eaten raw, cooked, powdered, juiced, taken as a tea, decoction, infusion, in food, and as an oil.

Used With Other Herbs?
Combines well with ginger, black pepper, cumin, coriander, eucalyptus.

HOW TO USE

Onion reduces kapha and vátha, and increases pitta. Its stimulating effects aid in the secretion of digestive juices. **Onion juice has been used to treat infected wounds, amebic dysentery, and, at one time, juice applied to the ear was said to cure deafness!** Onion may be used directly on the skin for natural relief from burns. Simply place slices of raw onion on the burned skin, or apply a homemade lotion of onion juice mixed with salt. This preparation is also effective for insect bites and stings. **For an antibiotic treatment, peel and eat (raw or cooked) one-quarter of one sweet white onion, two to four times a day. The onion must be chewed, crushed, chopped, or bruised to access its antibiotic properties.**

BELOW *Include onion in food as often as possible for its health-enhancing properties.*

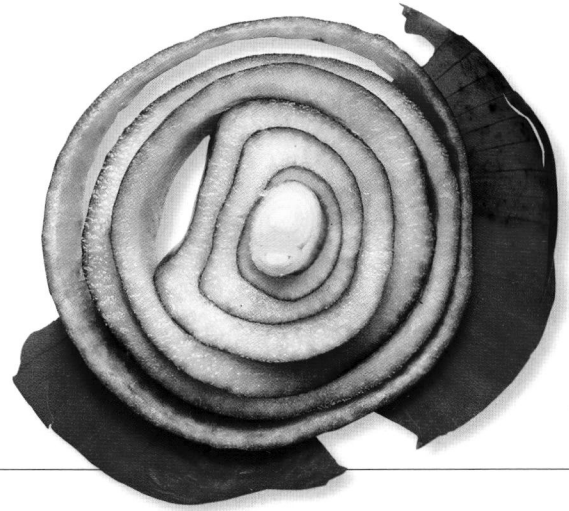

CAUTION
NURSING MOTHERS BEWARE: ONION IN YOUR BREAST MILK MAY CAUSE COLIC IN YOUR INFANT.

SOME PEOPLE HAVE ALLERGIES TO ONION AND MAY DEVELOP A SKIN RASH. IF ONE APPEARS, DISCONTINUE USE.

CONSULT A PHYSICIAN BEFORE CONSUMING LARGE QUANTITIES OF ONION FOR MEDICINAL PURPOSES.

SOME PEOPLE HAVE TROUBLE DIGESTING RAW ONION. IF THIS IS THE CASE, STEAM OR BLANCH THE ONION BEFORE EATING.

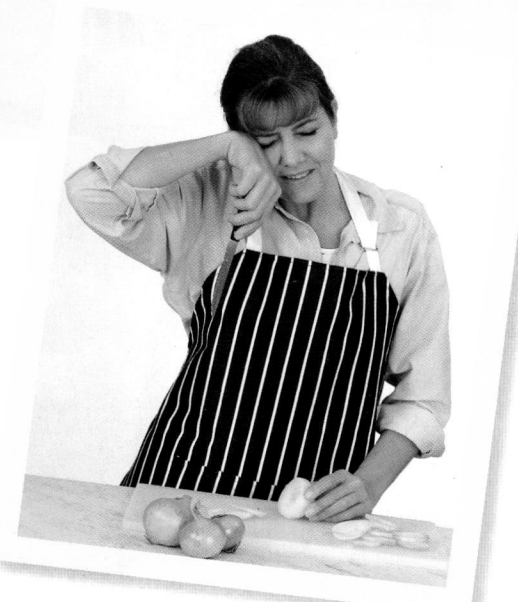

ABOVE *Tears – a well-known side-effect of chopping onions. Onions also stimulate the secretion of digestive juices.*

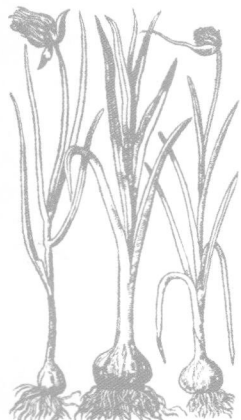

GARLIC
Allium sativum.

Allium sativum

GARLIC *LASHUNA*

Garlic is one of the oldest known medicinal plants. A remedy using garlic was found on a Sumerian clay tablet which dated back to 3000 B.C.E. Ayurvedic practitioners prescribed garlic liberally for cancer and leprosy. When the British came to India, leprosy became known as "peelgarlic," because of the frequent sight of lepers peeling and eating garlic cloves.

CAUTION

NURSING MOTHERS BEWARE: GARLIC IN YOUR BREAST MILK MAY CAUSE COLIC IN YOUR INFANT.

—◇—

SOME PEOPLE HAVE ALLERGIES TO GARLIC AND MAY DEVELOP A SKIN RASH. IF ONE APPEARS, DISCONTINUE GARLIC USE.

—◇—

CONSULT A PHYSICIAN BEFORE CONSUMING LARGE QUANTITIES OF GARLIC FOR MEDICINAL PURPOSES.

ABOVE *Grow your own garlic by planting individual cloves in the fall.*

DATA FILE

Properties

Garlic is a pungent, sweet bulb with heating and drying qualities. It is an excellent stimulant, carminative, and expectorant. The juice is disinfectant, rejuvenative, and antispasmodic. Garlic has a rejuvenating effect on all tissues and systems: digestive, respiratory, nervous, reproductive, and circulatory.

Part of Plant Used

The bulb.

Conditions Treated

Garlic has been used to treat a broad spectrum of ailments, including but not limited to nerve rejuvenation, colds, skin disease, parasites, joint problems and arthritis, cysts and growths, and fluid retention. Like onion, garlic helps eliminate lead and other heavy metals from the body. It is beneficial to diabetics and cancer patients.

Form Taken

Garlic cloves can be chewed, cooked, powdered, taken as a tea, decoction, infusion, in food, and as an infused oil.

Used With Other Herbs?

Ginger, black pepper, cumin, coriander, eucalyptus.

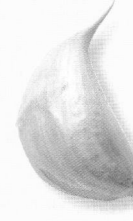

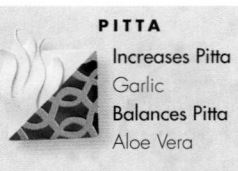
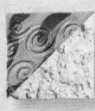
HOW TO USE

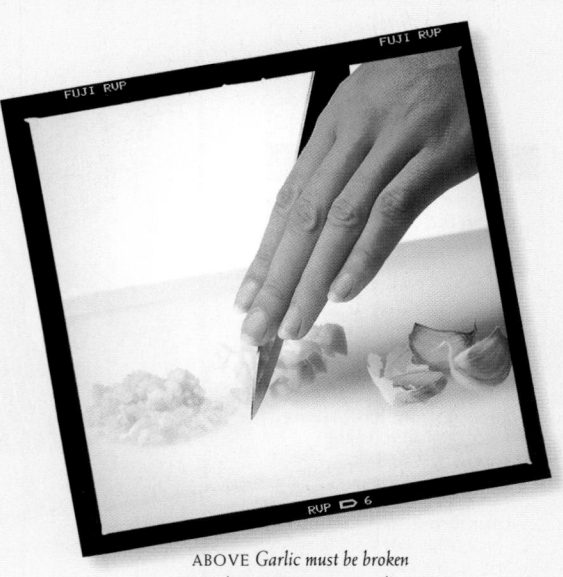

ABOVE *Garlic must be broken up in some way to access its healing properties.*

🍃 Garlic reduces kapha and vátha, and increases pitta. 🍃 **Its stimulating effect aids in the secretion of digestive juices.** 🍃 Garlic juice has been used to treat infected wounds and amebic dysentery. 🍃 **Garlic may be used as a natural antibiotic, and as a blood pressure and cholesterol reducer.** 🍃 To obtain antibiotic effects, 6–12 cloves of garlic a day are recommended. Peel and chew three cloves of garlic at a time, two to four times a day. 🍃 **The garlic must be chewed, crushed, chopped, or bruised to access its antibiotic properties.**

Aloe vera
ALOE VERA *KUMARI*

Aloe can be raised anywhere, and is often grown as a houseplant on the kitchen windowsill. Its fame as a treatment for burns and scalds goes back to Alexander the Great, who used an island off Somalia for the sole purpose of obtaining the "amazing wound-healing" plant. Another part of the aloe – the latex – is a powerful laxative, and is obtained in fresh aloe juice.

DATA FILE

Properties

Aloe vera has bitter, cooling, sweet qualities. It is astringent, and an excellent blood cleanser. Aloe vera alleviates all three doshas, and specifically reduces pitta (cooling pitta rashes, burns, and ulcers). Aloe vera works on the thyroid, the pituitary gland, and the ovaries.

Part of Plant Used

The leaf, the gel, the juice.

Conditions Treated

Aloe vera relieves inflammation, soothes muscle spasm, purifies the blood, and cleanses the liver. Fresh aloe gel scooped or expressed from the spongy leaves of the plant can be spread on the skin to heal burns, scalds, scrapes, sunburn, and wounds. Apply the gel directly to the outer eyelid for conjunctivitis. For cosmetic purposes, the gel can give skin a healthy glow – but use the fresh gel. Commercially packaged products use stabilized aloe, which has none of the fresh herb's healing properties.

Form Taken

Drink aloe juice for internal conditions, and apply the gel externally. To soothe wounds, clean the wound with soap and water. Cut several inches off an older leaf, slice it lengthwise, and apply the gel to the wound. Allow it to dry. You can leave the gel on the wound for several hours, or if it is painful, wash it off and reapply later.

Used With Other Herbs?

Barberry, cinnamon, cloves, licorice, St. John's wort.

HOW TO USE

🍃 Aloe Vera is good for all doshas; it will bring balance equally to kapha, pitta, and vátha.

🍃 Cover the leaves with vegetable oil. Any vegetable oil can be used as the base. Allow the mixture to soak for 60 days, then strain. Keep the oil in a dark glass container. Label the container, as the scent is subtle and will not be easy to identify. The oil will keep indefinitely.

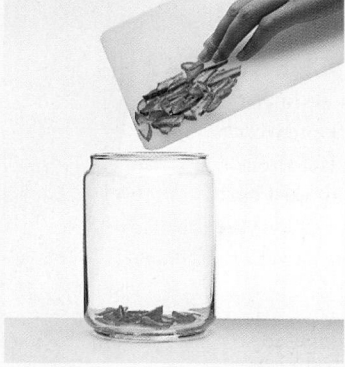

🍃 You can make your own aloe vera medicated oil by slicing up the leaves of the aloe vera plant, and placing them in a glass jar.

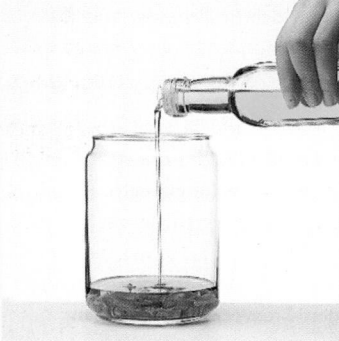

BELOW *Aloe vera gel helps to relieve the inflammation of conjunctivitis.*

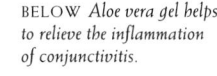

Rub gel on outer eyelid

Aloe vera gel

LEFT *Aloe vera is a succulent requiring a minimum temperature of 10°C (50°F).*

Angelica
ANGELICA *CHORAKA*

In the West, angelica has been associated with magic and sorcery for centuries. Necklaces of angelica leaf were thought to be protection against spells and illness, and its presence in a garden or cupboard was a defense against charges of witchcraft. Chinese angelica, or dong quai, has been used in Asia for thousands of years, and is enjoying renewed popularity as a gynecological aid. Ayurvedic practitioners prescribe the herb for menstrual problems, as well as arthritis, abdominal pains, and flu.

HOW TO USE

🍃 In general, angelica balances all three doshas. If used in excess, or in high pitta states, it will increase pitta.

🍃 **It is a wonderful expectorant and digestive aid.**

🍃 You can prepare the leaves and seeds as an infusion for a mild treatment, or use the root in a decoction for a stronger effect. For an infusion, use 1 teaspoon of the powdered leaves or seeds in a cup or teapot. Add 1 cup of boiling water. Steep for 10–15 minutes, then strain.

🍃 **For a decoction, take 3 teaspoons of the powdered root. Add 3 cups of water, and bring to a boil. Cover and simmer for 5 minutes. Remove from the heat and let stand for 15 minutes. Drink up to 2 cups a day. Sweeten with honey or anise if necessary.**

CAUTION

FRESH ANGELICA ROOTS ARE POISONOUS. DRYING ELIMINATES ALL DANGER.

DO NOT USE WITH HYPERTENSION, HEART DISEASE, OR HIGH PITTA CONDITIONS.

ANGELICA CAN INCREASE PHOTOSENSITIVITY; USE A SUNSCREEN IF SPENDING TIME OUTDOORS.

PREGNANT WOMEN SHOULD AVOID ANGELICA BECAUSE OF ITS HISTORY AS AN ABORTIFACIENT.

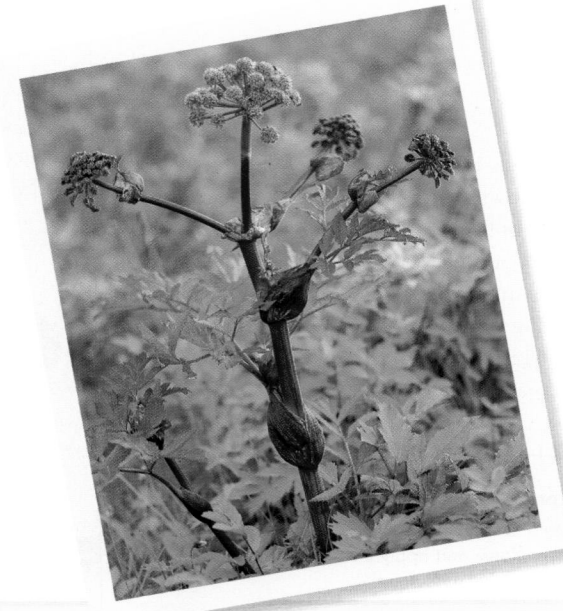

Cramping pains

THERAPY CONNECTIONS

ANGELICA

🍵 Chinese Herbal Medicine   *p.55*

✋ Herbalism   *p.115*

💧 Aromatherapy *p.146*

CELERY SEED

✋ Traditional Home and Folk Remedies *p.83*

💧 Aromatherapy *p.146*

LEFT *Most of the angelica plant is useful: collect the root, leaves and seeds. The plant is a biennial.*

DATA FILE

Properties

Angelica is pungent, sweet, heating, and moisturizing. It is stimulant, expectorant, tonic, emmenagogue, carminative, and diaphoretic. Angelica has antibacterial properties, and has been used to induce menstruation and abortion.

Part of Plant Used

The roots, leaves, and seeds.

Conditions Treated

Amenorrhea, menstrual cramps, PMS, anemia, headaches, colds, flu, hiccups, arthritis, rheumatism, poor circulation, adrenal excess, digestive disorders, heartburn, bronchitis, poor blood clotting, also poor liver function.

Form Taken

As an inhalant, nose drops, in a vaporizer, tea, tincture, massage oil.

Used With Other Herbs?

Rose, St. John's wort, yarrow, vetiver, fennel, cumin, chamomile.

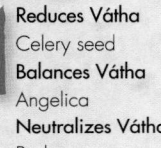

VÁTHA

Reduces Vátha
Celery seed
Balances Vátha
Angelica
Neutralizes Vátha
Barberry

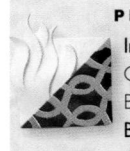

PITTA

Increases Pitta
Celery seed,
Barberry
Balances Pitta
Angelica

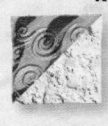

KAPHA

Reduces Kapha
Celery seed
Balances Kapha
Angelica,
Barberry

LEFT *Use angelica to treat painful menstrual cramps. Drink a cup of angelica decoction twice a day.*

Apium graveolens

CELERY SEED *AJWAN*

Celery seed, or *ajwan*, grows wild in India all year round. Traditional Ayurvedic practitioners prescribe celery seed to reduce high vátha states – indigestion, nervous stomach, and ungrounded emotions. In aromatherapy, celery seed oil can be used to counteract jet lag and exposure to smog and toxic environments. Celery seed is a strong diuretic, so you may want to drink extra water when taking this herb.

HOW TO USE

❧ Celery seed reduces kapha and vátha, and increases pitta. ❧ **It is most commonly used as a diuretic, since fluid retention aggravates high blood pressure, congestive heart conditions, premenstrual syndrome, arthritis, and gout.** ❧ For a mildly diuretic infusion, or to bring on menstruation, crush 1½ teaspoons of celery seeds. Add 1 cup of boiling water. Cover and let steep for 15–20 minutes. You may drink up to 3 cups of the infusion a day.

DATA FILE

Properties

Celery seed has pungent, salty qualities, and a heating/moisturizing effect. It is used as a stimulant and expectorant, an antispasmodic and lithotrophic (dispels stones). Celery seed is a strong diuretic. It also contains chemicals – phthalides – which have a sedative effect and can ease insomnia.

Part of Plant Used

The juice, roots, and seeds.

Conditions Treated

The common cold, coughs, sinus congestion, respiratory infections, bronchitis, laryngitis, arthritis, digestive problems, high blood pressure, insomnia, diseases of the liver and spleen, and irregular menstruation.

Form Taken

As a food, a tea or infusion, a steam, a powder, massage oil, or a gargle.

Used With Other Herbs?

Basil, black pepper, camphor, eucalyptus, sandalwood.

LEFT *Celery seed contains several oils, including apiol, a valuable curative.*

ABOVE RIGHT *Celery seed tea before bed lessens the risk of insomnia.*

CAUTION

CELERY SEED MAY CAUSE MINOR DISCOMFORT IN SOME PEOPLE. IF YOU ARE EXPERIENCING A STOMACH UPSET OR DIARRHEA WHILE TAKING CELERY SEED, DISCONTINUE USE.

PREGNANT WOMEN SHOULD NOT TAKE CELERY SEED WITHOUT A PHYSICIAN'S APPROVAL BECAUSE OF ITS STRONG DIURETIC PROPERTIES.

DO NOT GIVE CELERY SEED TO CHILDREN UNDER TWO YEARS OLD.

Berberis vulgaris

BARBERRY

Barberry has been in use as a healing herb for thousands of years. The Egyptians used it to prevent plagues – a testimony to its antibiotic properties. The Ayurvedics were more likely to prescribe it for dysentery, mouth ulcers, sore throats, and skin infections. Barberry has been proven to be a more powerful antibiotic and antibacterial agent than many current pharmaceutical products.

CAUTION

BARBERRY MAY STIMULATE THE UTERUS AND SHOULD NOT BE TAKEN BY PREGNANT WOMEN.

BARBERRY IS A VERY POWERFUL HERB, AND SHOULD BE USED IN SMALL DOSES AND UNDER THE SUPERVISION OF A PHYSICIAN OR ALTERNATIVE HEALTHCARE PRACTITIONER.

IF THE DOSAGE IS TOO HIGH, BARBERRY CAN CAUSE NAUSEA, VOMITING, HAZARDOUS DROPS IN BLOOD PRESSURE, AND DIZZINESS.

DATA FILE

Properties

Barberry is a stimulant, a respiratory aid, and is antibiotic, antibacterial, and antifungal. It decreases heart rate, shrinks tumors, stimulates intestinal movement, reduces bronchial constriction, and enlarges blood vessels.

Part of Plant Used

The berries, roots, and the ground bark.

Conditions Treated

Skin infections, urinary tract infections, diarrhea, dysentery, cholera, arthritis, conjunctivitis, high blood pressure, throat infections, mouth ulcers, abnormal uterine bleeding.

Form Taken

Tea or infusion, gargle, eyewash, douche, compress, and powder.

Used With Other Herbs?

Garlic, ginger, saffron, wild sunflower.

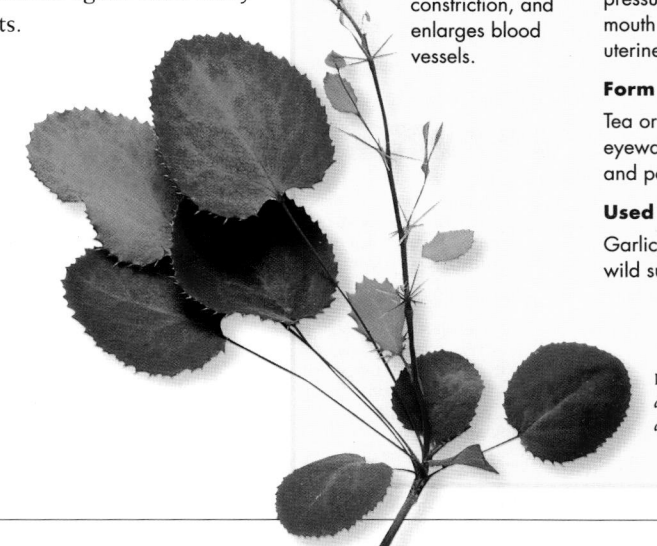

LEFT *Barberry makes a bitter tonic with strong antibiotic effects.*

HOW TO USE

❧ Barberry can be used to treat a variety of symptoms in its decoction form. Take 1 teaspoon of powdered root bark in a small enamel pan. Add 2 cups of water. Cover and boil for 15–30 minutes, with as little liquid loss as possible. Allow to cool. The taste will be quite bitter. Sweeten with honey to taste. Drink up to one cup a day. ❧ **For a compress to treat conjunctivitis, soak a clean cloth in the decoction (before you add any honey). Place over the eye.**

Brassica nigra
MUSTARD *RAI*

Mustard is an annual plant cultivated as a spice all over the world. It has been used for centuries as a pungent condiment and healing herb by the Chinese, the Greeks, and the Ayurvedics. Mustard is peculiar in that its strong taste develops only after the seeds are crushed and come into contact with water or saliva.

ABOVE *Ready-powdered mustard seeds can be mixed with warm water to form a thick paste. Spread on a piece of cloth to form a poultice.*

DATA FILE

Properties

Antiseptic, warming, carminative, antibacterial, antiseptic, and antiviral. Mustard aids digestion and eases gastric distention. It is an emetic, rubefacient, and a laxative. It acts as an irritant, encouraging blood flow toward the surface of the skin in cases of rheumatism, sciatica, peritonitis, and neuralgia, and for various muscle aches and pains.

Part of Plant Used

Seed, pods.

Conditions Treated

For centuries, mustard plasters have been used to treat chest colds and coughs. Mustard is also beneficial for backache, joint pain, digestive upsets, hiccups, and as a laxative. Mustard eases constipation, minor aches and pains, and muscle stiffness.

Form Taken

As a spice or oil, in compresses and poultices.

Used With Other Herbs?

Aloe vera, ginger, garlic, and onion.

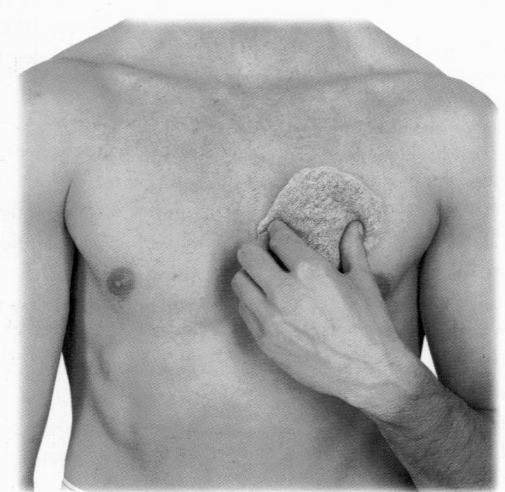

ABOVE *A mustard poultice, or plaster, helps to relieve the symptoms of a chest cold.*

HOW TO USE

🍃 Mustard reduces pitta and kapha, and has a neutral effect on vátha. 🍃 Mustard oil can be rectified with alcohol (1 part oil to 40 parts alcohol) and used as a lotion for joint pains, arthritis, and sluggish circulation. 🍃 A mustard foot bath will clear blood congestion in the head, warm up cold feet, and lower a fever in the early stages of illness. Put one-quarter of a cup of mustard seed in a small cloth bag or a large tea strainer. Steep in hot water for 5 minutes. Soak the feet until the water cools off.

CAUTION

LARGE AMOUNTS OF MUSTARD CAN CAUSE IRRITATION AND INFLAMMATION. DO NOT LET UNDILUTED MUSTARD OIL COME IN CONTACT WITH THE SKIN.

DO NOT USE MUSTARD PLASTERS FOR MORE THAN 10–15 MINUTES AT A TIME, OR BLISTERING AND IRRITATION CAN OCCUR.

Carum carvi
CARAWAY *SUSHAVI*

This perennial plant is found in the wild in North America, Europe, and Asia. Caraway is best known in Europe in the making of rye bread, where the addition of caraway seeds aids in the digestion of starch. It is also a favorite addition to laxative herbs, tempering their violent effects. Caraway seeds, infused and allowed to cool, soothe colicky children and can be added to desserts to speed digestion after a rich meal.

DATA FILE

Properties

Caraway is a pungent, heating/drying agent, known for its stimulant and carminative properties. As an antispasmodic, caraway will soothe the muscles in the digestive process. It can also relax uterine tissue and is therefore beneficial for menstrual cramps.

Part of Plant Used

Seed.

Conditions Treated

Caraway aids the digestive process, both internally and in external application. It soothes indigestion, gas, colic, flatulence, and accumulation of toxins and

fluids. It is also beneficial as a scalp treatment. The oil can be used as an enema for intestinal parasites. A stomach massage with a very small amount of the oil will reduce flatulence. Caraway seeds can be added to any laxative to temper its strength and to soothe the colon.

Form Taken

Teas, as an oil for stomach massage, in an inhaler, and as a spice to aid the digestion of starches.

Used With Other Herbs?

Caraway blends well with dill, fennel, anise, basil, cardamom, and jasmine.

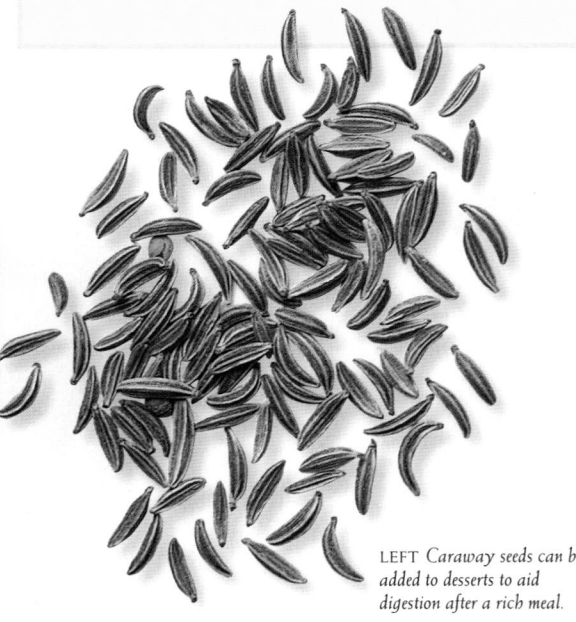

LEFT *Caraway seeds can be added to desserts to aid digestion after a rich meal.*

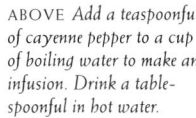

HOW TO USE

🌿 Caraway reduces vátha and kapha, and increases pitta. It clears kapha mucus build-up and soothes vátha emotion. Caraway increases pitta digestive fire. 🌿 Eat a teaspoonful of the seeds to aid digestion, or make an infusion.

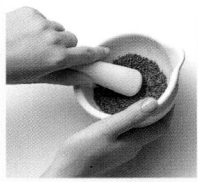

🌿 Finely crush 9 teaspoonsful of seeds using a pestle and mortar.

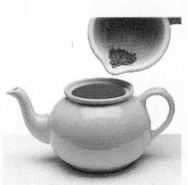

🌿 Place the seeds in a pot and add boiling water.

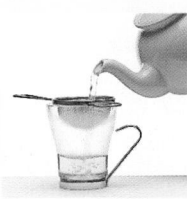

🌿 Allow the infusion to stand for 20 minutes, then strain and drink as needed, up to 3 cups a day.

THERAPY CONNECTIONS

MUSTARD
- Traditional and Folk Remedies   p.98
- Flower Remedies   p.239

CAYENNE PEPPER
- Herbalism   p.118

VÁTHA
Reduces Vátha
Caraway,
Cayenne Pepper
Neutralizes
Vátha
Mustard

PITTA
Reduces Pitta
Mustard
Increases Pitta
Caraway,
Cayenne pepper

KAPHA
Reduces Kapha
Caraway,
Mustard,
Cayenne pepper

Capsicum annuum
CAYENNE PEPPER *MERCHI*

This fiery red pepper, used the world over in cooking, is known to many Westerners by its Caribbean name, cayenne. Ironically, only a tiny amount of the world's red pepper supply comes from the Caribbean – India and Africa are the main producers. One traditional cayenne prescription is to put the powder into socks to warm cold feet!

DATA FILE

Properties
Cayenne pepper assists digestion by stimulating the flow of saliva and stomach secretions. It is analgesic and warming, increasing circulation. It has strong digestive, carminative, and emetic properties. Cayenne acts as a decongestant and an expectorant.

Part of Plant Used
The pod.

Conditions Treated
Cayenne alleviates colds, gastrointestinal and bowel problems, and is used as a digestive aid. Externally, cayenne treats arthritis and muscle soreness. Creams containing cayenne are frequently used in the treatment of shingles.

Form Taken
Raw, powdered, as a spice, oil, tea, or plaster.

Used With Other Herbs?
Garlic, onion, coriander, lemon, ginger.

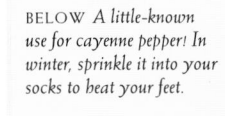

BELOW *A little-known use for cayenne pepper! In winter, sprinkle it into your socks to heat your feet.*

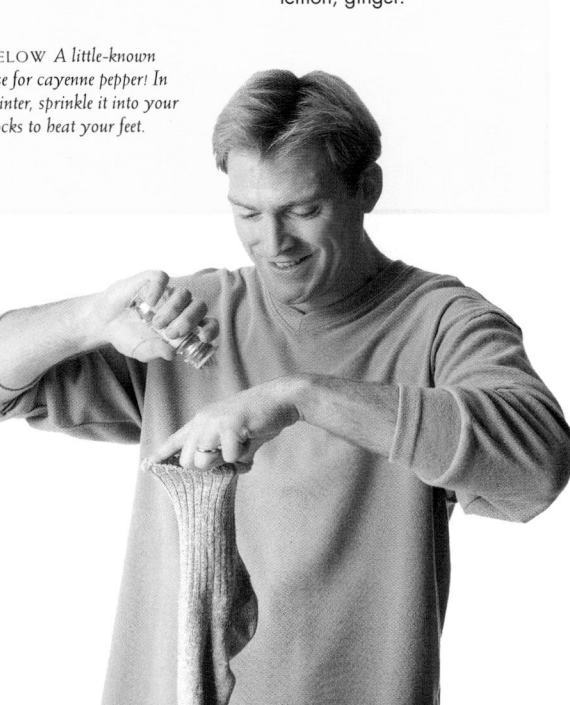

ABOVE *Add a teaspoonful of cayenne pepper to a cup of boiling water to make an infusion. Drink a table-spoonful in hot water.*

HOW TO USE

🌿 Cayenne, with its warming and mucus-relieving qualities, increases pitta and reduces kapha and vátha. Externally, cayenne can be used for arthritis and muscle soreness, and internally as a digestive aid and a treatment for colds, fever, toothache, diarrhea, and constipation. For a pain-relieving muscle rub, mix a half-teaspoon of cayenne powder or puréed fresh cayenne to 1 cup of warm vegetable oil.

CAUTION

DO NOT GIVE TO CHILDREN UNDER TWO YEARS OLD.

USE RUBBER GLOVES WHEN CHOPPING CAYENNE PEPPERS, AS THEY MAY BURN. IF BURNING DOES OCCUR, WASH WITH VINEGAR SEVERAL TIMES, RINSING CAREFULLY.

PEPPER OIL WILL CAUSE SEVERE PAIN ON CONTACT WITH SENSITIVE TISSUES, SUCH AS EYES OR GENITALS.

Cassia angustifolia
SENNA

The Chinese name for this herb is *Fan-Hsieh-Yeh*, or "foreign-country laxative herb." Senna has a very strong laxative effect on the body. Indian senna (*C. angustifolia*) is a close relative of North African and American senna, but its properties are much milder. Still a powerful laxative, it is gentler on the body. The seed pods can be used instead of the leaves for a still milder treatment.

DATA FILE

Properties

Bitter, pungent, cooling, and purging. It is cathartic, antiseptic, antispasmodic, cholagogue, and cleansing. Senna acts mostly on the lower half of the body.

Part of Plant Used

The leaves and the whole seed pods.

Conditions Treated

Senna is the most powerful herbal treatment for constipation, especially when it is chronic. Do not use if you suffer from hemorrhoids. Senna has sometimes been used to reduce fevers, and is an ingredient in sore throat remedies.

Form Taken

Used as a powder, a tea, or a supplement.

Used With Other Herbs?

Anise, cardamom, cinnamon, coriander, fennel, ginger, nutmeg, and orange.

BELOW *Only use North American and African senna with other herbs.*

HOW TO USE

❧ Senna reduces kapha and vátha, and increases pitta.
❧ A senna infusion will give you the benefits of senna's laxative power. Steep 3½ oz. (80g.) of senna leaves, ½ teaspoon of coriander, and ½ teaspoon of ginger in 1 quart (1l.) of hot water for 15 minutes. Take 1–4 tablespoons at a time. The infusion is more palatable cold than hot. ❧ For children or the elderly, senna pods have a more gentle laxative effect. Steep 3–4 pods in 4–5 tablespoons of cold water. Take 1 or 2 tablespoons at a time. ❧ For adults, use 6–12 pods for the same amount of water.

Cedrus deodara
CEDAR *DEVADARU*

The wood we know of for its insect repellent qualities (the cedar chest which protects woolens from moths) is also, according to the Ayurvedics, an excellent treatment for dandruff. Considered a soothing tonic to the skin, cedar is often used in men's perfumes and toiletries, particularly aftershave lotions.

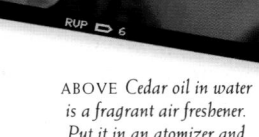

ABOVE *Cedar oil in water is a fragrant air freshener. Put it in an atomizer and spray your rooms.*

DATA FILE

Properties

Cedar is bitter and pungent, with antiseptic, diuretic qualities. It is useful as a nervine and expectorant. Cedar has a heating, drying effect on the body. The astringent, tonic qualities in cedar make it an excellent antidote to oily skin, oily scalp, and dandruff.

Part of Plant Used

The wood and bark.

Conditions Treated

Bronchitis, urinary infections, fear and nervous tension, oily hair, hair loss, oily skin, dandruff, sensitive skin, as a rub for sore joints and muscles, and to provoke sluggish menstrual cycles.

Form Taken

Oil for massage and inhalation; made into a tea or an infusion.

Used With Other Herbs?

Blends well with camphor, sandalwood, and vetiver.

HOW TO USE

❧ Cedar will reduce pitta and kapha, while increasing vátha.
❧ Cedar is an excellent air freshener, deodorizer, and insect repellent – add oil of cedar to water in an atomizer and spray the room, or add ten drops to a tablespoon of vegetable oil and rub it onto skin.

CAUTION

CEDAR SHOULD NOT BE TAKEN BY PREGNANT WOMEN, AS IT WILL STIMULATE THE MENSTRUAL CYCLE, AND ACTS AS A POSSIBLE ABORTIFACIENT.

RIGHT *Cedrus deodara grows quickly to reach a maximum height of 80ft. (25m.).*

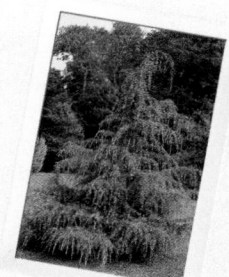

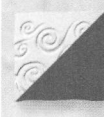

VÁTHA

Reduces Vátha
Senna, Camphor

Balances Vátha
Gotu Kola

Increases Vátha
Cedar

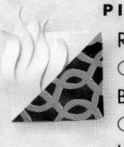

PITTA

Reduces Pitta
Cedar

Balances Pitta
Gotu Kola

Increases Pitta
Senna, Camphor

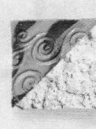

KAPHA

Reduces Kapha
Senna, Camphor, Cedar

Balances Kapha
Gotu Kola

Centella asiatica
GOTU KOLA *BRAHMI*

According to tradition, the natives of Sri Lanka were the first people to use gotu kola. They noticed that elephants, animals renowned for their longevity, loved to eat the rounded gotu kola leaves. Hence the proverb "Two leaves a day keeps old age away." The Ayurvedics used gotu kola like ginseng, as a tonic for longevity. Then they noticed it was beneficial for many skin diseases, including leprosy. Today it is used to aid a variety of conditions.

DATA FILE

Properties

Bitter, stimulating, cooling, and moistening. Gotu kola neutralizes blood acids and may lower body temperature. It acts as a nervine, a diuretic, and a rejuvenating tonic. It is excellent for hair growth and as a treatment for baldness.

Part of Plant Used

The seeds, nuts, and roots.

Conditions Treated

Gotu kola stimulates the central nervous system. It aids in the elimination of fluids, shrinks tissues, decreases fatigue and depression, and stimulates sexual appetite. Gotu kola

is recommended for rheumatism, blood disease, mental disorder, high blood pressure, a sore throat, tonsillitis, cystitis, venereal disease, insomnia, and to relieve stress.

Form Taken

Used as a massage oil, shampoo, poultice, tea, and skin cream.

Used With Other Herbs?

Sandalwood, lemon.

RIGHT *Gotu kola is reputed to prolong life, and acts as a general tonic.*

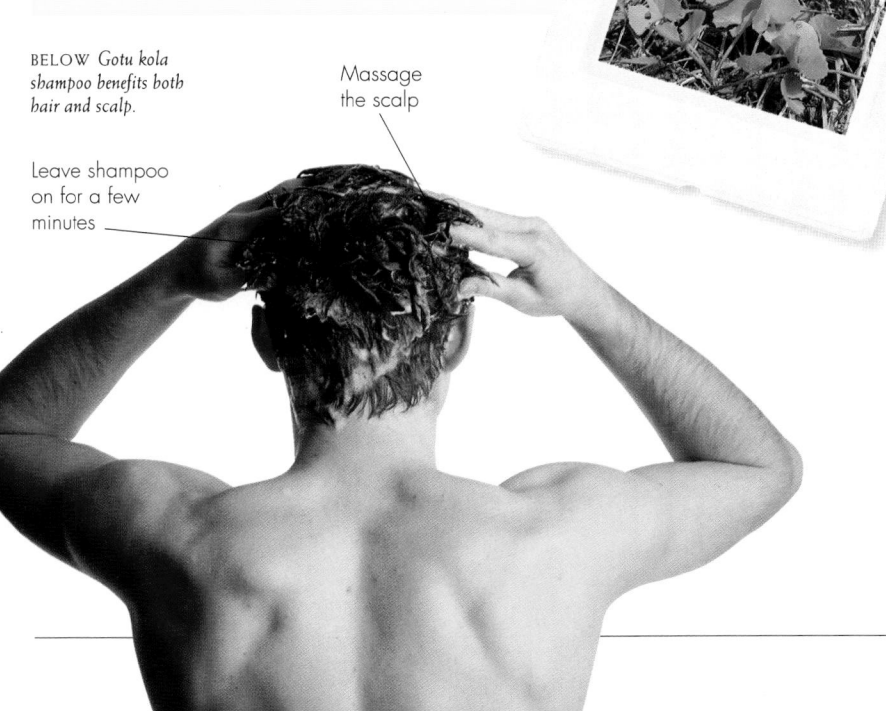

BELOW *Gotu kola shampoo benefits both hair and scalp.*

Massage the scalp

Leave shampoo on for a few minutes

HOW TO USE

Gotu kola has a balancing effect on all three doshas. Gotu kola infusions, taken as a beverage, will improve circulation in the legs and treat varicose veins.

They will also act as a soporific in cases of insomnia. Used as a compress, the infusion will relieve psoriasis.

To make an infusion, pour 2 cups of boiling water over 1 teaspoon of the herb. Let steep for 10 minutes. Drink up to 2 cups a day, adding lemon or honey to taste if desired.

If the results of a compress are disappointing, try strengthening the infusion used.

Cinnamomum camphora
CAMPHOR *KARPURA*

When camphor is steam-distilled, it is fractionalized into blue, brown, and white camphors. Blue camphor is the heaviest and weakest, and it is used mostly in perfume distillation. Brown camphor contains strong carcinogens and should be avoided. White camphor has medicinal qualities and is the most readily available.

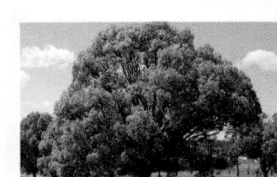

RIGHT *The camphor tree is a large evergreen grown in warm regions.*

HOW TO USE

Camphor reduces kapha and vátha, and it increases pitta when used in excess. For bronchitis and colds, try a camphor inhalation. Half-fill an enamel pan or heat-proof dish with just-boiled water. Add 7 drops of oil of camphor. Use a towel to form a "tent" over the bowl. Inhale deeply for several minutes. Stop if you feel dizzy or if the steam is too hot for your skin.

DATA FILE

Properties

Camphor is a pungent, sour, heating substance. It has moisturizing properties which recommend it for use as an expectorant, decongestant, and bronchial dilator. Camphor is frequently employed for its twin analgesic and antiseptic qualities.

Part of Plant Used

The twigs and the leaves. Both have a strong camphor smell. Make sure that you purchase camphor which has been steam-distilled from natural sources.

Conditions Treated

Camphor clears the mind and eases headaches. It alleviates joint and muscle pain. It acts on the nervous system and tissues, as well as the respiratory system. Camphor is indicated for bronchitis, asthma, coughs, arthritis, rheumatism, and gout. It also helps nasal and sinus congestion.

Form Taken

Use as a massage oil, compress, salve, steam inhalation, and in lotions.

Used With Other Herbs?

Use camphor in small doses only. Blends with rosemary, eucalyptus, and juniper.

Cinnamomum zeylanicum
CINNAMON *TWAK, TAJ*

Cinnamon originally grew in southern Asia. Ancient Ayurvedic practitioners used it as a treatment for fevers, diarrhea, and to mask unpleasant flavors in other healing herbs. The Greeks used cinnamon to treat bronchitis, but the Europeans championed the use of cinnamon in baking. Do not confuse cinnamon with cassia, or Chinese cinnamon, a more pungent herb which is frequently added to spiced meats.

DATA FILE

Properties

Cinnamon is a pungent, sweet astringent, with stimulating, heating qualities. It acts as a diaphoretic, parasiticide, antispasmodic, aphrodisiac, analgesic, and diuretic. Cinnamon's antiseptic, antibacterial, and antifungal qualities have frequently been utilized in toothpastes and as a treatment for gum disease. As an anti-yeast agent, cinnamon has been used to treat Candida and other yeast infections.

Part of Plant Used

The bark and the leaf.

Conditions Treated

Cinnamon is recommended for respiratory ailments such as colds, sinus congestion, and bronchitis. As a digestive aid, it relieves dyspepsia, intestinal infections, and parasites. It aids circulation and helps to alleviate anemia. Cinnamon is useful for the treatment of scabies and lice. Its benefits as an aid to circulation are especially powerful during the menopause, and cinnamon's properties will increase the appetite – both sexual and gastronomic.

Form Taken

As a tea, spice, inhalant, massage oil, or powder.

Used With Other Herbs?

Cardamom, orange, nutmeg, and licorice.

HOW TO USE

✦ Cinnamon reduces vátha and kapha, and increases pitta.
✦ **Because of its strong antibacterial effect, cinnamon can be used to treat minor scrapes and cuts.**
✦ Cinnamon contains the natural anesthetic oil eugenol, which will help relieve the pain of minor wounds. To treat cuts and scrapes, wash the affected area thoroughly. Pat dry. Sprinkle powdered cinnamon lightly over the area, then bind or bandage. Repeat treatment as needed until the area is healed.

CAUTION

DO NOT USE CINNAMON IN CASES OF HIGH PITTA.

CINNAMON WILL AGGRAVATE BLEEDING, AND CAN BE A SKIN IRRITANT AND A CONVULSIVE IN HIGH DOSES.

CINNAMON BARK OIL IN PARTICULAR CAN BE AN IRRITANT AND IS NOT RECOMMENDED FOR USE ON THE SKIN.

CINNAMON INFUSIONS SHOULD NOT BE GIVEN TO CHILDREN UNDER TWO.

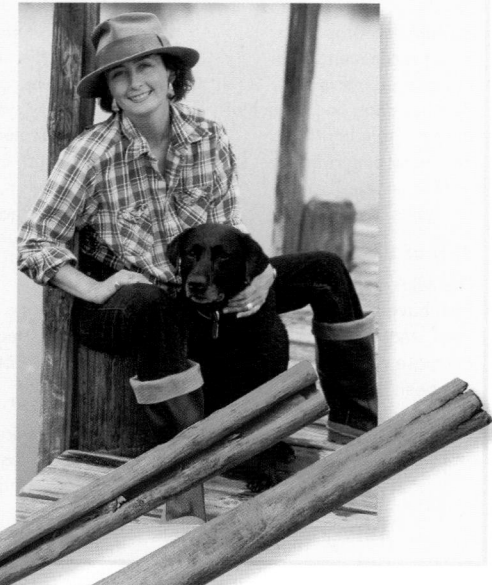

ABOVE LEFT *Cinnamon has powerful circulatory benefits during the menopause.*

BELOW LEFT *Cinnamon sticks are the dried inner bark of the shoots.*

Commiphora myrrha
MYRRH *BOLA*

Myrrh is the gum from a shrub native to northeastern Africa and southwestern Asia. The shrub can grow to 30ft. (9m.) tall. Myrrh exudes from natural cracks or man-made incisions in the bark. It leaves the tree as a pale yellow liquid, which hardens into a yellowish-red or reddish-brown substance which is collected for use. This resin or gum has been used for thousands of years for its healing properties. In the Bible, myrrh is one of the gifts the wise men brought to the Christ child.

ABOVE *Myrrh resin was used by the ancient Egyptians for embalming.*

DATA FILE

Properties

Myrrh is an alterative. It is analgesic, emmenagogic, rejuvenative, astringent, expectorant, antispasmodic, and antiseptic. Its tonic effects benefit all tissues of the body.

Part of Plant Used

The sap or gum.

Conditions Treated

Myrrh is a treatment for amenorrhea, dysmenorrhea, menopause, coughs, asthma, bronchitis, arthritis, rheumatism, traumatic injuries, ulcerated surfaces, anemia, pyorrhea, excessive weight, halitosis, gum disease, sore throat, canker sores, and mouth ulcers. Myrrh is used for embalming, to clean wounds, as a douche, to stimulate menstrual flow, to promote lung drainage, and to treat hemorrhoids.

Form Taken

As a lotion or salve, a massage oil, a gargle, an incense, plaster, or infusion.

Used With Other Herbs?

Frankincense, juniper, cypress, geranium, aloe, and pine.

HOW TO USE

✦ Myrrh reduces kapha and vátha, while increasing pitta. ✦ Its antiseptic and antifungal properties recommend it for sore throats, swollen gums, and cold sores. Myrrh oil can be used directly on sore gums, or to make a gargle.
✦ A gargle: mix 1 teaspoon of myrrh and 1 teaspoon of boric acid in 1pt. (500ml.) of boiling water. Stand for 30 minutes, then strain. Reheat and gargle. Do not swallow. Add 1 teaspoon of golden seal to cure bad breath.

CAUTION

DO NOT USE MYRRH IN CASES OF HIGH PITTA.

Coriandrum sativum

CORIANDER

DHANYAKA, DHANIA

By all accounts, coriander, or dhanyaka, originated in India. Two thousand years ago, it was imported to China. The herb was said to "stimulate arousal and confer immortality." A popular ingredient in curry spice blends, coriander retains its aphrodisiac status – but immortality has yet to be demonstrated!

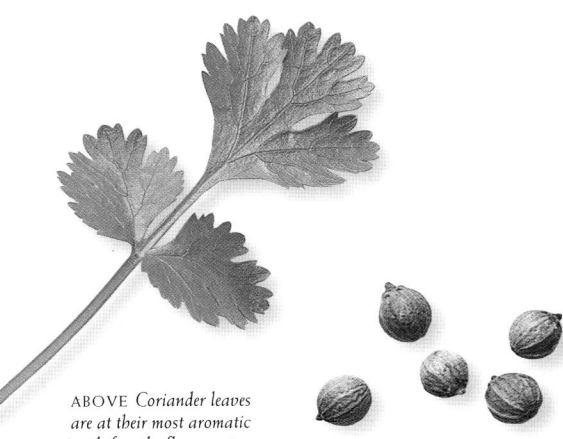

ABOVE *Coriander leaves are at their most aromatic just before the flowers open.*

DATA FILE

Properties

Coriander is a bitter, pungent herb, with a sweet, pleasant taste. Its energy is cooling and moisturizing. It has strong stimulant and alterative properties. Coriander acts as a diuretic and diaphoretic. Coriander stimulates the plasma, blood, and muscles. It is thought to be an aphrodisiac because of its phyto-estrogen content.

Part of Plant Used

The seeds and the leaves.

Conditions Treated

Coriander alleviates urinary infections, cystitis, rashes, hives, burns, digestive disorders such as gas pains, vomiting, and indigestion.

Coriander is beneficial for respiratory problems – it eases allergies and hay fever. It purifies the blood, decongests the liver, and reduces heat and fever in the body. As an anti-inflammatory, coriander benefits arthritis. Coriander is typically an ingredient in eyewashes for blindness, and has been indicated as a remedy for measles.

Form Taken

As a spice, a tea or infusion, a compress, douche, shampoo, and massage oil.

Used With Other Herbs?

Used with lemon, cajeput, lavender, cardamom, clove, nutmeg, jasmine, sandalwood, and cypress.

THERAPY CONNECTIONS

CINNAMON

Chinese Herbal Medicine   *p.59*

Aromatherapy *p.150*

MYRRH

Aromatherapy *p.155*

CORIANDER

Aromatherapy *p.156*

HOW TO USE

Coriander reduces all three doshas. **Its antifungal, antibacterial properties were noted by the Romans, who used coriander to preserve meats.** Like cinnamon, coriander powder can be sprinkled on cuts and scrapes to prevent infection. **The infusion makes an excellent digestive aid.** Bruise 1 teaspoon of the seeds (or use ½ teaspoon of the powder). Place in a cup, and add 1 cup boiling water. Let steep for 5 minutes. Drink up to 3 cups a day after meals. This same infusion, at half-strength, may be given, with caution, to children under two years of age for colic.

Drink up to 3 cups a day, after meals

CAUTION

IN HIGH DOSES, CORIANDER MAY CAUSE KIDNEY IRRITATION.

DURING PREGNANCY, USE ONLY UNDER RECOMMENDATION FROM YOUR PHYSICIAN.

RIGHT *Drinking coriander infusion helps with digestive problems.*

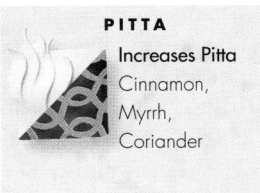

VÁTHA
Reduces Váta
Cinnamon, Myrrh, Coriander

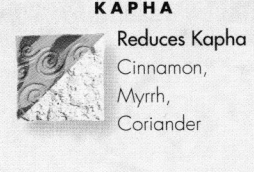

PITTA
Increases Pitta
Cinnamon, Myrrh, Coriander

KAPHA
Reduces Kapha
Cinnamon, Myrrh, Coriander

Crocus sativus
SAFFRON *KESAR, NAGAKESHARA*

Saffron is a small, perennial crocus with purple flowers cultivated in Spain, France, Sicily, Iran, and India. The young plant does not flower for the first few years. When it matures, it produces flowers with golden stigmas which are quite expensive to harvest. The stigmas, or threads, are highly valued for their medicinal and aphrodisiac properties, as well as their delicious flavor.

DATA FILE

Properties

Saffron is warming, digestive, stimulant, and rejuvenating. It has anodyne, antispasmodic properties; it is frequently used as an emmenagogue and expectorant. Saffron has been highly valued in Ayurvedic tradition for its aphrodisiac properties, especially its sweet, heavy aroma and taste.

Part of Plant Used

The stigmas or threads.

Conditions Treated

Aids digestion and improves appetite. Benefits menstrual pain and irregularity, menopause, impotence, infertility, anemia, enlarged liver, hysteria, depression, insomnia, neuralgia, lumbago, rheumatism, cough, asthma, gastro-intestinal complaints, colic, and chronic diarrhea.

Form Taken

Whole threads as a spice, in oils, infusions, and food. The oil can be used as a massage oil, a perfume, or a bath.

Used With Other Herbs?

Cedarwood, champa, lavender, rosewood, sandalwood.

HOW TO USE

🍂 Saffron can be used to balance all three doshas.
🍂 A saffron infusion can be helpful for irregular menstruation and menstrual pains. 🍂 Steep 6–10 stigmas in ½ cup of boiling water. Take 1 cup a day, unsweetened. 🍂 Saffron is prized for its aphrodisiac qualities. Try it to inspire your romantic encounters!

CAUTION

DO NOT USE DURING PREGNANCY, AS THE HERB CAN PROMOTE MISCARRIAGE.
—◇—
SAFFRON CAN BE NARCOTIC IN LARGE DOSES – DO NOT EXCEED THE MEDICINAL AMOUNT INDICATED. A DOSE OF ½OZ. (10–12G.) CAN BE FATAL FOR HUMANS.

BELOW *Saffron threads. Saffron comes from the iris family, and is used both as a spice and a yellow dye.*

Cuminum cyminum
CUMIN *JEERA*

Cumin seeds are pungent and savory brown seeds with a flavor common to Indian and Middle Eastern cooking. Heating the seeds, by cooking or infusing, aids the digestive power of the cumin. Cumin is very rich in vitamins and minerals, and is an antidote to weakness and fatigue.

CAUTION

AN EXCESS OF CUMIN MAY CAUSE NAUSEA.

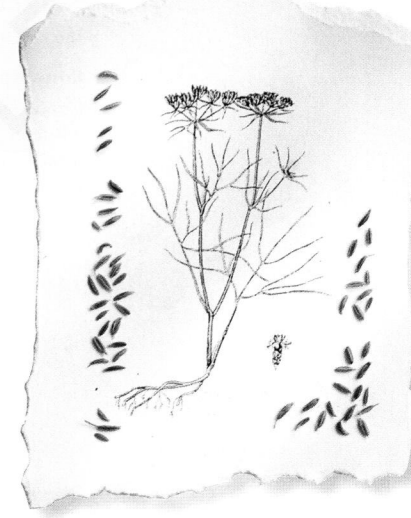

RIGHT *Cumin is an aromatic spice much used in Indian cooking to aid digestion.*

DATA FILE

Properties

Cumin has a pungent, bitter effect, with neutral to cooling properties. It acts as a blood cleanser, a carminative, aiding in the absorption of nutrients to the system. Cumin is a physical and sexual stimulant. It is antispasmodic, alterative, and acts as a lactagogue and immune builder.

Part of Plant Used

The seed.

Conditions Treated

Digestive disorders and gas pains, anemia, migraine, allergies, nervous conditions, low breast milk, and lack of sexual drive. Cumin builds up the immune system of people who suffer severe allergies.

Form Taken

In a compress, as a spice and infusion, in massage oil, and as an inhalation.

Used With Other Herbs?

Because of its overpowering smell, use cumin in small amounts when mixing with other herbs. Cumin is frequently used with lemon, black pepper, coriander, lavender, and rosemary.

HOW TO USE

🍂 Cumin reduces kapha and pitta, and increases vátha.
🍂 To relieve abdominal pain, add the seeds to food.
🍂 Abdominal pain can also be treated with a cumin seed poultice. First, soak 2 tablespoons of cumin seeds in hot water for two hours.

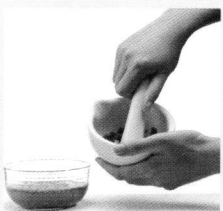

🍂 Strain, dry, then crush the seeds with a heavy object (a clean stone, rolling pin, or hammer).

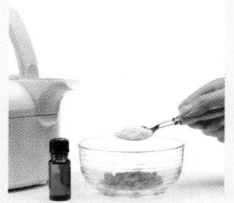

🍂 Add several drops of peppermint oil, a little flour and some hot water – just enough to make a paste. Mix well. Spread this mixture on a piece of muslin or thin cloth, and apply over the abdomen to relieve liver, stomach, and gall bladder pains.

Curcuma longa

TURMERIC *HARIDRA, HALDI*

Turmeric holds a place of honor in Ayurvedic medicine. It is a symbol of prosperity, and was believed to be a cleanser for all the systems in the body. Turmeric was prescribed as a digestive aid, a treatment for fever, infections, dysentery, arthritis, jaundice, and it has been used as a basic ingredient in curries for thousands of years.

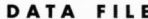

RIGHT *The leaves of the turmeric plant. Turmeric originates from south Asia.*

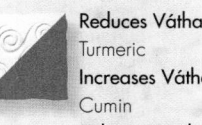

VÁTHA
Reduces Vátha
Turmeric
Increases Vátha
Cumin
Balances Vátha
Saffron

PITTA
Reduces Pitta
Cumin
Increases Pitta
Turmeric
Balances Pitta
Saffron

KAPHA
Reduces Kapha
Cumin, Turmeric
Balances Kapha
Saffron

CAUTION

DO NOT USE IN CASES OF HEPATITIS, EXTREMELY HIGH PITTA, OR PREGNANCY.

TURMERIC IS SAID TO REDUCE FERTILITY, AND WOULD NOT BE RECOMMENDED FOR SOMEONE TRYING TO CONCEIVE.

HOW TO USE

🍃 Reduces kapha and vátha, and increases pitta. 🍃 **Reduces fat, purifies blood, and aids circulation.** 🍃 It benefits digestion, and can help rid the body of intestinal parasites. 🍃 **A turmeric infusion will benefit all these conditions, and reduce arthritis pain.** 🍃 Warm 1 cup of milk and remove it from the heat before it boils. Stir in 1 teaspoon of turmeric powder. Drink up to 3 cups of this a day.

LEFT *Turmeric rhizomes are ground to make the familiar yellow powder.*

DATA FILE

Properties

Antiseptic, warming, pungent, bitter, and astringent. Turmeric acts as a stimulant, an alterative, and carminative, with vulnerary, antibacterial properties. Turmeric roots have a bright yellow color, and are sometimes used as a dye and a food coloring.

Part of Plant Used

The roots.

Conditions Treated

Indigestion, poor circulation, cough, amenorrhea, pharyngitis, skin disorders, diabetes, arthritis, anemia, wounds, bruises, and all immune system deficiencies. Because of its energizing effect on the immune system, turmeric is being studied for use in the treatment of HIV and AIDS.

Form Taken

As a massage oil, in facial creams and lotions, in compresses, or as a food or spice.

Used With Other Herbs?

Ginger, musk, wild sunflower.

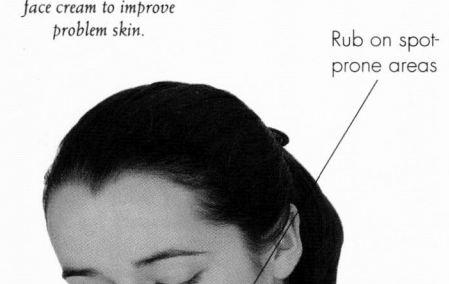

BELOW *Using turmeric face cream to improve problem skin.*

Rub on spot-prone areas

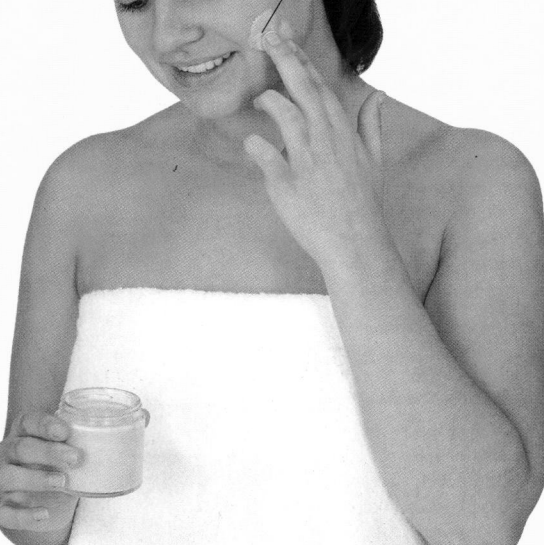

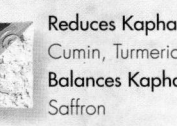

Elettaria cardamomum
CARDAMOM *ELAICHI*

Cardamom is a stimulating plant which eases the brain, the respiratory and the digestive systems. Its sweet, warming energy brings joy and clarity to the mind, and is particularly good for opening the flow of prana, or vital energy, through the body. Added to milk, cardamom will neutralize mucus-forming properties; added to coffee, it detoxifies caffeine.

LEFT *and* BELOW *Cardamom leaves and seeds. The main cardamom producers are Sri Lanka and India.*

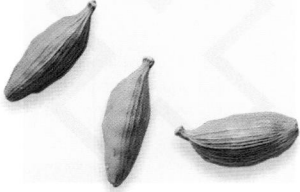

CAUTION
DO NOT USE WITH ULCERS, OR IN HIGH PITTA STATES.

DATA FILE

Properties

Cardamom is a stimulant, an expectorant, a diaphoretic, and has aphrodisiac properties. Its qualities are pungent and sweet, with heating/moisturizing effects on the doshas. Cardamom aids in the digestion of fats and starches, stimulates the spleen, and calms acid stomach and acid regurgitation. Cardamom suppresses vomiting when eaten with a banana.

Part of Plant Used

The seeds and root.

Conditions Treated

Cardamom aids respiratory problems such as coughs, colds, bronchitis, asthma, and loss of voice. It also benefits the digestive system in cases of vomiting, belching, and indigestion.

Cardamom's stimulating effects bring mental clarity and good humor.

Form Taken

Tea, as an additive to milk and food, as a bath, inhalation, or massage oil.

Used With Other Herbs?

Cardamom blends well with orange, anise, caraway, ginger, and coriander.

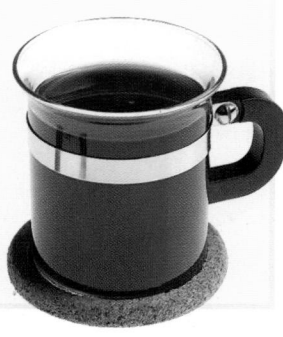

LEFT *Cardamom can be added to coffee to neutralize the caffeine.*

HOW TO USE

&. Cardamom reduces kapha and vátha, and stimulates pitta.

&. **Because of its soothing nervine properties, it will calm a fluttery high vátha state by kindling agni (fire).** &. Cardamom removes excess kapha mucus from the stomach and lungs.

&. Basundi, a milk-based digestive aid, is also a delicious dessert. To make this, take 2 cups of full cream milk, 2 teaspoons of cardamom powder, 2 tablespoons of ground almonds and pistachio, a pinch of saffron powder, and add honey to taste. Bring the milk to the boil and simmer until it thickens. Stir frequently to prevent burning. Add cardamom, chopped nuts, and a little honey. Continue to stir, and cook for another minute or two. Remove from heat, and add honey to taste. Let the mixture cool before eating. Serves two or three people.

Eugenia caryophyllata
CLOVES *LAVANGA*

Clove is the bud of a tropical evergreen tree. Now common as a kitchen spice, clove was a rare, prized substance for thousands of years. The demand for cloves and other Asian herbs spurred explorers like Magellan (who brought cloves to Spain) to circle the globe. Its sweetening, deodorizing properties have long been used externally in potpourris, incense, and air fresheners. Clove can also be used as an internal deodorizer, freshening the breath and reducing body odor.

ABOVE *Cloves: the dried flower buds of* Eugenia caryophyllata *which originated in Indonesia.*

DATA FILE

Properties

Clove has pungent and heating properties. It functions as an analgesic, expectorant, stimulant, and carminative. Clove has antifungal properties useful for treating athlete's foot, and it deodorizes the mouth and breath. As an anesthetic it has been used in treating toothache.

Part of Plant Used

Dried flower buds (either whole or powdered).

Conditions Treated

Clove is recommended for colds, coughs, asthma, laryngitis, pharyngitis, toothache, indigestion, vomiting, hiccups, low blood pressure, and impotence. Clove tones muscles, and expectant mothers are recommended to eat cloves in the last month of pregnancy to strengthen the uterus.

Form Taken

As an oil, a compress, inhalation, massage oil, lotion, spice, and tea.

Used With Other Herbs?

Cardamom, cinnamon, lavender, ginger, orange, bay leaf.

HOW TO USE

&. Cloves reduce kapha and vátha, and increase pitta.

&. **Clove has long been used to fight bacteria, tooth decay, and anesthetize dental pain.** &. For temporary relief of toothache prior to visiting your dentist, clean your teeth gently and thoroughly. Dip a Q-tip in pure clove oil. Apply it to the affected tooth and surrounding gum area.

CAUTION
CLOVE SHOULD NOT BE GIVEN TO CHILDREN UNDER TWO, NURSING MOTHERS, AND SHOULD BE USED WITH CARE BY PREGNANT WOMEN.

EXTERNAL USE OF THE OIL MAY CAUSE A RASH.

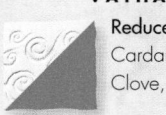
Glycyrrhiza glabra
LICORICE *MULATHI*

Licorice is one of the most popular healing herbs in Ayurvedic medicine. It has been used for ulcers and malaria, to treat throat and respiratory problems, and to soothe rashes and infections. Due to its strong, sweet taste, the herb is sometimes used in recipes to mask the unpleasant taste of another herb.

CAUTION

LICORICE MAY INCREASE
BLOOD PRESSURE SLIGHTLY
AND CAN CAUSE MILD
ADRENAL STIMULATION.

IN PREGNANT AND NURSING
WOMEN, CASES OF HIGH
BLOOD PRESSURE OR HIGH
ADRENAL FUNCTION, IT
SHOULD BE USED ONLY ON
THE ADVICE OF A PHYSICIAN.

RIGHT *Licorice root is sweet-tasting and used in confectionery and medicine.*

DATA FILE

Properties

Licorice is sweet and astringent. It is a demulcent, expectorant, and germicide, with laxative and alterative properties. It has been used with muscle problems because of its anti-inflammatory, antiarthritic properties. Licorice is antibacterial and antiviral.

Part of Plant Used

The root and the bark.

Conditions Treated

Strengthens the nerves, promotes the memory, treats asthma, bronchitis, throat problems, digestive disorders, disorders of the spleen, liver disease, Addison's disease, inflamed gall bladder, colds, coughs, constipation, ulcers, and gastritis. Licorice powder has also been used externally to treat genital herpes and cold sores.

Form Taken

As a powder, a tea or infusion, a food, or an oil.

Used With Other Herbs?

Black pepper, clove, fenugreek, ginger, long pepper, sage, turmeric.

VÁTHA

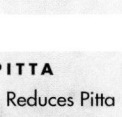 Reduces Vátha
Cardamom,
Clove, Licorice

PITTA

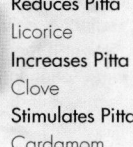 Reduces Pitta
Licorice
Increases Pitta
Clove
Stimulates Pitta
Cardamom

KAPHA

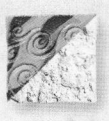 Reduces Kapha
Cardamom,
Clove

RIGHT *Licorice is a perennial growing to 4ft. (1.2m.) high with small, oval leaves.*

HOW TO USE

Licorice reduces both vátha and pitta. The herb, a common treatment for bronchitis and colds, may be chewed directly, taken as a tea, or made into a medicated ghee, or clarified butter, preparation. To make clarified butter, melt 1lb. (500g.) of unsalted butter, bringing it to a light boil and skimming off the foam until clear. Strain the clear butter through cheesecloth, and let it cool.

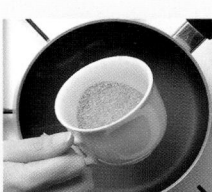

For licorice medicated ghee, you will need 2 cups of water, ¼ cup of licorice powder, and 2 tablespoons of pure ghee. Boil the water, add the licorice powder, then boil the mixture for 12 minutes.

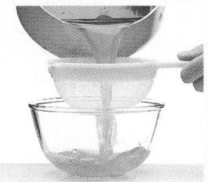

Remove from the heat and strain with a fine sieve.

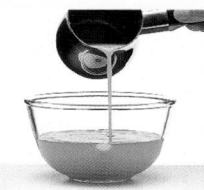

Add ghee to the remaining liquid, let it stand for 10 minutes, then administer externally or add it to food while it is still warm.

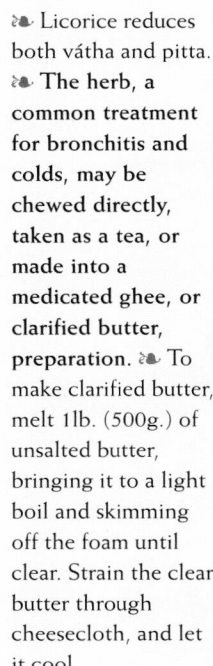

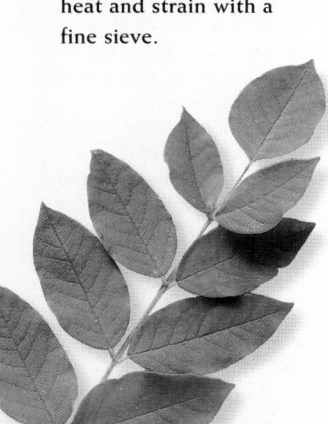

Inula helenium
WILD SUNFLOWER
ELECAMPANE, SURIA-MUKHI

Traditional Ayurvedic and Chinese herbalists have long used the dried root of the wild sunflower, or elecampane, to treat bronchial infections, asthma, and whooping cough. The Greeks were convinced of the healing properties of the herb for intestinal disorders such as dysentery, pinworm, and parasites. Today, elecampane is used to treat the respiratory and digestive systems, menstrual problems, and to aid kidney function.

ABOVE *The root of the wild sunflower is dug up in the fall and dried.*

HOW TO USE

🍂 Elecampane increases pitta, and reduces kapha and vátha with its warming, drying qualities.
A decoction treats both respiratory and digestive upsets. Put 3 cups of water and 2 teaspoons of powdered root into an enamel pan. Cover and boil gently for 30 minutes. Allow to cool. The taste will be bitter. Sweeten with honey if desired. Take 2 tablespoons at a time, up to 2 cups a day. Store the mixture in a refrigerator.

DATA FILE

Properties
Wild sunflower is a sweet, bitter, pungent herb with warming, drying qualities. It acts as an expectorant, a tonic for the nervous system, a rejuvenative, and a galactagogue (induces milk secretion). Elecampane's antibacterial and antifungal qualities support its use in the effective expulsion of intestinal parasites.

Part of Plant Used
The roots.

Conditions Treated
Colds, bronchial infections, coughs, lung congestion and infection. It aids digestive disorders such as amebic dysentery, pinworms, hookworms, and giardiasis. It stimulates the brain, kidneys, stomach, and uterus, and eases sciatica. Wild sunflower has been used to treat menstrual cramps.

Form Taken
Inhalations, massage oils, and lotions.

Used With Other Herbs?
Cedarwood, cinnamon, lavender, frankincense, musk, and tuberose.

Hypericum perforatum
ST. JOHN'S WORT

St. John's wort is a bushy, flowering shrub found the world over. The leaves and flowers have long been used for their diuretic, emmenagogic, and anti-depressant qualities. The Ancient Greek scholar, Galen, describes the herb as the antidote to intestinal worms. Scientists have recently discovered that the herb is a source of hypercin, which may counter the HIV virus.

HOW TO USE

🍂 St. John's wort reduces pitta and kapha, and increases vátha. An oil extract of St. John's wort can be used internally for stomach ache, colic, or intestinal disorders. Externally, the oil will soothe wounds, burns, and treat skin cancer. Put the fresh leaves and flowers in a glass jar, and fill it with olive oil. Close the jar and leave it for six to seven weeks, shaking it often. The oil will turn red. Strain the oil through a cloth. If a watery layer appears when the oil has stood for a while, decant or siphon it off. Stored in a dark container, the oil will keep for up to two years. Use the oil externally or take internally, 10–15 drops in water.

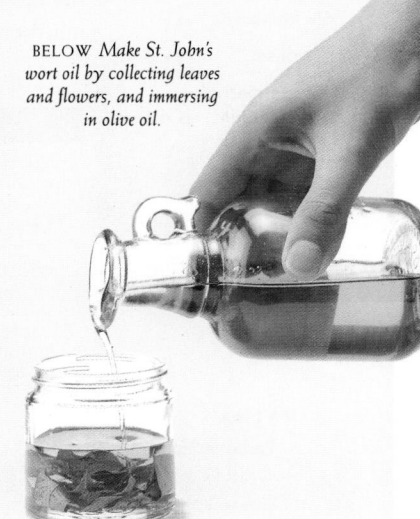

BELOW *Make St. John's wort oil by collecting leaves and flowers, and immersing in olive oil.*

BELOW *St. John's wort should be gathered when the plant is in flower.*

DATA FILE

Properties
Bitter, astringent, sweet, and cooling. St. John's wort has moisturizing, vulnerary, antispasmodic, anti-inflammatory properties. It is an expectorant, a nutritive tonic, and a nervine.

Part of Plant Used
The leaves and the flowers.

Conditions Treated
Spinal problems, skin problems, joint pain, problems associated with aging, trauma, and eczema. St. John's wort has been indicated for stomachache, colic, congestion in the lungs, insomnia, anemia, headache, jaundice, catarrh, burns, wounds, and sores. It can be used to treat carcinoma, bedwetting, melancholy, depression, uterine cramping, and menstrual problems.

Form Taken
As a massage lotion, compress, or salve; as a tea, tincture, or infusion.

Used With Other Herbs?
Angelica, chamomile, rosewood, yarrow.

THERAPY CONNECTIONS
ST. JOHN'S WORT
Herbalism   p.124
Homeopathy p.199

Medicago sativa
ALFALFA

Alfalfa is grown the world over, primarily as food for livestock. The ancient Chinese, noticing their cattle preferred grazing in alfalfa, started to sprout alfalfa shoots to use as a vegetable. Ancient Arabs fed it to their horses to increase speed and endurance. They called it al-fac-facah, "father of every food," and introduced it to the Spanish, who changed the name to alfalfa. Ayurvedics have used alfalfa to cleanse the liver, detoxify the blood, treat ulcers, arthritis, and fluid retention.

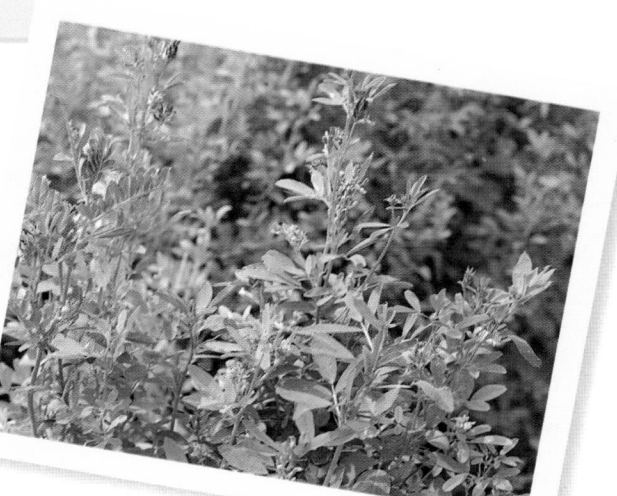

RIGHT *Alfalfa has deep roots and so is resistant to drought. It has mauve flowers in summer.*

DATA FILE

Properties

Alfalfa is bitter and astringent, with cooling properties. It is high in chlorophyll and nutrients. It alkalizes and detoxifies the body, aids the liver, and is good for anemia, ulcers, diabetes, hemorrhaging, and arthritis. Alfalfa promotes pituitary gland function and contains antifungal agents.

Part of Plant Used

The leaves, petals, flowers, and sprouts.

Conditions Treated

Ayurvedic medicine notes alfalfa's ability to soothe ulcers, as well as reduce arthritis and fluid retention. Alfalfa leaves help to reduce blood cholesterol levels and clean plaque deposits from arterial walls. The sprouts produce a similar but lesser effect; however, the sprouts help neutralize carcinogens in the colon, binding them and speeding their elimination from the body. Alfalfa has been used to treat anemia, colitis, sciatica, and rheumatism. Sip the infusion for a natural breath freshener.

Form Taken

Take as a tea, a supplement, or in sprouts.

Used With Other Herbs?

Fenugreek, garlic, ginger, saffron, turmeric.

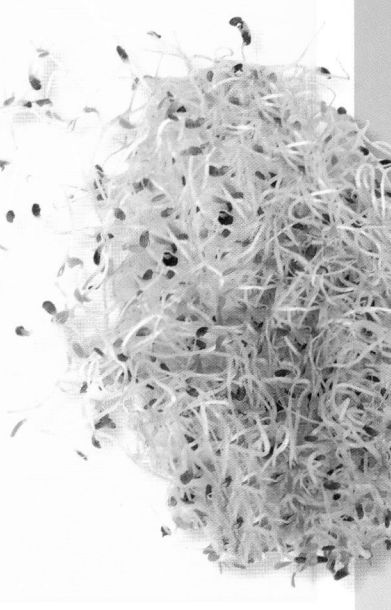

ABOVE *Originally from southwest Asia, alfalfa is now grown all over the world.*

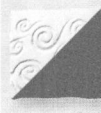
VÁTHA
Reduces Vátha
Alfalfa
Increases Vátha
St. John's wort

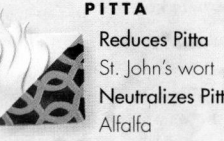
PITTA
Reduces Pitta
St. John's wort
Neutralizes Pitta
Alfalfa

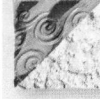
KAPHA
Reduces Kapha
St. John's wort
Increases Kapha
Alfalfa

HOW TO USE

Alfalfa reduces both kapha and vátha, and has a neutral effect on pitta. **It is a great detoxifier and can be used on a regular basis to cleanse the system and provide refreshing chlorophyll.** The tea can be used to reduce cholesterol. Use 2 teaspoons of the herb to 1 cup of boiling water. Let it steep for 15 minutes. Drink up to 3 cups of the tea a day.

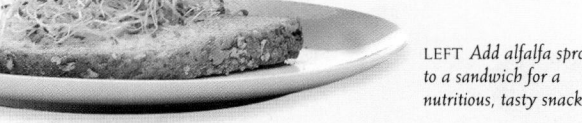

LEFT *Add alfalfa sprouts to a sandwich for a nutritious, tasty snack.*

CAUTION

NEVER EAT ALFALFA SEEDS BECAUSE THEY CONTAIN HIGH LEVELS OF THE TOXIC AMINO ACID CANAVANINE. OVER TIME, EATING THE SEEDS COULD RESULT IN IMPAIRED FUNCTIONING OF THE PLATELETS AND WHITE BLOOD CELLS.

THE ALFALFA PLANT ALSO CONTAINS SAPONINS, CHEMICALS WHICH MAY AFFECT RED BLOOD CELLS. IN RECOMMENDED DOSES, ALFALFA IS CONSIDERED COMPLETELY SAFE.

PREGNANT AND NURSING WOMEN SHOULD CONSULT A PHYSICIAN BEFORE USE.

Myristica fragrans
NUTMEG *JAIPHALA*

Nutmeg is a tropical evergreen tree native to Indonesia. The brown, wrinkled fruit contains a kernel which is covered by a bright red membrane. The membrane produces the spice mace. The 2–4in. (5–10cm.) kernel provides us with nutmeg. Many healing remedies use mace and nutmeg together.

DATA FILE

Properties

Warming, stimulant, rejuvenating. Nutmeg improves appetite and digestion. It is highly aromatic, carminative, and has strong hallucinogenic properties when ingested in large quantities. However, nutmeg is also highly toxic when ingested in large doses, and is only recommended for use in small doses of 1 teaspoonful or less.

Part of Plant Used

The kernel of the seed.

Conditions Treated

Nutmeg is calming and sleep-inducing, making it an excellent remedy for insomnia and other sleep disorders. It has been used to treat diarrhea and vomiting. Nutmeg strengthens the heart and eases menstruation. In small quantities, it acts on the stomach, improving digestion and appetite, while dispeling flatulence or acid stomach. Nutmeg has been used to ease kidney trouble.

Form Taken

Whole or as a powder, as a tea, a spice, a massage oil, or an inhalation.

Used With Other Herbs?

Balsam, bay, cinnamon, cumin, lavender.

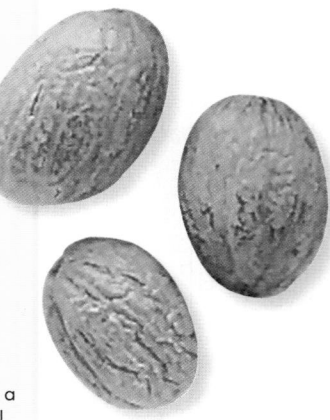

ABOVE *Whole nutmegs. The spice mace also comes from the* Myristica *plant.*

BELOW *Nutmeg helps to thwart insomnia. Drink nutmeg tea before going to bed.*

HOW TO USE

Nutmeg increases kapha and vátha, and has a neutral effect on pitta.

A nutmeg stomach tonic will relieve gas, nausea, and indigestion. Take 1½ teaspoons of powdered slippery elm bark, ½ teaspoon of nutmeg, and 1½ teaspoons of mace. Mix thoroughly and add a little cold water to make a smooth paste with no lumps. Bring 1pt. (500ml.) of light cream or ½pt. (250ml.) each of cream and water to the boiling point, remove from the heat, and quickly add the paste. Stir with a wooden spoon for 1 minute or until the powder is completely dissolved. Let cool until lukewarm. Drink ½ cup. You may take ½ cup up to three times daily, always warm, to help heal stomach problems.

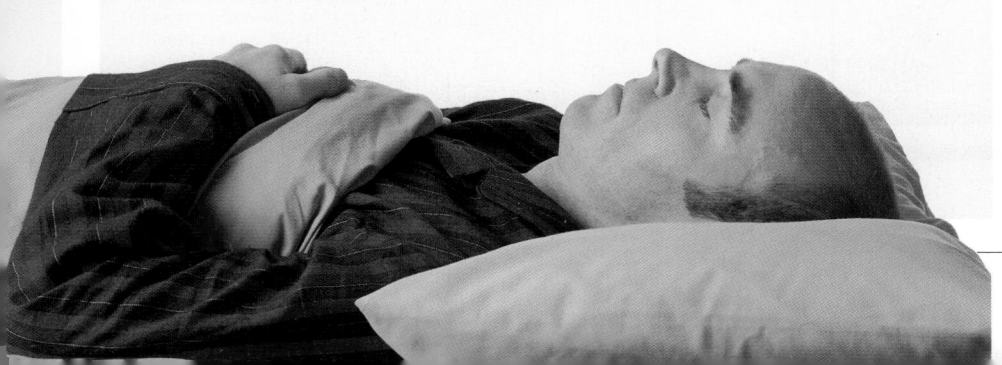

Ocymum basilicum
BASIL *TULSI*

There are many different varieties of basil. The Indian variety is also known as basil krishna, because it is said that Krishna wore garlands of this herb around his neck to increase his detachment and his faith. The faithful continue this practice, believing basil to be a protector in life and after death. Ayurvedics have used basil to treat stomach, kidney, and blood ailments.

ABOVE *Basil can be grown on a window-ledge if kept in a sunny position.*

HOW TO USE

Basil reduces kapha and vátha, and increases pitta.
It has a strong effect on the emotions, and can ease fear or sadness. Use a homemade infusion as an acne remedy. Steep 3 teaspoons of dried leaves in 1 cup of boiling water. Steep for 20 minutes. Apply with a cotton ball to freshly washed skin, or drink up to 3 cups of the tea per day as an internal antibacterial treatment.

DATA FILE

Properties

Basil acts as a diaphoretic, a febrifuge (a fever reducer), and a nervine. Basil is antibacterial, antiseptic, antifungal, and antispasmodic. Basil stimulates the immune system by increasing the production of antibodies.

Part of Plant Used

The leaves, the oil.

Conditions Treated

Basil can provide relief for colds, coughs, asthma, sinus congestion, headaches, arthritis, rheumatism, and fevers. Basil oil kills intestinal parasites, and as such is recommended for abdominal conditions, parasites, and stomachache. A basil poultice can be used to treat ringworm infections.

Form Taken

Basil can be drunk as a tea or juice, cooked into medicated ghee, used as an inhalation, massaged as a therapeutic oil, or made into a compress or poultice.

Used With Other Herbs?

Basil is wonderful when used in conjunction with camphor, rosemary, juniper, lemon, eucalyptus, myrtle, lavender, bergamot, lime, and clary sage. Great fragrances!

Piper longum
LONG PEPPER *PIPPALI*

Native to India and Java, these peppers are gathered and stored to ripen for use, in order to preserve the greatest heat potency. Long pepper, or pippali, is the primary ingredient in Ayurvedic medicine to treat kapha disorders. Together with ginger and black pepper, long pepper is used as a component in the Ayurvedic blend Trikatu.

CAUTION

LONG PEPPER SHOULD NOT BE GIVEN TO CHILDREN UNDER TWO YEARS OLD.

USE RUBBER GLOVES WHEN CHOPPING PEPPERS, AS IT MAY BURN THE FINGERTIPS. IF BURNING SHOULD OCCUR, WASH WITH VINEGAR SEVERAL TIMES, RINSING CAREFULLY.

PEPPER OIL CAN LINGER FOR SEVERAL HOURS, AND WILL CAUSE SEVERE PAIN IF IT COMES IN CONTACT WITH SENSITIVE TISSUES, SUCH AS EYES OR GENITALS.

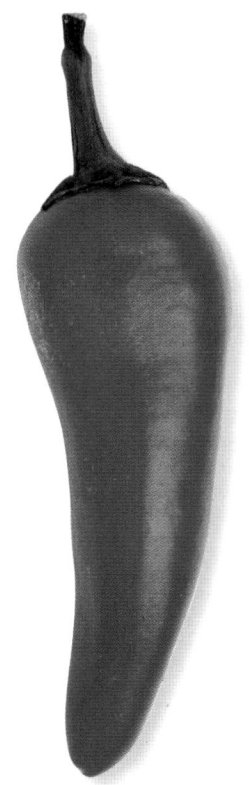

RIGHT *Long pepper obviously gets its name from its shape.*

HOW TO USE

🍃 Long pepper restores kapha and vátha to balance, invigorating sluggish kapha, and warming vátha's coolness. 🍃 **Its warming action increases pitta.** 🍃 Use a pippali and rock salt tea to clear sore throats, sinus congestion, coughs, and hiccups. 🍃 **To a large mug, add 1½ cups of boiling water, ½ teaspoon of long pepper powder, and ½ teaspoon of rock salt. Cover and let steep for 15 minutes. Pour the tea into another cup, leaving the sediment behind. Drink while warm.**

DATA FILE

Properties
Long pepper is a pungent, heating stimulant. It has strong digestive, carminative, and emetic properties. Long pepper acts as a decongestant and expectorant. It is analgesic and warming, and increases the circulation.

Part of Plant Used
The fruit (pepper).

Conditions Treated
Asthma, bronchitis, throat problems, digestive disorders, disorders of the spleen. Externally, long pepper can be used for arthritis and muscle soreness. Taken internally, it is useful as a digestive aid and a treatment for colds, fever, toothache, diarrhea, and constipation.

Form Taken
As a powder, a tea or infusion, a food, or an oil.

Used With Other Herbs?
Black pepper, fenugreek, ginger, turmeric.

BELOW *Pepper-infused oil's warming action benefits rheumatism and arthritis.*

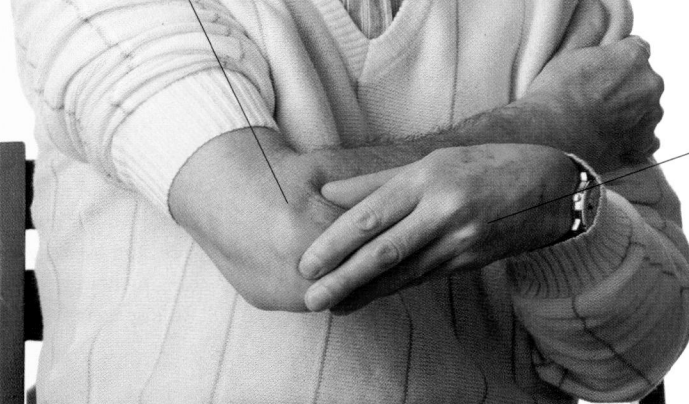

Painful joint

Rub in oil

THERAPY CONNECTIONS
BASIL
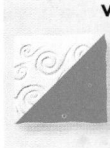 Aromatherapy p.164

VÁTHA

 Reduces Vátha
Basil
Balances Vátha
Long pepper
Increases Vátha
Nutmeg

PITTA

Increases Pitta
Basil,
Long pepper
Neutralizes Pitta
Nutmeg

KAPHA

Reduces Kapha
Basil
Balances Kapha
Long pepper
Increases Kapha
Nutmeg

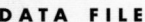

Piper nigrum
BLACK PEPPER
MARICH, MARI

In Ayurvedic traditions, black pepper or marich is named after the Sanskrit word for the sun. Black pepper contains very potent solar energy, and is a powerful digestive stimulant. Black pepper is rajasic, or energy-producing, in nature. The plant is native to South India, where the white-flowered shrub grows wild. The yellow berries, which are dried for peppercorns, turn red when they mature and are ready for harvesting.

ABOVE *Peppercorns are dried, unripe berries which are crushed to produce the oil.*

CAUTION

DO NOT USE IN HIGH PITTA STATE OR IN CASES OF INFLAMMATION OF THE DIGESTIVE ORGANS.

OVERUSE OF STIMULANT HERBS CAN IMPAIR YOUR BODY'S NATURAL BALANCING SYSTEMS.

IF YOU FIND YOU ARE ATTRACTED TO ADDING PEPPER TO MOST OF YOUR FOOD, THEN START CUTTING BACK.

DATA FILE

Properties

Black pepper has a heating and drying effect. The taste is pungent and bitter, both properties good for balancing an overabundance of kapha.

Part of Plant Used

The pepper kernel and the oil made from it.

Conditions Treated

Black pepper stimulates the plasma and the blood, the nervous system, the spleen, and reduces fat. It is beneficial for chronic indigestion, toxins in the colon, sinus congestion, and can stimulate the circulation to help warm cold hands and feet.

Form Taken

Take as a spice, as an oil, a tea, or a compress.

Used With Other Herbs?

Black pepper combines well with orange, ginger, cypress, anise, sandalwood, lemon, and basil.

HOW TO USE

🍃 Reduces kapha, increases pitta and vátha. 🍃 **Use in cooking as a stimulant – black pepper's qualities are enhanced by heating.** 🍃 The oil can be used to clear sinus congestion and stimulate fat reduction. To assist weight loss, blend 10 drops lavender oil, 10 drops black pepper oil, 5 drops sandalwood oil, 5 drops frankincense oil, and mix into 3fl. oz. (100ml.) almond oil. Store in a dark glass container. Clearly label the mixture to show it is for weight reduction use, and massage into areas where you want to lose weight.

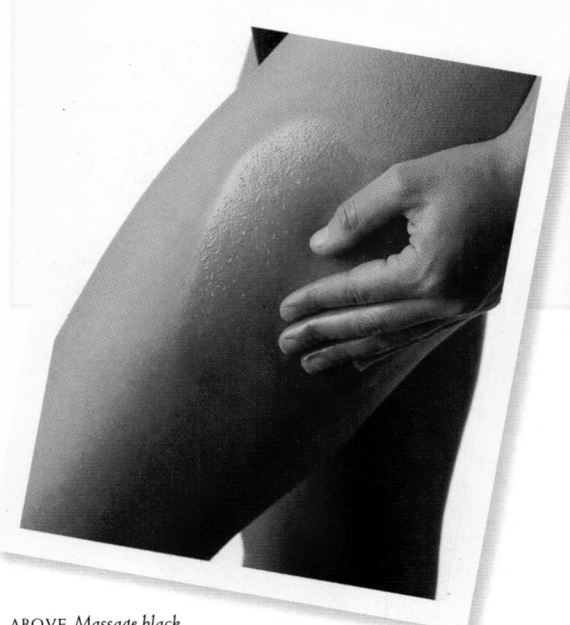

ABOVE *Massage black pepper oil into fat-prone areas to help weight loss.*

Santalum album
SANDALWOOD *CHANDANA*

Sandalwood is a small tree which grows primarily in southern Asia. While the aromatic wood is used to make scented carvings, the medicinal properties are in the oil, which can be pressed from the wood, or extracted with alcohol or water.

HOW TO USE

🍃 Reduces pitta and vátha, and has a neutral effect on kapha. 🍃 **A sandalwood decoction will reduce fever if taken internally; externally it can be used to treat acne and other skin problems.** 🍃 To make a decoction, boil 1 heaped teaspoon of sandalwood in 1 cup of water. Cover and boil for several minutes. Strain and cool. Drink 1 or 2 cups a day, a tablespoon at a time. For external use, apply to freshly washed skin, and let dry. Repeat three times a day or as needed.

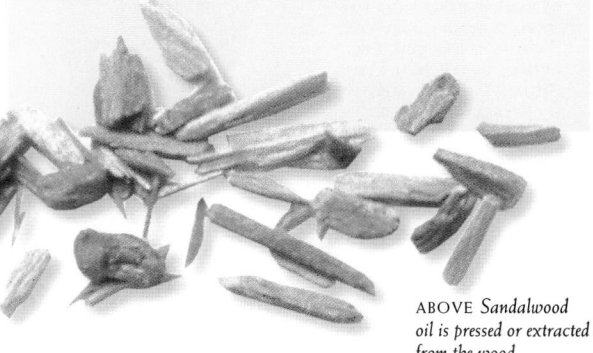

ABOVE *Sandalwood oil is pressed or extracted from the wood.*

DATA FILE

Properties

Bitter, sweet, astringent, cooling, moisturizing. Sandalwood is alterative, hemostatic, antipyretic, antiseptic, antibacterial, carminative, sedative, antispasmodic, and aphrodisiac. It works as a nervine, an expectorant, a diuretic, a disinfectant, and a moisturizer. It also helps to regenerate tissues.

Part of Plant Used

The wood.

Conditions Treated

Sandalwood has been used to treat cystitis, urethritis, vaginitis, acute dermatitis, herpes, bronchitis, palpitations, gonorrhea, sunstroke, dry skin, acne, laryngitis, nausea, tuberculosis, depression, insomnia, prostatitis, nervousness, anxiety, and impotence. Sandalwood can cure skin problems that are bacterial in origin.

Form Taken

In perfumes and massage oils; as a gargle, lotion, bath, inhalation, compress, or douche.

Used With Other Herbs?

Clove, geranium, musk, myrrh, tuberose, vetiver.

Trigonella foenum-graecum
FENUGREEK METHICA

Fenugreek is another healing herb whose qualities were brought to the attention of humans by animals. Farmers noticed that sick cattle would eat fenugreek plants even when they would not eat anything else. So fenugreek began to be used as a digestive aid and laxative. Fenugreek seeds contain a lot of bulk and mucilage, and, when mixed with water or saliva, become gelatinous and ease sluggish bowels.

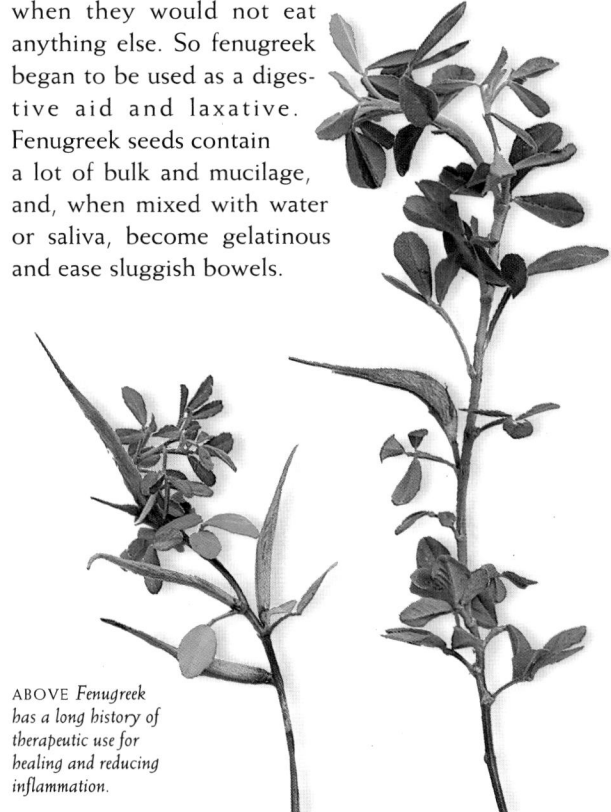

ABOVE *Fenugreek has a long history of therapeutic use for healing and reducing inflammation.*

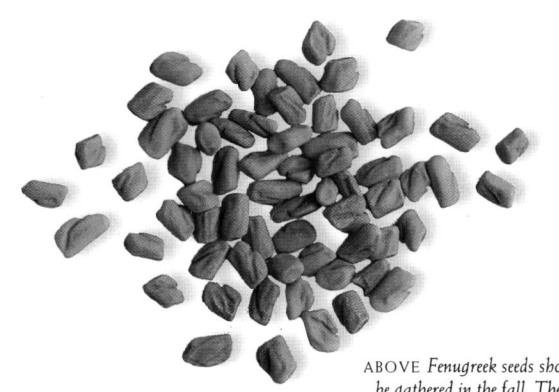

ABOVE *Fenugreek seeds should be gathered in the fall. Their bitterness soothes indigestion.*

DATA FILE

Properties

Antiseptic and warming. Fenugreek has expectorant qualities. It is anti-inflammatory, antiseptic, and soothing. The soothing expectorant qualities aid in promoting menstruation, as well as easing coughs, sore throats, and digestion (encouraging flow in the body).

Part of Plant Used

The seeds.

Conditions Treated

Constipation, digestive disorders, bronchitis, inflamed lungs, fevers, high cholesterol, eyestrain, sore throats, wounds, boils, rashes. It stimulates the uterus, promotes water retention and weight gain, reduces blood sugar levels, and lowers cholesterol.

Form Taken

As a spice, a tea, a massage oil, an inhalant, a poultice, or plaster.

Used With Other Herbs?

Peppermint, lemon, anise.

THERAPY CONNECTIONS

BLACK PEPPER

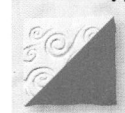 Traditional Home and Folk Remedies *p.97*

Aromatherapy *p.167*

SANDALWOOD

Aromatherapy *p.169*

VÁTHA

Reduces Vátha
Sandalwood, Fenugreek
Increases Vátha
Black pepper

PITTA

Reduces Pitta
Sandalwood
Increases Pitta
Black pepper, Fenugreek

KAPHA

Reduces Kapha
Black pepper
Fenugreek
Neutralizes Kapha
Sandalwood

HOW TO USE

🍃 Fenugreek reduces kapha and vátha, and increases pitta. 🍃 **Fenugreek helps asthma and sinus problems by reducing mucus.** 🍃 The seeds can be eaten by nursing mothers to increase milk production. 🍃 **A fenugreek poultice can be used to treat boils and rashes.** 🍃 Gargling a fenugreek decoction will soothe sore throats. 🍃 **Fenugreek decoctions have many healing uses: to treat arthritis and aching joints, to bring on menstruation, to lower cholesterol, or to ease sore throats and laryngitis.** 🍃 To make a decoction, bruise 2 tablespoons of fenugreek seeds. Add 4 cups of water. Bring to a boil, then cover and simmer for 10 minutes. Drink up to 3 cups a day. Add honey, lemon, or licorice to sweeten.

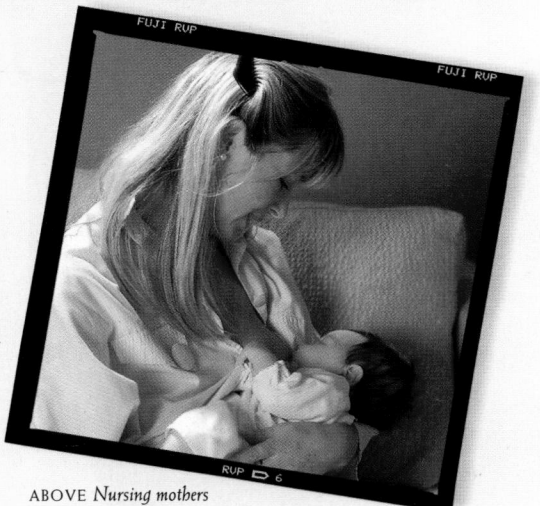

ABOVE *Nursing mothers can eat fenugreek seeds to increase their milk.*

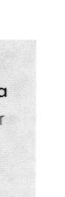

Vattiveria zizanoiodes
VETIVER

Vetiver is a grassy plant known for its grounding, centering properties. In India, it is sown wherever there is soil erosion, to hold down the earth and prevent further damage to the land. Modern herbalists use it to enable an individual to connect to the earth and feel his or her purpose. It is helpful during emotionally stressful times and has been used as a tonic for women suffering PMS.

ABOVE *Vetiver has aromatic roots which yield a fragrant oil used in perfumes.*

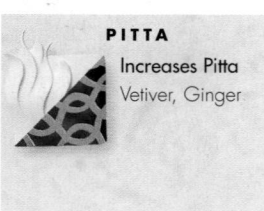

VÁTHA
Reduces Vátha
Vetiver, Ginger

PITTA
Increases Pitta
Vetiver, Ginger

KAPHA
Reduces Kapha
Ginger
Increases Kapha
Vetiver

DATA FILE

Properties
Warming, sweet, and bitter. Vetiver is an antiseptic tonic, grounding, regenerating, and strengthening. It is an aphrodisiac, and can be used to repel moths.

Part of Plant Used
The leaves and roots.

Conditions Treated
Arthritis, root chakra blockage, nervousness, insomnia, rheumatism, stress, disconnectedness, anorexia, postnatal depression, aging skin, fatigue, menopause, loss of appetite.

Form Taken
As a lotion, bath, massage oil, in patches and perfumes.

Used With Other Herbs?
Angelica, citrus, cinnamon, lavender, sandalwood, sage, yarrow.

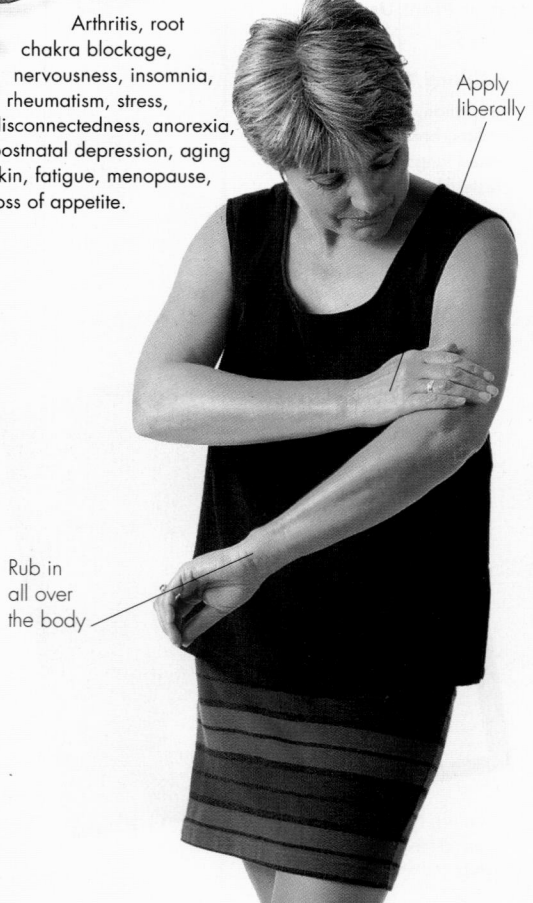

Apply liberally

Rub in all over the body

HOW TO USE

🍃 Vetiver reduces vátha, and increases both kapha and pitta. 🍃 **Vetiver oil is particularly useful for jet lag, and for grounding and clarity while traveling.**

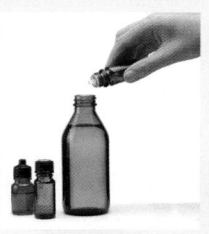

ABOVE *Add the essential oils to the base oil.*

🍃 Use as a base 2fl. oz. (60ml.) apricot kernel oil. Add 5 drops vetiver oil, 5 drops geranium oil, and 2 drops juniper or grapefruit oil. Apply this mixture liberally all over your skin before travel.
🍃 **Once traveling, reapply to as much of your body as possible every four or five hours.**
🍃 You may also carry a damp washcloth to which the oils have been added. If you are flying, the flight attendant may heat the washcloth in the microwave for you. Shower or bathe upon arrival, and reapply the oils. Enjoy your trip!

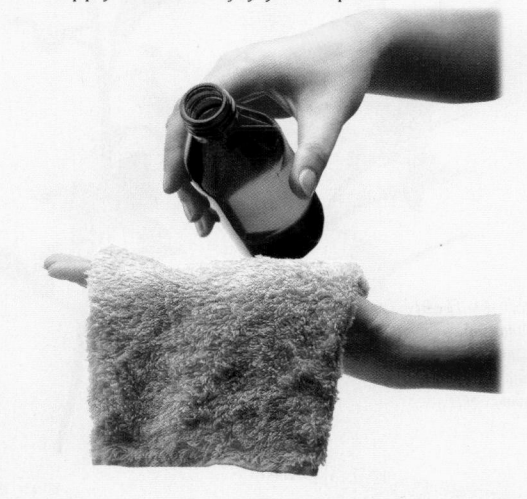

ABOVE *Apply the blend to a damp washcloth to pack and use during your journey.*

CAUTION
VETIVER HAS A VERY STRONG SMELL. DO NOT ALLOW IT TO OVERPOWER ANY BLEND YOU ARE MAKING WITH IT.

THERAPY CONNECTIONS

VETIVER
⬤ Aromatherapy *p.171*

GINGER
⬤ Aromatherapy *p.171*
⬤ Chinese Herbal Medicine *p.57*

LEFT *Massage vetiver travel oil blend into your skin to help the body cope with a journey.*

Zingiber officinalis

GINGER *ARDRAKA*

Ginger is native to India, where the ancient Ayurvedics used it to preserve food, as a digestive aid, and as a spiritual and physical cleanser. Garlic was shunned on the days leading up to religious festivities, but plenty of ginger would be consumed in order to be sweet-smelling and purified for the gods. The Greeks wrapped the root in a piece of bread and ate it after a heavy meal to prevent indigestion – this is the origin of gingerbread.

ABOVE *Children will enjoy making gingerbread – and eating the results of their handiwork!*

RIGHT *The fresh root of the ginger plant may be dried and powdered for convenience.*

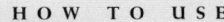

CAUTION

DO NOT USE IN CASES OF HIGH FEVER, BLEEDING, WITH INFLAMMATORY SKIN CONDITIONS, OR IF ULCERS ARE PRESENT.

◄◦►

GINGER IN LARGE DOSES CAN BRING ON MENSTRUATION.

◄◦►

PREGNANT WOMEN WITH A HISTORY OF MISCARRIAGE SHOULD EXERCISE CAUTION AND CONSULT THEIR PHYSICIAN BEFORE USE.

DATA FILE

Properties

Ginger is a pungent, sweet herb with warming/drying qualities. It acts as a stimulant, diaphoretic, antidepressant, and expectorant. Ginger stimulates all tissues of the body, and is highly recommended in cases where the illness is due to poor assimilation.

Part of Plant Used

The root.

Conditions Treated

Ginger is recommended for colds, coughs, flu, indigestion, vomiting, belching, abdominal pain, motion sickness, laryngitis, arthritis, hemorrhoids, headaches, impotence, diarrhea, heart disease, and memory loss.

Form Taken

As a food, a tea, a gargle, and a compress. Also used as a massage oil.

Used With Other Herbs?

Black pepper, eucalyptus, juniper, cedar, coriander, and all citrus fruits.

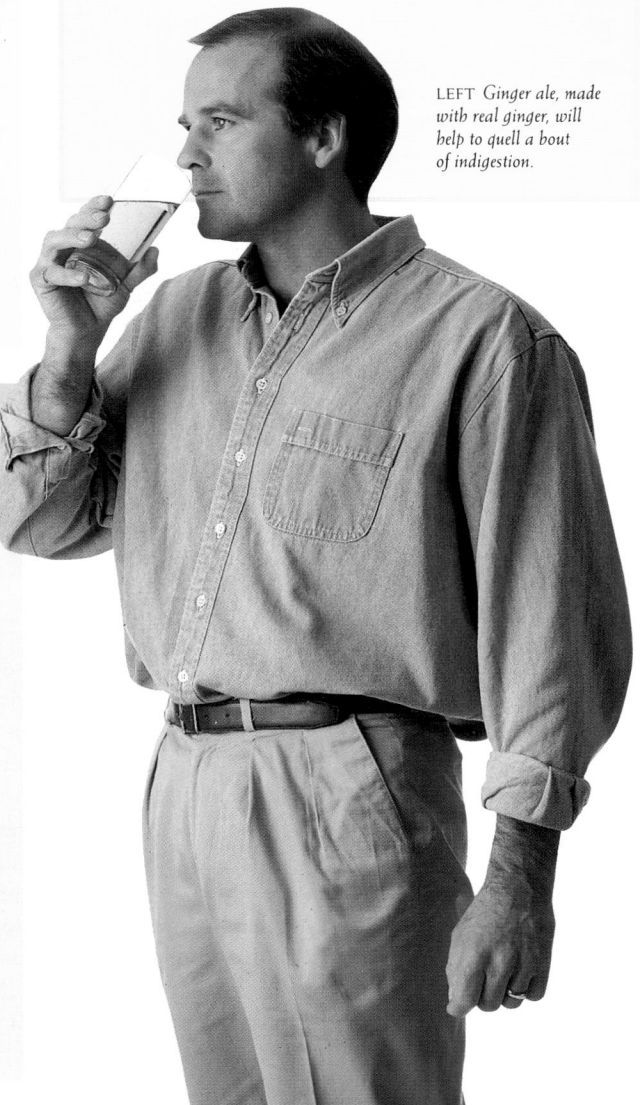

LEFT *Ginger ale, made with real ginger, will help to quell a bout of indigestion.*

HOW TO USE

🍂 Ginger increases pitta in the body, reducing both kapha and vátha. 🍂 **Its muscle-relaxant, heating pitta qualities can warm uterine walls, soothing menstrual cramps.** 🍂 It is also frequently used as an antidote to travel sickness. 🍂 **For motion sickness (on land, sea, or in the air), use a few drops of ginger oil on a small bandage and place behind the ear.**
🍂 Alternatively, you may take ginger capsules, or make a ginger tea with 2 teaspoons of the grated root to 1 cup of boiling water. Let it steep for 5 minutes. Of course, you could also sip a glass of ginger ale (provided it is made from real, not synthetic, ginger).

ABOVE *Motion sickness responds well to remedies made with ginger.*

CHINESE HERBAL MEDICINE

Chinese medicine is an ancient system of healing — acupuncture and Chinese herbal medicine grew up in tandem over 2,000 years. It is based on the philosophy of a very different civilization from our own, a civilization that perceived people as either "in harmony" or "out of harmony" with themselves and their surroundings. Traditional Chinese Medicine (TCM) sees disease in terms of patterns of disharmony, and so attempts to restore the balance in the person who is sick. Energy is believed to flow through channels called meridians, through which disease may be treated.

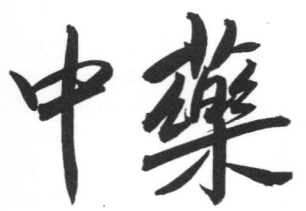

THE CHARACTERS FOR
CHINESE MEDICINE

WHAT IS CHINESE HERBAL MEDICINE?

TCM uses terminology that sounds strange to most Westerners. Instead of talking about rheumatic diseases or neurological diseases it classifies diseases as being caused by Wind, Heat, Dampness, or Cold. Instead of talking about rheumatism in the knee joint, it may classify it as Cold–Damp in the Stomach meridian *(see page 50)*. Western medicine focuses on a specific cause for a specific disease, and when it isolates that cause or agent it tries to control or destroy it. Chinese medicine is also concerned with the cause, but it focuses on the patient's response to that disease entity, both physiological and psychological. All the relevant information, including symptoms that may not seem related to the patient's main complaint, is collected together to enable the practitioner to discover the pattern of disharmony within that person, which can then be addressed by Chinese medicine. For instance, two patients coming with asthma may have completely different diagnoses according to Chinese medicine. The one with a pale face, prone to catching colds (Lung Qi Deficiency) will be given a completely different herbal formula to the patient who has a dry cough, thirst, and breathlessness on exertion (Lung Yin Deficiency). TCM does treat the same diseases – to a large extent people have the same problems the world over – it just perceives them in an entirely different way.

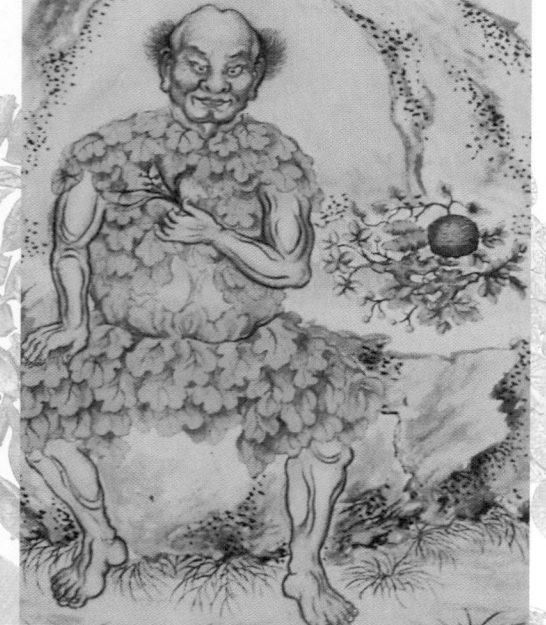

ABOVE *The Chinese
god of medicine. Chinese
medicine has an ancient
heritage.*

YIN AND YANG

Chinese medicine is based on the philosophy of yin and yang. These are the dual forces in the universe, seen both within nature and in human beings. They are used to explain the ongoing process of natural changes – yang is more prevalent during the day, while yin forces are more prevalent at night. There is no absolute yin or yang in living things – a cold yin-type illness may have aspects of yang, such as sharp, forceful contractions. Yin and yang both depend on each other and keep each other under control. However, it is when they go seriously out of balance and do not correct themselves that there is disease.

Everything has a yin and a yang aspect – for instance:

ITEM	YIN	YANG
Time	Night	Day
Season	Fall/Winter	Spring/Summer
Energy	Passivity/Stillness	Activity/Movement
Body	Front/Lower/Inside	Back/Upper/Outside
Breath	Inhalation	Exhalation
Temperature	Cold	Hot
Moisture	Wet/Damp	Dry
Direction	Downward	Upward

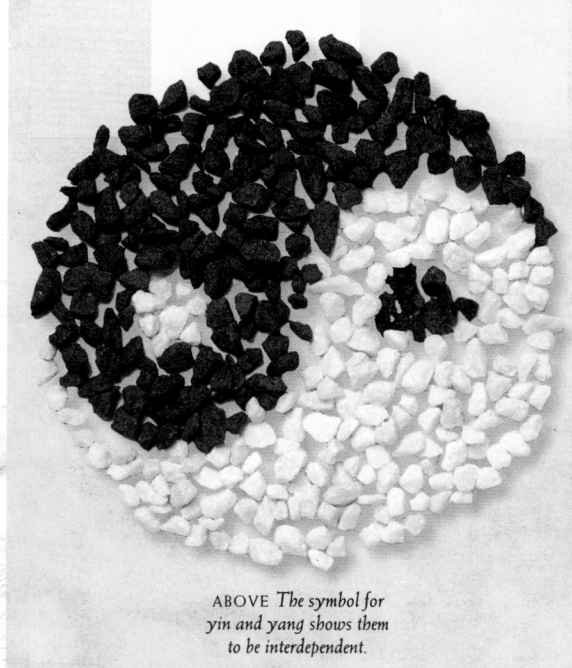

ABOVE *The symbol for
yin and yang shows them
to be interdependent.*

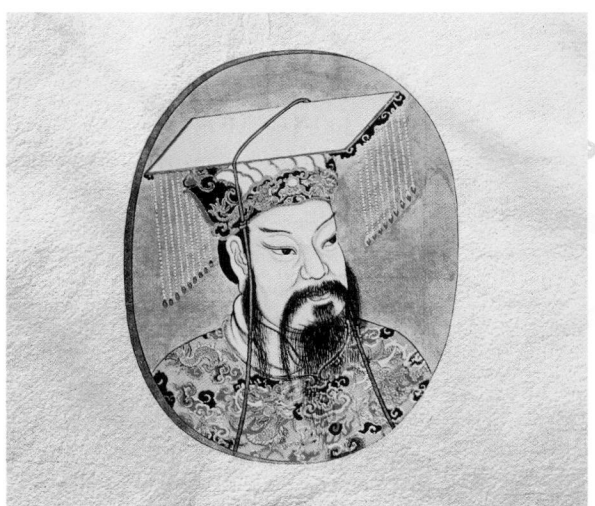

ABOVE *The* Inner Classic *takes the form of a dialog between the legendary Yellow Emperor and his minister Qi Bo on the topic of medicine.*

A SHORT HISTORY

The earliest herbal formulas in China were found to have been written down in the 3rd century B.C.E. In fact, the main book of the theory of Chinese medicine – the *Yellow Emperor's Inner Classic* – was compiled in the 1st century C.E., and is still taught in schools of TCM. Over the centuries, leading physicians have written down both herbal and acupuncture formulas, which explains the vast bulk of Chinese medicine reference books. The *Imperial Grace Formulary* of the Tai Pang Era (around 985 C.E.) for example, contains 16,834 entries, many of which are still commonly referred to today.

The early herbal formulas were very simple and elegant, while the later ones are much more complicated. Either type can be useful, depending on the patient and the physician's preferred manner of working. A practitioner of TCM, or someone practising Chinese herbal medicine specifically, will diagnose the patient's pattern of disharmony, find the tried and tested prescription which is closest to that patient's pattern, and add or subtract herbs to make it more suitable for that individual. Herbs are seldom used singly; they are usually combined in prescriptions containing 4–16 substances.

THE CHINESE THEORY OF LIFE

The Chinese believe that every living being is sustained by a basic Life Force, called "qi" (pronounced "chee"). Human beings receive their qi from a mixture of the influences of both Heaven and Earth. Therefore, we do have an element of the divine in us, which separates us from the animals. Chinese medicine works with the qi that we have to make us better. It may unblock the flow of qi in the body if it is stuck, or it may nourish qi if it is deficient.

We are born with a fixed amount of qi inherited from our parents (Yuan Qi – source or genetic qi). This is used both as our "reserve tank" and as a catalyst in most of the chemical processes of the body. We can nourish our Yuan Qi, though we cannot add to it. We may, however, deplete it through bad living practices – long-term lack of sleep or good food, drugs, drink, or years of excessive sex. The Chinese believe that this source qi is stored in the Kidneys (where its substance is called Jing or essence), and its functions include the control of sexual and reproductive activity in the body. We get our day-to-day qi from the air we breathe (Gong Qi) and the food we eat (Gu Qi).

Qi permeates the entire body; it directs the blood, nerve, and lymphatic systems (Ying Qi). It protects us from catching viruses (Wei Qi), and fights them if they get into the body. It transforms the food we eat into bodily substances – blood, tears, sweat, and urine – keeps organs in their proper place, and prevents excessive loss of sweat. Qi keeps the body warm and is naturally the source of movement and growth, as it has all these functions. We also use it in TCM to describe the functions of any Organ – for instance, Lung qi may be "weak" or Liver qi "blocked."

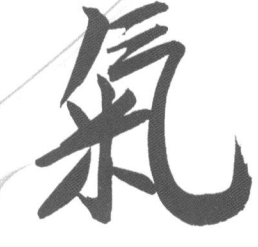

ABOVE *The Chinese character for qi. Qi is pronounced "chee," and often written as "chi."*

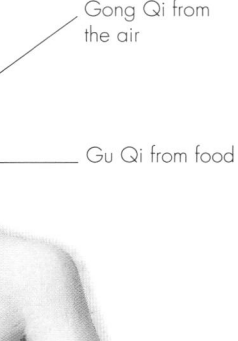

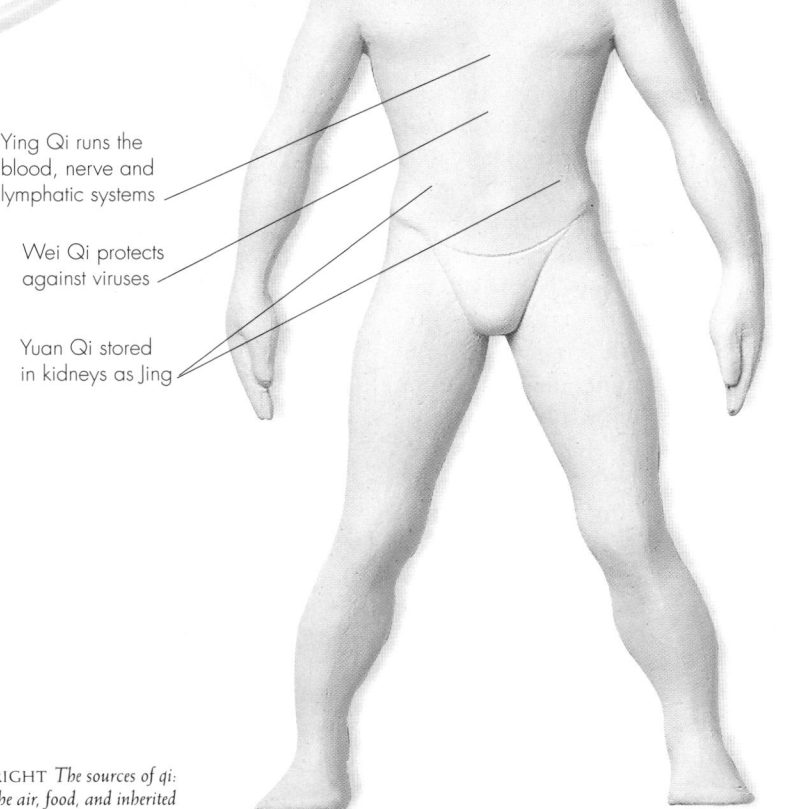

Gong Qi from the air

Gu Qi from food

Ying Qi runs the blood, nerve and lymphatic systems

Wei Qi protects against viruses

Yuan Qi stored in kidneys as Jing

RIGHT *The sources of qi: the air, food, and inherited genetic qi (Yuan Qi).*

MERIDIANS AND ORGANS

Although qi is everywhere in the body, it does have main pathways along which it flows, nourishing and warming the organs and body parts, and harmonizing their activity. These channels are called the meridian system (Jing-Luo). Most acupuncture points are sited along these channels, and most herbs that a practitioner of Chinese medicine prescribes enter one or more of the meridian pathways. There are 12 main meridians, and these correspond to the 12 main organs in the body, such as the Liver, Heart, Stomach, Kidneys, Spleen, and so on. These meridians are bilateral – there is an identical pair on each side of the body. Some are more yin meridians, with functions more to do with storing the vital essences of the body. These are the Kidneys, Liver, Spleen, Heart, Lungs, and Pericardium. The other six are more yang meridians, with functions more to do with transportation of fluids and food. These are the Bladder, Gall bladder, Stomach, Small Intestine, Large Intestine, and the Triple Burner (a mechanism which regulates the overall body temperature and the Upper, Middle, and Lower parts (Jiaos) of the body). There are also six Extra meridians, one of which runs up the front center line of the body – the Ren Mai or Conception Vessel, and one of which runs up the spine – the Du Mai or Governor Vessel.

When a practitioner of Chinese medicine talks about an organ being out of balance, he or she usually refers to the meridian related to that organ, not necessarily the physical organ itself. For instance, the Liver meridian runs from the big toe, up the inside of the leg, through the genitals, and then deep into the Liver organ itself. There can be problems along the course of the meridian, and there is also a sphere of influence which each organ has within the body. The Liver controls the free

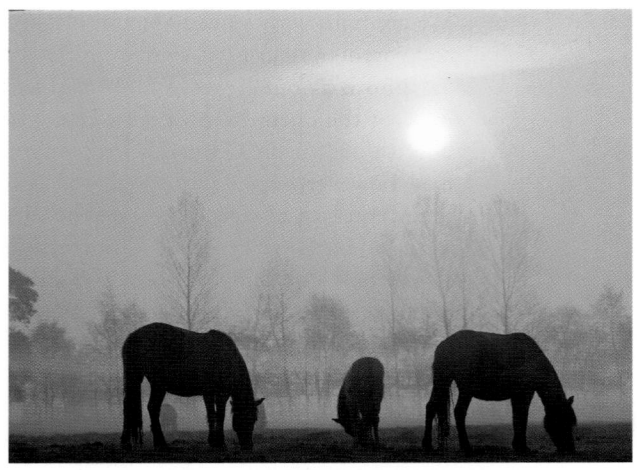

ABOVE *Chinese medicine sees harmony with nature and within ourselves as crucial for health.*

flow of qi generally in the body, including the evenness of emotions, digestion, and menstruation. It also stores the blood, rules circulation in the tendons, has the major influence on the eyes, and manifests in the nails. It is therefore possible to see how diseases in these areas of the body may be treated via the Liver meridian.

In illness, different meridians exhibit different tendencies of disharmony – for instance, the Spleen has a tendency to deficiency causing Damp. This creates symptoms such as diarrhea or lassitude (tiredness). The Liver, on the other hand, has a tendency toward Rising yang, creating red sore eyes, migraines, and high blood pressure. It is these disharmonies that Chinese herbal medicine can address.

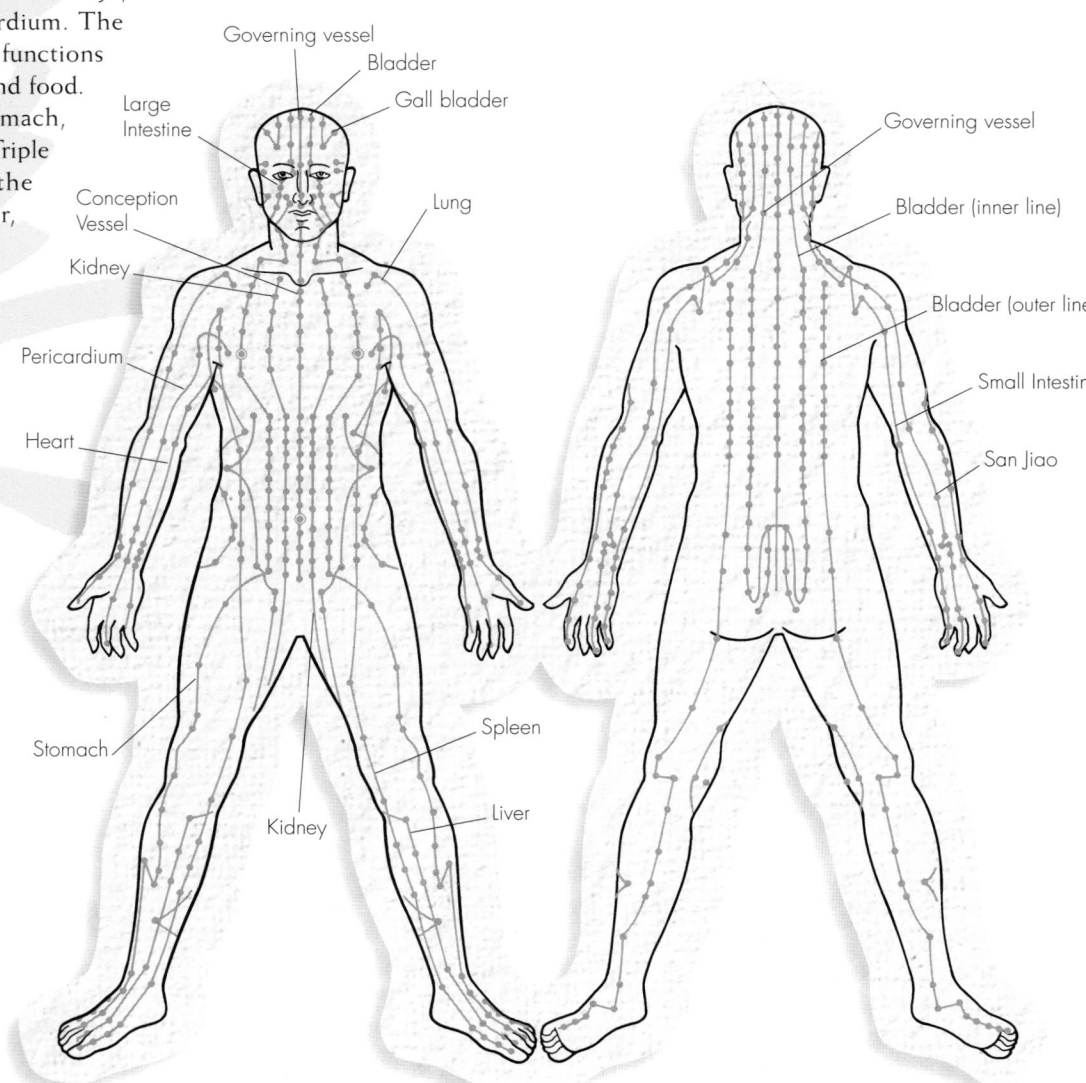

RIGHT *The 12 main meridians (energy channels) along which qi flows in the body.*

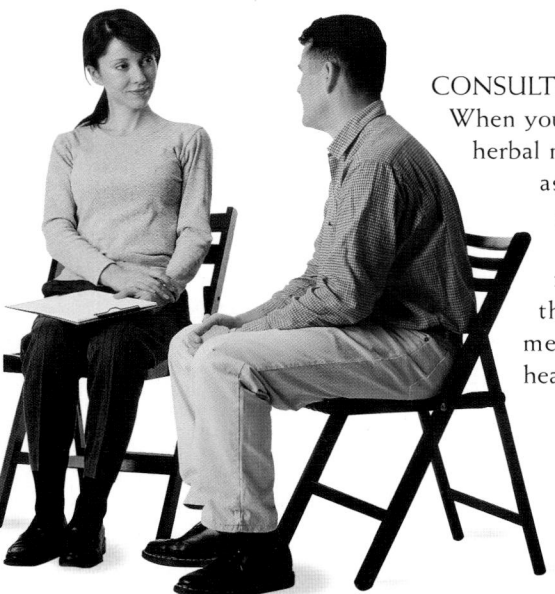

ABOVE *Find a registered practitioner from the national professional organization.*

CONSULTING A CHINESE HERBALIST

When you consult a practitioner of Chinese herbal medicine, he or she will first of all ask you in detail about your presenting condition – when it first appeared, your symptoms, what makes it worse or better. You will then be asked about your past medical history and your general health, for example:

◎ your appetite, diet, digestion, stools, and urination

◎ your sleep patterns, any pain – headaches, backache – ear, nose, and throat (ENT) problems

◎ intake of drugs, alcohol, nicotine

◎ body temperature (more hot or cold), circulation, and perspiration

◎ energy levels, mental, and emotional states

◎ gynecology – menstruation, pregnancies, menopause

Finally, your practitioner will take both radial (wrist) pulses and look at your tongue, in order to help him or her to make a diagnosis according to Chinese medicine. The practitioner may search through some books to check on the herbal prescription most suited to your condition, and will then write down a prescription. This will include anything from 4 to 20 herbs, and their dosages in grams or in *qian* (Chinese measurements). The names of the herbs will be in English, Latin, Pinyin (anglicized Chinese), or in Chinese characters. Your practitioner will then make up the prescription for you or refer you to a herbal supplier to have it made up elsewhere.

BELOW *A ginseng shop in Hong Kong. Ginseng is a useful but expensive herb.*

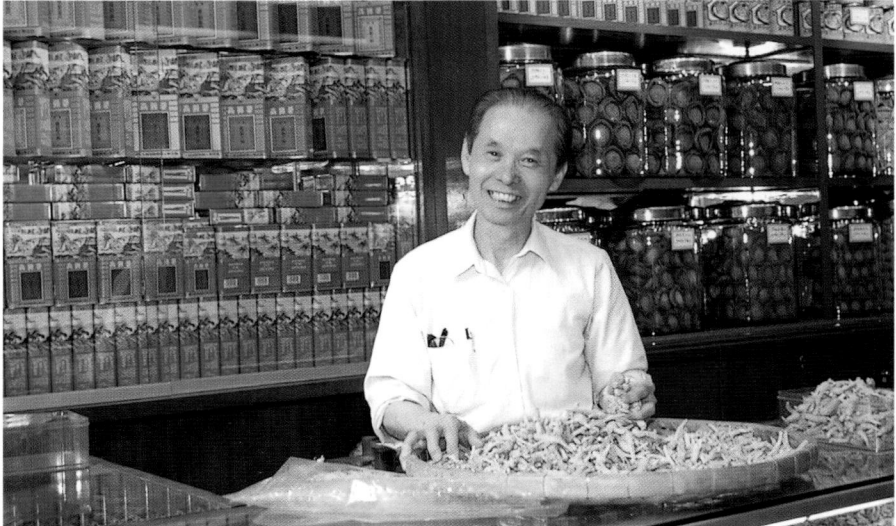

PREPARATIONS AND TREATMENT

There are many different ways of taking herbs. Individual herbs can be added to foods or taken as a tea, but Chinese herbs are rarely taken singly – they are much more effective when made into a composite prescription.

Decoctions Packets of dried herbs are boiled for around 30 minutes, down to 2 cups, and then often boiled again to last two days. They smell worse than they taste!

Powders One teaspoonful of cooked, freeze-dried herbs is taken two or three times a day, mixed with a little cold water to a paste; then a little boiling water is added. This is somewhat unpalatable but easy and effective.

Decoctions

Tinctures One teaspoon of liquid taken two or three times a day. These are more palatable but not as strong as decoctions or powders.

Pills and Capsules These are used for patent remedies (prescriptions which have not been changed to suit the individual). They are easy to swallow, but you have to take a lot more than with Western drugs – sometimes eight tablets at a time.

Syrups These are patent remedies, mainly good for coughs or children's tonics.

Plasters These are used for rheumatic ailments (Wind–Damp); they are very effective for relieving local pain and stiffness. Treatment generally means taking herbs two or three times a day until the problem is gone.

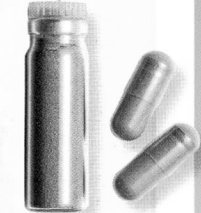

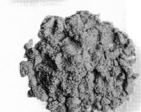

Powders and capsules

At first you will need to see your practitioner every one or two weeks so that he or she can alter the prescription as your symptoms improve. You may experience slight nausea, diarrhea, or digestive upset as your system becomes used to the herbs. In this case, you will need to halve your dosage and build it up again slowly; your practitioner may add more digestive herbs in order that you may tolerate it better. After that, you may be able to see or even telephone your practitioner once a month in order to report on progress, and so that the prescription can be changed accordingly. Herbal medicines should not be taken without review for more than 30 days.

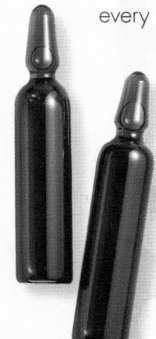

Tinctures

ABOVE *Chinese herbal preparations come in various forms, from raw and powdered herbs, to tinctures.*

THE HERBS USED

PLANTS

The medicinal use of herbs in China is believed to date back to about 2000 B.C.E., when Emperor Chi'en Nung wrote a book called the *Pen Tsao*, which listed the medicinal properties of over 300 plants. The Chinese word for herbalism, "Ben Cao," dates from about 500 B.C.E. "Ben" means a plant with a rigid stalk, and "Cao" means a grass-like plant. Herbalism developed to include the use of mineral and animal ingredients.

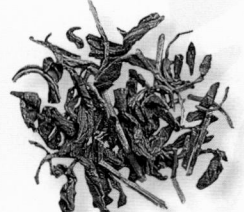

LEAF
Ren Shen (ginseng) leaf is sometimes used, but the root is more common.

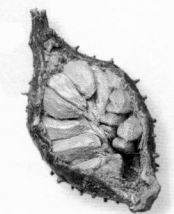

FLOWER
Jin Ying (rosehip) is an example of a flower that is used therapeutically.

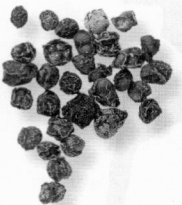

FRUIT
Wu Wei Zi (schisandra fruit) is sour and relieves sweating.

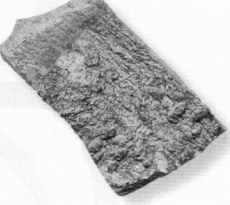

BARK
Rou Gui (cinnamon bark) is a warm herb and relieves Cold.

MINERAL
Shi Gao (gypsum) treats problems caused by excessive Heat.

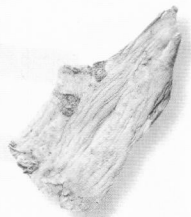

ROOT
Jie Geng (platycodon root) moves Lung Qi.

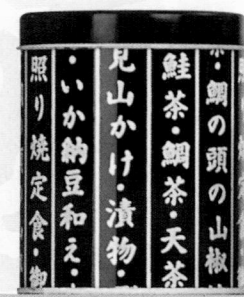

RIGHT *Herb storage jars. Herbs are kept separately to retain their individual properties.*

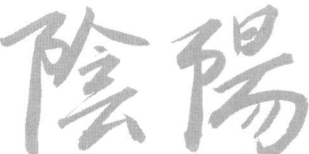

ABOVE *A prescription may contain an assortment of herbs.*

Chinese herbs are mostly made of plant parts – leaves, flowers, fruit, or fruit peel, twigs, roots, bark, or fungus. There are some minerals, such as gypsum, but these are less commonly used. There are also animal parts in Traditional Chinese Herbal Medicine, such as snake, mammal bones, or deer horn. However, their importation has now been forbidden, and herbal practitioners find alternatives to prescribe.

PATENT HERBAL PREPARATIONS

These are sold as over-the-counter remedies for colds and flu, coughs and phlegm, even strep throat infections; also for rheumatic ailments, pain, and bruising from trauma. Patent remedies used for anything else must be diagnosed by a herbal practitioner, even tonics; for instance, do you need to tonify the qi, blood, yin, or yang? It is important to consult a herbal practitioner if you intend to use a patent remedy over a long period of time, such as a long-term tonic for an elderly person. Tonics should not be taken during an episode of cold or flu (Wind Invasion), as they tend to drive Wind deeper into the body.

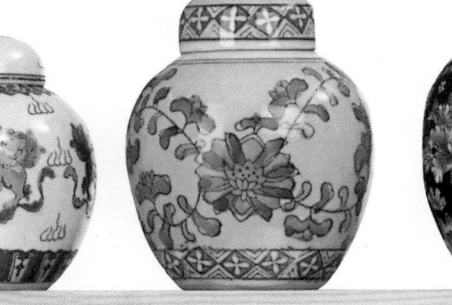

ABOVE *Patent medicines are useful for common problems.*

ABOVE *The Chinese characters for yin (left) and yang (right).*

NOTES

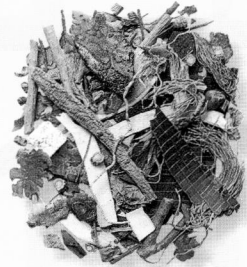

ABOVE *Herbal formulas have been developed over centuries, through both experiment and observation.*

☙ Mention of organs, functions, or causes of disease (e.g. Spleen, harmonize, Dampness) refer to particular Chinese concepts. *(See Glossary, page 472.)*

☙ Chinese herbs are hardly ever used singly – they are used mainly in combination with other herbs to make a balanced prescription. Some of the most commonly used herbs involved in those prescriptions follow in the next section. Each herb also has a particular range of dosages assigned to it – when comparing it to other herbs in a prescription, one can see whether it is used in an average dose, or whether one would use a smaller or larger dose in that prescription. Both these features mean that it is important to consult a qualified herbalist before using the herbs, either in a herbal pharmacy or privately through the Register of Chinese Herbal Medicine Practitioners (U.K.) or your state's Chinese Medicine Association.

A Brief Note About Tastes

In the next section, we will mention the taste of each herb. In TCM, taste partly determines therapeutic function, so it is important to know what it signifies:

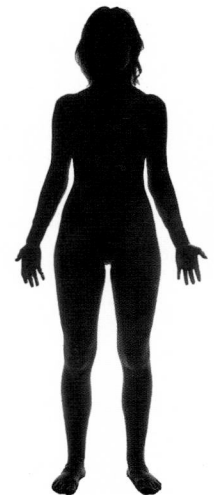

ABOVE *The taste of a herb relates to its action on qi in the body.*

HERB TASTES AND FUNCTIONS

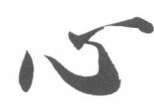

ACRID

☙ ACRID – Pungent or acrid substances disperse and move qi (energy).

☙ Acrid herbs mainly affect the Lung functions.

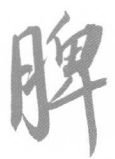

BITTER

☙ BITTER – These herbs reduce excess qi, drain and dry excess moisture.

☙ Bitter herbs mainly affect the Heart organ.

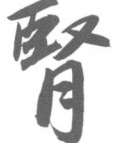

SALTY

☙ SALTY – these herbs purge (drain through the bowels) and soften.

☙ Salty herbs mainly affect the Kidney organ.

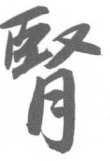

SWEET

☙ SWEET – Sweet substances tonify, harmonize, and strengthen qi, and may sometimes moisten.

☙ Sweet herbs mainly affect the Spleen organ.

SOUR

☙ SOUR – Sour substances are astringent and prevent or reverse the abnormal leakage of fluids and energy.

☙ Sour herbs mainly affect the Kidney organ.

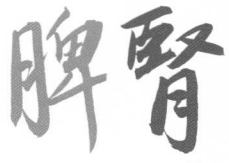

BLAND

☙ BLAND – Bland substances have none of these tastes. They primarily leech out Dampness and promote urination.

☙ This helps both the Spleen and the Kidneys.

CHILDREN AND BABIES

Chinese herbal medicine can be very effective for children and babies. Children's dosages are usually half or a quarter of those given for adults. There are ways of encouraging children to take the herbs, either by involving them in the preparation of the prescription, or by sweetening it with honey, or by offering a cookie afterward! There are certain herbal powders especially formulated for babies.

PREGNANCY

Many herbs are expressly forbidden in pregnancy, whilst some are especially good for pregnant women. There are several which may help to prevent miscarriage. Take only herbs prescribed by a qualified practitioner when pregnant.

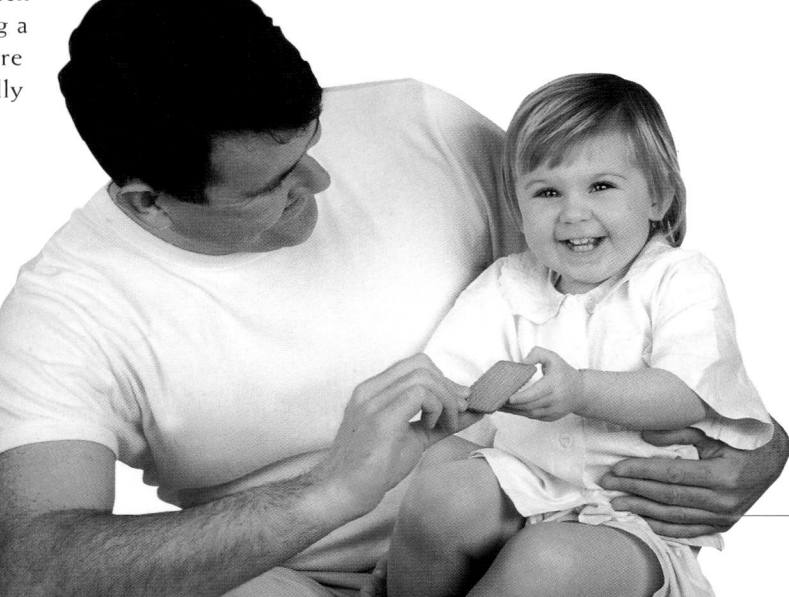

RIGHT *It can be difficult to persuade young children to take some Chinese remedies, due to their unfamiliar tastes. A reward will help!*

CHINESE HERBAL REMEDY SOURCES

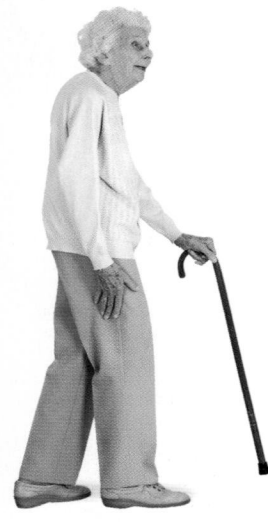

ABOVE *Arthritis, from Wind, Cold, and Damp, is treated through the Liver and Kidney meridians.*

Acanthopanax gracilistylus

WU JIA PI

This herb dispels Wind Dampness from the muscles, joints, and bones. Wind Dampness causes rheumatic and arthritic ailments. Wu Jia Pi also treats Damp Cold conditions where the circulation is obstructed, as in the swelling of the legs or stiff knee joints. The dried herb, or a decoction, can be taken in wine.

HOW TO USE

Wu Jia Pi is a warm drying (acrid) herb which tonifies the Liver and Kidneys. These meridians decline as we get older, so it is especially helpful in treating rheumatism, arthritis, or stiffness in the elderly or those suffering from long-term illness. It is particularly helpful when the smooth flow of qi and blood is obstructed. It is also good for developmental delays in the motor functions of children. It is also used for difficulties with urination, and edema.

CAUTION

USE WITH CAUTION IN YIN DEFICIENCY WITH HEAT SIGNS, AS IT DRIES AND HEATS FURTHER.

DATA FILE

Properties
Acrid, Warm

Channels
Liver, Kidney

Functions and Uses
Dispels Wind Dampness, and strengthens the sinews and bones: use for chronic Wind Cold Damp Painful Obstruction (Bi syndrome) when deficiency of the Liver and Kidneys causes weak sinews and bones.

Transforms Dampness and reduces swelling: use for water retention.

THERAPY CONNECTIONS

HYSSOP
Aromatherapy p.160

CARDAMOM
Ayurveda   p.38
Aromatherapy p.158

ANGELICA
Ayurveda   p.28
Herbalism   p.115
Aromatherapy p.146

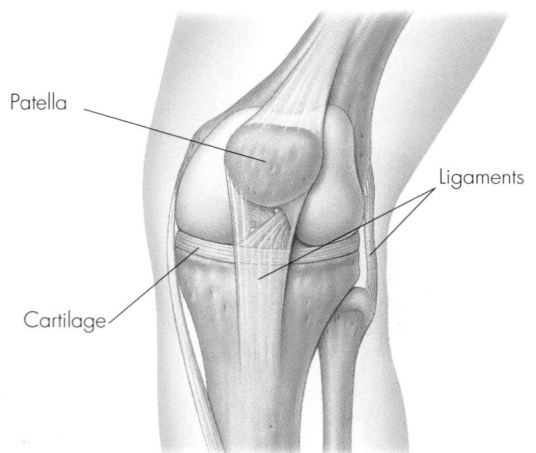

Patella

Ligaments

Cartilage

ABOVE *Wu Jia Pi has warming and drying qualities, and treats Damp conditions such as swollen or stiff joints.*

Agastache rugosa, wrinkled giant hyssop, patchouli

HUO XIANG

This herb transforms Dampness, a "pathogenic influence" which creates stagnation in the Middle Burner (Spleen and Stomach), with various digestive or fluid-retaining effects. Huo Xiang helps the Spleen to recover its function of transporting and transforming food in the body.

HOW TO USE

Huo Xiang is used specifically for stuck digestion, leading to bloating either above or below the navel, nausea, fatigue, lack of appetite, and a moist white coating on the tongue. It is the main herb in the patent formula Huo Xiang Zheng Qi Wan, which is used for gastric flu.

DATA FILE

Properties
Acrid, slightly Warm

Channels
Lung, Spleen, Stomach

Functions and Uses
Fragrantly transforms Dampness: this means that it tonifies the Spleen so that it transforms the Dampness obstructing the middle area, which is interfering with the Spleen's normal digestive functions.

Harmonizes the Middle Burner and stops vomiting; also used for morning sickness.

Releases the exterior and expels Dampness, as in gastric flu.

CAUTION

NO HERBS USED FOR GETTING RID OF DAMP (SHOWN BY A THICK TONGUE COATING OR BY THE PRESENCE OF PHLEGM) MAY BE USED IN DEFICIENT YIN WITH HEAT SIGNS (SHOWN BY A PEELED TONGUE) – THEY WILL FURTHER DRY THE PATIENT UP AND MAKE THE CONDITION WORSE.

BELOW *Huo Xiang comes from wrinkled giant hyssop, a summer-flowering perennial.*

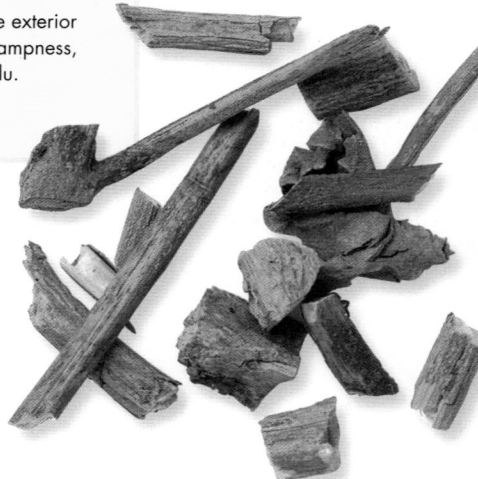

Alpinia oxyphylla, black cardamom
YI ZHI REN

This herb warms Internal Cold. Yi Zhi Ren is a cardamom, and all cardamoms warm the Middle area. Yi Zhi Ren also warms the Kidneys and controls fluids coming from that area – which makes it good for urinary incontinence, or frequency and enuresis (bedwetting) from Cold-Deficient Spleen and Kidneys.

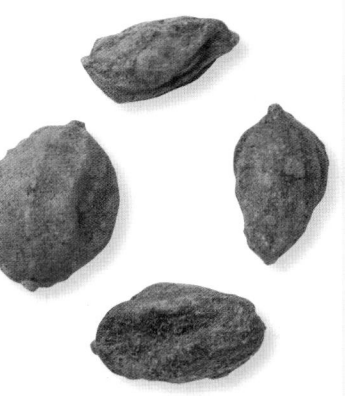

DATA FILE

Properties
Acrid, Warm

Channels
Kidney, Spleen

Functions and Uses

❧ Warms the Kidneys, firms the Jing-essence and holds in urine: this herb is used when the yang aspect of the Kidneys is Deficient and cannot hold sperm or urine in place.

❧ Warms the Spleen and stops diarrhea: Cold, Deficient Spleen or Stomach patterns causing diarrhea and other digestive symptoms.

CAUTION

CONTRAINDICATED FOR SPERMATORRHEA, FREQUENT URINATION, OR VAGINAL DISCHARGE DUE TO HEAT.

HOW TO USE

🍃 Yi Zhi Ren is helpful in spermatorrhea, when men cannot hold the sperm or when it leaks out. 🍃 When the Spleen yang is weak and Cold it does not transform the feces properly, leading to diarrhea. 🍃 **There may also be vomiting, Cold abdominal pain (better with warmth), excessive saliva, and a thick unpleasant taste in the mouth.** 🍃 It is very good to relieve drooling. 🍃 Yi Zhi Ren is a valuable herb for warming the system, from infancy to old age.

Angelica dahurica
BAI ZHI

Bai Zhi belongs to a group of Warm, Acrid herbs that release exterior conditions; that is, superficial illnesses caused by viruses, with symptoms in the skin or muscle layers. The herbs mainly affect the sweating mechanism, either causing the body to sweat, or if necessary stopping it from sweating.

HOW TO USE

🍃 Bai Zhi is used mainly for sudden headaches (Wind-caused headaches), especially those along the Stomach channel, i.e. the front of the head, the forehead.
🍃 **It is particularly good for headaches caused by sinusitis, and to help the sinusitis itself.** 🍃 It is very good for ulcerated boils in cases where the pus is not yet discharged – use it with Jie Geng. 🍃 **It is often added to prescriptions for vaginal discharge, especially for a white (Cold) discharge rather than a yellow, smelly one (Hot type).** However, with the right combinations, one could use Bai Zhi for other types of headaches or discharges.

LEFT *Yi Zhi Ren is the seed pod of Alpina oxophylla, an evergreen perennial.*

BELOW *A sudden headache will respond to treatment with Bai Zhi.*

ABOVE *Bai Zhi treats disorders via the Lung and Stomach meridians in the body.*

CAUTION

CONTRAINDICATED IN DEFICIENT BLOOD OR DEFICIENT YIN PATTERNS BECAUSE IT IS VERY DRYING. USE CAUTIOUSLY IF SORES HAVE ALREADY BURST.

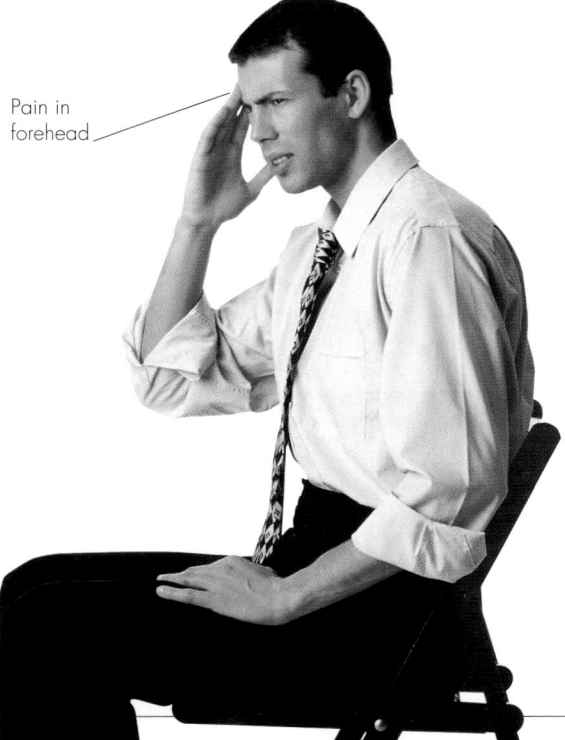

Pain in forehead

DATA FILE

Properties
Acrid, Warm

Channels
Lung, Stomach

Functions and Uses

❧ Expels Wind and alleviates pain: use for externally contracted Wind Cold patterns, especially those with head symptoms.

❧ Reduces swelling and expels pus: use in the early stages of a sore in order to reduce swelling.

❧ Expels Dampness and alleviates discharge. It is used for treating leukorrhea (vaginal discharge) from Damp Cold in the lower abdominal area.

❧ Helps to open up the nasal passages.

Angelica sinensis, Chinese angelica
DANG GUI

Dang Gui is such a widely used herb that it has entered the Western herbal pharmacy. In TCM it is used to treat patterns of Blood Deficiency, and therefore affects mostly the Heart and Liver, which direct and store the Blood, respectively.

HOW TO USE

Dan Gui is unusual among Blood-tonifying herbs in that it both nourishes and invigorates blood circulation, and is therefore not cloying, as Shu di Huang can be. It is good for Blood-Deficient symptoms such as pale complexion, tinnitus, blurred vision, and palpitations, and is commonly used for all menstrual disorders, such as irregular menstruation, amenorrhea, or dysmenorrhea (painful menstruation). It is essential for pain in general as it moves the Blood – abdominal pain, traumatic injury, and even arthritic pain associated with Blood Deficiency (pain according to TCM may be caused by Stagnant Blood). It is useful for dry stools and helps heal sores.

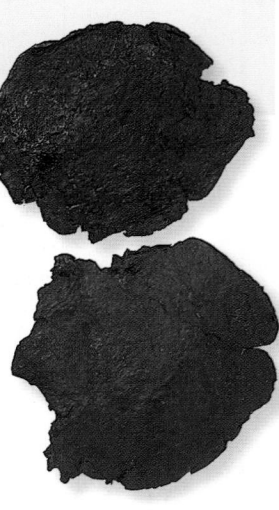

ABOVE *Dang Gui is recommended for all menstrual disorders.*

DATA FILE

Properties
Sweet, Acrid, Bitter, Warm

Channels
Heart, Liver, Spleen

Functions and Uses

Tonifies the Blood and regulates the menses.

Invigorates the Blood and disperses Cold: an important herb for stopping pain due to Blood stasis.

Moistens the intestines and unblocks the bowels: like all tonifying herbs, Dang Gui is moistening – in this case it is also directed to the intestines.

Reduces swelling, expels pus, generates new flesh, and alleviates pain: use for sores and abscesses.

CAUTION

USE WITH CAUTION FOR DIARRHEA OR ABDOMINAL SWELLING DUE TO DAMPNESS.

CONTRAINDICATED FOR YIN DEFICIENCY WITH HEAT SIGNS, AS IT IS WARMING.

Atractylodes macrocephala, atractylodes rhizome
BAI ZHU

This herb is one of a group that treat Qi Deficiency, and as we replenish our day-to-day energy from air and food, the two main organs involved are Lungs and Spleen.

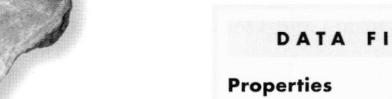

CAUTION

CONTRAINDICATED IN CASES OF YIN DEFICIENCY WITH HEAT SIGNS, OR INJURED FLUIDS.

ABOVE *Bai Zhu gives qi a boost when fatigue is experienced.*

HOW TO USE

Bai Zhu is a major tonifying qi herb in cases of diarrhea, vomiting, fatigue, lack of appetite, lack of strength in the limbs, and is one of the herbs in the seminal tonifying prescription of the "Four Gentlemen" (Si Jun Zi Wan). It also helps Damp disorders such as edema and reduced urination, and is used in the Jade Screen prescription for spontaneous sweating due to Qi Deficiency. It is used for any type of threatened miscarriage when combined with other appropriate herbs.

DATA FILE

Properties
Sweet, Bitter, Warm

Channels
Spleen, Stomach

Functions and Uses

Tonifies the Spleen and benefits the qi: use Bai Zhu to treat Spleen and Stomach Deficiency.

Strengthens the Spleen and dries Dampness: use for digestive disorders, water retention and even for treating Damp Painful Obstruction (rheumatic ailments).

Firms the exterior and stops sweating.

Strengthens the Spleen and calms the fetus: for restless fetus when due to Spleen Deficiency not holding the fetus in.

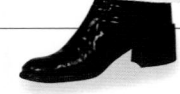

LEFT *Bai Zhu may be used to help women who run the risk of miscarriage.*

Astragalus membranaceus, milk-vetch root

HUANG QI

This herb treats Qi Deficiency, and as we replenish our day-to-day energy from air and food, the two main organs involved are Lungs and Spleen (the main digestive organ in TCM).

HOW TO USE

🍃 Huang Qi is for Spleen-Deficient symptoms such as lack of appetite, fatigue, and diarrhea. Its action is also upward and outward, so it helps prolapsed uterus or uterine bleeding, but is also used in prescriptions to help the immune system fight viruses. It is used for frequent colds and helps excessive sweating. It is good for edema and pus-filled sores that have not yet discharged, and is also used in postnatal fever from severe loss of blood.

DATA FILE

Properties

Sweet, slightly Warm

Channels

Lung, Spleen

Functions and Uses

🍃 Tonifies the Spleen and benefits the qi: use for all Deficient Spleen patterns.

🍃 Raises the yang qi of the Spleen and Stomach: use for prolapse – it makes things go up.

🍃 Tonifies the Protective Qi (Wei Qi) and firms the exterior: goes to the outside of the body, and regulates the opening and closing of the pores.

🍃 Benefits Water and reduces swelling.

🍃 Tonifies the qi and Blood: particularly for severe loss of blood.

ABOVE *Huang Qi is an ascending herb: it tends to move upward and outward.*

CAUTION

CONTRAINDICATED FOR FULL HEAT CONDITIONS OR YIN DEFICIENCY WITH FIRE – IT HEATS TOO MUCH.

DATA FILE

Properties

Acrid, slightly Bitter, Warm

Channels

Gall Bladder, Large Intestine, Spleen, Stomach

Functions and Uses

🍃 Promotes the movement of qi and alleviates pain: use for Spleen, Stomach, Liver, or Gall bladder Stagnant Qi (pain is always a result of Stagnant Qi or Blood).

🍃 Regulates Stagnant Qi in the Intestines.

🍃 Strengthens the Spleen and prevents Stagnation: use Huang Qi with tonifying herbs to prevent their cloying side-effects.

CAUTION

CONTRAINDICATED IN CASES OF YIN DEFICIENCY OR DEPLETED FLUIDS.

RIGHT *Mu Xiang helps to deal with lack of appetite, a symptom of Stomach Stagnation.*

Aucklandia lappa, costus root, saussurea

MU XIANG

Mu Xiang regulates and invigorates the qi when it becomes stuck or "stagnant," optimizing the function of the gastrointestinal tract and helping stop pain.

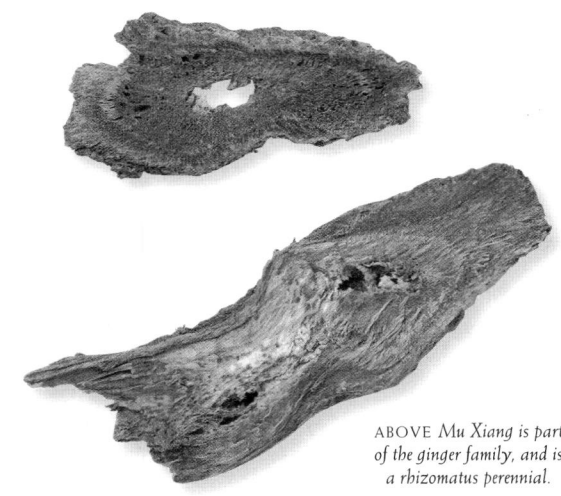

ABOVE *Mu Xiang is part of the ginger family, and is a rhizomatus perennial.*

HOW TO USE

🍃 Mu Xiang primarily helps digestive symptoms and pain. It is for Spleen or Stomach Stagnation symptoms such as lack of appetite, epigastric (above the navel) or abdominal pain or swelling, nausea, and vomiting. It is also used for Liver and Gall bladder Stagnation symptoms such as pain, swelling, or soreness in the flanks (sides). It is very good for diarrhea, dysentery, and tenesmus (a spasm of the rectum where one feels the need to defecate without being able to) due to Stagnation of qi in the Intestines rather than Deficiency. However, it also helps a Deficient Spleen regain its normal functions of transportation and transformation.

THERAPY CONNECTIONS

GINGER

🟢 Ayurveda   *p.47*

⚫ Aromatherapy *p.171*

Cannabis sativa, hemp, cannabis seeds
HUO MA REN

Huo Ma Ren comes into the category of Descending Downward: it facilitates the expulsion of the stool in cases of constipation. Huo Ma Ren is ungerminated cannabis seeds, but does not have the effects that smoking cannabis leaves or resin has.

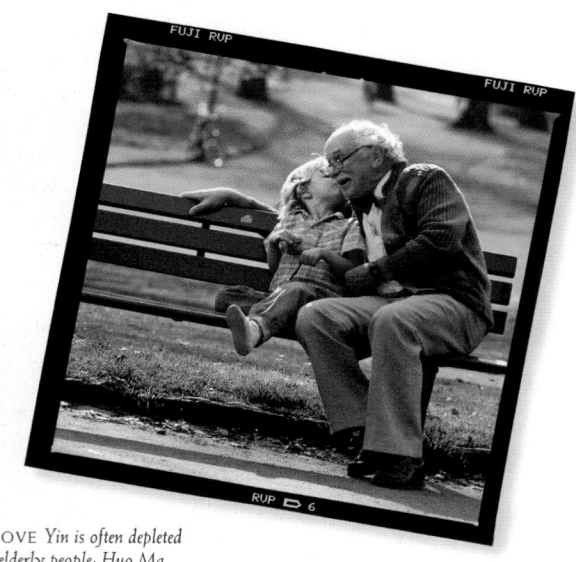

ABOVE *Yin is often depleted in elderly people: Huo Ma Ren helps to restore it.*

HOW TO USE

☙ Huo Ma Ren is a moist laxative and therefore works gently by lubricating the Intestines. As it is mild in nature it is suitable for debilitated patients, the elderly, and those who are weakened by a febrile (feverish) disease or after childbirth. Also, as it is moistening, it is good for Blood Deficiency and general lack of fluids. One would often add Blood-nourishing herbs, such as Shu di Huang and Dang Gui for constipation due to Blood Deficiency, as in the elderly.

CAUTION
LONG-TERM USE MAY POSSIBLY RESULT IN VAGINAL DISCHARGE.

OVERDOSE MAY LEAD TO NAUSEA, VOMITING, AND DIARRHEA.

RIGHT *A young cannabis plant. Huo Ma Ren is the ungerminated seeds of the plant.*

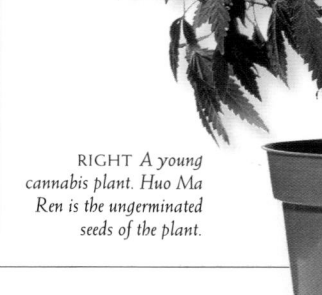

DATA FILE

Properties
Sweet, Neutral

Channels
Large Intestine, Spleen, Stomach

Functions and Uses

☙ Nourishes and moistens the Intestines: as it does not have a harsh effect, it is most suitable for constipation in the weak and elderly.

☙ Nourishes the yin: it mildly tonifies the yin and can be used in cases of Yin Deficiency with constipation. The yin is often depleted during a long illness like ME (or post-viral syndrome); also commonly in the elderly.

☙ Clears Heat and promotes healing of sores: use as an auxiliary herb for sores and ulcerations, taken orally or applied topically (locally).

Note: these seeds have been processed and therefore cannot germinate, so they cannot be considered an illegal drug.

Carthamus tinctorius, safflower flower
HONG HUA

This herb invigorates (or "regulates") the Blood, treating problems associated with Blood stasis. In TCM, these problems include pain and internal masses or growths.

HOW TO USE

☙ Hong Hua is used for any Blood stasis patterns. These may include such gynecological problems as amenorrhea, post-partum dizziness, or fibroids. It may also include other tumors if they are caused by congealed blood, and many skin diseases, such as Kaposi's sarcoma, and scarlet fever. As it helps stuck Blood pain it is good for wounds or painful sores. It helps to bring out a measles' rash fully, and is useful for pain in the limbs. It also helps joint pain in arthritis.

DATA FILE

Properties
Acrid, Warm

Channels
Heart, Liver

Functions and Uses

☙ Invigorates the Blood and unblocks menstruation: it expels congealed Blood in the meridians and is not just for menstrual problems.

☙ Dispels Blood stasis and alleviates pain: it enters the Blood level of the channels (as opposed to qi or organ level).

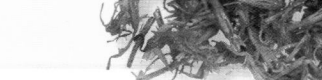

CAUTION
AS WITH MANY BLOOD-MOVING HERBS, DO NOT TAKE THIS DURING PREGNANCY.

ABOVE *Hong Hua is a pungent herb which helps move and invigorate the Blood.*

Cinnamomum cassia, cinnamon twigs

GUI ZHI

Gui Zhi belongs to a group of warm, acrid herbs that release exterior conditions; that is, superficial illnesses caused by viruses, with symptoms in the skin or muscle layers. These mainly cause sweating, or stop sweating where necessary.

HOW TO USE

🍃 Gui Zhi is used mainly for colds and flu, and commonly in combination with Bai Shao, when there is too much sweating in a cold condition and the patient is becoming weak. It is often added to prescriptions for rheumatic complaints in the joints and limbs, especially the shoulders, caused by Cold Obstruction causing pain, where it sends warmth through the channels. Use for edema, where it sends warm yang energy through the meridians to move and transform the settled fluid. It is often used with licorice (Gan Cao) for palpitations and shortness of breath due to Deficient Heart yang. It can be used for menstrual cramps or irregular menstruation caused by Cold.

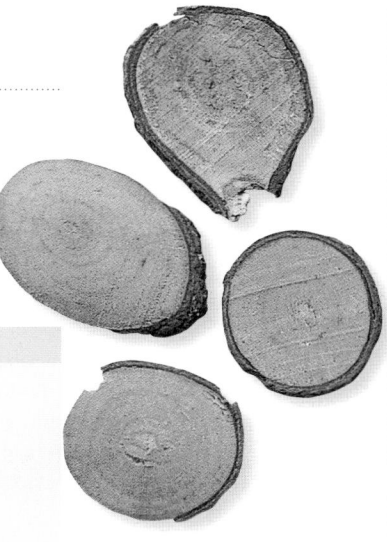

ABOVE *Gui Zhi is a warming herb, and is good for treating rheumatic complaints.*

CAUTION

CONTRAINDICATED IN WARM DISEASES, EITHER FROM FEVER, DEFICIENT YIN WITH HEAT SIGNS OR HEAT IN THE BLOOD WITH VOMITING.

BELOW *Gui Zhi is a good treatment for colds and flu, often combined with Bai Shao.*

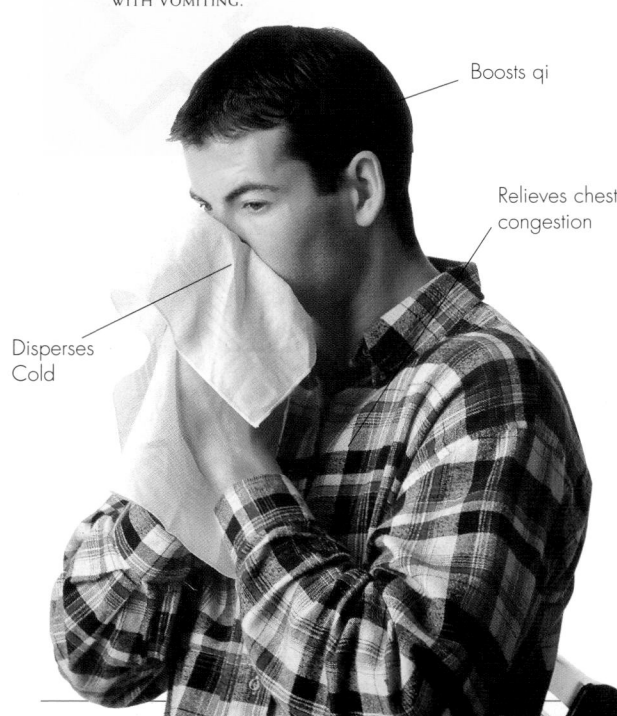

Boosts qi

Relieves chest congestion

Disperses Cold

DATA FILE

Properties

Sweet and warm

Channels:

Lung, Bladder

Functions and Uses

🍃 Adjusts the body's sweating in externally caused Cold conditions.

🍃 Warms the meridians and disperses Cold: use for rheumatic ailments; also for gynecological problems caused by Cold obstructing the Blood.

🍃 Moves the yang and transforms qi: use for water retention (edema) from Cold, where poor circulation of yang qi has failed to move the fluids in the body.

🍃 Strengthens the Heart yang: use for palpitations when the active functioning of the Heart is weak.

Citrus reticulata, tangerine peel

CHEN PI

This herb regulates and invigorates the qi when it becomes stuck or "stagnant," optimizing the function of the gastrointestinal tract and helping stop pain.

HOW TO USE

🍃 Chen Pi is a very important herb as it "awakens the Spleen." It is for stagnant qi patterns with symptoms like epigastric (above the navel) or abdominal bloating, fullness, belching, nausea, and vomiting. It is very good for a lot of sticky sputum and other Phlegm Damp symptoms such as loss of appetite, fatigue, loose stools, and a thick, greasy tongue coating. It is therefore used for disorders affecting both the Spleen and the Lungs. It is particularly important for putting into tonifying prescriptions to make them more digestible.

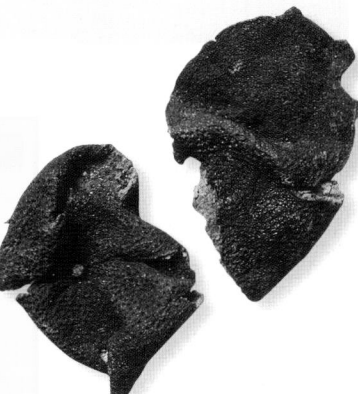

ABOVE *Chen Pi moves qi when it is stagnant, as revealed by Stomach disorders.*

DATA FILE

Properties

Acrid, Bitter, Warm, Fragrant

Channels

Spleen, Stomach, Lung

Functions and Uses

🍃 Regulates the qi and strengthens the transportation function of the Spleen: it promotes the movement of qi in general, while directing it down.

🍃 Dries Dampness and transforms Phlegm: use for a stuffy feeling in the chest and diaphragm.

🍃 Helps prevent stagnation.

CAUTION

CONTRAINDICATED IN DRY COUGH DUE TO YIN OR QI DEFICIENCY, AS IT IS DRYING (FRAGRANT) AND WARM.

USE WITH CAUTION WITH A RED TONGUE OR YELLOW PHLEGM (SYMPTOMS OF HEAT).

THERAPY CONNECTIONS

CINNAMON

🔲 Ayurveda   *p.34*

🔵 Aromatherapy *p.150*

YI YI REN

Codonopsis pilosula, codonopsis root
DANG SHEN

This herb is similar to Ren Shen: it treats Qi Deficiency, affecting primarily the Lungs and Spleen (the main digestive organ in TCM). It is less expensive than Ren Shen.

HOW TO USE

🍃 Dang Shen does basically the same work as Ren Shen, but is not as strong. In prescriptions it is used in place of Ginseng to tonify the qi of the Spleen and Lungs, while ginseng is preferred for more serious situations, such as a patient who is barely conscious.

🍃 It is used for lack of appetite, fatigue, tired limbs, diarrhea, vomiting, and prolapse – all symptoms of Spleen Qi Deficiency. It is also used for Lung Deficiency with chronic cough, shortness of breath, or copious sputum due to Spleen Deficiency. As it tonifies fluids, it is used in diabetes and the aftermath of febrile illnesses. It is the main herb in the seminal qi tonic prescription Si Jun Zi Wan ("Four Gentlemen"). Like all the qi tonics, it is sweet and cloying, and must therefore be combined with qi-moving herbs.

CAUTION

CONTRAINDICATED FOR PAINFUL URINATION OR DAMP–HEAT.

BELOW *Dang Shen enters all the channels, but especially the Lung and Spleen.*

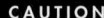

DATA FILE

Properties
Sweet, Neutral

Channels
Lung, Spleen

Functions and Uses
🌿 Tonifies the Middle area, benefits the qi and strengthens the Stomach and Spleen: use for all Deficient Qi patterns.

🌿 Tonifies the Lungs.

🌿 Strengthens the qi and nourishes fluids.

Coix lachryma jobi, seeds of Job's tears
YI YI REN

This is one of the Chinese herbs that transform Dampness, but it is more active on the Lower Burner than the Middle Burner.

HOW TO USE

🍃 Like Fu Ling, Yi Yi Ren clears Dampness by promoting urination, but its Spleen-strengthening function is not as strong, and it works more on the Lower Burner (Kidneys) than on the Middle Burner (Spleen and Stomach). Use with Spleen-tonifying herbs to get rid of water retention; it may be used for Lung or Intestinal abscesses to help get rid of pus.

CAUTION

USE WITH CAUTION DURING PREGNANCY.

DATA FILE

Properties
Sweet, Bland, slightly Cold

Channels
Spleen, Lung, Kidney

Functions and Uses
🌿 Promotes urination and leeches out Dampness: for edema or water retention in the legs.

🌿 Clears Wind Dampness: this means Painful Obstruction syndrome, such as arthritic conditions.

🌿 Clears Heat and expels pus: use when sores have become full of pus; pushes pus out.

🌿 Strengthens Spleen and stops diarrhea: use when the Spleen is deficient, causing Damp diarrhea.

🌿 Clears Damp Heat: for any digestive problems with a greasy yellow tongue coating.

Cornus officinalis, cornelian cherry fruit, dogwood fruit
SHAN ZHU YU

Shan Zhu Yu stabilizes and binds. It is sour and astringent, and helps keep in bodily substances which may leak, such as urine.

HOW TO USE

🍃 Shan Zhu Yu is used for leakage of fluids due to weak Jing-essence, with symptoms such as excessive urination, incontinence, spermatorrhea, and premature ejaculation. In shock, it helps Liver and Kidney Deficiency, with such symptoms as lightheadedness, dizziness, sore and weak low back and knees, or impotence. It is useful for excessive uterine bleeding when the cause is Deficiency. It is one of the six herbs in the basic yin-tonifying prescription Liu Wei di Huang Wan (Six Flavor prescription), so if carefully combined it may tonify yin or yang.

DATA FILE

Properties
Sour, slightly Warm

Channels
Kidney, Liver

Functions and Uses
🌿 Firms the Kidneys and retains the Jing-essence.

🌿 Absorbs sweating and supports collapse: use for devastated yang and qi, as in shock.

🌿 Tonifies and builds the Liver and Kidneys.

🌿 Stabilizes the menses and stops bleeding.

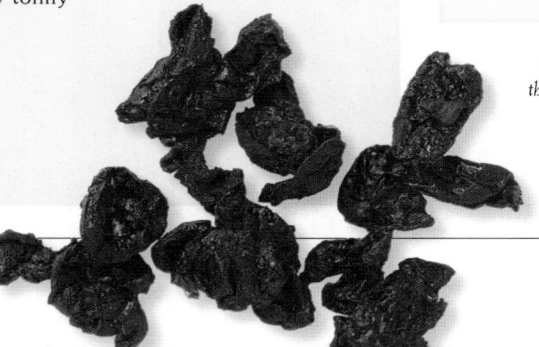

LEFT *Shan Zhu Yu is the fruit of the dogwood. It enters the Kidneys, where Jing is stored.*

BELOW Huang Lian is used to treat halitosis caused by Stomach problems.

Coptis chinensis, coptis rhizome, golden thread

HUANG LIAN

This herb clears Heat: this includes febrile conditions and any illnesses with Heat signs. It is one of the "Three Yellows," which are often used together for severe infections.

HOW TO USE

🍃 Huang Lian deals with Damp Heat in the Middle Burner (digestive organs), and also the Heart and Pericardium. This latter leads to symptoms such as very high fever with delirium and disorientation. It can also be used to treat painful, red eyes and sore throat. It is very good with the infectious diseases still prevalent in the developing world. It is used for violent diarrhea and acid regurgitation from Stomach Heat. A decoction may be placed on sore, red eyes, boils, anal fissures, conjunctivitis, and used locally it is very good for treating trichomoniasis, a protozoan infection of the vagina.

DATA FILE

Properties
Bitter, Cold

Channels
Heart, Liver, Stomach, Large Intestine

Functions and Uses

🍃 Clears Heat and detoxifies Fire Poison.

🍃 Clears Heat and drains Dampness, especially in the Stomach and Intestines – dysentery, vomiting.

🍃 Clears Heart Fire: symptoms such as irritability and insomnia.

🍃 Stops Hot bleeding.

🍃 Drains Stomach Fire: digestive dysfunction leading to bad breath and belching.

🍃 Clears Heat topically: use for red mouth ulcers, boils, and abscesses.

CAUTION

DO NOT USE FOR DEFICIENT YIN PATTERNS, WHERE THE FLUID MAY BE DEFICIENT ANYWAY – HUANG LIAN WOULD DRY IT OUT MORE. LIKE ALL THE CLEARING HEAT HERBS IT IS COLD IN ENERGY, SO IT IS CONTRAINDICATED IN ANY DISEASES CAUSED BY COLD.

LEFT Huang Lian decoction helps to soothe sore eyes and relieve redness.

Crataegus pinnatifida, hawthorn fruit, crataegus

SHAN ZHA

This herb relieves digestive problems resulting from over-indulgence in greasy foods, and helps to promote efficient digestion by increasing gastrointestinal secretions and enzymatic functions.

RIGHT Shan Zha deals with problems caused by an accumulation of greasy foods.

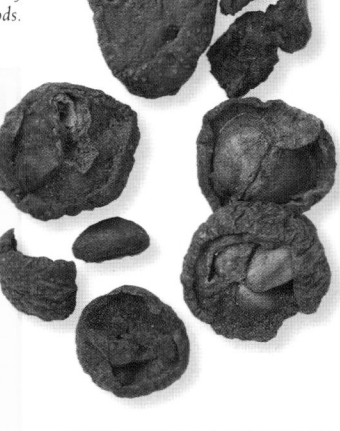

DATA FILE

Properties
Sour, Sweet, slightly Warm

Channels
Liver, Spleen, Stomach

Functions and Uses

🍃 Reduces and guides out food stagnation: for obstruction due to meat or greasy foods.

🍃 Transforms Blood stasis and dissipates knottedness: enters the Blood level and is used for treating Blood stagnation disorders.

🍃 Stops diarrhea: when the herb is slightly charred, it has an astringent effect.

THERAPY CONNECTIONS

HAWTHORN

🔘 Herbalism   *p.119*

HOW TO USE

🍃 Shan Zha is used for abdominal distention, belching, pain, and reduced appetite. It is also used for children who fail to thrive. It is especially useful if the symptoms are accompanied by diarrhea or chronic dysentery. It is particularly indicated for postnatal abdominal pain and menstrual pain when the cause is congealed Blood, and hernias with testicular pain and swelling. Recently it has also been used for hypertension (high blood pressure), coronary artery disease, and high cholesterol.

CAUTION

USE WITH CAUTION IN CASES OF SPLEEN AND STOMACH DEFICIENCY WITHOUT FOOD STAGNATION, AND IN DISEASES WITH ACID REGURGITATION.

Cuscuta chinensis, Chinese dodder seeds

TU SU ZI

This herb tonifies the yang, and as they are the basis of all the body's yang, it mainly affects the Kidneys. In TCM the Kidneys house the body's reserves, and the Kidney yang is also responsible for sexual and endocrine disorders.

HOW TO USE

🌿 Tu Su Zi helps the Jing-essence so is good for impotence, nocturnal emissions, and premature ejaculation, as well as such Kidney Yang Deficient symptoms as sore lower back and knees, frequent urination, incontinence, and vaginal discharge. It is used for such Liver and Kidney Deficient symptoms as tinnitus (ringing in the ears), dizziness, blurred vision, or spots in front of the eyes. It stops leaking, so it is good for diarrhea or loose stools from Deficiency, and it also helps prevent threatened or habitual miscarriage. It is added to Kidney Yang Deficient prescriptions to moisten the preparation.

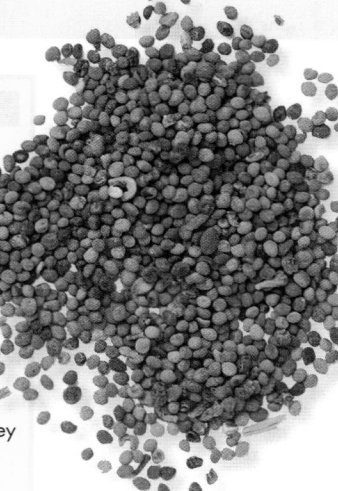

DATA FILE

Properties
Acrid, Sweet, Neutral

Channels
Kidney, Liver

Functions and Uses

🌿 Tonifies the Kidneys and benefits the Jing-essence: unlike most Kidney yang herbs, which are heating and therefore drying, Tu Su Zi is also moistening, so helps preserve the yin fluid.

🌿 Tonifies the Liver and Kidneys and improves vision: use for patterns of Deficient Liver and Kidney yin and yang.

🌿 Benefits the Spleen and Kidneys and stops persistent diarrhea.

🌿 Calms the fetus.

ABOVE *Tu Su Zi – Chinese dodder seed – is a moistening herb.*

CAUTION

ALTHOUGH THIS IS A NEUTRAL HERB, IT LEANS MORE TOWARD TONIFYING THE YANG AND SHOULD THEREFORE NOT BE USED FOR FIRE FROM YIN DEFICIENCY.

Cyperus rotundus, nut-grass rhizome

XIANG FU

This herb regulates and invigorates the qi when it becomes stuck or "stagnant," optimizing the function of the gastrointestinal tract and helping stop pain in various parts of the body, particularly menstrual and digestive pain.

HOW TO USE

🌿 Xiang Fu is a very widely used herb, as it has the ability to disperse stuck qi and to harmonize the energy, both in digestive and in gynecological disorders. It is particularly suitable for pain in the sides, fullness in the epigastrium (above the navel), pain and stuffiness in the chest, lack of appetite, wind and indigestion, as well as vomiting and diarrhea due to Liver Qi invading the Spleen. It is also for swollen, tender breasts (due to PMS), and is an important herb for breast lumps. It is essential in prescriptions for dysmenorrhea (menstrual cramps) or irregular menstruation, and can be used in pregnancy for treating Liver Qi stagnation patterns.

CAUTION

CONTRAINDICATED IN QI DEFICIENCY WITHOUT STAGNATION, AND IN YIN DEFICIENCY OR HEAT IN THE BLOOD.

LEFT *Xiang Fu is useful for treating gynecological disorders.*

DATA FILE

Properties
Acrid, slightly Bitter, slightly Sweet, Neutral

Channels
Liver, Triple Burner

Functions and Uses

🌿 Moves qi and regulates Liver Qi: in pathology, the Liver energy has a tendency to become "constrained," resulting in pain above the navel and around the ribs.

🌿 Regulates menstruation and alleviates pain: according to TCM, the Liver is one of the main organs involved in gynecology, and the cause of menstrual pain is frequently due to "constrained Liver Qi."

Gastrodia elata, gastrodia rhizome

TIAN MA

This herb has a sinking action – that is to say it takes qi down strongly.

HOW TO USE

🌿 Tian Ma is a very important herb for treating internal Liver Wind, with symptoms such as childhood convulsions or tantrums, epilepsy, spasms, or seizures. It is used for headaches, dizziness, and migraines caused by Wind Phlegm patterns, as well as Wind Stroke (stroke) with hemiplegia and numbness in the extremities. It is also good for rheumatic ailments in the lower back and limbs.

CAUTION

MAY BE TOXIC IN LARGE DOSES.

RIGHT *Tian Ma is a sweet herb which tonifies qi and treats the Liver.*

DATA FILE

Properties
Sweet, Neutral

Channels
Liver

Functions and Uses

🌿 Calms the Liver, extinguishes Wind, and controls tremors. There are two kinds of Wind in TCM, external – which brings in cold or flu, or arthritic symptoms, and internal – which is generated by dysfunction of the Liver. This herb treats the second.

🌿 Extinguishes Wind and alleviates pain: especially Wind Mucus head pain.

🌿 Disperses painful obstruction caused by Wind Damp.

Eucommia ulmoides, eucommia bark
DU ZHONG

This herb belongs to a group that tonify the yang, and as the Kidneys are the basis of all the body's yang, it mainly affects the Kidneys. In TCM the Kidneys house the body's reserves, and the Kidney yang is also responsible for sexual and endocrine disorders.

BELOW *Du Zhong is the bark of Eucommia ulmoides, a 40ft. (12m.) deciduous, wide-spreading tree.*

DATA FILE

Properties
Sweet, slightly Acrid, Warm

Channels
Kidney, Liver

Functions and Uses
🌿 Tonifies the Liver and Kidneys, strengthens the tendons and bones.

🌿 Aids the smooth flow of qi and Blood: use to promote circulation.

🌿 Calms the fetus: use for Cold (lack of yang) Deficient Kidney patterns during pregnancy.

HOW TO USE

🌿 Du Zhong is an expensive herb – it is necessary to kill the tree in order to get the bark. The Liver rules the sinews, the Kidneys rule the bones, so it is used for weak, sore, or painful lower back and knees, chronic fatigue, spermatorrhea (leaking of sperm), and frequent urination. Yang Deficient symptoms are always accompanied by Cold. It is the main herb for lower back pain caused by qi and Blood stagnation. It helps prevent miscarriage with bleeding during pregnancy, or when the fetus is restless, and it has recently been used for dizziness and lightheadedness due to hypertension from rising Liver yang.

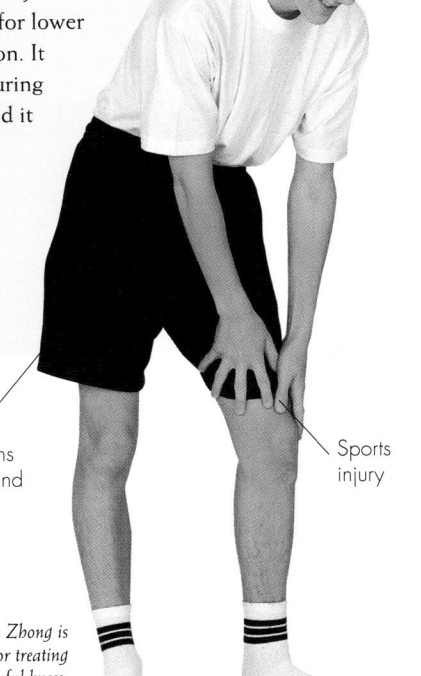

Strengthens tendons and bones

Sports injury

RIGHT *Du Zhong is indicated for treating painful knees.*

CAUTION

CONTRAINDICATED FOR HEAT FROM YIN DEFICIENCY.

Fritillaria thunbergii, fritillaria bulb
ZHE BEI MU

Like Ban Xia, this herb transforms Phlegm, which in TCM is the accumulation of thick fluid mainly in the respiratory and digestive tracts, but which may occur in the muscles and other body tissues.

HOW TO USE

🌿 Zhe Bei Mu is a Cold herb which treats Phlegm Heat (as opposed to Ban Xia, which is warming), characterized by yellow sputum or sputum which is difficult to bring up. It is also indicated for Phlegm Fire coagulating and causing lumps in the breast or neck, and for Lung abscesses. Chuan Bei Mu is another form of this herb which is milder and not so cooling, and may be used for many types of cough, including dry yin-deficient ones.

BELOW *Zhe Bei Mu disperses the stubborn Phlegm of a heavy cold.*

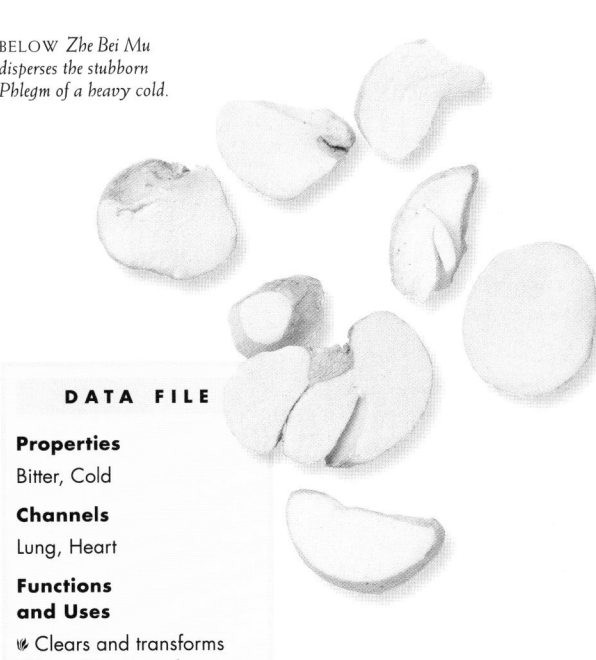

DATA FILE

Properties
Bitter, Cold

Channels
Lung, Heart

Functions and Uses
🌿 Clears and transforms Phlegm Heat: use for acute Lung Heat patterns with productive yellow sputum.

🌿 Clears Heat and dissipates nodules: use for Phlegm Fire which congeals and causes neck swellings.

CAUTION

INEFFECTIVE IN COUGHS DUE TO PHLEGM COLD.

Glycyrrhiza uralensis, licorice root

GAN CAO

This herb is one of a group that treat qi Deficiency and tonifies the Spleen. As we replenish our day-to-day energy levels by breathing in air and eating food, the two main organs involved are Lungs and Spleen (the main digestive organ in TCM).

HOW TO USE

🍃 Gan Cao is a very useful herb, primarily because it is sweet and mild, so that it moderates the violent properties of other herbs in a prescription and makes them more digestible. Furthermore, it enters all 12 channels, so it can lead other herbs into those channels. It is used for Spleen Deficiency with shortness of breath, tiredness, and loose stools, and for Blood Deficiency with an irregular pulse and palpitations. It is used for any coughing and wheezing, and is good for spasms or cramps in the abdomen or legs. It is also useful for strep throat infections.

DATA FILE

Properties
Sweet, Neutral (raw), Warm (toasted)

Channels
All 12 channels

Functions and Uses

❧ Tonifies the Spleen and benefits the qi.

❧ Moistens the Lungs and stops coughing: because it is neutral it can be used to treat either Heat or Cold in the Lungs.

❧ Clears Heat and detoxifies Fire-Poison: use Gan Cao for sores or sore throats with pus.

THERAPY CONNECTIONS

LICORICE

Ayurveda   *p.39*

Traditional Home and Folk Remedies   *p.91*

Herbalism   *p.122*

Moderates spasms

Moistens the Lungs

❧ Moderates spasms and alleviates pain.

❧ Antidote for toxic substances, applied either internally or externally.

❧ Moderates and harmonizes the effects of other herbs.

RIGHT *Gan Cao stops coughing and soothes a sore throat.*

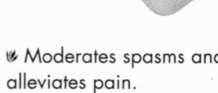

ABOVE *Gan Cao is useful for regulating the pulse.*

Ledebouriella sesloides

FANG FENG

Fang Feng belongs to a group of warm, acrid herbs that release exterior conditions; that is, superficial illnesses caused by viruses, with symptoms in the skin or muscle layers. These herbs mainly cause sweating, or stop sweating where necessary.

HOW TO USE

🍃 Fang Feng means in English "guard against wind," so it is used particularly in ailments where Wind is predominant, according to TCM. This means it causes sweating (Acrid quality) in colds and flu. It is also useful in arthritis, where the pain moves about from joint to joint (Wind type of arthritis). It treats numbness and trembling caused by Wind and Phlegm blocking the channels – for instance in convulsions associated with rabies or, more commonly, Parkinson's disease.

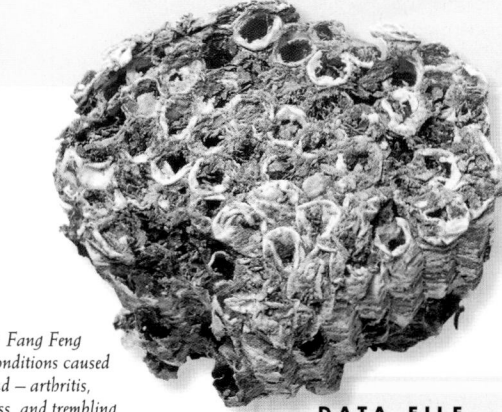

RIGHT *Fang Feng treats conditions caused by Wind – arthritis, numbness, and trembling.*

DATA FILE

Properties
Acrid, Sweet, slightly Warm

Channels
Bladder, Liver, Spleen

Functions and Uses

❧ Releases the Exterior and expels Wind: use for headaches, chills, and body aches from externally contracted Wind Cold.

❧ Expels Wind Dampness and alleviates pain: use for Exterior Wind Damp Painful Obstruction (rheumatic ailments).

❧ Expels Wind: Fang Feng alleviates trembling of the hands and feet.

Ligusticum chuanxiong,
Szechuan lovage root, cnidium

CHUAN XIONG

This herb invigorates (or "regulates") the Blood, treating disorders associated with Blood stasis. In TCM these problems include pain and internal masses or growths.

DATA FILE

Properties

Acrid, Warm

Channels

Liver, Gall bladder, Pericardium

Functions and Uses

❦ Invigorates the Blood and promotes the circulation of qi: use for any Blood stasis patterns, especially in gynecology.

❦ Expels Wind and alleviates pain: it goes to the top and exterior parts of the body.

Itching caused by Wind

Enters Liver, Gall bladder and Pericardium

CAUTION

CONTRAINDICATED IN YIN DEFICIENCY WITH HEAT SIGNS (IT IS WARMING), HEADACHES DUE TO RISING LIVER YANG (UNLESS COMBINED CAREFULLY), QI DEFICIENCY (IT DOES NOT TONIFY), OR EXCESSIVE MENSTRUAL BLEEDING (IT MOVES BLOOD FURTHER).

HOW TO USE

❧ Chuan Xiong is an important herb for gynecology, as many gynecological problems are caused by stagnant Blood circulation – problems such as dysmenorrhea (menstrual cramps), amenorrhea (lack of menstruation), difficult labor, or retained placenta. It is also used for chest, flank, and epigastric (above the navel) pain caused by Stagnant Qi and Blood. It is a leading herb for externally caught Wind disorders (viruses) with symptoms such as headaches, migraines, and dizziness. It is useful for arthritis and a variety of skin problems caused by Wind, including itching. As it moves the qi upward it is an essential herb used in combinations for treating all types of headaches.

ABOVE *Itchy skin problems can be improved by taking Chuan Xiong.*

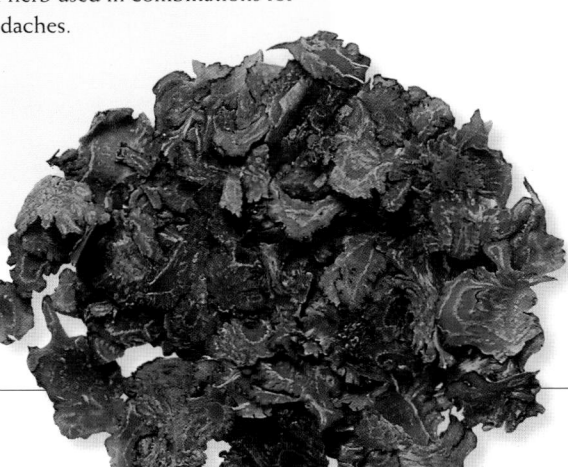

RIGHT *Chuan Xiong moves Stagnant Blood, and therefore eases painful periods.*

Lonicera japonica, honeysuckle flower,
"Gold Silver flower"

JIN YIN HUA

Jin Yin Hua is one of a group of herbs that clear Heat: this includes febrile conditions and any illnesses with Heat signs, such as fever, inflammation, red eyes, aversion to heat, and hot skin eruptions.

HOW TO USE

❧ Jin Yin Hua has a strong effect against many pathogenic bacteria. It is especially useful against Salmonella (food poisoning), and is effective against many streptococcus or staphylococcus infections. It is good for painful, hot swellings, particularly of the breast (mastitis), throat (viral or bacterial tonsillitis), or eyes (conjunctivitis). It is also used in "summer-heat diseases," where the hot weather produces fevers, sweating, and thirst. It is used for bad dysentery and bacterial urinary tract infections.

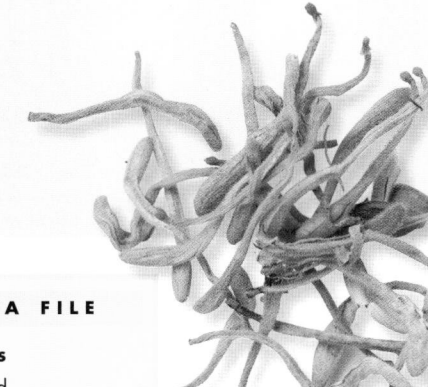

DATA FILE

Properties

Sweet, Cold

Channels

Large Intestine, Lung, Stomach

Functions and Uses

❦ Clears Heat and relieves toxicity: use Jin Yin Hua for hot, painful sores.

❦ Expels External Wind Heat: use for the early stages of febrile illnesses.

❦ Clears Damp Heat from Lower Burner: use for dysentery or cystitis.

ABOVE *Jin Yin Hua is useful against food poisoning and throat infections.*

CAUTION

CONTRAINDICATED IN CASES OF DIARRHEA DUE TO SPLEEN AND STOMACH DEFICIENCY – IT IS FOR STRONG INFECTIONS AND DOES NOT TONIFY WEAKNESS.

CONTRAINDICATED IN SORES WHICH DO NOT HAVE INFECTED PUS, BUT CLEAR LIQUID INSIDE.

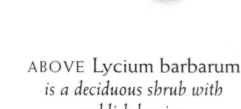

Lycium barbarum, Chinese wolfberry fruit, matrimony vine fruit
GOU QI ZI

This herb treats patterns of Blood Deficiency, and in TCM the two organs most affected by this disorder are the Heart and Liver, which direct and store the Blood, respectively.

HOW TO USE

🍂 Gou Qi Zi is used for such Liver and Kidney Deficient symptoms as sore back and weak knees, impotence, leaking of sperm, and diabetes, particularly in the elderly, when the yin is in decline. It is used for Liver and Kidney Deficiency which leads to Blood and essence failing to nourish the eyes, so is good for failing or blurred vision, dizziness, dry, or sore eyes. As it enriches the yin of the Lungs, it is good for consumptive coughs.

ABOVE *Lycium barbarum is a deciduous shrub with reddish berries.*

CAUTION

CONTRAINDICATED IN FULL HEAT DISORDERS, ESPECIALLY EXTERNAL (VIRUSES), AND IN CASES OF SPLEEN DEFICIENCY WITH LOOSE STOOLS.

DATA FILE

Properties
Sweet, Neutral

Channels
Liver, Lung, Kidney

Functions and Uses

🌿 Nourishes and tonifies the Liver and Kidneys: because this herb is neither Hot nor Cold, it is commonly used in treating Liver and Kidney Deficiency with patterns of Yin and Blood Deficiency.

🌿 Benefits the Jing-essence and brightens the eyes: Jing (ancestral qi) is held in the Kidneys, while the Liver meridian goes to the eyes.

🌿 Moistens the Lungs.

BELOW *Gou Qi Zi helps treat conditions in the elderly caused by depleted yin.*

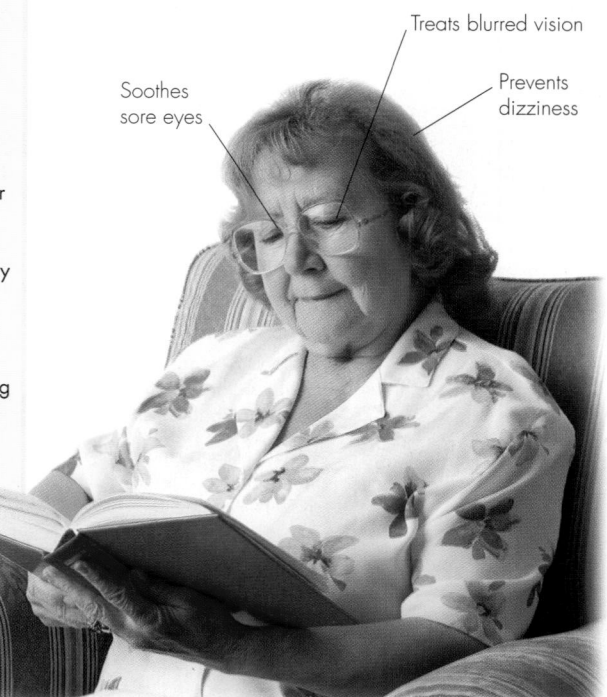

Soothes sore eyes

Treats blurred vision

Prevents dizziness

Ophiopogon japonicus, ophiopogon tuber
MAI MEN DONG

This herb tonifies the yin, and it therefore moistens and nourishes fluid. Any of the major organs may suffer from a Yin Deficiency, so Mai Men Dong is an important herb for their revitalization.

HOW TO USE

🍂 Mai Men Dong particularly strengthens the yin in the Upper part of the body, so it is good after febrile illness when the mouth is parched, and there is severe thirst or recurring fever. It is used for an irregular pulse and palpitations from the same causes of injury to the fluids or Blood. It is particularly for a dry cough, with or without mucus, and for Stomach Yin Deficiency, which includes stomach aches, "dry" vomiting, and a shiny tongue with little coating. It is also for diabetes, as well as being used to brighten the vision and strengthen the lower back. Like Tu Su Zi, it is added to prescriptions to moisten, but only in yin-deficient patterns.

DATA FILE

Properties
Sweet, Bitter, slightly Cold

Channels
Lung, Stomach, Heart

Functions and Uses

🌿 Moistens the Lungs and stops coughing.

🌿 Tonifies the Stomach Yin and generates fluid.

CAUTION

CONTRAINDICATED IN CASES OF DEFICIENCY WITHOUT HEAT SIGNS.

LIKE ALL TONIFYING YIN HERBS, IT AIDS DAMPNESS AND SHOULD THEREFORE NOT BE USED FOR COLD PHLEGMY COUGHING OR DEFICIENT SPLEEN WITH LOOSE STOOLS OR A THICK, GREASY TONGUE COATING.

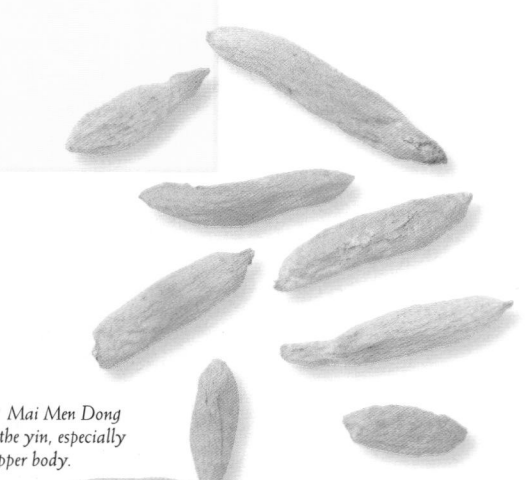

RIGHT *Mai Men Dong tonifies the yin, especially in the upper body.*

Paeonia lactiflora, white peony root

BAI SHAO

Bai Shao is a cooling herb with a sinking action – which means it takes qi down strongly. It is useful when the Liver is not fulfilling its function of making the Blood and qi flow smoothly.

HOW TO USE

❧ Bai Shao has many uses and is an important herb. It treats headaches and dizziness due to rising Liver yang, and flank, chest, and abdominal pain from constrained (stuck) Liver Qi, or disharmony between the Liver and Spleen, which normally have a close relationship in the upper abdomen. Generally, this herb "softens" the Liver, treating spasms in the abdomen, or cramps in the hands or feet. It is good for menstrual irregularity or pain, or uterine bleeding, and, as it preserves the yin fluids, treats vaginal discharge and leaking of sperm. It treats excessive sweating in an external illness, or night sweating in Yin Deficiency.

DATA FILE

Properties

Bitter, Sour, Cool

Channels

Liver, Spleen

Functions and Uses

❧ Pacifies the Liver yang and alleviates pain: use for patterns of Liver yang rising, constrained Liver Qi or disharmonies between the Liver and the Spleen.

❧ Nourishes the Blood and regulates the menses.

❧ Preserves the yin.

❧ Adjusts the Ying and Wei: this refers to the balance between the inner and outer qi levels, which control the opening and closing of the pores.

CAUTION

EXERCISE CAUTION WITH DIARRHEA DUE TO COLD FROM DEFICIENCY, AS IT IS A COLD HERB.

BELOW *Bai Shao harmonizes the functions of the Liver and preserves the yin.*

Panax ginseng, ginseng root, "man root"

REN SHEN

Ren Shen is an expensive herb as it takes six or seven years to cultivate. It is calming and has a proven effect on stress.

HOW TO USE

❧ Ren Shen is invaluable because it tonifies both the qi (lack of energy) and the yin (lack of fluid). It is used after shock, with shallow respiration, shortness of breath, cold limbs, profuse sweating, and a weak pulse. It is good for Lung problems such as labored breathing and wheezing, and Spleen Qi deficient problems such as lethargy, lack of appetite, bloating, and diarrhea, or, more severely, prolapse of the stomach, uterus, or rectum. It calms the Heart when there are palpitations, and in cases of anxiety, insomnia, or forgetfulness. As it is so expensive, it is usually substituted by Dang Shen in prescriptions.

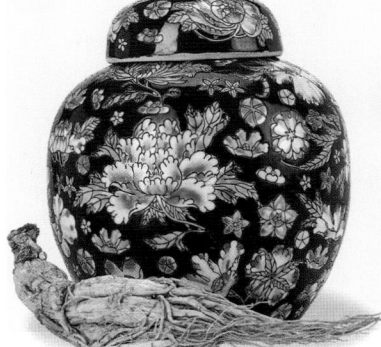

ABOVE *Ren Shen calms anxiety and works on Heart Qi.*

ABOVE *Ginseng should not be taken over an extended period.*

CAUTION

CONTRAINDICATED FOR YIN DEFICIENCY WITH HEAT SIGNS (IT IS SLIGHTLY WARMING), HEAT EXCESS OR NO SIGNIFICANT QI DEFICIENCY.

OVERDOSE CAN LEAD TO HEADACHE, INSOMNIA, AND A RISE IN BLOOD PRESSURE.

THERAPY CONNECTIONS

GINSENG

◎ Herbalism   p.126

DATA FILE

Properties

Sweet, slightly Bitter, slightly Warm

Channels

Lung, Spleen

Functions and Uses

❧ Strong tonifier of Root Qi: helps to revive an unconscious person.

❧ Tonifies the Lungs and benefits the qi.

❧ Strengthens the Spleen and tonifies the Stomach.

❧ Ren Shen generates fluid and stops thirst: use for diabetes when the qi and Blood have been injured by high fever and sweating.

❧ Benefits the Heart Qi and calms the spirit.

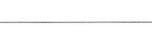

Panax notoginseng,
notoginseng root, pseudoginseng root

SAN QI

This herb is used for bleeding or hemorrhage. Generally this herb is not used alone, but with other herbs that treat the cause of the bleeding, such as Hot Blood, Yin Deficiency, Spleen Deficiency, or stasis of the Blood.

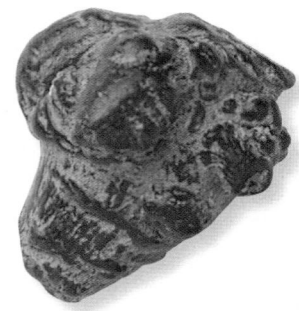

LEFT *San Qi treats pain in both the chest and the abdomen.*

HOW TO USE

San Qi has long been used in battle – soldiers carried this black powder with them to stem wounds. It may be taken on its own or in a prescription. It is used for all kinds of internal and external bleeding, such as vomiting blood, nosebleed, blood in the urine or stool, uterine bleeding, or trauma-induced bleeding. It is good for chest and abdominal pain, as well as joint pain caused by congealed Blood. It can also be used after heart attacks to get rid of debris in the coronary artery, and is very useful after injuries, for swelling and pain due to falls, fractures, bruises, and sprains.

BELOW *Soldiers used to carry San Qi to stop bleeding wounds.*

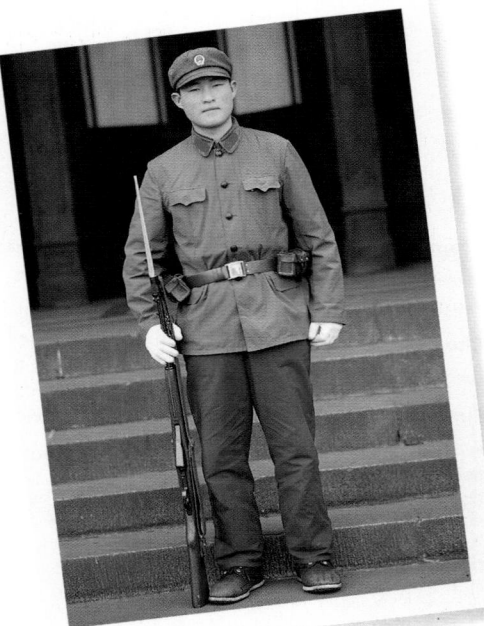

DATA FILE

Properties
Sweet, slightly Bitter, Warm

Channels
Liver, Stomach, Large Intestine

Functions and Uses
🗘 Stops bleeding and transforms Blood stasis: because this herb can stop bleeding without causing Blood stasis, it is very widely used.

🗘 Reduces swelling and alleviates pain: San Qi is a first choice for traumatic injuries.

CAUTION

CONTRAINDICATED
DURING PREGNANCY.
◦◦◦
USE WITH CAUTION IN
PATIENTS WITH BLOOD OR
YIN DEFICIENCY.

Phellodendron amurense, amur cork-tree bark,
Cypress Rotundis, "Yellow Fir"

HUANG BAI, HUANG BO

This herb is one that clears Heat: this includes febrile conditions and any illnesses with Heat signs. It is one of the "Three Yellows," which are often used together for severe infections.

HOW TO USE

🗘 Huang Bai is particularly good for Damp Heat symptoms in the bottom third of the body, such as yellow, smelly vaginal discharge, foul-smelling diarrhea or dysentery. It is also used for red, swollen, and painful legs, and Damp Heat jaundice. It can be used for menopausal symptoms of hot sweats, or for afternoon fevers at the end of a long illness or when withdrawing from illicit drugs. It is good for leg ulcers which require antibiotics. It is a weaker (and cheaper) version of Huang Lian in its antimicrobial effects.

CAUTION

CONTRAINDICATED IN CASES
OF SPLEEN DEFICIENCY, WITH
OR WITHOUT DIARRHEA
(SPLEEN DEFICIENCY MUST BE
DIAGNOSED BY A QUALIFIED
TCM PRACTITIONER).

DATA FILE

Properties
Bitter, Cold

Channels
Kidney, Bladder

Functions and Uses
🗘 Drains Damp Heat, particularly in the Lower Burner: use Huang Bai for Damp Heat leukorrhea (vaginal discharge).

🗘 Drains Kidney Fire: Ascending Kidney Fire with deficient yin signs, such as night sweating and a feeling of Heat in the patient's bones.

🗘 Detoxifies Fire Poison, i.e. toxic sores with pus in them.

BELOW Phellodendron amurense *has dark, cork-like bark when the tree is old.*

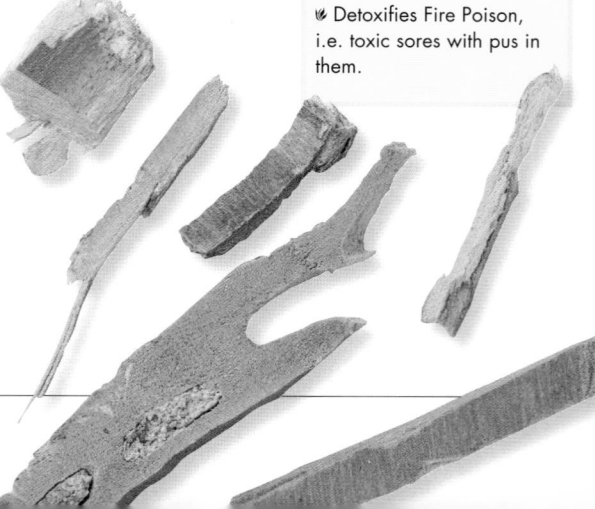

Pinellia ternata, pinellia rhizome
BAN XIA

This herb is one that transforms Phlegm, which in TCM is the accumulation of thick fluid mainly in the respiratory and digestive tracts, but which may occur in the muscles and other body tissues.

HOW TO USE

Ban Xia is one of the main herbs for drying Damp, and is used for abdominal and epigastric (upper abdominal) bloating and nausea, or for a stifling feeling in the chest due to Phlegm Damp – it is often used with Chen Pi. It can be added to prescriptions to avoid nausea from other herbs. It reduces any lumps or obstructions caused by Phlegm in the body.

DATA FILE

Properties

Acrid, Warm

Channels

Lung, Spleen, Stomach

Functions and Uses

Dries Dampness, transforms Phlegm, and helps rebellious qi to descend; it is one of the main herbs for coughs with sputum. It helps the Spleen to dry out and so produce less mucus.

Harmonizes the Stomach and stops vomiting: it takes qi down so helps Phlegm Dampness in the Stomach that rebels upward and causes vomiting.

Dissipates nodules and reduces lumps: use for nodules caused by Phlegm lingering, such as goiter or lumps in the breast.

ABOVE *Ban Xia is used to treat an enlarged thyroid gland.*

CAUTION

CONTRAINDICATED IN BLEEDING, COUGHS DUE TO YIN DEFICIENCY (DRY COUGHS) OR DEPLETED FLUIDS – IT IS VERY DRYING.

USE WITH CAUTION IN HEAT CASES.

IN VERY LARGE AMOUNTS, IT IS SOMEWHAT TOXIC (CAUSING NAUSEA), BUT CAN BE CURED BY GINGER.

Platycodon grandiflorum, balloon flower root
JIE GENG

This herb relieves coughing and wheezing. Like other cough remedies it treats the manifestation (presenting symptoms) of the problem, and therefore needs to be combined with other herbs that treat the root cause.

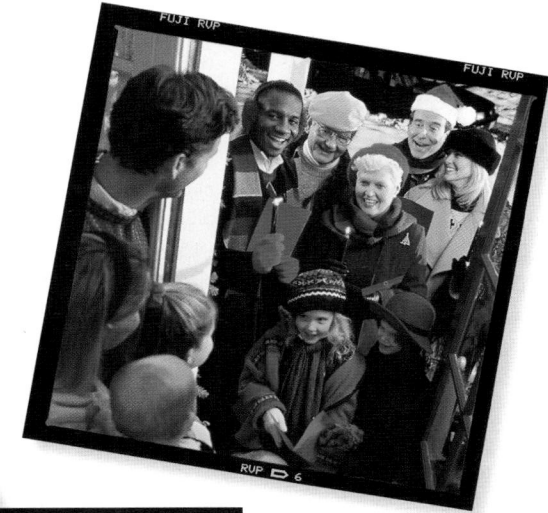

CAUTION

CONTRAINDICATED IN COUGHING BLOOD (HEMOPTYSIS), AS IT MAKES THINGS GO UP AND WOULD MAKE THE CONDITION WORSE.

ABOVE *Carol singers in full voice. Jie Geng opens the voice and benefits the throat.*

HOW TO USE

Like Xing Ren, Jie Geng can be used for a wide variety of coughs, especially for coughs caused by external pathogens, either Wind Cold or Wind Heat. It is useful for loss of voice, especially when this is caused by external Heat drying up the fluids in the throat. However, when combined carefully, it can be used for loss of voice due to Phlegm Heat or Yin Deficiency. It is often put into other prescriptions to direct herbs to the chest and head areas.

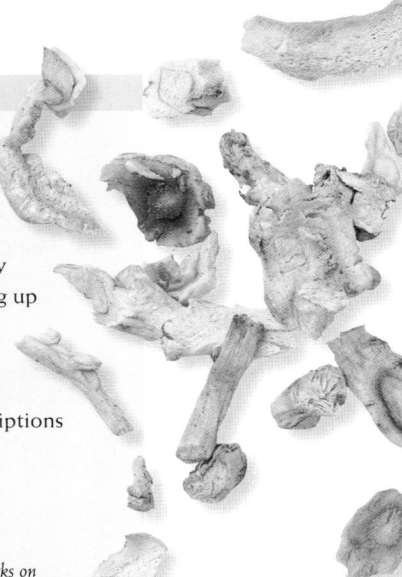

RIGHT *Jie Geng works on the Lung meridian, treating chest complaints.*

DATA FILE

Properties

Bitter, Acrid, Neutral

Channels

Lung

Functions and Uses

Circulates the Lung qi, expels Phlegm and stops coughing: Jie Geng can be used to treat a wide variety of coughs, depending on the other herbs with which it is combined.

Benefits the throat and opens the voice: used in many cases of sore throat and loss of voice, especially those caused by external Heat.

Promotes the discharge of pus: use for expelling pus associated with Lung abscess or throat abscess.

Makes herbs go to the upper body.

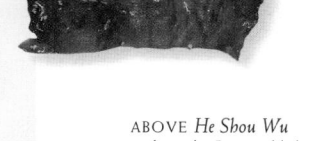

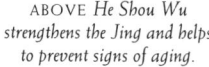

Polygala tenuifolia, Chinese senega root, polygala
YUAN ZHI

Yuan Zhi nourishes the Heart and calms the Spirit, or Shen, which is said to reside in the Heart. When the Shen is calm, personality is at its most potent.

HOW TO USE

🍂 Yuan Zhi is used for insomnia, anxiety, palpitations, and forgetfulness. However, it differs from Suan Zao Ren in that it is most effective in cases when the patient thinks too much (excessive brooding), or for restlessness and disorientation. "Phlegm misting the Heart" implies quite serious psychological or psychiatric disturbances, when the Spirit is not clear and the patient loses touch with reality. It is also used for seizures and epilepsy. It is useful for coughs with copious sputum, especially when difficult to expectorate, and is applied topically for abscesses, sores, and swollen and painful breasts.

Polygonum multiflorum, fleeceflower root
HE SHOU WU

This herb treats patterns of Blood Deficiency, and in TCM the two organs most affected by this disorder are the Heart and Liver, which direct and store the Blood, respectively.

HOW TO USE

🍂 He Shou Wu is very commonly used, as it both tonifies and preserves the Kidney Jing-essence without being cloying. It is particularly used for premature graying or when the hair falls out (the name means "black hair"), as well as for dizziness, blurred vision, spots in front of the eyes, and a weak lower back and knees. It stops premature ejaculation, leaking of sperm, and vaginal discharge. Used raw, it is good for goiter and neck lumps – and as it moistens, is useful for constipation. It treats chronic malaria and prevents hardening of the arteries.

ABOVE *He Shou Wu strengthens the Jing and helps to prevent signs of aging.*

DATA FILE

Properties
Bitter, Acrid, slightly Warm

Channels
Heart, Lung, Kidney

Functions and Uses

🍃 Calms the Spirit and quietens the Heart: use for pent-up emotions.

🍃 Expels Phlegm and clears the orifices: when "mucus envelops the orifices of the Heart," with consequent emotional problems.

🍃 Helps expel Phlegm from the Lungs.

🍃 Reduces abscesses and dissipates swellings: use in powdered form, applied topically or mixed into a glass of wine.

ABOVE *Yuan Zhi is a good herb for treating emotional problems.*

CAUTION

CONTRAINDICATED FOR YIN DEFICIENCY WITH HEAT SIGNS.

◦

CAUTION SHOULD BE EXERCISED WITH ULCERS OR GASTRITIS.

CAUTION

CONTRAINDICATED FOR SPLEEN DEFICIENCY, PHLEGM OR DIARRHEA.

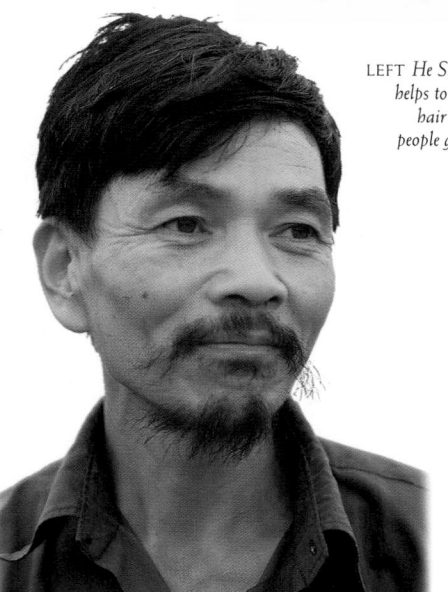

LEFT *He Shou Wu helps to preserve hair color as people get older.*

DATA FILE

Properties
Bitter, Sweet, Astringent, slightly Warm

Channels
Liver, Kidney

Functions and Uses

🍃 Tonifies the Liver and Kidneys, nourishes the Blood and Jing-essence: used for treating Yin and Blood Deficiency.

🍃 Firms the Jing and stops leakage: this refers to male sexual problems.

🍃 Relieves Fire toxicity: use He Shou Wu raw for carbuncles and sores.

🍃 Moistens the Intestines and unblocks the bowels.

🍃 Expels Wind from the skin by nourishing the Blood: use for rashes that appear suddenly.

YE JIAO TENG
Polygonus multiflorum, fleeceflower vine

Ye Jiao Teng nourishes the Heart and calms the Spirit, which is said to reside in the Heart. It is therefore useful in tackling disturbed emotions.

HOW TO USE

🍃 Ye Jiao Teng is good for yin or Blood Deficiency patterns with insomnia, irritability, or emotional and nervous patients who cannot eat. It is especially useful for dream-disturbed sleep, and helps one feel comfortable in oneself. It also nourishes the Blood in the four limbs when the circulation is blocked or weak due to Blood Deficiency, and is used for such symptoms as generalized weakness, soreness, and aching or numb limbs. As it nourishes the Blood in the channels (meridians), it is also used externally as a wash for itching and skin rashes.

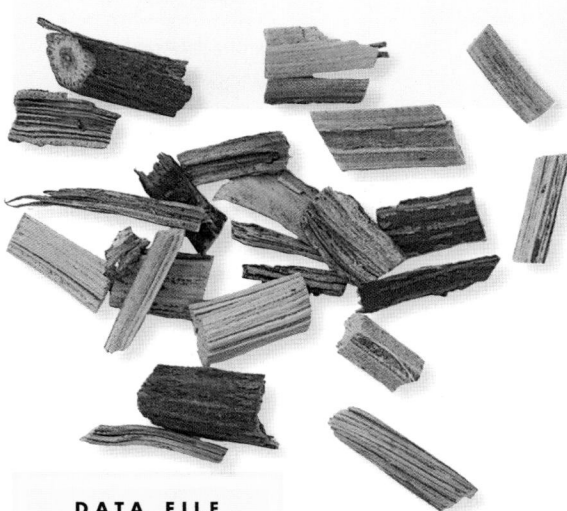

DATA FILE

Properties
Sweet, slightly Bitter, Neutral

Channels
Heart, Liver

Functions and Uses

🌿 Nourishes the Heart and Blood, and calms the Spirit.

🌿 Activates Blood circulation and unblocks the channels.

🌿 Alleviates itching: use as an external wash.

ABOVE *Ye Jiao Teng can be made into a decoction and applied to itchy skin rashes.*

CAUTION
CONTRAINDICATED WITH DIARRHEA.

FU LING
Poria cocos, tuckahoe, hoelen, bread root

Fu Ling is a widely used herb that transforms Dampness, a "pathogenic influence" which creates stagnation in the Middle Burner, with various digestive or fluid-retaining effects.

HOW TO USE

🍃 Fu Ling both strengthens the Spleen and gets rid of Dampness. It is good for difficulty with urination, diarrhea or edema (water retention), all symptoms of Dampness in the system. It helps with loss of appetite or bloating. Other symptoms of Phlegm include headaches or dizziness, and as it calms the Spirit it is good for palpitations, insomnia, or forgetfulness. It is a main ingredient in the qi-strengthening prescription Si Jun Zi Wan ("Four Gentlemen") and is also essential in the main Yin-tonifying prescription, where it stops a person becoming too moist from the yin (fluid) tonifying herbs.

CAUTION
CONTRAINDICATED FOR COPIOUS URINE FROM DEFICIENT COLD.

ABOVE *Fu Ling is a neutral herb which is added to many prescription mixes.*

DATA FILE

Properties
Sweet, Bland, Neutral

Channels
Heart, Spleen, Lung

Functions and Uses

🌿 Promotes urination and leeches out Dampness by causing urination.

🌿 Strengthens the Spleen and harmonizes the Middle area: helps prevent Dampness building up.

🌿 Strengthens the Spleen and transforms Phlegm (congested fluids which can cause Heart palpitations and other symptoms).

🌿 Quietens the Heart and calms the Spirit.

XING REN
Prunus armenica, apricot kernel

This herb is primarily used to treat coughing and wheezing. As it treats the manifestation (presenting symptoms) of the problem, it needs to be combined with other herbs that treat the root cause.

HOW TO USE

🍃 Xing Ren may be used for many kinds of coughing, whether from Heat or Cold, Exterior or Interior, depending on the combination with other herbs. Because the herb is moist in nature, it is useful for externally caught dry cough. It can be combined with Huo Ma Ren or Dang Gui for constipation due to Deficient Qi and dry Intestines.

CAUTION
USE WITH CAUTION FOR CHILDREN AND IN CASES OF DIARRHEA.

DATA FILE

Properties
Bitter, slightly Warm, slightly Toxic

Channels
Lung, Large Intestine

Functions and Uses

🌿 Stops coughing and calms wheezing: Xing Ren is used widely for many kinds of cough.

🌿 Moistens Intestines and unblocks the bowels: a secondary benefit due to the high oil content of Xing Ren.

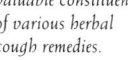

LEFT *Xing Ren is a valuable constituent of various herbal cough remedies.*

Prunus persica, peach kernel

TAO REN

This herb invigorates (or "regulates") the Blood, treating problems associated with Blood stasis. In TCM these disorders include pain and internal masses or growths.

HOW TO USE

🌰 Tao Ren is a very strong herb. It breaks through Blood and is an important herb for hard abdominal masses and tumors, and for epigastric lumps such as enlarged Liver or Spleen, if there is Stagnant Blood present. It also treats congealed Blood amenorrhea and abdominal pain, or pain from injuries. It is good for psychosis caused by congealed Blood (according to TCM) or post-partum psychosis, and treats Lung and Intestinal abscesses. Like many seeds it is useful for constipation caused by dry Intestines.

ABOVE *Tao Ren, the peach kernel, treats disorders of the Blood.*

DATA FILE

Properties

Bitter, Sweet, Neutral

Channels

Heart, Liver, Lung, Large Intestine

Functions and Uses

🌿 Breaks up Blood stasis: it is a stronger herb than Hong Hua.

🌿 Moistens the Intestines and moves stools.

Radix rehmannia glutinosa, Chinese foxglove root

SHENG DI HUANG

Sheng di Huang is one of a group of herbs that clear Heat: this includes febrile conditions and any illnesses with Heat signs. It can be used to treat diabetes by addressing the Heat cause.

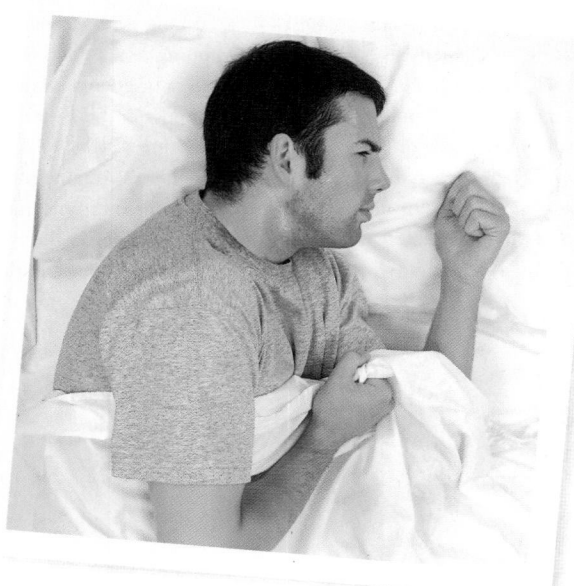

ABOVE *Feverish illnesses respond to treatment with Sheng di Huang, which is a cooling herb.*

DATA FILE

Properties

Sweet, Bitter, Cold

Channels

Heart, Liver, Kidney

Functions and Uses

🌿 Clears Heat and cools the Blood: use in all febrile conditions where there is a very high fever, thirst, and a scarlet tongue. Also in hemorrhage when Heat enters the Blood level.

🌿 Nourishes the yin and generates fluids: treats low-grade long-term fever with dry mouth, constipation, night sweats.

🌿 Cools Heart Fire blazing: mouth and tongue ulcers, irritability, insomnia.

🌿 Wasting–Thirsting syndrome, i.e. diabetes.

HOW TO USE

🌰 Sheng di Huang is a very moistening as well as cooling herb. Therefore it is used in febrile illnesses where the Heat over a period has dried up the fluids in the body, causing thirst, irritability, and a scarlet tongue. It is also used, often with Bai Shao, when Heat in the Blood level causes hemorrhage from the vessels, leading to bloody urine, nosebleeds, and vomiting of blood. Untreated diabetes causes excessive thirst and urine – Sheng di Huang treats the Heat cause and helps the body replace the fluids.

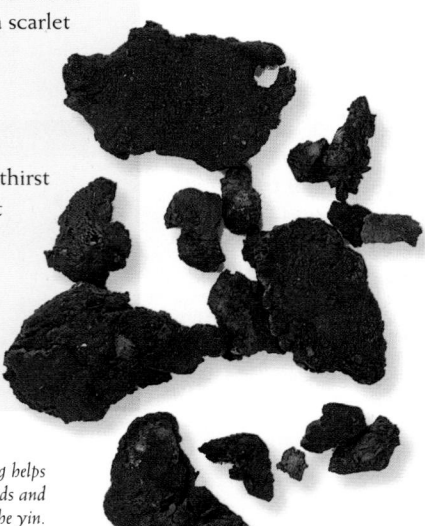

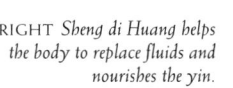

RIGHT *Sheng di Huang helps the body to replace fluids and nourishes the yin.*

Rehmannia glutinosa,
Chinese foxglove root cooked in wine
SHU DI HUANG

This herb treats patterns of Blood Deficiency, and in TCM the two organs most affected by this disorder are the Heart and Liver, which direct and store the Blood, respectively.

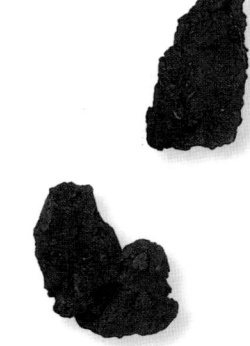

LEFT *Shu di Huang is Sheng di Huang which has been cooked in red wine.*

HOW TO USE

Shu di Huang is a very important herb – it is both a Blood and a yin tonic. Blood Deficient symptoms include a pale complexion, dizziness, palpitations, and insomnia; also menstrual problems such as irregular bleeding, uterine bleeding, and amenorrhea (no menstruation). Kidney Yin Deficient patterns include night sweats, heat in the bones, nocturnal emissions (wet dreams), diabetes, and tinnitus (ringing in the ears). Jing Deficiency includes such Kidney symptoms as low back pain, weakness of the knees and legs, lightheadedness, deafness, and also premature graying of the hair.

DATA FILE

Properties

Sweet, slightly Warm

Channels

Heart, Kidney, Liver

Functions and Uses

Tonifies the Blood: Blood deficient symptoms are similar to those of anemia.

Nourishes the yin: use for treating Kidney yin deficient patterns.

Nourishes the Blood and tonifies the Kidney essence (Jing) together: use it to treat Jing Deficient symptoms.

BELOW *Shu di Huang treats the symptoms caused by Blood Deficiency.*

CAUTION

USE WITH CAUTION IN CASES OF SPLEEN AND STOMACH DEFICIENCY, OR STAGNANT QI OR PHLEGM.

AS WITH MANY TONIFYING HERBS, IT NOURISHES THE MOIST SUBSTANCES IN THE BODY, SO OVERUSE CAN LEAD TO BLOATING AND LOOSE STOOLS: IT MUST BE CAREFULLY COMBINED.

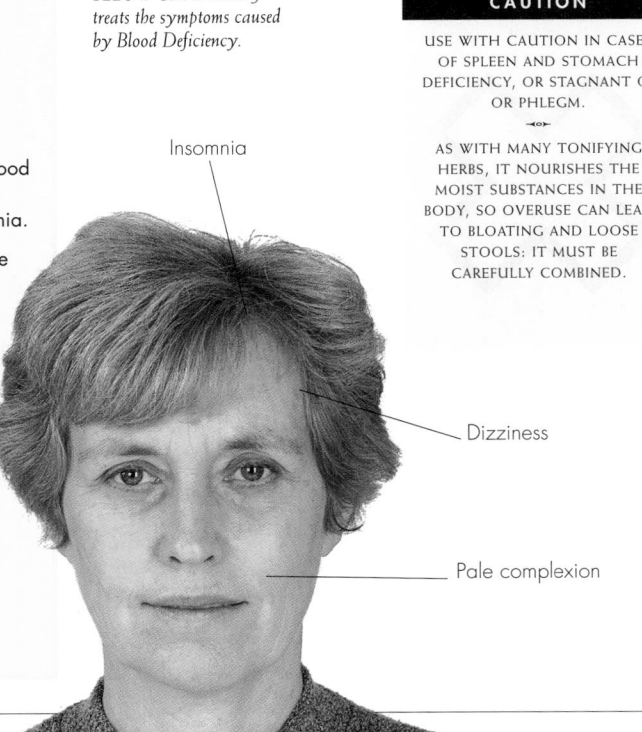

Insomnia

Dizziness

Pale complexion

Rheum palmatum, rhubarb root and rhizome
DA HUANG

Da Huang comes into the category of Descending Downward: it facilitates the expulsion of stools in cases of constipation. This downward action clears Heat.

HOW TO USE

Da Huang (rhubarb) is a purgative. It has a strong downward action and clears Heat by acting as a powerful laxative. It treats Damp Heat jaundice, dysentery, and cystitis in the same way. It is good for Stagnant Blood complaints such as endometriosis, amenorrhea (lack of menstruation), and appendicitis.

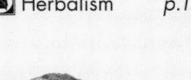

THERAPY CONNECTIONS

RHUBARB

Herbalism   *p.127*

DATA FILE

Properties

Bitter, Cold

Channels

Heart, Large Intestine, Liver, Stomach

Functions and Uses

Drains Heat and purges accumulations: use for Full Heat conditions where there is fever, thirst, constipation, abdominal pain, a full pulse, and yellow fur on the patient's tongue.

Drains Damp Heat via the stools.

Clears Full Heat from the Blood: use for "reckless" bright red Blood that is flowing strongly, e.g. bleeding hemorrhoids (piles), nosebleeds.

Invigorates the Blood: dispels Blood stagnation. Blood stasis can occur after traumatic injury, leading to a fixed pain.

Clears Heat, resolves Fire Poison: use either topically or internally for boils, sores, burns, or Hot skin lesions (red lesions, giving off heat).

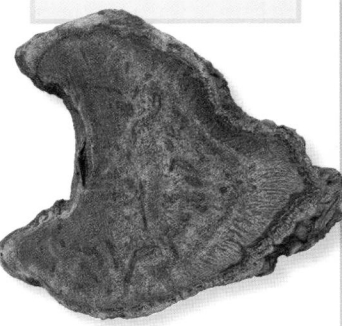

ABOVE *Da Huang is a Cold herb, used to treat Heat conditions by purging the body.*

CAUTION

CONTRAINDICATED IN THE FIRST STAGE OF INFECTIOUS DISEASES.

ALSO CONTRAINDICATED FOR QI OR BLOOD DEFICIENCY – IT DOESN'T TONIFY WEAKNESS BUT MAY BE ADDED TO A TONIFYING PRESCRIPTION TO CLEAR HEAT.

CONTRAINDICATED FOR COLD – IT IS A COLD HERB.

EXTREME CAUTION SHOULD BE EXERCISED DURING PREGNANCY, DURING MENSTRUATION, AND POST-PARTUM (AFTER BIRTH): IT HAS A STRONG DOWNWARD ACTION.

Schisandra chinensis, schisandra fruit
WU WEI ZI

Wu Wei Zi stabilizes and binds. It is a sour and astringent herb, and helps to keep leaking fluids and other substances within the body.

HOW TO USE

🍃 Wu Wei Zi is used for chronic coughs, wheezing, and asthma, especially with mucus, although it can also be used for dry coughs, as it nourishes the yin fluid. At the other end of the body, it is used for leaking of sperm, and urinary frequency or incontinence, vaginal discharges, especially watery and white (Cold), and daybreak diarrhea due to Spleen and Kidney Deficiency. It is indicated for excessive day or night sweating, with thirst and dry throat, but in common with other herbs in this category, it is not for sweat caused by outside infections. It also treats diabetes, the "wasting–thirsting" syndrome. Furthermore, it "holds the Heart yin in place," treating symptoms such as palpitations, irritability, dream-disturbed sleep, insomnia, forgetfulness, fear of ghosts, and of going outside. Basically, it helps keep a person feeling sane and calm.

ABOVE *Wu Wei Zi's uses include treatment of mental and physical disorders.*

BELOW *Wu Wei Zi helps to alleviate panic attacks of any kind.*

CAUTION

CONTRAINDICATED FOR EXTERNAL CONDITIONS, AND THE EARLY STAGES OF COUGHS AND RASHES – IT WILL KEEP THE "EXTERIOR PATHOGENIC FACTOR" INSIDE.

THERAPY CONNECTIONS

SCHISANDRA

🔘 Herbalism   *p.130*

SKULLCAP

🔘 Herbalism   *p.131*

DATA FILE

Properties

Sour, Warm

Channels

Heart, Kidney, Lung

Functions and Uses

🍃 Absorbs the leakage of Lung Qi and stops attacks of coughing.

🍃 Firms the Kidneys, binds up Jing-essence and stops bouts of diarrhea.

🍃 Absorbs sweating and generates fluids.

🍃 Quietens the Spirit and calms the Heart.

Scutellaria baicalensis, skullcap root
HUANG QIN

This herb is one that clears Heat: this includes febrile conditions and any illnesses with Heat signs. It is one of the "Three Yellows," which are often used together for severe infections.

HOW TO USE

🍃 Huang Qin mainly clears Heat in the chest and abdominal areas, so it is used for virulent diseases with high fever, irritability, thirst, cough, and expectoration (coughing up) of thick, yellow sputum. It can also be used topically on a dressing to clear red, hot swellings. It is used for dysentery and smelly diarrhea; also for febrile diseases which have a Damp element – symptoms such as a feeling of heaviness on the chest, and thirst with no desire to drink. It may be used for Damp Heat jaundice. It is one of the main herbs used in pregnancy to prevent miscarriage, and if toasted can stop Hot Bleeding from the nose, uterus, chest area, or in stools.

DATA FILE

Properties

Bitter, Cold

Channels

Heart, Lung, Gall bladder, Large Intestine

Functions and Uses

🍃 Clears Heat, particularly in the Upper Burner (the upper third of the body, chest area).

🍃 Clears Damp Heat: especially in the Stomach or Intestines. It is also used for Damp Heat in the Lower Burner, with symptoms such as cystitis.

🍃 Clears Heat and calms the fetus.

🍃 Stops bleeding due to Hot Blood: characterized as "the Blood becomes reckless with Heat and bursts out of its vessels."

CAUTION

CONTRAINDICATED FOR TUBERCULOSIS, WHICH IS A HEAT DEFICIENCY OF THE LUNGS, NOT A FULL HEAT, COLD DIARRHEA OR ANY COLD IN THE ABDOMEN, THREATENED MISCARRIAGE FROM A COLD CONDITION.

BELOW *Huang Qin comes from skullcap, a summer-flowering perennial.*

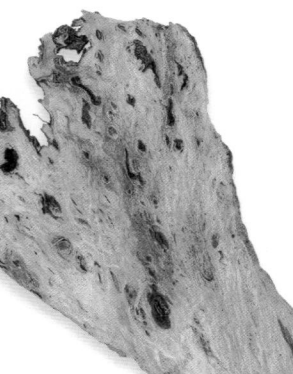

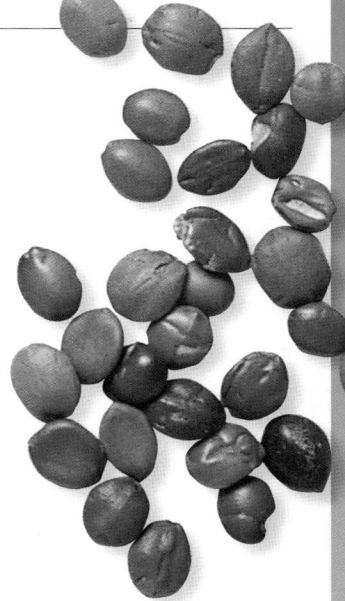

Stephania tetrandra, stephania root
HAN FANG JI

Like Wu Jia Pi, this herb dispels Wind Dampness from the muscles, joints, and bones. Whereas Wu Jia Pi is a Warm herb, however, Han Fang Ji is Cold. Wind Damp causes rheumatic and arthritic ailments.

CAUTION

USE WITH CAUTION IN CASES OF YIN DEFICIENCY, AS IT IS VERY DRYING.

DATA FILE

Properties

Bitter, Acrid, Cold

Channels

Bladder, Spleen, Kidney

Functions and Uses

❧ Expels Wind Dampness and alleviates pain: use for Wind–Damp–Heat in the channels, causing painful hot joints.

❧ Promotes urination; very effective at reducing edema – use Han Fang Ji whenever Damp collects.

BELOW *A colored X-ray of hands suffering from severe rheumatoid arthritis. Han Fang Ji relieves this condition.*

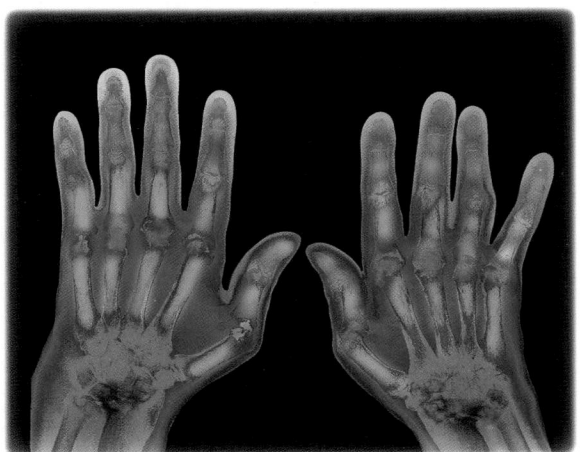

HOW TO USE

❧ As a Cold herb, Han Fang Ji treats hot, painful swollen joints, such as in an acute attack of rheumatoid arthritis. It has an analgesic (pain relieving) and anti-inflammatory effect. It is very good in treating edema, especially of the lower body and legs, gurgling or ascites in the abdomen. It may also treat acute edema of the upper body (water on the lung).

Ziziphus spinosa, sour jujube seed
SUAN ZAO REN

This herb nourishes the Heart and calms the Spirit, which is said to reside in the Heart. Laboratory tests have proved that Suan Zao Ren has a sedative effect. It is used to treat emotional problems.

HOW TO USE

❧ Suan Zao Ren is one of the main herbs used for calming the Heart by nourishing the Blood, treating symptoms such as irritability, insomnia, palpitations, and anxiety. It is also very good for both spontaneous and night sweating, and is used both in menopausal syndromes and withdrawal from addictive drugs, as well as many kinds of emotional problems.

ABOVE *Suan Zao Ren acts via the Heart, Spleen, Gall-bladder, and Liver.*

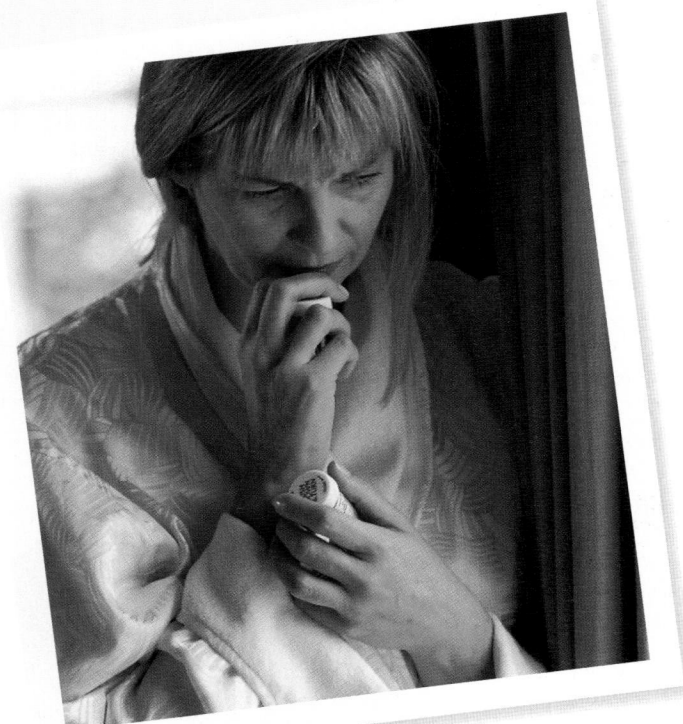

ABOVE *Suan Zao Ren is useful for fighting dependence or addictive drugs.*

DATA FILE

Properties

Sweet, Sour, Neutral

Channels

Liver, Gall Bladder, Heart, Spleen

Functions and Uses

❧ Nourishes the Heart yin and the Liver Blood, and calms the Spirit.

❧ Prevents occurrence of abnormal sweating.

CAUTION

CAUTION SHOULD BE EXERCISED IN CASES OF SEVERE DIARRHEA OR HEAT EXCESS.

TRADITIONAL HOME AND FOLK REMEDIES

Every culture, across the centuries, has had its own understanding and ways of healing. Local plants, customs, and beliefs determined the form it took, which varied not only across countries but also between villages. Even today, away from the convenience of conventional physicians, local communities around the world practise their own form of medicinal healing using plants, age-old wisdom, and an instinctive and learned knowledge of their bodies as the tools.

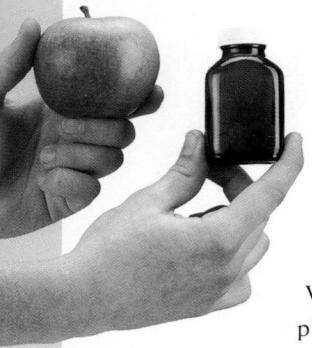

ABOVE *It's our choice: relying on conventional drugs, or reinvestigating alternative methods used for hundreds of years.*

A RETURN TO OLD WAYS

With the advent of technology and the growing dependence upon the miracles of modern medicine, most of us have lost the art of looking after ourselves. We have become dependent upon physicians, prescription drugs, store-bought preparations, and, through that, have lost an understanding of our bodies and how they work. Somewhere along the line we have put not only our faith but our independence in the hands of others. When we have a cold, a rash, even painful joints, we go straight to the medicine cabinet, or ring to arrange an appointment at the physician's surgery. The use of natural preparations, and the number of people addressing minor complaints in their own homes, hit an all-time low over the past decades, and only now are we experiencing a renaissance of natural healing and home remedies, as it becomes clear that conventional medicine, for all its wonders, is not the answer to everything.

Busy Western physicians have little time to spend diagnosing their patients, and our Western approach to pathology and anatomy is based on the theory that we are all the same. Individual personalities, lifestyles, emotions, spirituality, and indeed physical bodies are not taken into consideration for most conventional treatment, but we have now learnt that it is the complex combination of these very things that can make us sick or well. Treatment, therefore, needs to examine a wider picture.

In the past, many of us had the knowledge and the wherewithal to treat ourselves, using foodstuffs in our larders, and plants growing in our yards and fields. There would have been a village healer or physician who could be called upon in times of emergency, but for day-to-day and common ailments, treatment was undertaken at home.

While our understanding of biochemistry could not match that of a modern physician, our knowledge of how plants and various substances work in our bodies, and, indeed, how our bodies respond in various situations, and to different treatments, was much more profound. Women instinctively treated their children and their families – recognizing a bad temper as the onset of illness, perhaps, and being capable of addressing the cause of an illness according to a more general knowledge of our holistic being.

Today, most drugs on the market tend to deal with symptoms, rather than the root cause of an illness. Conditions and symptoms such as asthma, eczema, ME (CFS), headaches, and menstrual problems are controlled rather than cured. We take a tablet to ease the pain of a headache, but we do not stop and consider why we have a headache. We apply creams to stop the itching of eczema, but we do nothing to address the cause. In the past, we had a much greater general understanding of the causes and effects of illness, and a much more instinctive approach to treatment. Folk medicine and home remedies kept the majority of people healthy and it is that tradition to which many people are increasingly returning today.

ABOVE *Exercise and diet are important when aspiring to adopt a more holistic lifestyle.*

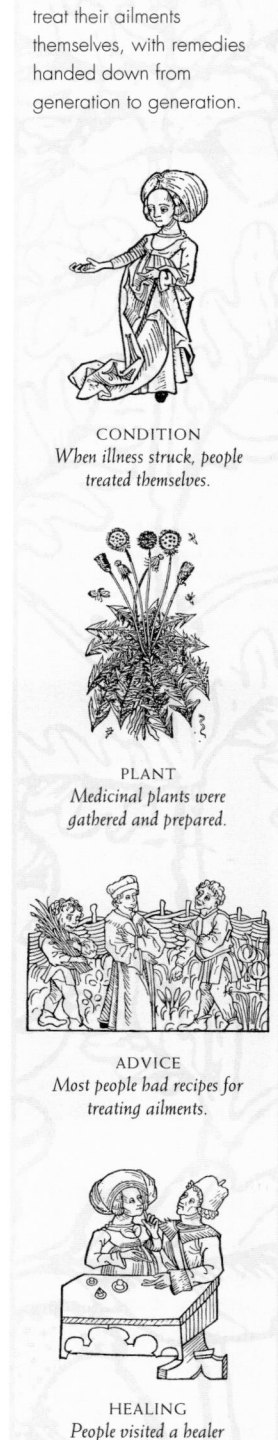

TRADITIONAL REMEDIES

In times gone by, people more commonly tried to treat their ailments themselves, with remedies handed down from generation to generation.

CONDITION
When illness struck, people treated themselves.

PLANT
Medicinal plants were gathered and prepared.

ADVICE
Most people had recipes for treating ailments.

HEALING
People visited a healer if self-treatment failed.

CONVENTIONAL MEDICINE AND THE FOLK TRADITION

Physicians' offices are overwhelmed by the constant needs and demands of people suffering from minor illnesses. Conventional medicine has its place, and no one can deny that it has extended our lifespans and improved our chances of surviving serious illnesses. But it has its own drawbacks, one of the first and foremost being our dependence upon it. The majority of us are not able to listen to our bodies, and to take responsibility for our own health, in our own environment. Even conventional physicians welcome simple remedies to deal with the recurrent hazards of everyday life – coughs and colds, sore throats, cuts, bruises, skin infections, and many others – because it takes the pressure off medical systems and allows them to spend more time with more serious cases.

In the past, when conventional medicine did not have as much to offer and people could not afford to visit a physician, there was a commonsense approach to minor ailments. Indeed, many of the same remedies used have been adopted and adapted by conventional Western medicine. The popularity of these remedies is, quite simply, due to the fact that they are effective. They do, on many occasions, work better or at least as well as some of the pharmaceuticals of the modern age, and treatment is less likely to be complicated by side-effects. Their wider use means that we are less dependent upon conventional medical expertise and more self-confident. The power shifts from the physician back to the patient, which is both time- and cost-effective for everyone, and gives us a stake in our own health. Once learned, folk and home remedies can be used again and again.

PREVENTING ILLNESS

Natural medicine in the home is more than just first aid for common and minor ailments. It can be preventive, using some of the most common items in the larder – onions, garlic, thyme, mint, sage, chamomile – to protect against many illnesses. Modern research – particularly over the last three decades – is now justifying the use of plants and household items, things that have been used for centuries in both folk medicine and traditional cookery. For example, mint calms the digestive system, lemon is a great detoxifier, helping the liver and kidneys to function effectively, rosemary has profound antiseptic powers and is a natural stimulant, and caraway seeds will prevent flatulence.

By incorporating some of these elements in your day-to-day meals, you not only add flavor and variety, but

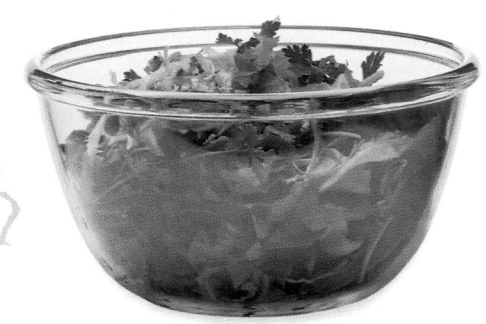

ABOVE *Adding beneficial herbs, such as mint, sage, and thyme to a salad, is an easy way to maintain health.*

also provide the systems of your body with nourishment and support. These remedies have a beneficial effect on our general health and deal with specific problems, something that conventional drugs do not. Most available drugs work to address specific systems and do nothing for our overall health; many of them have side-effects that are more dangerous than the symptoms they are addressing. Traditional folk and home remedies tend to work with our bodies, allowing them to heal themselves by keeping them strong and healthy.

BELOW *The cottage garden was designed to provide a source of medicinal plants, as well as vegetables and beautiful flowers.*

WHAT IS FOLK MEDICINE?

The term "folk medicine" refers to the traditional beliefs, practices, and materials that people use to maintain health and cope with disease, outside of an organized relationship with academic, professionally recognized, and established medical systems and treatments.

The beliefs and practices that make up a system of folk medicine are very closely related to the history, traditions, and life of a recognizable social group. Many people practise folk medicine today, generally working in an environment where they share the belief system of their patients, and their approach to maintaining health and treating disease.

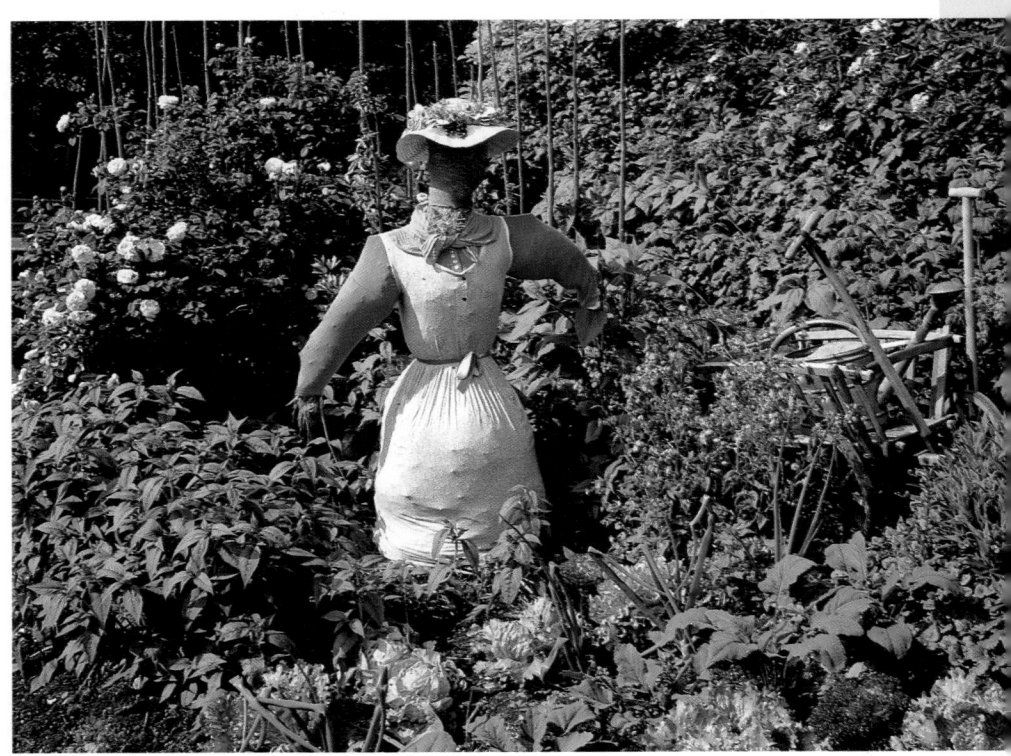

A HISTORICAL PERSPECTIVE

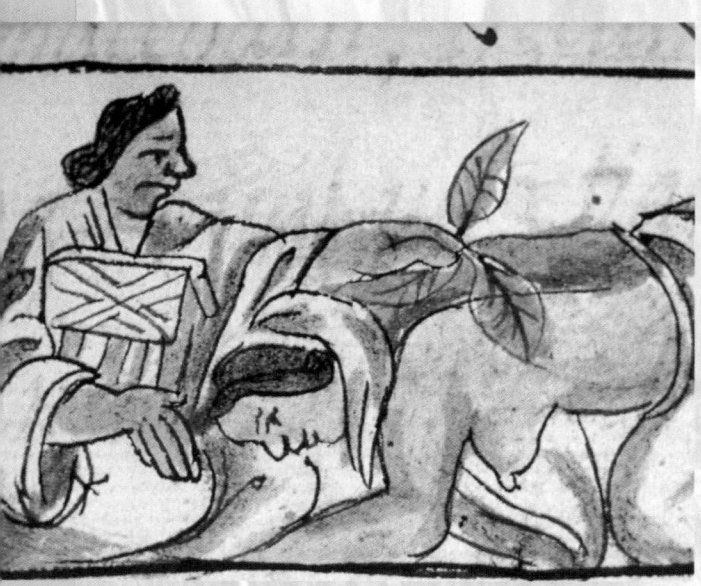

ABOVE *The Aztecs used certain plants to numb the pain of childbirth.*

Whenever possible, a system of folk medicine is best understood as a dynamic in a historical context. The Aztecs in Mexico provide a good example of how conventional medical systems can go hand in hand with folk medicine, feeding from one another and allowing both to grow according to the needs of the population.

Aztec establishment (as opposed to folk) medicine was highly organized, with a herbarium, a zoo, an intellectual elite, and a training and certification academy. It was based on a complex theoretical structure and experimental research. Some segments of the population, however, had only limited access to this medicine. They relied instead on traditional treatments and medicines.

Aztec establishment medicine was eliminated when the Spanish conquerors killed the medical personnel and introduced their own medicine. This intrusive system became the new medicine of the Aztec establishment. The system still offered limited access. Some elements of the European approach, however, were compatible with the folk medical practice of the Native Americans and were therefore incorporated into a new folk system. Mexican folk medicine thrived and continued to incorporate elements of the new establishment medicine.

Similarly, Native North American systems, while not highly organized and academic, were the establishment medicine in their own societies before conquest. Europeans brought diseases that decimated populations and challenged indigenous medical systems. The social and moral bases of the systems came under attack by missionaries and governments, even as immigrants began to adopt the ideas and materials from native systems. Again, this intrusive medicine became the establishment medicine, and Native American medicine, incorporating some Euro-American elements, became folk medicine.

DISCOVERING PLANT BENEFITS

But the history of using plants for medicine and healing goes back to the beginning of humankind. In their search for nourishment, primitive humans sampled many kinds of plants. Those that were palatable were used for food, while plants with toxic or unpleasant effects were avoided or used against enemies. Other plants that produced physiological effects such as perspiration, defecation, healing, or hallucinations were saved for medicinal purposes and divination. Over the course of thousands of years, people have learnt to use a wide variety of plants as medicines for different ailments.

More than 4,000 years ago, the Chinese emperor Qien Nong (Chi'en Nung) put together a book of medicinal plants called *Ben Zao (Pen Tsao)*. It contained descriptions of more than 300 plants, several of which are still used in medicine. The Sumerians, at the same time and later, were recording prescriptions on clay tablets, and the Egyptians were writing their medical systems on rolls of papyrus. The oldest such document, known as the *Papyrus Kahun*, dates from the time of King Amenemhet III (1840–1792 B.C.E.) and contains information about women's diseases and medical conditions.

The most famous of these medical papyri, the so-called *Ebers Papyrus*, reports voluminously on the pharmaceutical prescriptions of the era. It includes specific information on how plants are to be used, for example, in the treatment of parasite worms or of stomach ailments. Some of these plants are still used today – in folk and conventional medicine.

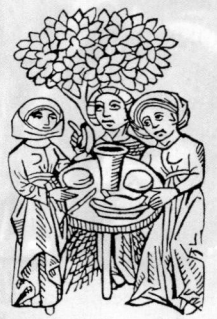

ABOVE *Medieval herbalists studying the properties of medicinal plants.*

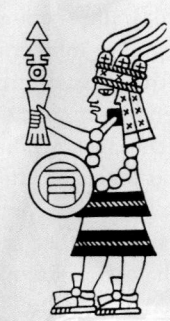

ABOVE *Aztec healers from the upper classes were highly trained.*

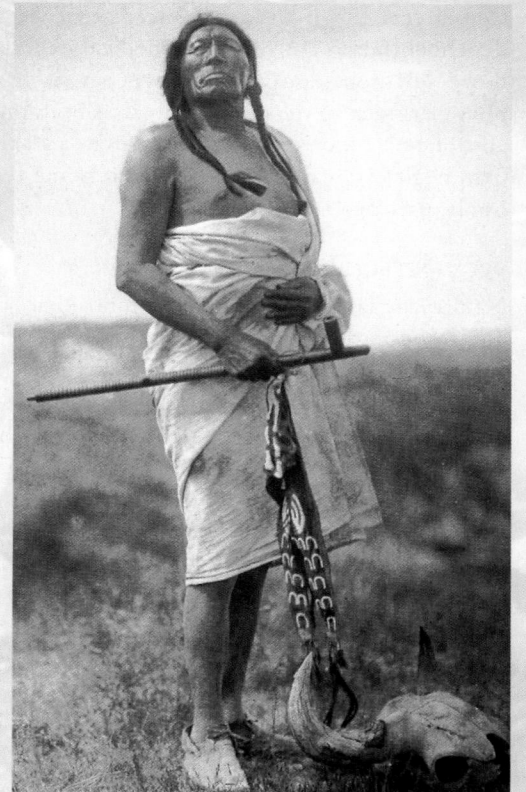

RIGHT *In Native North American tribes, healing was the domain of a shaman.*

TRADITIONAL FOLK MEDICINE TODAY

The growing concern about the side-effects of medicinal drugs, including the tragedies caused by compounds like thalidomide, has meant that herbalism has been called upon once more to provide natural medicines. In particular, pregnant women, children, people with chronic conditions (including chronic stress) that have refused to be shifted by orthodox

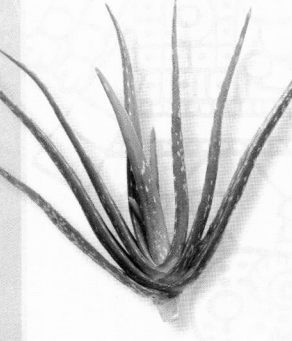

ALOE VERA

medicine, and those with immunosuppressed conditions have had successful – and, most importantly, safe – treatment without the use of toxic drugs. Environmental pollution, food additives, contaminated water, and many other factors put massive stress on our bodies and on our immune systems, and it is now more important than ever to take a step back from chemical preparations and find ways to support our bodies against the demands of contemporary living.

As research into the active constituents of herbs continues, increasing numbers of ancient treatments and tonics are being rediscovered and recognized, and brought back into widespread use. The global transport network means that we now have access to treatments used in countries around the world – bringing us a variety of

amazing plants such as ginseng, guarana, tea tree oil, aloe vera, and ginkgo biloba.

Much of the pharmacopeia of academic medicine – including aspirin (from the white willow) – has been derived from folk remedies, even as academic medicine has disparaged the folk reasons for their use. In the past this process has mostly been haphazard, but since the Second World War there has been an intensified, systematic investigation of tribal and folk medicines in the search for new preparations. More than 120 current prescription drugs are obtained from plants, and about 25 percent of all prescriptions contain one or more active ingredients from plants. There are plenty of herbal remedies already in use within orthodox medicine; for example, components of the yew tree have been used successfully to halt cancer, and

the rosy periwinkle is used to control leukemia, especially leukemia in children.

Comparison and evaluation of folk and academic medical systems and practices is difficult. On the one hand, indiscriminate interpretation of folk medicine may result in inappropriate rejection of proven establishment methods – for example, some immunization, and drugs required to treat chronic and serious illness that may not have existed in the past. On the other hand, the dangerous aspects of folk medicine have often been emphasized, usually without recognizing the contributions of folk to conventional medicine and the similarities between them.

Today, there is a greater understanding of the power of natural remedies, and their use is being slowly accepted and

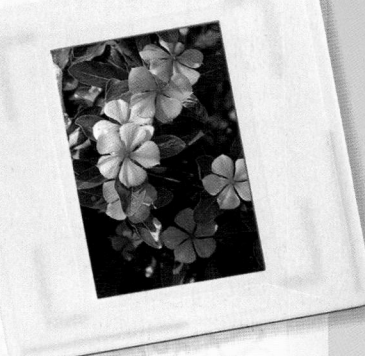

ROSY PERIWINKLE

indeed encouraged – particularly for ailments that people can safely and appropriately treat at home, such as headaches and upset stomachs, or sore throats. Disorders of the liver, heart, kidneys, etc., as well as severe illness – particularly in small children – are too serious for home treatment, and should be referred to a professional practitioner.

The Greeks and the Romans derived some of their herbal knowledge from these early civilizations. Their contributions are recorded in Dioscorides' *De Materia Medica* and the 37-volume natural history written by Pliny the Elder. Some of these works are known to us through translations into Arabic by Rhazes and Avicenna. The knowledge of medicinal plants was further nurtured by monks in Europe, who grew medicinal plants and translated the Arabic works. The first recognized apothecaries opened in Baghdad in the 9th century. By the 13th century, London became a major trading center in herbs and spices.

In the Dark Ages, the belief of the Christian Church that disease was a punishment for sin caused a great setback in medical progress. Women in childbirth welcomed the pain as an opportunity to atone for their sins. Only in monasteries did herbals and other documented sources of natural medicine continue to be painstakingly translated.

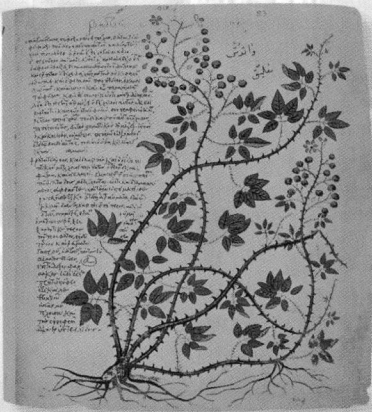

The Renaissance provided a new forum for the development of the folk tradition. William Caxton printed dozens of medical manuals and Nicholas Culpeper translated the entire physicians' pharmacopoeia *The English Physician and Complete Herbals* in 1653. It is still in print.

The advent of alchemy, and the split between the "new philosophy" of reason and experiment, and the previous tradition of "science" (ancient medical doctrines, herbalism, astrology, and the occult) ended the golden age of herbals. Witch hunts disposed of village "healing women"; women were forbidden to study and all nonprofessional healers were declared heretics. The use of herbs became associated with magic and the occult, an uneasy alliance that has been difficult to shake. Herbalism was effectively dropped from mainstream medical training, though folk advice and treatment from the apothecary herbalist continued to be available, especially in less well-off areas.

LEFT *A page from* De Materia Medica, *written by Dioscorides. Herbal knowledge was passed on from one civilization to another and expanded.*

CAUTION

THERE ARE SYMPTOMS WHICH COULD INDICATE A SERIOUS MEDICAL PROBLEM, AND FOR WHICH PROFESSIONAL ADVICE SHOULD BE SOUGHT IMMEDIATELY. THESE INCLUDE UNUSUAL OR PERSISTENT HEADACHES, CHRONIC PAIN, BLOOD IN THE URINE, FECES, OR MUCUS, PERSISTENT FATIGUE OR WEIGHT LOSS, AND BLEEDING BETWEEN MENSTRUAL PERIODS. THAT IS NOT TO SAY THAT HOME REMEDIES CANNOT BE USED TO TREAT THE PAIN AND DISCOMFORT OF SERIOUS PROBLEMS – FOLK AND HOME TREATMENT CAN GO HAND IN HAND WITH CONVENTIONAL MEDICINE, AND MANY REMEDIES ARE SAFE TO TAKE ALONGSIDE MEDICATION.

LEARNING ABOUT FOLK MEDICINE

Take time to learn about the various properties of the products available, and experiment until you find remedies that suit you and your family. Retrain yourself to consider the underlying causes of illness before seeking an instant relief from symptoms. Many of the home remedies work as fast as conventional drugs to bring relief, but the treatment of chronic disorders, such as bronchitis or rheumatism, will be slow, gentle, and cumulative, working to strengthen and stimulate various parts of the body over a long period of time. It is important to remember that the fresher or more recently picked the herb, the stronger its active properties. Dried herbs are more readily available and are about one-third as strong as the fresh product – and in some cases are better for the condition.

WHO CAN BENEFIT?

Folk medicine and home remedies do not provide a miracle cure, but almost anyone can benefit from the prudent use of herbs, plants, and household items as a form of restorative and preventive medicine. Most plants offer a rich source of vitamins and minerals, aside from having healing properties, and can be an important part of the daily diet, eaten fresh, or perhaps drunk as a tisane. A herbal tonic is useful, for example, in the winter months, when fresh fruit and green vegetables are not a regular part of our diets. Or plants like echinacea or garlic can be taken daily to improve the general efficiency of the immune system.

Some of the most common conditions that respond to home treatment include: hay fever, colds and respiratory disorders, digestive disorders (like constipation and ulcers), cardiovascular disease, headaches, anxiety, depression, chronic infections, rheumatism, arthritis, skin problems, anemia, and many hormonal, menstrual, menopausal, and pregnancy problems. On top of that are minor ailments such as scrapes, bruises, burns, swellings, sprains, and bites and stings.

Herbs do influence the way in which the body works, and although they are natural, they will have a profound effect on its functions. It is essential that you read the labels of any herbal products you have purchased, and follow carefully the advice of your herbalist. More is not better; although herbs don't have the side-effects of orthodox drugs, they have equally strong medicinal properties and can be toxic when taken in excess, causing liver failure, miscarriage, and heart attack, among other things.

TREATING YOURSELF AT HOME

Treatment is designed to help our bodies as a whole, and to stimulate their responses in order to cure disease. There are a variety of forms in which treatment can be offered, depending on the condition and your individual needs. Look at the "Preparing Remedies" box alongside. Many remedies are easily and quickly made. Some can be prepared in advance and stored for future use.

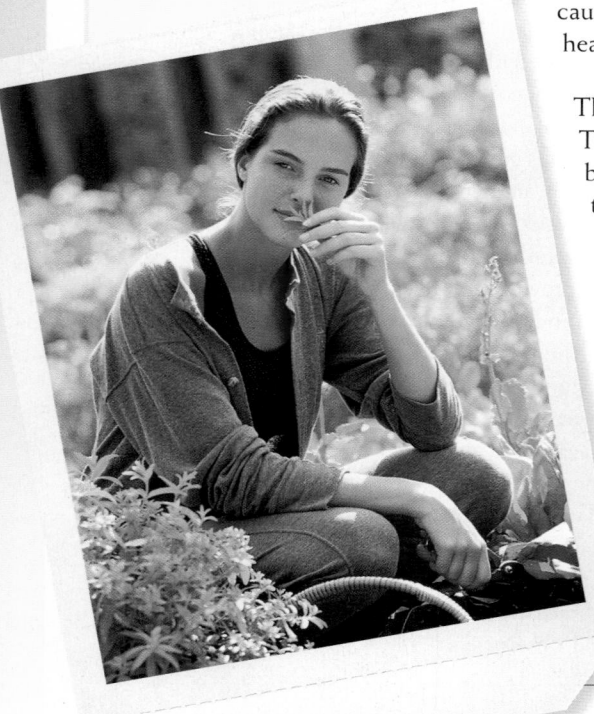

LEFT *Everybody can use traditional home remedies, along with conventional medicine if necessary.*

PREPARING REMEDIES

❁ **TISANES** Tisanes are mild infusions, usually prepackaged and sold in the form of a tea bag, which are boiled for a much shorter period than an infusion.

❁ **POWDERS** Plants in this form can be added to food or drinks, or put into capsules for easier consumption. Make your own powder by crushing dried plant parts.

❁ **PILLS** Plant remedies only rarely take this form since it is difficult to mix more than one herb and control the quantities. Some of the more common remedies will be available from professional herbalists or health food stores, or you can press your own with a domestic press.

❁ **COMPRESSES AND POULTICES** Compresses and poultices are for external use, and can be extremely effective; the active parts of the herb reach the affected area without being altered by the digestive process.

A **poultice** is made up of a plant which has been crushed and then applied whole to the affected areas. You can also boil crushed plant parts for a few minutes to make a pulp, which will act as a poultice, or use a powdered herb and mix with boiling water. Because they are most often applied with heat and use fresh parts of the plant, they are more potent than compresses (*see below*). Poultices are particularly useful for conditions like bruises, wounds, and abscesses, helping to soothe and to draw out impurities.

A **compress** is usually made from an infusion or decoction, which is used to soak a linen or muslin cloth. The cloth is then placed on the affected area, where it can be held in place by a bandage or plastic wrap. Compresses can be hot or cold and are generally milder than poultices.

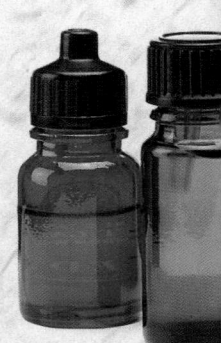

ESSENTIAL OILS

❁ **ESSENTIAL OILS** Often used in other therapies, like aromatherapy (*see page 140*), the essential oils of a plant are those which contain its "essence," or some of its most active principles. Useful for making tinctures and ointments.

❁ **BATHS** Plants and other items can be added to bath water for therapeutic effect – inhalation (through the steam) and by entering the bloodstream through the skin. An oatmeal bath, for instance, would work topically on eczema, and a chamomile bath would both soothe skin, and calm and relax.

❁ **INHALATIONS** Warm moist air can relieve many respiratory problems and allow the healing properties of plants and other products to enter the bloodstream through the lungs. To prepare an inhalation, half fill a big bowl with steaming water, and add a herbal infusion or decoction, or 2–3 drops of an essential oil.

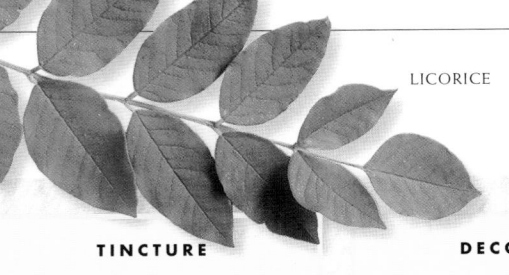

TINCTURE

Powdered, fresh, or dried herbs are placed in an airtight container with alcohol and left for a period of time. Alcohol extracts the valuable or essential parts of the plant and preserves them for the longest possible time.

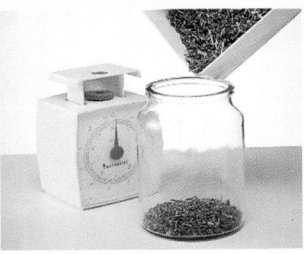

1 You can make your own tincture at home by crushing the parts of the plants you wish to use (about 1oz. [25g.] will do).

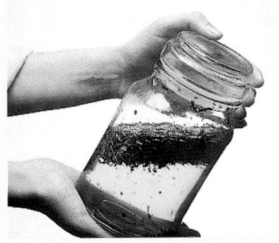

2 Suspend the plants in alcohol (about 1–1⅓pt. [600ml.] of vodka or any 40 percent spirit) for about two weeks, shaking occasionally. Dried or powdered herbs (about 4oz. [100g.]) may also be used, with the same amount of alcohol.

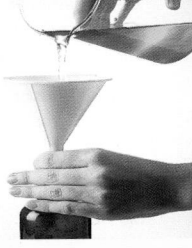

3 After straining, the tincture should be stored in a dark glass airtight jar. Doses are usually 5–20 drops, which can be taken directly or added to water.

DECOCTION

The roots, twigs, berries, seeds, and bark of a plant are used, and much like an infusion, they are boiled in water to extract the plants' ingredients. The liquid is strained and taken with honey or brown sugar as prescribed.

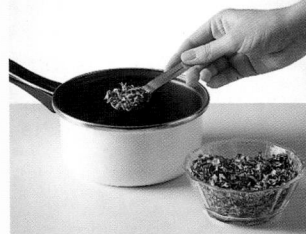

1 Put 1 teaspoonful of dried herb or 3 teaspoonfuls of fresh herb (for each cup) into a pan. Fresh herbs should be cut into small pieces.

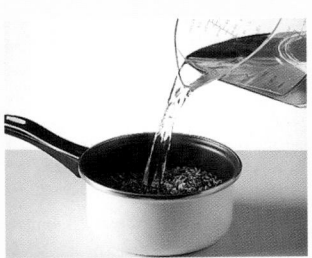

2 Add some water to the herbs. If making large quantities, use 1oz. (30g.) dried herb for each 1pt. (500ml.) of water. The container should be glass, ceramic, or earthenware. Metal pans should be enameled. Do not use aluminum.

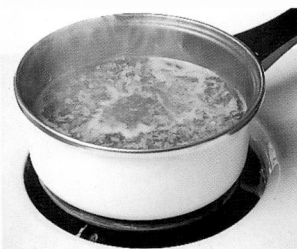

3 Bring to the boil and simmer for 10–15 minutes. If the herb contains volatile oils, cover the pan. Strain, cool, and refrigerate. The decoction will keep for about three days.

INFUSION

Effectively another word for tea, an infusion uses dried herbs, or in some instances fresh, which are steeped in boiled water for about 10 minutes. Infusions may be drunk hot, which is normally best for medicinal teas, or cold, with ice.

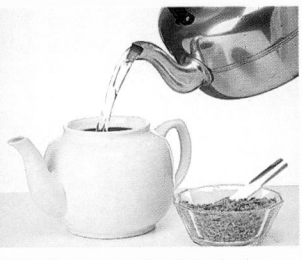

1 Put 1 teaspoonful of the herb or herb mixture into a china or glass teapot, for each cup of tea that is required. Add boiling water.

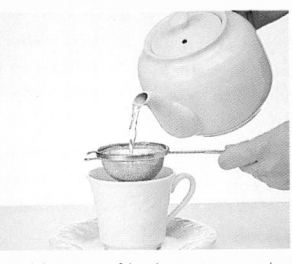

2 Add 1 cup of boiling water to the pot for each teaspoonful of herb that has been used. Keep the pot covered and always use the purest water available, which will ensure that the medicinal properties of the plant are effectively obtained. Strain the infusion and drink hot or cold – either sweetened or unsweetened. Use licorice root, honey, or brown sugar to sweeten. Infusions should be made fresh each day, if possible. Infusions are most suitable for plants from which the leaves and flowers have been used, since their properties are more easily extracted by gentle boiling.

OINTMENT

For external use, ointments and creams are often prescribed. You can make your own by boiling the plant parts to extract the active properties, and adding a few ounces (grams) of pure oils (such as olive or sunflower).

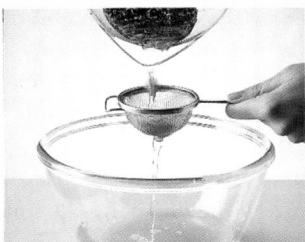

1 Make 1pt. (500ml.) of infusion or decoction (depending on what is appropriate for the herb), and strain. Reserve the liquid.

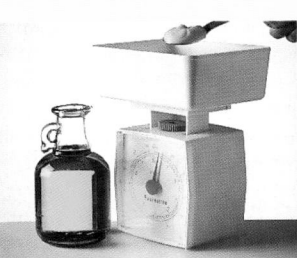

2 Pour 3fl.oz. oil (90ml.) into a pan. Mix 3oz. of fat into the oil. If a perishable base fat is used (such as lard), a drop of tincture of benzoin should be added for each 1oz. (30g.) of base. Add the liquid.

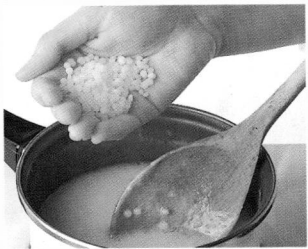

3 Simmer until the water has evaporated. Stiffen the mixture with a little beeswax or cocoa butter to make a cream. Melt in slowly.

OINTMENT

TRADITIONAL HOME AND FOLK REMEDY SOURCES

Allium cepa
ONIONS

The onion is by far the most important bulb vegetable in terms of its healing properties. It is used both in its green stage as a scallion, or green onion, and in its mature stage as a bulb – the tightly packed globe of food-storage leaves containing the volatile oil that is the source of the onion's pungent flavor. Thought to have originated in Asia, the onion has been cultivated since ancient times. The bulb of the onion is used in cooking and medicinally; like garlic, it warms the body and stimulates the circulation. Onions have long been considered the mainstay of every household remedy chest.

ABOVE *Grow your own: onions can be harvested 22 weeks after sowing.*

BELOW *Macerated raw onion can be used to heal a painful burn. It stimulates circulation and is antiseptic.*

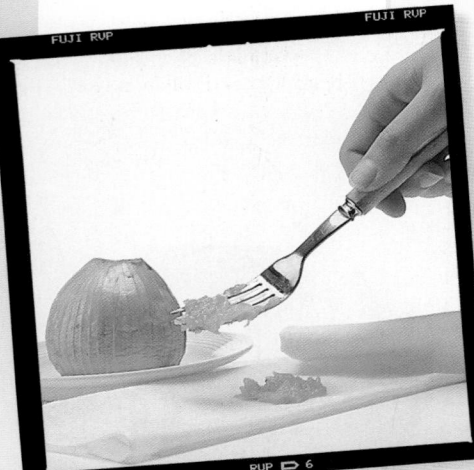

DATA FILE

Properties
❧ Onions cause the body to "weep," which helps to release toxins

❧ Onion increases blood circulation and can relax the muscles

❧ Expectorant and diuretic

❧ Helps to reduce serum cholesterol after a fatty meal

❧ May provide some protection against cancer

❧ Antibiotic, draws out infection

❧ Warming

❧ Strengthens the lungs

❧ Cleanses the intestines and helps to maintain balance of bacteria

and help to encourage circulation to the area, which will facilitate quick healing.

❧ Mix onion juice with honey to relieve the symptoms of a cold.

❧ Taken daily, onions can help to prevent cancers of the digestive tract.

❧ The regular consumption of onions can reduce nervous debility.

❧ Onion poultices are used to treat bronchitis and can also help in the treatment of acne and boils.

❧ Onions are often recommended for gastric infections; onions will be effective cooked and raw.

❧ Use a poultice of roasted onion for earaches.

❧ Apply raw, macerated onions on sprains, bruises, and unbroken chilblains.

❧ Eat daily if you are at risk of heart disease or circulatory disorders.

Uses
❧ Apply fresh onion to an abscessed tooth or a boil to draw out infection

Allium sativum
GARLIC

Garlic belongs to the onion family, and is one of the best-known and most-used medicinal plants. It has a strong odor, which many people find off-putting, but its health-giving and preventive properties make it well worth suffering the effects. Garlic has been shown to lower total serum cholesterol as well as LDL cholesterol in human clinical trials. Effective herbal preparations of garlic can be used at less cost and with fewer side-effects than most pharmaceutical drugs, and its use has recently been applauded by the conventional medical establishment.

DATA FILE

Properties
❧ Cleanses the blood and helps to create and maintain healthy bacteria population (flora) in the gut

❧ Helps to bring down fever

❧ Antiseptic

❧ Antibiotic

❧ Antifungal

❧ Tones the heart and circulatory system

❧ Boosts the immune system

❧ May help to reduce high blood pressure

❧ May prevent some cancers, in particular stomach cancer

❧ Treats infections of the stomach and respiratory system

❧ Helps prevent heart disease and reduces the risk of atherosclerosis

❧ Antioxidant

❧ Decongestant

Uses
❧ Fresh garlic, eaten daily, can reduce chronic acidity of the stomach.

❧ Eat crushed garlic for sexual debility.

❧ May help to reduce attacks of allergic asthma and hay fever.

❧ Garlic-infused oil can be used as a chest rub for respiratory or digestive ailments, or in the ear to reduce inflammation.

❧ Fresh garlic, eaten regularly, will reduce the need for antibiotics.

❧ Garlic syrup can be used to treat bronchitis, lung infections, and digestive disorders.

❧ Fresh garlic juice is antifungal, and can be applied neat to infections such as athlete's foot.

❧ Chew whole roasted garlic cloves to improve circulation.

❧ The intestinal tract can be cleansed by adding several mashed, raw garlic cloves to salads. Excellent in combination with red onion.

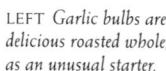

LEFT *Garlic bulbs are delicious roasted whole, as an unusual starter.*

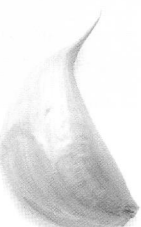

GARLIC CLOVE

GARLIC SYRUP

Garlic syrup relieves bronchitis, and lung infections. You need some honey and a fresh garlic bulb.

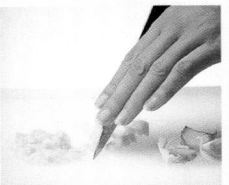

Peel and chop 6–8 cloves of fresh garlic.

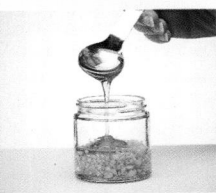

Place the chopped garlic in a jar, and cover with 8 tablespoons of honey. Let it stand for several days, and then strain. The garlic-infused honey can be given by the teaspoonful (1 for children, 4 for adults) to boost the immune system and treat infections.

Apium graveolens
CELERY

Hippocrates, the father of medicine, wrote that celery could be used to calm the nerves, and, indeed, its very high calcium level is likely to be the reason for this phenomenon. The seeds, leaves, and edible root of the plant are used. Celery is best eaten raw, and its juice is particularly useful. The seeds are rich in iron and many vitamins, including A, B, and C, and can be used in the treatment of liver problems and high blood pressure.

LEFT *Celery seeds are rich in vitamins and iron.*

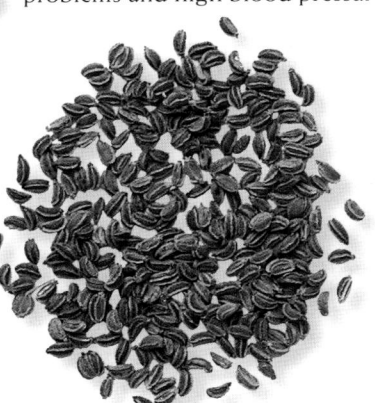

ABOVE *Celery is a popular vegetable; the leaves may also be used in cooking.*

DATA FILE

Properties

- Celery helps to reduce high blood pressure

- Digestive, reducing spasm in the muscle of the intestinal tract and acting as an anti-inflammatory agent

- Purifies the blood

- May help in the treatment of arthritis and rheumatic disorders; in Japan, rheumatic patients are sometimes put on a celery-only diet

- Celery seeds also have anti-inflammatory properties

- Stimulates the thyroid and pituitary glands

- Possibly antioxidant

- Celery clears uric acid from painful joints

- Acts on the kidneys and is a mild diuretic

Uses

- Eat the seeds to treat arthritis (for which they act as an anti-inflammatory) and to relieve muscle spasms (antispasmodic action).

- Grated, raw celery can be used as a poultice to apply to swollen glands.

- Raw, whole celery can be eaten regularly to reduce high blood pressure, and to act as a tonic for the liver.

- Celery juice or an infusion of celery seeds may be drunk to alleviate sciatica.

- Drink celery juice before meals to suppress the appetite. Chew celery seeds after a meal as a digestive.

- Celery root is said to be an aphrodisiac.

THERAPY CONNECTIONS

CELERY
- Ayurveda — p.29
- Aromatherapy — p.146

ONION
- Ayurveda — p.25
- Homeopathy — p.178

GARLIC
- Ayurveda — p.26
- Herbalism — p.113

CELERY TONIC

Celery seeds can be used to make a tonic that benefits the kidneys. You will need a bottle of brandy, and celery seeds.

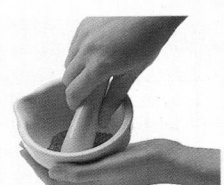

Steep 2 tablespoons of bruised celery seeds in 1pt. (500ml.) of brandy.

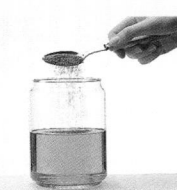

Take 1 tablespoon of the infused brandy, mixed with 2 tablespoons of water, three times daily.

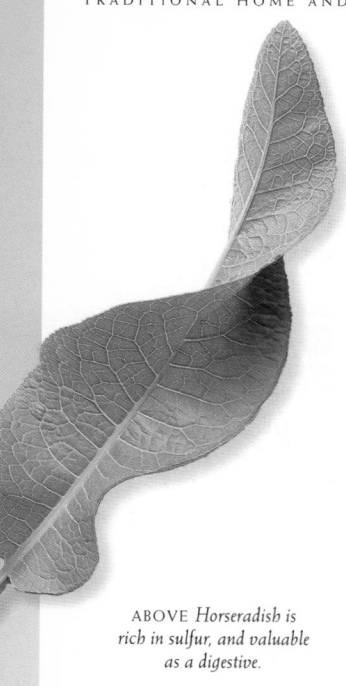

ABOVE *Horseradish is rich in sulfur, and valuable as a digestive.*

Armoracia rusticana
HORSERADISH

Horseradish is a member of the mustard family, and is native to southeastern Europe. It is widely cultivated for its pungent, fleshy root. Japanese horseradish, or wasabi (*Wasabid japonica*), is used both for cooking and for therapeutic purposes, and the grated rhizomes are often sold as a dry, green-colored powder. Horseradish root has been used for centuries in folk medicine, particularly to clear nasal passages. It also has a powerful diuretic effect.

CAUTION

TOO MUCH HORSERADISH TAKEN INTERNALLY CAN CAUSE NIGHT SWEATS, AND OCCASIONALLY DIARRHEA AND ABDOMINAL CRAMPING.

DATA FILE

Properties
- Diuretic
- Stimulant
- Clears nasal passages
- Warming
- Antiseptic
- Stimulates blood flow

Uses
- Apply tincture of horseradish root to skin eruptions, including those associated with acne, to draw out the infection and encourage healing.
- Add some horseradish root to your toothpaste to clean teeth effectively, kill bacteria, and control mouth ulcers.
- Eat fresh horseradish, mixed with a little lemon juice, for the relief of sinus infections and nasal blockages.
- Eat freshly grated horseradish root for the edema and swelling associated with PMS.
- A horseradish poultice can be applied to chilblains and hemorrhoids to encourage healing and improve the circulation of the blood.
- Chronic rheumatism may respond to an old remedy: eat tiny pieces of horseradish root without chewing, and continue for several weeks.

Avena sativum
OATS

Oats are a cereal plant, and are both extremely nutritious and useful therapeutically. Oats are one of the best sources of inositol, which is important for maintaining optimum blood cholesterol levels. Eaten daily, they provide a wealth of excellent effects.

DATA FILE

Properties
- A tonic for general debility, and used in the treatment of anorexia, also helpful for convalescence and fatigue
- Oats lower blood cholesterol levels
- Oats help to control hormonal activity
- Cleansing – internally and externally; may protect against bowel cancer when taken internally
- Used in the treatment of eczema
- Extremely rich in B vitamins and minerals
- Antidepressant, and can be used to treat depression, stress, and nervous disorders
- Often used in the treatment of addictions

Uses
- Eat raw oats as a source of fiber to ease constipation.
- Oatmeal (unrefined) can be eaten on a regular basis to reduce the effects of stress and nervous disorders.
- Cooked oats will relieve fatigue.
- A compress of oatmeal or an oatmeal bath soothes eczema and other problem skin conditions.
- Boil a tablespoon of oats in ½pt. (250ml.) of water for several minutes and drain; use as a nerve tonic and for its nourishing properties.
- Use the tincture for stress, addictions, eating disorders, and depression.
- Eat oats daily to lower blood cholesterol and to experience tonic effects.

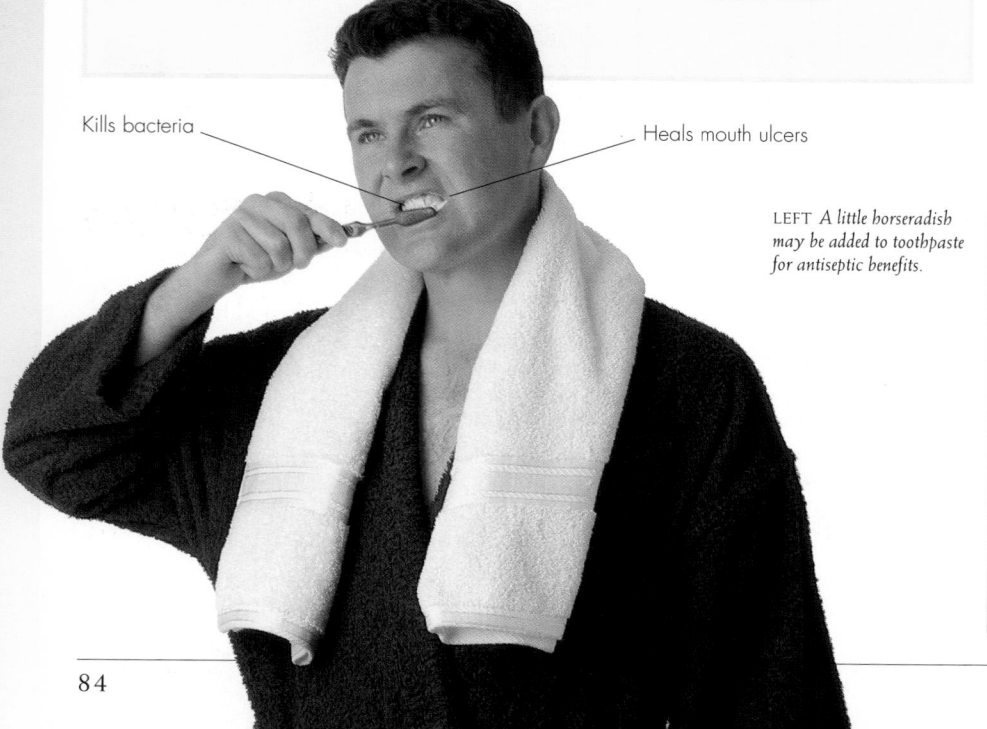

Kills bacteria

Heals mouth ulcers

LEFT *A little horseradish may be added to toothpaste for antiseptic benefits.*

CAUTION

OATS CONTAIN GLUTEN WHICH CAUSES AN ALLERGIC REACTION IN SOME INDIVIDUALS.

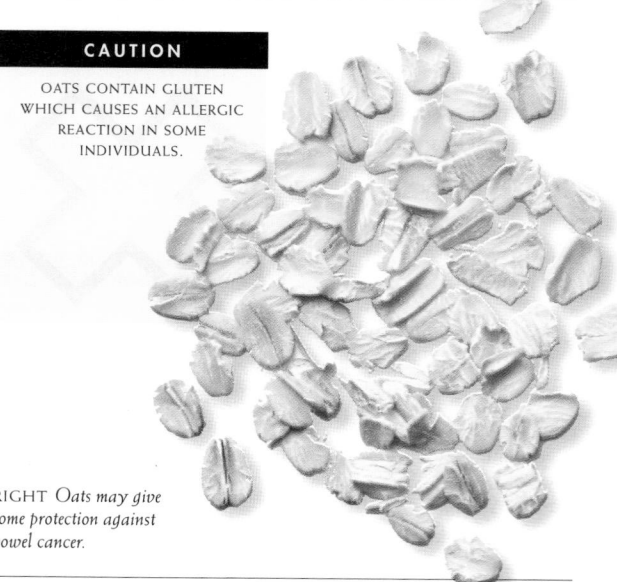

RIGHT *Oats may give some protection against bowel cancer.*

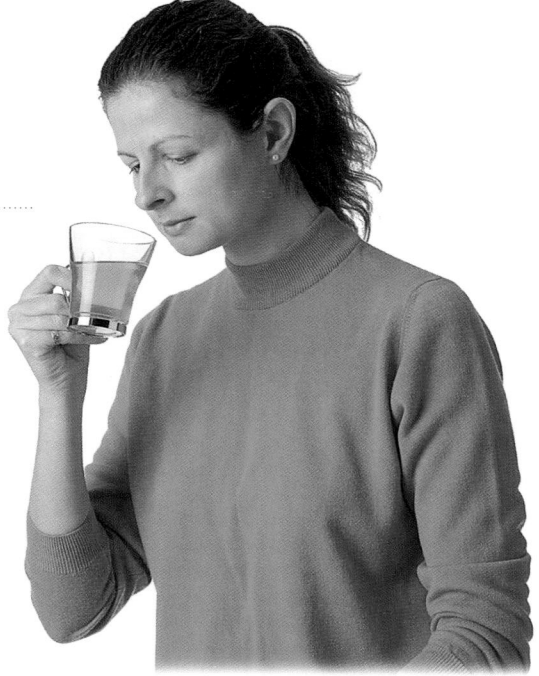

Asparagus officinalis
ASPARAGUS

A herbaceous perennial of the *Liliaceae* family, asparagus is cultivated for its tender shoots, which appear in early spring. In 1806 the French chemist Louis Nicolas Vauquelin, who discovered the elements chromium and beryllium, isolated asparagine, the first amino acid to be discovered, from the asparagus plant. Asparagus is a liver tonic, and promotes elimination (through the urine).

ABOVE *The water left after cooking asparagus treats urinary problems.*

CAUTION

ASPARAGUS IS HIGH IN PURINES, AND ANYONE SUFFERING FROM GOUT SHOULD AVOID IT.

DATA FILE

Properties

❧ Encourages the flow of urine, making asparagus a useful diuretic

❧ Acts as a tonic to the liver

❧ Aids digestion

❧ May help control the symptoms of PMS, including breast tenderness and abdominal bloating

Uses

❧ Drink asparagus water (the water remaining after steaming asparagus spears) for urinary complaints, arthritis, and rheumatism.

❧ Freshly cooked asparagus will tonify the liver, and may be used in cases of liver congestion and conditions such as hepatitis to encourage healing.

❧ Asparagus tincture can be added to food and drinks to encourage the elimination of urine.

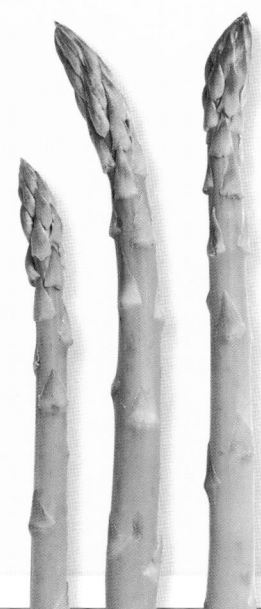

ASPARAGUS

Brassica oleracea
CABBAGE

Cabbage has traditionally been used for medicinal purposes as well as for cooking. It has anti-inflammatory properties, and contains chemicals which can prevent cancer. The ancient Greeks used fresh white cabbage juice to relieve sore or infected eyes, and juice from the cabbage stem is a good remedy for ulcers. Traditionally, the Romans and Egyptians would drink cabbage juice before big dinners to prevent intoxication; cabbage seeds are said to prevent hangovers.

DATA FILE

Properties

❧ An excellent anti-inflammatory

❧ Cabbage contains lactic acid, which acts to disinfect the colon

❧ Used to reduce the pain of headaches and rheumatic disorders

❧ Soothes eczema and other itching or weeping skin conditions

❧ Anticancer

❧ Draws out infection

❧ Red cabbage leaves are the basic ingredient of a good cough syrup

Uses

❧ Make cabbage a regular part of your diet to reduce the risk of cancer.

❧ A cabbage poultice can be applied to boils and infected cuts to draw out the infection and disperse pus.

❧ Applied to bruises and swelling, macerated cabbage leaves will encourage healing.

❧ Dab white cabbage juice on mouth ulcers, and gargle for sore throats.

❧ A warm cabbage compress, on the affected area, reduces the pain of headaches and some kinds of neuralgia.

❧ Drink fresh cabbage juice daily to reduce the discomfort of gastric ulcers and bronchial infections.

❧ A cabbage leaf, lightly pounded, can be placed directly on the breast to relieve mastitis.

❧ Raw cabbage juice is said to be useful for the treatment of ulcers, psoriasis, chronic headaches, asthma, cystitis, and bronchitis. Drink 1–2fl. oz. (25–50ml.) daily to get the best effects.

ABOVE *Cabbage leaves are excellent for bringing down swelling and drawing out infection.*

CAUTION

DO NOT EAT RED CABBAGE RAW, BECAUSE THE HIGH LEVELS OF IRON CAN INTERFERE WITH GUT ABSORPTION AND IRRITATE THE GUT, CAUSING CONSTIPATION.

AVOID CABBAGE IF YOU SUFFER FROM GOITER, OR TAKE MAOI ANTIDEPRESSANTS.

RED CABBAGE (COOKED) CAN CAUSE CONSTIPATION AND IRRITATION OF THE COLON, DUE TO THE LARGE QUANTITIES OF IRON.

Camellia sinensis
TEA

Tea is the beverage made when the processed leaves of the tea plant are infused with boiling water. Native to Southeast Asia, the tea plant is a small, shrub-like, evergreen tree that belongs to the family *Theaceae*; its seeds contain a volatile oil, and its leaves contain the chemicals caffeine and tannin. Green tea is made from the tips, or shoots, of the shrub *Camellia sinensis*; black tea is made from the fermented dried leaves. An essential oil, called tea absolute, is distilled from black tea. Both the leaves and the oil are used for medicinal purposes. Fruit teas do not actually contain tea but can also be beneficial to the health.

ABOVE *Tea contains caffeine, which is a stimulant.*

DATA FILE

Properties

❦ Provides folic acid (vitamin B9), some potassium, and also magnesium

❦ Contains fluoride (a trace)

❦ Acts on the nervous system to control the respiratory and digestive systems

❦ Diuretic and astringent

❦ Antioxidants called polyphenols have beneficial effects on the circulatory system, while flavonoids act on the immune system

❦ Tannins may help to prevent heart disease and halt the course of, and prevent, some cancers

Uses

❦ The fluoride in tea may be beneficial in preventing dental caries.

❦ Tea may help in the treatment of diarrhea, dysentery, hepatitis, and gastroenteritis.

❦ The flavonoids contained in tea may destroy harmful bacteria and viruses.

❦ Cold, steeped tea bags placed over the eyes will soothe soreness and irritation. Tea's astringent properties also make tea bags useful for treating minor injuries and insect bites.

❦ The leaves of green and black tea may be beneficial in the prevention of heart disease and stroke.

❦ Raspberry leaf tea is a well-known tonic when taken during pregnancy. It also helps prepare the breasts for breast-feeding.

❦ Green tea may help to prevent cancer if it is drunk on a regular basis.

CAUTION

TEA CAN INTERFERE WITH THE EFFECTIVENESS OF DRUGS SUCH AS ALLOPURINOL (FOR THE TREATMENT OF GOUT), ANTIBIOTICS, ANTIULCER DRUGS, AND THE DRUG THEOPHYLKLINE, PRESCRIBED FOR ASTHMA.

IT CAN PREVENT THE ABSORPTION OF IRON AND INTERFERE WITH THE EFFECTIVENESS OF SEDATIVE DRUGS.

DRINKING TEA TO EXCESS CAN CAUSE CONSTIPATION, INDIGESTION, DIZZINESS, PALPITATIONS, IRRITABILITY, AND INSOMNIA.

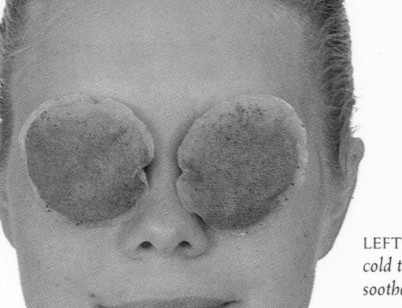

LEFT *A resourceful use of cold tea bags! They will soothe sore eyes.*

Capsicum annuum var. annuum
RED PEPPER

The red pepper is also known variously as bell pepper, sweet pepper, and capsicum. It is one of five different types (grossum type) of Capsicum *annuum var. annuum*; the peppers from which the spices cayenne and chili are produced are longum peppers. Red peppers, which are the ripened fruit (some varieties ripen to yellow or purple), are used in the manufacture of paprika, cayenne, and chili powder. Green peppers are immature fruit. Other related peppers used for culinary and therapeutic purposes include *C. baccatum*, *C. chines* and *C. frutescens*, the Tabasco or hot pepper.

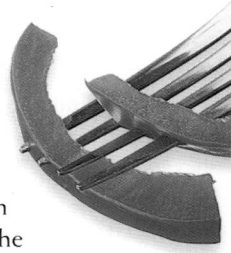

ABOVE *Peppers are rich in vitamins A and C. Add them to salads.*

CAUTION

PUNGENT PEPPERS SUCH AS CHILI PEPPERS MAY CAUSE SKIN IRRITATION AND PAINFUL INFLAMMATION WHEN USED IN EXCESS OR WHEN IN CONTACT WITH THE EYES AND BROKEN SKIN.

THE SEEDS ARE PARTICULARLY POWERFUL. STRONG PEPPERS MAY ALSO TEMPORARILY IRRITATE THE URINARY SYSTEM AS THE OILS ARE EXCRETED IN URINE.

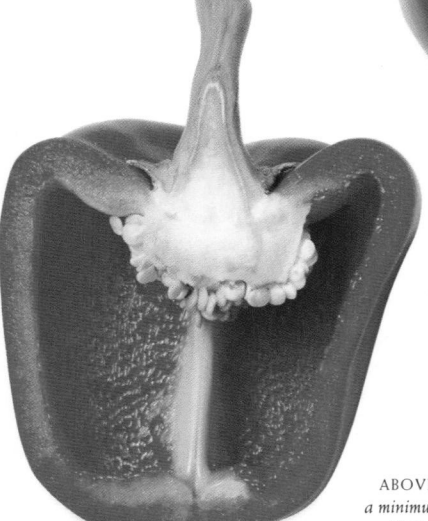

ABOVE *Peppers need a minimum temperature of 4°C (39°F) to grow.*

DATA FILE

Properties

❧ Peppers are an excellent source of vitamin C (a fresh green pepper contains 10 percent vitamin C)

❧ All peppers also contribute small amounts of iron and vitamin A: the largest amounts of vitamin A are found in fresh red peppers, while paprika and chili powder are also very rich in this vitamin

❧ Peppers are a good source of potassium, and have low levels of sodium and fiber

❧ They act as a tonic, have antiseptic effects, and are stimulating to the circulatory and digestive systems

❧ Peppers also have anesthetic properties

Uses

❧ Peppers increase perspiration and therefore have a cooling effect on the body.

❧ They may be effective in the treatment of varicose veins, asthma, and digestive complaints.

❧ Peppers reduce sensitivity to pain by irritating the tissues and increasing blood supply to the affected area, which then effectively numbs the pain.

❧ Cayenne acts as a tonic for those suffering from tiredness and cold. It can also induce a feeling of well-being. It is an expectorant and has been effective in treating catarrh and sinus problems.

❧ Peppers also help to eliminate various toxins from the body.

Citrus limon

LEMON

Lemons are the most widely grown acid species belonging to the citrus group of fruits. They rank third among all citrus fruits in tonnage produced, and have been used for generations for their therapeutic properties. Lemons are rich in vitamin C, and have a cleansing effect on the digestive system. They have a wide range of therapeutic properties, making them the mainstay of any good home remedy chest. The leaves and the whole fruit may be used, according to requirements.

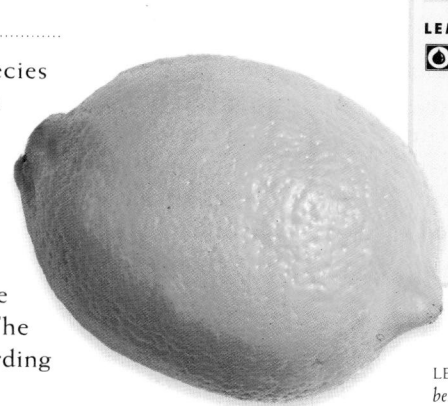

LEFT *Neat lemon juice can be dabbed on cold sores.*

DATA FILE

Properties

❧ Blood purifier, improves the body's ability to expel toxins; useful for skin problems like acne and boils

❧ Rich in vitamins B and C

❧ Antifungal

❧ Antacid

❧ Antiseptic

❧ Aids digestion

❧ One of the most powerful natural styptics; use on cuts and grazes to stop bleeding

❧ Antibacterial and antiviral properties. Lemons are excellent for halting the progression of infections

❧ Controls bladder and kidney infections

Uses

❧ The high potassium content of lemons will encourage the heart action, so lemons are a useful tonic for anyone with heart problems.

❧ Lemons are a natural insecticide and will discourage mosquitoes, black flies, and house flies.

❧ Drink fresh lemon juice (lemon in hot water will do) to cleanse the system.

❧ Drink lemon juice in hot or warm water first thing in the morning as a liver tonic.

❧ Lemon juice taken in hot water will ease stomach acidity; when drunk before going to bed it may help to relieve cramp and "restless legs" syndrome.

❧ Lemon strengthens the immune system and helps relieve the symptoms of colds and flu. It can also be beneficial in the treatment of other infections.

❧ Add slices of lemon to food on a daily basis to strengthen the circulatory system.

❧ Apply pure lemon juice to a wasp sting to relieve the pain.

❧ Regular intake of fresh lemons may be useful in the treatment of hemorrhoids and kidney stones; also for varicose veins.

❧ Drinking lemon juice mixed with olive oil may help to dissolve gallstones.

❧ To help cure cold sores, put a few drops of undiluted lemon juice on the affected area. Repeat several times a day until the sore goes.

❧ A drop of lemon juice will also benefit ulcers on the tongue and in the mouth.

BELOW *For a lemon drink, boil 3 sliced lemons in 1pt. (600ml.) water, until the liquid is reduced by half. Add honey to taste.*

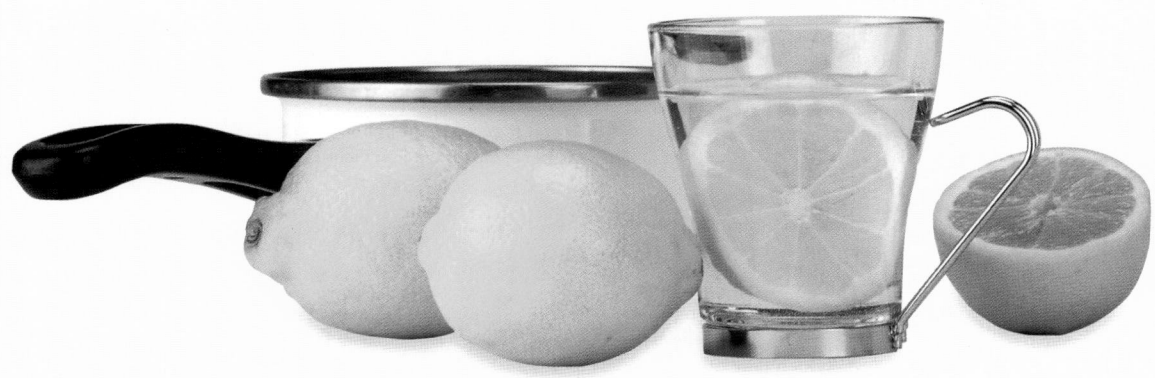

Citrus paradisi

GRAPEFRUIT

The grapefruit is an evergreen tree, *Citrus paradisi*, of the *Rutaceae* family, and its fruit is the largest of the commercially grown citrus fruits. Like all citrus fruit, grapefruit is rich in vitamin C and potassium. Pink grapefruit is rich in vitamin A, and acts as a natural antioxidant. Grapefruit is an excellent cleanser for the digestive and urinary systems, and the peel has many therapeutic properties.

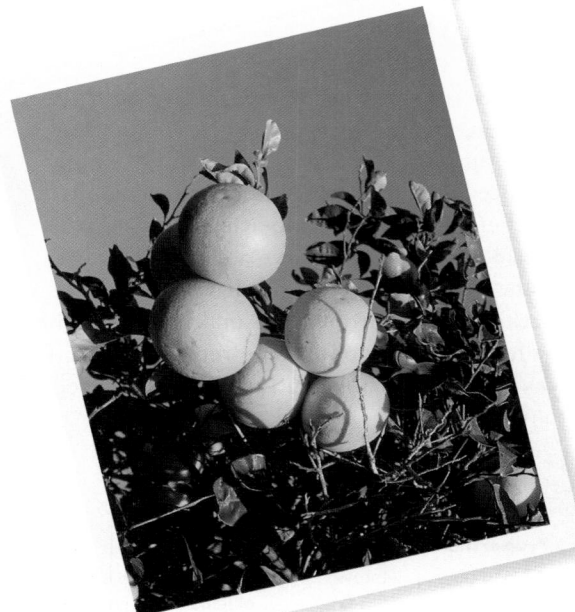

LEFT *Citrus requires a temperature of 15–30°C to grow well.*

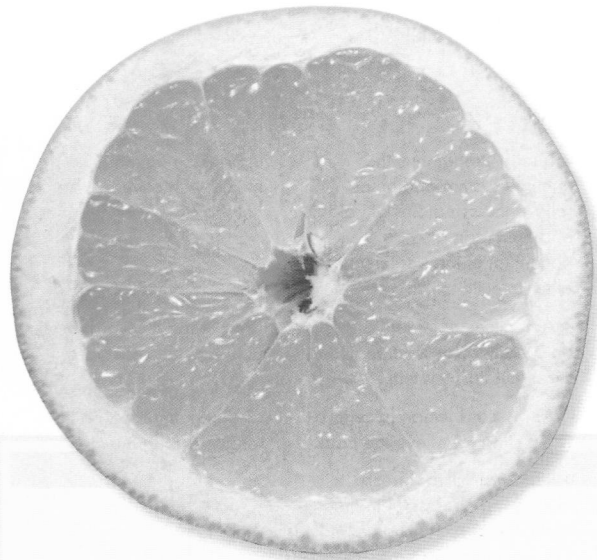

LEFT *Start the day the healthy way. Grapefruit is high in vitamin C and helps ward off colds.*

THERAPY CONNECTIONS

GRAPEFRUIT

Aromatherapy *p.155*

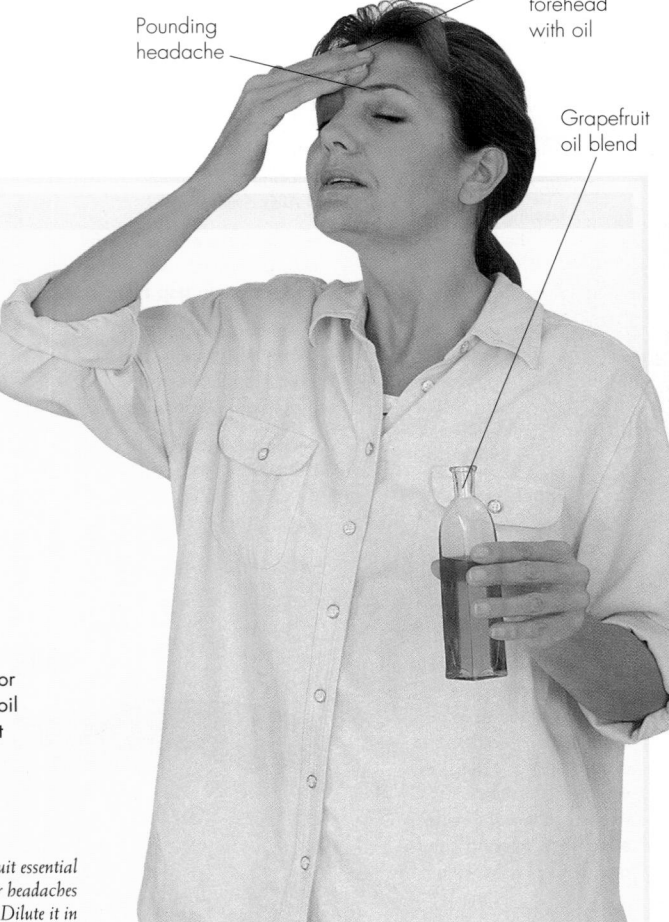

Massage forehead with oil

Pounding headache

Grapefruit oil blend

RIGHT *Grapefruit essential oil is excellent for headaches and hangovers. Dilute it in a carrier oil for massage.*

Properties

❦ Grapefruit cleanses the digestive and urinary systems, and is therefore often recommended by naturopaths

❦ Reduces appetite

❦ Aids in the breakdown of fats in the body

❦ Strengthens the respiratory system and aids respiration

❦ Invigorating tonic

❦ Relieves symptoms of colds and flu

❦ May help in the treatment of osteoarthritis

❦ Helps to balance the nervous system

Uses

❦ Eat grapefruit seeds to rid the body of worms.

❦ Grapefruit pith and membranes lower cholesterol in the blood.

❦ Drinking grapefruit juice can encourage healthy skin; used in the treatment of acne for its mild exfoliating properties.

❦ Grapefruit juice cleanses the kidneys and helps to eliminate toxins from the body.

❦ Aromatherapy massage with grapefruit oil is invigorating and uplifting, and may help to treat depression.

❦ Local massage, with a few drops of essential oil blended in a carrier oil, will relieve the severity of a headache.

DATA FILE

❦ Drinking grapefruit juice with iron supplements or foods rich in iron increases the absorption of iron in the body.

❦ Detoxifies the liver, and can ease chronic liver conditions. May help to reduce the severity of a hangover.

❦ Massage with grapefruit essential oil stimulates the immune system, which is particularly useful when suffering from infections.

❦ Used in steam inhalation or burnt in a room, grapefruit oil is beneficial in the treatment of colds, flu, and general respiratory problems.

Cucumis sativis

CUCUMBER

The cucumber, *Cucumis sativis*, is a vine fruit that can be eaten fresh or pickled. A member of the *Cucurbitaceae* family, it is related to melons and squash. Cucumbers were native to northwestern India but have long been distributed throughout Asia, Europe, and Africa. Cucumber is a popular vegetable, which has been widely used in folk medicine to reduce heat and inflammation. It is a rich source of vitamin C, and can be used externally to cool and cleanse.

LEFT *To soothe the eyes, lie down for half an hour with a slice of cucumber on each eye.*

DATA FILE

Properties

- Diuretic
- Cooling
- Cleansing, particularly for skin disorders
- Used in the treatment of gout and arthritis
- Anti-inflammatory – soothes inflamed skin
- May help to treat lung and chest disorders
- Drink cucumber juice for inflammatory conditions such as arthritis

Uses

- Drink cucumber juice or eat fresh cucumber to soothe heartburn or to improve an acid stomach.
- Drink 3–5fl. oz. (100–150ml.) of cucumber juice every two hours for a gastric or duodenal ulcer.
- For strained or inflamed eyes, place a slice of cucumber on each eyelid to reduce swelling and soothe.
- Apply fresh cucumber or cucumber juice to sunburned skin to cool it down.
- Ground dried cucumber seeds are used to treat tapeworm.
- Cucumber juice, drunk daily, may help to control eczema, arthritis, and gout.
- Skin conditions respond to cucumber. Include fresh cucumber in your diet as much as possible.
- Cucumber juice acts as a kidney tonic.
- Use cucumber ointment externally on inflammatory skin conditions.
- Fresh cucumber juice, or the whole raw vegetable, is a mild diuretic and is cleansing. Use to treat lung and chest infections, and to bring down fever.

Daucus carota

CARROT

The carrot is a member of the *Umbelliferae* family, which also includes celery and parsnip. Carrots were first used as medicinal herbs rather than as vegetables, and they have the dual purpose of acting as therapeutic agents, and providing the best source of beta carotene (a form of vitamin A) in the human diet. They are rich in vitamins A, B, C, and E, and the minerals phosphorus, potassium, and calcium. Chinese medical practitioners suggest eating carrots for Liver energy.

DATA FILE

Properties

- Energizing
- Carrot cleanses the system of impurities
- Contains calcium, which will encourage health of skin, hair, and bones
- May help in the treatment of eye problems
- Useful in the treatment of respiratory conditions
- Carrot may help to relieve skin disorders
- May help to overcome many glandular disorders
- Taken daily, carrots may help to regulate the menstrual cycle
- Anti-inflammatory
- Antiseptic

Uses

- Drink fresh, raw carrot juice daily to energize and cleanse the body. It will help to relieve the effects of stress and fatigue, and boost the body after illness.
- Carrot soup is a traditional home remedy for infant diarrhea – it soothes the bowel and slows down bacterial growth.
- Raw, grated carrots or cooked, mashed carrots can be applied to wounds, cuts, inflammations, and abscesses to discourage infection and encourage healing.
- Dried carrot powder will restore energy, and can help to treat infections, glandular problems, headaches, or joint problems.
- The antioxidant qualities of carrots (see Glossary, page 472) will help to prevent some of the damage caused by smoking.

(see Glossary, page 472)

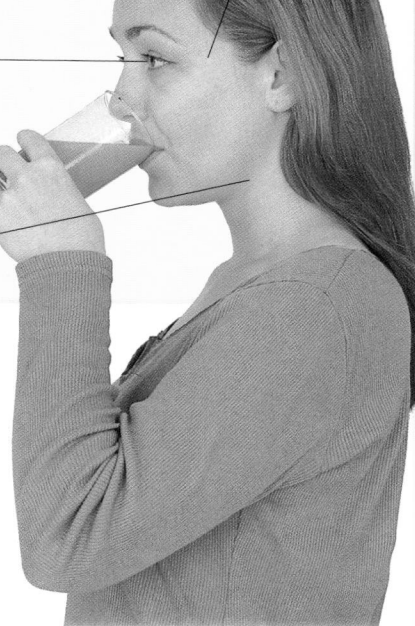

Relieves stress

Improves skin

Traditionally recommended for eyes

Treats glandular problems

ABOVE *Carrots contain beta carotene, an antioxidant which protects the body against cancer.*

RIGHT *Make your own carrot juice daily for a cleansing, nutritious, energizing drink.*

CAUTION

EATING AN EXCESSIVE QUANTITY OF CARROTS MAY CAUSE THE SKIN TO YELLOW - TEMPORARILY.

CARROT SEEDS ARE A NERVE TONIC AND WILL ALSO INDUCE ABORTION; AVOID DURING PREGNANCY.

Eugenica caryophyllata
CLOVES

Cloves are the dried buds of a tree of the myrtle family, *Syzygium aromaticum*. The tree, which may reach a height of 40ft. (12m.), produces abundant clusters of small red flower buds that are gathered before opening and dried to produce the dark brown, nail-shaped spice, clove. Whole and ground cloves used as food seasonings account for half the world production of cloves. Ground cloves are also used in a type of tobacco popular in Asia. Almost 20 percent of the clove's weight is essential oil, obtained by distilling, and used in perfumes, blends of spices, medications, and candies.

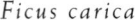

DATA FILE

Properties

❧ Antiseptic and powerfully analgesic – particularly to the gums and teeth

❧ Cloves are warming, and useful for people who are prone to colds

❧ Anti-inflammatory, when used locally on swellings

❧ Cloves are calming to the digestive system

❧ Eliminate parasites from the body

Uses

❧ Oil of cloves can be placed directly on a sore tooth or mouth abscess to draw out the infection and ease the pain. Chew cloves for the same effect.

❧ Dab a tiny amount of neat oil on insect bites.

❧ Clove tea is warming, and can encourage the body to sweat, which is helpful for high fever or vomiting.

❧ Oil of cloves may be used during a long labor to hasten birth.

❧ Clove tea can be used to soothe wind and ease nausea – particularly the nausea of travel sickness.

❧ Inhale an infusion of cloves to clear the lungs and refresh the airways.

❧ A clove and orange pomander can be hung in cupboards as an effective insect repellent.

❧ Steep cloves in boiling water and then simmer. Strain and use the remaining liquid as a mild sedative and to soothe an acid stomach.

❧ Clove tea may be used in the treatment of depression – a cup a day can be uplifting for sufferers.

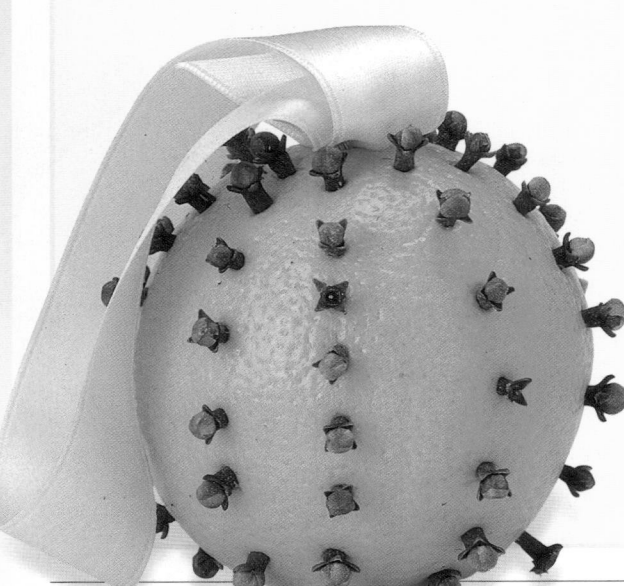

LEFT *Make a fragrant pomander by pushing cloves into an orange. Attach a piece of ribbon to hang it up.*

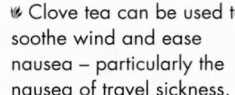

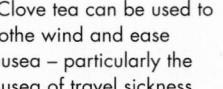

Ficus carica
FIG

Figs comprise a large family of deciduous and evergreen tropical and subtropical trees, shrubs, and vines belonging to the mulberry family, *Moraceae*. The most important fig is *Ficus carica*, the tree that produces the edible fig fruit. Figs are a nutritious and sustaining food, with a long history of medicinal use. For example, there are several references in the Bible to figs being used to treat infections.

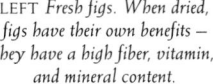

LEFT *Fresh figs. When dried, figs have their own benefits – they have a high fiber, vitamin, and mineral content.*

DATA FILE

Properties

❧ Highly alkaline

❧ Contains a powerful healing agent

❧ Soothes mucous membranes, particularly in the respiratory system

❧ The stem of the fresh fruit is antifungal, and can be used to treat warts

❧ Anticancer

❧ Contains ficin, which aids the digestion

❧ Contains a bactericide

❧ Reduces body heat, and helps to ease inflammation

Uses

❧ Eat dried figs to ease constipation.

❧ To bring a boil to a head, split a fig, heat it, and place it directly on the boil. This is a particularly good method for treating boils and ulcers in the mouth.

❧ Fig juice can be drunk daily as a cancer preventive.

❧ Digestive troubles can be eased by eating fresh figs after light meals or just prior to heavy meals.

❧ Roasted figs can be used as a poultice on boils and hemorrhoids in order to encourage healing and to draw out infection.

❧ Fresh figs can soothe respiratory ailments by acting as an anti-inflammatory agent.

❧ Boil four or five fresh figs in about 1pt. (500ml.) of water; bring to the boil, strain, cool, and drink the liquid for sore throats.

Glycyrrhiza glabra
LICORICE

Licorice is a pretty blue-flowered perennial, grown mainly in Europe. The roots are crushed, ground, and boiled to extract the juice, which is then thickened to produce hard black sticks of paste known as black sugar. The bittersweet flavoring is used in candy and tobacco, as a soothing ingredient in cough lozenges and syrups, as a laxative, and in the manufacture of shoe polish. Licorice is also an excellent source of iron.

LEFT *The leaves of the licorice plant, a perennial. The root of the plant is used for treatments.*

DATA FILE

Properties

❦ Expectorant and anti-inflammatory, making it excellent for stubborn coughs and lung infections

❦ Mild laxative

❦ Adrenal tonic

❦ Detoxifies the body. In the Far East, licorice is used to rid the body of poisons such as salmonella or as an antidote to overuse of drugs

❦ Raises blood pressure. Can be used in the treatment of low blood pressure

❦ Inhibits gastric secretions, making it useful in the treatment of gastric ulcers

❦ Stimulates the kidneys and the bowels

Uses

❦ Licorice syrup can be used to treat persistent coughs, and to reduce the incidence of asthma attacks.

❦ A strong infusion can protect against and heal ulcers. Drink it three times each day.

❦ Steep licorice root with a blend of other soothing herb teas to treat gastric disorders, and to stimulate kidneys and bowel.

❦ Used with other strengthening herbs such as ginseng for exhaustion.

❦ Licorice is used in creams or pastes for the relief of inflamed psoriasis and hot and weepy skin conditions.

THERAPY CONNECTIONS

CLOVES

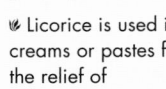 Ayurveda   *p.38*

LICORICE

Ayurveda   *p.39*

Herbalism   *p.122*

Chinese Herbal Medicine   *p.64*

WITCH HAZEL

Herbalism   *p.123*

Homeopathy   *p.197*

CAUTION

LARGE DOSES OF LICORICE CAN CAUSE WATER RETENTION AND EXACERBATE HIGH BLOOD PRESSURE.

AVOID IN PREGNANCY.

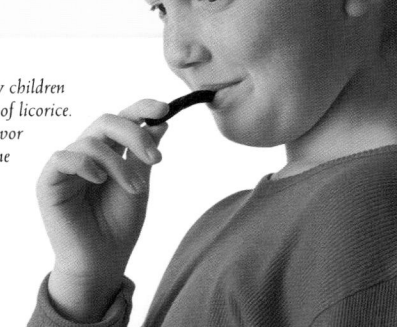
RIGHT *Many children enjoy the taste of licorice. It is used to flavor candy and some medicines.*

Hamamelis virginiana
WITCH HAZEL

Witch hazel is a common tree grown in the U.S. Its leaves or roots are used for medicinal purposes. The common name arose as a result of the remarkable medicinal properties of the alcoholic extract from the leaves and bark of the plant, which is used on bruises and inflammations, and as a rubbing lotion.

RIGHT *Both the leaves and the bark of witch hazel have beneficial properties. The shrub grows to 12ft. (3.6m).*

DATA FILE

Properties

❦ Analgesic

❦ Antiseptic – witch hazel can be used as a facial wash, and diluted to wash cuts and grazes

❦ Helps to control diarrhea when taken internally, and can encourage the health of the digestive tract

❦ Witch hazel soothes swellings, and reduces inflammation and bleeding, internally and externally

❦ Will encourage healing of bruises, sprains, and bleeding hemorrhoids

Uses

❦ Drink an infusion two or three times daily when there is inflammation (such as that of arthritis or rheumatism,

sprains, or bruising) and for internal bleeding.

❦ Apply externally (as a decoction, tincture, or cream) for the treatment of bruising, hemorrhoids, or varicose veins.

❦ Use as a compress for sprains and strains.

❦ Dilute one part witch hazel to 20 parts boiled, cooled water, and use as an eyewash for sore and inflamed eyes.

❦ Add to the bath to reduce the aches and pains of rheumatic conditions.

❦ Witch hazel ointment can be used for painful joints, bruising (applied very gently), and local pain.

Hordeum sativum vulgare
BARLEY

Barley is rich in minerals (calcium and potassium) and B-complex vitamins, which makes it useful for convalescents or people suffering from stress. Barley has been used for its restorative qualities, in medicine and in cooking, for thousands of years. Malt is produced from barley.

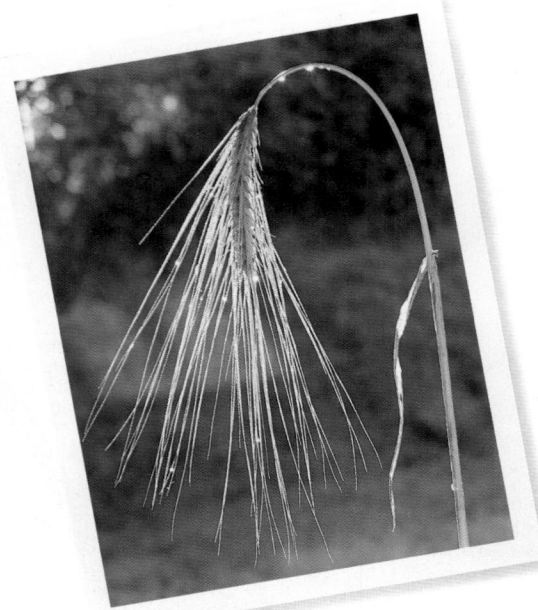

RECIPE
Barley Water

Add 2 tablespoons of pearl barley to 1pt. (500ml.) of water and boil for 10 minutes. ❧ Strain, and add barley to a fresh pint of water. ❧ Boil for another 10 minutes. ❧ Strain barley and serve water warm or cold, with lemon and honey.

ABOVE *Barley is a cereal crop cultivated for humans and animals.*

RIGHT *Barley water is delicious served with lemon. It helps relieve cystitis.*

THERAPY CONNECTIONS
WALNUT
Flower Remedies   *p.232*

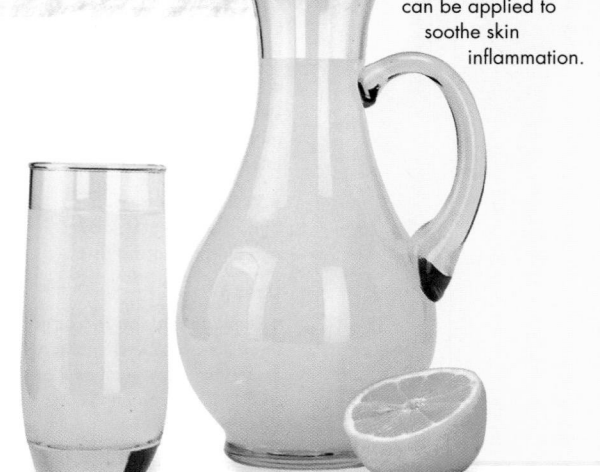

DATA FILE

Properties

❧ Nutritious

❧ Anti-inflammatory, particularly to the urinary and digestive systems

❧ Used in the treatment of respiratory disorders

❧ Taken daily, it may lower cholesterol levels

Uses

❧ Barley water can be used in the treatment of respiratory disorders, and eases dry, tickling coughs.

❧ Barley water can be used for urinary tract infections and cystitis, and can ease flatulence and colic.

❧ Cooked barley is easily digested and nutritious, and is a traditional remedy for constipation and diarrhea.

❧ Barley water reduces acid in the spleen if drunk twice a day for a month.

❧ Make a poultice of barley flour to reduce inflammation of the skin.

❧ Barley may help to prevent heart disease, as it promotes the normal functioning of the heart and is able to stabilize blood pressure.

❧ Eat in soups and stews when convalescing.

❧ Barley poultices can be applied to soothe skin inflammation.

Juglans regia
WALNUT

Walnut is the common name for about 20 species of deciduous trees in the walnut family, *Juglandaceae*. The fruit has an outer leathery husk and an inner hard and furrowed stone, or nut. Walnuts are rich in protein, and high in potassium and other minerals such as zinc and iron. The bark of the walnut tree is used to treat gum disease, among other things.

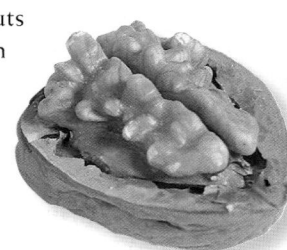

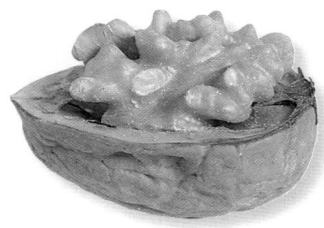

ABOVE *Walnuts are the fruit of a 50ft. (15m.) deciduous tree. Walnut leaves can be rubbed on a pet's coat to repel fleas.*

DATA FILE

Properties

❧ The bark of the walnut tree is astringent and cleansing

❧ Walnut bark strengthens the gums and acts as an anti-inflammatory

❧ The bark discourages milk flow in nursing mothers

❧ The nuts are aphrodisiac and mildly laxative

❧ The nuts prevent worms

❧ The nuts are soothing and a natural digestive

Uses

❧ Eat daily while convalescing to relieve fatigue and generally strengthen the body.

❧ Fresh walnuts and walnut oil can encourage circulation, and because they are rich in potassium, will keep the heart healthy.

❧ Add walnut bark to the bath for rheumatism, and sore and aching muscles and joints.

❧ Apply walnut bark tincture, in a little carrier oil, to swellings and skin problems, in order to encourage healing.

❧ Eat walnuts for heartburn and diarrhea.

❧ Fresh walnuts can help to soothe colic and dispel gas in the abdomen.

❧ Walnut oil, added to salads and vegetables, will help to ease the discomfort of irritable bowel syndrome and act as a mild laxative.

Lactobacillus
YOGURT

Yogurt is a fermented, slightly acidic food product made from milk. Its origins are unknown (although the name is Turkish), and it resembles the many other fermented milk foods made throughout the world, such as kefir and kumiss. Unlike many of these foods, however, yogurt is usually made from a concentrated milk and is soured by a specific bacillus, *Lactobacillus bulgaricus*. As a food, yogurt is a rich source of protein, and contains all of the vitamins and minerals found in milk. Live yogurt, which contains active bacteria, is most often used therapeutically, and should be eaten to increase the healthy bacteria in the body, to help it fight infection.

ABOVE *Make your own yogurt. Add 3 teaspoons of live yogurt to 1pt. (600ml.) of milk. Leave to set.*

> **CAUTION**
>
> LIVE YOGURT IS NOT EFFECTIVE WHEN MIXED WITH SWEETENERS; FOR BEST EFFECT MAKE YOUR OWN YOGURT AND FLAVOR WITH A LITTLE UNPASTEURIZED HONEY AND A BANANA.

BELOW *Natural yogurt is a good facial cleanser and moisturizer. Apply to the skin with cotton wool.*

DATA FILE

Properties

- Live yogurt is antifungal, and can be used in the treatment of thrush
- Live yogurt may help to reduce cholesterol levels
- Encourages the growth of healthy bacteria in the bowels, which aids absorption of nutrients and helps to prevent infection
- Helps to produce vitamin B
- Yogurt stimulates bowel movements
- Helps to prevent and control the growth of cancerous cells
- Aids digestion

Uses

- Live yogurt should be eaten to increase beneficial bacteria following a course of antibiotics. Eat daily for two to three weeks.
- Apply live yogurt to areas affected by thrush; it can also be used internally as a douche.

- Daily intake of yogurt may prevent heart disease.
- Cleanse the skin with yogurt, which is a natural moisturizer.
- Eat live yogurt for chronic constipation and dyspepsia.
- Eat daily as a cancer preventive.

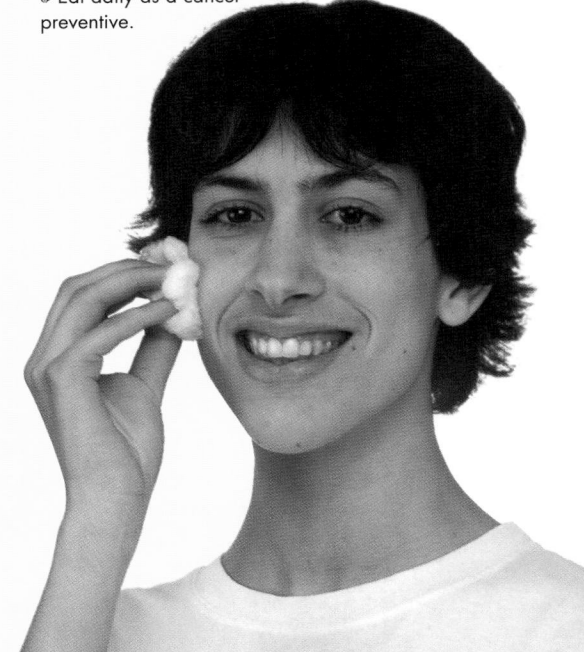

Linum usitatissimum
FLAXSEED

Flax is a group of annual and perennial plants from the *Linaceae* family. Several varieties of one species, *L. usitatissimum*, are grown primarily for their fiber, used in making linen, or for their seeds, the source of linseed oil. The seeds contain a remarkable healing oil which can be used both internally and externally. Flaxseed is also known as linseed, but should not be confused with the "boiled" linseed oil available from building merchants. As far back as Hippocrates, flaxseed tea has been used to treat sore throats, hoarseness, and bronchial spasms.

> **CAUTION**
>
> COMMERCIALLY PRODUCED LINSEED OIL IS USED IN PROTECTIVE COATINGS SUCH AS PAINTS AND VARNISHES BECAUSE IT HAS A DRYING ACTION. IT IS NOT SUITABLE FOR HUMAN CONSUMPTION!

RIGHT *A field of flax grown for commercial purposes. Flax is used to make linen and linseed oil.*

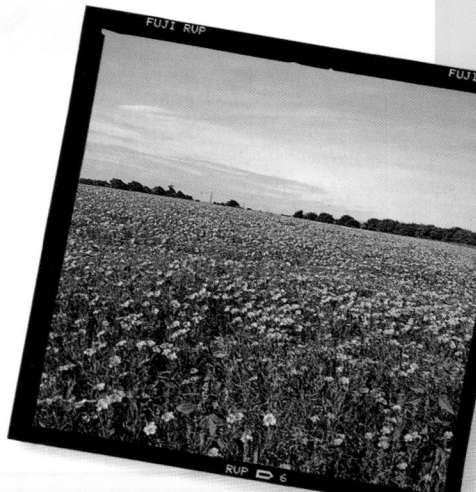

DATA FILE

Properties

- Mildly laxative
- Tonic for the kidneys and encourages their action
- Encourages healing
- Analgesic
- Antispasmodic

Uses

- Apply the oil to sprains to reduce inflammation and ease the pain.
- Mix flaxseed with lime water to reduce the pain of burns.

- Flaxseed (linseed) tea can be used for mild constipation, and to encourage kidney function. The tea also works to ease kidney pains and cramping.
- The tea can be drunk during bouts of bronchitis to reduce inflammation of the lungs and prevent spasm.
- Add lemon and honey to flaxseed tea to encourage its action and improve taste.

Malus species, including Malus pumila

APPLE

The apple has many uses in traditional medicine, and the old adage "To eat an apple going to bed will make the physician beg his bread" has been justified by its many health-giving properties. Research shows that apples are excellent detoxifiers, and apple juice – even store bought – can destroy viruses in the body.

Nasturtium officinalis

WATERCRESS

Watercress is a floating or creeping water plant of the mustard family, *Cruciferae*. A perennial, it grows best in fresh water, particularly in cool streams and ponds, and in wet soil. Its round, edible leaves are pungent to the taste, and commonly used as salad greens or as a garnish. It is a rich source of vitamin C.

DATA FILE

Properties

- Cleans teeth and strengthens gums
- Lowers cholesterol levels
- Antiviral action
- Detoxifies
- Protects from pollution, binding to toxins in the body and carrying them out
- Neutralizes indigestion
- Prevents constipation
- Soothing and antiseptic

Uses

- Eat raw apples regularly, as a detoxificant, for gout and rheumatism.

- To prevent viruses from settling in, and to reduce their duration, eat an apple (or drink a glass of apple juice) three times a day.

- Raw, peeled, and grated apples can be used as a poultice for sprains.

- For indigestion, heartburn, and other digestive disorders, eat an apple with meals.

- Use an apple poultice for treating rheumatic and weak eyes.

- Two apples a day can reduce cholesterol levels by up to 10 percent.

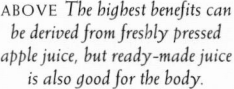

ABOVE *The highest benefits can be derived from freshly pressed apple juice, but ready-made juice is also good for the body.*

- As a treatment for intestinal infections, hoarseness, rheumatism, and fatigue, increase your daily intake to as much as 2lb. (1kg.).

- For curative purposes, as an alternative to eating the whole fruit, drink 1pt. (500ml.) of naturally sweet apple juice a day.

- Grated apple, mixed with live yogurt, may be helpful in cases of diarrhea.

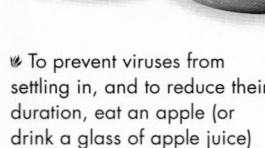

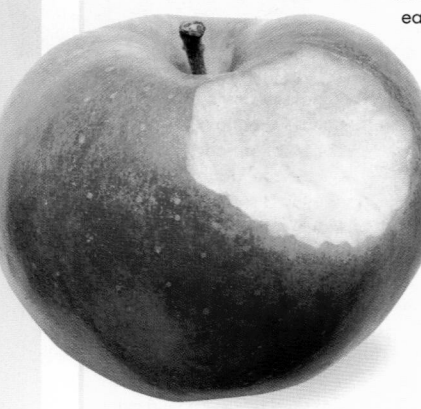

ABOVE *Apples have long been known to be beneficial to health and should be eaten regularly.*

DATA FILE

Properties

- Contains benzyl mustard oil, which is powerfully antibiotic, but does not harm our healthy bacteria (flora)
- Beneficial to the health of the intestines
- Encourages immune activity in the body
- Provides good supplies of the vitamins C, A, and B (thiamine and riboflavin), iron, potassium, and calcium
- Stimulates digestion
- Anti-inflammatory, diuretic, expectorant, antiseptic

Uses

- Sometimes recommended for gall bladder complaints and anemia.

- The bruised leaves are said to remove pimples and to fade freckling. Eat to help skin eruptions.

- Eat fresh daily: may help to prevent migraine. Eat with a meal if you have a tendency towards heartburn or dyspepsia.

- High levels of potassium may help to prevent insomnia – eat some fresh leaves an hour before bedtime, and often throughout the day.

- Watercress may help in the treatment of edema.

- It is used to treat respiratory ailments such as coughs, catarrh, and bronchitis – eat fresh until symptoms improve. It can be useful as a preventive measure for chronic respiratory conditions.

- Watercress may strengthen the whole body system in cases of debility caused by chronic illness. It can also help to relieve stress.

THERAPY CONNECTIONS

APPLE
- Flower Remedies   *p.234*

OLIVE
- Flower Remedies   *p.235*

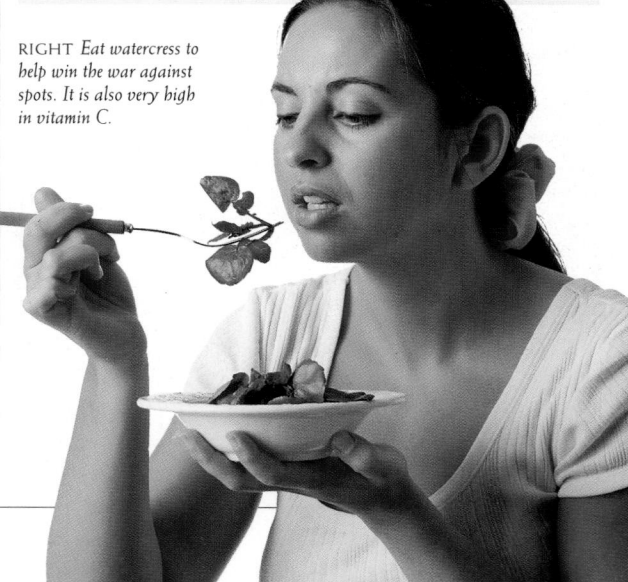

RIGHT *Eat watercress to help win the war against spots. It is also very high in vitamin C.*

Olea europea
OLIVE

The olive is a handsome, long-lived, evergreen, subtropical tree, and has been cultivated for at least 4,000 years for its edible fruit and its valuable oil. It is native to the eastern Mediterranean region, where its culture may have been begun by Semitic people as long ago as 3500 B.C.E. Its leaves and the oil of its fruit are used in cooking and medicinally, and studies show that it has powerful anticholesterol action in the body, making it a useful addition to any home medicine cabinet. Only cold-pressed olive oil is suitable for therapeutic use.

RIGHT *The olive branch is an ancient symbol of peace. Olive is reputed to calm nervous disorders.*

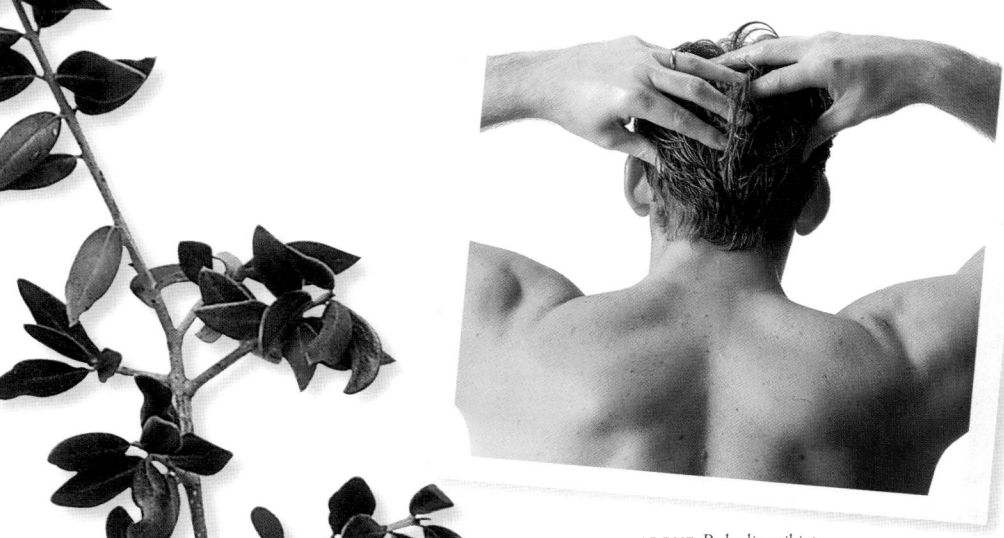

ABOVE *Rub olive oil into the scalp to improve problems such as itchy dandruff, eczema, and psoriasis.*

DATA FILE

Properties

❧ Antioxidant

❧ Anticancer

❧ Emollient – particularly useful for skin conditions

❧ Olive oil can be used to treat constipation

❧ Soothes the itching of eczema, and moisturizes dry skin, hair, and scalp

❧ Olive oil is rich in vitamin E, and is now known to help lower cholesterol levels in the body

❧ It may reduce the risk of circulatory disease and nervous disorders

❧ Useful in the treatment of gastric disorders because it reduces the secretion of gastric juices

Uses

❧ Rub olive oil into patches of eczema, dandruff, and psoriasis to reduce itching and encourage healing.

❧ Olive oil, taken daily, can reduce the risk of heart disease and help to slow down the degenerative effects of aging.

❧ Drink a little extra virgin olive oil to cure a hangover.

❧ Olives and olive oil, as part of a daily diet, will help to prevent and treat circulatory problems, and lower cholesterol levels.

❧ Eat olives for constipation.

❧ Olives are said to counteract poisoning from mushrooms or fish – drink a little extra virgin, cold-pressed oil when symptoms present themselves.

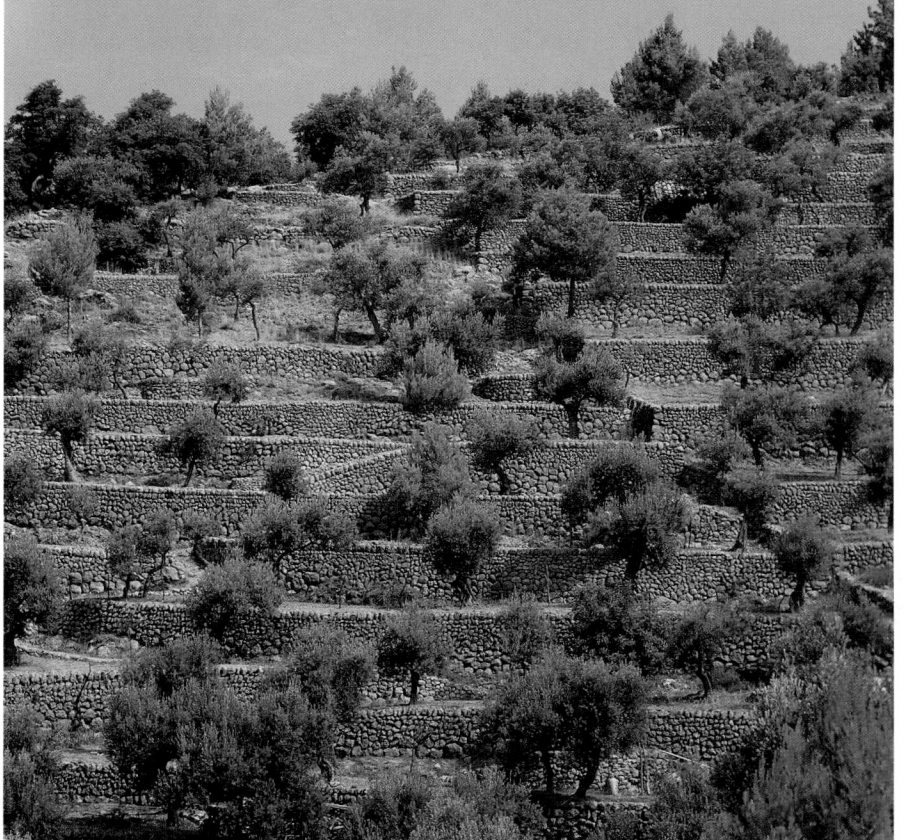

LEFT *A Mediterranean olive grove. The slow-growing trees thrive in a warm, sunny climate.*

Oyrza sativa
RICE

Rice is the cereal that is a
staple food to more than
half of the world's peoples.
It also has important medicinal uses,
for which the rhizomes, seeds (the grains), and
germinated seeds are used. White rice is the grain that
is left after the bran and germ have been removed;
brown rice retains the bran and germ. Rice is available
as a breakfast cereal (the grains are "puffed" during
manufacture), and is fermented to produce rice wine,
called *saki* by the Japanese.

DATA FILE

Properties

❧ Rice contains high levels of carbohydrates (87 percent of white, uncooked rice)

❧ Rich in B vitamins (folic acid and pyridoxine), iron, and potassium. Brown rice also contains the B vitamin thiamine, which is present in the bran.

❧ White rice has 1 percent of fat; in brown rice the amount of fat is higher

❧ Rice contains low amounts of sodium and is also free from cholesterol

❧ A natural tonic

❧ Diuretic

❧ Digestive

❧ Controls sweating

❧ Lowers blood pressure

❧ Anti-inflammatory

Uses

❧ Eat rice daily if you suffer from chronic dyspepsia – excellent for heartburn, particularly that associated with pregnancy.

❧ Use rice bran for the treatment of hyperalcuria.

❧ Use rice flour to make a poultice for relieving inflammation of the skin, including acne, measles, burns, and hemorrhoids.

❧ A natural diuretic – increase your intake prior to menstruation if you suffer from bloating and symptoms of PMS. Eaten regularly, rice can prevent edema.

❧ The seeds are used to treat urinary ailments.

❧ Rice water helps to overcome stomach upsets.

❧ Rice and rice flour are used as substitutes for wheat and some other cereals by people who cannot tolerate gluten and gliadin, such as those with celiac disease.

❧ Germinated rice seeds may help in the treatment of abdominal bloating, lack of appetite, and indigestion.

LEFT and ABOVE Brown rice and white rice. Brown, unpolished rice contains more vitamins and fiber.

Persica americana gratissima
AVOCADO

Avocados are the fruit of a small, subtropical tree.
They are rich in vitamins A, some B-complex, C, and E
vitamins, and potassium, and because they contain
some protein and starch, as well as being a good
source of monounsaturated fats, they are considered to
be a perfect – or complete – food. Traditionally
avocados have been used for skin problems. The pulp
has both antibacterial and antifungal properties.

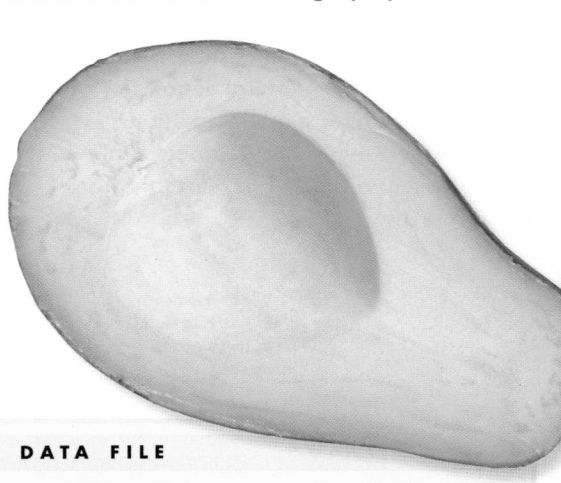

RIGHT Avocados are full of vitamins and minerals, but they also have a high fat content.

DATA FILE

Properties

❧ Excellent restorative food, particularly during convalescence

❧ Traditionally used for sexual problems

❧ Helps with skin disorders

❧ Antioxidant

❧ Used to treat circulatory problems

❧ Digestive

❧ Antibacterial

❧ Antifungal

Uses

❧ An avocado paste can be applied to rashes and rough skin to soothe and smooth.

❧ Avocado oil can be used as a base oil for massage.

❧ Eat an avocado each day when convalescing.

❧ The pulp, applied to grazes and shallow cuts, and covered with sterile gauze, can prevent infection entering the body and encourage healing.

❧ Eat regularly for digestive and circulatory problems.

❧ The flesh of a ripe avocado soothes sunburned skin. Cut an avocado in half and rub gently over the affected area.

BELOW To make a face mask, mash a ripe avocado with a little olive oil and apply to the skin.

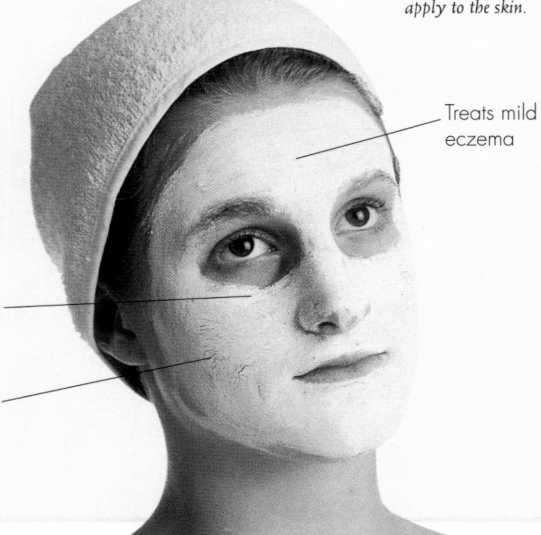

Treats mild eczema

Antibacterial

Leave on for 15 minutes

Piper negrum
BLACK PEPPER

Black pepper, a traditional seasoning for food, is a warm, aromatic, and comforting spice with therapeutic uses. The fruit, or corns, of the vine and the essential oil extracted from them are used. Black pepper is the whole, sun-dried, unripened fruit of the vine; white pepper is the ripe fruit, from which the skins have been removed.

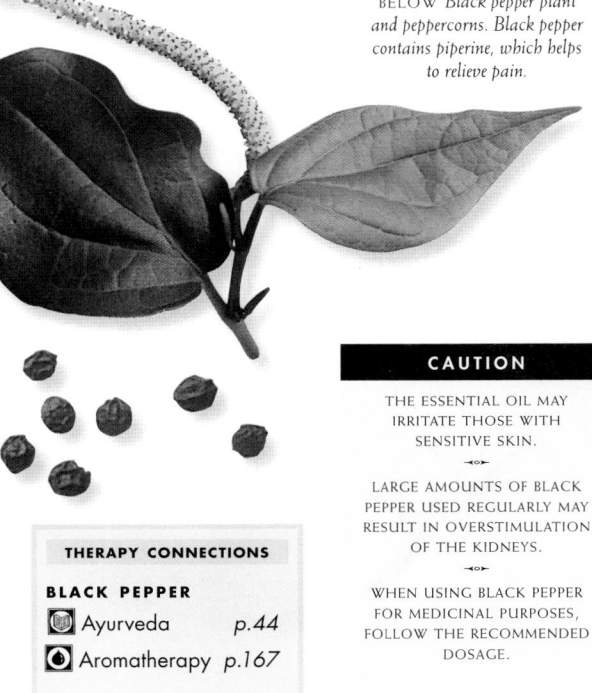

BELOW *Black pepper plant and peppercorns. Black pepper contains piperine, which helps to relieve pain.*

THERAPY CONNECTIONS

BLACK PEPPER

Ayurveda   *p.44*

Aromatherapy   *p.167*

DATA FILE

Properties

- Stimulating
- Expectorant
- Anesthetic
- Tranquilizing
- Analgesic

Uses

- Black pepper is useful for treating indigestion and flatulence – add to food daily for preventive action.

- Its essential oil eases muscular aches and pains, and is used to treat colds and flu.

- When used as a homeopathic remedy for fever, pepper can help to lower the body temperature.

- Pepper is an effective emetic and expectorant, and can be taken internally, or rubbed onto the chest (a tiny amount of oil in a suitable carrier oil) to prevent catarrh and to encourage healing.

- In Ayurvedic medicine, black pepper mixed with ghee is used to treat nasal congestion, sinusitis, and inflammation of the skin.

Prunus amygdalmus dulcis and
Prunus amygdalmus amara
ALMOND

The almond tree produces the oldest and most widely grown of all of the world's nut crops, and is indigenous to western Asia and North Africa. Of the two major types of almonds grown, the sweet almond (*P. dulcis*) is cultivated for its edible nut. The bitter almond (*P. amara*) is inedible but contains an oil – also present in the sweet almond, and in the ripe kernels of the apricot and peach – which, when combined with water, yields hydrocyanic (prussic) acid and benzaldehyde, the essential oil of bitter almonds. The oil is used in making flavoring extracts and in some sedative medicines.

Almonds have been used for centuries to heal the body internally, and may be used ground in water to prevent fevers.

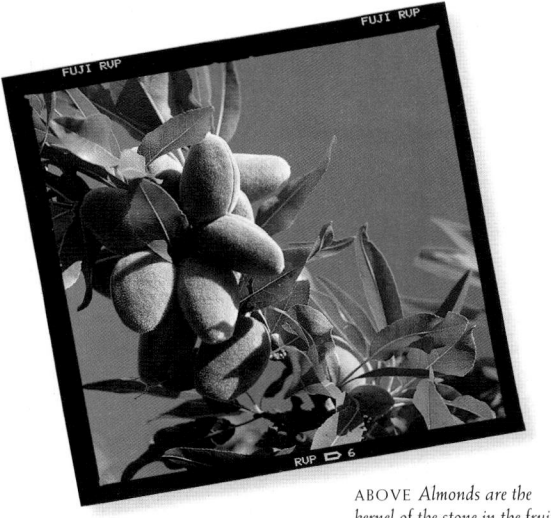

ABOVE *Almonds are the kernel of the stone in the fruit of the almond tree.*

DATA FILE

Properties

- Sweet almonds are high in protein

- Almonds reduce inflammation: used in the treatment of bronchitis

- Rich in protein, fat, zinc, potassium, iron, B vitamins, and magnesium

- Aids respiration

- Acts as a digestive

Uses

- Combine almond milk *(see right)* with barley water for urinary problems.

- Almond milk is an excellent tonic during convalescence.

- Drink almond milk daily to reduce frequency of digestive disorders, and to relieve respiratory problems.

ALMOND MILK

Almond milk helps digestive, respiratory, and urinary problems. Drink it every day for the best results.

You will need almonds (6 tablespoonsful), water, and honey.

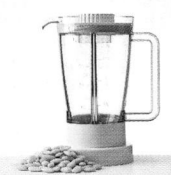

Blend the almonds in a food processor with 1pt. (500ml.) water. Grind until smooth.

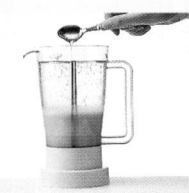

Add 1 teaspoonful of honey for flavor.

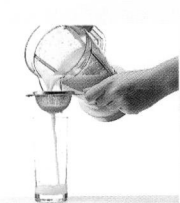

Strain the mixture through a sieve or fine cloth to drink. Store in a refrigerator.

Sinapis alba, Brassica nigra
MUSTARD

Black and white mustards are used for culinary and medicinal purposes. The leaves, flowers, seeds, and oils of the black mustard are used, while only the seeds of the white mustard are useful. Black mustard powder is an important herbal remedy because it draws blood to the surface of the skin quickly, which means that it is "rubefacient," and warming. Mustard oil is used as an ingredient in liniments, stomach stimulants, and emetics.

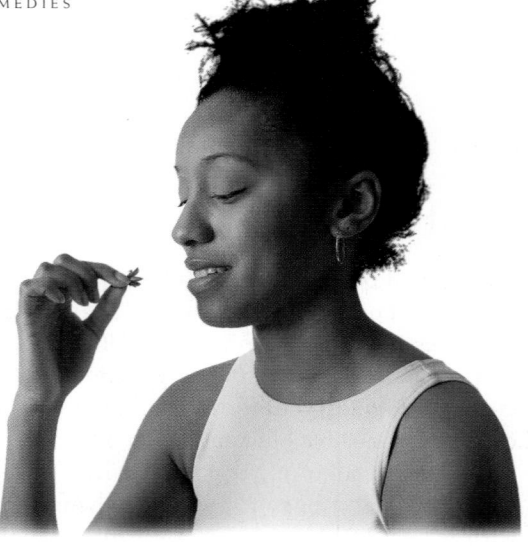

ABOVE *Mustard leaves are very nutritious, containing vitamin A, iron, and zinc.*

CAUTION

MUSTARD SEEDS CAN BURN THE SKIN; USE CAREFULLY.

AVOID CONTACT WITH THE MUCOUS MEMBRANES, AND WITH SENSITIVE SKIN.

THERAPY CONNECTIONS

MUSTARD
Ayurveda	p.30
Flower Remedies	p.239

BELOW *Powdered mustard seeds have no smell until water is added, when a pungent odor is released.*

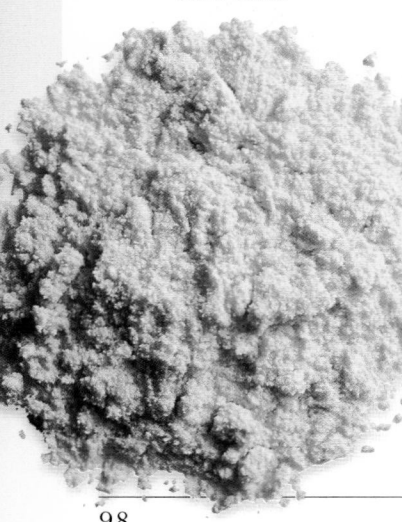

DATA FILE

Properties
- Rich in calcium and iron
- Mustard helps to restore bacterial balance in the intestines
- Mustard greens are rich in vitamin A, iron, and zinc
- White mustard relieves pain, and is a diuretic and an antibiotic
- Mustard flour is an antiseptic and a deodorizer
- Mustard oil can be used for pain relief of arthritic conditions and chilblains
- An excellent expectorant
- A powerful emetic
- Black mustard and white mustard are warming and can be used to draw infection or congestion away from its source for nasal congestion, or for relief of an abscess
- Rubefacient qualities help respiratory and circulatory disorders, including heart problems

Uses
- Taken internally, mustard encourages the circulation, eases stomach and liver problems, and is able to stimulate the heart.
- Eat fresh mustard leaves when convalescing – they are nutritious and will help to encourage healing.
- A mustard foot bath (1 teaspoon of mustard powder added to a bowl of hot water) is a traditional remedy for colds, circulatory problems, and headaches.
- A mustard poultice on the chest relieves infection and congestion.
- Mustard essential oil can be used externally for neuralgia; massage a little oil gently into the affected area a few times a day.
- A poultice of mustard seeds or mustard essential oil is helpful when applied to areas of the body troubled by pain from rheumatism, sciatica, and lumbago.

Solanum tuberosum
POTATO

The potato plant is native to the Americas. It was supposedly endowed with powers such as the ability to cure impotence, and so long as the plant remained rare in Europe, its price often reached astronomical heights. Potatoes have been used for medicinal purposes for hundreds of years, and are extremely nutritious, supplying fiber, B vitamins, minerals, and vitamin C. The peels are high in potassium, and potato-peel tea has been traditionally used around the world for high blood pressure. The juice of raw potatoes is most useful, and can be added to soups, juices, or stews to disguise the taste.

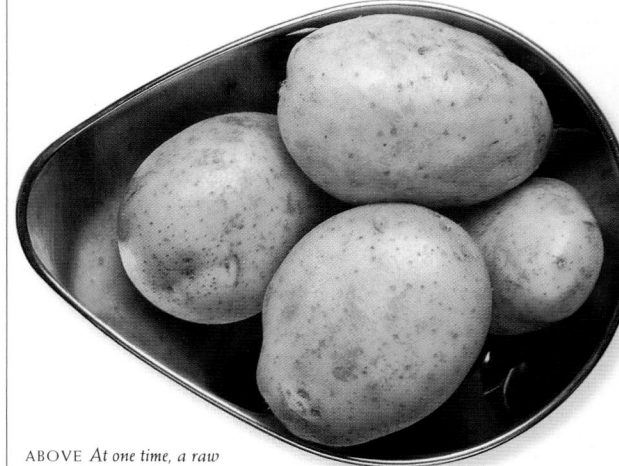

ABOVE *At one time, a raw potato was carried in a garment pocket to protect against rheumatism.*

CAUTION

POISONOUS ALKALOIDS ARE PRESENT IN MOST NIGHTSHADE PLANTS, INCLUDING THE COMMON POTATO, BUT IT IS PERFECTLY SAFE TO EAT IF COOKED, AND IN SMALL AMOUNTS WHEN RAW.

SPROUTING POTATOES ARE POISONOUS AND SHOULD NOT BE EATEN.

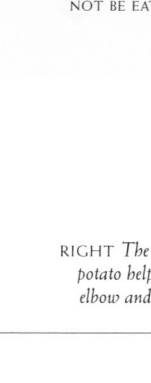

Potato pulp

RIGHT *The pulp of a hot baked potato helps to relieve tennis elbow and other joint pain.*

Vaccinium oxycoccus var. palustris

CRANBERRY

Cranberries are small acidic berries which are rich in vitamins C and A, and contain an excellent infection-fighting ingredient. The commercial cranberry, *Vaccinium macrocarpon*, is a creeping evergreen plant of the heath family, whose red, acidic fruit is used in sauces and jellies served with savory and sweet foods and in a variety of fruit juice beverages.

DATA FILE

Properties

❧ An antiseptic action on the urinary system

❧ Used to control asthma

❧ Improves the health of the circulatory system

❧ Aids in the treatment of kidney stones

Uses

❧ Cranberries contain a substance which affects the acidity of the urine and acts as a bactericide. A daily glass of cranberry juice will prevent and treat cystitis, and discourage kidney stones. Fresh cranberries and cranberry juice are used in the treatment of prostate problems, and urinary tract infections.

❧ Crushed cranberries, boiled in distilled water and skinned, can be added to a cup of warm water to overcome an asthma attack. The berries contain an active ingredient similar to that in the drugs used to control asthma.

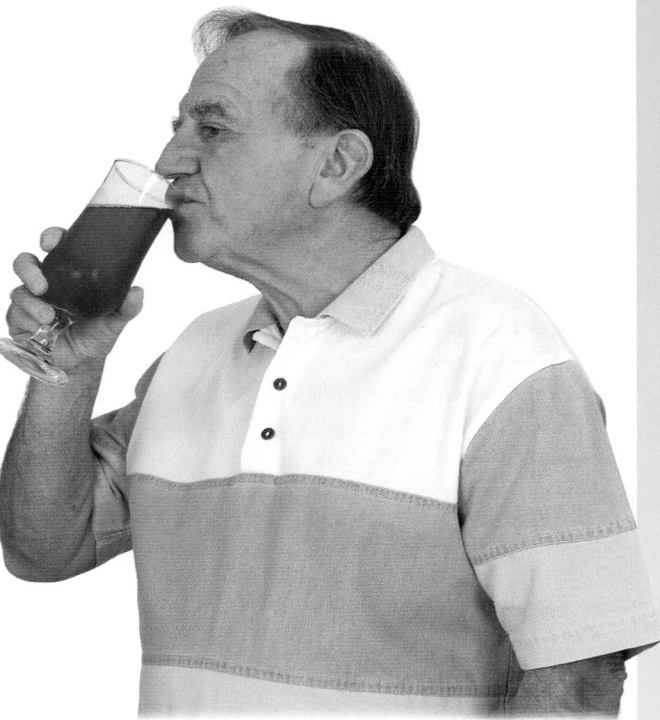

ABOVE *The prostate gland may cause urinary problems in later life. Fresh cranberry juice will help.*

CAUTION

CRANBERRIES CONTAIN LARGE AMOUNTS OF OXALIC ACID, AND SHOULD NOT BE EATEN RAW.

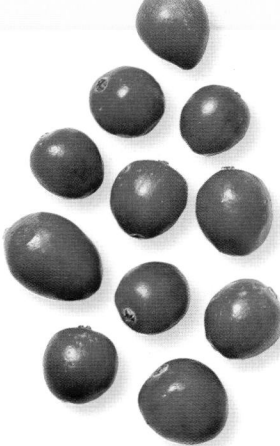

ABOVE *Cranberries are the fruits of an ericaceous shrub. They prevent harmful bacteria attaching to the bladder walls.*

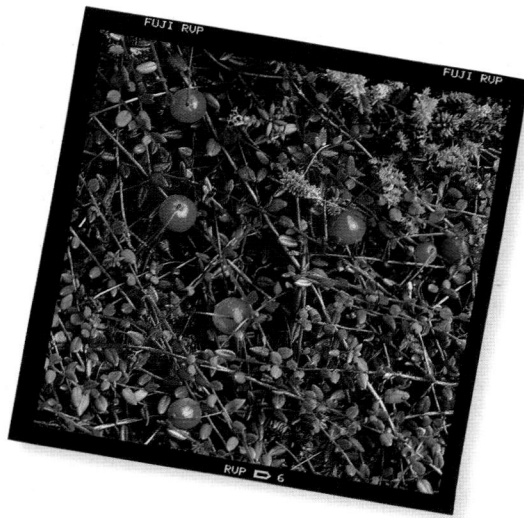

ABOVE *The juice extracted from cranberries contains oxalic acid, which discourages the formation of kidney stones.*

Zea mays
CORN

Archeological evidence indicates that a type of primitive corn was used as a food in Mexico at least 7,000 years ago. The kernels of corn have a translucent, horny appearance when immature and are wrinkled when dry. The ears are eaten fresh or frozen, or are canned. Corn, or maize, is known primarily as a staple food, but it also has therapeutic properties. The corn silk (stigmas and styles of female flowers), fruit, seeds, and oil are used. Corn is particularly useful as a remedy for urinary problems.

CAUTION

PEOPLE SUFFERING FROM PELLAGRA (A NIACIN-DEFICIENCY DISEASE) MAY BE ADVISED TO ELIMINATE CORN AND CORN PRODUCTS FROM THEIR DIET.

SOME PEOPLE ARE ALLERGIC TO CORN – IF YOU SUFFER A RASH, HEADACHES, OR ANY OTHER SYMPTOMS, AVOID CORN AND CORN PRODUCTS.

ABOVE *Corn silk refers to the hairs covering the corn: save these for making into herbal tea.*

DATA FILE

Properties

❧ Corn provides carbohydrates, B vitamins (thiamine and riboflavin), vitamin C, vitamin A, potassium, and zinc

❧ Stimulating and cooling

❧ Used in Chinese medicine for treating urinary and kidney problems

❧ Corn silk cleanses the kidneys and the urinary tract

Uses

❧ A tea made by infusing corn silk in hot water may help in the treatment of kidney stones. Drink three times a day.

❧ Corn silk is also a good cleanser of the urinary tract. A little of it eaten raw, with or without the corn kernels, will benefit the whole urinary system and may help to prevent cystitis.

❧ Corn and its products may be beneficial in the treatment of bedwetting in children, disorders of the prostate and cystitis, and inflammation of the urethra.

❧ Cornstarch, manufactured from the inner part of the corn kernel, makes a fine powder suitable for use as a face or bath powder.

Bicarbonate of soda
BAKING SODA

Baking soda is a white powder that is traditionally used as a raising agent for baking. It is used in many natural remedies, and on its own for its soothing and neutralizing properties.

DATA FILE

Properties

❧ Anti-inflammatory, particularly useful for skin conditions

❧ Natural bleach for teeth

❧ Alkaline (neutralizes acids)

Uses

❧ Salt and baking soda in the bath may reduce the effect of minor exposure to X-rays.

❧ A paste of baking soda and water can be applied to diaper rash to reduce skin inflammation and irritation.

❧ Drink a solution of baking soda and hot water (1 teaspoon to ½pt. [250ml.]) to reduce flatulence and ease indigestion.

❧ For bee stings, extract the sting and apply a paste of baking soda and water to neutralize it.

❧ The juice of half a lemon mixed with 1 teaspoon of baking soda and warm water will help ease a headache. Drink every 15 minutes until the pain begins to recede.

❧ Brush your teeth with baking soda, a natural whitener which reduces agents causing bad breath.

ABOVE *Take a teaspoonful of bicarbonate of soda in water to treat cystitis.*

RIGHT *Baking soda toothpaste helps to whiten the teeth.*

CAUTION

BAKING SODA SHOULD BE USED ONLY EXTERNALLY ON CHILDREN AND BABIES.

CONSULT A PHYSICIAN BEFORE TAKING BICARBONATE OF SODA IF YOU HAVE HIGH BLOOD PRESSURE OR HEART TROUBLE.

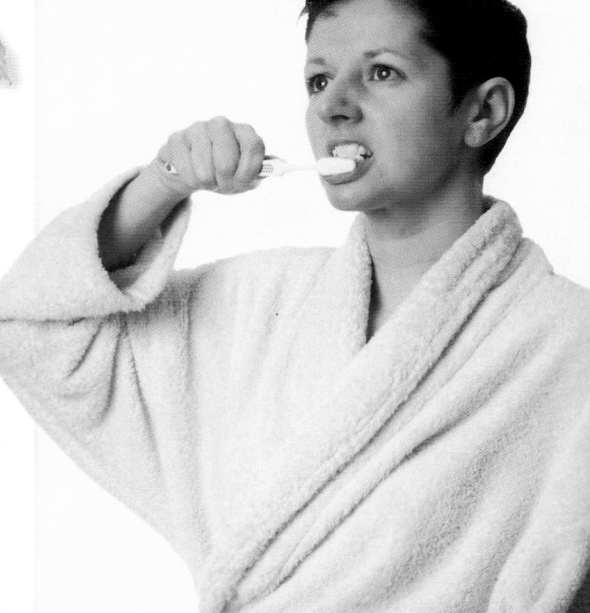

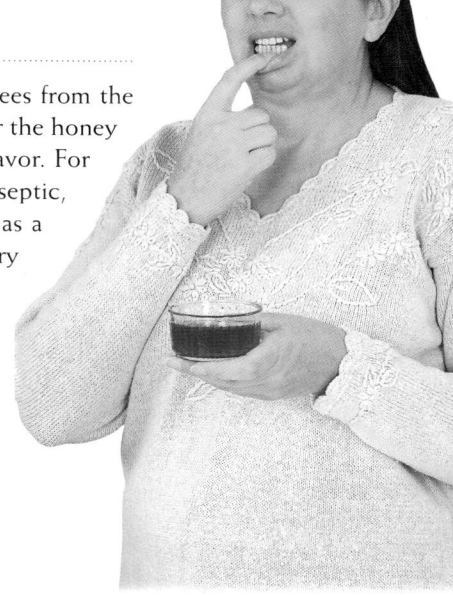

HONEY

Honey is the sweet liquid produced by bees from the nectar of flowers. The source of the nectar the honey is made from determines its color and flavor. For centuries honey has been used as an antiseptic, for external and internal conditions, and as a tonic for overall good health. Each country has a distinctive type of honey, dependent on the local flowers upon which the bees feed. All honeys are complex mixtures of the sugars fructose and glucose with water, organic acids, and mineral and vitamin traces, as well as some plant pigments.

ABOVE AND BELOW Wholegrain bread contains three times as much fiber as white bread.

BREAD

Bread – particularly wholegrain bread – is an excellent source of carbohydrates and B-complex vitamins, which maintain the health of the nervous system and ensure the healthy functioning of body systems. Traditionally, bread was used as a poultice, and applied as a styptic to stop the bleeding of wounds.

CAUTION

UNPASTEURIZED HONEY SHOULD NOT BE EATEN BY PREGNANT WOMEN, AND ONLY SPARINGLY BY CHILDREN. HOWEVER, ENSURE THAT YOU BUY COLD-PRESSED HONEY, BECAUSE HEATED HONEY CONTAINS ADDITIVES AND LOSES ITS HEALING PROPERTIES.

ABOVE Honey ointment helps to heal sore places in the mouth.

LEFT Bees make honeycomb – where honey is stored, and eggs are laid.

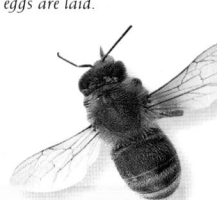

DATA FILE

Properties
- Nutritious
- Anti-inflammatory
- Styptic (stops bleeding)

Uses
- Apply cold bread to closed eyes to reduce the inflammation of conjunctivitis and soothe itching.
- Apply a warm bread poultice to infected cuts to reduce itching and pain.
- Apply fresh bread to shallow wounds to help stop the bleeding.
- Ease the pain, and help to bring out a boil by applying a hot bread poultice.
- Eat wholegrain bread while convalescing and when under stress – it is rich in B vitamins that feed the nervous system.

DATA FILE

Properties
- Soothes raw tissues
- Helps to retain calcium in the body
- Honey helps to balance acid accumulations in the body (because of the significant amount of potassium it contains)
- Sedative
- Antifungal
- Possibly aphrodisiac
- Nourishing – some minerals and vitamins, along with amino acids
- Antibacterial, for external and internal infections; unpasteurized honey has antibiotic properties

Uses
- Honey water can be used as an eye lotion (particularly good for conjunctivitis and other infectious conditions).
- Gargle with honey water to soothe a sore throat and ease respiratory problems.
- Honey and lemon mixed together are a traditional remedy for coughs.
- Mix with apple cider vinegar as a tonic or "rebalancer." This may also help to relieve the symptoms of arthritis and reduce arthritic deposits.
- Honey ointment can soothe and encourage healing of sores in the mouth or vagina.
- Honey is an excellent moisturizer, and can be rubbed into the skin as a revitalizing mask.
- Honey warmed with a little milk can be used as a gentle sedative.
- Eating a little local honey will sensitize you to pollens in the area – acting as a natural remedy for hay fever and all its symptoms.
- Apply a honey compress to cuts and bruises to soothe, encourage healing, and prevent infection.
- Smear set honey on ringworm or athlete's foot several times a day. Leave the foot uncovered.

Acetic acid
VINEGAR

Vinegar (from the French *vinaigre*, "sour wine") is an acidic liquid obtained from the fermentation of alcohol, and used either as a condiment or a preservative. Vinegar usually has an acid content of 4–8 percent; in flavor it may be sharp, rich, or mellow. Vinegar is often used to preserve herbs, and used on its own for medicinal purposes. Apple cider vinegar is the most useful medicinally.

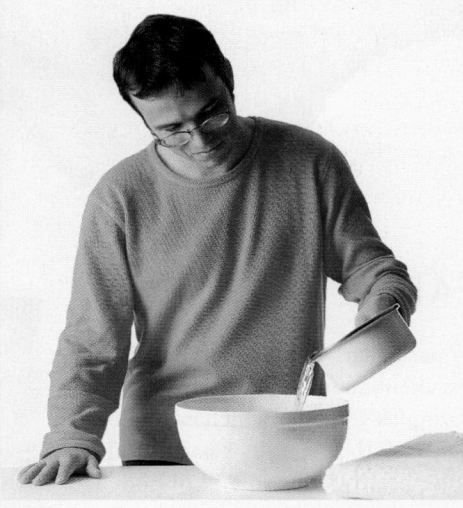

INHALATION

Vinegar is antispasmodic, and is useful for treating the bronchospasms common to bronchitis sufferers. Bronchitis is the inflammation of the bronchi, which link the windpipe to the lungs. It causes production of thick phlegm, and gives rise to bouts of coughing.

Inhaling the steam given off by hot cider vinegar will soothe spasms. Pour some apple cider vinegar into a pan and put it on the cooker to heat. Bring to the boil and simmer for a few minutes. Remove from the heat and pour into a medium-sized bowl.

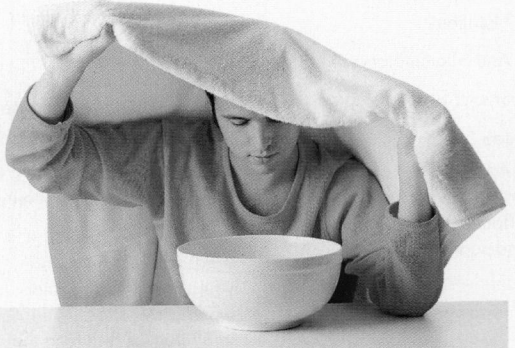

Take the bowl to your kitchen table and sit down with it in front of you. Drape a large towel over your head and the bowl, making a tent. Inhale deeply while the steam continues to be produced. This will also help catarrh.

DATA FILE

Properties

❧ Helps to make more efficient use of calcium in the body, and can help to encourage strong bones, hair, and nails

❧ Vinegar is antiseptic, astringent, and excellent for urinary tract infections

❧ Antispasmodic

❧ Antibacterial

❧ Improves functioning and adjustment of the body so that there is efficient use of the food you eat (i.e. it balances metabolic activity)

❧ Antifungal, used in the treatment of thrush

❧ Apple cider is a good tonic, and can help to relieve a sore throat

Uses

❧ Sip first thing in the morning, and just prior to meals to reduce appetite and encourage efficient digestion.

❧ Simmer cider vinegar in a pan, cover with a towel, and inhale to reduce the spasms of bronchitis and to help reduce any excess catarrh.

❧ Drink a glass of warm apple cider vinegar with honey a half-hour before bed to encourage restful sleep.

❧ Vinegar can be drunk (warm with a little honey) to treat digestive disorders and urinary infections.

❧ Apply vinegar to wasp stings to reduce swelling and ease discomfort.

❧ Coughs, colds, and infections will respond to a cup of warm water with 2

tablespoons of vinegar and some honey. Arthritis and asthma may also be treated with the same drink, adding slightly more vinegar.

❧ Apply cider vinegar to the skin to treat athlete's foot, ringworm, and eczema.

❧ Drink vinegar daily to treat thrush, and apply to the exterior of the vagina (mixed with a little warm water) to ease itching.

❧ Add vinegar to bath water to soothe skin problems, help to draw out toxins from the skin, and ease thrush.

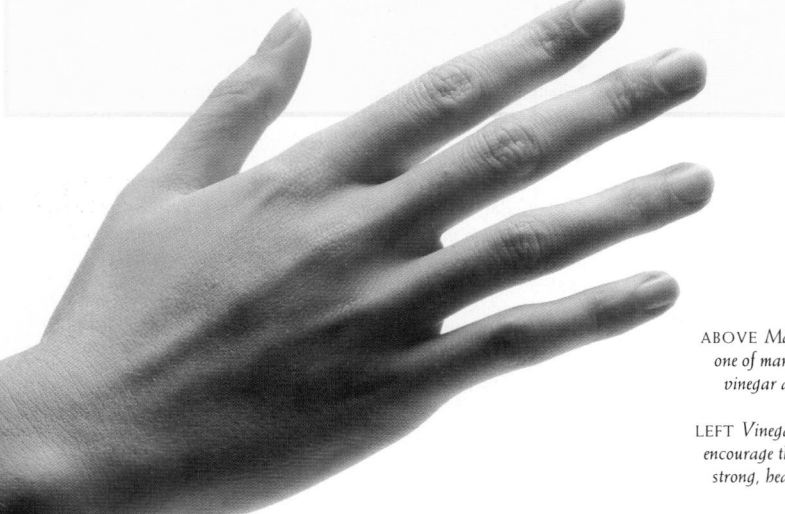

ABOVE *Malt vinegar is one of many types of vinegar available.*

LEFT *Vinegar can help to encourage the growth of strong, healthy nails.*

Hydrogen dioxide
WATER

Pure water is a clear, colorless liquid made up of oxygen and hydrogen. Water is the most common substance on the Earth's surface, covering more than 70 percent of the planet. It is also present in the atmosphere as a gas (water vapor or steam). Water is essential to life on Earth and constitutes a large part of most living things. Human beings are comprised of about 75 percent water. Water is necessary for maintaining the correct osmotic pressure in cells, and is needed for many other body processes, such as transporting nutrients and waste products around the body in the blood (blood is about 80 percent water). Water that has been cooled or heated to form ice, hot water, or steam can be used to treat minor complaints.

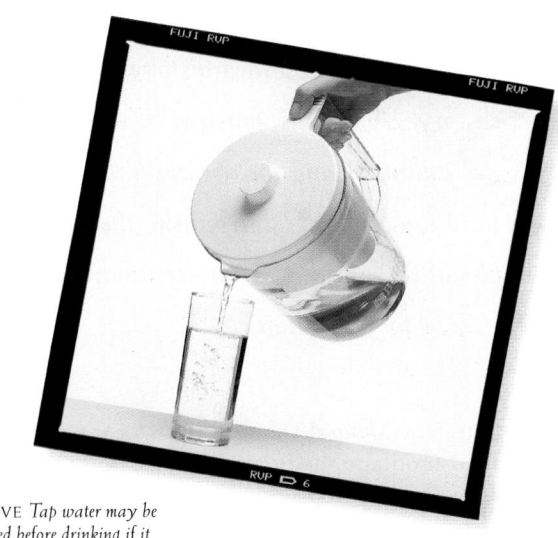

ABOVE *Tap water may be filtered before drinking if it is thought to contain a lot of impurities.*

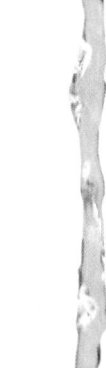

DATA FILE

Properties

- Essential for life
- Dilutes toxins in the body, and expels them
- A natural diuretic
- Salt water is antiseptic
- Aids kidney action
- Prevents constipation
- May contain some naturally occurring fluoride
- Prevents dehydration

Uses

- Drink plenty of fresh water if you suffer from edema.
- Drink water to counter the effects of a hangover, and during illness to encourage the expulsion of toxins. People who drink excessive amounts of alcohol or coffee, or who smoke, should drink at least eight glasses of water daily.

- It can help to prevent tooth decay when sufficient fluoride is present.
- Water acts as a diuretic and a mild laxative – it adds water to stools and may stimulate muscle contraction in the digestive tract.
- Hard water may play a role in preventing hypertension and heart disease.

- Ice reduces swellings and is particularly beneficial for sprains. Ice packs help to relieve backache.
- Cold compresses placed around the throat may ease an attack of croup.
- Children suffering from croup will get relief when placed in a steamy bathroom. This is best achieved by running the hot water faucet or the shower.
- Swallowing cracked ice may be beneficial in relieving morning sickness and motion sickness.
- A hot compress can help to reduce skin inflammations caused by infection. Dip a face cloth or other thick cloth in hot water and wring out before applying.
- Bathing in warm water can encourage relaxation. Hot baths may help to soothe muscular aches and pains. A cool bath can be soothing for sufferers of prickly heat.

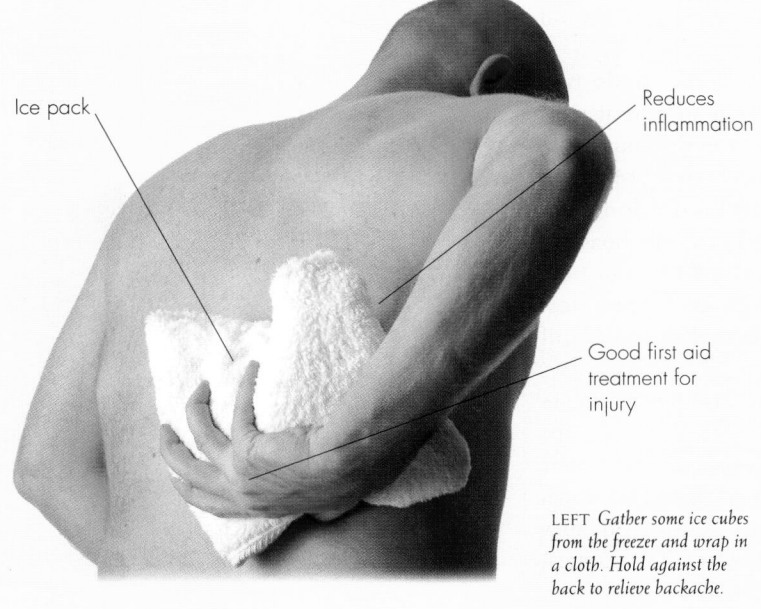

Ice pack

Reduces inflammation

Good first aid treatment for injury

LEFT *Gather some ice cubes from the freezer and wrap in a cloth. Hold against the back to relieve backache.*

CAUTION

WATER SHOULD BE FILTERED BEFORE IT IS DRUNK IF IT CONTAINS IMPURITIES.

BOTTLED MINERAL WATERS MAY BE HIGH IN SODIUM.

HERBALISM

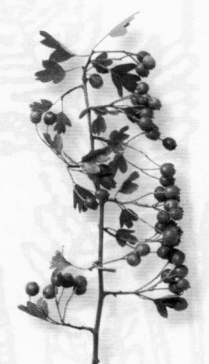

HAWTHORN
Hawthorn berries work to improve the functioning of the heart.

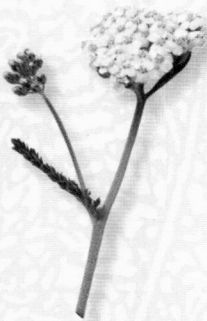

YARROW
Yarrow reduces fever, heals wounds, and lowers blood pressure.

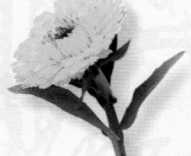

MARIGOLD
Calendula is antifungal, and treats wounds, burns, and indigestion.

*S*ince before recorded history humans have used plants for food, medicines, shelter, clothing, dyes, weapons, musical instruments, and transportation. The cultural development of different countries and the rise and fall of empires have often been linked to the understanding and exploitation of plants. Herbalism, the use of plants for medicinal purposes, has been common to all peoples of the world. Our understanding of herbalism has been passed down by word of mouth from generation to generation.

It is the most natural thing in the world to use local flora for food and medicine, and list this knowledge for posterity. All native cultures have a well-developed understanding of local plants, and most of the world, even today, relies on herbal expertise for its primary healthcare. Shamans, wise women, bush doctors, traditional healers, and native medicine workers carry on a tradition thousands of years old.

Herbalism is the oldest, most tested, and proven form of medicine in the world. The *Ebers Papyrus* of the ancient Egyptians lists 85 herbs, some of which, like mint, are used in a similar way today. The Chinese herbal, *Pen Tsao*, contains over a thousand herbal remedies. The Assyrian and Babylonian scribes wrote herbal recipes on clay tablets. The Greek Hippocrates (477–360 B.C.E) mentions herbs, remedies, and treatment stratagems which are still valid. Indeed, there is much practical and theoretical knowledge to be rediscovered. Globally, herbal lore is a treasure chest beyond price.

In the West, the Saxons wrote the *Leech Book of Bald*, a mixture of remedies and ritual. Their nine sacred herbs included yarrow, marigold, and hawthorn. A modern practitioner of herbal medicine would rate them equally highly. The golden age of herbals was precipitated by the development of the printing press. Culpeper printed the *London Dispensary* (1653) in English (it had previously been printed in Latin), and later published his *Complete Herbal* – a book, he boasted, from which any man (or woman) could find out how to cure themselves for less than three pennies! Culpeper's herbal was immensely popular and is still available, having gone through over 40 reprints.

Botanical medicine was regarded as fringe medicine for many years. It was valued as a starting place for modern research, but thought to have nothing to offer Western society as a therapy in itself. Pharmaceutical companies identified the active therapeutic principles of many plants, synthesized commercial analogues, and patented new drugs. But in doing so they often missed the major principles of using natural sources for therapeutic purposes. Herbalism, when practised properly, is marked by a completely different attitude from orthodox medicine. It is a holistic system that uses plants, or plant parts, in a nonintrusive way. Herbalists believe that the constituents of a plant work synergistically to stimulate the natural healing process.

THE TENETS OF HERBALISM

- ❧ The whole plant is better than an isolated extract.
- ❧ Treat the whole person not just the symptoms.
- ❧ Practise minimum effective treatment and minimum intervention.
- ❧ Strengthen the body and encourage it to heal itself.

Today there is a worldwide renaissance in therapeutic systems which use herbs as their major source of medicines. Modern science is validating traditional practices, precipitating a general reappraisal. Tibetan, Chinese, Native American, Indian, and Western systems are all examining their philosophical roots in a cross-cultural examination which is enriching to all. Many people now use herbs because they are felt to be safer, cheaper, more natural, and to have fewer side-effects. This is not always the case. Any substance can trigger an idiosyncratic response. Herbs must be given with knowledge and responsibility. But by following a few rules and using common sense, we add to our health, our sense of belonging, and our pleasure at being on the planet.

RIGHT *Really getting to know plants and the therapeutic actions of the remedies they provide is crucial to a sound practice of herbalism.*

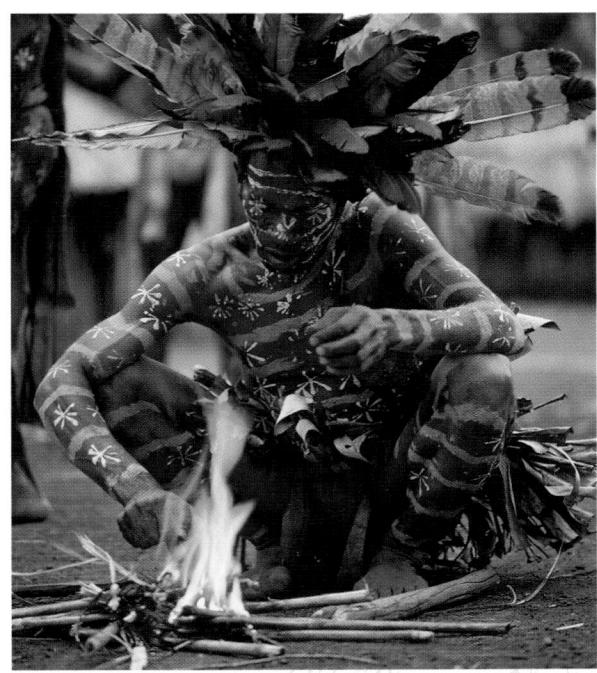

ABOVE *Native cultures have preserved the knowledge and practice of herbal treatments.*

THE TWO LEVELS IN MODERN HERBALISM

Modern herbalism is practised on two levels. These differ in the range of herbs which can be used, the results that can be achieved, and the amount of responsibility taken for treatment:

AS A PROFESSION

Western consultant medical herbalists act in just the same way as orthodox practitioners. They are trained in orthodox medical diagnosis and can provide a complete alternative. They also work with physicians to offer a complementary service. A medical herbalist will sometimes use some powerful herbs which are restricted by law, or only available after a personal consultation, in the same way as an orthodox practitioner will use prescription-only medicines. A good medical herbalist will have undergone extensive training and he or she will certainly belong to an established body of practitioners. (*For a list of organizations which keep a register of qualified herbal practitioners, see* Useful Addresses, *page* 487.)

AS A SELF-HELP SYSTEM

Herbs are ideal as a simple system of home care for first aid, everyday ailments, the management of chronic conditions, strengthening of the body, and preventive treatment. Herbs can be safely taken as long as a few simple rules are followed (*see* The Rules of Safe Home Treatment, *page* 106).

HERBALISM AND CONSERVATION

One hundred years ago, a person could have walked into the garden or local woods and returned with a remedy for the baby's gripe, a stomach ache, sprained ankle, stiffening gout, or any number of ailments. Today we can walk into the local store and find the shelves full of natural ingredients from all corners of the world – from carrots and cabbage to precious spices like cinnamon. This array would have been the envy of a medieval apothecary; but while the stock is available, the knowledge is scarce. The culture of responsibility, self-care, and interaction with nature has largely been lost. It must be rediscovered if herbs and their proper uses are to be properly understood.

A herb has a taste, color, smell, texture, and history. The antiseptic calendula lotion applied to a spot was once an orange marigold growing clear and open-faced in a sunny meadow. The lavender used to reduce the tension of a pounding headache and bring sleep once shimmered in a soporific violet-purple haze on a French mountainside. Such pictures are part of the heritage of healing, and help us to remember and understand the actions of herbs and the way they work within the body.

Part of the beauty of herbalism lies in the many different possible methods of taking herbs. The skill in choosing the best method for a specific individual and condition is part of the art of caring. Hand baths, foot baths, skin washes, rubs, massage oils, eye baths, compresses, and fomentations are undervalued. Local treatments allow the herb to act exactly where it is needed, avoid affecting the whole system, and are comforting and effective. Remember that in all herbal preparations it is best to use organic herbs.

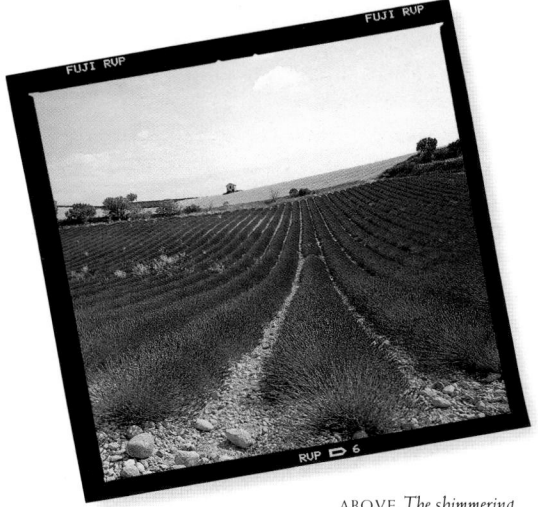

ABOVE *The shimmering violet-purple haze of a lavender field.*

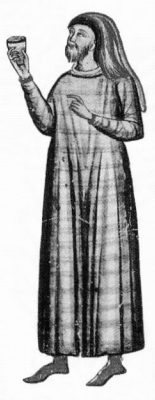
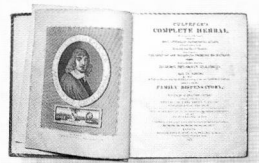
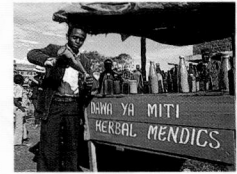

USING HERBS AT HOME

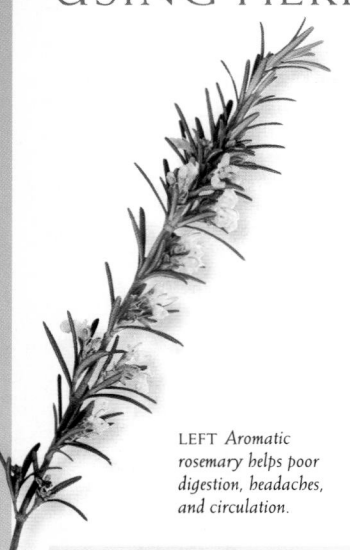

To be able to care for yourself and your family by making natural remedies is a pleasure, and the benefits are legion. The organic chemistry of remedy-making is an extension of cooking, and the same principles and skills apply. For success, use the best-quality ingredients, practise absolute cleanliness, and follow the instructions carefully.

It is important to remember that several herbs may be recommended for a particular ailment; all are slightly different. For example, would rose, lavender, rosemary, or chamomile be best for your headache? Would a cool compress be best, or a long soak in a rosemary bath? Knowledge of the herb, the individual, and the different methods must be combined to prescribe remedies that will be really effective.

LEFT *Aromatic rosemary helps poor digestion, headaches, and circulation.*

THE RULES OF SAFE HOME TREATMENT

🌿 Consider the whole body and person first. Is medication needed? Consider a change of rest, diet, or exercise before prescribing the patient any remedy.

🌿 Use simple remedies internally and externally. This will encourage the body to heal itself.

🌿 Make a list. Know what you are taking and what to expect. Keep a note of all remedies taken. This will be useful if you need help later.

🌿 Take as recommended. Remember the herbal tenet of minimum effective dosage and intervention. Stick to the standard dosages. Doubling does not double effectiveness; it may put an extra burden on a body that is already sick.

🌿 TLC. Use lots of Tender Loving Care. A positive and loving attitude helps to make the illness more bearable, and may even speed up the healing process.

🌿 Monitor progress after a few days.

🌿 Stop treatment if there is any adverse reaction.

Remember, people are all individuals; children, especially, respond quickly, so be alert for changes or new symptoms.

🌿 Seek professional help if in any doubt. Assessing your own symptoms is different from making a diagnosis, which needs an objective eye.

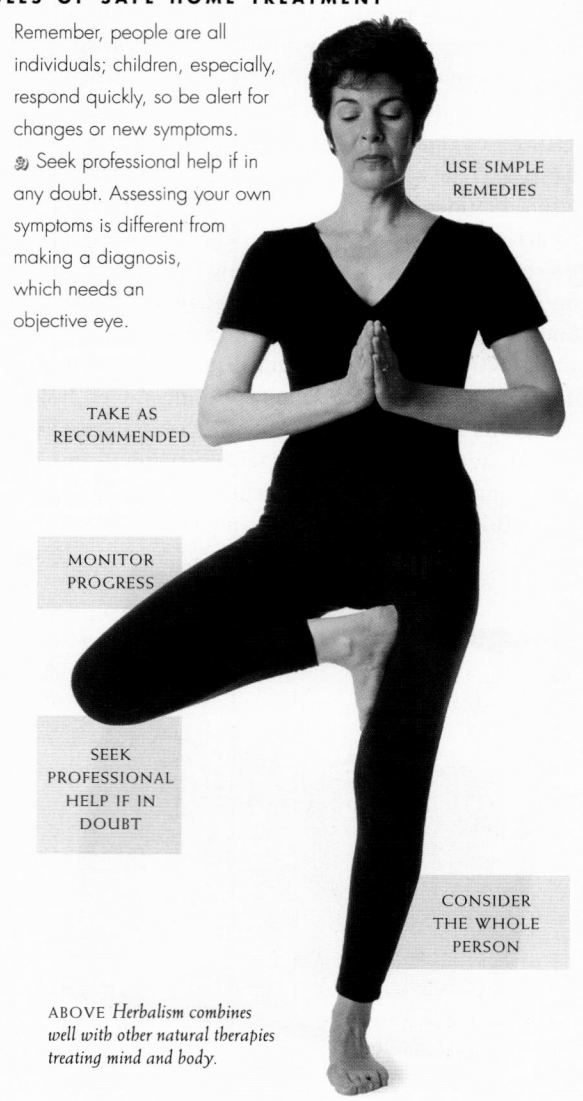

USE SIMPLE REMEDIES

TAKE AS RECOMMENDED

MONITOR PROGRESS

SEEK PROFESSIONAL HELP IF IN DOUBT

CONSIDER THE WHOLE PERSON

ABOVE *Herbalism combines well with other natural therapies treating mind and body.*

WHAT IS A HERB?

Herbage, like foliage, refers to plants with green leaves, but in herbal remedies more than leaves are used. Indeed, any part of a plant can be used:

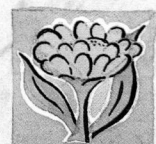

FLOWERS
Chamomile, marigold, linden, St. John's wort

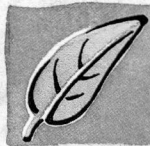

LEAVES
Peppermint, sage, thyme, comfrey

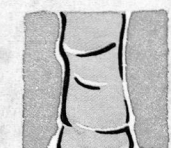

BARK
Willow, oak, cinnamon

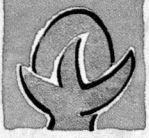

BUDS
Cloves

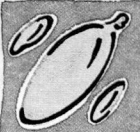

SEEDS
Fennel, cardamom

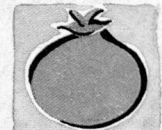

FRUITS
Cayenne, rose hips

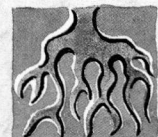

ROOT
Dandelion, marshmallow

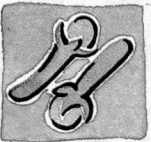

INNER SAP/GEL
Clove, Aloe Vera

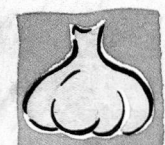

BULB
Garlic

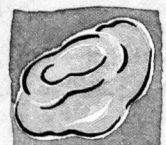

WOOD
Pau D'arco

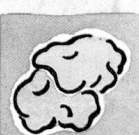

RESIN
Myrrh, frankincense

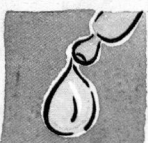

ESSENTIAL OIL
Rose, rosemary, lavender

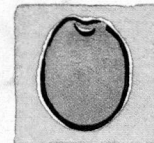

FIXED OIL
Olive oil, St. John's wort

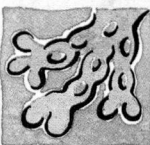

SEAWEED
Kelp, bladderwrack

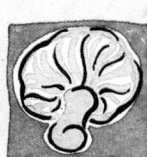

MUSHROOMS
Ganoderma (reishi), oyster

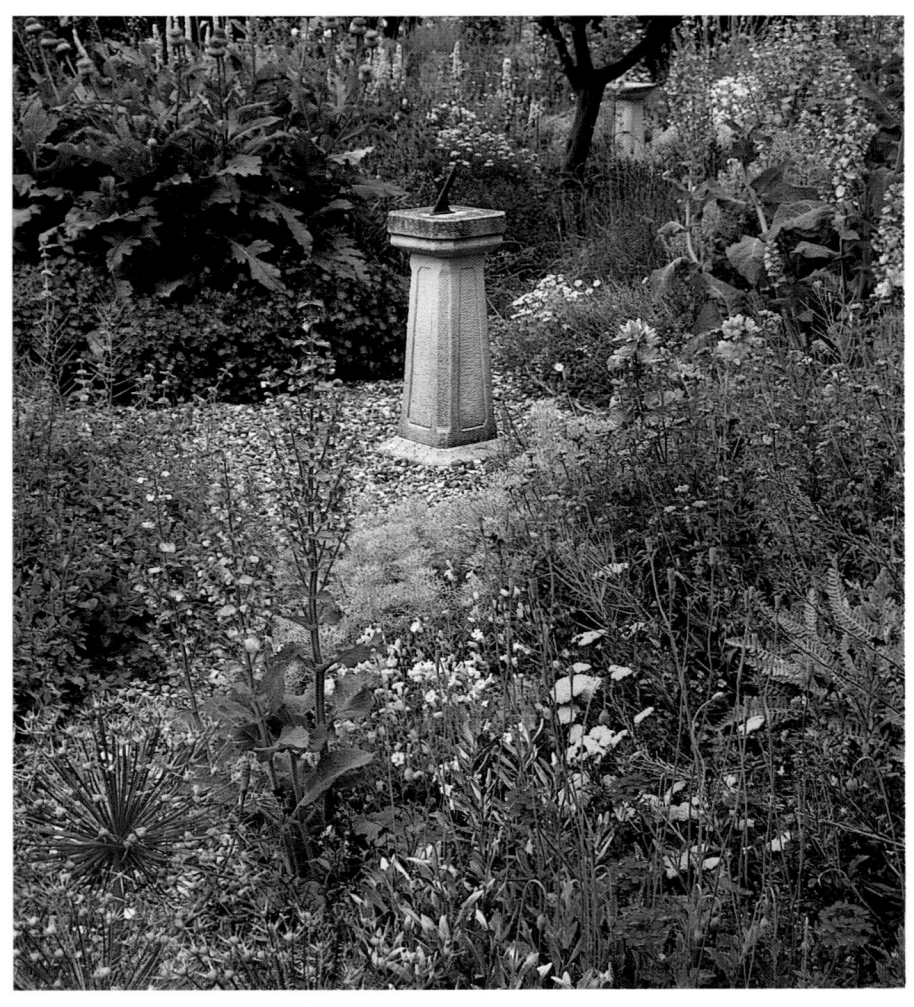

ABOVE *A dedicated herb garden close to the house is the best way to grow herbs.*

WHERE TO GET HERBS

❉ Many herbs and herbal products are freely available. Plants or seeds can be bought from garden centers (always check the Latin name) and grown in the garden or in a window-box.

❉ Dried herbs are available from herb stores and some wholefood outlets. Always specify the herb (the Latin name if possible) and the part of the plant to be used — root, bark, leaf, or flower.

❉ Herbal products, remedies, tinctures, tablets, etc. are available from wholefood stores, and some pharmacies and general food stores. Read the label and instructions carefully.

❉ Regarding plants picked from the wild, countries have different rules and some plants are protected by law. Check the legal situation and get permission from the landowner. Check identification carefully and pick the minimum required, with proper regard for conservation. Never gather roots from the side of the road, by recently sprayed crops or foliage, or from sick-looking plants.

PREPARATION

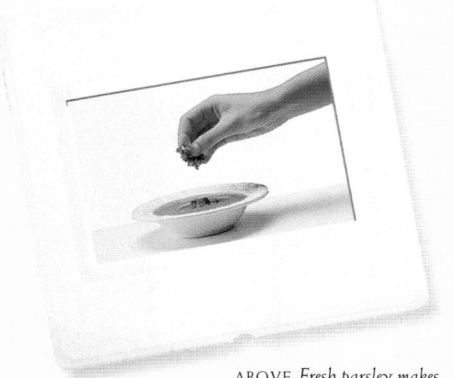

ABOVE *Fresh parsley makes a tasty addition to soup, and is high in vitamin C.*

THE FRESH PLANT

The easiest way to take a herb is to pick it directly from the plant.

Leaves can be used in salads, sandwiches, or soups. Chickweed, chicory, dandelion, and marigold make excellent salad additions. Nettle is traditional for green soup. Elderflower fritters are fun.

Chewing a few fresh leaves of marjoram will help clear the head. Horseradish leaves will clear sinuses. Sage eases mouth sores and sore throats.

Fresh leaves can also be used to make water infusions (teas), decoctions, tinctures, infused oils, and creams. Follow standard recipes and dosages. Most recipes give the amounts for dried herbs. When using fresh material add one-third more, as fresh plants contain a considerable amount of water.

IMMEDIATE RESPONSE

For cuts, grazes, and stings, pick four or five leaves (dock is traditional when stung on countryside walks as it is so readily available) and rub the leaves together between the hands to bruise them and release the juices. When damp, apply to the affected area and hold in place. Poultices can be made in the same way.

Rub together to release juices

Dock leaves

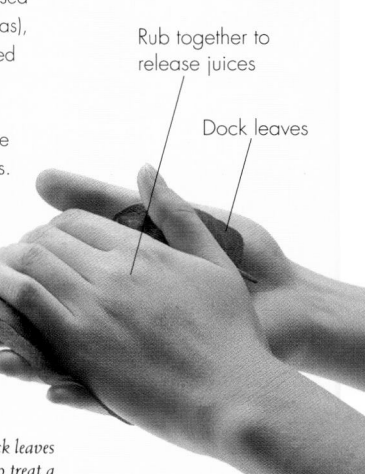

RIGHT *Dock leaves can be used to treat a sting. Bruise and apply.*

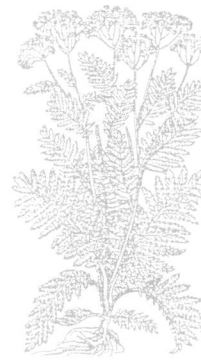

PREPARATIONS

Most herbs are sold in dried form. In this form they can simply be powdered and sprinkled on to food (half a flat teaspoon twice daily), but most are prepared further. Herbs are prepared for:

* AVAILABILITY AND PRESERVATION – so that seasonal plants are available all year round.
* CONVENIENCE, EASE OF USE – compressed tablets are often more convenient to take than a cup of tea.
* SPECIFIC USE, TO AID THE ACTION OF THE HERB – for example infused oils for rubs, honey for adding a soothing and demulcent quality to thyme.

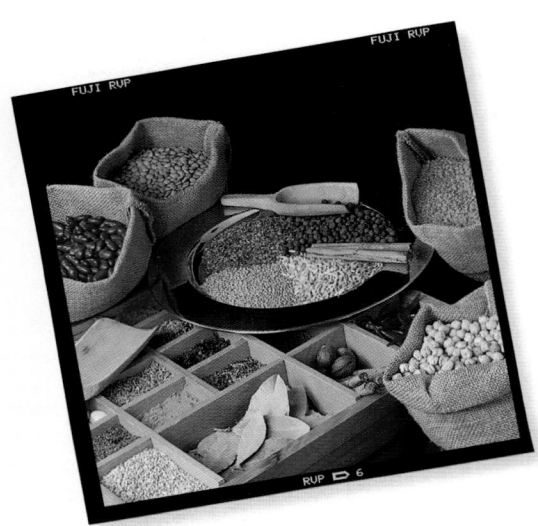

ABOVE *Dried herbs are most convenient for medicinal use, as they are readily available all year round.*

There are three main carriers for herbs, each of which adds a different quality:

* WATER – Infusions (teas). For flowers, leaves, some seeds, and fruit. Quickly assimilated and utilized by the body. Gentle for children, convalescents, and those with a delicate digestion. Ideal for diuretic, diaphoretic, cooling, and cleaning regimes. Decoctions are used for harder parts, like roots, and for stronger preparations.
* ALCOHOL – Tinctures and spiced wines. For all plant parts, especially hard parts. Alcohol adds some temporary heat and stimulation. It is convenient, although not for those intolerant of alcohol or for babies. Keeps indefinitely.
* OIL – Herbs infused in oil. For all parts of the plant. For rubs, massage oils, and liniments. Infused oils can be thickened with beeswax to make soothing and nourishing ointments and salves.

METHODS AND DOSAGES

WATER~INFUSIONS (TEAS)

STANDARD STRENGTH

1oz. (25g.) herb to 1pt. (500ml.) water; or 1 teaspoon herb to 1 cup water

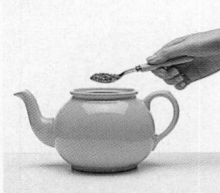

Use 1 teaspoon dried herb or (1½ teaspoon fresh) per cup required. Put the herb into a teapot.

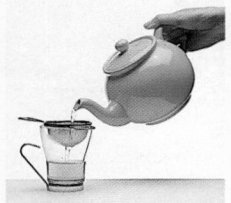

Pour on boiling water. Put on a tight lid. Brew for the required time (see below). Strain and use.

DOSE

Some herbs have specific indications and dosages; other herbs are not recommended at certain times, for example early pregnancy or when breast-feeding. Read the indications and contraindications of each herb carefully.

STANDARD ADULT DOSE

* 1 cup three times a day for normal conditions
* 1 cup up to six times a day, or every two hours, for acute conditions
* Drink 1 cup twice a day as a long-term strengthening tonic

CHILDREN'S DOSE

Reduce proportionally. Give a child of seven half the standard adult dose. At six months use 1 teaspoon of the standard strength tea. For breast-feeding infants give the remedy to the mother.

BREWING TIMES

To some extent this depends on personal taste, but the following is a good guide:

* up to 3 minutes for flowers and soft leaves
* up to 5 minutes for seeds and leaves
* up to 10 minutes for hard seeds, roots, and various barks

Water infusions at the standard strength are used as teas, gargles, as lotions for the skin, as compresses, and for fomentations. Dilute with an equal amount of water for hand or foot baths, douches, and enemas.

WATER~DECOCTIONS

STANDARD STRENGTH

* 1½oz. (40g.) herb to 1½pt. (750ml.) water

METHOD

* Put herb in saucepan
* Add 1½pt. (750ml.) water
* Put on a tight lid
* Bring to the boil, then turn down as low as possible and simmer for 10–15 minutes
* Strain thoroughly
* Discard herb
* Pour decoction into a clean bottle
* Will keep in a refrigerator for two or three days

DOSE

* ⅓ cup twice a day for normal conditions, and as a tonic
* ⅓ cup three to six times a day for acute conditions

Decoctions can be diluted with an equal amount of water and used in the same ways as water infusions for hand baths, gargles, etc.

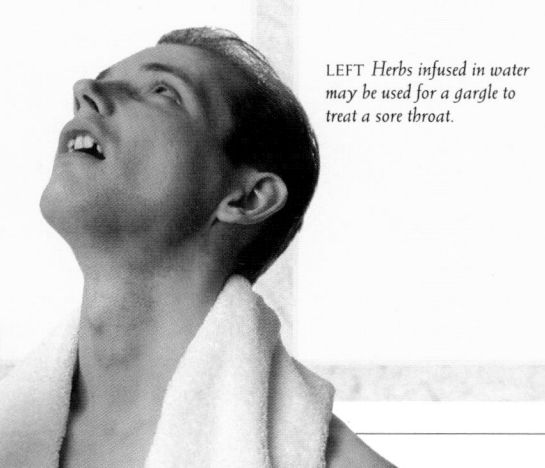

LEFT *Herbs infused in water may be used for a gargle to treat a sore throat.*

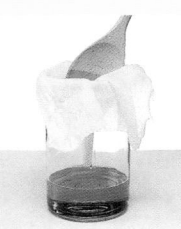

BEARBERRY

WATER~SIMPLE SYRUPS AND HONEYS

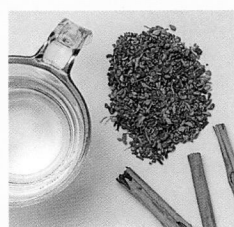

ABOVE *Ingredients for a laxative syrup: yellow dock root, cinnamon, and water.*

METHOD

🍃 Make standard decoction with 1½oz. (40g.) herb and 1½pt. (750ml.) water
🍃 Return to heat, remove lid, and simmer gently till liquid is reduced to ½pt. (250ml.), which may take a few hours
🍃 Add 1¼lb. (600g.) honey or 1lb. (500g.) sugar, stirring until completely dissolved
🍃 Pour into clean bottle, label, and date

STANDARD ADULT DOSE

🍃 1 dessertspoon 3 to 6 times a day

CHILDREN UNDER FIVE

🍃 1 teaspoon three times a day

Syrups and honeys can be used to sweeten other herbal preparations, or added to food or drink. They are ideal for children because they are sweet.

ALCOHOL~ TINCTURES

A tincture is an alcohol-based herbal preparation. Tinctures can be made with fresh or dried herbs. The absolute strength of the alcohol needed varies slightly depending on the herb, but the method given below is sufficient for standard home use.

METHOD

To make 9fl.oz. (300ml.) of tincture:
🍃 Chop ½oz. (12g.) dried or 1oz. (25g.) fresh herb
🍃 Put in large glass jar
🍃 Cover with 6fl.oz. (200ml.) alcohol, such as vodka or brandy, and 3fl.oz. (100ml.) water
🍃 Put on a lid and leave for two weeks
🍃 Shake occasionally
🍃 After 2 weeks, strain well through a muslin bag
🍃 Squeeze out the liquid
🍃 Pour into clean, amber glass bottle
🍃 Label and date
🍃 Keep in a cool place away from children
🍃 Will keep indefinitely

STANDARD ADULT DOSE

🍃 1 teaspoon 3 times a day, standard
🍃 5 drops to 1 teaspoon a day as a tonic
🍃 1 teaspoon 6 times a day for acute conditions

A tincture can be diluted with water: 1 dessertspoon to 1 cup water can be used as skin lotion, a wash, footbath, gargle, compress, or douche.

OIL~LINIMENT

A liniment is a soothing rub to relieve fatigued and stiff muscles and joints.

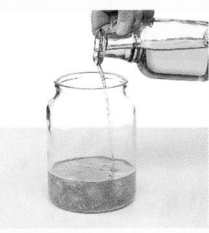

Put the fresh herb in a jar and cover with olive oil. Leave for up to 6 weeks.

Strain the mixture through a cloth. Stand until the oil separates off: use this.

RHUBARB ROOT

OIL

Oil is soothing and nourishing for the skin, and acts as a lubricant to carry the active principles of the herbs in rubs, massage oils, and salves. There are two methods of infusion, hot and cold. Hot is used for thyme, rosemary, comfrey root, and spices such as cayenne, mustard, and ginger.
Cold is used for flowers (see St. John's wort, step-by-step, page 124).

INFUSED OIL
METHOD

To make ½pt. (250ml.):
🍃 Chop 2–3oz. (50–75g.) dried herbs or spices, or 3–4oz. (75–100g.) fresh herbs
🍃 Put half into a clean pan with a lid

🍃 Cover with ½pt. (250ml.) pure vegetable oil (a pure and light vegetable oil is best).
🍃 Put in a water bath and simmer gently for 2 hours (it is important that direct heat is not used, as this might burn the oil)
🍃 Strain
🍃 Throw away used herbs
🍃 Put remaining half of unused herbs in pan
🍃 Cover these with the oil (it will have changed color, having picked up some of the quality of the herbs)
🍃 Replace lid and return pan to water bath for another couple of hours
🍃 Strain
🍃 Pour oil into clean bottles, label, and date

ALCOHOL~SPICED OR TONIC WINE

A good way to make a strengthening remedy for everyday use is to make a tonic wine. Spiced wines make good aperitifs, to stimulate and improve digestion.

METHOD

🍃 1oz. (25g.) herb(s)
🍃 1–2oz. (25–50g.) spices, depending on taste
🍃 4¼pt. (2l.) of wine
🍃 Stand for two weeks
🍃 Strain and bottle

DOSE

¼ cup twice a day before meals (warm water can be added)

This double method makes a strong infused oil which can be used as it is, mixed with tincture for a liniment, or thickened with beeswax (for a thin cream, use 1 part beeswax to 10 parts infused oil; for a thick salve, use 1 part beeswax to 5 parts infused oil).

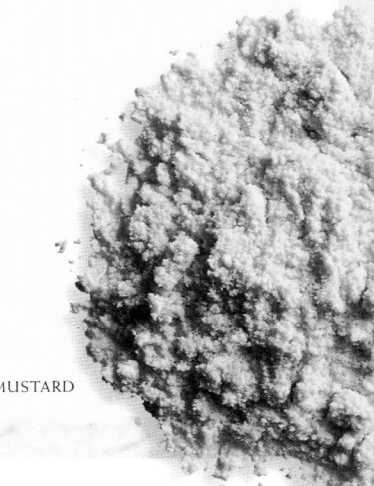

MUSTARD

THE REMEDIES

HERBAL REMEDY CARRIERS

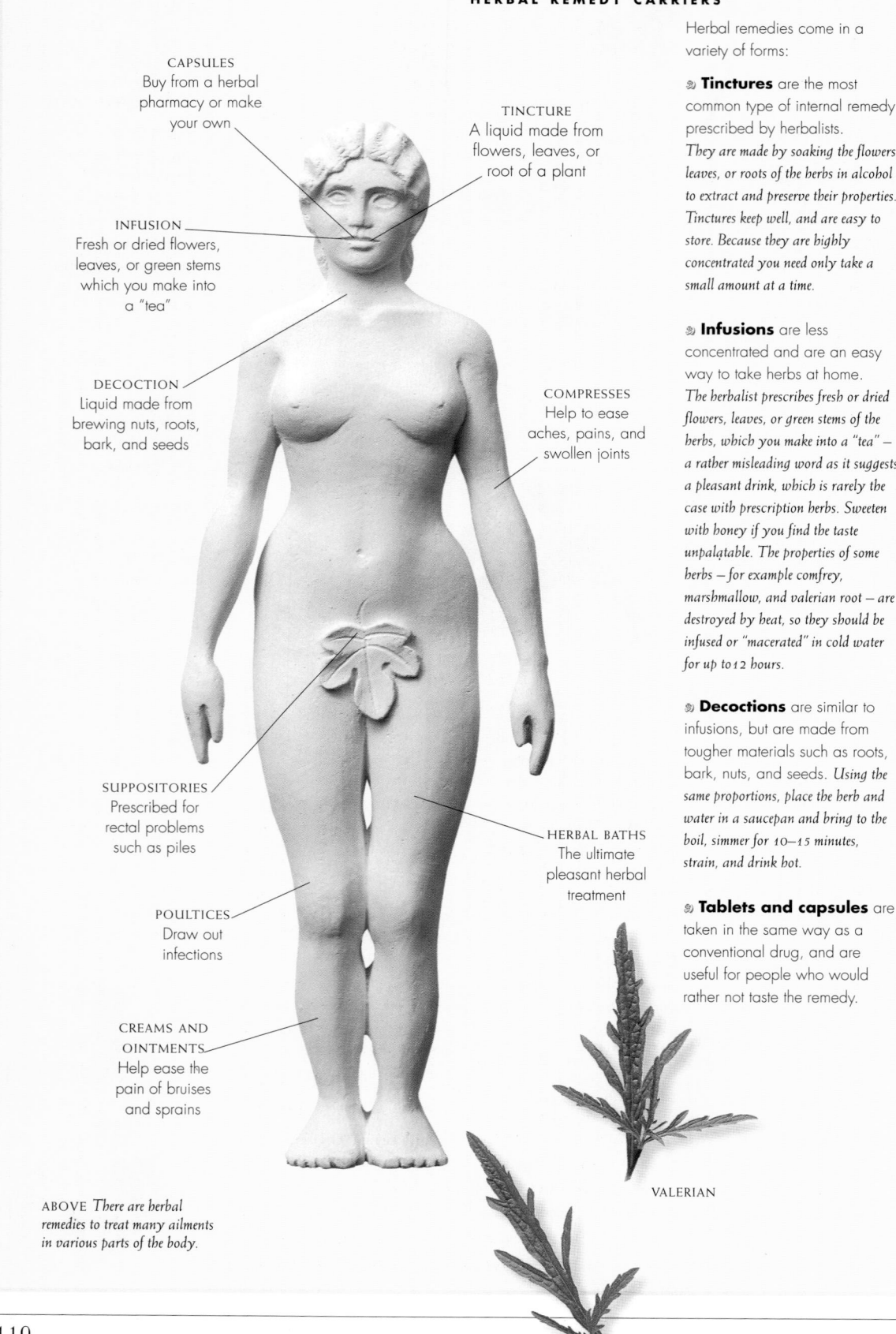

CAPSULES
Buy from a herbal pharmacy or make your own

TINCTURE
A liquid made from flowers, leaves, or root of a plant

INFUSION
Fresh or dried flowers, leaves, or green stems which you make into a "tea"

DECOCTION
Liquid made from brewing nuts, roots, bark, and seeds

COMPRESSES
Help to ease aches, pains, and swollen joints

SUPPOSITORIES
Prescribed for rectal problems such as piles

POULTICES
Draw out infections

CREAMS AND OINTMENTS
Help ease the pain of bruises and sprains

HERBAL BATHS
The ultimate pleasant herbal treatment

ABOVE *There are herbal remedies to treat many ailments in various parts of the body.*

VALERIAN

Herbal remedies come in a variety of forms:

Tinctures are the most common type of internal remedy prescribed by herbalists. *They are made by soaking the flowers, leaves, or roots of the herbs in alcohol to extract and preserve their properties. Tinctures keep well, and are easy to store. Because they are highly concentrated you need only take a small amount at a time.*

Infusions are less concentrated and are an easy way to take herbs at home. *The herbalist prescribes fresh or dried flowers, leaves, or green stems of the herbs, which you make into a "tea" — a rather misleading word as it suggests a pleasant drink, which is rarely the case with prescription herbs. Sweeten with honey if you find the taste unpalatable. The properties of some herbs — for example comfrey, marshmallow, and valerian root — are destroyed by heat, so they should be infused or "macerated" in cold water for up to 12 hours.*

Decoctions are similar to infusions, but are made from tougher materials such as roots, bark, nuts, and seeds. *Using the same proportions, place the herb and water in a saucepan and bring to the boil, simmer for 10–15 minutes, strain, and drink hot.*

Tablets and capsules are taken in the same way as a conventional drug, and are useful for people who would rather not taste the remedy.

Creams and ointments are applied externally to soothe irritated or inflamed skin conditions, or ease the pain of sprains or bruises. *Cream moistens dry or cracked skin, and massaging the ointment into bruises and sprains helps to ease the pain. In both cases the active ingredients of the herb pass through the pores of the skin into the blood stream to encourage healing.*

Compresses, either hot or cold, help with aches, pains, and swollen joints. *Fold a clean piece of cotton into an infusion of the prescribed herb and apply to the point of pain. Repeat as the compress cools or, in the case of cold compresses, until the pain eases.*

Poultices, made from bruised fresh herbs or dried herbs moistened into a paste with hot water, are also good for painful joints or drawing out infection from boils, spots, or wounds. *Place the herb on a clean piece of cotton and bandage on to the affected area. Leave in place for around two hours or until the symptoms ease.*

Suppositories and douches are sometimes prescribed for rectal problems such as piles, or vaginal infections, respectively. *The suppositories will come ready-made for you to insert. Douches are made from an infusion or decoction that has been allowed to cool.*

Herbal baths are perhaps the most pleasant of the herbal remedies, and are a useful supplement to other forms of treatment. *The heat of the water activates the properties of the volatile oils so that they are absorbed through the pores of the skin and inhaled through the nose. In both cases they pass into the bloodstream, and when inhaled they also pass through the nervous system to the brain, exerting a healing effect on both mind and body.*

SEEING A PROFESSIONAL

Professional consultant medical herbalists are usually trained in orthodox diagnosis and can treat all of the ailments treated by a family physician or general practitioner. Accredited members of organizations such as the National Institute of Medical Herbalists have undergone four years of university or university-standard study and two years of supervision. They will understand all the indications and contraindications of herbs, and any problems which may arise from taking orthodox drugs. They will refer to other specialists if necessary. (*For a list of organizations which keep a register of qualified herbal practitioners, see Useful Addresses, page 487.*)

It is becoming more common for a patient to register with a herbalist in the same way as one would register with a physician – for a check-up and then to be on the books should the need arise. Such patients have yearly checks to maintain optimum health. Whole families register, as herbalism is especially suited to children and the elderly.

A consultation will take about an hour and consider all aspects of health, diet, exercise, and lifestyle. Your herbalist will take a "holistic" view, which means taking into consideration everything that affects your health on a physical, mental, and spiritual level.

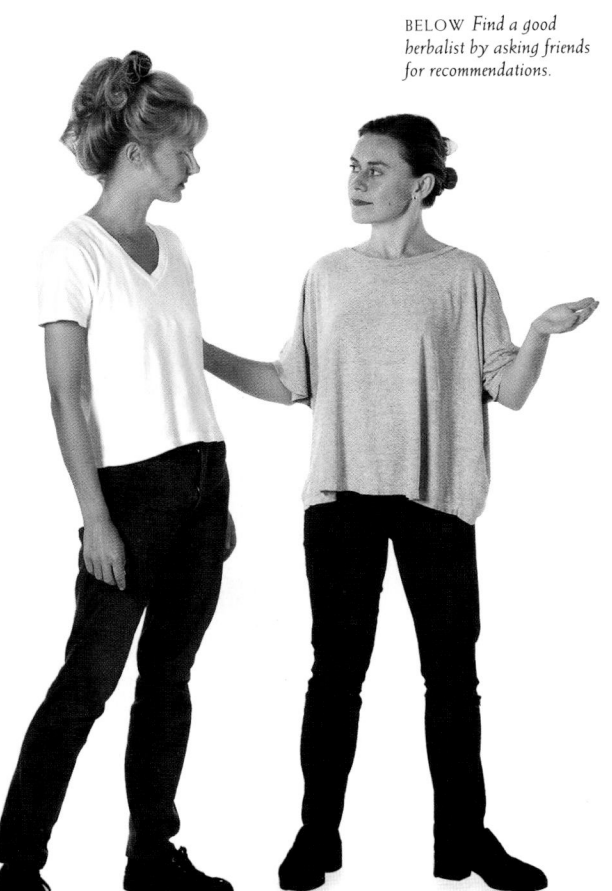
BELOW *Find a good herbalist by asking friends for recommendations.*

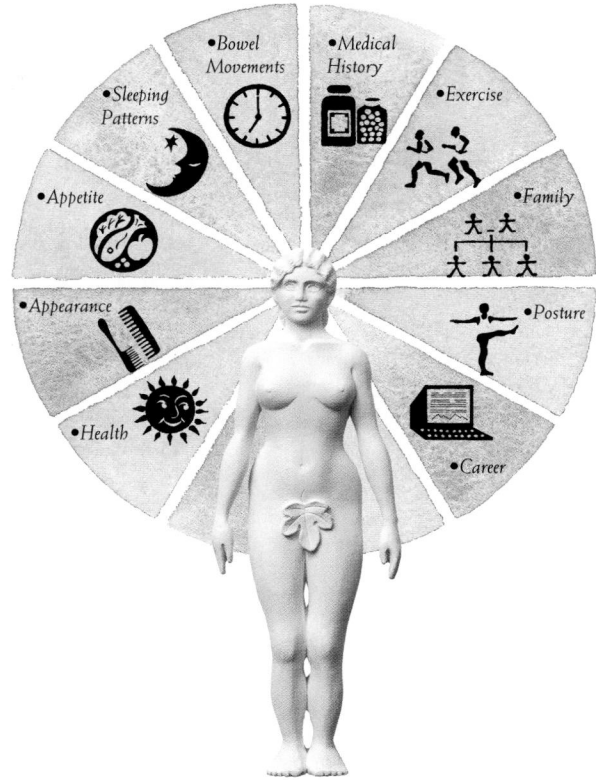
ABOVE *A consultation with a herbalist will cover a range of areas.*

You will be asked questions about:
age ❧ career ❧ personality and what is important to you ❧ concerns ❧ appetite ❧ sleeping patterns ❧ previous medicines and illnesses ❧ bowel movements ❧ family ❧ symptoms ❧ any other aspect that is relevant.

As well as what you say, your therapist will want to know how you feel and will note your appearance. The condition of your hair, skin, and facial expression, your posture, and how you move all provide important clues that will help with the diagnosis. There may also be a physical examination. Treatment will then be prescribed by the therapist.

Before a first visit it is worth spending some time considering your health and your expectations. It is useful to make a list of relevant points in your medical history and questions you want to ask, as these can easily be missed or forgotten in the stress of a first meeting. If for any reason you do not get on with the practitioner, try another one. It is important that there is a relationship of mutual trust and respect.

Many of the herbs prescribed will be familiar, but some will be unknown to you. After a consultation, a herbalist is able to prescribe herbs which are limited by law and not freely available over the counter to the general public.

WHO CAN IT HELP?

Every member of the family can benefit from herbal treatments.

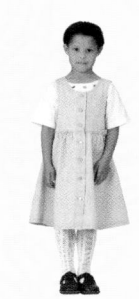
CHILDREN
Children respond especially well to herbal remedies.

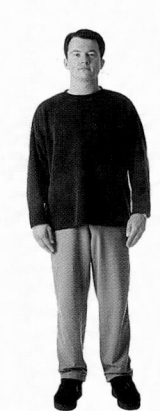
ADULTS
More and more people favor a return to natural treatments.

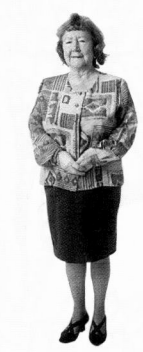
THE ELDERLY
Older people welcome the opportunity to cut down on prescribed drugs.

HERBAL REMEDY SOURCES

Achillea millefolium
YARROW

A common wild plant with feathery leaves and white or pink flowers. Often found on lawns. In Greek myth, *achillea* is said to have been used by Achilles to treat his army's wounds.

DATA FILE

Properties
- Diaphoretic
- Anti-inflammatory
- Antiseptic
- Antispasmodic
- Styptic
- Gentle bitter tonic

Uses
- Early stages of fevers, especially with hot, dry skin.
- Catarrh, sinusitis, hay fever, and dust allergies.
- For high blood pressure, with hawthorn and linden.
- With a little ginger for cold feet.
- Internal and external use for varicose veins and spontaneous bruising.
- Useful for thrombosis, to prevent blood clots.
- Supportive for people undergoing radiotherapy and intestinal infections.
- Diarrhea, liverishness, colic, and weak digestion.
- Irregular menstrual bleeding, cramps, and vaginal discharges.
- Helps pelvic circulation.
- With sage and marigold for pelvic infections and pelvic congestion with menstrual cramps, and pain before menstruation.
- Tea or tincture to disinfect wounds and stop bleeding.
- As a cream or compress for bleeding piles.
- Apply the infused oil to inflammations associated with varicose veins.
- In the bath to relieve aches and pains.

THERAPY CONNECTIONS

YARROW
- Ayurveda   *p.24*

AGRIMONY
- Flower Remedies   *p.225*

GARLIC
- Ayurveda   *p.26*
- Traditional Home and Folk Remedies   *p.82*

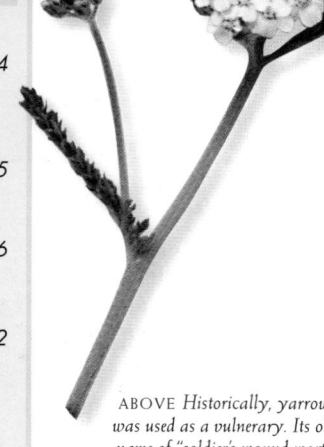

ABOVE *Historically, yarrow was used as a vulnerary. Its old name of "soldier's wound wort" gives a clue to this.*

NOTES AND DOSAGES

- **Standard doses** *(see pages 108–9)*. **Take freely for fevers and acute complaints.**

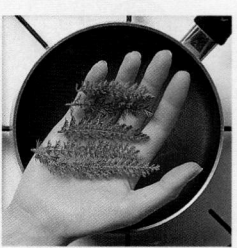

- For a bath, simmer a handful of fresh leaves in 1pt. (500ml.) water for 15 minutes.
- Strain and add to your bath water.
- Chew a fresh leaf and apply to cuts to stop bleeding.
- Wash fresh root and chew for toothache.
- It is said that one famous herbalist, when asked for suggestions for various ailments, said, "Go to bed with Yarrow tea and a hot brick." Yarrow is very versatile. The tea is excellent, on its own, for all feverish conditions, and can be mixed with other herbs, such as elderflower and peppermint, to treat colds and flu.

CAUTION

AVOID LARGE DOSES IN PREGNANCY. SMALL AMOUNTS ARE SAFE, BUT IF IN DOUBT CONSULT A PROFESSIONAL HERBALIST.

SOME PEOPLE DEVELOP AN ALLERGIC RASH IF THEY HANDLE THE FRESH HERB IN SUNLIGHT.

Agrimonia eupatoria
AGRIMONY

A common wild plant with slender spikes of bright yellow flowers. The whole herb is used. Culpeper recommended it for gout "used outwardly in an oil or ointment, or inwardly, in a syrup or juice."

RECIPE

Agrimony Digestive Tonic

Combine equal parts of agrimony, raspberry leaf, and lemon balm *(Melissa officinalis)*. Store away from the light. Make a tea from 1 teaspoon of the mixture to 1 cup of boiling water, and drink freely for colicky pains with looseness and nervous diarrhea.

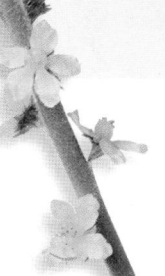

DATA FILE

Properties
- Astringent and tonic
- Tones and strengthens the digestive system and liver
- A wound herb

Uses
- As a tea or tincture for indigestion, heartburn, diarrhea, and liverish feelings. Especially helpful for people suffering from food allergies – on a long-term basis.
- With St. John's wort and horsetail for bedwetting and chronic cystitis.
- As a lotion for the cleansing of wounds.
- As an eyewash for sore and inflamed eyes.

NOTES AND DOSAGES

- Standard doses *(see pages 108–9)*.
- **Agrimony makes a tasty substitute for ordinary tea.**

ABOVE *The word "agrimony" comes from a Greek word describing plants which heal the eyes.*

CAUTION

MAY AGGRAVATE CONSTIPATION, BUT OTHERWISE A SAFE AND GENTLE HERB TO USE.

Alchemilla vulgaris

LADY'S MANTLE

A wild plant of wayside and meadows. Grows well in shady gardens, and bears sprays of greenish-yellow flowers.

CAUTION

DO NOT USE IN PREGNANCY EXCEPT UNDER PROFESSIONAL GUIDANCE, BUT OTHERWISE A SAFE HERB.

ALWAYS SEEK MEDICAL ADVICE FOR BLEEDING IN MID-MENSTRUAL CYCLE.

DATA FILE

Properties

- Astringent
- Tones and strengthens the womb

Uses

- Heavy menstrual bleeding, either alone or with an equal part of shepherd's purse or yarrow. Also for bleeding in the middle of the menstrual cycle and for irregular menstruation.

- To prevent menstrual cramps and for PMS, taken during the second half of the menstrual cycle.

- Thrush and other vaginal discharges, taken as a tea or douche.

- Traditional treatment for infertility in women with no obvious cause.

- Children's diarrhea.

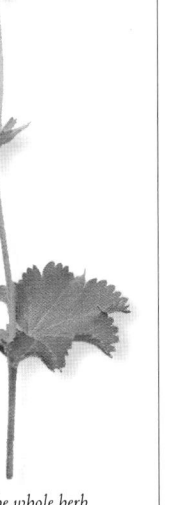

ABOVE *The whole herb is gathered when the plant is in flower.*

RECIPE

Lady's Mantle and Chamomile Wash

Make a strong tea with 1 cup of boiling water to 1 teaspoon of lady's mantle and 2 teaspoons of chamomile flowers. Infuse in a covered vessel for 15 minutes. Use this as a soothing wash for itchy genitals, in men and women.

NOTES AND DOSAGES

- Standard doses. It is a pleasant drinking tea.

Allium sativum

GARLIC

The familiar cooking herb. Garlic can be harvested about six to eight months after planting, in the summer. Bulbs not needed immediately can be dried in the sun and stored.

DATA FILE

Properties

- Antiseptic
- Antibiotic
- Expectorant
- Fungicide
- Antihistamine
- Lowers blood pressure and cholesterol

Uses

- Beneficial in cases of thrombosis, hardening of the arteries, high blood pressure, and high cholesterol.

- For chest infections, asthma, flu, colds, and ear infections. Combines well with echinacea.

- For intestinal worms and fungal infections.

ABOVE RIGHT *The active properties of garlic are due to its volatile oil.*

CAUTION

SAFE TO USE BUT MAY BE TOO HOT FOR SOME CONSTITUTIONS, IN WHICH CASE USE WITH MILK.

ENTERIC-COATED TABLETS ARE AVAILABLE. THESE ARE EASIER ON THE DIGESTION.

RECIPE

Garlic or Onion Milk

Put 1 onion or 3 cloves of garlic, thinly sliced, into a pan with 2 cups of milk (cow's, goat's, sheep's, soy milk, or nut milk). Simmer over a very low heat for 20 minutes. Strain. Can be stored in a refrigerator for 2 or 3 days. *Dose:* Infants 1 or 2 dessertspoons every four hours. Young children can drink freely if feverish and croupy.

NOTES AND DOSAGES

- Tablets are easy to take. Follow the instructions on the box. **Mix chopped garlic with an equal amount of honey and take 1 teaspoon 3 to 6 times daily. Half dose for children.** The infused oil can be applied to the skin, ear, and chest, to fight infections. **Regular dietary use benefits the circulation.**

- Garlic is an exceptional respiratory disinfectant, but it is often too strong for young children. **Onions and leek are in the same family and have similar but milder actions.** Onion or garlic milk is an ideal remedy for infants and small children.

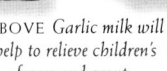

ABOVE *Garlic milk will help to relieve children's fevers and croup.*

Aloe vera
ALOE VERA

A succulent, tropical plant that has been used for centuries to heal both externally and internally. Aloes are resistant to drought, taking in water very easily and losing moisture very slowly.

DATA FILE

Properties
- Soothing
- Cooling
- Antiseptic
- Antifungal

Uses
- Applied to burns and sunburn, ringworm, infected cuts, acne, shingles, eczema, wrinkles, and areas of dry, itchy skin.
- Use as a mouthwash for sore gums.
- As an internal medicine for candidiasis (thrush).

NOTES AND DOSAGES

Aloes are easily grown as a house plant. Cut the leaf and apply the gel directly to the skin, or take 1 tablespoon, twice daily, as an internal medicine. The cut leaves will keep and can be used again. There are many excellent preparations of aloe in the stores — follow the instructions on the packet.

The fresh aloe is unsurpassed for burns, irritable rashes, and sunburn. Keep some in the freezer for immediate use.

CAUTION

THE GEL IS SAFE, BUT PREPARATIONS OF THE WHOLE LEAF ARE STRONGLY LAXATIVE AND SHOULD NOT BE USED FOR LONG PERIODS OR IN PREGNANCY.

LEFT *Grow aloe inside, in a sunny position with a minimum temperature of 10°C (50°F).*

RECIPE
Aloe Gel

Wash the leaves. Cut into 2in. (5cm.) lengths. Slice each piece in half, to expose the largest amount of gel. Wrap each piece in plastic wrap and date. To use: remove plastic and apply the gel side of the leaf to the skin; smear over the affected area, or hold in place with a bandage.

Althea officinalis
MARSHMALLOW

A wild plant easily grown in gardens. Use the root and leaves. It grows up to 4ft. (1.5m.) tall, with pale pink flowers. Its name comes from the Greek word *altho,* meaning "to cure."

DATA FILE

Properties
- Soothing
- Mucilaginous

Uses
- For acid stomach, heartburn, ulcers, hiatus hernia, and irritable bowel.

- Helps nonproductive and dry coughs.
- Irritable bladder.
- Dry skin, taken as a tea.
- Powdered root mixed into a cream or added to water to make a paste for insect bites and weeping eczema.

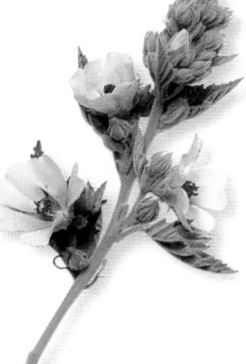

LEFT AND BELOW
Marshmallow leaves and root are used. Both have a high mucilage (a glutinous substance) content.

NOTES AND DOSAGES

Can be taken freely. For best results soak 1oz. (25g.) cut root or leaf in 1pt. (500ml.) cold water overnight. Strain and drink 3 cups daily.

RECIPE
Marshmallow Paste

THIS IS AN ESPECIALLY EFFECTIVE PREPARATION FOR INSECT BITES AND STINGS.

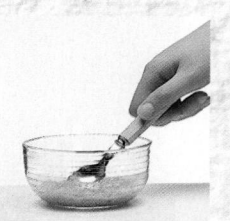

Take enough marshmallow root powder to cover the affected area, and add cold water to make a stiff paste.

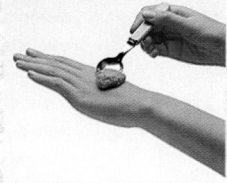

Apply thickly and allow to dry. Wash off and replace the paste every 2 or 3 hours.

Angelica archangelica and *Angelica sinensis*

ANGELICA ROOT

A tall, stately plant, popular in large gardens. The root should be dug up in the fall of the plant's first year, dried quickly, and stored in an airtight container. It will retain its medicinal properties for several years.

RECIPE

Candied Angelica

Cut the stems into 1in. (2.5cm.) lengths and simmer in sugar water until they are soft. Strain. Simmer in a sugar syrup (1lb. [500g.] sugar in ½pt. [250ml.] water) for an hour. Strain and allow to dry. Sprinkle with confectioner's sugar and store in an airtight tin. Dose: 2in. (5cm.) strip every few hours.

DATA FILE

Properties

- Warming and restorative
- Antiseptic
- Diuretic
- Diaphoretic
- Expectorant
- Relaxes spasm and strengthens digestion
- An excellent general tonic for those run down by chronic disease

Uses

- Tincture or decoction for convalescence, persistent fevers, indigestion, and weak digestion in general, colic and cramping pains, coughs, poor circulation, and general weakness with feelings of cold.
- Chinese angelica (Dang gui or *Angelica sinensis*) is an especially good tonic for women. In China it is called the "women's ginseng." It is used for menstrual cramps and pains, anemia, and general debility in women.

THERAPY CONNECTIONS

ALOE VERA

Ayurveda		p.27

ANGELICA

Ayurveda		p.28
Chinese Herbal Medicine		p.55
Aromatherapy		p.146

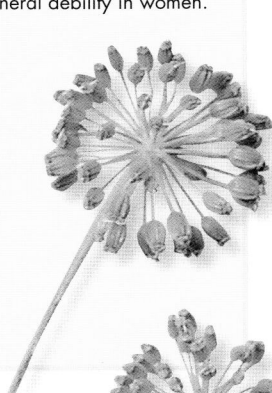

ABOVE *Angelica archangelica bears large umbels of yellow flowers from late spring to summer.*

CAUTION

ANGELICA ROOT IS CONTRAINDICATED IN DIABETES, AS IT INCREASES THE SUGAR LEVEL IN THE BLOOD.

AVOID LARGE DOSES IN PREGNANCY, EXCEPT AS ADVISED BY A QUALIFIED HERBALIST.

THE AMOUNTS TAKEN IN FOOD ARE HARMLESS.

SOME PEOPLE'S SKINS ARE SENSITIVE TO HANDLING THE FRESH PLANT.

NOTES AND DOSAGES

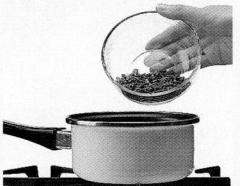

- Decoct 1oz. (30g.) of the root to 1pt. (500ml.) of water and take 2 or 3 times daily, or take up to ½ teaspoon (1–2ml.) diluted in water 3 times a day.
- **Crystallizing angelica preserves its fresh qualities for winter. When chewed it soothes the throat, and warms the chest and digestion.**

Arctium lappa or *Arctium minus*

BURDOCK

A common wayside plant with large leaves and purple flowers. The root is commonly used. Combined with yellow dock and sarsaparilla, it treats eczema.

NOTES AND DOSAGES

- Take 2 teaspoons of dried root, decocted, daily, or 1 teaspoon of the tincture twice daily for some months. For lack of appetite take the tincture 3 times daily, before meals, in a little water or fruit juice, 5–10 drops for children and 20 drops for adults.

Pickled burdock root makes a good daily tonic, digestive, and blood strengthener. It is a useful way to use the roots after weeding.

ABOVE *Burdock has large wavy leaves and round heads of purple flowers.*

CAUTION

LARGE DOSES MAY CAUSE A CLEANSING RASH. IT IS BEST TO START WITH SMALL DOSES AND THEN SLOWLY INCREASE THEM.

AVOID IN EARLY PREGNANCY EXCEPT WITH EXPERT ADVICE.

DATA FILE

Properties

- Blood cleanser
- Alterative
- Diuretic
- Lymphatic cleanser

Uses

- For "eruptive" and stubborn skin conditions, especially when hot and inflamed-looking – for example acne, spots, boils, rashes, psoriasis, rheumatism, and gout.
- With dandelion root for skin and liver problems.
- Chronic cystitis and loss of appetite.

RECIPE

Pickled Burdock Root

Wash the root and cut into small rounds. Simmer in water until soft. Strain and put into a clean jar. Pour hot cider vinegar over the root. Label and date. Dose: As a tonic chew a piece first thing every morning. As a digestive, chew a piece 20 minutes before your meals.

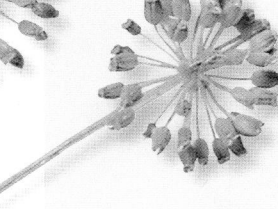

Arctostaphylos uva-ursi
UVA URSI LEAVES

A small evergreen shrub of moors and mountains, also known as bearberry. The leaves are astringent and have a high tannin content.

DATA FILE

Properties
- Diuretic
- Urinary antiseptic
- Astringent

Uses
- For cystitis, together with soothing herbal remedies such as marshmallow.
- With horsetail or nettle for irritable bladder with persistent frequency.
- With lady's mantle or shepherd's purse for thick, white vaginal discharges.
- Take along with agrimony for diarrhea.

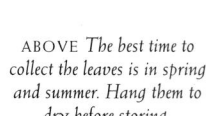

ABOVE *The best time to collect the leaves is in spring and summer. Hang them to dry before storing.*

CAUTION

DO NOT USE DURING PREGNANCY OR BREAST-FEEDING, OR DURING KIDNEY DISEASE.

DO NOT USE FOR MORE THAN TWO WEEKS WITHOUT CONSULTING A PROFESSIONAL HERBALIST.

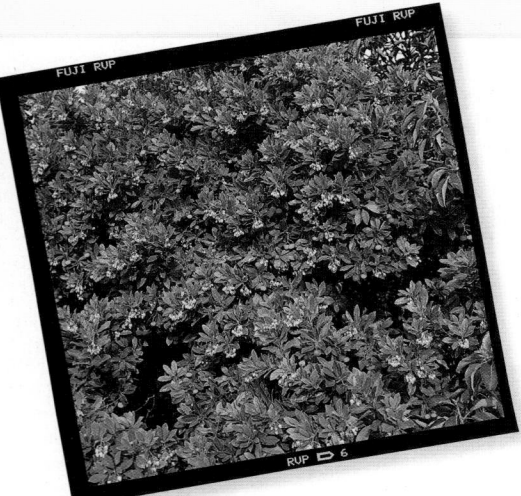

ABOVE *Bearberry leaves can be collected all year round, but are best in spring and summer.*

NOTES AND DOSAGES

For tea, use 1 teaspoon dried leaves to 1 cup water and infuse for 10 minutes. **For acute cystitis, take 1 cup of tea, or 1 teaspoon of tincture, 2 or 3 times daily for up to a week.** Take in combination with the suggested herbs for long-term use.

RECIPE
Tincture of Bearberries

Fill a jamjar with fresh or dried bearberries. Pour vodka over the berries until they are well covered. Store in a cool place for three weeks. Shake well every few days. Strain and store in a dark bottle. Dose: 30 drops. Use for bladder and intestinal infections. Blueberries or cranberries can also be used.

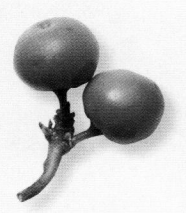

BEARBERRIES

Astragalus membranaceus
ASTRAGALUS

A herbaceous perennial plant of the pea family. The root is used for therapeutic purposes.

NOTES AND DOSAGES

Standard doses (*see pages 108–9*). Called Huang Qi. **The root can be bought in Chinese herb stores.** It is often used as a soup stock with other nourishing herbs for people with severe immune deficiencies.

Immune-enhancing soups can be made using astragalus root, which has a mild, sweet taste.

ABOVE *Dried astragalus root, sold in Chinese herb stores as Huang Qi. Use for decoctions.*

CAUTION

A SAFE HERB FOR HOME USE, BUT SEVERELY DEBILITATED PATIENTS SHOULD ALWAYS BE SEEN BY A PROFESSIONAL HERBALIST, WHO WILL PRESCRIBE ACCORDING TO THE INDIVIDUAL'S CONDITION AND CIRCUMSTANCES.

ALWAYS TELL THE HOSPITAL IF YOU ARE TAKING HERBAL MEDICINE IN CONJUNCTION WITH THEIR TREATMENT.

DATA FILE

Properties
- Helps to strengthen the immune system
- A famous Chinese tonic

Uses
- Decoction or tincture for chronic fatigue, persistent infections, night sweats, multiple allergies, and glandular fever.
- Modern research shows that the herb helps to counteract tiredness and lack of appetite in patients undergoing chemotherapy and radiotherapy for cancer.
- Soothing and healing for stomach ulcers.

RECIPE
Immune-enhancing Soup

Put 1oz. (25g.) of the chopped root in a pan. Simmer for one hour in 1pt. (500ml.) of water. Use as a stock for vegetable soups or for cooking brown rice. Take this every day. The soup has a mild, sweet taste that goes well with a range of vegetables.

Calendula officinalis
MARIGOLD FLOWERS

A popular garden plant with orange or yellow flowers. Do not confuse it with French and African marigolds (*Tagetes* species), which must not be taken internally.

NOTES AND DOSAGES

🌿 Add 2 or 3 flowers to 1 cup of boiling water. Infuse for 10 minutes. Drink 3 cups a day, or 1 cup every 3 hours for acute complaints. Half dose for children over five years old. Give infants 3 or 4 teaspoons of a weak tea in fruit juice.

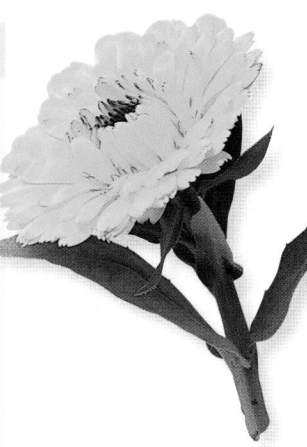

ABOVE *Calendula-infused oil helps cradle cap. Add a few teaspoonsful to the bath, for dry skin.*

DATA FILE

Properties

🌿 Lifts the spirits

🌿 Antispasmodic

🌿 Antiseptic

🌿 Antifungal

🌿 Healing and anti-inflammatory

Uses

🌿 Digestive colic, stomach, and duodenal ulcers.

🌿 Speeds post-operative healing, reduces adhesions.

🌿 Children's infections and fevers; as a gargle for sore throats, and tonsillitis.

🌿 Wash, cream, or compress for boils, spots, inflamed wounds, painful varicose veins, leg ulcers, sore nipples in nursing mothers, and sore eyes.

🌿 Douche or bath for thrush and vaginal infections.

🌿 Lotion or cream for itchy skin rashes, grazes, cuts, broken chilblains, eczema, and fungal infections.

🌿 Ideal first-aid remedy.

RECIPE
Marigold Tincture
🌿 🌿 🌿 🌿

Also sold as calendula lotion. Compresses and fomentations: 1 dessertspoon tincture to 1 cup water. Dip cloth into water, wring out. Use cold water to soothe and draw heat, for sprains, congestive pain, and hot joints. Use hot water (compress is called a fomentation) to relax and encourage circulation. For spasm, stiffness, and cold joints. Wrap around affected part. Cover.

Avena futua
WILD OATS

A wild grass, and the origin of cultivated oats (*Avena sativa*). The whole plant (called oat straw) is used, picked while still green. Cultivated oats may be substituted. Groats, or oat grains, may be substituted, although they are not quite as good.

DATA FILE

Properties

🌿 Nourishing and restorative to nerves and reproductive organs

🌿 Antidepressant

🌿 Strengthening

Uses

🌿 Weakness and nervous exhaustion. A good remedy for helping to "keep on the go."

🌿 Restless sleep from overexcitement.

🌿 With valerian to ease the symptoms of withdrawal from tranquilizers.

🌿 With vervain for weakness following illness.

🌿 PMS with scanty menstruation and cramps.

🌿 For exhaustion after childbirth and during breast-feeding.

🌿 Addresses loss of libido in both sexes.

🌿 With horsetail to strengthen the bones of children and the elderly.

🌿 Baths and lotions are very soothing for eczema.

BELOW *The wild oat grass benefits the nervous system.*

NOTES AND DOSAGES

🌿 For oat straw, make a tea with 2 teaspoons to 1 cup of water. Infuse for 15 minutes. 🌿 **For oats in general, buy the tincture. Use 20 drops every 2 hours when you need to keep going or 1 teaspoon 3 times daily for weakened states.** 🌿 Eating porridge is beneficial to the nervous system and helps lower cholesterol levels. 🌿 **For a bath, fill a muslin bag with porridge oats and hang it under the hot faucet, so that the water flows through it.** 🌿 Preparations of oats for making baths can also be bought at general and herbal pharmacies.

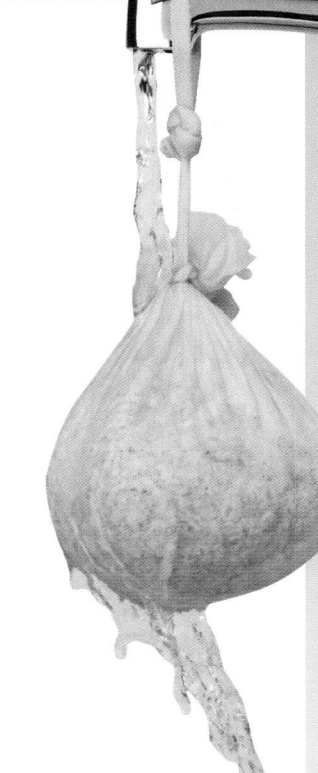

ABOVE *For an oat bath, fill a muslin bag with oats and run water through it.*

THERAPY CONNECTIONS

MARIGOLD

🌀 Aromatherapy p.148

☯ Homeopathy p.187

WILD OATS

✹ Flower Remedies p.226

RECIPE
Oat Water
🌿 🌿 🌿 🌿

Take 1 dessertspoon of porridge oats and rub well between your fingers. Add to 1 cup of cold water. Stir well and leave for 20 minutes. Stir again and pass through a tea strainer. Makes a soothing drink for diarrhea, cystitis, and stomach upsets caused by antibiotics.

Capsicum minimum
CAYENNE

The kitchen spice, also called chili pepper. There are many different types of pepper spices made from red peppers, varying in strength from the mild paprika to the hottest cayenne.

NOTES AND DOSAGES

People with poor circulation can add capsicum to any herbal medicines, with benefit. **Capsicum-based creams, liniments, and infused oils should only be used on small areas and rubbed in well.** Post-shingles neuralgia and chronic back pain may take a week or two to improve. **Useful for unbroken chilblains.** Hot oil is so called because it is hot to the taste and not because it is applied hot. It is a warming antispasmodic rub, improving circulation, and relaxing tension and spasm.

DATA FILE

Properties

- Circulatory stimulant
- Antispasmodic
- Carminative

Uses

- Poor circulation, chills, and inefficient digestion in the elderly.
- Externally for cramps and muscle spasm, aches and pains, cold and stiff joints, post-shingles neuralgia, and for unbroken chilblains.

CAUTION

USE ONLY IN VERY SMALL QUANTITIES. A SMALL PINCH OF THE POWDER OR 5–10 DROPS OF THE TINCTURE IS SUFFICIENT FOR A SINGLE DOSE.

AVOID APPLYING TO INFLAMED AREAS. AVOID GETTING IT INTO YOUR EYES.

CAN AGGRAVATE ACIDITY AND HEARTBURN.

RECIPE
Hot Oil

Make an infused oil using: 1 dessertspoon cayenne pepper, 2 dessertspoons powdered mustard seed, 2 teaspoons powdered ginger root, 1 cup unblended vegetable oil, sunflower or grapeseed oil. Use as a rub for cold joints and muscle spasm.

BELOW *Blend together these ingredients for a warming muscle rub.*

VEGETABLE OIL

CAYENNE PEPPER

GINGER

MUSTARD

THERAPY CONNECTIONS

CAYENNE PEPPER
Ayurveda   *p.31*

CHAMOMILE
Aromatherapy *p.150*
Homeopathy *p.204*

HAWTHORN
Chinese Herbal Medicine   *p.61*

Codonopsis pilosula
CODONOPSIS

A sprawling herb with yellow, bell-shaped flowers, grown in China. The roots of this plant are used for medicinal purposes. Codonopsis can be purchased in Chinese herbal pharmacies as Dang Shen.

DATA FILE

Properties

- Soothing and strengthening
- An immune system tonic

Uses

- For general debility, exhaustion, weakness, lack of appetite, chronic diarrhea, excessive perspiration, acidity, chronic coughs, asthma, and shortness of breath.

- Used as a decoction, a tincture, or as a powder sprinkled on food.

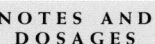

ABOVE *Codonopsis root. In Chinese medicine it is used for digestive problems and as a tonic.*

CAUTION

SAFE BUT BEST USED FOR LONG-TERM DEBILITY. USE OTHER HERBS IN ACUTE CONDITIONS.

NOTES AND DOSAGES

Take 1oz. (25g.) of the powder daily, sprinkled onto soups or made into a decoction. **Also called Dang Shen in Chinese herb stores.** Codonopsis is also known as the poor man's ginseng.

RECIPE
Soup of the "Four Gentlemen"

This is a famous traditional Chinese digestive and energy tonic. It is made from codonopsis, white atractylodes (Bai Zhu), Chinese angelica (Dang Gui), poria (Fu Ling), and licorice. Add 1oz. (25g.) of the herb mixture to 1pt. (500ml.) of water. Simmer for 15 minutes, strain, and drink daily.

Chamomilla recutita
CHAMOMILE

A wild plant with small, daisy-like flowers. It is the flowers that are most often used for therapeutic purposes. Chamomile is an aromatic plant, and it was used as a strewing herb in the Middle Ages.

NOTES AND DOSAGES

May be taken freely. As a sedative make a double-strength tea, using 2 teaspoons of flowers or 2 tea bags. Use a covered vessel, so the steam does not escape. Linden flowers, chamomile, and four cloves makes an effective drink before bed, relaxing the body and the mind, and bringing satisfying sleep. For infants, make an ordinary strength tea and give them 2 or 3 teaspoons to drink, either directly or in some pure fruit juice. For times of severe stress make a mixture of three parts chamomile to two parts sage and one part basil (a pinch of ginger powder is optional). Take twice a day to reduce tension and husband resources.

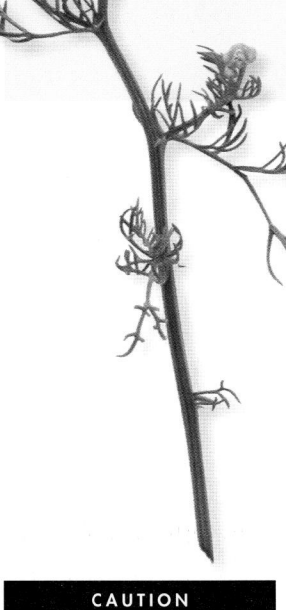

CAUTION

CAN CAUSE AN ALLERGIC RASH, BUT THIS DISAPPEARS ON STOPPING USE OF THE HERB.

DATA FILE

Properties
- Calming and soothing
- Anti-inflammatory
- Antiseptic
- Antispasmodic
- Digestive

Uses
- Anxiety, tension, headaches, and insomnia.
- For any kind of digestive upset – acidity, heartburn, wind, and colic.
- Lotion, cream, or bath for itchy skin conditions.
- For restless and overexcitable children, and for most children's complaints, including fevers and teething troubles. Especially helpful for infants.
- Although chamomile is sold in tea bags as a herbal drink for everyday use, it should not be overlooked as a medicinal herb, for it is gentle but very powerful.

LEFT *Chamomile has a long history. The Egyptians used it to cure fever.*

RECIPE
Chamomile Compress for Sore and Inflamed Eyes or Skin

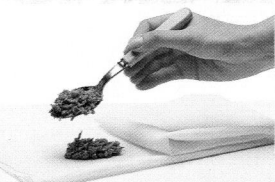

Put a handful of dried chamomile flowers into a bowl. Slowly pour on boiled water, stirring all the time until they make a mush. Allow to cool. Wrap in a length of cotton and apply. Leave on for at least 15 minutes.

Crataegus oxycantha or *Crataegus monogyna*
HAWTHORN BERRIES AND FLOWERING TOPS

The berries and flowering tops of the common may tree. Hawthorn's Latin name comes from Greek words meaning hard (wood), sharp, and thorn.

DATA FILE

Properties
- Strengthens the heart
- Lowers blood pressure
- Relaxes arteries

Uses
- Heart failure. If you are taking drugs for heart problems, seek professional advice before taking any herbal medicine.
- Irregular heartbeat.
- Helpful for angina and high blood pressure, as part of an overall strategy.
- With nervine herbs such as valerian and linden, for anxiety with palpitations.

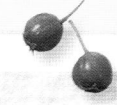

RECIPE
Hawthorn Brandy

This is the nicest way of taking hawthorn as a heart-strengthening tonic. Pick the flowering shoots (with flowers and leaves), wash, dry, and pack into a large jar. Cover with brandy and leave in a cool place for two weeks. Strain off the liquid, bottle, and label. Dose: 2 dessertspoons daily.

NOTES AND DOSAGES

Standard dose (*see pages 108–9*). Make a tea of the flowering tops or a decoction of the berries. Tincture: take 1 teaspoon in a little water twice daily. For heart disease, take this dosage for at least 6 months.

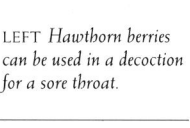

LEFT *Hawthorn berries can be used in a decoction for a sore throat.*

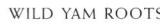

Dioscorea villosa
WILD YAMS

The rhizome of a Mexican wild yam. The dried root retains its medicinal value for up to a year.

WILD YAM ROOTS

DATA FILE

Properties
- Anti-inflammatory
- Antispasmodic

Uses
- Stomach cramps, nausea, vomiting, hiccups, recurrent colicky pains, pain of diverticulitis, and gall-bladder pains. With a little ginger for a quicker action.
- Menstrual cramps, and pain on ovulation.
- Menopausal symptoms, vaginal dryness.
- Useful for the treatment of rheumatoid arthritis.

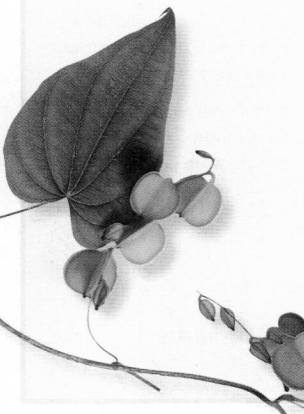

ABOVE *Dried wild yam root, leaves, and fruit. The plant is dug up in the fall to harvest the root.*

NOTES AND DOSAGES

- Standard doses (*see pages 108–9*). **Works especially well on persistent and recurrent problems.**
- Wild yam is the starting point for synthesization of hormones for the contraceptive pill and for "natural progesterone," used in a prescription cream for the menopause.

RECIPE
Decoction for Arthritic Pains

Take 1oz. (25g.) each of wild yam root and willow bark. Add to 3pt. (1.5l.) water. Simmer together for 20 minutes. Strain. The decoction will keep in the refrigerator for two or three days. Dose: ½ cup 3 times daily, adding honey to taste.

Echinacea angustifolia and Echinacea purpurea
ECHINACEA ROOT

Purple cone flower, a native plant of the U.S. Echinacea is the best way of ridding the body of microbial infections. It is effective against both bacteria and viruses.

DATA FILE

Properties
- Antiseptic
- Stimulates the immune system

Uses
- For a weak immune system where patient suffers chronic tiredness and is susceptible to minor infections.
- For boils, acne, duodenal ulcers, flu, herpes, and persistent infections.
- As a gargle and mouthwash for sore throats, tonsillitis, mouth ulcers, and gum infections.

NOTES AND DOSAGES

- For acute conditions take large doses, 1 cup of the decoction or 1 teaspoon of the tincture every two hours for ten days.
- **For chronic conditions use in combinations and take ½ cup of the combined decoction or 1 teaspoon of the combined tincture, 3 times daily.**

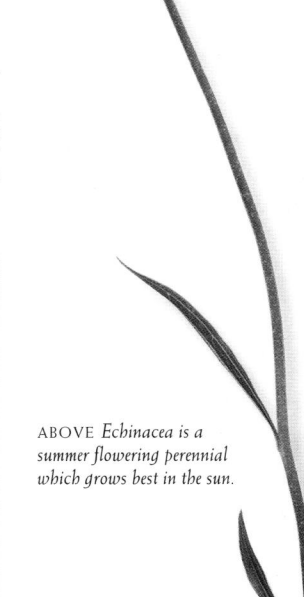

ABOVE *Echinacea is a summer flowering perennial which grows best in the sun.*

Equisetium arvense
HORSETAIL

A weed which is common on damp ground. Horsetail reproduces by spores, like ferns. Galen, a physician of Ancient Greece, used horsetail to heal sinews.

BELOW *Collect horsetail in early summer. Hang in large bunches and leave it to dry.*

CAUTION
AVOID LARGE DOSES IN EARLY PREGNANCY.

NOTES AND DOSAGES

- The healing properties of horsetail are due to its high content of silica and zinc. **For a decoction, simmer 1 teaspoon in 2 cups of water for half an hour.** Drink twice daily for one month. **Make up a pitcher and keep it in the refrigerator.**

DATA FILE

Properties
- Styptic
- Diuretic
- Strengthens the bladder
- Antifungal

Uses
- For irritable bladder with urgency and frequency.
- For blood in the urine.
- For bedwetting problems, with cramp bark or St. John's wort.
- For arthritis.
- Strengthens nails and hair.
- Speeds healing after surgery.
- Compress for infected, weepy skin conditions.

Filipendula ulmaria
MEADOWSWEET

The leaves, stalks, and flowers of a wild plant common in damp meadows. The flowers are very fragrant, and the plant was a medieval strewing herb. Culpeper described it as a help to acquiring a "merry heart."

DATA FILE

Properties

- Antacid
- Astringent
- Anti-inflammatory
- Diuretic
- Calming for overactive digestive systems

Uses

- Acid stomach, heartburn, ulcers, and hiatus hernia. Combines well with comfrey, marshmallow, and chamomile.
- With peppermint or chamomile for indigestion, diverticulitis, and wind.
- Helpful for rheumatism and arthritis. Clears sandy deposits in the urine.
- Excellent for summer diarrhea and fevers with an upset stomach in children.

RECIPE
Tea for Acid Stomachs

Take equal parts of meadowsweet, chamomile flowers, and comfrey leaves, dried. Mix together and store in a clean jar. Use 1 teaspoon of the mixture to 1 cup boiling water. Allow the tea to draw for 10 minutes. Drink 3–6 cups daily.

CAUTION

LARGE DOSES AND STRONG TEAS MAY CAUSE NAUSEA IN SOME PEOPLE.

NOTES AND DOSAGES

- Standard doses. Half dosages for children and elderly people. Will give quick relief for stomach pains, but best results come from long-term use.

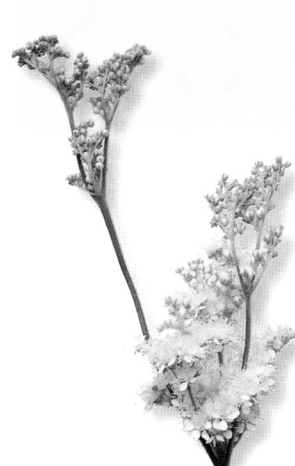

RIGHT *Filipendula bears cream flowers in summer and should be picked at this time.*

Foeniculum vulgare
FENNEL

A familiar cooking herb – the leaves and seeds are used. Fennel has feathery leaves and grows to about 6ft. (2m.). It was traditionally reputed to instil strength and courage.

DATA FILE

Properties

- Warming
- Carminative
- Antispasmodic
- Antidepressant
- Promotes milk flow in nursing mothers

Uses

- For colic, wind, and irritable bowel.
- For breast-feeding; helps milk flow and reduces colic.
- For anxiety, depression, and disturbed spirits.
- For arthritis and water retention or edema.
- For griping in infants, give the tea in teaspoon doses, as much as they will take, or add 2 teaspoons to milk formulas.

ABOVE *Fennel seeds have an anise-like flavor, and help digestion.*

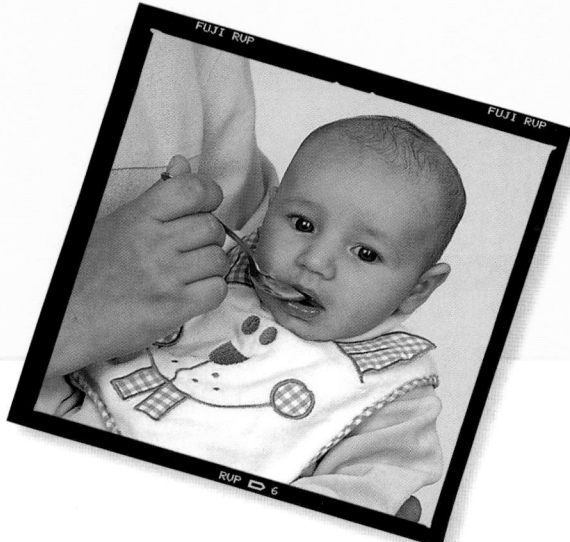

RIGHT *Fennel tea will soothe a baby's colic. Give by the teaspoonful.*

NOTES AND DOSAGES

- Standard doses.
- Fennel seed tea bags are easily available – remember to cover the cup to avoid losing any goodness.
- Traditionally taken during fasts to reduce hunger.

RECIPE
Fennel Eye Bath

Fennel tea, diluted 1:1 with water and with the addition of a pinch of salt helps ease tired, dry eyes and maintain clear vision. As with any liquid used for the eyes, absolute cleanliness must be observed. Strain the tea through a very fine strainer before use, and make fresh every day.

THERAPY CONNECTIONS

FENNEL

- Aromatherapy *p.159*

CAUTION

REMEMBER THAT ANY BLOOD IN THE URINE SHOULD ALWAYS BE INVESTIGATED BY YOUR PHYSICIAN.

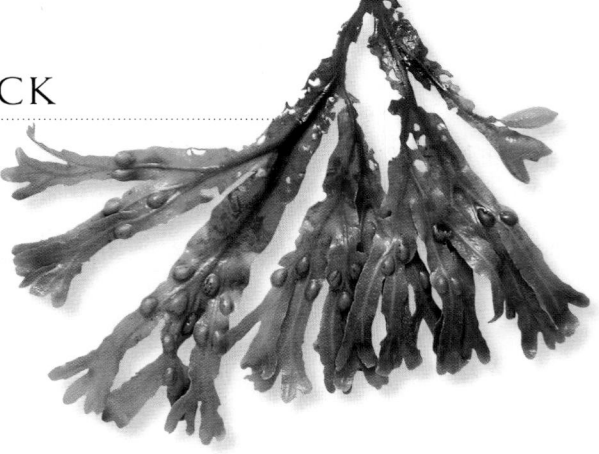

Fucus vesiculosis
BLADDERWRACK

A common dark brown seaweed found in the U.S and Europe. Also called kelp.

NOTES AND DOSAGES

🍂 Take 1 tablet 3 times a day, or follow the instructions on the packet.

🍂 **When using powder, 1 or 2 teaspoons may be sprinkled on to cooked meals or soups.**

🍂 Half doses for children.

CAUTION

AVOID IN OVERACTIVE THYROID CONDITIONS, EXCEPT WITH PROFESSIONAL GUIDANCE.

NOT RECOMMENDED FOR CHILDREN UNDER FIVE.

IT IS BEST TO SEEK ADVICE BEFORE USING HERBS FOR WEIGHT LOSS.

DATA FILE

Properties

🌿 Nourishing and soothing.

🌿 Stimulates the thyroid gland.

Uses

🌿 A nourishing tonic.

🌿 Obesity with tiredness and dry skin.

🌿 Cellulite, chronic dry skin, and stubborn constipation. Regular use will delay the progress of arthritis and hardening of the arteries. A good tonic for old age.

🌿 For children with slow mental and physical development.

ABOVE *Gather bladderwrack from clean beaches, keeping away from sewage outlets.*

RECIPE
Bladderwrack Liniment
🌿 🌿 🌿 🌿

To make an excellent liniment for rheumatism and arthritis add 1oz. (25g.) of dried bladderwrack to 1pt. (500ml.) of water. Simmer for a half-hour. Strain and add to an equal amount of comfrey infused oil *(see page 132)*. Shake before use and rub in well twice daily.

Ginkgo biloba
GINKGO LEAVES

Leaves of the maidenhair tree, originally from China and often grown in parks. The tea, tincture, and tablets treat poor circulation, thrombosis, and varicose veins.

DATA FILE

Properties

🌿 Improves blood flow

🌿 Strengthens blood vessels

🌿 Anti-inflammatory

🌿 Relaxes the lungs

Uses

🌿 For poor circulation, thrombosis, varicose veins, cramp which comes on walking, white finger, and spontaneous bruising.

🌿 Especially helpful for failing circulation to the brain in elderly people.

🌿 Strengthens memory.

🌿 Often improves deafness, tinnitus, vertigo, and early senile dementia.

🌿 Helpful in asthma.

NOTES AND DOSAGES

🍂 The tea is best taken in large doses – at least 3 cups a day for some months. It is a pleasant drinking tea. Tablets are available – follow the dose on the packet.

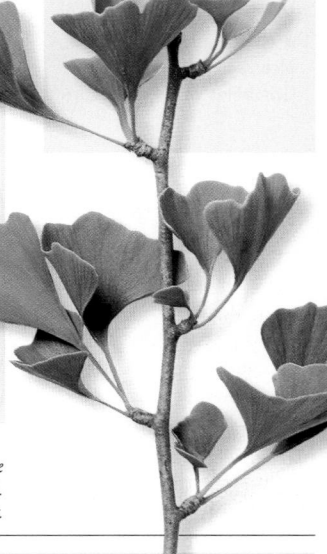

RIGHT *The ginkgo tree grows to almost 100ft. (30m.). It is a deciduous conifer.*

Glycyrrhiza glabra
LICORICE ROOT

A sweet root used in confectionery and medicine (often mixed with other herbs for long-term use).

CAUTION

CAN CAUSE WATER RETENTION AND RAISED BLOOD PRESSURE.

LARGE DOSES CAN BE LAXATIVE.

PROLONGED USE SHOULD BE AVOIDED IF YOU SUFFER FROM HIGH BLOOD PRESSURE.

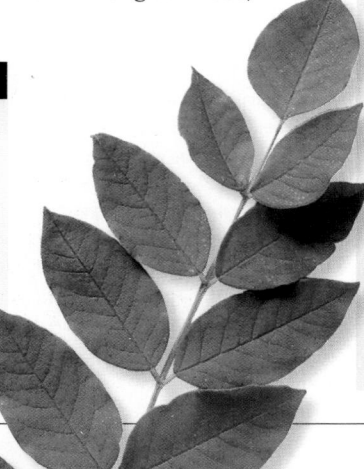

NOTES AND DOSAGES

🍂 For bronchitis take ¼oz. (5g.) of the powdered root 3 times daily with honey or in capsules, for up to 2 weeks. For a decoction use ½ teaspoon to 1 cup of water – take 3 cups daily. Half this for long-term use. Boiling the decoction for an hour and then drying it out in a low oven produces an extract that is easy to take.

DATA FILE

Properties

🌿 Soothing and anti-inflammatory

🌿 Strengthening and up-building

🌿 Expectorant

Uses

🌿 Irritable, dry coughs and bronchitis.

🌿 Stomach, acidity, heartburn, ulcers, colitis, and intestinal infections.

🌿 With other strengthening herbs for exhaustion.

🌿 In creams for inflamed psoriasis and hot and weepy skin conditions.

LEFT *The Greeks were using licorice in 3 B.C.E. for asthma and a dry cough.*

Harpagophytum procumbens
DEVIL'S CLAW

The tuber from a South African plant, which survives in very arid conditions. Devil's claw contains a glycoside called harpagoside that helps to reduce inflammation in the joints.

DATA FILE

Properties

✿ Bitter tonic and anti-inflammatory

Uses

✿ Decoction or tincture for all types of arthritis, especially for inflamed joints and arthritis affecting a number of joints.

✿ For gout, lumbago, sciatica, and rheumatism.

✿ For gall-bladder inflammation, piles, and phlebitis (internally).

✿ For itchy skin with no obvious cause.

NOTES AND DOSAGES

✿ Decoction: ½ teaspoon to 1 cup of water, 2 cups a day. Tincture: 1 teaspoon twice daily. Tablets are available in most health food stores – follow the dosage on the box. For acute flare-ups double the dosage for a week or two.

CAUTION

AVOID IN PREGNANCY.

◆—◆

MAY AGGRAVATE STOMACH ACIDITY.

◆—◆

DO NOT USE IN GASTRITIS AND WITH ULCERS.

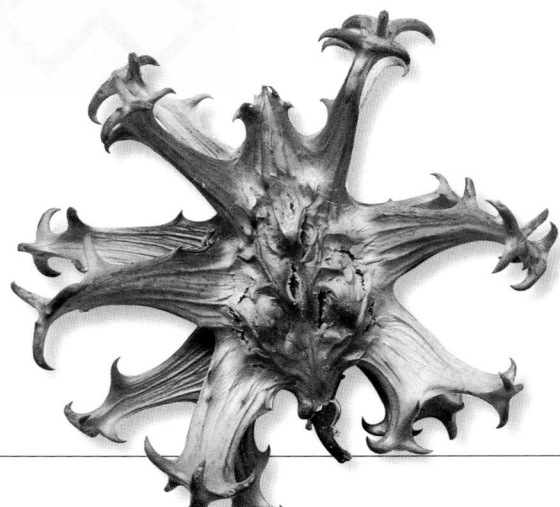
BELOW *Devil's claw tubers are dug up at the end of the rainy season and dried.*

RECIPE
Devil's Claw Capsules
✿ ✿ ✿ ✿

Capsules are a good way of producing a customized remedy, and useful if you do not want to take a lot of liquid decoctions.

Dose: two capsules three times daily.

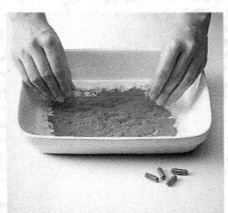

Buy 120 empty gelatin capsules from a herb store. Get out a flat dish and a coffee grinder.

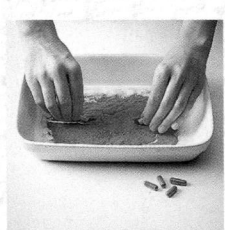

Powder 1oz. (25g.) chopped devil's claw in the coffee grinder (some stores sell it pre-ground).

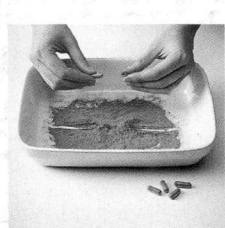

Put the powder in the dish. Fill each capsule by pushing the halves through the powder.

Hamamelis virginiana
WITCH HAZEL BARK AND LEAVES

A small U.S. tree often grown in gardens for its fragrant yellow spring flowers. The bark and leaves are used.

DATA FILE

Properties

✿ Astringent

✿ Anti-inflammatory

✿ Antiseptic

✿ Styptic

Uses

✿ External use only for bruises, cuts, oily skin, spots, broken capillaries, piles, and painful varicose veins.

✿ As a compress for sprains, phlebitis, sunburn, and hot swollen joints.

✿ As a compress and wash for hot and tired eyes.

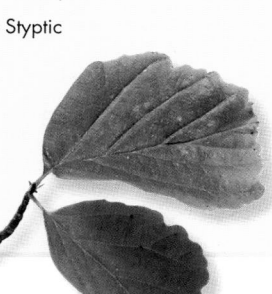
ABOVE *and* LEFT *Witch hazel's oval leaves turn yellow in the fall.*

NOTES AND DOSAGES

✿ Distilled witch hazel and other preparations are easily available. The decoction and tincture are stronger but tend to stain clothes. Dilute the tincture with 3 parts of water to use as a compress or lotion.

THERAPY CONNECTIONS

WITCH HAZEL

✋ Traditional Home and Folk Remedies p.91

☺ Homeopathy p.197

LICORICE

☗ Ayurveda p.39

☗ Chinese Herbal Medicine p.64

✋ Traditional Home and Folk Remedies p.91

RECIPE
Witch Hazel Compress
✿ ✿ ✿ ✿

Take 1oz. (25g.) cut bark and 1pt. (500ml.) water. Simmer together for 10 minutes. Strain and allow to cool. Dip a cloth into the decoction, wring, and apply for a half-hour, wetting it again as needed. Suitable for sunburn, swollen and inflamed joints, and aching varicose veins.

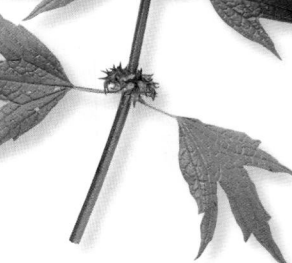

Hypericum perforatum
ST. JOHN'S WORT

A common European wild plant, now a weed in many parts of the world. The tops of the plant are picked in full flower. It is easy to grow, but make sure you get the right species – *perforatum* has oil glands in the leaves which show up as transparent dots against the light.

DATA FILE

Properties

❦ Strengthens the nervous system and speeds healing

❦ Analgesic

❦ Antiviral

❦ Anti-inflammatory

Uses

❦ Neuralgia, sciatica, and back pain.

❦ Pain from deep wounds.

❦ Mild depression. (Not for severe depression.)

❦ Tincture for shingles, cold sores, and herpes.

❦ Cream for sore skin, inflamed rashes, and cuts.

❦ Infused oil as base oil for aromatherapy back massage, and with lavender essential oil for neuralgia.

Leonurus cardiaca
MOTHERWORT

A European wild plant with a tall spike of small pink flowers. Self-seeds readily in the garden. Culpeper wrote, "...there is no better herb to drive melancholy vapours from the heart ... and make the mind cheerful, blithe and merry."

DATA FILE

Properties

❦ Calms the heart and relaxes the womb

❦ Antispasmodic

❦ Emmenagogue

Uses

❦ Anxiety with palpitations and irregular heartbeat.

❦ Tachycardia from an overactive thyroid.

❦ With skullcap or valerian, for tranquilizer withdrawal.

❦ With vervain for anxiety from stress and overwork.

❦ With sage for menopausal hot flushes.

❦ For menstrual cramps, taken on a regular basis.

❦ Take daily during the last two weeks of pregnancy to help with the birth.

ABOVE *Motherwort is especially good for female disorders – hence its name.*

NOTES AND DOSAGES

🍂 Standard doses. It may be a week before depression begins to lift. 🍂 The best preparations for external use are the infused oil and creams based on the infused oil (*see box*). For nerve damage you may need to continue use for some months.

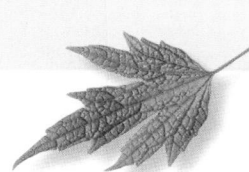

LEFT *St. John's wort oil can cause photosensitivity in direct sunlight.*

NOTES AND DOSAGES

🍂 Standard doses of decoction or tincture. May take a few weeks to work.

RECIPE
Motherwort and Lemon Balm Tea
❦ ❦ ❦ ❦

Make an infusion, or tea, by pouring a cup of boiling water on to 1–2 teaspoonsful of the dried herb. Leave to infuse for 10–15 minutes. The tea should be drunk 3 times a day. Motherwort and lemon balm tea combines motherwort's sedative effect and lemon balm's antidepressant qualities.

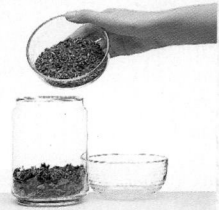

Mix together equal amounts of dried motherwort and lemon balm (*Melissa officinalis*) herbs. Store in a clean jar and label.

Take as a regular tea for depression.

CAUTION

AVOID IN PREGNANCY, EXCEPT DURING THE LAST TWO WEEKS.

RECIPE
St. John's Wort Oil
❦ ❦ ❦

Pick the flowering tops. Put into a pestle, add a small amount of a pure, light vegetable oil such as sunflower oil. Pour just enough to cover, then pound together to crush, bruise, and start releasing the oil. Put into a large clear glass jar. Cover with more oil so that all of the herb is well covered. Shake well. Then add another inch of oil. Leave outside in direct sunlight for 20 days. The oil will turn red when it is ready. Use for skin, healing nerve damage, as a base for massage oils, or as a salve.

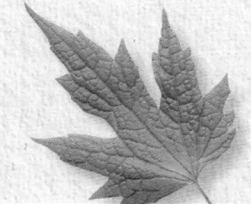

Lycium barbarum or *Lycium chinense*
LYCIUM FRUIT

The bright red fruit of a Chinese shrub, grown in Europe as a hedging plant. It is a deciduous shrub, growing to 8ft. (2.5m.) tall and spreading to about 15ft. (5m.). Lycium bears pinkish flowers and grows well even in poor soil.

Mentha piperita
PEPPERMINT LEAVES

One of the most popular herb teas in the world. Easily grown in gardens, but is a rather invasive plant. Try growing it in a bucket buried in the ground, with the bottom knocked out.

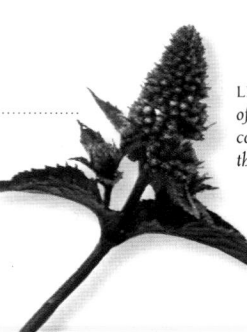

LEFT *The leaves of peppermint are collected just before the flowers open.*

DATA FILE

Properties
- Tonic for old age and associated weakness

Uses
- General weakness with vertigo, tinnitus, and recurrent headaches.
- For impotence and premature ejaculation.
- Convalescence, with equal parts of schisandra; improves skin color and restores strength.
- Failing eyesight.
- Aches and pains, especially backache, particularly in old age.

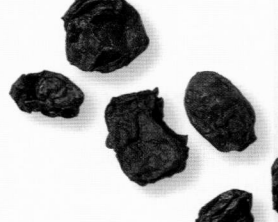

CAUTION

AVOID LARGE DOSES IN PREGNANCY.

THE AMOUNTS TAKEN IN FOOD ARE HARMLESS.

NOT SUITED TO INFANTS; USE CATMINT, WHICH HAS THE SAME PROPERTIES AND IS MORE SUITABLE.

DATA FILE

Properties
- Digestive
- Carminative
- Antispasmodic
- Mild stimulant
- Emmenagogue
- Cooling on the skin

Uses
- Indigestion, colic, wind, nausea, vomiting, depressed appetite, menstrual cramps, and gall bladder pain. Adding a couple of drops of the essential oil to hot water, and drinking it, or sucking a strong peppermint sweet, is also effective.
- With elderflower and yarrow for colds, sinus problems, and blocked nose. Inhale the steam as you drink.
- For hot, itchy skin problems, a strong tea used as a lotion.

RECIPE
Eye-strengthening Soup

Take 1oz. (25g.) lycium fruit, 3 chopped carrots, and a sliced onion. Add to 1pt. (500ml.) soup stock made with chicken or vegetable stock cubes. Simmer until the vegetables are cooked. Strain and blend. Take regularly to "nourish the vital essence and benefit vision."

RIGHT *and* ABOVE *Lycium leaves and dried berries. The berries are favored for problems of old age.*

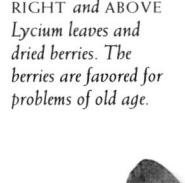

NOTES AND DOSAGES

Take freely. A small amount of peppermint may be added to most herb teas for flavor.

NOTES AND DOSAGES

Also called wolfberry and the Duke of Argyle's tea plant. Chinese herbalists call the berries Gou-qi-zi. Tincture: ½fl.oz. (15ml.) with a little water daily. Dried fruit, ½oz. (10g.) daily chewed or in decoction. Traditionally the berries are added to soup to help strengthen eyesight.

RECIPE
Cooling Peppermint Drink for Hot Weather

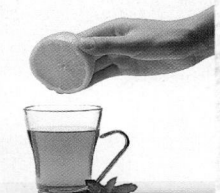

Make a weak peppermint tea using ½oz. (12g.) peppermint and 1pt. (500ml.) water. Add the juice of one lemon. Cool in the refrigerator, add ice and a sprig of fresh mint. Drink freely to avoid the debilitating effects of heat.

THERAPY CONNECTIONS
ST. JOHN'S WORT
Ayurveda   p.40
Homeopathy   p.199

PEPPERMINT
Aromatherapy p.164

Panax ginseng and *Eleutherococcus senticosus*

GINSENG AND SIBERIAN GINSENG ROOT

A famous tonic of the Far East, where it is very widely used. The word "ginseng" is said to mean "the wonder of the world."

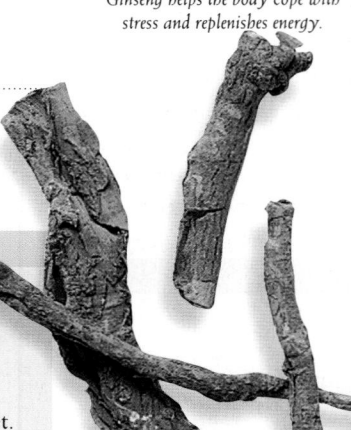

BELOW *Siberian ginseng root. Ginseng helps the body cope with stress and replenishes energy.*

NOTES AND DOSAGES

🍃 Dose: 100mg. of powdered root, 300mg. of cut root in decoction, or 20–30 drops of the tincture twice daily. 🍃 **Best suited to old and weakened people.** 🍃 Many preparations are available in the stores – follow the dose on the packet.

CAUTION

NOT TO BE TAKEN IN PREGNANCY.

—◦—

MAY AGGRAVATE ANXIETY AND IRRITABILITY.

—◦—

AVOID WITH HIGH BLOOD PRESSURE.

—◦—

DO NOT TAKE LARGE DOSES IN CONJUNCTION WITH STIMULANTS.

—◦—

DO NOT TAKE CONSISTENTLY WITHOUT PROFESSIONAL ADVICE.

—◦—

NOT FOR CHILDREN, EXCEPT UNDER PROFESSIONAL GUIDANCE.

THERAPY CONNECTIONS

GINSENG

🔘 Chinese Herbal Medicine   *p.67*

RHUBARB

🔘 Chinese Herbal Medicine   *p.73*

ROSEMARY

🔘 Aromatherapy *p.168*

DATA FILE

Properties

🍃 Replenishes vital energy

🍃 Strengthens the immune system

🍃 Adaptogenic

🍃 Increases concentration

Uses

🍃 Convalescence, exhaustion, lack of concentration, weakness in old age.

🍃 With other strengthening herbs for getting rid of persistent infections.

🍃 Loss of sex drive in men.

🍃 Helps the body to cope with the side-effects of chemotherapy for cancer.

🍃 Jet lag.

RECIPE

Ginseng Tonic Wine

🍃 🍃 🍃 🍃

You can make a reviving tonic wine using this simple recipe.

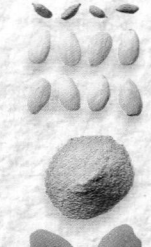

1oz. (25g.) powdered ginseng, 4 dried apricots, 8 blanched almonds, 4 cardamom pods (optional), 2pt. (1l.) red or white wine to taste. Put ingredients together, stand for 2 weeks, and strain. Drink a small glass (¼ cup) daily.

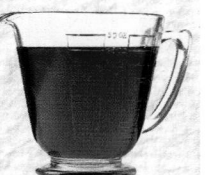

Plantago major or *Plantago lanceolata*

PLANTAIN LEAF

The broad-leaved plantain or the ribwort plantain are common weeds of pathways and lawns. It was said to spring up wherever the English established a colony, giving rise to its common name of "white man's foot."

DATA FILE

Properties

🍃 Soothing

🍃 Healing

🍃 Astringent

Uses

🍃 Running nose from allergies, irritation, and colds.

🍃 Irritable bowel and irritable bladder.

🍃 Compress or lotion for insect bites, allergic rashes, and infected eczema,

cleaning wounds, drawing stings, and splinters.

🍃 Soothes neuralgic pains and shingles rash.

🍃 Cream or ointment for bleeding piles.

🍃 The tea is a cooling drink for persistent fevers and is a useful addition to any medicine given to "hot" people.

🍃 Mouthwash for sore and bleeding gums.

RECIPE

Plantain Lotion

🍃 🍃 🍃

Finely chop sufficient fresh plantain leaves to fill a small jar. Add sufficient glycerin to cover the leaves. Stand for 2 weeks, stirring from time to time. Strain and store in a dark bottle. Makes a soothing and healing lotion for weeping and itchy rashes, and insect bites.

BELOW *In times past, plantain was reputed to cure mad dogs and snakebites.*

NOTES AND DOSAGES

🍃 Double-strength tea (2 teaspoons per cup) for most purposes. Take it freely.

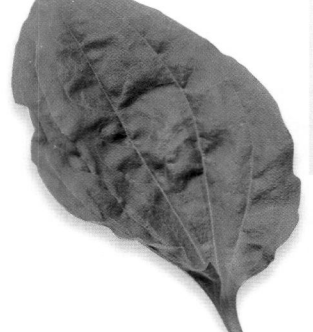

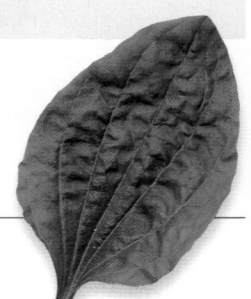

Rheum palmatum and *Rheum officinale*
RHUBARB ROOT

Chinese rhubarb, also called turkey rhubarb. Edible garden rhubarb is a hybrid of this. *Rheum palmatum* is a perennial growing to a height of 6ft. (2m.), with 2ft. (60cm.) leaves.

DATA FILE

Properties
- Laxative
- Astringent
- Bitter tonic
- Cooling

Uses
- Constipation, acute liver and gall bladder diseases.
- Feelings of congestion and fullness in the stomach.
- Stomach acidity.
- Gastroenteritis and diarrhea from food poisoning.
- Gout.
- Traditionally used in cancer.
- As a poultice for abscesses.

NOTES AND DOSAGES

Half the standard dose: ½ teaspoon to 1 cup of water for decoction, or 30–40 drops of the tincture, 3 times daily.

ABOVE *Rhubarb root may cause the urine to take on a reddish tinge.*

RECIPE
Laxative Wine

Warm a glass of white wine (don't boil). Pour on to 1 teaspoon of chopped rhubarb root. Add a good pinch of cinnamon powder and stand overnight. Strain and drink.

CAUTION

AVOID IN PREGNANCY, EXCEPT AS ADVISED BY A QUALIFIED HERBALIST.

NOT USED IN BOWEL SPASM OR WHEN COLICKY PAINS ARE PRESENT.

AVOID TAKING LAXATIVES FOR LONG PERIODS.

DO NOT EAT RHUBARB LEAVES.

Rosmarinus officinalis
ROSEMARY LEAVES

Late-flowering woody shrub. The whole plant smells, and it is almost impossible to pass by a rosemary bush without pinching a few leaves and rubbing them between the fingers to release the smell. Rosemary has many traditional uses and stories. It is planted in cemeteries for remembrance, and it does enhance the memory by improving the circulation. Rosemary vinegar is a powerful disinfectant.

NOTES AND DOSAGES

Standard doses used freely. Add 15 drops of essential oil to a bath to ease muscular tension, improve circulation, and boost spirits. **Rosemary tea can be used as a conditioning hair rinse.** For dandruff but also for gloriously glossy hair (especially for dark hair), use rosemary vinegar.

CAUTION

AVOID LARGE DOSES IN PREGNANCY, EXCEPT AS ADVISED BY A QUALIFIED HERBALIST.

DO NOT USE FOR TREATING HEADACHES AND MIGRAINES THAT FEEL "HOT."

THE AMOUNTS TAKEN IN FOOD ARE HARMLESS.

BELOW *In times of plague, rosemary was carried to ward off infection.*

RECIPE
Rosemary Vinegar

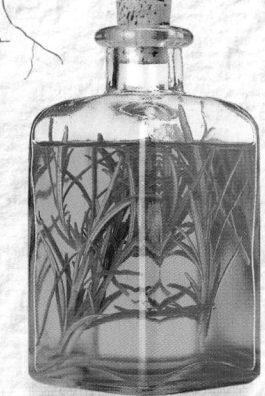

Take 1oz. (25g.) rosemary and 2pt. (1l.) cider vinegar. Leave the rosemary to steep in the vinegar for two weeks. Shake occasionally. After two weeks, strain, bottle, label, and date.
Use 1–2 dessertspoons in the final rinsing water when washing hair. For dandruff, massage rosemary vinegar thoroughly into the scalp 20 minutes before washing.

DATA FILE

Properties
- Lifts the spirits
- Improves circulation
- Carminative
- Gentle bitter tonic

Uses
- Depression.
- Headaches associated with gastric upsets. Take rosemary with chamomile for stress-related headaches.
- Poor circulation, taken regularly. A useful addition to any herbal medicine for conditions associated with cold and poor circulation.
- Poor digestion, gall bladder inflammation, gallstones, and general feeling of liverishness.
- As a gargle for sore throats. Useful substitute for sage during pregnancy.
- With horsetail for hair loss due to stress and worry.
- As an infused oil for massage of cold limbs and aches and pains.
- Rosemary will encourage the circulation.
- Good circulation to the head strengthens the brain and improves the quality and strength of hair. Two cups of rosemary tea a day will prevent hair loss through poor circulation and restimulate growth after chemotherapy.

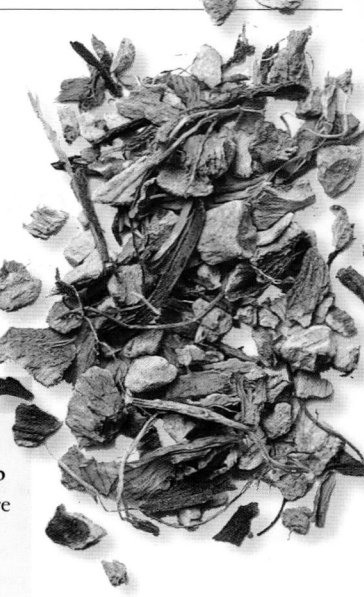

Rubus idaeus
RASPBERRY LEAVES

The leaves from the raspberry bush. Raspberries grow best in rich, moist, well-drained soil, and prefer a sunny position.

DATA FILE

Properties

✿ Astringent

✿ Antispasmodic

✿ Especially applicable to the womb

Uses

✿ To promote an easy birth by tonifying the uterus.

✿ A mouthwash for sore mouths, sore throats, weak gums, and mouth ulcers.

✿ With marshmallow and peppermint for diverticulitis.

✿ Children's diarrhea and oral thrush. For infants put raspberry leaf tea in a sterilized spray bottle and spray into the mouth 3 or 4 times daily.

LEFT *When picking, make sure that the bush has not been sprayed with pesticide.*

NOTES AND DOSAGES

✿ Standard doses. For tablets, follow the dose on the packet. ✿ **To prepare for birth, the herb needs to be taken for at least 2 months.** ✿ Continue for 3 or 4 weeks afterward to re-tone the womb quickly.

CAUTION

AVOID IN EARLY PREGNANCY EXCEPT WITH PROFESSIONAL ADVICE – BEST TAKEN DURING THE LAST THREE MONTHS. OTHERWISE A SAFE HERB.

RECIPE
Raspberry Vinegar
✿ ✿ ✿ ✿

This is made with the raspberry fruit. Fill a large jar with fresh raspberries. Cover with cider vinegar and stand in a cool place for two weeks. Strain and store in clean bottles. As a gargle for throats, dilute the vinegar with two parts of water to use.

Rumex crispus
YELLOW DOCK ROOT

A common wild plant, often used for blood and skin diseases. It contains anthraquinones, which act on the bowel and relieve constipation.

NOTES AND DOSAGES

✿ Make the decoction using ½oz. (12g.) yellow dock root to 1pt. (500ml.) water. ✿ **For constipation, 1 cup of decoction or 2 teaspoons of tincture daily.** ✿ More might be needed for short periods. ✿ **Use half this dose for chronic conditions, for children, and for constipation in pregnancy.**

ABOVE *Dried yellow dock root. It is dug up in the fall.*

RECIPE
Laxative Syrup
✿ ✿ ✿ ✿

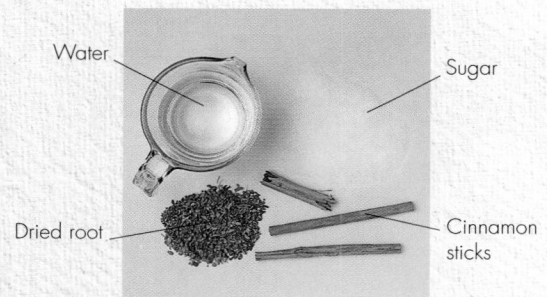

Water

Sugar

Dried root

Cinnamon sticks

Take ½oz. (12g.) dried root, ½pt. (250ml.) of water and one stick of cinnamon. Simmer together for 20 minutes, then strain. Reduce over low heat to 2fl. oz. (50ml.). Add 4oz. (100g.) sugar. Stir over low heat until dissolved. Dose: 6 dessertspoons for adults, 3 for children and pregnant women.

CAUTION

ALWAYS CONSIDER DIETARY CHANGES FOR STUBBORN CONSTIPATION.

DATA FILE

Properties

✿ Astringent

✿ Laxative

✿ Bitter tonic

✿ Alterative

Uses

✿ Chronic constipation.

✿ Liver congestion with poor fat digestion, and for feelings of heaviness which come on after eating.

✿ Stomach acidity, and for irritable bowel syndrome with constipation.

✿ Food poisoning and intestinal infections, to clear the source of irritation out of the digestive system.

✿ With burdock for the relief of chronic, hot, and itchy skin diseases.

LEFT *Yellow dock is also known as curled dock, as evident from its leaves.*

Salix alba
WHITE WILLOW BARK

Bark from the willow tree. *Salix alba* is a 50ft. (15m.) silver-gray deciduous tree. A decoction or tincture of white willow treats arthritis, back pain, and lessens sexual desire.

DATA FILE

Properties
- Anti-inflammatory
- Mild painkiller
- Anaphrodisiac
- Tonic

Uses
- All types of arthritis, especially with inflamed joints, and for gout. With celery seed for multiple painful joints.
- With cramp bark for inflammatory back pain, and lumbago.
- Chronic diarrhea.
- Take together with rosemary for headaches.
- Sexual overstimulation, wet dreams, and for premature ejaculation.
- Convalescence and low-grade recurrent fevers; feeling of being overheated in the evenings.

NOTES AND DOSAGES

🍂 Take standard doses (*see pages 108–9*) and persist.
🍂 **Willow bark contains aspirin-like compounds, but it does not upset the stomach.** 🍂 It can be used to reduce dependency on aspirin and other anti-inflammatories.

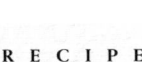

ABOVE *Do not take willow bark when pregnant or breast-feeding.*

RECIPE
Willow Bark and Ginger Decoction
❦ ❦ ❦ ❦

Take 2 heaped teaspoons dried willow bark and 1 heaped teaspoon ginger powder. Add to 2 cups of water. Simmer together for 10 minutes. Strain. Add honey to taste and drink. Take freely, as needed, for chills, chronic diarrhea, and as a strengthening drink in convalescence.

Salvia officinalis
SAGE LEAVES

The common garden and cooking herb. The purple or red variety is stronger, but any variety will suffice. Sow seeds in late spring, in well-drained soil. Choose a sunny position. The plant grows to about 2ft. (60cm.).

NOTES AND DOSAGES

🍂 Standard doses (*see pages 108–9*). Traditionally, 1 cup a day maintains health in old age. 🍂 **For an extra strength gargle add 5 drops of tincture of myrrh (from pharmacies or herb stores) to 1 cup of sage tea.** 🍂 Sage tincture can be taken, instead of the cold tea, for stopping night sweats – 4 teaspoons daily, in a little water.

ABOVE RIGHT *Sage leaves may be added to meat, fish, egg, and vegetable dishes.*

DATA FILE

Properties
- Astringent
- Stimulant
- Antiseptic
- Carminative
- Antispasmodic
- Nervine
- Generally strengthening
- A woman's tonic

Uses
- Depression and nervous exhaustion, post-viral fatigue, general debility.
- Anxiety and confusion in elderly people, or accompanying exhaustion and weakened states.
- For indigestion, wind, loss of appetite, and mucus on the stomach.
- Excessive sweating and night sweats, tincture taken cold.
- Weak lungs with persistent and recurrent coughs and allergies.
- Menopausal hot flushes, menstrual cramps, and premenstrual painful breasts (as a tea and compress).
- Cold sage tea taken every few hours will usually dry up breast milk.
- As a gargle and mouthwash for sore throats, laryngitis, tonsillitis, mouth ulcers, and inflamed and tender gums.
- As an antiseptic wash for dirty wounds which are slow to heal.

RECIPE
Sage and Vinegar Poultice
❦ ❦ ❦ ❦

Bruise a handful of fresh sage leaves by flattening them with a rolling pin. Place in a pan and cover with cider vinegar. Simmer very gently until the leaves are soft. Wrap the leaves in a cloth and apply warm for bruises, swellings, and stings.

CAUTION

AVOID IF ALLERGIC TO SALICYLATES (ASPIRIN).
◦—◦—◦
NOT SUITABLE FOR CHILDREN.

THERAPY CONNECTIONS

WILLOW
⊛ Flower Remedies   *p.239*

RIGHT *Sage tea wards off anxiety and exhaustion in the elderly.*

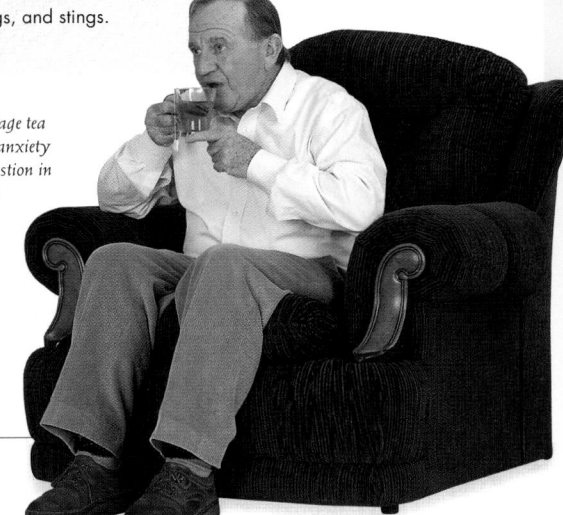

Sambucus nigra
ELDERFLOWERS

The creamy white flowers from a small tree common in hedgerows and on wasteland. The tree is in flower for only three weeks in summer. Elderflower ointment has long been a remedy for chilblains and chapped hands.

NOTES AND DOSAGES

❧ The hot tea is taken freely, up to 1 cup every 2 hours, for colds and fevers; 3 cups a day for chronic colds and sinusitis. ❧ **For children over five use half doses.** ❧ Eating fresh elderflowers will relieve the symptoms of hay fever, as will drinking a tea made with equal parts of elderflowers and eyebright (*Euphrasia officinalis*). ❧ **To prevent hay fever take 3 cups a day, starting two months before your regular season.** ❧ For colds and runny noses in infants add 3 or 4 cups of elderflower tea to their daily bath.

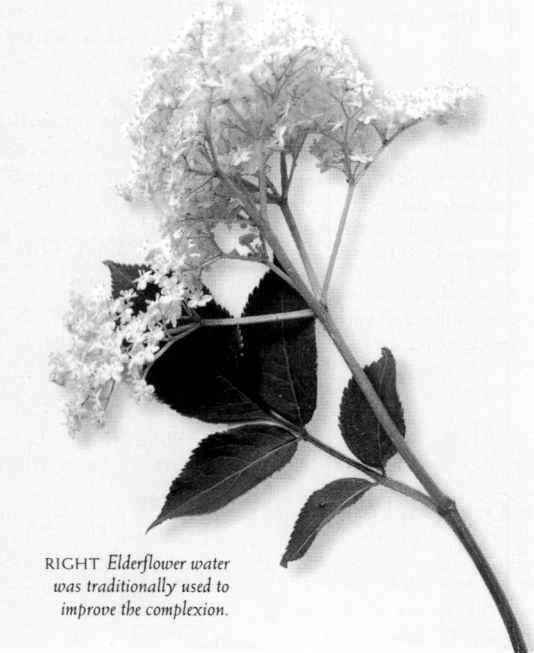

RIGHT *Elderflower water was traditionally used to improve the complexion.*

DATA FILE

Properties

❧ Restorative for mucous membrane and sinuses

❧ Diaphoretic

❧ Diuretic

❧ Anti-inflammatory

Uses

❧ Take the tea or tincture for sinusitis, colds, running nose, hay fever, and flu.

❧ To break a fever with hot, dry skin – it will induce sweating, bring down the temperature, and protect the kidneys.

❧ Suitable for use in children's fevers as a tea and as a lotion to soothe the rashes that often come with them.

❧ Lotion or compress for sore and runny eyes, eyestrain, and sunburn.

❧ Cream for chapped and discolored skin.

THERAPY CONNECTIONS

SCHISANDRA

▣ Chinese Herbal Medicine *p.74*

SKULLCAP

▣ Chinese Herbal Medicine *p.74*

RECIPE
Elderflower Nose Wash
❧ ❧ ❧ ❧

Elderflower nose wash is useful for sinusitis and hay fever. Make a cupful of a strong infusion, allow it to cool to blood heat, and add a pinch of salt. Sniff the mixture up each nostril in turn, then allow it to run out or use a special nasal bath. Use daily during the hay fever season.

Schisandra chinensis
SCHISANDRA BERRIES

The red berries of an ornamental vine grown in China. The Chinese use schisandra berries to relieve spontaneous sweating.

NOTES AND DOSAGES

❧ Called Wu Wei Zi in Chinese herbalism. ❧ **Also available from specialist herb stores.** ❧ Dose: tincture – take 1 teaspoon three times daily; dried berries – take ½oz. (10g.) daily by decoction.

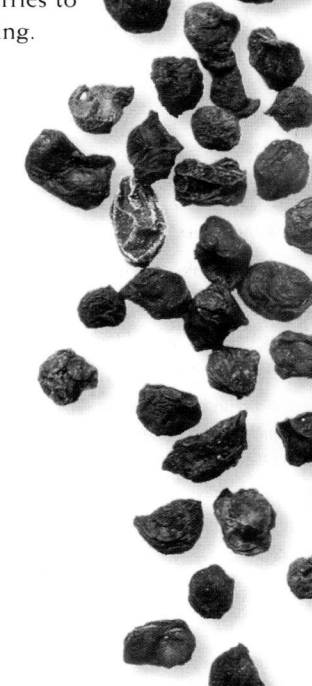

RIGHT *Dried schisandra berries are valued as a skin beautifier.*

DATA FILE

Properties

❧ Astringent

❧ Nourishing

❧ Soothing expectorant

Uses

❧ Weakness with nervous exhaustion and sleeplessness; exhaustion from prolonged hard work.

❧ Loss of sex drive in women and men; restores softness to the skin.

❧ Dry and chronic coughs, and asthma.

❧ Night sweats.

RECIPE
Schisandra Wine
❧ ❧ ❧ ❧

Add 4oz. (100g.) dried schisandra berries to a bottle of rice wine. Store in a cool place for four weeks. Drink a small wine glass twice daily. For weak lungs with recurrent coughs, and to keep skin soft in old age.

Serenoa serrulata
SAW PALMETTO BERRIES

The fruit of a small palm-like plant grown in the West Indies and the U.S. The berries are gathered from early fall to the middle of winter, and dried for storage.

DATA FILE

Properties

- Strengthening tonic
- Urinary antiseptic
- Alterative
- Stimulates sex hormones

Uses

- Prostate enlargement and cystitis.
- With damiana for weakness and impotence in men.
- Helps restore weight after severe illness.
- Failure to thrive in children, with marshmallow; take 10–15 drops of the combined tincture three times daily in fruit juice.

NOTES AND DOSAGES

- Decoction: ½ teaspoon of the crushed berries to 1 cup water. **Adult dose: 1 or 2 cups daily.** Tincture: 20–40 drops, in water, 3 times daily.

CAUTION

AVOID IN EARLY PREGNANCY, EXCEPT WITH PROFESSIONAL ADVICE.

ALWAYS HAVE SUSPECTED PROSTATE PROBLEMS MEDICALLY CHECKED.

RECIPE
Saw Palmetto and Nettle Root Tincture

Dig up, wash, and finely chop two or three handfuls of fresh nettle roots. Place in a jar and cover with saw palmetto tincture (available from specialist herb stores). Leave for two weeks, shaking from time to time. Strain and bottle. Dose: 30 drops, 3 times daily, for prostate problems.

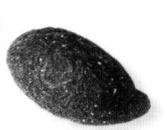
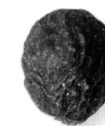
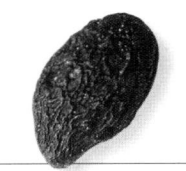

BELOW *Saw palmetto berries are a diuretic and tissue builder.*

Silybum marianum
MILK THISTLE SEED

A tall, beautiful thistle that can easily be grown. The seeds resemble sunflower seeds. The seedheads are stored in a warm place to release the seeds.

NOTES AND DOSAGES

- Standard decoction: ½ cup 3 times daily for at least six months.
- Tablets are also available – follow the instructions on the box. Recent research indicates it may be useful in hepatitis C.

BELOW *Milk thistle gets its name because it promotes milk production in nursing mothers.*

CAUTION

LIVER DISEASE SHOULD BE TREATED BY A PROFESSIONAL.

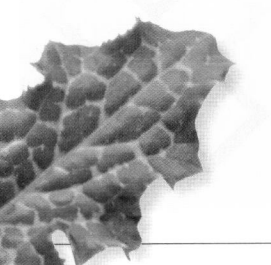

DATA FILE

Properties

- Strengthens and clears the liver and gall bladder.

Uses

- For "liverishness" and liver disease, poor fat tolerance, pale stools, and to protect the liver when taking strong drugs and medicines.
- Depression which comes on following hepatitis.
- For treating gallstones and for inflammation.
- Useful for Candida and food allergies.
- High blood pressure with liverish symptoms.

Scutellaria laterifolia or *Scutellaria galericulata*
SKULLCAP

U.S. skullcap, which is easily grown in gardens, or European skullcap, which grows wild on river banks.

DATA FILE

Properties

- Strengthens and calms the nervous system
- Antispasmodic

Uses

- Anxiety, tension headaches, PMS; for examination nerves, and to help fight off post-examination depression.
- With valerian or chamomile and linden flowers for insomnia and disturbed sleep, and for tranquilizer withdrawal.
- With vervain for workaholics, the mixture being relaxing without sedative effects.
- Supportive treatment in epilepsy and for people on major tranquilizers. Reduces anxiety without interfering with medication.

RIGHT *Skullcap prefers a sunny, open position in ordinary soil. The plant lives for about three years.*

CAUTION

SOME YEARS AGO COMMERCIAL PREPARATIONS WERE FOUND TO CONTAIN GERMANDER, WHICH IS POISONOUS. ALWAYS BUY YOUR HERBS AND HERBAL PREPARATIONS FROM A REPUTABLE FIRM.

NOTES AND DOSAGES

- Standard doses (*see pages 108–9*).
- **There are many relaxing tablets available at various stores containing skullcap and other herbs** Follow the dosage on the box.

RECIPE
Examination Tea

Mix together equal parts of dried skullcap, linden flowers, and sage leaf. Store in a jar in a dark place. Make a tea in the normal way, using 1 teaspoon of the mixture to 1 cup of boiling water. Drink 1 cup before examinations or 3 cups a day whilst studying.

Symphytum officinale
COMFREY

A common wild plant with large, bristly leaves and clusters of purple flowers. Comfrey root is used for treatment. One common name for comfrey is "knitbone," testifying to its healing powers.

DATA FILE

Properties
- Healing
- Mucilaginous

Uses
- Comfrey promotes rapid healing of cuts, wounds, sprains, and broken bones when taken as a tea or tincture, or used in poultices, creams, and liniments.
- Clean wounds well before applying comfrey.
- As a cream for cracked, dry skin.
- With chamomile and meadowsweet for hiatus hernia and stomach ulcers.

RIGHT *Comfrey grows to about 3ft. (1m.) high and bears purplish or cream flowers.*

NOTES AND DOSAGES

- Standard doses (*see pages 108–9*).
- Add a few drops of a warming essential oil such as black pepper to the infused oil to make a good liniment for arthritis, bunions, and aches and pains arising from old injuries. - Comfrey ointment is a traditional soothing and healing preparation for sprains, and aches and pains.

CAUTION

THERE HAS BEEN SUSPICION OF LIVER DAMAGE FROM USING COMFREY ROOT AND FROM EATING LARGE AMOUNTS OF THE HERB.

THE HERB TEA AND TINCTURE ARE SAFE TO USE, BUT IT IS SENSIBLE TO AVOID THEM IN PREGNANCY, DURING BREAST-FEEDING, AND FOR INFANTS.

PREPARATIONS OF THE ROOT ARE NOT TAKEN INTERNALLY.

DATA FILE

Properties
- Immune tonic
- Antibiotic
- Antifungal

Uses
- Immune deficiency with susceptibility to infections.
- Good for diarrhea and intestinal infections.
- Traditionally used for cancer. Recent research has shown that the herb may be helpful for breast, liver, and prostate cancers. May be taken in conjunction with orthodox cancer treatment.
- For oral thrush, as a mouthwash; and to treat candidiasis, when taken as a decoction.

CAUTION

LARGE DOSES MAY CAUSE NAUSEA.

PEOPLE WITH BLOOD-CLOTTING DISORDERS SHOULD SEEK PROFESSIONAL ADVICE BEFORE TAKING THE HERB.

RIGHT *The inner bark of Pau D'arco is known to be an excellent antifungal agent.*

Tabebuia avellanedae
PAU D'ARCO

A tree from the South American rainforest. Also called lapacho and the Taheebo tree. It is particularly useful in the treatment of immunodeficiency diseases.

RECIPE
Tonic Soup

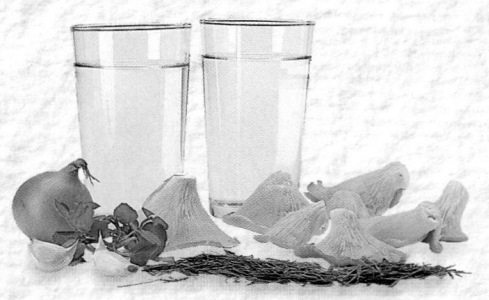

Make a decoction with ½oz. (12g.) Pau D'arco and 2pt. (1l.) water. Strain. Chop a small onion, two cloves of garlic, and a dozen oyster fungi. Simmer in the decoction until soft. Chop a small bunch of watercress and add to the soup just before serving. Eat daily for a weak immune system.

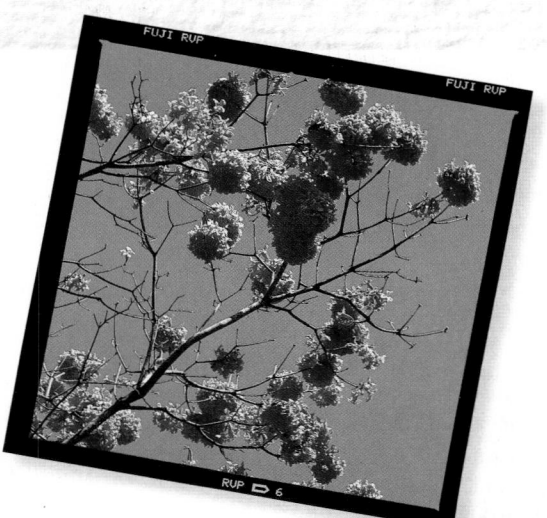

NOTES AND DOSAGES

- Make half-strength decoctions, ½oz. (12g.) Pau D'arco to 1pt. (500ml.) water. - **Drink 3 cups daily.**
- Tablets and capsules are available – follow the doses on the packet.

Tanacetum parthenium
FEVERFEW

A small-flowered daisy, easily grown in gardens. Use the leaves, which should be picked just before the plant flowers. Feverfew is good for period pains, vertigo, and arthritis. The name is a corruption of the word "febrifuge."

DATA FILE

Properties
- Anti-inflammatory
- Antispasmodic
- Emmenagogue

Uses
- For migraine and arthritis.
- Combined with valerian for migraine linked with anxiety and tension.

ABOVE *Combined with skullcap, feverfew relieves persistent headaches.*

NOTES AND DOSAGES

The best preparation is the tincture made from the fresh plant. **Dose: 1 teaspoon in a little water at the first signs of a migraine; repeat after 2 hours if necessary.** For repeated attacks and as a treatment for arthritis, take 1 teaspoon every morning. If you have a plant, 2 or 3 medium-sized leaves equal 1 teaspoon of tincture.

CAUTION

NOT TO BE TAKEN IN PREGNANCY OR DURING BREAST-FEEDING.

AVOID GIVING TO SMALL CHILDREN.

DO NOT TAKE IF USING BLOOD-THINNING DRUGS SUCH AS WARFARIN.

CHEWING THE LEAF CAN CAUSE MOUTH ULCERS IN SOME PEOPLE; IF THIS IS THE CASE, USE THE TINCTURE OR CAPSULES.

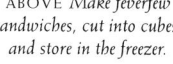

ABOVE *Make feverfew sandwiches, cut into cubes, and store in the freezer.*

RECIPE
Feverfew Preparations

There are many preparations of feverfew on the market, although many people still find that the fresh plant is the most effective. If it is not possible to keep a feverfew plant, make fresh feverfew sandwiches and keep them in the freezer.

Butter the bread. Cover one slice with a double layer of fresh feverfew leaves. Put on the top slice and press. Cut the sandwiches into small cubes. Each cube should have two or three medium-sized feverfew leaves. Wrap each cube in plastic wrap. Label, date, and freeze. Dose: one cube at the first sign of headache, then every two hours until the headache is over.

Taraxacum officinalis
DANDELION LEAF

The leaves from the familiar weed, which can be picked at any time. The leaves can be cooked and eaten like spinach, and are good for a springtime cleansing tonic. Dandelion leaf tea relieves edema and water retention.

DATA FILE

Properties
- A powerful diuretic
- Nourishing

Uses
- Tea for all types of water retention and edema, especially for swollen ankles

which are associated with circulatory problems.
- Take with uva ursi or thyme for cystitis.

NOTES AND DOSAGES

Use 2 or 3 teaspoons of the dried herb to 1 cup of boiling water. **Drink freely. Take sufficient to produce a good flow of urine.** Contains vitamins A and C and many trace minerals, and is especially high in potassium. The fresh leaves are a tasty salad ingredient.

RECIPE
Blanched Dandelion Leaf

This stimulates digestion and is excellent to include in daily salad for cases of poor appetite, weak digestion, and liver, and for general convalescence. Put a large pot upside down over a growing plant to keep out the light. Leave for two weeks or until the leaves are white. Dose: two leaves daily.

Taraxacum officinalis
DANDELION ROOT

The bitter dandelion root is a favorite in folk medicine, and particularly useful for stimulating a sluggish liver. The root of the dandelion is more effective than the leaves and stem in the treatment of liver problems. Coffee made from dandelion root is available, and it is thought to have a tonic effect on the pancreas, spleen, and female organs.

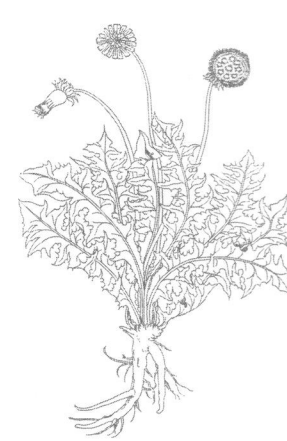

RIGHT *Dandelion root is a safe diuretic herb.*

DATA FILE

Properties

⚘ Liver tonic

⚘ Promotes good digestion

⚘ Alterative

Uses

⚘ For all types of liver and gall bladder problems.

⚘ For indigestion, loss of appetite, and constipation in pregnancy.

⚘ For arthritis and stubborn skin disease in combination with burdock.

⚘ Research shows that regular use helps reduce blood cholesterol.

⚘ The liver plays a crucial role in detoxification and nutrition, hence dandelion root is helpful in most chronic and wasting diseases, and helps the body to cope with strong chemical drugs.

RECIPE
Dandelion Coffee
⚘ ⚘ ⚘ ⚘

Although dandelion is a wonderful plant it does not always grow where it is wanted. When weeding, keep the long taproots. Scrub all the dirt off the roots, chop into pieces, and roast in a medium oven until dry and slightly burnt. Make a decoction and take 1 or 2 cups a day as a liver strengthener and tonic.

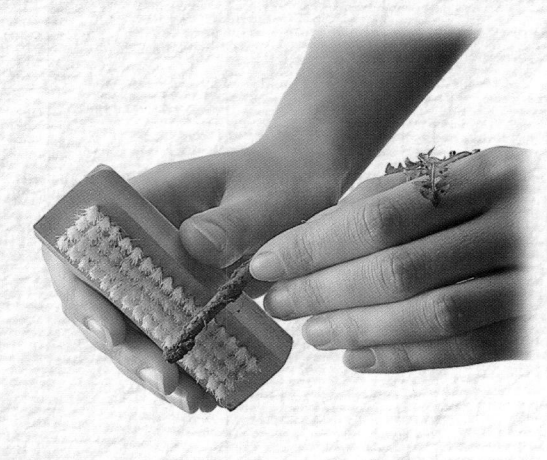

NOTES AND DOSAGES

🌿 At least 3 cups of decoction a day for 6 months. 🌿 **Tincture: 4–6 teaspoons daily.** 🌿 The decoction is best for liver problems.

ABOVE *Do not slice the roots when you gather them, or the valuable sap will be lost.*

Tilia europea
LINDEN

A tree often grown in parks and along streets. Its wood is good for carving, as it will take fine detail. Use the flowers, which are also called limeflowers. *Tilea europea* grows to 35m. (120 ft.). Its flowers are toxic to bees.

RIGHT *Limeflowers combined with elderflowers treat colds, and with hops treat nervous tension.*

DATA FILE

Properties

⚘ Calming and soothing

⚘ Strengthens nerves

⚘ Antispasmodic

⚘ Diaphoretic

Uses

⚘ For anxiety, irritability, and insomnia. Long-term use strengthens the nervous system and improves tolerance of stress.

⚘ Improves digestion, nervous indigestion.

⚘ Induces sweating and reduces temperature in fevers. Suitable for children. Use at standard tea strength and take freely.

⚘ Take linden with hawthorn tops as a tea for mild high blood pressure.

CAUTION

OLD OR IMPROPERLY DRIED FLOWERS ARE SAID TO BE SOMEWHAT NARCOTIC. REJECT STALE-SMELLING AND DISCOLORED FLOWERS. STORE CAREFULLY.

NOTES AND DOSAGES

🌿 Standard doses (*see pages 108–9*). May be taken freely.
🌿 **A popular everyday tea in France.**
🌿 Linden mixes well with other herb teas.

RECIPE
Linden Flower Bath for Infants
⚘ ⚘ ⚘ ⚘

Especially good for dry skin and eczema with irritability. Take ½oz. (12g.) dried linden flowers and 1pt. (500ml.) water. Put into pan and bring to the boil, cover, and allow to stand for 15 minutes. Add to the baby's bath.

Turnera diffusa

DAMIANA

A small, strongly aromatic shrub grown in South America. The leaves are used for therapeutic purposes. They treat depression, anxiety, poor digestion, cystitis, and are a tonic for the reproductive system.

DATA FILE

Properties

🌿 Stimulant tonic for the nerves and reproductive system in both sexes

🌿 Aphrodisiac

Uses

🌿 For impotence and sterility associated with anxiety, especially in men.

🌿 For physical weakness, depression, mental stupor, and nervous exhaustion in both sexes.

🌿 For prostatitis and relief of chronic cystitis.

🌿 For poor digestion with constipation and lack of appetite.

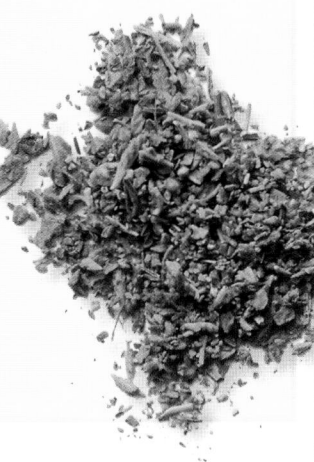

ABOVE *Dried damiana leaves and stems. These are gathered when the plant is in flower.*

CAUTION

SAFE BUT QUITE STIMULATING.

—◇—

DO NOT EXCEED THE RECOMMENDED DOSE.

NOTES AND DOSAGES

🌿 Take ½ cup of the tea or 1 teaspoon of the tincture twice daily.
🌿 Alternatively combine damiana with other herbs, such as wild oats or saw palmetto, and use 1 cup of the combination tea, or 1 teaspoon of tincture, twice daily.

RECIPE

Damiana Combination for Herpes

🌿 🌿 🌿 🌿

Combine equal parts of tinctures of damiana and echinacea. Dose: 1 teaspoon every four hours. This will often avert an attack, if taken at the first signs. Alternatively, make a decoction with equal parts of the herbs and take ½ cup every four hours.

Thymus vulgaris

THYME

The popular thyme used in cooking recipes. Thyme is an attractive small perennial herb. It is easy to grow and thrives in the rock garden or a sunny well-drained border. There are many different garden varieties.

NOTES AND DOSAGES

🌿 Take freely. 🌿 Large doses might be needed for coughs. 🌿 For infants' coughs, 2 or 3 teaspoons of syrup up to 4 times daily. Make a chest rub from the infused oil. For children's worms, ¼–½ cup strong tea before breakfast, for 2 weeks.

CAUTION

AVOID LARGE DOSES IN PREGNANCY, EXCEPT AS ADVISED BY A QUALIFIED HERBALIST.

—◇—

THE AMOUNTS TAKEN IN FOOD ARE HARMLESS.

—◇—

ASTHMA CAN BE SERIOUS AND SHOULD BE TREATED BY A PROFESSIONAL.

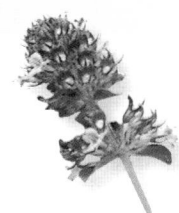

RECIPE

Thyme Syrup

🌿 🌿 🌿 🌿

Thyme makes an ideal antiseptic expectorant cough syrup. This recipe is for a tight chest and restless unproductive cough. Take ½oz. (12g.) thyme, 1oz. (25g.) chamomile, 1 teaspoon cinnamon, a pinch of cayenne or ginger (optional). Make a decoction, reduce, and add sugar or honey. Take as directed.

DATA FILE

Properties

🌿 Antiseptic

🌿 Antibacterial

🌿 Antifungal

🌿 Expectorant

🌿 Digestive tonic

Uses

🌿 For any cough with infected or tough phlegm.

🌿 Helpful, if taken regularly, in asthma.

🌿 Specific for the treatment of whooping cough.

🌿 Indigestion, wind, and intestinal infections.

🌿 Take along with marshmallow for cystitis.

🌿 Fights distressing intestinal worms in children.

🌿 Weak tea for nightmares.

🌿 Thyme vinegar is antifungal for athlete's foot.

🌿 Use thyme vinegar, diluted with an equal amount of water, for washes and douches for thrush.

THERAPY CONNECTIONS

THYME

⬤ Aromatherapy *p.170*

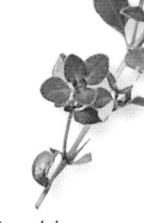

ABOVE *Ground thyme, with sage and chamomile, inhaled on a charcoal block, helps asthma.*

LEFT *Thyme cough syrup tastes pleasant and appeals to children.*

Ulmus fulva
SLIPPERY ELM BARK

The inner bark of a small U.S. tree, usually sold powdered. It smells rather like fenugreek, but tastes bland. It is very nutritious, as well as having healing properties.

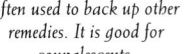

BELOW Slippery elm is often used to back up other remedies. It is good for convalescents.

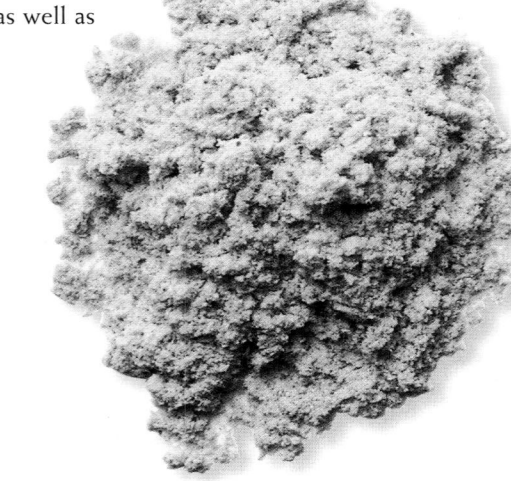

DATA FILE

Properties

❧ Soothing

❧ Mucilaginous

Uses

❧ Any sort of inflammation or irritation in the digestive tract: nausea, indigestion, wind, food allergies, stomach ulcers, acidity, heartburn, hiatus hernia, colitis, diverticulitis, and diarrhea. One of the most useful herbs for treating digestive problems.

❧ Mix with sufficient water to make a paste for drawing splinters.

RECIPE
Slippery Elm and Chamomile Poultice
❧ ❧ ❧ ❧

Mix together 2 dessertspoons each of slippery elm powder and dried chamomile flowers. Add hot water, slowly, stirring all the time to make a paste. Wrap the warm paste in light cotton and apply. Leave in place for a half-hour. Soothing and healing for any kind of painful swelling.

BELOW Stir slippery elm powder into a glass of milk, and drink before meals to help digestion.

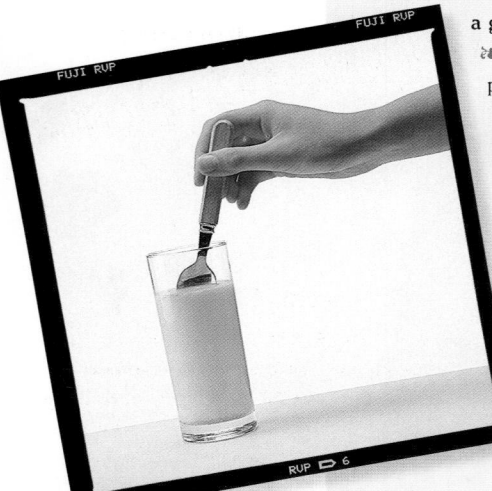

NOTES AND DOSAGES

❧ Tablets flavored with carminative herbs are especially useful. ❧ **Take 1 or 2 with a glass of water or milk before meals.** ❧ For travel sickness and nausea in pregnancy, suck one tablet slowly. ❧ **Stir 1 level teaspoon of powder into a drink, and take 3 times daily before meals.**

Valeriana officinalis
VALERIAN ROOT

The root of a wild plant with pretty pink flowers. In the Middle Ages, it was used as a spice and a perfume, as well as a medicine.

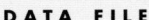

ABOVE Valerian leaves. The roots of the plant are used, and are dug up in the fall.

NOTES AND DOSAGES

❧ The cold decoction is best: soak 1 teaspoon in 1 cup of cold water overnight. ❧ **Dose: ½–1 cup.** ❧ **Tincture: 20–60 drops 3 times daily.** ❧ **More may be needed to help with tranquilizer withdrawal.** ❧ Relaxing tablets containing valerian are widely available.

CAUTION

A SAFE HERB IN GENERAL USE.

CAUSES HYPERACTIVITY IN SOME PEOPLE.

VERY LARGE DOSES CAN CAUSE TEMPORARY GIDDINESS.

DO NOT TAKE FOR LONG PERIODS WITHOUT EXAMINING WHY YOU ARE SO TENSE.

TRANQUILIZER WITHDRAWAL SHOULD ONLY BE UNDERTAKEN WITH PSYCHOLOGICAL SUPPORT.

DATA FILE

Properties

❧ Sedative

❧ Nerve restorative

❧ Calms the heart

❧ Antispasmodic

❧ Carminative

Uses

❧ Anxiety, confusion, migraines, insomnia, and depression with anxiety.

❧ Useful when flying.

❧ Palpitations.

❧ Helpful for withdrawal from tranquilizers.

❧ Good for high blood pressure from stress.

❧ With chamomile for colic and nervous indigestion.

BELOW Valerian grows in damp ground, reaching 3ft. (1m.).

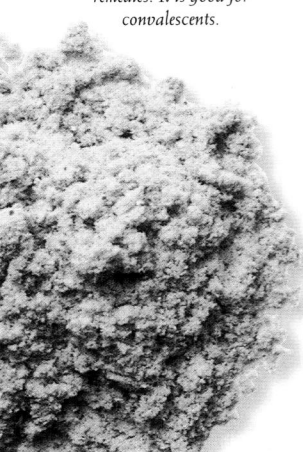

RECIPE
Valerian Sleeping Mixture
❧ ❧ ❧ ❧

Mix together equal amounts of tinctures of valerian root, dandelion root, and chamomile flowers (some specialist stores will make up the mixture for you). Store in a dark bottle and label. Adult dose: 1–3 teaspoons in a little water before bed for sleeplessness with tension or from indigestion.

Urtica dioica
NETTLE

The common stinging nettle, which grows all over the world. Plants have either male or female flowers, which is suggested by the name *dioica*, meaning "two houses." Nettles produce a good textile fiber.

DATA FILE

Properties

❦ Iron tonic

❦ Mild diuretic

❦ Antihistamine

❦ Strengthening

❦ Styptic

Uses

❦ Iron deficiency anemia. Nourishing and building, good to take in pregnancy.

❦ For lethargy, weakness, and feelings of heaviness in the body.

❦ Nettle rash, allergies to strawberries, and insect bites; as tea and lotion, and nervous eczema.

❦ Treats urinary gravel and water retention.

❦ Helpful for arthritis.

❦ Taken with cleavers as a spring tonic.

CAUTION

MAY BE TOO DRYING FOR SOME PEOPLE, IN WHICH CASE TAKE WITH MARSHMALLOW.

RIGHT *The juice of a nettle will relieve a nettle sting, strangely enough!*

RECIPE
Nettle Soup
❦ ❦ ❦ ❦

Young nettle tops gathered in spring provide an unusual vegetable, which can be made into a nourishing soup. Pick 1pt. (500ml.) of the tops of young nettles, avoiding too much stem. Chop two medium potatoes, a carrot, and a small onion. Add the ingredients to twice as much water and boil until the potatoes are soft. Blend in a food processor. Serve seasoned to taste.

NOTES AND DOSAGES

❧ Standard doses (*see pages 108–9*). ❧ **Leave to infuse for 15 minutes for best effect.** ❧ The tops can be cooked as spinach or made into soup. ❧ Rubbing stiff joints with fresh nettles gives instant relief.

Verbascum thaspus
MULLEIN

A beautiful wild flower with a tall, thick spike of yellow flowers. Use the leaves and flowers. Mullein is demulcent, emollient, and astringent, good for lung complaints and diarrhea.

DATA FILE

Properties

❦ A soothing expectorant

❦ Clears mucus

❦ Heals wounds

Uses

❦ For deep and ticklish coughs and bronchitis. Helpful in asthma, by clearing sticky mucus.

❦ Mullein flower infused oil as ear drops for itchy ears and chronic earache, and as a salve for itchy eyelids.

❦ Mullein and garlic infused oil to soothe the pain of acute earache.

❦ Two drops of mullein flower infused oil, in a little juice, three times daily, is helpful for bedwetting.

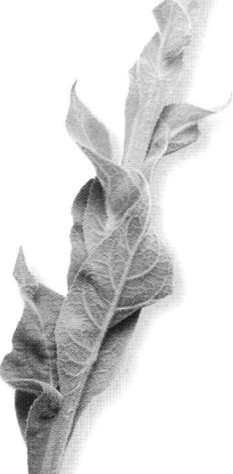

RIGHT *Mullein was also known as "bullock's lungwort" – because it cured cattle's lung diseases.*

NOTES AND DOSAGES

❧ The tea gives the best results for coughs. ❧ Allow the mullein to infuse for a long time and drink freely.

CAUTION

DO NOT USE EARDROPS IF THE EARDRUM HAS BURST.

THERAPY CONNECTIONS

NETTLE

☺ Homeopathy *p.217*

RECIPE
Mullein and Garlic Infused Oil
❦ ❦ ❦ ❦

Pick the spike from a mullein in full flower. Make an infused oil (*see the instructions on page 109*). This is used for itchy ears. Fill a small jar with chopped garlic and cover it with the mullein oil. Leave overnight. Strain and use as drops for ear infections.

Verbena officinalis
VERVAIN

An unprepossessing wild plant with a spike of small, pale pink flowers. Often missed. Vervain is a nourishing tonic.

RECIPE
Combined Vervain Remedy
❦ ❦ ❦

Prepare a vervain flower remedy *(see page 241)*, or buy a bottle of the prepared flower remedy stock. Add 4 drops of this remedy to 1 cup of vervain tea, standard strength. Drink 2 or 3 cups daily to relieve tiredness and tension resulting from overwork.

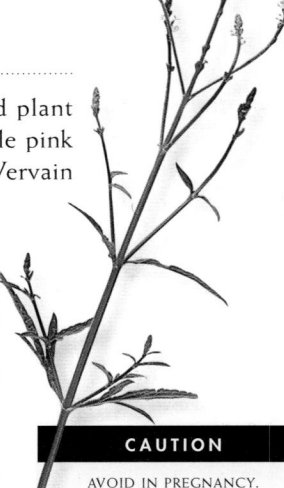

CAUTION

AVOID IN PREGNANCY.
—◦—
SAFE FOR CHILDREN AND WHEN BREAST-FEEDING.
—◦—
LARGE DOSES OF THE TEA CAN CAUSE NAUSEA.

DATA FILE

Properties
- ❦ Tonic
- ❦ Fever herb
- ❦ Nerve restorative
- ❦ Antispasmodic
- ❦ Carminative
- ❦ Diuretic
- ❦ Promotes milk flow
- ❦ Emmenagogue

Uses
- ❦ Exhaustion and post-viral fatigue. Exhaustion from overwork. Vervain is a useful general tonic.
- ❦ Nervous depression.
- ❦ Fevers and flu, especially accompanied by headaches and nervous symptoms.
- ❦ Insomnia and excessive dreaming; also for feelings of paranoia.
- ❦ Good for "letting go."

- ❦ Indigestion, worms, and parasites; digestive discomfort following treatment for parasites.
- ❦ "Liverishness" with nausea, heavy headaches, and depression.
- ❦ Irritable bowel syndrome with mucus in the stools.
- ❦ Helpful in asthma – relieves chest tension.
- ❦ Sip the tea throughout labor to encourage regular contractions. Continue taking it after the birth to encourage milk flow.
- ❦ Post-natal depression.
- ❦ Menstrual cramps and to restore menstruation stopped by stress.
- ❦ Post-operative tiredness and depression.
- ❦ As a compress for inflamed eyes.

NOTES AND DOSAGES

🍃 Standard-strength teas taken every two hours in fevers, or 3 cups a day for chronic complaints. For worms and parasites, make double-strength tea and drink before breakfast for some weeks or until better. Vervain tea is an ideal restorative for people strained by overwork, especially mental work.

ABOVE LEFT Both the leaves and the flowers of the vervain plant are used to make herbal remedies.

BELOW Vervain helps to treat depression and exhaustion.

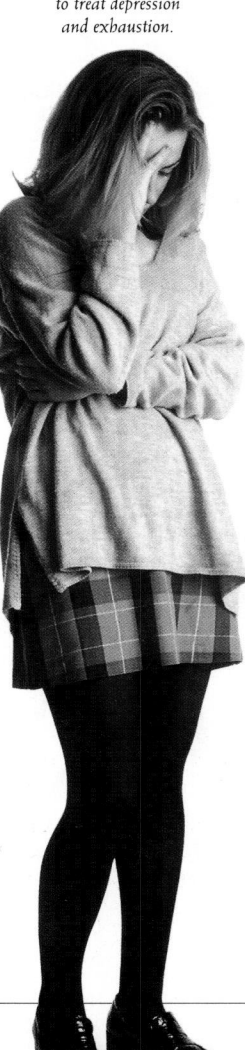

Viburnum opulus
CRAMP BARK

The bark from the wild form of the guelder rose. Treats nervous complaints, cramp, spasms, heart disease, and rheumatism.

ABOVE The bark has a strong smell and is sold in thin strips. It is produced mainly in northern Europe.

DATA FILE

Properties
- ❦ Relaxant
- ❦ Antispasmodic
- ❦ Mildly sedative

Uses
- ❦ For any sort of cramping pains, colic, menstrual cramps, muscle spasm, and shoulder and neck tension.

- ❦ Back pain usually involves some muscle spasm – often a dramatic improvement with cramp bark.
- ❦ For children when bedwetting is associated with tension and anxiety.

NOTES AND DOSAGES

🍃 Best taken freely, 1 cup of the decoction or 1–2 teaspoons of the tincture 4 or 5 times daily. May be improved by the addition of a little ginger. For children, give 30 drops of tincture, in fruit juice, three times daily.

CAUTION

SAFE IN GENERAL USE.
—◦—
SOME PEOPLE FIND THAT LARGE DOSES WILL LOWER THEIR BLOOD PRESSURE, MAKING THEM FEEL A LITTLE FAINT.

RECIPE
Cramp Bark Capsules for Menstrual Cramps
❦ ❦ ❦ ❦

Grind 1oz. (30g.) cramp bark and 1 teaspoon ginger powder together in a coffee grinder until you have a fine powder. Fill standard-sized gelatin capsules, available from herb suppliers. Take 2 or 3 capsules as required for quick relief from pain.

Vitex agnus-castus
AGNUS CASTUS BERRIES

The fruit of a pretty, half-hardy Mediterranean shrub. *Vitex agnus-castus* is also known as chaste tree, and is reputed both to increase sex drive, and also to damp it down, as indicated by its name!

DATA FILE

Properties

❧ Balances hormones

Uses

❧ PMS with irritability, breast pain, and water retention.

❧ Menopausal symptoms, especially with mood swings and depression. With sage for hot flushes.

❧ Helps restore a regular menstrual cycle when coming off the contraceptive pill or when the cycle has been disrupted.

CAUTION

MAY CAUSE CHANGES IN THE MENSTRUAL CYCLE. THIS IS A NATURAL PART OF THE WAY THE HERB WORKS.

AGNUS CASTUS MAY BE TAKEN IN CONJUNCTION WITH HORMONE DRUGS, BUT IT IS BEST TO SEEK THE ADVICE OF A PROFESSIONAL HERBALIST BEFORE DOING SO. NOT TO BE TAKEN WITH PROGESTERONE.

NOTES AND DOSAGES

❧ The best time to take the berries is first thing in the morning, before breakfast. One cup of the decoction or 20–30 drops of the tincture in a little water, taken daily, will usually suffice.

RECIPE
Agnus Castus Pepper

The dried berries have a pleasant, peppery taste, and may be powdered in a coffee grinder and sprinkled on to meals. Dose: two good pinches or ¼ flat teaspoon.

Agnus castus is still used in monasteries to help the monks keep to their vows of chastity, by balancing excess male hormones.

RIGHT *The leaves of the chaste tree. Berries should be picked in the fall and dried.*

Zingiber officinale
GINGER

Ginger is the spice made from the rhizome, or enlarged underground stem, of the herbaceous perennial plant *Zingiber officinale*, a member of the ginger family. Native to southern Asia, ginger is widely cultivated in Africa, Asia, Australia, and the West Indies, particularly Jamaica. Ginger is a warming, stimulating herb which is especially good for the circulation. The Chinese regularly use it in cooking.

RECIPE
Crystallized Ginger for Travel Sickness and Nausea

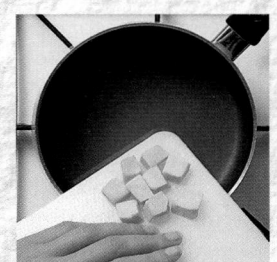

Peel a large piece of fresh ginger and chop it into small cubes. Make a syrup by dissolving 1 cup of sugar in 4 cups of water. Add the ginger and simmer gently until the root is soft. Leave in the syrup overnight, drain, and pack in sterilized jars.

DATA FILE

Properties

❧ Warming

❧ Carminative

❧ Antispasmodic

❧ Diaphoretic

❧ Anti-emetic

Uses

❧ For nausea and the nausea of pregnancy and travel sickness.

❧ For wind, colic, and irritable bowel.

❧ Good for chills, colds, and poor circulation.

❧ For fevers, added to elderflower or yarrow tea.

❧ For menstrual cramps, with cramp bark and as a compress of grated root.

CAUTION

AVOID TAKING GINGER IN ACUTE INFLAMMATORY CONDITIONS OR USING LOCALLY ON HOT AND INFLAMED AREAS. IT WILL BE TOO HEATING.

THERAPY CONNECTIONS

VERVAIN

◉ Flower Remedies   *p.241*

NOTES AND DOSAGES

❧ More easily tolerated than cayenne. May be added to most remedies to improve absorption and activity. A mixture of ½ teaspoon of powder to 1 cup boiling water may be taken freely. Tincture: 5–20 drops in any herb tea. Crystallized ginger helps with the control of travel sickness.

ABOVE *Ginger root is dug up when the leaves have dried. It is then thoroughly washed.*

AROMATHERAPY

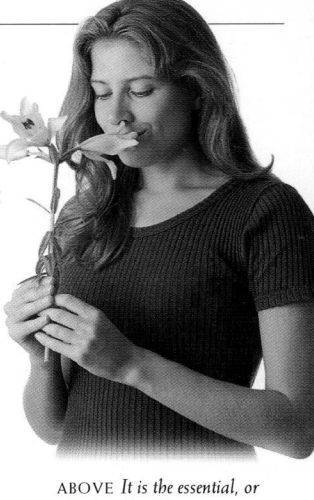

ABOVE *It is the essential, or volatile, oils of flowers, spices, and herbs that give them their unique fragrance.*

ESSENTIAL OILS

The practice of aromatherapy is based on the use of essential oils. The oils work on the whole body to treat specific ailments and restore the natural balance on both the physical and mental levels.

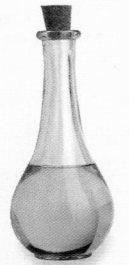

Each essential oil has its own individual scent and healing properties.

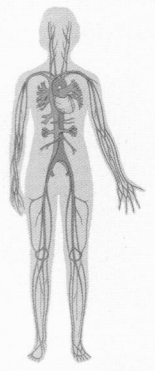

The oil molecules enter the bloodstream and are carried to every part of the body.

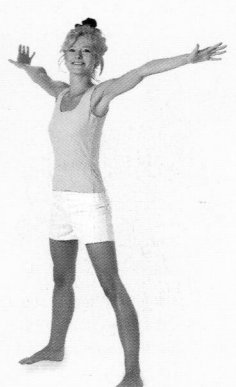

Oils affect both mind and spirit, restoring physical health and lifting the spirits.

The word aromatherapy means "treatment using scents." It refers to a particular branch of herbal medicine that uses concentrated plant oils called essential oils to improve physical and emotional health, and to restore balance to the whole person. Unlike the herbs used in herbal medicine, essential oils are not taken internally, but are inhaled or applied to the skin. Each oil has its own natural fragrance, and a gentle healing action that makes aromatherapy one of the most pleasant and popular of all the available complementary therapies.

HOW AROMATHERAPY WORKS

Aromatherapy is subtle but effective when used correctly and given time to work. While one treatment may prove immediately relaxing or reviving, the effects tend to be short-lived. Regular treatments are needed to rebalance body systems and if you have been stressed or ill, it could take several weeks of treatment before you notice an improvement. The practice of aromatherapy involves using more than just the aroma of certain plant oils to treat mind and body. It is concerned with getting essential oils into the body in order to alter body chemistry, support body systems, and improve moods and emotions. This is done most effectively by massaging oils into the skin. Manipulating the soft tissues of the body has been shown to release emotional and physical tension, relieve pain, promote healthy circulation, and restore the whole person to a balanced state of health. Massage is the method of choice for professional aromatherapists. However, for home use oils can also be added to bathwater, or applied on hot or cold compresses to swollen, painful, or bruised areas.

When applied to the skin, essential oils start to work immediately on body tissues. The molecules in the oils are so small that they can be absorbed through the pores of the skin and into the bloodstream, by which means they are carried to every part of the body.

LEFT *Essential oils are blended with a carrier oil for massage.*

However, aroma is important. Inhalation can reinforce the effects of oils applied to the skin, and it is a safe way to benefit from the healing properties of oils that could cause irritation. No one knows exactly how aromas affect the mind, but it has been theorized that receptors in the nose convert smells into electrical impulses which are transmitted to the limbic system of the brain. Smells reaching the limbic system can directly affect our moods and emotions, and improve mental alertness and concentration.

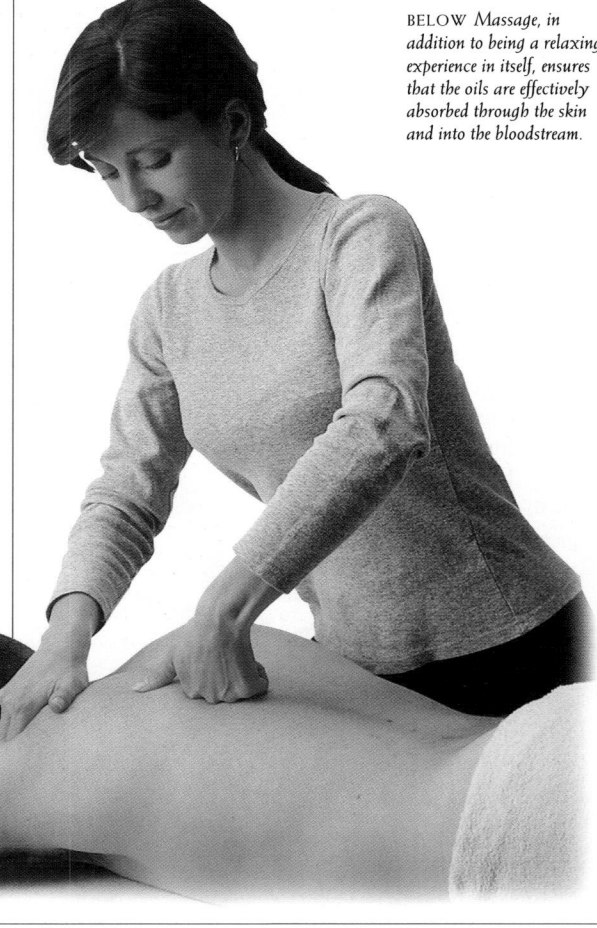

BELOW *Massage, in addition to being a relaxing experience in itself, ensures that the oils are effectively absorbed through the skin and into the bloodstream.*

THE BENEFITS OF AROMATHERAPY

Aromatherapy benefits people rather than illnesses. It is gentle enough to be used by people of all ages and states of health. It is nurturing for babies and children, and offers comfort and care to the elderly. Pregnant women and even seriously ill patients with cancer or AIDS can benefit from professional treatment. Aromatherapy is not recommended as a cure for any disease. Its most potent effect is that it relaxes mind and body, relieves pain, and restores body systems to a state of balance in which healing can best take place. It is also most effective when used as a preventive or to alleviate subclinical symptoms before they escalate into disease. The therapy has been shown to be particularly effective in preventing and treating stress and anxiety-related disorders, muscular and rheumatic pains, digestive problems, menstrual irregularities, menopausal complaints, insomnia, and depression.

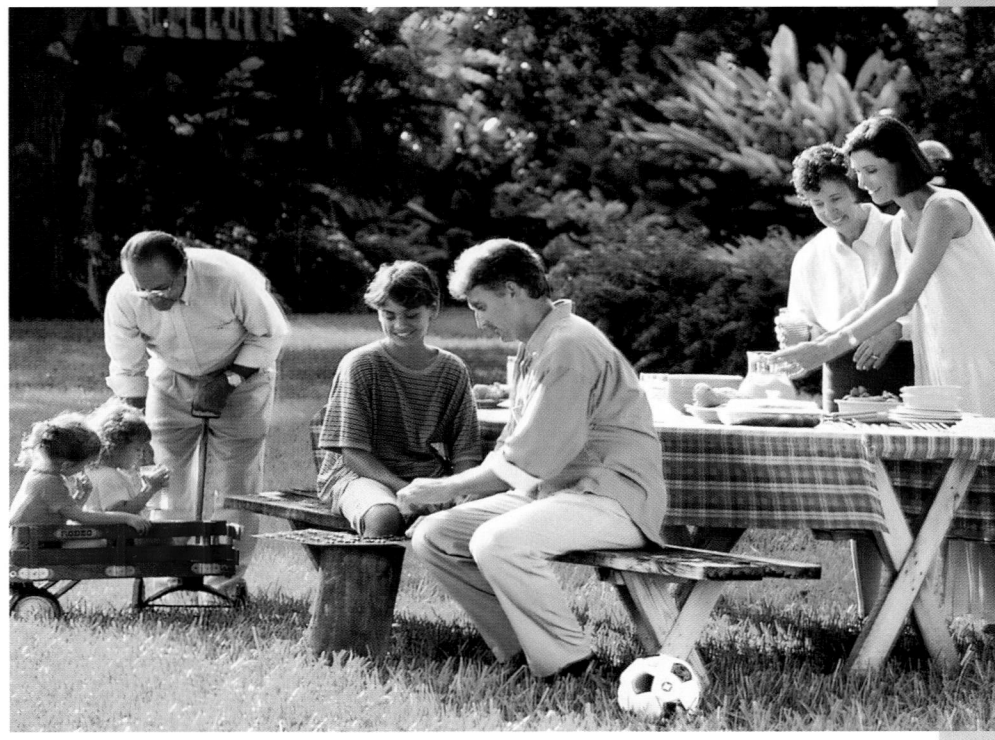

RIGHT *Aromatherapy is a safe, natural treatment that can benefit everyone, no matter what age or state of health.*

ANCIENT ORIGINS OF A MODERN THERAPY

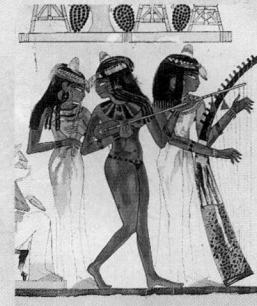

ABOVE *An ancient Egyptian wall painting showing women wearing perfume cones on their heads.*

Aromatic plant oils have been used therapeutically for thousands of years. The ancient Vedic literature of India, and historic Chinese and Arabic medical texts document the importance of aromatic oils for health and spirituality. In ancient Greece, Hippocrates, the "father of medicine," used fragrant fumigations to rid Athens of plague, and Roman soldiers kept up their strength by bathing in scented oil and having regular massages. However, the Egyptians were the most noted of the ancient aromatherapists. Physicians from all over the world are reputed to have traveled to Egypt to learn aromatic techniques.

Aromatherapy is believed to have come west at the time of the Crusades. Historical records show that essential oils were used during the plague in the 14th century. In the 16th and 17th centuries aromatherapy was popular among the great European herbalists. But it was not until the 18th and 19th centuries that scientists were able to identify many of the individual components of plant chemistry.

Research enabled scientists to extract the active components of medicinal plants. Ironically, this led to the development of pharmaceutical drugs and a rejection of plant medicine. However, in the 1920s the devotion of a French chemist, René Maurice Gattefossé, initiated a modest revival in plant oils. Gattefossé discovered that lavender oil quickly healed a burn on his hand, and went on to show that many essential oils were better antiseptics than their synthetic counterparts.

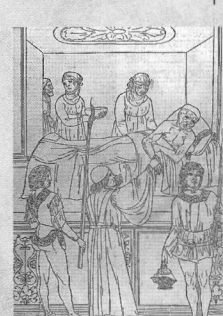

ABOVE *In the Middle Ages exotic essences, introduced into Europe by the Crusaders returning from the East, were used to treat many illnesses.*

He coined the term "aromathérapie" to encapsulate the healing effect of scented oils. Later, a French army surgeon, Dr. Jean Valnet, successfully used essential oils to treat soldiers wounded in battle and patients in a psychiatric hospital. In 1964 Valnet published *Aromathérapie*, still considered by many to be the bible of aromatherapy.

In the 1950s Marguérite Maury, an Austrian beauty therapist and biochemist, introduced the concept of using essential oils in massage, and established the first aroma-therapy clinics in Britain, France, and Switzerland. From this varied history, aromatherapy has evolved to become one of the most valued of modern complementary therapies.

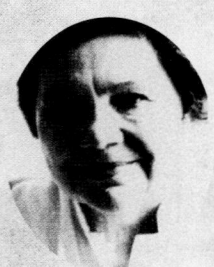

ABOVE *Marguérite Maury used aromatherapy in herbal beauty treatments to revitalize her clients.*

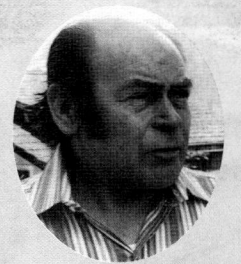

ABOVE *Jean Valnet used essential oils to treat specific medical and psychiatric disorders.*

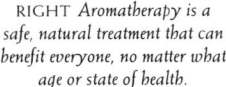

ESSENTIAL OILS AND HOW THEY WORK

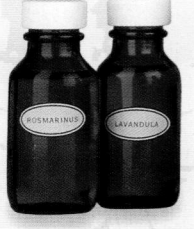

Essential oils should be stored in dark, well-stoppered, glass bottles, away from light and heat in order to maintain their potency.

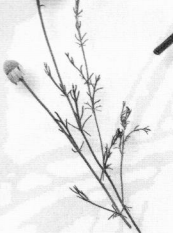

CHAMOMILE
Chamomile has long been appreciated for its calming and soothing properties.

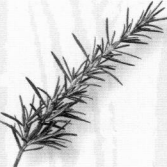

ROSEMARY
The dominant characteristic of rosemary oil is its stimulating effect.

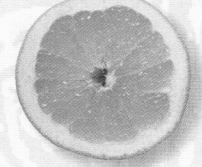

GRAPEFRUIT
Grapefruit oil, which is expressed from the peel of the fruit, refreshes the body and enlivens the mind.

Essential oils are extracted from the aromatic essences of certain plants, trees, fruit, flowers, herbs, and spices. They are natural volatile oils with identifiable chemical and medicinal properties. Over 150 essential oils have been extracted, each one with its own scent and unique healing properties. Oils are sourced from plants as commonplace as parsley and as exquisite as jasmine. For optimum benefits, essential oils must be extracted from natural raw ingredients and remain as pure as possible.

ESSENTIAL OILS IN ACTION

Despite considerable research, the chemistry of essential oils is not fully understood. Each oil is composed of at least 100 different chemical constituents, which are classified as aldehydes, phenols, oxides, esters, ketones, alcohols, and terpenes. There may also be many chemical compounds that have yet to be identified.

The oils and their actions are extremely complex. All the oils are antiseptic, but each one also has individual properties; for example, they may be analgesic, fungicidal, diuretic, or expectorant. The collective components of each oil also work together to give the oil a dominant characteristic. It can be relaxing, as in the case of chamomile, refreshing, like the citrus grapefruit, or stimulating, like the aromatic rosemary.

Within the body, essential oils are able to operate in three ways: pharmacologically, physiologically, and psychologically. From a pharmacological perspective, the chemical components of the oils react with body chemistry in a way that is similar to drugs, but slower, more sympathetic, and with fewer side-effects. Essential oils also have notable physiological effects. Certain oils have an affinity with particular areas of the body. For example, rose has an affinity with the female reproductive system, while spice oils tend to benefit the digestive system. The oil may also sedate an overactive system, or stimulate a different part of the body that is sluggish.

ABOVE Jasmine, highly valued for its exquisite floral fragrance, is widely used in cosmetics and perfumes.

RIGHT Rose, a perennial favorite as a perfume ingredient and cosmetic oil, also has an affinity with the female reproductive system.

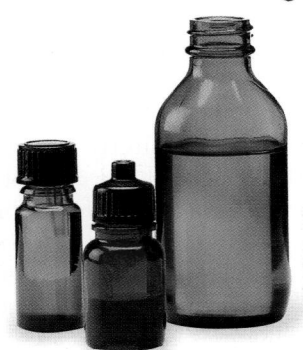

LEFT Essential oils that share a high proportion of common constituents generally blend well together.

Some oils, such as lavender, are known as adaptogens, meaning they do whatever the body requires of them at the time. The psychological response is triggered by the effect that the aromatic molecules have on the brain.

Essential oils are not all absorbed into the body at the same rate. They can take 20 minutes or several hours, depending on the oil and the individual body chemistry of the person being treated. On average, absorption takes about 90 minutes. After several hours, the oils leave the body. Most oils are exhaled, others are eliminated in urine, feces, and perspiration.

BLENDING AND USING ESSENTIAL OILS

Essential oils can be used alone or blended together. Oils are blended for two reasons: to create a more sophisticated fragrance, or to enhance or change the medicinal actions of the oils. Blending changes the molecular structure of essential oils, and when they are blended well therapists can create a "synergistic" blend, where the oils work in harmony and to great effect. To create a blend, the therapist considers not only the symptoms and underlying causes of a patient's particular problem, but also the individual's biological and psychological make-up, and personal fragrance preferences. For therapeutic purposes it is usual to mix only three or four oils together.

ABOVE Lavender is one of the most versatile essential oils because it responds to the body's particular needs at the time.

METHODS OF EXTRACTION

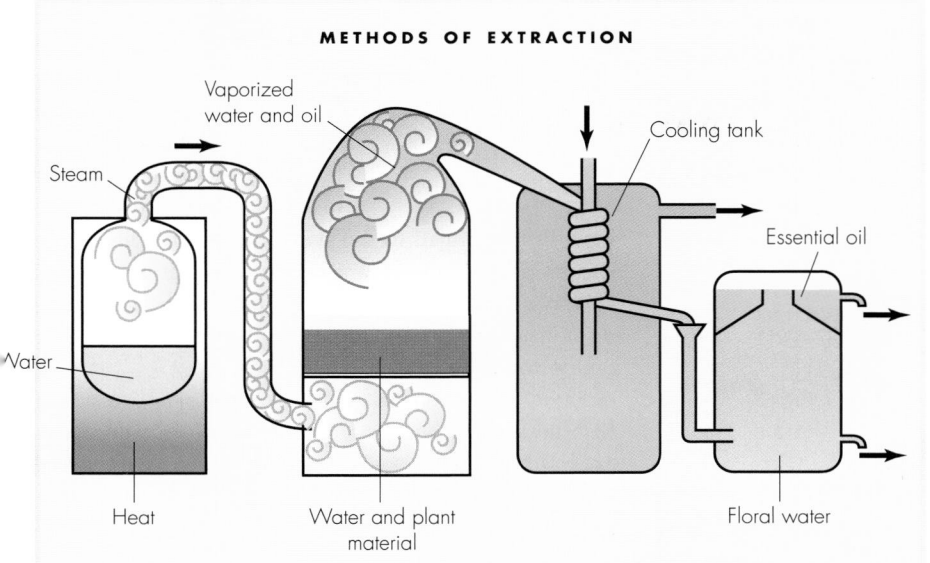

Steam

Vaporized water and oil

Cooling tank

Essential oil

Water

Heat

Water and plant material

Floral water

Essential oils are extracted from plants by a simple form of pressure known as expression, or by distillation. Most oils are extracted by steam distillation (*see above*). This involves steaming the parts of the plant to be used in order to break down the walls of the cells that store the essence. The released essence, combined with the steam, passes to cooling tanks, where the steam condenses to a watery liquid, and the essential oil floats on top. The oil is skimmed off and bottled, and the remaining liquid is sometimes used as flower or herbal water.

If you want to blend oils at home, choose two or three oils which you believe complement each other. In general, oils from the same groups (citrus, floral, spicy, etc.), and those which share similar constituents, blend well. Using the proportions detailed overleaf, mix a blend using small amounts of the strongest scented oils and more of the lighter fragrances. You can use the recipes for suggested blends in the remedies section, or create some of your own. Be guided by your own likes and dislikes – the best blend for you is often the one you find most appealing.

CREATING BLENDS

To use oils on the skin, choose a light cold-pressed vegetable oil such as grapeseed, sweet almond, or sunflower oil. For hair treatments choose a more penetrative oil, such as olive oil or jojoba. Where you need a slightly astringent oil, try hazelnut. Add your essential oils to the base oil a little at a time. Shake the bottle well and rub a little on the back of your hand to test the scent. Adjust the quantities until you achieve the blend you want. Add about 5 percent wheat germ oil to preserve the blend. Store blended oils in labeled dark bottles, out of children's reach, and use within three months.

BELOW Essential oils can be used to treat skin disorders, but they are also appreciated purely for their unique scents.

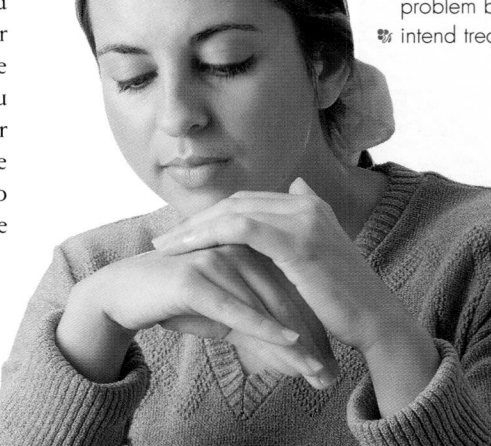

USING ESSENTIAL OILS SAFELY

Aromatherapy is compatible with conventional medicine and most other forms of holistic treatment. However, if you are taking medication consult your physician. Some oils are not compatible with homeopathic treatment. Aromatherapy is safe to use at home for minor or short-term problems, providing you follow certain guidelines.

* Do not take essential oils internally.
* Do not put essential oils in the eyes.
* Keep all oils away from children.
* Do not apply oils undiluted to the skin, unless it is stated that it is safe to do so.

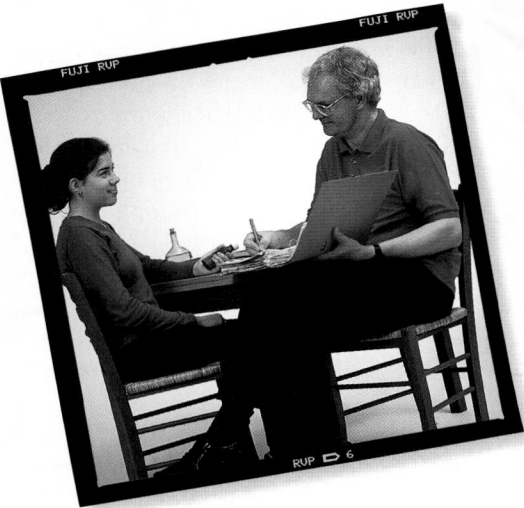

ABOVE Aromatherapy is generally a safe form of home treatment, but there are certain situations when it is best to consult a qualified practitioner.

Consult a qualified practitioner for advice and treatment if you:

* are pregnant;
* have an allergy;
* have a chronic medical condition such as high blood pressure or epilepsy;
* are receiving medical or psychiatric treatment;
* are taking homeopathic remedies;
* have a chronic or serious health problem, or if a problem becomes severe or persistent;
* intend treating babies or very young children.

AROMATHERAPY TECHNIQUES

There are many ways to use essential oils to good effect. The most common form of treatment among professional aromatherapists is to apply diluted essential oils to the body in a full body massage. But therapists also encourage the use of essential oils at home. When massage is not possible or appropriate, there are many other ways for people to benefit from aromatherapy.

MASSAGE

Massage in itself is nurturing and therapeutic, and the rubbing action releases the fragrance of the oils and ensures that they are well absorbed into the skin. When combined with the medicinal properties of the oils, massage forms a potent healing treatment that can be relaxing or energizing; it can soothe the nervous system, or stimulate the blood and lymphatic systems to improve physical and psychological functioning. It eases pain and tension from tired, taut, or overworked muscles, and lifts the spirits. Whenever possible, try to include massage in your home aromatherapy treatments.

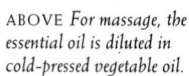

ABOVE *For massage, the essential oil is diluted in cold-pressed vegetable oil.*

❀ BASIC MEASUREMENTS *Dilute the essential oil in a cold-pressed vegetable carrier oil such as grapeseed, sweet almond, or sunflower oil. Use up to 5 drops of essential oil to 1 teaspoon of carrier oil for adults, half that strength for children under seven, and a quarter of the strength for children under three. The only essential oils suitable for babies are chamomile, rose, or lavender. Use only 1 drop to 1 teaspoon of carrier oil.*

BATHS

Aromatic baths are a simple, useful, and versatile way to use essential oils at home. They can be used to enhance moods, relax or stimulate body systems, treat skin disorders, and ease musculoskeletal pain. Essential oils do not dissolve in water, but form a thin film on the surface. The heat of the water releases their vapor and aids absorption into the skin.

❀ BASIC MEASUREMENTS *Fill the bath with warm water before you add the oils. For adults add 5–10 drops of essential oil to a full bath. Use less than 4 drops for children over two, and 1 drop for babies. Stir through the water with your hand.*

RIGHT *When used for skin care, the oils are best added to a cream or lotion.*

Oils can be used in a variety of ways, depending on individual preferences and the type of ailment being treated.

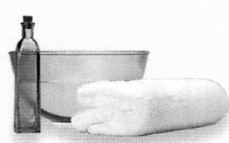

MASSAGE
Massage is one of the most popular and relaxing aromatherapy treatments.

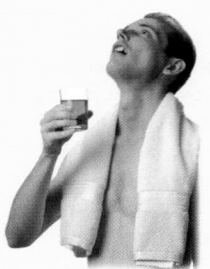

GARGLE
Antiseptic mouthwashes and gargles can be made with essential oils.

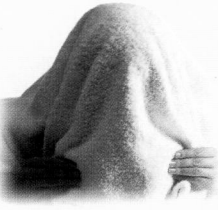

INHALATION
Steam inhalation of essential oils is suitable for sinus, throat, and chest problems.

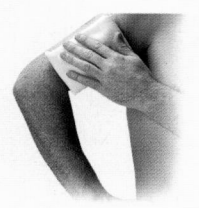

COMPRESS
Oils added to hot and cold compresses offer effective relief from pain and reduce inflammations.

ABOVE *A few drops of oil can be added directly to a bowl of boiling water for a steam inhalation.*

STEAM INHALATIONS

Inhalations are most beneficial for throat and respiratory infections, sinus and catarrhal congestion, and headaches. They are also effective for those oils that could cause irritation if applied to the skin. The steam releases the vapors of the oils. Steam inhalations are not always suitable for asthmatics or people with breathing difficulties, and they are not appropriate for treating children and infants.

❀ BASIC MEASUREMENTS *Add 3–4 drops of oil to a bowl of boiling water. Bend over the bowl, cover your head with a towel, and breathe deeply for a few minutes. You can also use this method as a facial sauna.*

VAPORIZERS

These can be electric, or a ceramic ring that is heated by a light bulb, but most are ceramic pots warmed by a small candle. They are a natural way to scent, deodorize, or disinfect a room, and are one of the best ways to use oils for enhancing mood and balancing the mind. Vaporizers are also useful for when young children have breathing difficulties.

❀ BASIC MEASUREMENTS *Add water and 6–8 drops of oil to the vaporizer. Alternatively, add the oil to a bowl of water and place by a radiator.*

CREAMS, LOTIONS, SHAMPOOS, AND GELS

One of the best ways to use oils for skin care and chronic skin complaints is to add them to a cream or lotion. This is more convenient and less greasy than massage, and it also means the oils can be applied when needed to wounds, bruises, or itchy skin. Adding oils to shampoos helps with everyday hair-care problems, and using essential oils with shower gels is excellent for fatigue and hangovers.

❀ BASIC MEASUREMENTS *Add 1 or 2 drops of essential oil to creams, lotions, and shampoos, and massage into the skin or scalp. Choose unscented products that are lanolin-free and made from good-quality natural ingredients.*

GARGLES AND MOUTHWASHES

Although essential oils should not be swallowed, mouthwashes and gargles are excellent ways to use antiseptic oils to treat mouth ulcers, gum disease, throat infections, and bad breath. These methods are not suitable for children.

❀ BASIC MEASUREMENTS *Dilute 4–5 drops of essential oil in a teaspoon of brandy. Mix into a glass of warm water and swish around the mouth or use as a gargle. Do not swallow.*

AROMATHERAPY

HOT AND COLD COMPRESSES

Compresses are an effective way of using essential oils to relieve pain and inflammation. They can be either hot or cold. Hot compresses are good for muscle pain, arthritis, rheumatism, toothache, earache, boils, and abscesses. Cold compresses benefit headaches, sprains, and swelling.

❀ BASIC MEASUREMENTS *Add 4–5 drops of essential oil to a bowl of hot or cold water. Soak a folded clean cotton cloth in the water, wring it out, and apply over the affected area. If using a hot compress, cover with a warm towel and repeat when it cools.*

❀ NEAT: *A few essential oils – such as lavender, tea tree oil, and sandalwood – can be applied undiluted to the skin. Most oils should not be used neat as they can cause irritation.*

❀ NOTE: **These are average safe dilutions for essential oils. In some of the following blends these measurements may vary slightly, but are still within safe guidelines.**

SEEING A PROFESSIONAL

A first appointment with an aromatherapist lasts between 60–90 minutes. It should take place in a warm, comfortable, subtly lit treatment room, containing a massage table, clean towels, and the therapist's stock of oils. The therapist may play soft music to create a relaxing atmosphere.

Every consultation begins with the therapist taking your case history. In order to provide safe, effective, holistic treatment he or she needs to know about your medical history and if you have come with a particular problem. As well as finding out which oils would be best to use, aromatherapists need to know which to avoid. If you are pregnant, have sensitive skin, high blood pressure, epilepsy, or have recently had an operation, some oils would be unsuitable to use. Pregnant women, for example, should avoid certain oils including thyme, basil, rosemary, clary sage, and juniper, because they may harm the fetus or induce miscarriage. The therapist will ask about your stress levels, and if you are using medication or taking homeopathic remedies. It is also important for the aromatherapist to know what sort of mood you are in and what kind of day you have had. This interview takes about 20 minutes and you may be asked to sign a consent form at the end of it.

Treatment usually involves massage. For this you will be asked to undress down to your underwear and lie on the massage table covered with a towel to keep you warm and prevent you from feeling exposed. The aromatherapist will move the towel as he or she works around your body, but will not remove it completely.

The therapist uses the information you have provided when deciding on a suitable blend of oils. Generally, the oils you like best are the ones that work best for

AROMATHERAPY MASSAGE

The techniques of massage as we know it today in the West were developed in the 19th century by a Swedish professor, Pier Heidrich Ling, and his work is the basis for massage treatment today. Different strokes are appropriate to different areas of the body. Gentle strokes are used to commence a session to relax the superficial muscles, and more vigorous strokes then stimulate the deeper muscles.

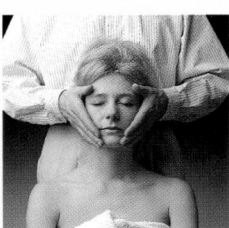

EFFLEURAGE

Effleurage is designed to sensitize your partner and prepare for the later strokes. It is particularly effective for the face. Place your hands on your partner's cheeks, fingers downward. Then stroke gently toward the ears, using the minimum pressure required to maintain contact. You can use this sliding stroke to massage the whole body if you vary the pressure and speed.

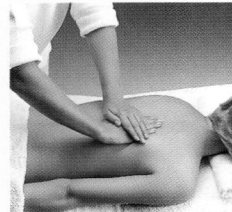

CIRCLING

Place both hands on your partner, a few inches apart, and stroke in a wide circular movement. Press into the upward stroke and glide back down. Your arms will cross as you make the circle, so just lift one hand over the other to continue. Circle lightly in a clockwise direction over the stomach to aid digestion.

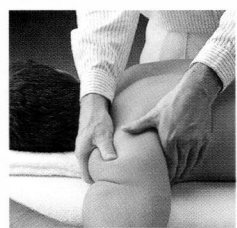

KNEADING

Place both hands on the area to be massaged with your fingers pointing away from you. Press into the body with the palm of one hand, pick up the flesh between your thumb and fingers, and press it toward the resting hand. Release and repeat with the other hand, as if you were kneading dough.

you. Using the chosen blend the aromatherapist will begin your massage using gentle massage strokes and may also work on pressure points of the body. During the 30–45 minutes that it takes to give a full body massage the therapist will talk very little if at all, allowing you to relax completely.

At the end of your massage, you may be advised not to bathe or shower for several hours so that the oils can be fully absorbed. The therapist may conclude the visit by giving you oils to use at home.

BELOW The essential oils used for massage are always diluted in a carrier oil or lotion.

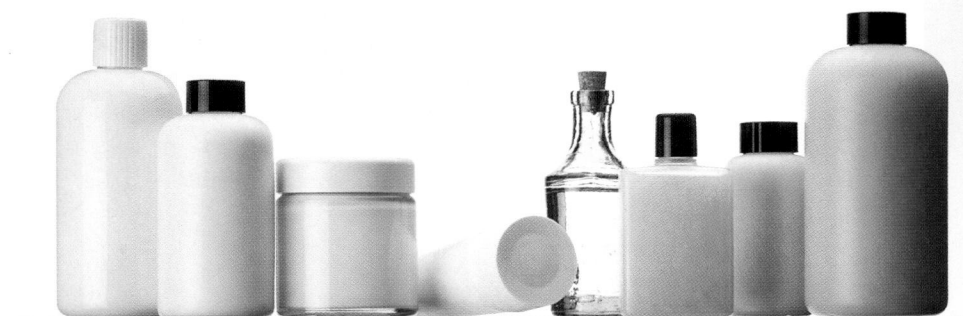

ESSENTIAL OILS

Angelica archangelica
ANGELICA

The healing properties of angelica were so revered in antiquity that it was called the root of the Holy Spirit. There are over 30 varieties of angelica grown around the world; at least 10 are highly valued in Traditional Chinese Medicine. Angelica root and the seeds are used to produce the essential oil, which has a musky, sweet, woody scent.

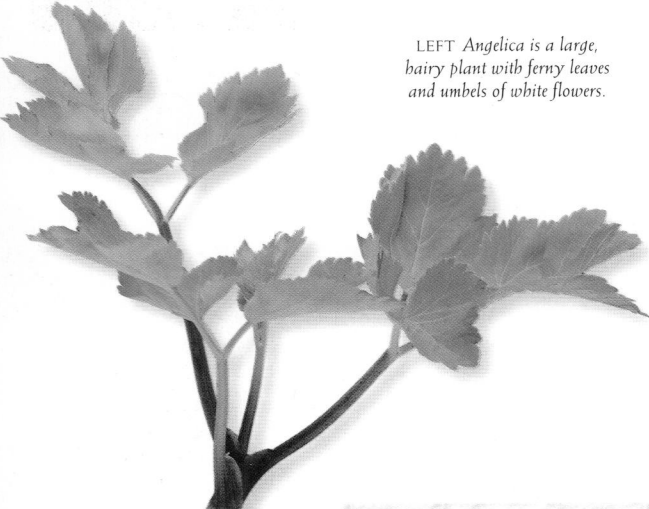

LEFT *Angelica is a large, hairy plant with ferny leaves and umbels of white flowers.*

RECIPE
Angelica Travel Oil
🌿 🌿 🌿 🌿

Add 5 drops angelica, 5 drops melissa, 5 drops peppermint, and 5 drops ginger to a small dropper bottle containing 1fl.oz. (30ml.) of sweet almond oil. Inhale or massage a few drops into the temples or around the back of the neck to relieve jet lag or headaches. A few drops massaged in a clockwise direction around the abdomen can ease stomach ache.

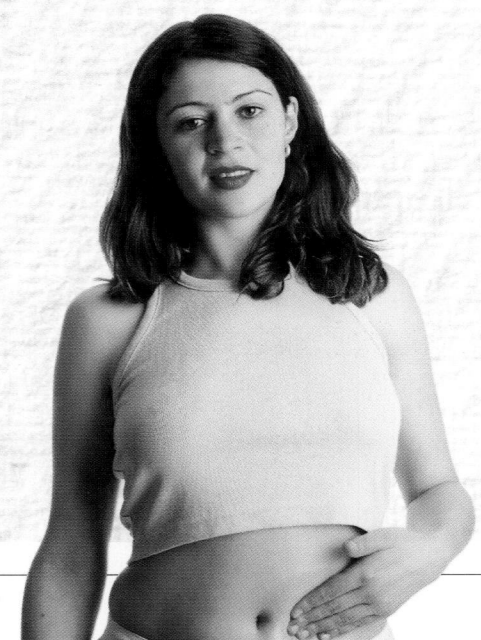

CAUTION

DO NOT USE DURING PREGNANCY OR IF YOU ARE A DIABETIC.

DO NOT USE ON SKIN EXPOSED TO SUNLIGHT.

ANGELICA OIL ATTRACTS INSECTS.

INFORMATION

BLENDS WELL WITH CLARY SAGE, PATCHOULI, SANDALWOOD, VETIVER, BENZOIN, LEMON, AND OTHER CITRUS OILS.

RIGHT *A few drops of blended angelica oil massaged around the abdomen soothes stomach ache.*

Apium graveolens
CELERY SEED

Best known as a salad vegetable in Europe, celery is grown in India, China, the Netherlands, and Hungary for its essential oil. Celery seeds are crushed to produce the warm, spicy, scented essential oil. Celery has been valued throughout history for its use as a diuretic and a digestive aid.

RECIPE
Detoxifying Massage Blend
🌿 🌿 🌿 🌿

Add 4 drops celery, 3 drops juniper, 3 drops lemon to 4 teaspoons (20ml.) grapeseed oil, and use for a full body massage.

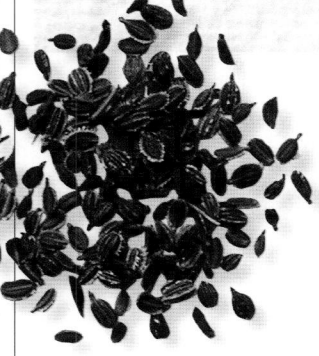

ABOVE *and* BELOW *Celery is a popular salad vegetable, and the seeds are widely used as a cooking spice.*

THERAPY CONNECTIONS

ANGELICA

🔶 Ayurveda		p.28
🔷 Chinese Herbal Medicine		p.55
🔶 Herbalism		p.115

CELERY

🔶 Ayurveda		p.29
✋ Traditional Home and Folk Remedies		p.83

INFORMATION

BLENDS WELL WITH LEMON, PEPPERMINT, JUNIPER, FENNEL, LAVENDER, BERGAMOT, PINE, TEA TREE, CINNAMON, AND OTHER SPICE OILS.

CAUTION

DO NOT USE DURING PREGNANCY.

Aniba rosaeodora

ROSEWOOD

Most rosewood oil comes from Brazil, where it is distilled from the heartwood of the rosewood tree. Although distillation from wild trees contributes to the destruction of the rainforest, cultivated trees are also used in the production of rosewood essential oil. But for the sake of preserving the rainforests, it may be best to keep this oil, with its subtle woody floral fragrance, for special occasions, or for when no other oil is suitable.

BELOW Rosewood is especially beneficial for skin care.

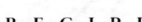

DATA FILE

Properties and Uses

Rosewood is a tonic and an immune stimulant, useful for infections or viruses such as colds or glandular fever. It can be used as a mild painkiller, an antidepressant, and an aphrodisiac. As a tissue regenerator it diminishes scars, wrinkles, and stretch marks. Because it is such a gentle oil rosewood benefits sensitive or irritated skin, and its antiseptic and bactericidal properties make it suitable for acne and wounds. The oil is also used to treat coughs and headaches, especially when they are accompanied by nausea. Rosewood is an emotionally uplifting and comforting oil that helps to rebalance the nervous system in times of stress. Rosewood is nonirritant, nontoxic, and nonsensitizing.

RECIPE

Replenishing Skin Care Oil

❦ ❦ ❦

Pour 4 teaspoons sweet almond oil into a small, dark glass bottle. Add 4 drops rosewood, 3 drops sandalwood, 3 drops frankincense. Seal and shake well. Smooth over face, neck, and dry skin patches, using gentle circular movements.

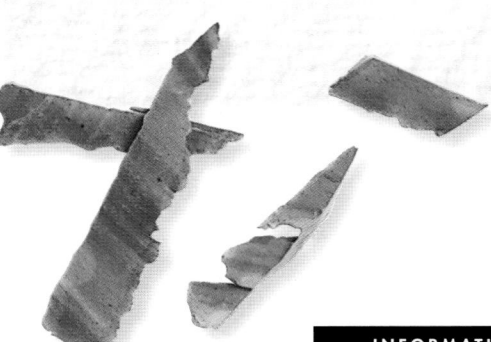

ABOVE Rosewood oil is extracted by steam distillation from the wood chippings.

INFORMATION

BLENDS WELL WITH LAVENDER, SANDALWOOD, FRANKINCENSE, BASIL, PATCHOULI, CEDARWOOD, AND MOST WOODY, CITRUS, AND FLORAL OILS.

Boswellia carteri

FRANKINCENSE

Frankincense, also known as olibanum, is distilled from the resin produced by the bark of a small North African tree. Wonderfully calming and richly fragrant, the oil has a history of use as a fumigant, in embalming, and as incense. It is considered a spiritual oil, used by many to encourage meditation.

DATA FILE

Properties and Uses

Frankincense slows the breathing and calms the nervous and digestive systems, relieving anxiety, depression, nervous tension, emotional upsets, and stress-related digestive problems. As an immune stimulant and an expectorant it can help respiratory and catarrhal conditions such as asthma, colds, chest infections, and chronic bronchitis. Frankincense has wound-healing, astringent, antiseptic, and anti-inflammatory properties, making it ideal for treating cuts, scars, blemishes, and inflammation, and it is recommended for firming aging skin. Frankincense is helpful for cystitis, as it has an affinity with the genitourinary system. Irregular or heavy menstrual bleeding and nosebleeds can also benefit from its gentle healing properties.

CAUTION

SAFE TO USE DURING PREGNANCY.

◦◦◦◦

DO NOT TAKE IT INTERNALLY AND KEEP IT OUT OF CHILDREN'S REACH.

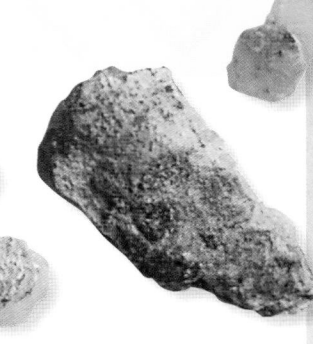

ABOVE The gum resin used to make frankincense oozes out from the tree as a milky-white liquid and then solidifies into tear-shaped, amber to orange-brown lumps.

INFORMATION

BLENDS WELL WITH ROSE, LAVENDER, GERANIUM, NEROLI, ORANGE, BERGAMOT, MANDARIN, SANDALWOOD, PINE, BLACK PEPPER, CINNAMON, AND OTHER SPICE OILS.

RECIPE

Inhalation for Dry Coughs

❦ ❦ ❦ ❦

Add 2 drops frankincense, 2 drops lavender, 2 drops cypress to a bowl of steaming hot water. Lean over the bowl, cover your head with a towel, and inhale the aroma for 5–10 minutes.

Calendula officinalis
MARIGOLD

Calendula essential oil is not widely available, as the bright orange flowers of the common pot marigold yield only small amounts of oil. More common is infused oil of calendula, where the flowers are infused in warm oil, macerated, and strained. Marigold has had a variety of historical uses, treating anything from snake bites to toothache. The famous herbalists Nicholas Culpeper and John Gerard called the flower a "comforter of the heart and spirits."

INFORMATION

BLENDS WELL WITH MOST FLORAL AND CITRUS OILS.

DATA FILE

Properties and Uses

As a soothing anti-inflammatory, antiseptic, and gentle astringent, calendula-infused oil is good for dry, cracked, or chapped skin, eczema, diaper rash, cracked nipples, and varicose veins. Because it helps to stop bleeding and has valuable wound-healing properties, it is a first-aid kit essential for cuts, grazes, wounds, and insect bites. Calendula has an affinity with the female reproductive system and has properties which help to regulate the menstrual cycle. The oil can also be used as a base for blending other essential oils.

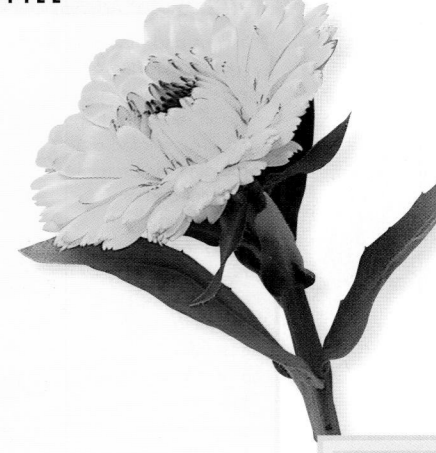

ABOVE *Marigold is an annual herb with bright orange, daisylike flowers; it has become naturalized throughout temperate regions of the world.*

THERAPY CONNECTIONS

MARIGOLD

Herbalism   *p.117*

Homeopathy   *p.187*

RECIPE
Calendula Cream

To make a soothing skin cream, add calendula oil drop by drop to any ready-made unperfumed pure plant cream, and blend thoroughly. Stop adding the oil when the cream reaches a soft usable consistency. Do not worry about adding too much calendula oil. Pure plant creams are often available from the suppliers of essential oils.

LEFT *Calendula cream is easy to make and is a valuable treatment for various skin disorders.*

Cananga odorata var. genuina
YLANG YLANG

This is extracted from a tropical tree that grows in the Philippines, Indonesia, the Comoros, and Madagascar. The name ylang ylang means "flower of flowers." The name suits the heady floral fragrance of this oil, which is distilled from the freshly picked flowers. Ylang ylang is a traditional tropical remedy for infections and skin diseases, but is also well known for its use in the Victorian hair preparation, Macassar oil.

DATA FILE

Properties and Uses

Ylang ylang is a sedative, an antidepressant, and a tonic for the nervous system. Depression, anxiety, tension, irritability, and stress-related insomnia can all benefit from its soothing properties. It helps to rebalance sebum production in oily skin, acne, and both dry and greasy scalps. It can also be used to calm irritated skin, as well as bites and stings. Ylang ylang is reputed to be an aphrodisiac. It can be used to treat sexual problems. It acts as a circulatory tonic and generally rebalances body functions. It can help to reduce blood pressure, and slow down breathing and heart rate in cases of shock, panic, or rage.

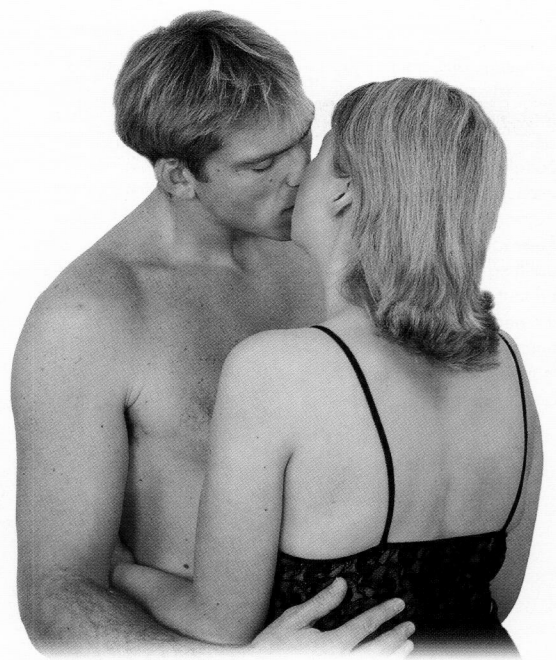

ABOVE *Ylang ylang is highly regarded as an aphrodisiac. In Indonesia, the ylang ylang flowers are spread out on the marriage bed of the bride and groom.*

RECIPE

Bath Blend for Nervous Tension

Add 3 drops ylang ylang, 2 drops rosewood, 3 drops lavender to 1½ teaspoons (8ml.) of a dispersible bath oil such as red turkey oil, and add to a warm bath; or drip the oils directly into the bath water and disperse with your hand. Relax in the bath for 10 minutes.

INFORMATION

BLENDS WELL WITH ROSEWOOD, ROSE, BERGAMOT, VETIVER, FRANKINCENSE, CHAMOMILE, LAVENDER, CEDARWOOD.

CAUTION

CAN CAUSE NAUSEA OR HEADACHES IN HIGH CONCENTRATIONS.

MAY IRRITATE THE SKIN OF SOME HYPERSENSITIVE PEOPLE.

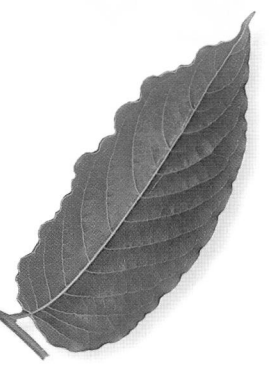

ABOVE *Leaves from the tropical ylang ylang tree.*

Cedrus atlantica
CEDARWOOD

The aromatic oil from the evergreen cedar tree was one of the first oils to be used in ancient medicine and ritual. Used by the ancient Egyptians for embalming, and by the people of the Middle East since biblical times, the wood still provides Tibetan monks with incense, burnt to aid meditation. Cedarwood oil is extracted by steam distillation from the wood chips. It has a rich, woody, masculine scent that is warming, physically cleansing, and emotionally grounding.

DATA FILE

Properties and Uses

The antiseptic, anti-seborrheic, and mild astringent properties of cedarwood make it a popular choice for treating acne, oily skin eruptions, and dandruff. It has diuretic properties which benefit the urinary system and help to relieve cystitis, and it is also used for vaginal infections and discharges. Cedarwood is an expectorant and mucolytic, which explains its traditional use in the treatment of catarrhal problems, especially bronchial congestion and infections. The oil is also valued for its ability both to stimulate the circulation and relax the nervous system, while having a tonic effect on the whole body.

On an emotional level, cedarwood can dispel gloomy or scattered thoughts, anxiety, obsessions, and fears.

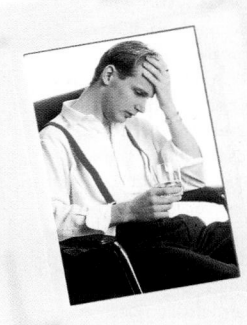

BELOW *Cedarwood oil helps to relieve nervous tension and stress-related conditions.*

CAUTION

DO NOT USE DURING PREGNANCY.

SEVERAL VARIETIES OF CEDAR TREES ARE USED TO PRODUCE OIL THAT IS SOLD AS CEDARWOOD. SOME OF THIS OIL IS VERY DIFFERENT FROM *CEDRUS ATLANTICA.* ALWAYS MAKE SURE YOU BUY ATLAS CEDARWOOD OIL.

RIGHT *Cedarwood oil is used to treat dandruff.*

INFORMATION

BLENDS WELL WITH NEROLI, JASMINE, JUNIPER, CHAMOMILE, GERANIUM, LAVENDER, FRANKINCENSE, ROSEMARY, YLANG YLANG, ROSEWOOD, VETIVER.

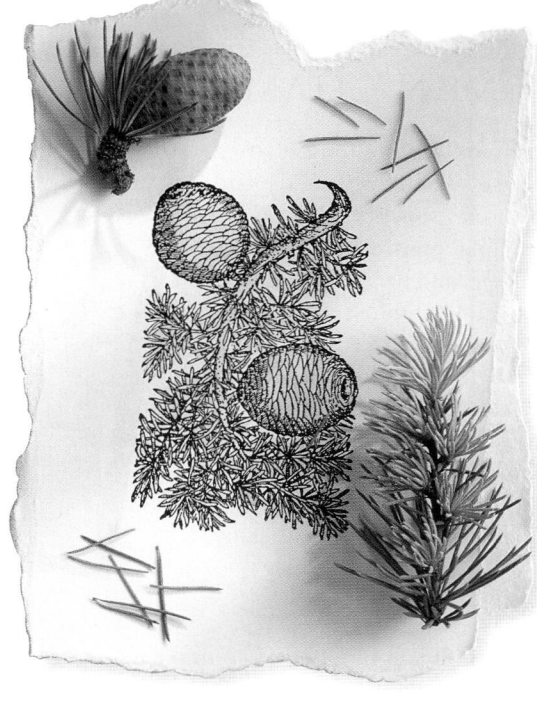

ABOVE *Cedar is a pyramid-shaped evergreen tree, up to 130 ft. (40m.) high. Its strongly aromatic wood contains a high percentage of essential oil.*

RECIPE

Antidandruff Treatment

Add 6 drops cedarwood, 6 drops rosemary, 4 drops cypress oil to 1½fl. oz. (50ml.) olive oil. Massage into the scalp with your fingertips, cover, and leave overnight, if possible. Shampoo thoroughly. Use half the recipe for children.

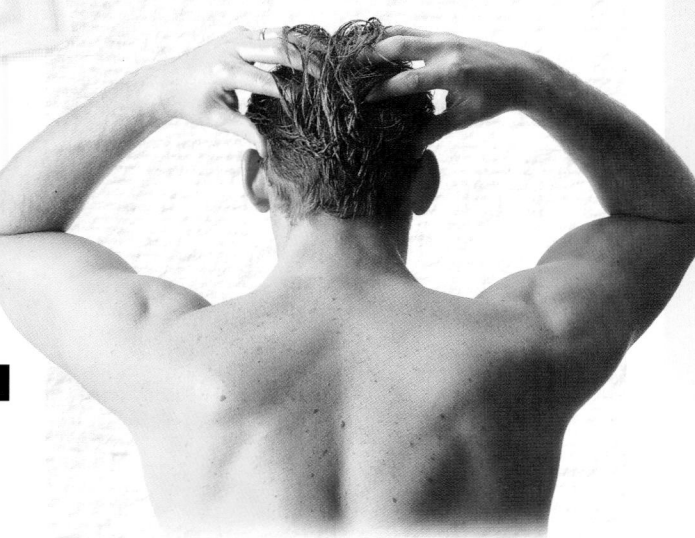

Chamaemelum nobile
ROMAN CHAMOMILE

Chamomile has a long history of use as a physical and emotional soother. It is one of the most gentle essential oils available, and particularly suitable for treating children. Massage can soothe fretful or colicky babies, and the diluted oil can be rubbed into the cheek to relieve teething pain. Of the many varieties of chamomile available, Roman chamomile is one of the most commonly used in aromatherapy.

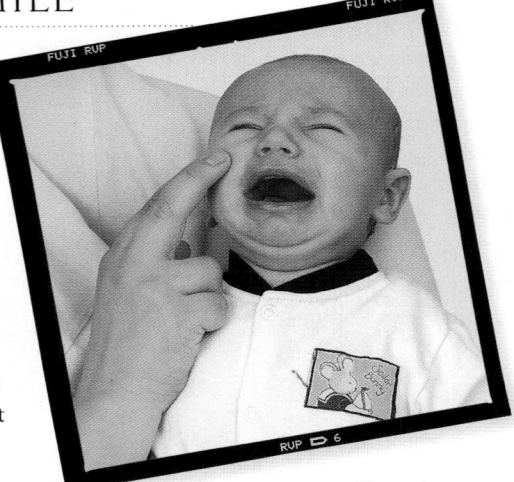

ABOVE *Chamomile is suitable for treating children and infants.*

RECIPE
Chamomile Compress

Fill a bowl with ice-cold or hot water and add 4–5 drops of chamomile oil. Soak a clean face cloth or folded piece of clean cotton in the bowl, and wring it out. Apply the compress to the affected area until it has cooled or warmed to body temperature. Repeat. *Note*: Use a cold compress for rashes, cuts, headaches, sprains, or swellings; a hot compress for arthritic or rheumatic pain, boils, abscesses, earache, or toothache.

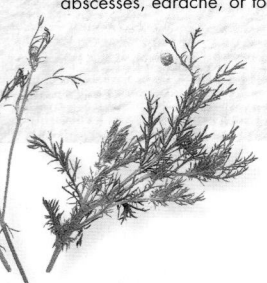

LEFT *Chamomile is a small perennial herb with daisy-like white flowers and feathery pennate leaves.*

CAUTION

DO NOT USE IN THE FIRST THREE MONTHS OF PREGNANCY.

DO NOT ALLOW CHAMOMILE ESSENTIAL OIL TO GET INTO THE EYES.

CAN CAUSE DERMATITIS IN SOME PEOPLE.

GERMAN CHAMOMILE MAY BE USED INSTEAD OF ROMAN CHAMOMILE, BUT NOT CHAMOMILE *MAROC ORMENIS MULTICAULIS*, WHICH IS NOT TRUE CHAMOMILE.

DATA FILE

Properties and Uses

Chamomile calms the nervous system and induces sleep. It has valuable anti-inflammatory, antiseptic, and bactericidal properties. Chamomile prevents and eases spasms, relieves pain, settles digestion, and acts as a liver tonic. It can be used to relieve headaches, toothache, menstrual cramps, arthritis, and neuralgia. Indigestion, nausea, and flatulence can also benefit, and all manner of skin problems such as rashes, inflammation, cuts, boils, allergies, insect bites, and chilblains can be helped by a chamomile compress or bath. It also has a balancing effect on the menstrual cycle, reduces fluid retention, and acts as a gentle antidepressant and stress reliever. Chamomile also helps to reduce fever.

INFORMATION

BLENDS WELL WITH LAVENDER, GERANIUM, BERGAMOT, JASMINE, ROSE, NEROLI, CLARY SAGE, SANDALWOOD, MANDARIN.

Cinnamomum zeylanicum
CINNAMON LEAF

Cinnamon is grown in India, Sri Lanka, the Comoros, and the Seychelles, but the best cinnamon oil is believed to come from Madagascar. Cinnamon was used by the Greeks, Romans, and ancient Egyptians, and its medicinal properties have long been valued by the people of India and of China. The familiar warm, spicy fragrance is also reputed to enhance psychic ability.

RECIPE
Cinnamon Room Freshener

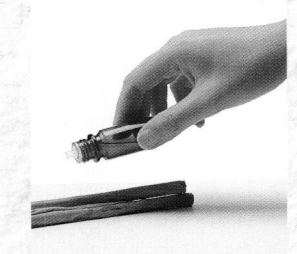

Sprinkle a few drops on rolled cinnamon sticks and add to potpourri made from dried orange peel, orange oil, and basil for a room freshener that stimulates and refreshes the mind, relieves tension, and soothes the nerves.

CAUTION

CINNAMON LEAF OIL MAY CAUSE SKIN IRRITATION.

USE ONLY IN A 1 PER CENT DILUTION, AND IN MODERATION.

DO NOT CONFUSE WITH CINNAMON BARK OIL, WHICH IS AN IRRITANT AND SHOULD NOT BE USED IN AROMATHERAPY.

INFORMATION

BLENDS WELL WITH YLANG YLANG, FRANKINCENSE, ORANGE, BENZOIN, MANDARIN, LEMON, BASIL, MYRRH, LAVENDER, GINGER.

BELOW *The inner bark of the new shoots of the cinnamon tree is gathered every two years and sold in the form of cinnamon sticks.*

DATA FILE

Properties and Uses

Cinnamon stimulates a sluggish digestion, relieves flatulence and spasms, and combats intestinal infection. It acts as a respiratory and circulatory stimulant, helping with rheumatic problems and chest infections. It helps to fortify the immune system against chills and infections, and has a cooling effect on fevers. Cinnamon also has antiseptic, antimicrobial, and parasiticidal properties, making it good for head lice, scabies, and other skin infections. Cinnamon can relieve mental fatigue, improve poor concentration and nervous exhaustion, and help to lift depression.

Citrus aurantifolia
LIME

Limes were traditionally used as a digestive remedy and to prevent scurvy among sailors. Lime has a fairly wide application in modern aromatherapy. It has properties similar to those of lemon, and the two oils are often used interchangeably. The essential oil is expressed from the peel of the fruit, or steam-distilled from the whole fruit.

DATA FILE

Properties and Uses

Lime acts as an appetite and digestive stimulant, and also helps to treat the symptoms of dyspepsia. Its antiseptic, anti-viral, bactericidal, and fever-reducing properties make it valuable in fighting colds, flu, fever, and chest and throat infections. It also helps to strengthen the immune system. Oily skin and conditions such as acne, boils, and warts can also benefit from these properties. Lime has a restorative, tonic effect on the whole person. It also has notable anti-rheumatic properties, and is known to increase mental alertness and assertiveness.

RECIPE
Stay-alert Diffuser Blend

Fill the dish of a pottery burner with water and add 4 drops lime, 2 drops black pepper, 2 drops peppermint. Light the night light and let the heat diffuse the oil into the air.

CAUTION

LIME INCREASES THE SKIN'S SENSITIVITY TO SUNLIGHT. DO NOT APPLY TO THE SKIN WITHIN TWO DAYS OF EXPOSURE TO SUNLIGHT

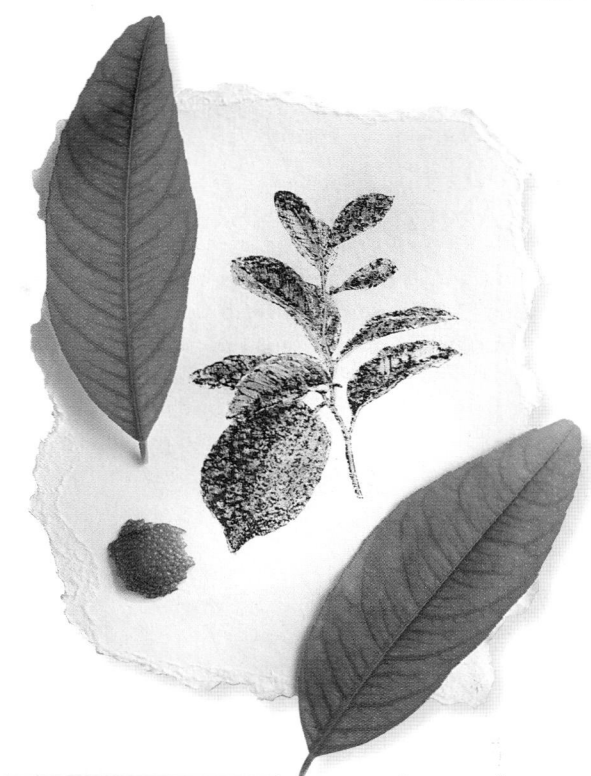

INFORMATION

BLENDS WELL WITH LAVENDER, ROSEMARY, CLARY SAGE, BLACK PEPPER, BERGAMOT, AND OTHER CITRUS OILS.

ABOVE *Lime is a small evergreen tree, up to 15 ft. (4.5 m.) tall, with stiff, sharp spines, smooth ovate leaves, and small white flowers. The pale green fruit is the size of a small lemon.*

Citrus aurantium var. amara, Citrus sinensis
ORANGE

Originally from China, oranges have a history of use in Traditional Chinese Medicine. Dried sweet orange is used to treat coughs and colds, while bitter orange is used to treat diarrhea. The outer peel of both bitter and sweet oranges is pressed to produce the sweet, fruity orange essential oil.

RECIPE
Massage Blend for Constipation

Mix 3 drops orange, 3 drops black pepper, 4 drops rosemary, 3 teaspoons (15ml.) sweet almond or grapeseed oil. Warm a little oil in the hands; massage into the abdomen clockwise.

CAUTION

ORANGE OIL CAN INCREASE SKIN SENSITIVITY TO THE SUN.

MAY CAUSE CONTACT DERMATITIS IN SOME PEOPLE.

DO NOT USE MORE THAN FOUR DROPS IN THE BATH.

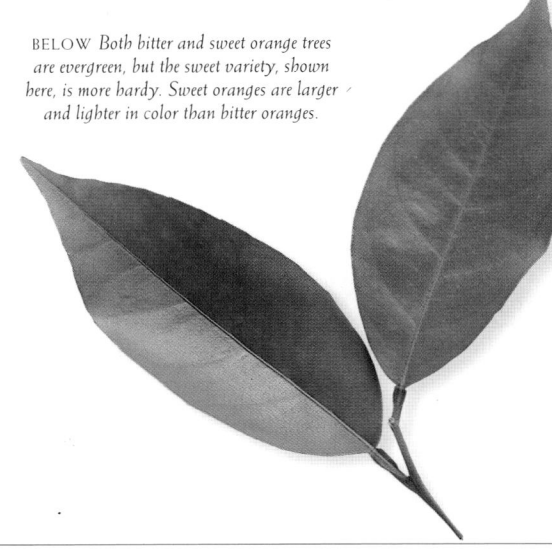

BELOW *Both bitter and sweet orange trees are evergreen, but the sweet variety, shown here, is more hardy. Sweet oranges are larger and lighter in color than bitter oranges.*

DATA FILE

Properties and Uses

As a sedative orange is good for nervous tension and related insomnia, either blended with lavender, or alternated with lavender or sandalwood. It is also a cheering oil, which enlivens the mind and dispels depression. Orange has a normalizing effect on intestinal peristalsis, making it beneficial for painful spasms, constipation, and diarrhea. It also helps to normalize blood pressure and circulation, and stimulates the lymphatic system to relieve water retention. Orange helps to fight chills, bronchitis, colds, and flu, especially when mixed with complementary winter spice oils such as cinnamon and clove.

THERAPY CONNECTIONS

CHAMOMILE

Herbalism   p.119
Homeopathy   p.204

CINNAMON

Ayurveda   p.34
Chinese Herbal Medicine   p.59

INFORMATION

BLENDS WELL WITH LAVENDER, YLANG YLANG, NEROLI, CINNAMON, BLACK PEPPER, CLARY SAGE, LEMON, MYRRH, CINNAMON, CLOVE.

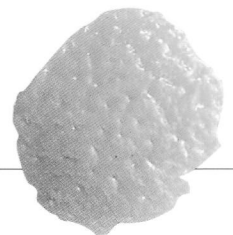

Citrus aurantium var. amara
NEROLI
(ORANGE BLOSSOM)

The blossoms of the bitter orange tree yield this oil, which has an exquisite fresh floral fragrance. Neroli is named after an Italian princess, Anne-Marie of Nerola, who used it as a perfume. In folk traditions, orange flowers were included in bridal bouquets as a symbol of innocence and fertility, and to calm nervous couples on their wedding night.

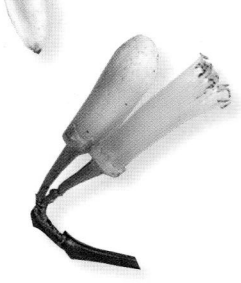

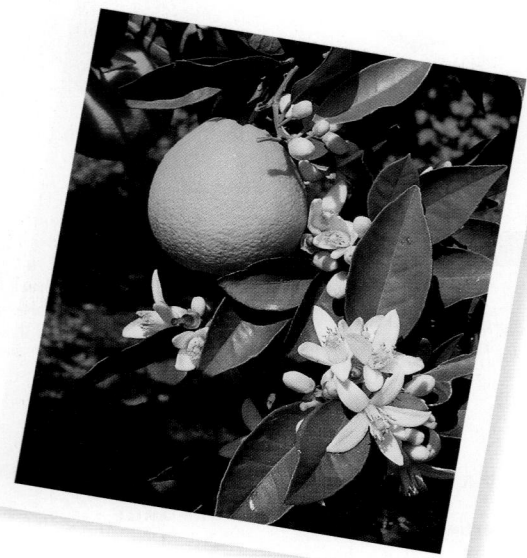

ABOVE *Orange blossoms and weddings have had a long association in folk tradition.*

Massage Blend for High Blood Pressure

❦ ❦ ❦

Add 3 drops neroli, 3 drops celery, 4 drops rose to 1fl. oz. (25ml.) or 5 teaspoons grapeseed or other vegetable oil and use for gentle massage.

DATA FILE

Properties and Uses

Neroli tones the heart and circulatory system, and its carminative and antispasmodic properties can relieve digestive problems such as indigestion, diarrhea, flatulence, and stomach cramps. Neroli helps to tone the skin and improve elasticity. Added to cream or diluted in oil, it is used to prevent stretch marks, scarring, wrinkles, and to soothe sensitive skin. It is a gentle antidepressant and a nerve tonic, perhaps most helpful in treating anxiety, depression, nervous tension, and stress-related problems. As a sedative it can also help to combat associated insomnia.

CAUTION

KEEP ALL ESSENTIAL OILS OUT OF THE EYES AND NEVER TAKE THEM INTERNALLY.

INFORMATION

BLENDS WELL WITH LAVENDER, LEMON, BERGAMOT, ROSEMARY, ROSE, YLANG YLANG, CHAMOMILE, GERANIUM, BENZOIN, AND MOST OILS.

Citrus aurantium var. amara
PETITGRAIN

Fresh and flowery petitgrain is often regarded as a cheaper alternative to neroli. It is distilled from the leaves and twigs of the bitter orange tree, whereas neroli comes from the blossom. Both oils have similar properties and fragrances, but petitgrain is also a valuable oil in its own right, with a revitalizing and restorative character.

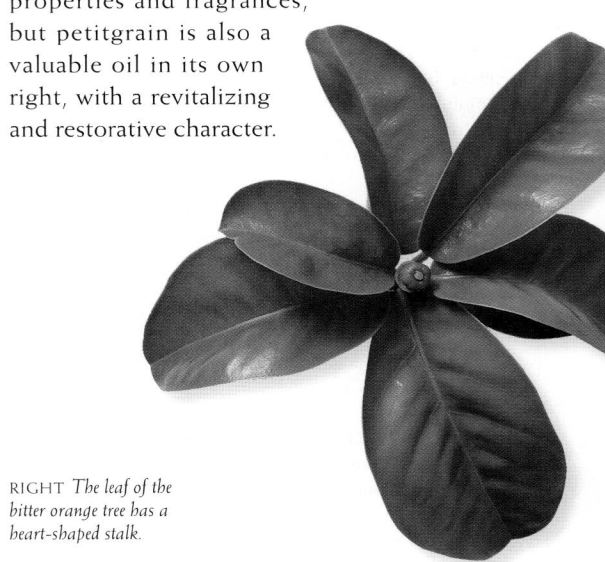

RIGHT *The leaf of the bitter orange tree has a heart-shaped stalk.*

RECIPE

Invigorating Room Fragrancer

❦ ❦ ❦

Add 3 drops petitgrain, 3 drops lime, 2 drops cypress to a vaporizer dish filled with water. Light and burn for 10–15 minutes.

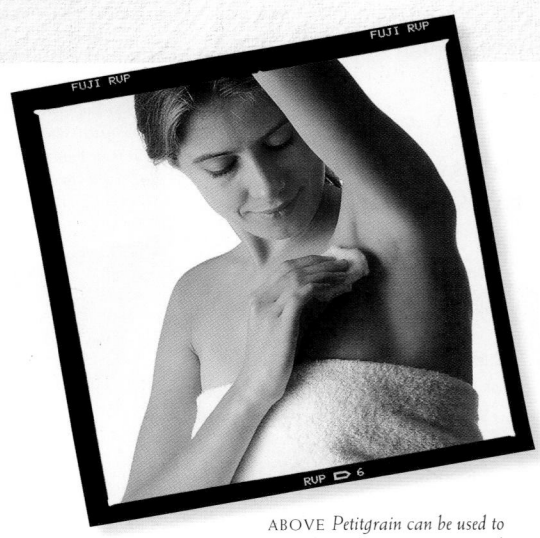

ABOVE *Petitgrain can be used to control excessive perspiration and is a gentle antiseptic.*

DATA FILE

Properties and Uses

Petitgrain can refresh or relax, depending on which oils it is blended with. It strengthens and tones the nervous system, and as such it can soothe many stress-related problems, such as nervous exhaustion and insomnia. Feelings of apathy, irritability, mild depression, anxiety, loneliness, and pessimism can all get a lift from petitgrain's antidepressant properties. This oil also has a tonic effect during convalescence, or when one is feeling "run down." It has a notable antispasmodic effect and helps to tone the digestive system, relieving flatulence and indigestion. Petitgrain is a deodorant, sometimes used to control excessive perspiration. It is also used to control the over-production of sebum in the skin and has gentle antiseptic properties, making it ideal for many greasy skin and scalp conditions, especially acne and greasy hair.

INFORMATION

BLENDS WELL WITH LAVENDER, GERANIUM, BERGAMOT, JASMINE, CLOVE, PALMAROSA, CLARY SAGE, AND OTHER ORANGE OILS.

CAUTION

KEEP OUT OF THE REACH OF CHILDREN.

Citrus bergamia

BERGAMOT

The bergamot tree was originally cultivated in Italy, where the fruit has a history of use in folk medicine. The refreshing essential oil is expressed from the peel of the fruit, which resembles a small yellow orange, when it is nearly ripe. Outside Italy, bergamot is perhaps best known as an ingredient in both Earl Grey tea and eau de Cologne.

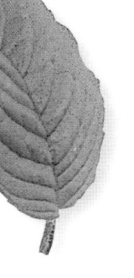

CAUTION

BERGAMOT INCREASES THE SKIN'S SENSITIVITY TO SUNLIGHT. NEVER USE UNDILUTED ON THE SKIN. AVOID IT IF YOU HAVE SENSITIVE SKIN.

MIX WITH A CARRIER OIL BEFORE ADDING TO BATH WATER TO ENSURE IT DISPERSES WELL IN THE WATER.

RECIPE

Bergamot Wash for Cystitis Relief

Cystitis is a bacterial infection causing inflammation of the bladder. This soothing wash will ease the characteristic burning sensation that occurs while urinating. You can also use absorbent cotton soaked in the solution to swab the opening of the urethra after passing water.

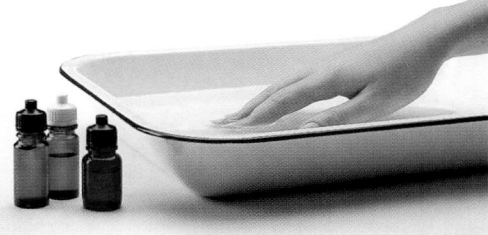

Add 3 drops bergamot, 3 drops lavender, 3 drops niaouli to a warm bath and soak for at least 10 minutes, or fill a bowl that is big enough to sit in with lukewarm water and add 1 drop of each oil. Agitate the water thoroughly with your hand to disperse the oil.

INFORMATION

BLENDS WELL WITH CHAMOMILE, GERANIUM, LEMON, SANDALWOOD, MYRRH, JUNIPER, LAVENDER, NEROLI, CYPRESS, JASMINE, TEA TREE.

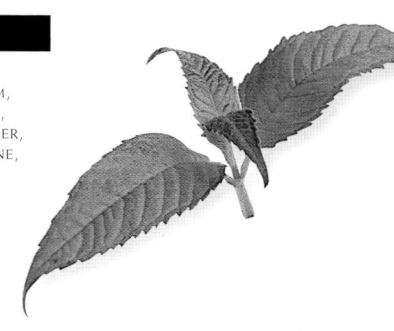

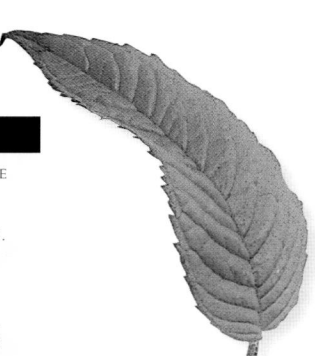

ABOVE *The bergamot is a small tree with fruits which are yellow when ripe.*

DATA FILE

Properties and Uses

Joyous and uplifting, bergamot is a powerful antidepressant which has a wonderfully balancing effect on moods. As an antiseptic it is good for acne and boils. Other skin complaints, such as oily skin, eczema, and psoriasis, cuts, and insect bites, can also respond well to bergamot. The oil inhibits viral activity; when diluted in alcohol it can be dabbed on cold sores, chicken pox, and shingles. The fragrance repels insects and the oil can be used to expel worms. Bergamot has an affinity with the genitourinary system. It is a diuretic and a powerful urinary disinfectant, particularly good for cystitis. It can also be used for thrush and other types of vaginal itching and discharge. As a digestive, bergamot is sometimes used to encourage appetite. It is also used to cool fevers.

Citrus limon
LEMON

The ancient Greeks and Romans included lemon in their medicine chest and it has a history of use in European folk medicine. The essential oil which is expressed from the fresh peel has many varied applications, making it invaluable in the home aromatherapy kit.

RECIPE
Hangover Bath Oil

Add 4 drops lemon, 2 drops fennel, 2 drops lavender to a warm bath and agitate the water with your hand. Relax for 10 minutes and inhale deeply.

INFORMATION

BLENDS WELL WITH GERANIUM, FENNEL, JUNIPER, EUCALYPTUS, SANDALWOOD, FRANKINCENSE, CHAMOMILE, LAVENDER, YLANG YLANG, ROSE, NEROLI, AND OTHER CITRUS OILS.

CAUTION

CAN IRRITATE SENSITIVE SKIN.

DO NOT USE BEFORE SUNBATHING.

DILUTE WELL FOR MASSAGE AND BATH BLENDS, AND DO NOT USE FOR MORE THAN A FEW DAYS AT A TIME.

RIGHT *Lemon essential oil is expressed from the peel of the fresh fruit.*

DATA FILE

Properties and Uses

Lemon can stimulate the body's defenses to fight all kinds of infection. It is beneficial in treating inflamed or diseased gums, mouth ulcers, sore throats, and acne. It helps to clear colds, flu, and bronchitis, and can be used to remove warts and verrucas, and to clear herpes blisters. The oil has a tonic effect on the circulation and is often used to treat varicose veins, poor circulation, high blood pressure, and fluid retention. Lemon is both diuretic and laxative, and has the ability to stop bleeding in minor cuts and nosebleeds. As an astringent it benefits greasy skin and can also be used to reduce a fever. Because it also counteracts acidity in the body, lemon helps to relieve acid indigestion, arthritis, and rheumatism. On an emotional level, refreshing lemon dispels depression and indecision.

Citrus reticulata
MANDARIN

As the name suggests, mandarin oil originated in China, where the small, sweet fruit was traditionally given as a gift to the Mandarin. The essential oil is expressed from the peel. It has a delicate, fruity, floral aroma and a gentle healing action.

CAUTION

MANDARIN MAY INCREASE THE SKIN'S SENSITIVITY TO THE SUN.

INFORMATION

BLENDS WELL WITH FRANKINCENSE, CHAMOMILE, LAVENDER, ROSEWOOD, NEROLI, AND OTHER CITRUS OILS AND SPICE OILS, SUCH AS CLOVE AND CINNAMON.

LEFT *The mandarin tree was brought to Europe in 1805 and to the U.S. 40 years later, where it was renamed tangerine.*

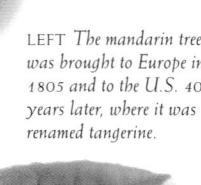

RECIPE
Oil to Prevent Stretch Marks

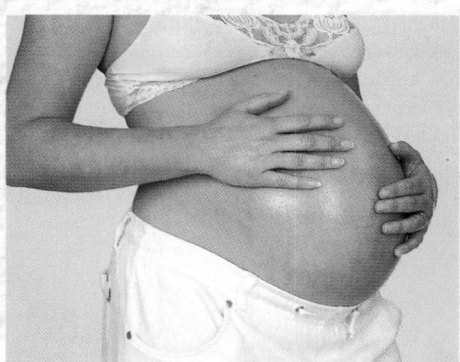

Add 4 drops mandarin, 3 drops neroli, 3 drops lavender to a bottle containing 1fl.oz. (25ml.) or 5 teaspoonsful sweet almond oil and 1 teaspoonful wheat germ oil. Massage into the abdomen twice a day from the fifth month of pregnancy.

DATA FILE

Properties and Uses

Mandarin is used mostly for treating digestive problems. It soothes indigestion and relieves intestinal spasms. It has a mild laxative effect and acts as a tonic for the stomach. It is gentle enough for children's digestive problems and hiccups. Mandarin also tones the liver, the body's main chemical processing and elimination organ. Because it is also a mild diuretic, mandarin can help to relieve fluid retention and stored toxins. The oil can be used as a skin toner for oily skin, acne, or congested pores. As a sedative it is also used to relieve nervous tension and insomnia during pregnancy, and can help to settle restless children.

Citrus x paradisi
GRAPEFRUIT

Refreshing grapefruit oil is expressed from the peel of the fruit, cultivated mainly in California, Florida, Brazil, and Israel. It has a fresh, tangy citrus scent that enlivens the mind and disperses feelings of gloom. Unlike many citrus oils, grapefruit does not increase the skin's sensitivity to sunlight.

RECIPE
Wake-up Shower Gel

Mix 2 drops grapefruit, 2 drops petitgrain, 1 drop rosemary with a dollop of unscented shower gel and work to a lather with a sponge.

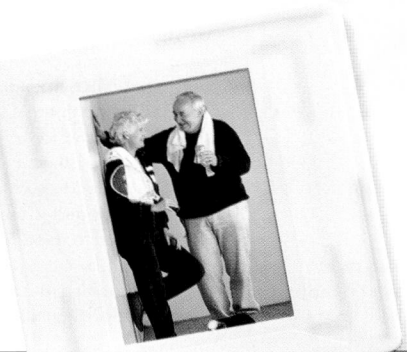

BELOW *A grapefruit oil massage helps to ease stiff muscles after exercise.*

DATA FILE

Properties and Uses

Grapefruit is diuretic, detoxifying, and cleansing to the kidneys. It also has a stimulating effect on the lymphatic system. Because of these properties it helps to relieve fluid retention and eliminate the toxins that cause cellulite. It is also beneficial in a massage blend to ease stiff muscles after exercise. Grapefruit tones an oily skin and scalp, is helpful in treating acne and congested pores, and can be applied neat to cold sores. It also stimulates digestion and improves immunity to infection. As an antidepressant, grapefruit oil enlivens the mind, relieves anxiety, and combats nervous exhaustion.

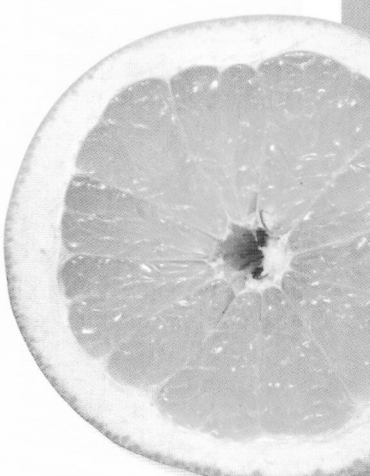

ABOVE *Like other citrus species, grapefruit is high in vitamin C and is a good protection against infectious illnesses.*

Commiphora myrrha
MYRRH

Perhaps best known as one of the three gifts brought to the infant Jesus, myrrh was valued in ancient times as an ingredient in embalming preparations, incense, and as a medicine. According to legend, the soldiers of ancient Greece took myrrh ointment into battle to treat their wounds. Essential oil of myrrh has a musty, balsamic odor and is closely related to frankincense, with which it is often linked.

RECIPE
Chapped Skin Cream

Add 5 drops myrrh, 5 drops benzoin, 4 drops geranium to 1oz. (30g.) of good unperfumed, lanolin-free cream. Mix well and apply to the skin.

RIGHT *Myrrh is the hardened oleoresin from shrubs and small trees of the* Commiphora *species.*

DATA FILE

Properties and Uses

Myrrh has an excellent soothing, antiseptic, and healing effect on sore or inflamed gums, mouth ulcers, wounds, and cracked or chapped skin. It can speed the healing of weepy eczema, and because of its antifungal properties it can be used as a vaginal wash for thrush or in a foot bath for athlete's foot. Myrrh is also an expectorant and a lung tonic, good for coughs, colds, bronchitis, and flu. It stimulates, tones, and soothes the digestive system, and is often used for diarrhea, hemorrhoids, and indigestion. The oil is a uterine tonic, which can be helpful for menstrual irregularities. Myrrh relieves agitation, calms fears and uncertainties, and has a positive, balancing effect on the emotions.

THERAPY CONNECTIONS

LEMON
Traditional Home and Folk Remedies *p.87*

GRAPEFRUIT
Traditional Home and Folk Remedies *p.88*

MYRRH
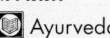 Ayurveda *p.34*

Coriandrum sativum
CORIANDER

Coriander is a highly aromatic annual herb. Coriander seeds were used by the ancient Greeks and have also been found in Egyptian tombs. The seeds and leaves are both used in cooking, and the Chinese use the whole herb for medicinal purposes. The essential oil, distilled from the crushed seeds, has a sweet and slightly musky, spicy, and woody aroma.

ABOVE *Coriander, also known as cilantro, is an annual herb with bright green, delicate leaves.*

INFORMATION

BLENDS WELL WITH BERGAMOT, SANDALWOOD, PETITGRAIN, PINE, CITRONELLA, CLARY SAGE, GINGER, AND OTHER SPICE OILS.

DATA FILE

Properties and Uses

Coriander's pain-relieving properties make it suitable for headaches and neuralgia. It has a warming, antirheumatic effect, good for muscular pain and stiffness, arthritis, and rheumatism. Coriander is an effective digestive stimulant and tonic, used to relieve diarrhea, flatulence, nausea, painful spasms, and to stimulate appetite in cases of anorexia. It is also a nervous stimulant, beneficial for apathy, nervous exhaustion, and fatigue. The oil's stimulatory properties also work on the circulation. As such it is useful for hemorrhoids, poor circulation, and fluid retention. Coriander is an aphrodisiac which has a warming, stimulatory effect on the emotions.

THERAPY CONNECTIONS

CORIANDER

Ayurveda   *p.35*

RECIPE

Coriander Muscle Rub

Add 2 drops coriander, 4 drops juniper, 4 drops black pepper to 4 teaspoons (20ml.) grapeseed oil, and massage into tired and aching muscles.

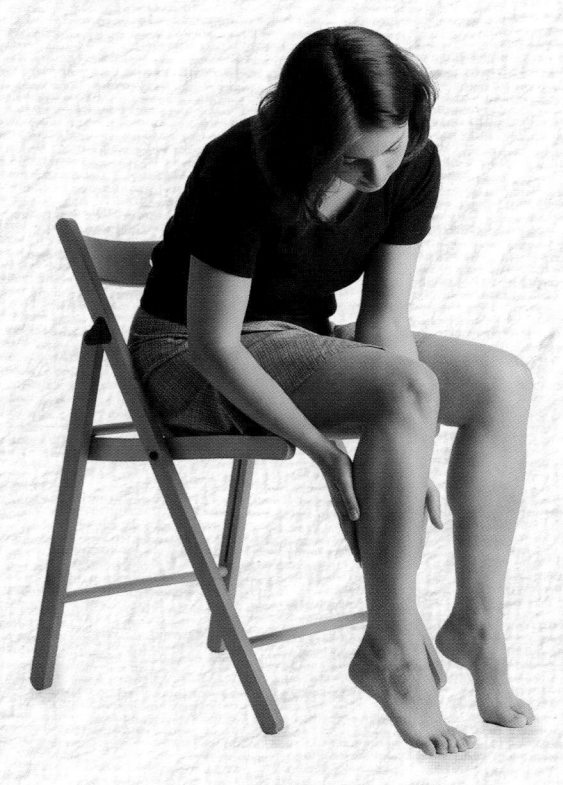

Cupresses sempervirens
CYPRESS

Ancient civilizations used the tall evergreen cypress tree as a source of incense for religious ceremonies and for medicinal purposes. The oil, which is distilled from the twigs and needles of the cypress, has a pleasant, smoky, wood aroma, and a number of therapeutic uses.

DATA FILE

Properties and Uses

Cypress is an anti-spasmodic, useful in a vaporizer for respiratory problems such as bronchitis or asthma, or to prevent coughing attacks. Astringent properties make it suitable for use in a wash for hemorrhoids and for excessively oily skin. It can also be applied to cuts to stop bleeding and is used as a mouthwash for bleeding gums. Cypress is a circulatory tonic, which can improve poor circulation, relieve fluid retention, and soothe muscular cramp, and can be applied gently to varicose veins. In a foot bath it counteracts excessively sweating and smelly feet. The oil is used to treat PMS, regulate the menstrual cycle, and counteract heavy bleeding. Menopausal symptoms such as hot flushes and irritability can also be alleviated by cypress.

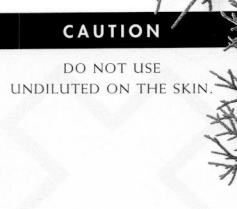

ABOVE *Cypress bears small flowers and round, brownish-gray cones or nuts.*

RECIPE

Varicose Vein Toner

Add 5 drops cypress and 10 drops geranium oil to 5 teaspoons (25ml.) vegetable oil. Starting at the ankle, gently stroke up the legs towards the heart.

INFORMATION

BLENDS WELL WITH JUNIPER, PINE, LAVENDER, SANDALWOOD, LEMON, MANDARIN, ORANGE, BERGAMOT, CLARY SAGE.

Cymbopogon citratus
LEMONGRASS

Lemongrass is a tall, aromatic grass. It is used as a flavoring in Thai cuisine and has been used in traditional Indian medicine for centuries. The essential oil is distilled from the grass leaves. It has a strong refreshing citrus smell that has many aromatherapy and domestic uses.

LEFT *The long, thin leaves of lemongrass are the source for its essential oil.*

DATA FILE

Properties and Uses

Lemongrass has a tonic effect on the nervous system and the body in general. It is also painkilling and antidepressant, good for headaches, lethargy, symptoms of stress, and beneficial for muscular pain and poor muscle tone. It has fever-reducing properties and helps the immune system to fight infections. As a deodorant, lemongrass can be used for excessive perspiration and sweaty feet, and its astringent properties make it an effective skin toner which helps to close open pores. Lemongrass is also an effective flea, lice, and tick repellent. Use it in a vaporizer to keep flies out of the kitchen in summer and to get rid of pet smells from the home.

INFORMATION

BLENDS WELL WITH LAVENDER, ORANGE, GERANIUM, JASMINE, ROSEMARY, NEROLI, BASIL, SANDALWOOD, EUCALYPTUS.

CAUTION

DILUTE WELL, AS LEMONGRASS MAY CAUSE SKIN IRRITATION IN SOME PEOPLE.

—◆—

DO NOT USE ON BABIES OR CHILDREN.

—◆—

DO NOT USE AROUND THE EYES.

RECIPE
Greasy Hair Shampoo

Add 2 drops of lemongrass to a normal dollop of mild, unscented shampoo, rub between your palms, and wash your hair as normal.

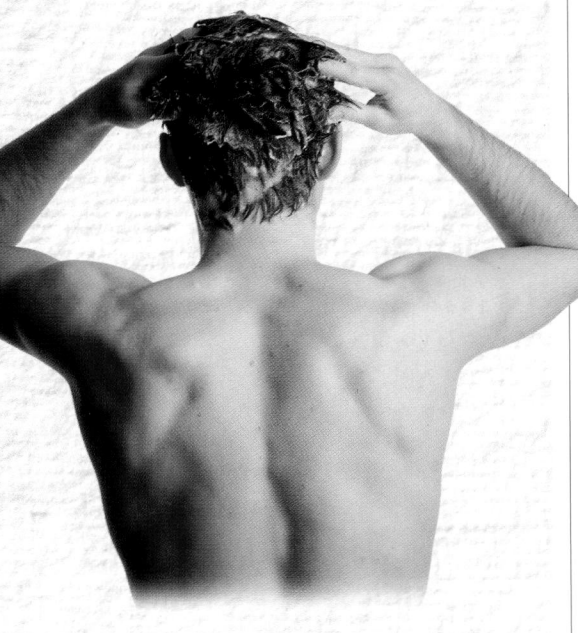

RIGHT *A few drops of lemongrass added to shampoo make an ideal greasy-hair formula.*

Cymbopogon martinii var. martinii
PALMAROSA

In Indian Ayurvedic medicine palmarosa has long been used to combat infectious diseases. Distilled from a fresh scented grass, similar to lemongrass, palmarosa has a gentle floral fragrance like a mix of rose and geranium. In the past it was also known as Indian or Turkish geranium.

RECIPE
Skin Rejuvenator

Add 6 drops palmarosa, 3 drops rose, 3 drops frankincense to a small bottle containing 5 drops evening primrose and 3 teaspoons (15ml.) apricot kernel oil. Shake well. Gently massage into the face at night.

DATA FILE

Properties and Uses

Palmarosa is a valuable oil in skin care. The diluted oil applied to the skin rebalances sebum production, thereby hydrating dry skin conditions. It also rejuvenates wrinkled or aging skin by promoting cellular regeneration, and it helps to heal wounds. Palmarosa is beneficial for acne, dermatitis, and skin infections because of its antiseptic properties. It has a stimulatory effect on the circulatory and digestive systems, helping to increase appetite and activate a sluggish digestion. As a bactericide, the oil prevents and treats intestinal infections. Used in a massage blend, palmarosa is good for nervous exhaustion and stress-related problems.

RIGHT *Palmarosa is a perennial plant with long stems and terminal flowering tops.*

INFORMATION

BLENDS WELL WITH SANDALWOOD, LAVENDER, GERANIUM, ROSEWOOD, CEDARWOOD, FRANKINCENSE, LEMON, FLORAL, CITRUS OILS, AND WOODY OILS.

Cymbopogon nardus

CITRONELLA

The leaves of this tropical scented grass are valued in many countries for their medicinal properties. The essential oil, which is distilled from the dried leaves, has a strong, fresh, lemony scent. Although it is not widely used in aromatherapy, it is highly valued as a household disinfectant and insecticide.

RECIPE

Refreshing Foot Soak

Add 4 drops citronella, 2 drops tea tree, 3 drops cypress to a foot bath to refresh hot and sweaty feet.

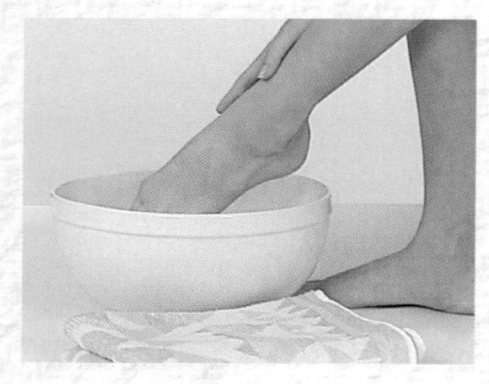

DATA FILE

Properties and Uses

Refreshing and uplifting, citronella helps to combat headaches, fatigue, and feelings of depression. It has strong deodorant properties, which make it suitable for refreshing tired or sweaty feet, and for treating fungal infections such as athlete's foot. In Eastern cultures it is used to settle digestion and menstrual problems, and as a rub for rheumatic pain. It makes an excellent insect repellent, either used in a room spray, vaporizer, or dropped on to a square of cotton and added to a linen cupboard to keep clothes fresh and free from moths. Cats dislike the smell of citronella, so it can be used to keep them away from areas of the garden.

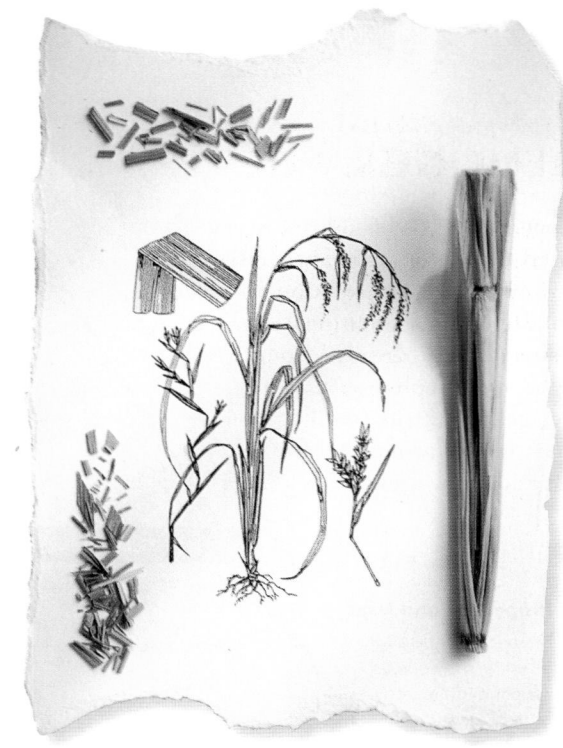

ABOVE *Citronella is a tall, aromatic, perennial grass derived from wild "managrass" found in Sri Lanka.*

CAUTION

DO NOT USE DURING PREGNANCY.

DILUTE WELL, AS IT MAY CAUSE IRRITATION TO SOME PEOPLE WITH SENSITIVE SKIN.

INFORMATION

BLENDS WELL WITH GERANIUM, LEMON, ORANGE, CEDARWOOD, CYPRESS, TEA TREE, BERGAMOT, EUCALYPTUS, PINE.

Elettaria cardamonum

CARDAMOM

This spice has been used since antiquity as a food flavoring, but it has also played a part in Indian Ayurvedic medicine for thousands of years. Hippocrates, a famous Greek physician known as the father of medicine, also acknowledged the therapeutic benefits of cardamom. The essential oil distilled from the seeds has a warm, sweet, spicy aroma and a warming quality similar to ginger.

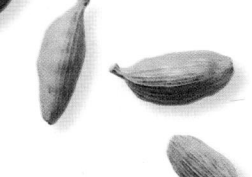

BELOW *and* ABOVE *Cardamom is a reedlike herb with long, blade-shaped leaves and yellowish flowers with purple tips, ripening into oblong seed pods.*

RECIPE

Massage Oil for Stomach Cramps

Add 1 drop cardamom, 1 drop basil, 2 drops marjoram to 2 teaspoons (10ml.) vegetable oil and massage in a clockwise direction over the stomach and abdominal area.

DATA FILE

Properties and Uses

Mainly used as a digestive remedy because of its soothing, antispasmodic, and digestive properties, cardamom is good for indigestion, flatulence, abdominal pain, heartburn, bloating, nausea, and bad breath. It has a diuretic effect which can help to relieve water retention. Cardamom also has a wonderful, stimulating, and tonic effect on mind and body; it makes a refreshing bath which can relieve fatigue and soothe strained nerves, and helps to clear the mind of confusion. In India cardamom is reputed to be an aphrodisiac.

INFORMATION

BLENDS WELL WITH BERGAMOT, ROSE, FRANKINCENSE, CLOVE, YLANG YLANG, NEROLI, BASIL, CEDARWOOD, FENNEL, LEMON, AND GINGER.

CAUTION

DO NOT TAKE INTERNALLY.

USE SPARINGLY, AS SPICY OILS MAY CAUSE IRRITATION IN SOME PEOPLE.

Eucalyptus globulus
BLUE GUM EUCALYPTUS

Several of the 700 species of eucalyptus are used to distill medicinal-quality essential oil, but the Australian "blue gum" is by far the most widely used. Eucalyptus is a traditional remedy in Australia and a familiar ingredient in numerous chest rubs and decongestants. The oil also eradicates lice and fleas.

BELOW *This evergreen tree bears long, narrow, yellowish leaves. Eucalyptus oil is extracted from the leaves and young twigs.*

RECIPE
Disinfectant Wash for Insect Bites

Add 3 drops eucalyptus, 3 drops thyme, 3 drops lavender to a bowl of clean water. Use cotton wool or a clean cotton cloth to dab repeatedly on the affected area.

CAUTION

DO NOT TAKE WHEN USING HOMEOPATHIC REMEDIES.

DO NOT USE FOR MORE THAN A FEW DAYS AT A TIME BECAUSE OF THE RISK OF TOXICITY.

DO NOT USE ON BABIES OR VERY YOUNG CHILDREN.

INFORMATION

BLENDS WELL WITH PEPPERMINT, TEA TREE, ROSEMARY, THYME, LAVENDER, CEDARWOOD, LEMON, PINE.

DATA FILE

Properties and Uses

Eucalyptus is a powerful antiseptic and renowned decongestant, used mostly for coughs, colds, chest infections, and sinusitis. It alleviates inflammation generally, and is helpful in treating rheumatism, muscular aches and pains, and fibrositis. It is a diuretic and a deodorant, with strong antiviral and immune-stimulating properties, and is an effective local painkiller, especially for nerve pain. Urinary tract problems such as cystitis respond well to eucalyptus. The oil is also used to reduce fevers and treat skin infections, cuts, and blisters, genital and oral herpes, chicken pox, and shingles. Eucalyptus eases the pain of burns and helps new tissue to form. It is used to prevent and relieve insect bites and is an effective mosquito repellent.

Foeniculum vulgare
FENNEL

In folklore fennel was believed to convey courage and strength and contribute to a long life. It also has a history of use as an antidote to poisons. The essential oil, distilled from the crushed seeds, is still valued for its detoxifying properties.

RECIPE
Anticellulite Massage Oil

Add 8 drops fennel, 8 drops juniper, 10 drops grapefruit oil to 5 teaspoons (25ml.) sweet almond oil and 5 drops jojoba oil. Store in a dark glass bottle and massage into the affected area every day after your bath or shower.

LEFT *Fennel is a biennial or perennial herb with feathery leaves.*

DATA FILE

Properties and Uses

Fennel appears to have a rebalancing effect on hormones, probably due to an estrogen-like plant hormone. As such it helps to stabilize hormone activity during the menopause and has traditionally been used to increase milk flow in breast-feeding mothers. It is a good diuretic, antimicrobial, and antiseptic which can help with premenstrual water retention and urinary tract infections. It helps to eliminate toxic wastes from the body, making it valuable in treating arthritis and cellulite. It reduces digestive spasms, calms and tones the stomach and digestive system, and has a slightly laxative effect, benefiting nausea, indigestion, constipation, and stomach cramps. Fennel also makes a good mouthwash for gum disease or infections.

THERAPY CONNECTIONS

CARDAMOM

Ayurveda — p.38

Chinese Herbal Medicine — p.55

FENNEL

Herbalism — p.121

CAUTION

USE ONLY SWEET FENNEL (ALSO KNOWN AS ROMAN OR FRENCH FENNEL), AS BITTER FENNEL SHOULD NOT BE USED ON THE SKIN.

DO NOT USE DURING PREGNANCY.

NOT SUITABLE FOR EPILEPTICS OR CHILDREN UNDER SIX YEARS OLD.

NARCOTIC IN LARGE DOSES.

INFORMATION

BLENDS WELL WITH LAVENDER, LEMON, ORANGE, PEPPERMINT, ROSE, GERANIUM, JUNIPER, SANDALWOOD, ROSEMARY CYPRESS, CLARY SAGE.

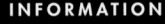

LEFT *Fennel is used in mouthwashes to treat gum diseases and infections.*

Hyssopus officinalis
HYSSOP

Revered as a sacred cleansing herb by the Hebrews and the ancient Greeks, hyssop has also long been valued by herbalists for its medicinal properties. Both the leaves and the small blue or mauve flowers are distilled for their essential oil, which has a strong, spicy, herbaceous scent.

RECIPE
Inhalation for Chest Infections

Add 2 drops hyssop, 2 drops lavender, 2 drops benzoin to a bowl of steaming water. Cover your head with a towel, bend over the bowl, and inhale.

CAUTION

DILUTE WELL AND USE FOR NO MORE THAN A FEW DAYS AT A TIME BECAUSE THERE IS SOME RISK OF TOXICITY.

DO NOT USE DURING PREGNANCY.

DO NOT USE IF YOU ARE EPILEPTIC.

FOR PEOPLE WITH HIGH BLOOD PRESSURE HYSSOP SHOULD ONLY BE USED AS DIRECTED BY A QUALIFIED AROMATHERAPIST.

DATA FILE

Properties and Uses

Hyssop is an expectorant with antispasmodic, bactericidal, and antiseptic properties, which can be helpful for coughing, whooping cough, catarrh, sore throats, and chest infections. It can be used in skin care for cuts, bruises, and inflammation. Hyssop has hypertensive properties, making it useful in the treatment of low blood pressure, and has a general tonic effect on circulation. As an emmenagogue it can be used for scanty or no menstrual bleeding. The oil can also soothe indigestion and relieve colicky cramps. Hyssop's sedative and tonic properties can benefit stress- or anxiety-related problems. It helps to relieve fatigue, and increase alertness.

INFORMATION

BLENDS WELL WITH SANDALWOOD, LAVENDER, YLANG YLANG, ROSEMARY, CLARY SAGE, CYPRESS, GERANIUM, LEMON, AND OTHER CITRUS OILS.

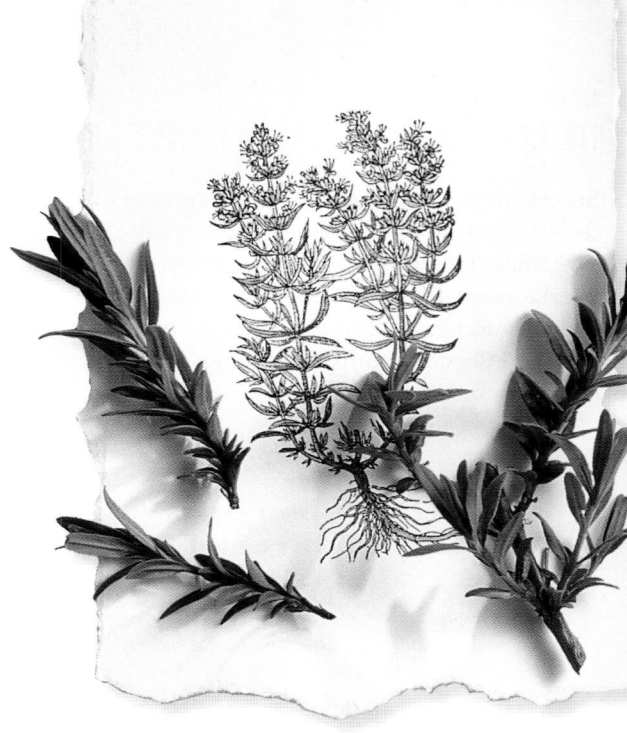

ABOVE *Hyssop is a perennial, almost evergreen shrub, with woody stems and small, lance-shaped leaves.*

Juniperus communis
JUNIPER

Used in ancient Greece and Egypt to combat the spread of disease, juniper was still being used in French hospitals during the First World War. This warm woody-scented oil can be distilled from juniper berries and twigs, but the best oil is produced by distilling the ripe berries only.

CAUTION

DO NOT USE DURING PREGNANCY.

NOT SUITABLE FOR PEOPLE WITH KIDNEY DISEASE.

INFORMATION

BLENDS WELL WITH PINE, LAVENDER, CYPRESS, CLARY SAGE, SANDALWOOD, VETIVER, BENZOIN, ROSEMARY, FENNEL, GERANIUM, BERGAMOT, AND OTHER CITRUS OILS.

LEFT *Juniper is an evergreen shrub with bluish-green stiff needles.*

RIGHT *A hair and scalp tonic can be made with juniper oil.*

RECIPE
Hair and Scalp Tonic

Add 10 drops juniper, 8 drops rosemary, 7 drops cedarwood to 1½fl.oz. (50ml.) or 10 teaspoons olive oil and massage into your hair and scalp before you wash it. Wrap your hair in a warm towel and leave for about 2 hours. Wash out with a mild shampoo, massaging the shampoo into the hair before you wet it to remove all the oil.

DATA FILE

Properties and Uses

Juniper is physically and emotionally cleansing. It helps to detoxify the body of harmful waste products that contribute to problems such as rheumatoid arthritis and cellulite, and clears the mind of confusion and exhaustion. Juniper is also diuretic, has an affinity with the genitourinary system, and is excellent for treating cystitis. Skin problems, especially weepy eczema and acne, respond well to its toning, astringent, and antiseptic properties. Juniper is also good for hemorrhoids and hair loss, and assists with wound healing. In addition, it stimulates appetite, relieves nervous tension, and is an excellent disinfectant.

Jasminum officinale

JASMINE

It takes huge quantities of jasmine flowers to produce a small amount of this very expensive essential oil. However, very little is needed to produce an effect, and the sensual floral perfume makes it a highly prized oil. In China the flowers and the root are used to treat conditions as diverse as liver cirrhosis and headaches.

RECIPE

Jasmine Massage for Menstrual Cramps

Add 4 drops jasmine, 4 drops clary sage, 2 drops lavender to 5 teaspoons (25ml.) sweet almond oil. Start the massage by sliding your hands from your hips across your abdomen. Gently stroke around the abdomen in a clockwise direction, sliding one hand after the other. Stroke your hands back up and around your hips, and around to the small of your back. Repeat.

CAUTION

JASMINE MAY CAUSE AN ALLERGIC REACTION IN RARE CASES.

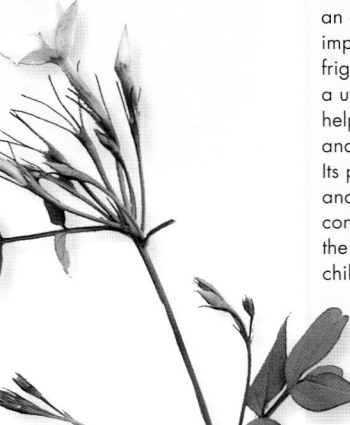

ABOVE *Jasmine is an evergreen shrub or vine, up to 33 ft. (10m.) high, with delicate leaves and highly fragrant flowers.*

DATA FILE

Properties and Uses

Jasmine has a reputation as an aphrodisiac, benefiting impotence in men and frigidity in women. It is also a uterine tonic which can help with menstrual cramp and disorders of the uterus. Its pain-relieving properties and ability to strengthen contractions make it one of the best oils to use during childbirth. It is also believed to strengthen male sex organs and has been used for prostate problems. Its relaxing and antidepressant effect helps to clear postnatal depression. It is excellent for stress relief and is uplifting during times of lethargy. Jasmine has a soothing, warming, and anti-inflammatory effect on joints and a rejuvenating effect on dry, wrinkled, or aging skin. Its antiseptic and expectorant properties also make it applicable for catarrh, and infections of the chest and throat.

INFORMATION

BLENDS WELL WITH LAVENDER, GERANIUM, CHAMOMILE, CLARY SAGE, SANDALWOOD, ROSE, NEROLI, AND OTHER CITRUS OILS.

THERAPY CONNECTIONS

HYSSOP

Chinese Herbal Medicine   *p.54*

JASMINE

Homeopathy   *p.195*

Lavendula augustifolia

LAVENDER

Of the several varieties of lavender used medicinally, *Lavendula augustifolia* is the most important. Lavender is the most versatile, best loved, and most widely therapeutic of all essential oils. Both the flowers and the leaves are highly aromatic, but only the flowers are used to make essential oil.

DATA FILE

Properties and Uses

Lavender is calming, soothing, antidepressant, and emotionally balancing. Its antiseptic, antibacterial, and painkilling properties make it valuable in treating cuts, wounds, burns, bruises, spots, allergies, insect bites, and throat infections. Because it is a decongestant it is also effective against colds, flu, and catarrhal conditions. Lavender lowers blood pressure, prevents and eases digestive spasms, nausea, and indigestion. It is antirheumatic and a tonic. Tension, depression, insomnia, headaches, stress, and hypertension respond particularly well to its soothing properties.

CAUTION

LAVENDER IS USUALLY SAFE FOR ALL AGE GROUPS, BUT SOME HAY FEVER OR ASTHMA SUFFERERS MAY BE ALLERGIC.

DILUTE WELL IF TAKING HOMEOPATHIC REMEDIES.

INFORMATION

BLENDS WELL WITH FLORALS SUCH AS ROSE, GERANIUM, YLANG YLANG, CHAMOMILE, JASMINE, CITRUS OILS SUCH AS ORANGE, LEMON, BERGAMOT, AND GRAPEFRUIT, ROSEMARY, MARJORAM, PATCHOULI, CLARY SAGE, CEDARWOOD, CLOVE, AND TEA TREE.

LEFT *Lavender is an evergreen woody shrub up to 3ft. (1m.) tall.*

RIGHT *Lavender is a reviving yet soothing oil, an ideal ingredient for the bath or in a blend for massage.*

RECIPE

Bath or Massage Blend for Irritability

Add 3 drops lavender, 3 drops chamomile, 2 drops neroli directly to a warm bath and disperse with your hand. Alternatively, add to 3 teaspoons (15ml.) grapeseed or sweet almond oil for a soothing massage.

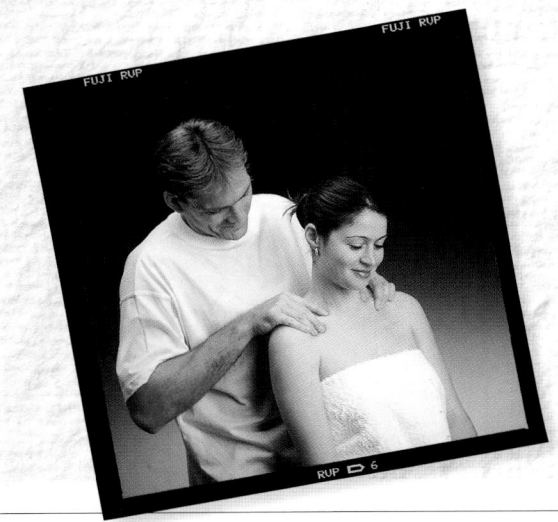

Melaleuca alternifolia
TEA TREE

This small tree or shrub is a traditional remedy among the Aboriginal people of Australia. Originally, the leaves were made into a tea, and hence its name. More recently, scientific research has shown that tea tree oil can combat all types of infection.

DATA FILE

Properties and Uses

Primarily an anti-infection oil, tea tree has antifungal, antibacterial, and antiviral properties. It is frequently used for skin problems such as spots, acne, warts, verrucae, athlete's foot, rashes, insect bites, burns, and blisters. It is used to clean cuts and infected wounds, and it helps skin to heal by encouraging the formation of scar tissue. Tea tree is effective against dandruff, cold sores, and urinary or genital infections such as cystitis and thrush. It is an expectorant that also alleviates inflammation and is a valuable immune stimulant. It is an excellent choice when fighting colds, flu, respiratory infections, catarrhal problems, and infectious illnesses. Tea tree is also used to bring down a fever, to kill fleas and lice, and as a deodorant.

RECIPE
Treatment Oil for Acne

Add 4 drops tea tree, 3 drops bergamot, 3 drops lavender to 2 teaspoons (10ml.) jojoba oil, which is excellent for inflamed or acne-prone skin. Dab onto the affected areas.

INFORMATION

BLENDS WELL WITH LAVENDER, GERANIUM, CHAMOMILE, MYRRH, LEMON, ROSEMARY, MARJORAM, CLARY SAGE, PINE, AND SPICE OILS SUCH AS CLOVE AND CINNAMON.

CAUTION

PEOPLE WITH SENSITIVE SKIN SHOULD INTRODUCE THE OIL WITH CAUTION.

DO NOT SWALLOW MOUTHWASHES OR GARGLES.

BELOW *Tea tree is a small tree or shrub, with needlelike leaves similar to those of cypress, and stalkless yellow or purple flowers.*

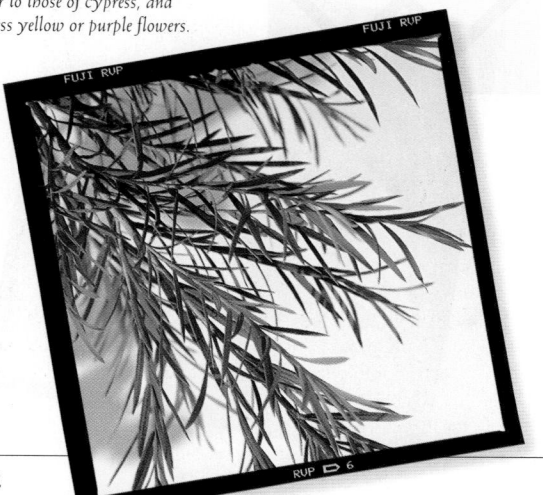

Melaleuca cajeputi
CAJEPUT

In Malaysia, the Philippines, Indonesia, and Australia, wild cajeput is used extensively for all manner of ills, from colds to toothache. Closely related to tea tree, this oil is distilled from the leaves and buds of cajeput, and has a distinctly medicinal camphorous odor.

RECIPE
Inhalation for Colds and Flu

Add 4 drops cajeput, 3 drops rosemary, 2 drops eucalyptus to a bowl of steaming water, cover your head with a towel, bend over the bowl, and inhale for 5–10 minutes.

DATA FILE

Properties and Uses

Cajeput is antiseptic, antimicrobial, and it clears mucus. It is good to use in steam inhalations for colds, flu, sinusitis, asthma, bronchitis, and other respiratory infections. It has painkilling properties which can ease headaches and sore throats, and can be used to good effect on muscular and arthritic pain. The oil is also a urinary antiseptic.

Used with care, it is effective against cystitis and other urinary infections. Cajeput can be used to soothe the stomach, counteract digestive spasms, and kill infections in the gastro-intestinal system. It is widely used for minor conditions such as insect bites and spots. Inhalation, which is one of the best ways to use this oil, helps to dispel mental fatigue and apathy.

BELOW *Cajeput is a tall, evergreen tree, up to 100ft. (30 m.) high, with thick pointed leaves and white flowers.*

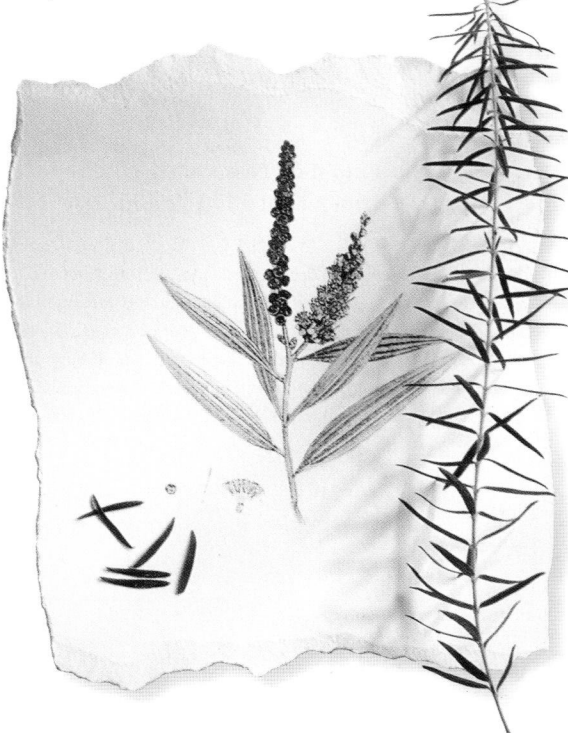

CAUTION

DILUTE WELL, AS CAJEPUT IS A SKIN IRRITANT.

DO NOT USE AS A GARGLE OR AS A VAGINAL WASH AS THE OIL CAN IRRITATE THE MUCOUS MEMBRANES.

CAJEPUT IS A STIMULANT, AND SO IS BEST AVOIDED IN THE LATE EVENING.

INFORMATION

BLENDS WELL WITH SANDALWOOD, JUNIPER, HYSSOP, LAVENDER, ROSEMARY, PINE, LEMON, EUCALYPTUS, MARJORAM.

Origanum marjorana
SWEET MARJORAM

In ancient times marjoram was reputed to promote longevity, a belief that encouraged the ancient Greeks to include it in perfumes, cosmetics, and medicine. In folk tradition marjoram was believed to bring joy to newlyweds and peace to the dead. The essential oil, with its warm spicy scent, is still used to relieve agitation, dispel grief, and restore calm.

INFORMATION
BLENDS WELL WITH BERGAMOT, CHAMOMILE, FRANKINCENSE, ROSE, SANDALWOOD, LAVENDER, ROSEMARY, CEDARWOOD, JUNIPER, EUCALYPTUS, TEA TREE.

CAUTION
DO NOT USE DURING PREGNANCY.

DATA FILE

Properties and Uses
Marjoram is warming and pain-relieving. It also has antispasmodic properties, making it good for muscle spasms and strains. It is a sedative and nerve tonic which works to relieve nervous tension and promote restful sleep. Inhaling marjoram can help to relieve headaches and migraine. Antiviral and bactericidal properties help to fend off colds and infections, and its expectorant properties make it a useful oil to include in a steam inhalation for chest infections. Massaged into the chest or throat, marjoram can also relieve painful coughs. The oil is a vasodilator which is beneficial in treating high blood pressure and improving circulation. It also calms digestion, strengthens intestinal peristalsis, and eases menstrual cramps. Marjoram is a comforting oil that reduces sexual desire.

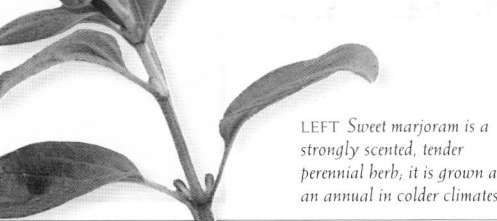

LEFT *Sweet marjoram is a strongly scented, tender perennial herb; it is grown as an annual in colder climates.*

RECIPE
Marjoram Cold Cure
Add 4 drops marjoram and 2 drops eucalyptus to a hot bath to relieve cold symptoms, or add 2 drops to 1 teaspoon (5ml.) of vegetable oil and use as a chest rub.

Pelargonium graveolens
GERANIUM

Potted geraniums have a long history of medicinal use. Over 700 varieties exist, and their essential oils differ depending on where the plant is grown. Fresh and floral in fragrance, geranium was traditionally regarded as a feminine oil, a powerful healer, and a valuable insect repellent.

CAUTION
DO NOT USE DURING THE FIRST THREE MONTHS OF PREGNANCY AND NOT AT ALL IF THERE IS A HISTORY OF MISCARRIAGE.

INFORMATION
BLENDS WELL WITH LAVENDER, BERGAMOT, ROSE, ROSEWOOD, SANDALWOOD, PATCHOULI, FRANKINCENSE, LEMON, JASMINE, JUNIPER, TEA TREE, BENZOIN, BASIL, BLACK PEPPER.

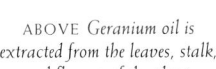

ABOVE *Geranium oil is extracted from the leaves, stalk, and flowers of the plant.*

RECIPE
Massage Blend for PMS
Add 10 drops geranium, 10 drops clary sage, 10 drops bergamot to a bottle containing 1fl. oz. (30ml.) or 6 teaspoons vegetable oil and shake well. Put 6–8 drops in your bath and use a little as a body oil to massage around your abdomen, hips, and lower back.

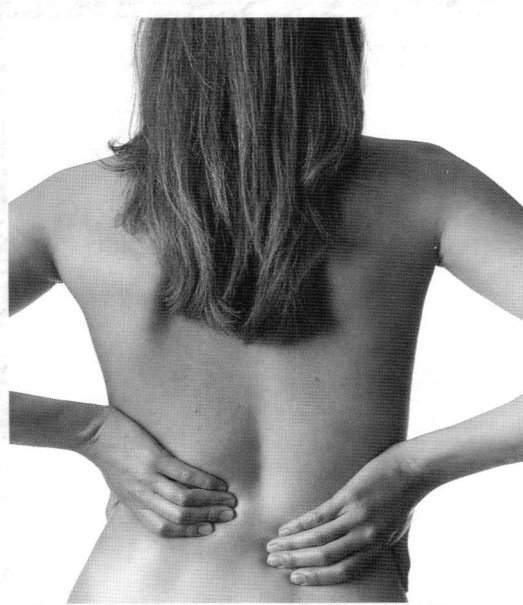

RIGHT *A massage with geranium oil helps to relieve premenstrual pain and tension.*

DATA FILE

Properties and Uses
Geranium is mentally uplifting and refreshing. It has a balancing effect on the nervous system, helping to alleviate apathy, anxiety, stress, hyperactivity, and depression. The anti-inflammatory, soothing, and astringent properties of geranium account for its success in treating arthritis, acne, diaper rash, burns, blisters, eczema, cuts, and congested pores. Antiseptic properties make it useful for cuts and infections, sore throats, and mouth ulcers. It is also a diuretic, used to relieve swollen breasts and fluid retention, and to stimulate sluggish lymph and blood circulation. Geranium helps to stop bleeding, and acts as a tonic for the liver and kidneys. It is used to treat PMS and menopausal problems, and has a balancing effect on mind and body.

Petroselinum sativum
PARSLEY

Common garden parsley is not only rich in vitamins, but also has significant therapeutic properties. The root is used in herbalism for digestive disorders, while the herb and seeds are used mainly for kidney and bladder problems. The essential oil, distilled mainly from the seeds, has a warm, spicy, herbaceous scent.

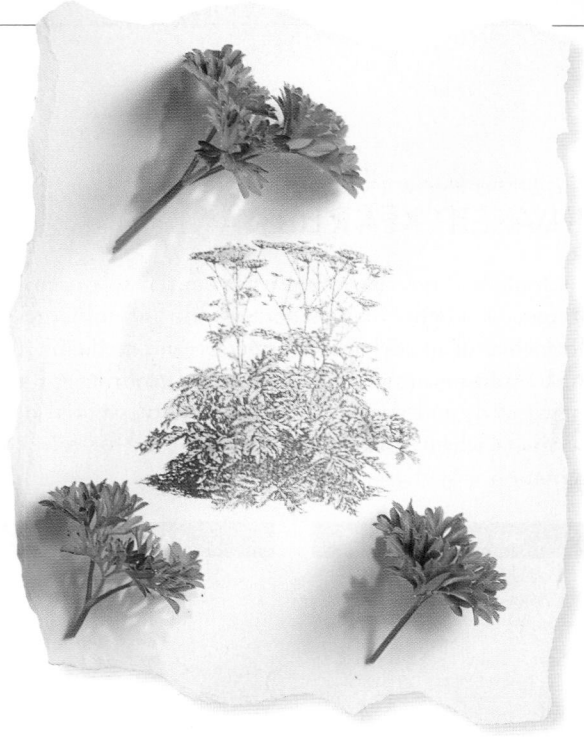

ABOVE *Parsley has crinkly green foliage and small greenish-yellow flowers that produce small brown seeds.*

RECIPE
Parsley Bath for Water Retention

Add 2 drops parsley, 3 drops geranium, 3 drops fennel to a warm bath and swirl through the water with your hand.

CAUTION

USE IN MODERATION, AS PARSLEY CAN BE TOXIC AND IRRITANT.

DO NOT USE DURING PREGNANCY.

DATA FILE

Properties and Uses

Used mainly as a diuretic, parsley is good for fluid retention, PMS, and cellulite, and because of its antiseptic effect it also helps with cystitis. Parsley has a tonic effect on the reproductive system. It is sometimes used during labor and it helps to regulate the menstrual cycle.

It has the ability to shrink small blood vessels and is helpful in treating piles, broken or thread veins, and bruising. Parsley is also used to stimulate appetite; it has a laxative effect on sluggish digestion, and it relieves flatulence, stomach cramps, and indigestion. Parsley has antirheumatic properties.

INFORMATION

BLENDS WELL WITH GERANIUM, ROSE, ROSEMARY, LAVENDER, BERGAMOT, LEMON, NEROLI, CLARY SAGE, TEA TREE, SPICE OILS.

Pinus sylvestris
SCOTCH PINE

Perhaps one of the best-known natural fragrances is the fresh, invigorating aroma of pine. The Arabs, Greeks, and Romans all made use of its medicinal properties, while Native Americans are believed to have used pine to prevent scurvy and infestation with lice and fleas.

CAUTION

USE ONLY SMALL AMOUNTS IN THE BATH OR IN MASSAGE.

DO NOT USE IF YOU HAVE AN ALLERGIC SKIN CONDITION.

ALWAYS CHECK THE SOURCE OF YOUR OIL, AS OILS ARE DISTILLED FROM SEVERAL SPECIES OF PINE, SOME OF WHICH ARE UNSUITABLE FOR USE IN AROMATHERAPY.

INFORMATION

BLENDS WELL WITH LAVENDER, ROSEMARY, CEDARWOOD, EUCALYPTUS, TEA TREE, JUNIPER, SANDALWOOD.

RECIPE
Inhalation for Sinusitis and Stuffy Colds

Add 2 drops pine, 2 drops eucalyptus, 2 drops peppermint to a bowl of steaming hot water. Bend your head over the bowl and cover with a towel to keep in the steam. Inhale for 5–10 minutes. Do this five or six times a day.

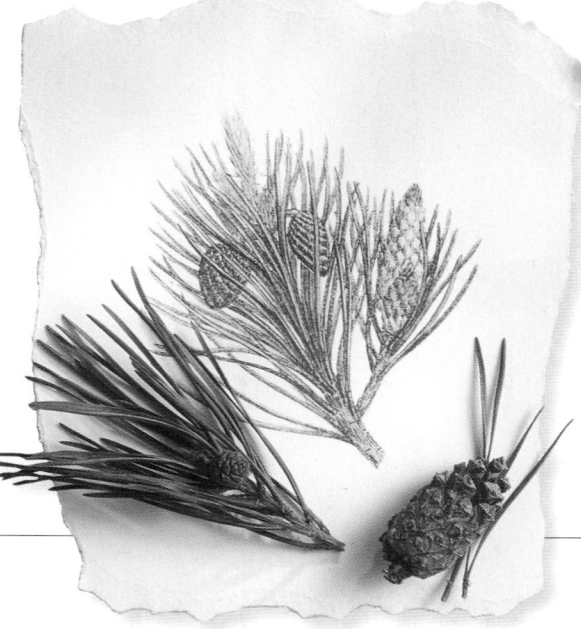

LEFT *Scotch pine has long, stiff needles that grow in pairs and pointed, brown cones.*

THERAPY CONNECTIONS

PINE
- Flower Remedies *p.236*

BLACK PEPPER
- Ayurveda *p.44*
- Traditional Home and Folk Remedies *p.97*

DATA FILE

Properties and Uses

Inhalations of pine are wonderful for colds, catarrhal conditions, including hay fever, and sore throats. The oil, which is expectorant, antiseptic, and antiviral, helps to clear chest infections, sinuses, and ease breathing. Pine stimulates the circulation and helps to relieve rheumatic and muscular aches, pains, and stiffness. Pine is also deodorizing and insecticidal, good for excessive perspiration, and for clearing lice and scabies. The invigorating, refreshing aroma dispels apathy, relieves mental fatigue, nervous exhaustion, and stress-related problems.

Piper nigrum
BLACK PEPPER

Best known for its use in cooking, black pepper also has a 4,000-year-old medicinal history. Prized by the Chinese, the Romans, and the Greeks, pepper was one of the earliest spices ever used. The spicy-scented essential oil is extracted from dried, crushed black peppercorns.

DATA FILE

Properties and Uses

Black pepper stimulates the nervous, digestive, and circulatory systems, which makes it good for poor circulation, constipation, sluggish digestion, and drowsiness. It also has a laxative effect, tones the muscles of the colon, soothes the stomach, helps to prevent food poisoning, and stimulates the appetite.

As a rubefacient it helps with rheumatic and arthritic pain, poor muscle tone, and muscular aches and pains. It helps the immune system fight off infections and viruses, warms against chills, and as an expectorant it clear mucus from the chest. Black pepper helps prevent anemia and is credited with aphrodisiac properties.

RECIPE
Compress for Painful Joints

Add 3 drops black pepper, 2 drops chamomile, 2 drops marjoram to a bowl of hot or cold water and apply to the affected area as directed.

ABOVE *The berries of the pepper vine turn from red to black as they mature.*

CAUTION

DILUTE WELL WHEN USING ON THE SKIN.

DO NOT USE WHILE TAKING HOMEOPATHIC REMEDIES.

INFORMATION

BLENDS WELL WITH FRANKINCENSE, LAVENDER, ROSEMARY, MARJORAM, LAVENDER, LEMON, BENZOIN, CEDARWOOD, PARSLEY, FENNEL, SPICES, AND FLORALS.

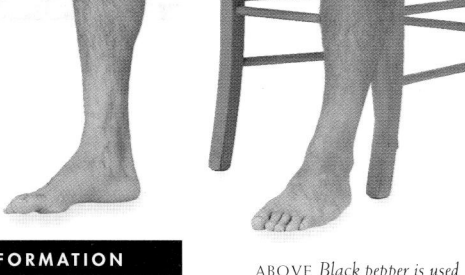

ABOVE *Black pepper is used in hot or cold compresses to ease painful joints.*

Pogostemon cablin
PATCHOULI

The distinctive exotic and earthy aroma of patchouli is one that you either love or hate. Smell is important to the success of aromatherapy, so only use this oil if you like its scent. Patchouli has many uses, and is especially pleasant when used as part of a blend. It is an intense odor, which improves with age.

ABOVE *Patchouli is a perennial herb with large, fragrant, furry leaves.*

RIGHT *The oil extracted from dried patchouli leaves is good for aging skin.*

CAUTION

KEEP ALL ESSENTIAL OILS OUT OF THE REACH OF CHILDREN.

INFORMATION

BLENDS WELL WITH ROSE, GERANIUM, BERGAMOT, NEROLI, YLANG YLANG, LEMON, SANDALWOOD, CLARY SAGE, CLOVE, CEDARWOOD, LAVENDER.

RECIPE
Antiwrinkle Night Oil

Add 2 drops patchouli, 3 drops lemon, 5 drops rose to 2 drops evening primrose oil and 1 teaspoon (10ml.) sweet almond or hazelnut oil. Blend well and apply to the face and neck at night.

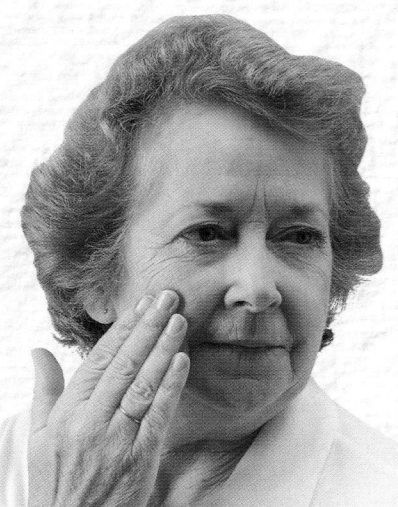

DATA FILE

Properties and Uses

An important anti-depressant, nervous tonic, and reputedly an aphrodisiac, patchouli is valued in treating depression, anxiety, nervous exhaustion, lack of interest in sex, and stress-related problems. It is astringent, antiviral, antiseptic, and anti-inflammatory, good for chapped or cracked skin and open pores, and is also effective for acne, eczema, and dermatitis. It is one of the best choices for dandruff and fungal infections of the skin. It is a cell regenerator, good for aging skins, and it promotes wound-healing. Patchouli acts as a diuretic. It is often recommended for cellulite and as a general tonic.

Rosa centifolia, Rosa damascena
ROSE

Most of the rose oil used in aromatherapy is produced from two types of rose. They vary slightly in color and fragrance, but have similar properties and uses. Rose oil is expensive, but you need only use a little of this complex oil to reap the benefits.

DATA FILE

Properties and Uses

A renowned aphrodisiac, sedative, and a tonic with antidepressant properties, rose has an affinity with the female reproductive system, helping to regulate the menstrual cycle and alleviate PMS or post-natal depression. It benefits stress-related conditions such as insomnia and nervous tension, and is a powerful antiseptic against viruses and bacteria. Rose oil acts as a tonic for the heart, circulation, liver, stomach, and uterus, and helps to detoxify the blood and organs. It regulates the appetite, and prevents and relieves digestive spasms, constipation, and nausea. It soothes cracked, chapped, sensitive, dry, inflamed, or allergy-prone skin, stops bleeding, and encourages wound-healing. Broken veins, and aging or wrinkled skin also benefit. Rose is also useful in treating headaches, earache, conjunctivitis, coughs, and hay fever.

BELOW The healing virtues of the rose have been known since antiquity.

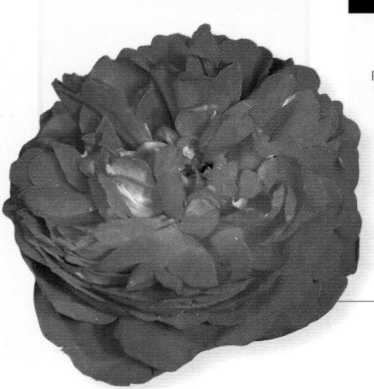

THERAPY CONNECTIONS

ROSE
🌸 Flower Remedies   *p.238*

ROSEMARY
🌿 Herbalism   *p.127*

SANDALWOOD
🪷 Ayurveda   *p.44*

RECIPE
Comforting Massage Blend for Grief
🌿 🌿 🌿 🌿

Add 4 drops rose, 2 drops frankincense, 4 drops chamomile to 3 teaspoons (15ml.) sweet almond or grapeseed oil.

INFORMATION

BLENDS WELL WITH MOST OILS, ESPECIALLY CLARY SAGE, LAVENDER, SANDALWOOD, GERANIUM, BERGAMOT, PATCHOULI, YLANG YLANG.

CAUTION

DO NOT USE DURING THE FIRST THREE MONTHS OF PREGNANCY AND NOT AT ALL IF THERE IS A HISTORY OF MISCARRIAGE.

CAUTION

DO NOT USE DURING PREGNANCY.

ROSEMARY IS NOT SUITABLE FOR PEOPLE WITH EPILEPSY OR HIGH BLOOD PRESSURE.

RIGHT Rosemary is an aromatic, evergreen bush, with silvery green leaves and pale blue flowers. The oil is usually extracted from fresh flowering tops.

RECIPE
After-sport Shower Formula
🌿 🌿 🌿 🌿

Add 2 drops rosemary, 2 drops pine, 4 drops lemon to a large dollop of a gentle, unscented shower gel. Step into a hot shower and work into a lather using a sponge or flannel.

Rosmarinus officinalis
ROSEMARY

Rosemary was one of the first herbs to be used medicinally. Traditionally it was used to ward off evil, to offer protection from the plague, and to preserve and flavor meat. This strong ,distinctively scented oil is one of the most valuable of all essential oils.

INFORMATION

BLENDS WELL WITH FRANKINCENSE, PETITGRAIN, BASIL, THYME, BERGAMOT, LAVENDER, PEPPERMINT, PINE, CEDARWOOD, CYPRESS, SPICE OILS SUCH AS CINNAMON, CLOVE, GINGER, AND BLACK PEPPER.

DATA FILE

Properties and Uses

Refreshing rosemary is a circulation stimulant, excellent for low blood pressure, muscle fatigue, poor circulation, aches, pains, and strains. It acts as a tonic for the nervous system and is anti-depressant. It relieves stress-related disorders, mental exhaustion, and promotes mental clarity. It also tones the skin, liver, and gall bladder. It is used for acne, eczema, dandruff, lice, and hair loss. Antiseptic and antibacterial, antifungal, and a diuretic, it is generally cleansing, and useful for fluid retention. It has properties that help to relieve painful menstruation and clear vaginal discharge, flatulence, indigestion, and constipation. Rosemary prevents and reduces digestive spasms, relieves wind, and regulates digestion. It helps to clear catarrh, coughs, colds, and headaches.

BELOW Rosemary oil's stimulating effect on the circulatory system makes it an ideal remedy for muscle fatigue.

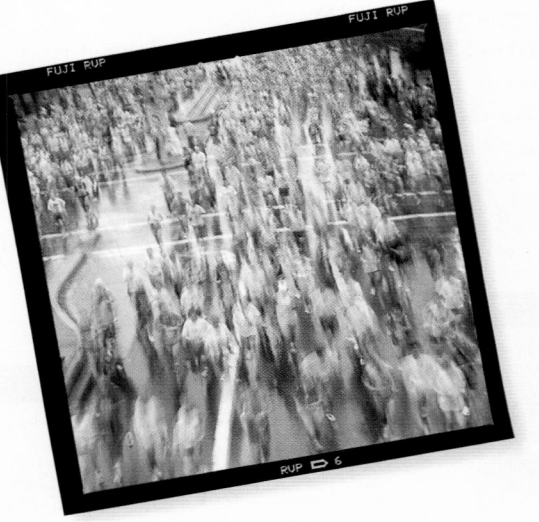

Salvia sclarea
CLARY SAGE

Affectionately known as "clear eye," clary sage was used in medieval times for clearing foreign bodies from the eyes. It remains popular in aromatherapy because of its gentle action and pleasant nutty fragrance. The oil is extracted from the flowering tops and leaves.

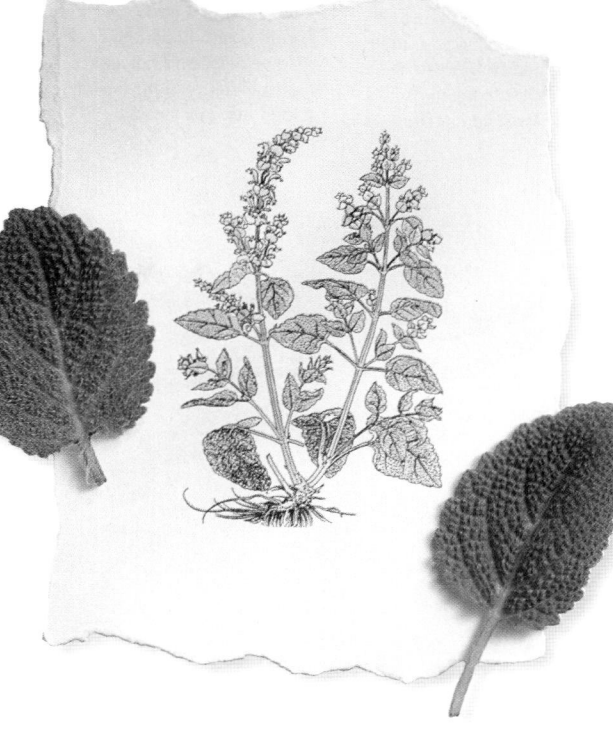

ABOVE *Clary sage is a biennial or perennial herb with large, hairy leaves, green with a hint of purple, and small blue flowers.*

DATA FILE

Properties and Uses

Clary is antidepressant, and sometimes described as euphoric. It helps to regulate the nervous system and is most beneficial in treating anxiety, depression, and stress-related problems. It acts as a powerful muscle relaxant, helping to ease muscular aches and pains, and benefits digestion, relieving indigestion and flatulence. Its astringent properties make it useful for oily skin and scalp

conditions. Clary helps to prevent and arrest convulsions. It is antibacterial, and useful for throat and respiratory infections. Clary helps to lower blood pressure. It is recommended for absent or scanty menstruation and PMS, and is a renowned aphrodisiac that can benefit frigidity and impotence.

CAUTION

DO NOT USE DURING PREGNANCY.

DO NOT USE WHEN DRINKING ALCOHOL, AS IT CAN MAKE YOU DRUNK, DROWSY, AND CAN CAUSE NIGHTMARES.

INFORMATION

BLENDS WELL WITH LAVENDER, FRANKINCENSE, SANDALWOOD, CEDARWOOD, CITRUS OILS SUCH AS LEMON, ORANGE, AND BERGAMOT, GERANIUM, YLANG YLANG, JUNIPER, CORIANDER.

RECIPE

Premenstrual Bath Blend

❧ ❧ ❧ ❧

Add 3 drops clary sage, 2 drops chamomile, 2 drops geranium to a warm bath, disperse with your hand, and relax for at least 10 minutes.

Santalum album
SANDALWOOD

The sweet, woody, oriental smell of sandalwood is one of the most appealing fragrances of all essential oils. The best sandalwood oil comes from India, where it has been used for at least 4,000 years for medicinal and religious purposes.

DATA FILE

Properties and Uses

Sandalwood is an antiseptic, especially effective for all urinary disorders, above all cystitis. It is bactericidal, astringent, and a trusted insect repellent. It clears catarrh and is effective for respiratory conditions such as bronchitis, dry coughs, and sore throats. The oil contains constituents that soothe the stomach, reduce digestive spasms, relieve fluid retention, and reduce inflammation. Sandalwood encourages wound-healing, and skin problems such as dry, chapped skin, acne, psoriasis, eczema, and shaving rash can all benefit from its soothing, rehydrating and antiseptic action. It is an anti-depressant oil that calms the nervous system. The fragrance can also help to lift depression and banish feelings of anxiety and lack of sexual desire.

BELOW *Sandalwood oil is extracted from the powdered and dried roots and heartwood of this small evergreen tree.*

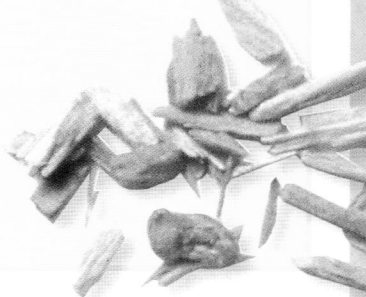

RECIPE

Aftershave Soother

❧ ❧ ❧ ❧

Add 4 drops sandalwood, 6 drops benzoin, 4 drops chamomile to a bottle containing 4 teaspoons (20ml.) hazelnut oil. Warm a tiny amount in your hands and smooth into the face after shaving.

CAUTION

DO NOT USE UNDILUTED ON THE SKIN.

INFORMATION

BLENDS WELL WITH LAVENDER, ROSE, YLANG YLANG, GERANIUM, CHAMOMILE, PATCHOULI, BERGAMOT, FRANKINCENSE, BLACK PEPPER, BENZOIN, TEA TREE, JUNIPER, MYRRH, CYPRESS.

LEFT *Sandalwood is often used to fragrance cosmetics but its essential oil has the added benefit when used in aftershave of soothing the skin.*

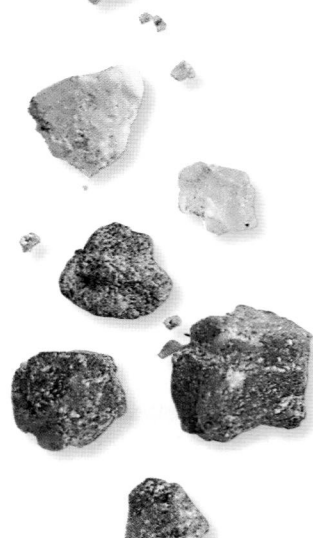

Styrax benzoin
BENZOIN

Benzoin has been used in the East since antiquity as a medicine and as incense. It came into use in the West in the Middle Ages as a remedy for respiratory complaints. The oil, which has a sweet vanilla-like scent, is extracted from the resin of the tropical benzoin tree. It is not strictly an essential oil, but a resinoid dissolved in alcohol.

CAUTION

CAN CAUSE IRRITATION IN SOME SENSITIVE INDIVIDUALS.

RIGHT *Crude benzoin is collected from the tree directly and made into benzoin resinoid using solvents, which are then removed.*

INFORMATION

BLENDS WELL WITH SANDALWOOD, LEMON, ROSE, JUNIPER, MYRRH, FRANKINCENSE, JASMINE, CYPRESS, SPICE OILS.

RECIPE
Warming Winter Bath

Add 2 drops benzoin, 3 drops marjoram, 2 drops clary sage to a warm bath. Disperse with your hand, close the bathroom door to keep in the steam, and soak for at least 10 minutes.

DATA FILE

Properties and Uses

Warming and decongestant, benzoin is helpful for colds and flu, and for clearing mucus from the system. Inhaled, it can soothe sore throats and help to restore a lost voice. Benzoin blended with cream or oil and rubbed into the skin soothes chapped or irritated skin on the hands, as well as cuts and skin inflammation. As a diuretic and antiseptic, benzoin is good for urinary tract infections. It also stimulates the circulation, and its anti-inflammatory action helps to alleviate arthritis and rheumatism. Benzoin is emotionally calming in a crisis, warming and comforting in times of loneliness, and helps to dispel depression, anxiety, and nervous tension.

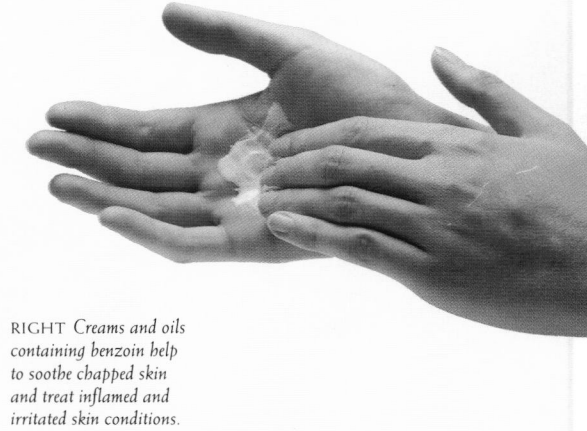

RIGHT *Creams and oils containing benzoin help to soothe chapped skin and treat inflamed and irritated skin conditions.*

Thymus vulgaris
THYME

One of the most useful medicinal herbs in natural healthcare, thyme was also one of the first plants to be used for its healing properties. The oil, distilled from the leaves and tiny purple flowering tops of this sub-shrub, has a fresh green scent.

RECIPE
Antiseptic Mouthwash

Add 10 drops thyme, 15 drops peppermint, 5 drops fennel, and 5 drops myrrh to a bottle containing 4fl.oz. (125ml.) of cheap brandy. Shake well and add 2 teaspoons (10ml.) of the mix to a glass of warm water. Rinse the mouth thoroughly, but do not swallow.

CAUTION

DILUTE WELL, AS THYME MAY CAUSE IRRITATION AND SENSITIZATION IN SOME PEOPLE.

DO NOT USE IF YOU HAVE HIGH BLOOD PRESSURE.

AVOID DURING PREGNANCY.

DO NOT USE IF YOU ARE TAKING HOMEOPATHIC REMEDIES.

INFORMATION

BLENDS WELL WITH LEMON, BERGAMOT, ROSEMARY, LEMON BALM, LAVENDER, PINE, BLACK PEPPER, TEA TREE, LIME, CEDARWOOD, GRAPEFRUIT.

RIGHT *Thyme was used by the ancient Egyptians in the embalming process and by the ancient Greeks to fumigate against infectious diseases.*

DATA FILE

Properties and Uses

Thyme is antiseptic and antibiotic, disinfectant, and strongly germicidal. It is valuable for all infections, especially gastric and bladder infections, as it also has digestive and diuretic properties. The oil's antirheumatic and antitoxic properties are beneficial in treating arthritis, gout, and cellulite. Rubefacient and stimulant actions also help with muscle and joint pain, and poor circulation. Thyme stimulates the immune system to effectively fight off colds, flu, and catarrh, and ease coughing. The diluted oil is good for cleaning wounds, burns, bruises, and clearing lice. Used as a mouthwash it helps to soothe and heal abscesses and gum infections. Thyme has an uplifting fragrance, which can relieve depression, headaches, and stress.

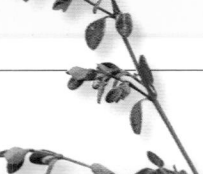

Vetiveria zizanioides
VETIVER

In India and Sri Lanka, where vetiver grows, the essential oil is known as "the oil of tranquility." The tall grass is also cultivated in other countries, and the essential oil is distilled from the dried roots. The deep, smoky, earthy aroma of vetiver is wonderfully grounding and relaxing.

RIGHT *Vetiver is a tall, tufted, perennial, scented grass with straight stems and long, narrow leaves.*

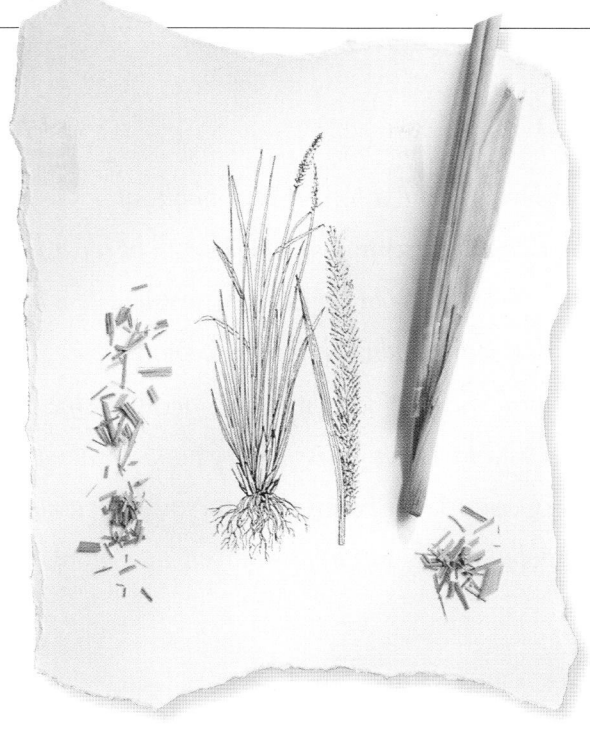

DATA FILE

Properties and Uses

Valued most for its sedative properties, vetiver is used in massage and in baths to relieve stress, anxiety, nervous tension, and insomnia. It also helps to ground people who live too much in their head, or who need to feel stable after shock or a period of insecurity. Vetiver is a circulation stimulant and rubefacient, so it can provide relief from arthritis or rheumatism, and general muscular aches and pains. It is useful in skin care as an antiseptic, tonic, and detoxifier. It helps to clear acne, and because it promotes skin regeneration and strengthens the connective tissue, it assists with wound-healing and benefits aging skin.

THERAPY CONNECTIONS

THYME

🔾 Herbalism p.135

VETIVER

⬡ Ayurveda p.46

GINGER

⬡ Ayurveda p.47

🔾 Chinese Herbal Medicine p.57

INFORMATION

BLENDS WELL WITH JASMINE, CEDARWOOD, LAVENDER, SANDALWOOD, ROSE, YLANG YLANG, CLARY SAGE, PETITGRAIN, MANDARIN.

CAUTION

KEEP OUT OF THE EYES.

DO NOT TAKE INTERNALLY.

KEEP AWAY FROM CHILDREN.

RECIPE
Tranquility Bath Oil
🌿 🌿 🌿 🌿

Add 2 drops vetiver, 2 drops lavender, 4 drops rose to 2 teaspoons (10ml.) of sweet almond oil. Add to a running bath and disperse with your hand. Relax for at least 10 minutes.

Zingiber officinale
GINGER

Originally from India and China, warm, spicy ginger is now grown commercially throughout the tropics. It is a perennial herb with a thick, rhizomatus root. It has been used both to flavor food, and in medicine, for thousands of years, particularly by the Chinese. The essential oil distilled from the root smells similar to fresh root ginger.

RECIPE
Ginger Throat Gargle
🌿 🌿 🌿 🌿

Add 2 drops of ginger oil to 1 teaspoon (5ml.) of vodka and dilute with hot water. When it has cooled sufficiently, use it as a gargle for a sore throat.

DATA FILE

Properties and Uses

Ginger is a rubefacient which can effectively ease painful conditions such as arthritis, rheumatism, or muscle pain, and improve poor circulation. Massaged around the stomach and abdomen, diluted ginger calms the digestion, tones and soothes the stomach, and stimulates the appetite. It helps to alleviate nausea, travel sickness, indigestion, pain, and diarrhea. Ginger is pain-relieving, antiseptic, and antioxidant, valuable for preventing and treating colds, sore throats, and catarrhal congestion. It also eases coughing, and because it promotes sweating, it can be useful for flu. When inhaled, the warming ginger essence eases mental confusion, and helps to relieve fatigue and nervous exhaustion.

CAUTION

USE SPARINGLY, AS HIGH CONCENTRATIONS OF GINGER CAN CAUSE IRRITATION IN SENSITIVE PEOPLE.

DO NOT USE IN EXCESSIVELY HOT OR INFLAMED CONDITIONS.

INFORMATION

BLENDS WELL WITH ROSE, CEDARWOOD, ROSEWOOD, FRANKINCENSE, VETIVER, PATCHOULI, PETITGRAIN, NEROLI, LIME, AND OTHER CITRUS OILS.

RIGHT *Ginger is used to prevent and treat colds and sore throats.*

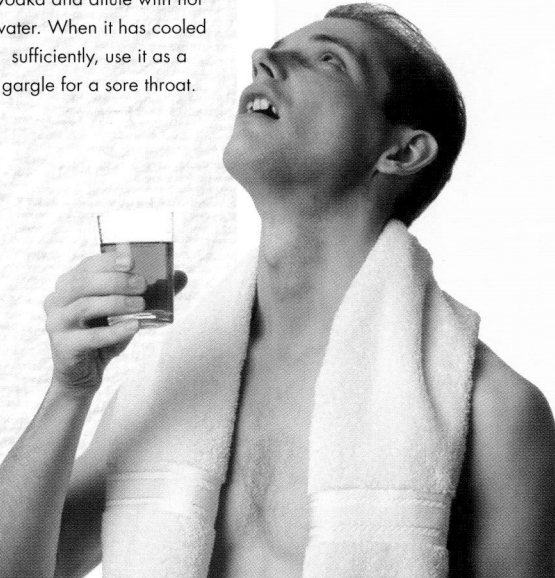

HOMEOPATHY

Homeopathy works by treating a person as a whole, or holistically, so although presenting symptoms will be looked at, the individual person — his or her mental, physical, emotional, and spiritual health — will also be taken into account. Homeopathy is based on the principle that "like cures like", meaning the treatment given is similar in substance to the illness it is helping. Although it has roots that go back many centuries, it began in its present form a mere 200 years ago and today is popular as a safe and effective treatment of many problems.

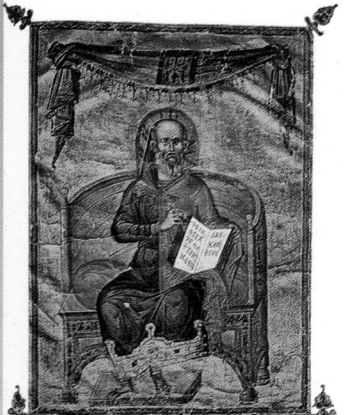

ABOVE *The Ancient Greek physician Hippocrates, whose theories had similarities with those of homeopathy.*

BELOW *Medical practices in the 18th century involved debilitating blood-letting as well as harsh drugs.*

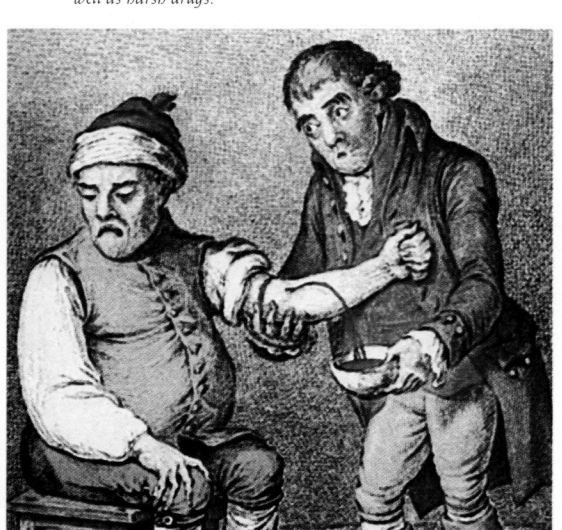

THE ORIGINS OF HOMEOPATHY

It was the Greek physician Hippocrates, known as the "father of medicine," who, in the 5th century B.C.E., was the first to understand the principle of treating the body with a remedy which will produce similar symptoms to the ailment suffered. He also believed that symptoms specific to an individual, that person's reactions to an ailment, and a person's own powers of healing were important in diagnosing and choosing a cure. On this basis, he built up his own medicine chest of homeopathic remedies. But it was the German physician Samuel Hahnemann (1755–1843) who first developed homeopathy as it is known and practised today. A prominent physician, chemist, and author, Hahnemann had become increasingly disillusioned with the methods of treatment of the day. These included harsh practices such as blood-letting and purging, and large doses of medicines that were often more debilitating than the illness itself. Yet it was obvious these practices were not working — disease was rampant. Hahnemann was one of the first physicians to advocate the improvement of poor hygiene, both in the home and in public places, and he stressed the importance of a good diet, fresh air, and higher standards of living for all. But disillusionment with the lack of response to his initiatives meant that he eventually decided to give up medical practice. In 1789 he moved to Leipzig, where he became a translator of medical texts.

HOMEOPATHY V. ALLOPATHY

Homeopathy works on the principle of stimulating the body's defense mechanism by treating it with minute doses of a substance that produces symptoms similar to those of the illness. Allopathic, or conventional, treatment works by suppressing symptoms, so that diarrhea is treated by a substance that causes constipation and insomnia is treated with sedatives.

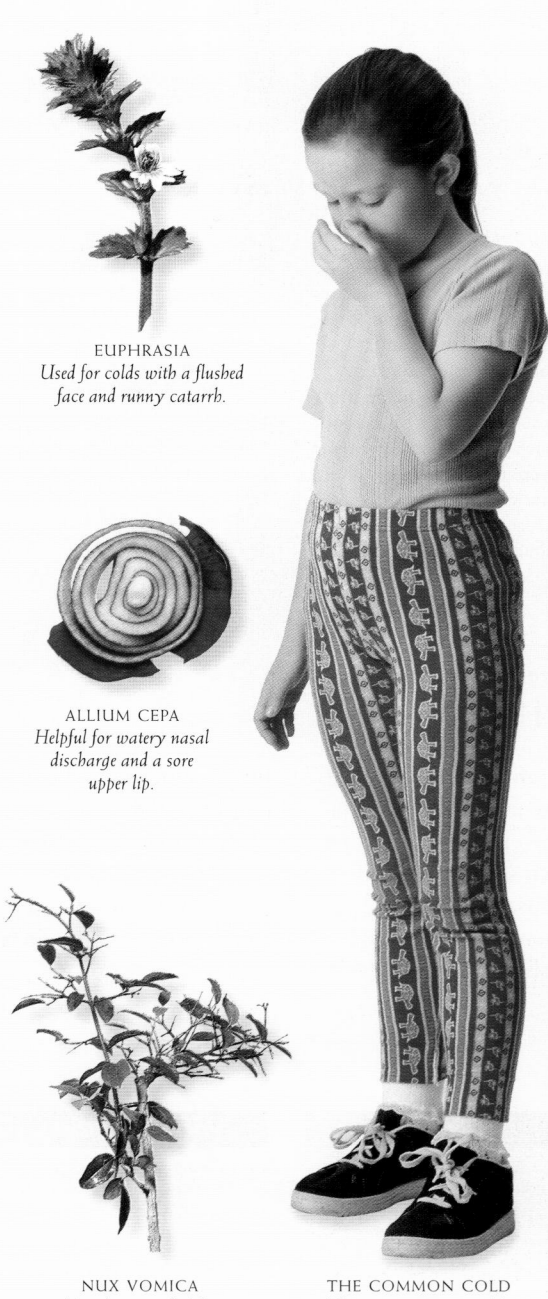

EUPHRASIA
Used for colds with a flushed face and runny catarrh.

ALLIUM CEPA
Helpful for watery nasal discharge and a sore upper lip.

NUX VOMICA
May be prescribed for patients who have a blocked nose at night and a runny nose during the day.

THE COMMON COLD
There are various possible homeopathic remedies for the common cold and the homeopath will select the most appropriate one in each case.

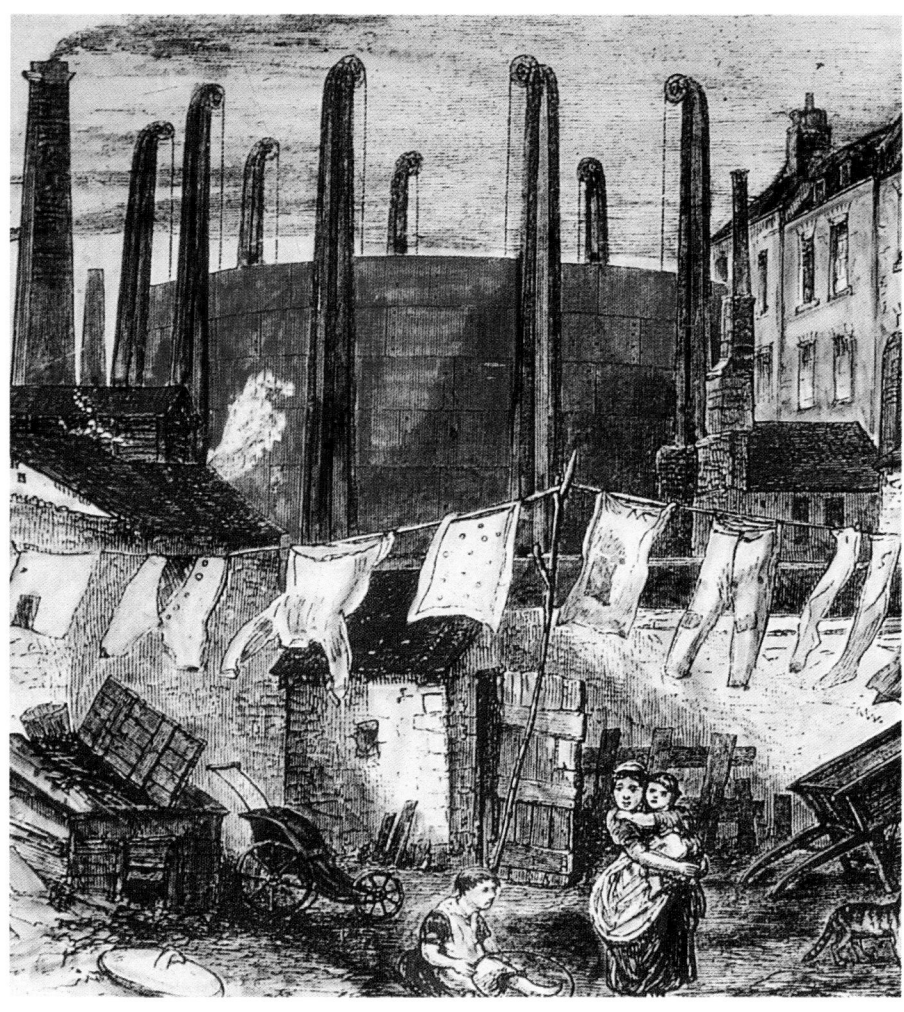

ABOVE *As Hippocrates had shown many centuries earlier, Hahnemann saw that the patient's circumstances can both cause and exacerbate disease.*

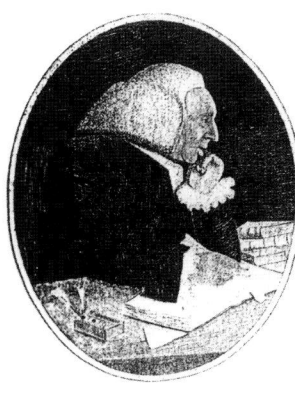

BELOW *Dr. William Cullen, a Scottish physician whose observations about the therapeutic effects of quinine stimulated Hahnemann's homeopathic experiments.*

While translating one of these texts in 1790, *A Treatise on Materia Medica,* by Dr. William Cullen of London University, Hahnemann noticed an entry which was to set him on a path which would lead to the founding of homeopathic practice.

Cullen wrote that quinine (an extract of Peruvian bark) was an effective treatment for malaria because of its astringent qualities. As a chemist, Hahnemann knew quinine was effective against the disease, but doubted this was due to its astringency. He decided to explore this further and for days took doses of quinine himself and recorded his reactions. He found that he developed all the symptoms of malaria – palpitating heart, irregular pulse, drowsiness, and thirst – although he did not have the disease. Each time he took a new dose, the symptoms recurred. He speculated that it was the quinine's ability to induce the malarial symptoms that made it effective as a treatment. To back up his theory, he gave doses of quinine to volunteers, whom he called "provings," recorded their reactions, and found similar results.

A PICTURE OF SYMPTOMS

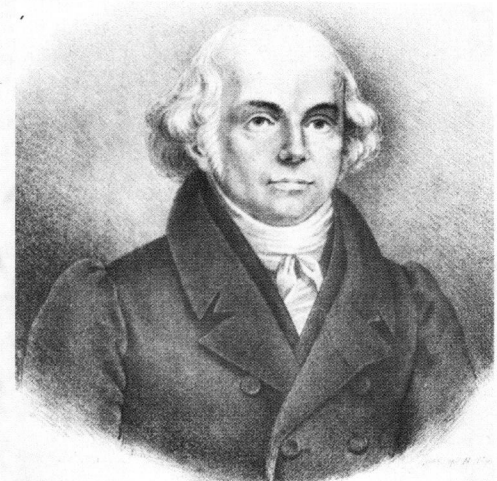

ABOVE *Samuel Hahnemann (1755–1843), who founded the system of homeopathy.*

Hahnemann experimented with other substances, as well as quinine, which were used as medicines at the time, such as arsenic, belladonna, and mercury. With each new substance given, he noted that individuals differed in their severity of symptoms and how they healed. Some showed few symptoms, while others suffered badly.

He found that some symptoms were commonly found after giving a substance. He called these first-line, or keynote, symptoms. The less common symptoms he called second-line, and those that were more rare he called third-line symptoms. The combination of all these types of symptoms enabled him to build up a "drug picture" for each substance that he tested.

Following this, Hahnemann went on to develop a "symptoms picture" of his patients. This included a physical examination, questions about their symptoms and general health, what made them feel better or worse, their likes and dislikes, and their lifestyle. He found that the more information he had about the patient, the more accurately he could match up the symptom picture to the remedy picture before prescribing, and therefore the more successful the eventual treatment. Hahnemann believed he had developed a new system of medicine – a system that worked on the principle that a substance and a disease that produce similar symptoms can negate each other, resulting in the full health of the patient. He called his new system "homeopathy," from the Greek words *homios,* meaning like, and *pathos,* meaning suffering.

WHAT IS HOMEOPATHY?

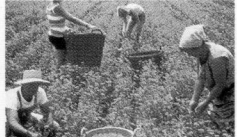

INGREDIENTS
Many remedies are prepared from plant material. After harvesting, the ingredients are steeped in alcohol to produce a tincture, which is then repeatedly diluted.

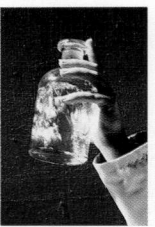

SUCCUSSION
Each time the tincture is further diluted it is subjected to succussion (vibration or shaking) to release its potency.

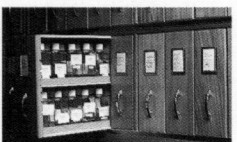

DISPENSARY
The dilution and succussion may be repeated up to 30 times to make a remedy of greater potency. The remedies are stored in sealed dark glass bottles in the dispensary.

The efficacy of homeopathy is proven by the popularity it has across the world, the number of practitioners and hospitals dedicated to homeopathic care, and the clinical trials that have been undertaken. Even so, it can be difficult to understand exactly how the principles of homeopathy actually work in practice, leading some modern doctors to remain skeptical about its effectiveness.

WHAT IS HOMEOPATHY?

From Hahnemann's first experiment with quinine, he went on to prove the efficacy of around 100 homeopathic remedies. There are now more than 2,000 available, with new ones continually being added. The remedies are made from animal, vegetable, and mineral sources, which are as varied as honey bees (including the sting), snake venom, and poison ivy leaves, onions, coffee beans, and daisies. But the amounts used are so minute that no substance can be tasted or side effects experienced, however poisonous or toxic the substance might be.

In his "provings," Hahnemann had been worried by some patients who got worse before they got better after taking the substances given to them. To prevent this happening, he developed a new system of diluting the remedies. He diluted each remedy and then "succussed" or shook it. He believed that doing this released the energy of the substance. He found not only that the new system of diluting prevented the worsening of symptoms, but also, to his astonishment, that the more diluted the substance, the better its effects. He called this method "potentization."

BELOW Homeopathic remedies are usually offered as pills or powders, so they are very easy to take.

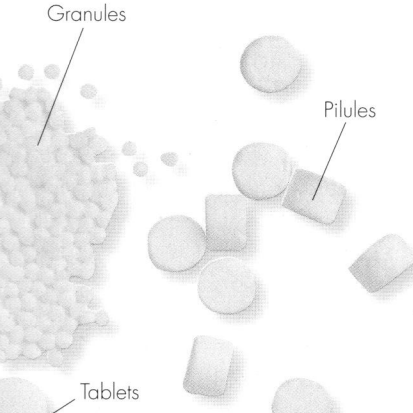

Powder

Granules

Pilules

Tablets

REMEDY SOURCES

Many of the ingredients used to make homeopathic remedies would be extremely harmful if ingested in their crude form. As well as plant material, substances of animal and mineral origin are used.

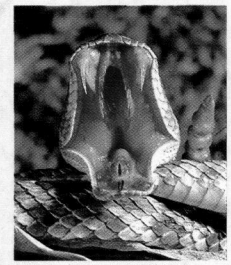

SNAKE VENOM
The venom of the North American rattlesnake is used to make a remedy known as Crotalis horridus, *used for shock and festering wounds.*

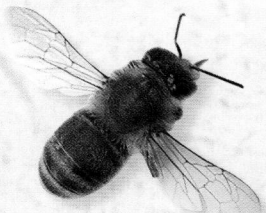

HONEY BEE
Whole bees and their stings are used to produce a remedy known as Apis mellifica. This can be helpful in treating patients with rashes, especially where there is burning or stinging.

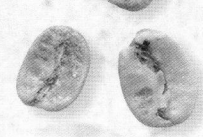

COFFEE
Coffee beans are used in the preparation of Coffea. This treats people who are mentally and physically overactive for any reason.

ACONITUM NAPELLUS
Aconitum napellus, *or monkshood, is the source for Aconite. This is used for healthy-looking people who are struck by sudden acute conditions.*

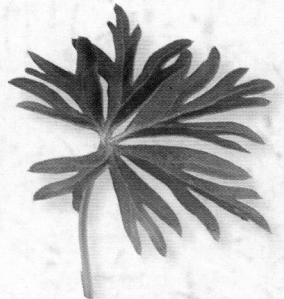

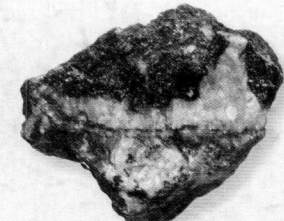

COPPER
Mineral sources include copper, which can be used to treat spasms, cramps, and convulsions.

DILUTION

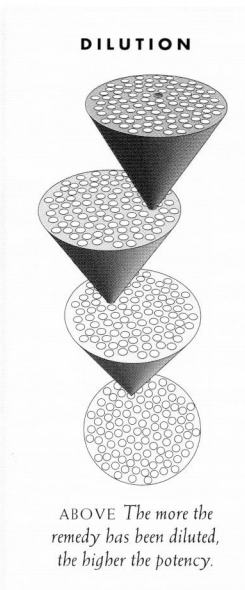

ABOVE *The more the remedy has been diluted, the higher the potency.*

The process of making the remedies is very precise. Soluble substances such as plant and animal extracts are dissolved in a solution of about 90 percent alcohol and 10 percent distilled water, depending on the substance. The mixture is kept in an airtight container and left to stand for two to four weeks, occasionally being shaken. Insoluble substances, such as gold, are first ground down into a fine powder until they become soluble, and then undergo the same process. The mixture is then strained, and the resulting solution is known as the mother tincture.

The mother tincture is then diluted again to produce the different potencies which make up the homeopathic remedies. The dilution is measured as either decimal (x) or centesimal (c). Decimal remedies are diluted to the ratio 1:10, while the centesimal ratio is 1:100. So to produce a 1c potency, one drop of the mother tincture is added to 99 drops of an alcohol and water solution, and then succussed. To produce a 2c potency, one drop of the 1c solution is mixed with an alcohol and water solution, and then succussed. By the time the remedy reaches a 12c potency it is unlikely that any of the original substance remains in the solution, and yet it remains effective. This is why some skeptics find it difficult to accept the efficacy of homeopathy. But the therapy's supporters believe that physics is not yet developed enough to explain the phenomenon. However, one theory is that the dilution process triggers an electromagnetic imprint which affects our own electromagnetic field; another is that the method of succussion creates and stores an electrochemical pattern in the solution which then spreads through the patient when taken. Once the solution has been succussed and diluted to a certain level, the potentized remedy is then added to lactose, or milk sugar, in the form of tablets, pilules, granules, or powder, and stored in a dark glass bottle, away from direct sunlight. For treatment purposes, different potencies are prescribed. For an acute illness, a low-potency remedy is recommended; for a chronic disease, a higher potency is more useful.

THE 12 TISSUE SALTS

In the 19th century Wilhelm Schussler identified 12 minerals that he believed to be vital to human health. When these are lacking they can be taken in the form of homeopathically prepared tissue salts.

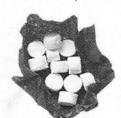

CALC. PHOS.
Produced from calcium phosphate

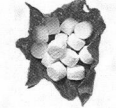

CALC. SULF.
Produced from calcium sulfate

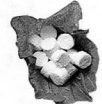

FERR. PHOS.
Produced from iron phosphate

SIL.
Produced from silicon dioxide

KALI MUR.
Produced from potassium chloride

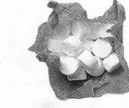

KALI PHOS.
Produced from potassium phosphate

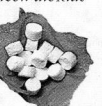
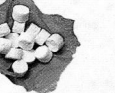

KALI SULF.
Produced from potassium sulfate

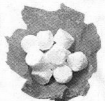

MAG. PHOS.
Produced from magnesium phosphate

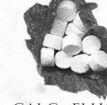

CALC. FLUOR.
Produced from calcium fluoride

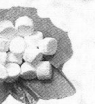

NAT. MUR.
From sodium chloride (common salt)

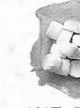

NAT. PHOS.
Produced from sodium phosphate

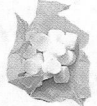

NAT. SULF.
Produced from sodium sulfate

THE 12 TISSUE SALTS

Biochemic tissue salts are homeopathically prepared ingredients which were introduced at the end of the 19th century by a German physician, Wilhelm Schussler. He believed that many diseases were caused by a deficiency of one or more of 12 vital minerals. A deficiency in each salt would manifest as particular symptoms. Lack of calcarea phosphorica (Calc. phos.), for example, would show up as teething problems or an inability to absorb nutrients properly, while lack of magnesium phosphate (Mag. phos.) would affect nerve endings and muscles. Replacing the missing mineral with a minute dose of the tissue salt can correct the problem. Tissue salts are prepared only from mineral sources such as calcium, iron, and salt, but homeopathic remedies are made from animal, vegetable, and mineral sources. These can be as exotic and deadly as snake's venom or as common as the stinging nettle, but in all cases they are diluted to such an extent that there can be no possible side effects from even the most toxic substances.

THE VITAL FORCE

Hahnemann believed that we all have our own energy, or vital force. The force, which stimulates the body mentally, physically, and emotionally, can be disrupted by poor diet, stress, lack of exercise, pollution, and hereditary problems, weakening it so that illness results. The remedies stimulate the force, enabling the body to heal itself.

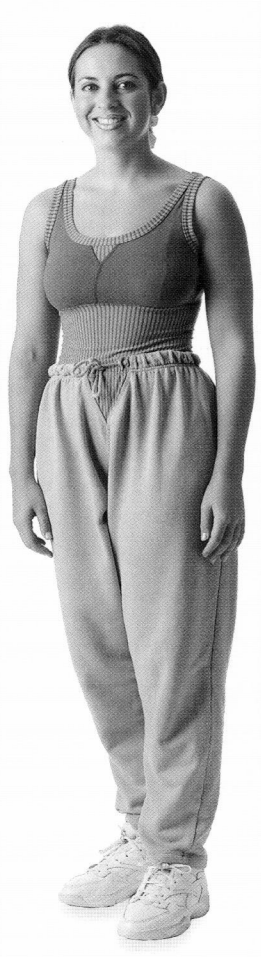

ABOVE *A healthy person has strong powers of self-healing. Illness is a sign that this vital force has been weakened.*

HOMEOPATHIC TECHNIQUES

Homeopathy can be safely used by anyone, from pregnant women to babies and the elderly. Its popularity has grown in the U.K. since the first homeopathic hospital opened in 1849. It is widely used in Europe, particularly France and Germany, and in South America. It has spread, too, across continents, to Asia and India, where it is now officially recognized as a branch of medicine. In the U.S. homeopathy is becoming a recognized alternative to conventional healthcare, and homeopathic remedies are widely available in health stores.

HOW HOMEOPATHY WORKS

Homeopathy sees symptoms of disease as a positive outward sign that the body is trying to heal itself. Therefore, it holds that the symptoms should not be suppressed (as they are in allopathic medicine), and remedies are used which will help stimulate and support the healing process. In some cases, the symptoms will worsen before they improve.

A homeopath prescribes remedies for the "whole" person, basing his or her decision on Hahnemann's principles – the law of similars, the principle of minimum dose, and prescribing for the individual.

❋ THE LAW OF SIMILARS Formulated in 1796, it states that a substance that, in large doses, can produce symptoms of illness in a healthy person can cure similar symptoms in a sick person if used in minute doses. Hahnemann believed this was because nature allows for the existence of two similar diseases in the body at the same time. Homeopathic remedies work by introducing a similar artificial disease that negates the original disease, and yet its own effects are so minimal it causes no suffering.

❋ THE MINIMUM DOSE This states that successive dilutions enhance the curative properties of a substance, while eradicating any side effects. This means only the most minute dose of the substance is needed to help heal.

❋ WHOLE-PERSON PRESCRIBING Homeopaths believe that symptoms, pain, or diseases do not occur in isolation, but are an overall reflection of a person. They therefore do not just look at the problem presented to them, but at the person as a "whole." Each person is treated as an individual, and the homeopath will consider the patient's personality, temperament, emotional and physical state, and likes and dislikes before prescribing a treatment. In this way, a homeopath might see two people with similar symptoms, but would treat them totally differently.

Homeopaths also believe treatment works according to a set of three rules known as the Laws of Cure. These are:

> ❋ *A remedy starts healing from the top of the body and works downward.*
> ❋ *It starts from within the body, working outward, and from major to minor organs.*
> ❋ *Symptoms clear up in reverse order to their manner of appearance.*

Homeopaths also believe that treatment should be prescribed according to a person's constitution, which is made up of inherited and acquired mental, physical, and emotional characteristics. These are matched to a remedy which will improve all-round health, no matter what illness the individual is suffering. This constitutional profile corresponds to a particular remedy, and a person might therefore be known as a Sepia type, or a Lachesis type.

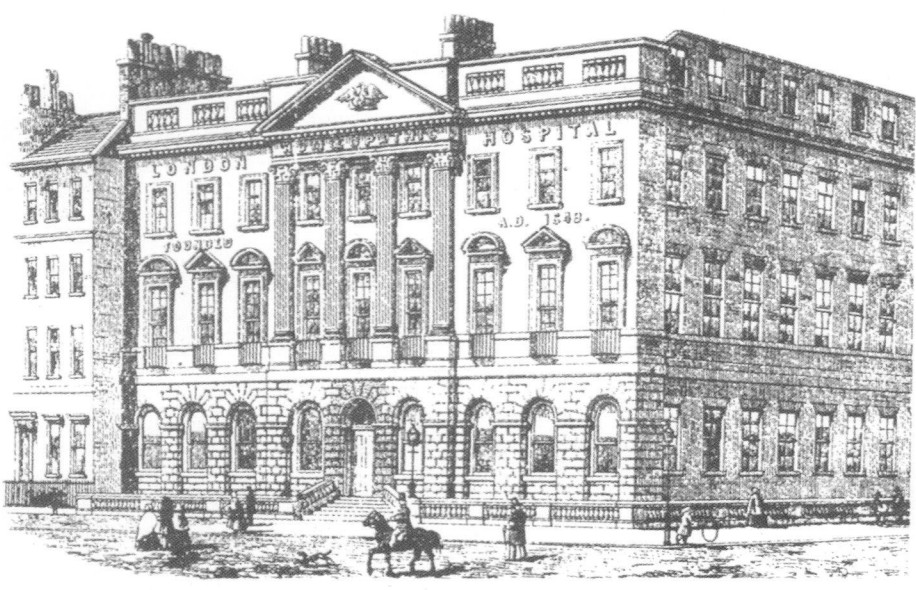

HAHNEMANN'S CASE

Hahnemann used this wooden case to store hundreds of remedies in small glass vials. He continued to treat patients for many years, and died in 1843 at the age of 88.

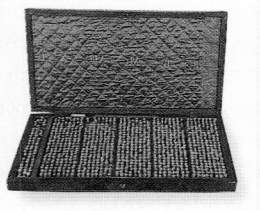

ABOVE *An illness and its remedies are affected by the constitution, character, diet, and lifestyle of the individual concerned.*

LEFT *The first homeopathic hospital in the U.K. opened in London in 1849, and the therapy has become steadily more popular across Europe and the U.S.*

VISITING A HOMEOPATH

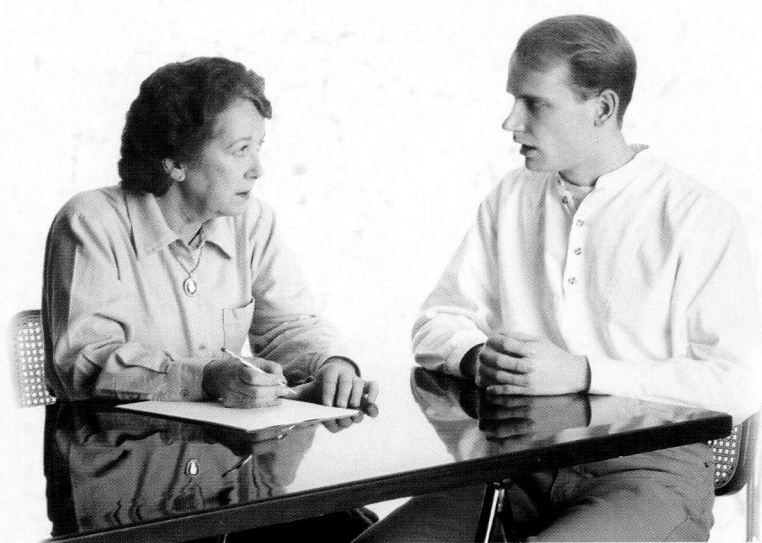

ABOVE *The first consultation with a homeopath involves many questions that will be seemingly unrelated to the health problem concerned. These enable the consultant to form a complete picture of the patient.*

A first visit may last around an hour, as the homeopath asks detailed questions to build up an overall picture of your mental, physical, emotional, spiritual, and general health. As well as questions about any inherited problems, past illnesses, and diet, you may also be asked which side you sleep on, what type of weather you prefer, and whether you have food preferences. Only then will the homeopath prescribe a remedy specifically to suit you. One remedy at a time is usually given, although the prescription may change as your symptoms change. You may not be told which remedy has been prescribed. This is because some people are not happy with the constitutional character type attributed to them. Diet and lifestyle changes may also be recommended.

The remedies should be handled as little as possible, so are usually taken on a spoon and slipped under the tongue to dissolve. Food and drink should be avoided for a half-hour before and afterward. You may also be advised to avoid coffee and peppermints as they may counteract the remedies.

A follow-up appointment will be made for about a month later to assess progress. You may only need two appointments, but chronic conditions tend to take longer. If there is no improvement after around four visits, think about trying alternative treatment. Once symptoms improve, the remedy should be stopped. The remedies are perfectly safe, and although "overdosing" will do no harm, as with any medicine it is best avoided. Treatment can be given alongside conventional medicine, although some drugs may affect the efficacy of homeopathic remedies.

HOME USE

The remedies can be used at home for simple ailments and first aid, but should not be taken as a substitute for professional care. As a general rule, low potencies (e.g. 6c) are used for chronic conditions, and higher potencies (e.g. 30c) for acute conditions such as a cold. Remedies for acute conditions are usually taken on a half-hourly basis at first, and then the intervals spread out to about 8–12 hours. More chronic conditions may combine both low and high potencies.

HOW TO TAKE AND STORE REMEDIES

❖ Take only one remedy at a time.
❖ Do not touch the remedies; empty them onto a teaspoon and put under the tongue, or tip them into the cap of the bottle to transfer them to the mouth.
❖ Take in a "clean mouth" at least 30 minutes after meals. If you need to take them sooner rinse your mouth out first with water. Avoid alcoholic drinks and cigarettes, spicy or minty foods while taking the remedies.
❖ Store in a cool dark place in tightly closed bottle away from strong smells such as perfumes, air fresheners, or essential oils. Stored correctly, remedies will keep for around five years.

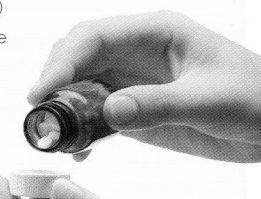
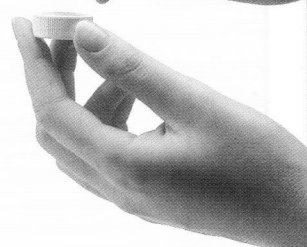

ABOVE *Remedies should not be touched by hand. Tap them out into the container lid or transfer them to a clean teaspoon.*

WHICH PROBLEMS CAN BE TREATED?

Homeopathy can successfully treat most complaints – physical, mental, and emotional – although some people respond better than others. Minor problems such as colds, diarrhea, and allergies, and more serious conditions such as rheumatoid arthritis, psoriasis, and depression can all improve with homeopathic treatment.

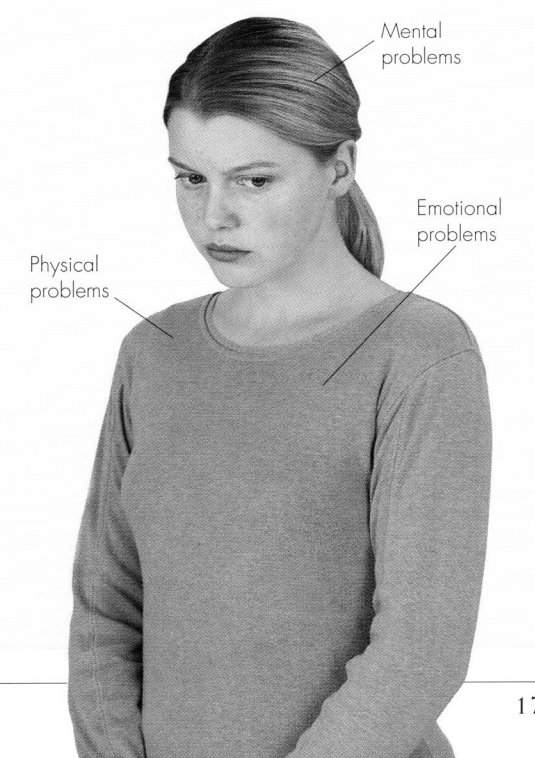

Mental problems

Emotional problems

Physical problems

HOMEOPATHIC REMEDIES

Aconitum napellus, wolfsbane,
blue monkshood, blue aconite
ACONITE

This deadly plant has been used for its poison for centuries. Saxon hunters dipped the tips of their arrows into its juice before hunting wolves, giving it one of its common names, wolfsbane – although its original title comes from the Latin word *acon*, meaning dart. It is grown in the European mountains, and the flowers, root, and leaves are used.

DATA FILE

Relieves

❧ acute conditions which begin suddenly and after shock or exposure to abrupt changes of climate

❧ skin irritations

❧ fears

Uses

Works well when given in the early stages of infections and inflammation, such as sore throats, coughs, and ear and eye problems and when the skin becomes hot, dry, and burning. Used for complaints which come on suddenly, for instance after shock or exposure to

weather extremes. Also, when restlessness and fear accompany an illness or complaint, resulting in palpitations, panic attacks, or agoraphobia.

Which type of person?

❧ strong, full-blooded, healthy-looking

❧ when well, happiest in company, but may be malicious and insensitive to cover a lack of self-esteem

❧ when ill, avoid company

❧ do not handle shock well and fear dying, even to the extent of predicting their own time of death

SYMPTOMS

MENTAL

🐾 mainly fears – general anxiety, of crowds, of dying

PHYSICAL

🐾 infections or inflammation due to injury

🐾 sudden fevers, accompanied by hot, dry skin

🐾 tingling in hands and feet

🐾 thirst

Symptoms improve in warmth and fresh air but worsen when listening to music, lying on the affected side, at night, and in airless rooms.

RIGHT *Aconite is one of Hahnemann's original remedies and is derived from the poisonous plant Aconitum napellus, or monkshood.*

Allium cepa, red onion
ALLIUM

The onion, grown worldwide, has been used across many continents and by many religions for its healing properties. The whole red onion bulb is used, and its potent oil stimulates the tear glands and nasal mucous membranes, causing the eyes and nose to water. In homeopathy it is used to treat any condition which includes these symptoms, such as colds, allergies, and hay fever.

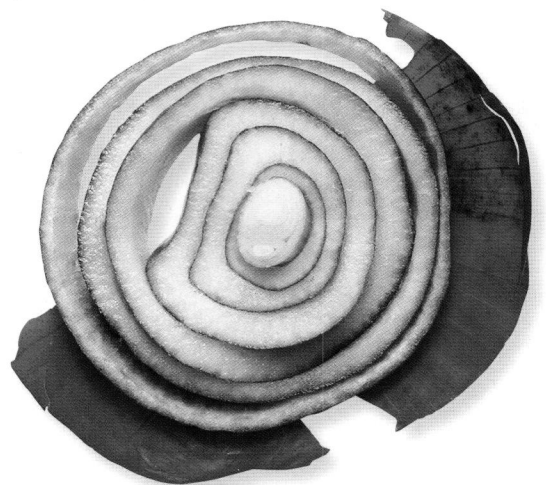

ABOVE *The red onion used in cooking is the source of the Allium remedy, used to treat coughs, colds, and hay fever.*

RIGHT *Allium is often used to treat earache and toothache in children, as well as the acute symptoms of a cold and related headaches.*

DATA FILE

Relieves

❧ streaming eyes and nose

❧ headaches, burning pain, and neuralgia

❧ pains that move from side to side, commonly from left to right

Uses

Particularly good for cold and hay fever symptoms – profuse discharge, smarting and swollen eyes, sneezing, sore nose and upper lip from irritation due to streaming. Also for burning or neuralgic pain that moves from side to side. Also, in children, neuralgic pain which accompanies earache, molar toothache which moves around, and headaches behind the forehead. Coughing and the early stages of laryngitis can also be helped.

Which type of person?

❧ no particular type

SYMPTOMS

MENTAL

🐾 fear of pain

PHYSICAL

🐾 profuse discharge from eyes and nose

🐾 headache, toothache, earache in children, stuffiness, cough, neuralgia, colic in babies.

Symptoms improve in fresh, cool air, and worsen in warm, stuffy rooms, and in the cold and damp.

THERAPY CONNECTIONS

ONION

🔲 Ayurveda   p.25

✋ Traditional Home and Folk Remedies   p.82

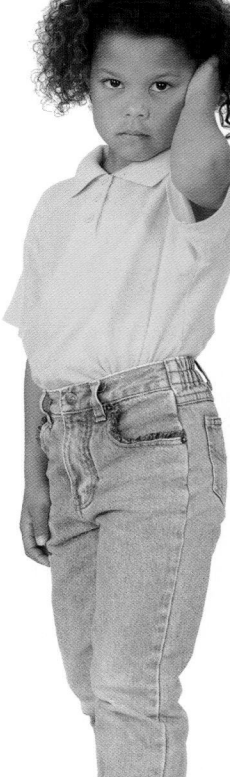

Anacardium orientale,
Semecarpus anacardium, marking nut tree
ANACARD. OR.

Grown in the East Indies; the Hindus use the acrid black juice of this nut to burn away moles, warts, and other skin complaints. They also use it, mixed with ink, to make markings on linen. The Arabs used the juice for a number of conditions, such as mental illness, memory loss, and paralysis. Homeopathically, cardol, the juice extracted from the pith between the shell and kernel, is used to make the remedy which is given for "tight" feelings of pain.

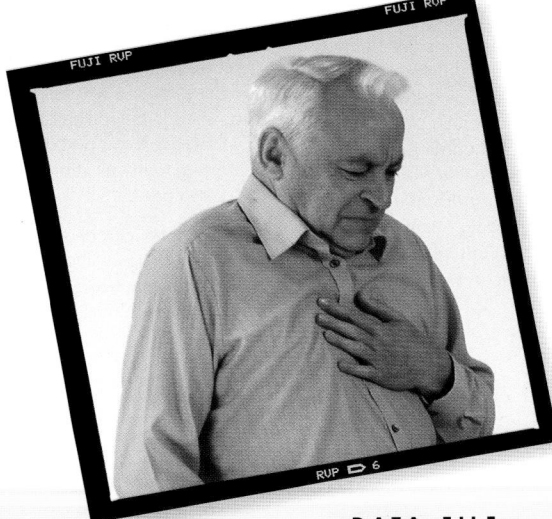

MENTAL

- loss of memory, leading to instances of harsh behavior
- obsessive behavior
- fixations
- irritability
- nervous exhaustion

PHYSICAL

- tight feeling of constriction
- duodenal ulcers
- blocked gut or anus

Symptoms improve immediately after eating, when lying on the affected part, after rubbing, and worsen around midnight, after washing in hot water and using a compress.

LEFT *Anacard. or. is used to treat "tight" feelings of pain or constriction.*

DATA FILE

Relieves

- constricted pain
- plugged ear, nose, or back passage
- inferiority complex

RIGHT *A liking for dairy products may suggest that a person will respond well to Anacard. or.*

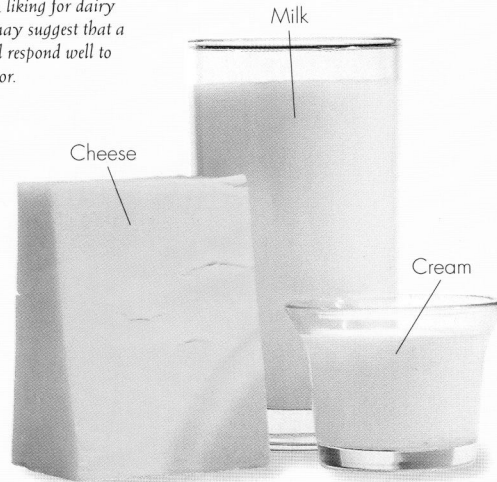

Cheese

Milk

Cream

Uses

This remedy is useful when there is a feeling of tightness or constricted pain. Other conditions that may be relieved are itchy skin; piles; constipation; indigestion; rheumatism and duodenal ulcers which feel better immediately after eating, but cause discomfort two hours later. It is particularly beneficial for those who suffer an inferiority complex and who want to prove themselves, for those who feel possessed, or those who just don't quite feel themselves.

Which type of person?

- pale face
- blue rings around the eyes
- strong moral sense, so feel guilt acutely
- easily offended
- lack self-confidence
- like dairy products

Antimonium tartaricum, antimony potassium
tartrate, tartar emetic
ANT. TART.

Antimony potassium tartrate is a poisonous crystalline salt which has no color or odor and is used as a fix for leather and textiles, and in insecticides. In the past it was used in conventional medicine as an emetic, and as an expectorant. Homeopathically, it is used to treat gastric disorders and chest complaints.

DATA FILE

Relieves

- chest conditions
- gastric or bowel complaints

Uses

This remedy is particularly good in the very young or very old who are too feeble or weak to help themselves, for instance by coughing up phlegm. Wet, cold conditions bring on excess thick mucus in the air passages, leading to rattling breathing. Sour food or drink can lead to gastric problems, intense nausea, and lack of thirst. Other symptoms treated include headaches with the feeling that there is a tight band around the head; a face cold to the touch; a thickly coated tongue; fluid retention leading to bloated legs; nausea.

Which type of person?

- pale, sickly looking
- dark rings around the eyes
- cold sweat on face
- look run down
- do not like being fussed over or interfered with when ill
- do not like being disturbed
- babies who whine, moan, or always want to be carried

BELOW *Tartar emetic is the source for Antimonium tartaricum, used for people who feel anxious and weak, especially old people and the very young.*

MENTAL

- irritable and anxious
- despairing

PHYSICAL

- stomach upsets
- sweats
- build-up of mucus and phlegm
- off food and do not want to drink
- drowsy

Symptoms improve when sitting up, after vomiting, and in cold air, and worsen in stuffy rooms, if wearing too much, with movement, or when lying down.

Apis mellifica, Apis mellifera, honey bee

APIS

The bee is known for its unique ability to produce honey and for its painful sting. Bee products – honey, beeswax, propolis (resin used in the building of hives), and royal jelly (fed to queen bees) – are used in complementary medicine. In homeopathy, Apis is used to treat stinging pain and inflamed, burning skin which has swollen and is painful to touch. The honey bee is commonly found in Europe, Canada, and America. Homeopathically, the whole live bee is used, including the sting, and dissolved in alcohol. The remedy was first "proved" in the U.S., at the Central New York State Homeopathic Society.

BELOW *The Apis type will often spend hours trying irritably to achieve something without success.*

DATA FILE

Relieves

🐝 hot, stinging pain

🐝 smarting, watery swellings, which are sensitive to the touch

🐝 fever with dry skin

🐝 violent headache

🐝 lack of thirst

Uses

Used for complaints such as bites, stings, and urticaria, when the skin becomes swollen, dry, and itchy, or burns and is sensitive to the touch. Also used for urinary tract infections, such as cystitis, and for urine and fluid retention. Allergic reactions which affect the nose, eyes, and throat, such as anaphylactic shock, when watery swelling occurs, and complaints where joints become swollen, such as arthritis, can also be treated. Also good for fever, accompanied by dry skin, sore throat, severe headache, and lack of thirst.

Which type of person?

🐝 protective of own territory, resentful of outsiders

🐝 irritable, agitated, and difficult to please

🐝 love trying to organize other people's lives but have a "sting in the tail" for those who cross them, perhaps leading to the nickname "queen bee"

🐝 spend hours trying to achieve things without making much headway

BELOW *This remedy is derived from the bodies of honey bees, including their stings.*

SYMPTOMS

MENTAL

🐝 restlessness

🐝 jealousy

🐝 irritability

🐝 sensitivity

🐝 depression

🐝 unpredictability

PHYSICAL

🐝 watery swellings, from stings to edema

🐝 fevers with dry, sensitive skin

🐝 intense headaches

🐝 lack of urination

Symptoms improve under cool conditions, but worsen when touched, in heat, or during sleep.

CAUTION

DURING PREGNANCY, AVOID APIS BELOW 30C POTENCY.

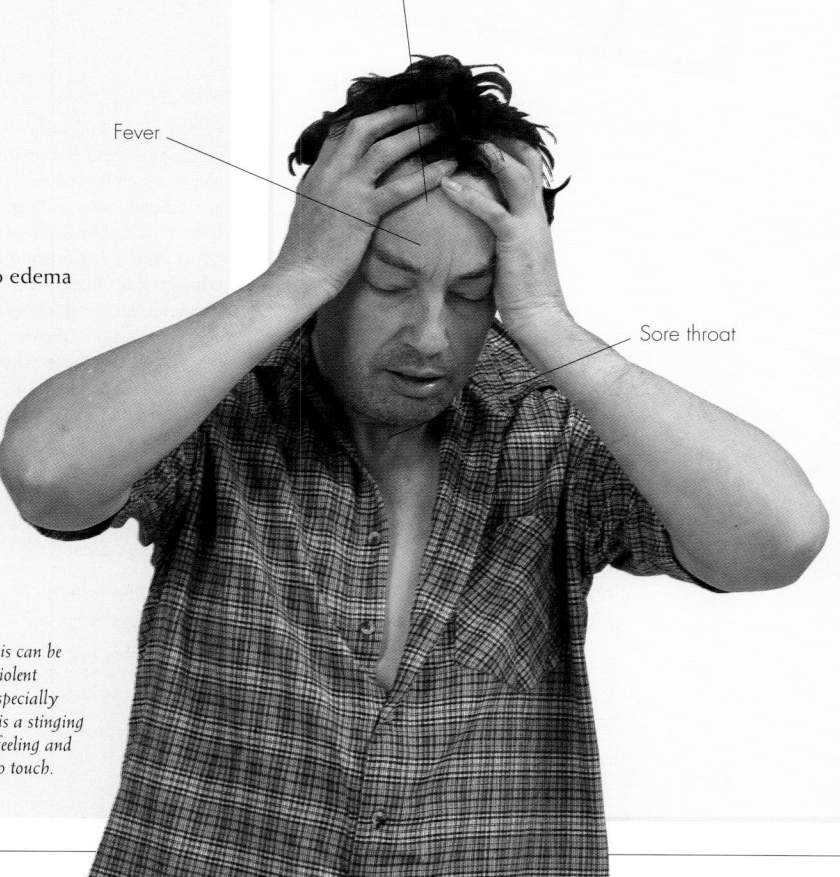

Severe headache

Fever

Sore throat

RIGHT *Apis can be tried for a violent headache, especially where there is a stinging or burning feeling and sensitivity to touch.*

Argentum nitricum, hell stone,
devil's stone, lunar caustic

ARG. NIT.

Silver nitrate, the source of this remedy, was given the names "hell stone" or "devil's stone" because of its corrosive effect. Silver nitrate is extracted from the mineral acanthite, the main ore of silver, and is produced mainly in the U.S., South America, and Norway. In the past, due to its caustic and antibacterial qualities, it was used in medicine to cauterize wounds after surgery and treat conditions such as warts and eye infections. Although it is safe in small doses, large amounts are poisonous, causing breathing problems and damaging the kidneys, liver, spleen, and aorta, and overdosing affects the skin, turning it permanently blue. It has also long had a less lethal use – for making the backs of mirrors. In homeopathy, the remedy is most often used for nervous and digestive complaints.

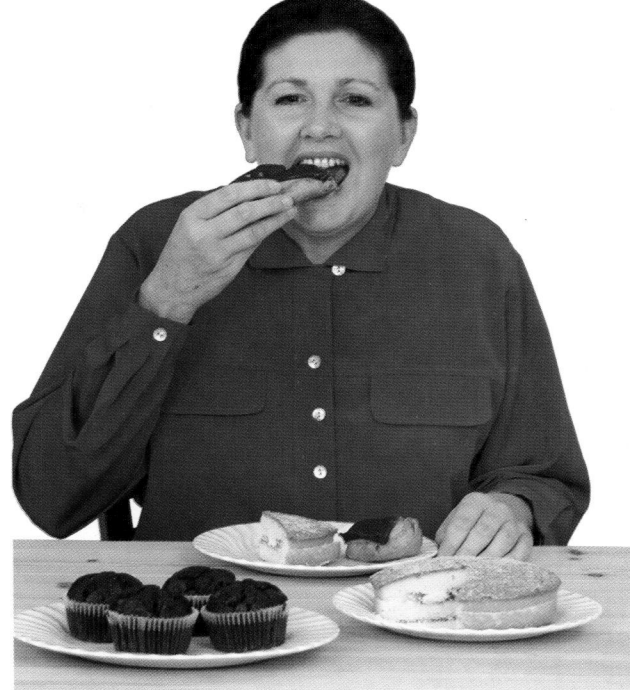

RIGHT *This treatment may suit impulsive people who can be irrational when under stress and binge on sweet foods.*

BELOW LEFT *Fears and anxiety, headache and neck tension, especially when under pressure, may be treated by Arg. nit.*

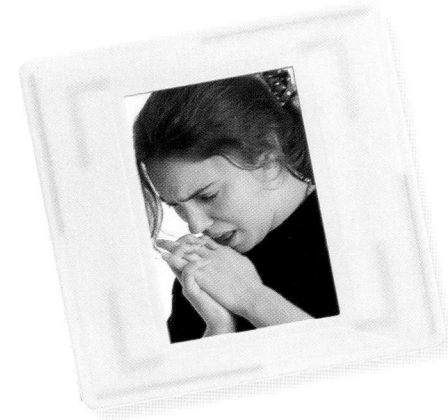

SYMPTOMS

MENTAL

🍃 under stress, find it hard to control emotions, leading to irrational thoughts and impulses

🍃 under pressure, and push themselves, because of a fear of failing

PHYSICAL

🍃 headaches, brought on by overwork, excitement, and sweet foods, will be slow in onset then disappear

🍃 tension in the neck

🍃 weak areas: nerves, lining of the stomach, the left side of the body.

Symptoms improve in fresh air and in coolness, and if pressure is applied, but worsen in heat, at night, under stress, and if lying on the left side.

DATA FILE

Relieves

🌿 fears, anxiety, phobias

🌿 palpitations, sweating

🌿 mental exhaustion

🌿 digestive complaints brought on by nerves and other tension

🌿 problems due to overconsumption of sweet, sugary foods

🌿 vertigo

Uses

Arg. nit. is mainly used for fear and anxiety, usually brought on by stress, and can help with problems such as claustrophobia, dangerous impulses, such as throwing oneself off a bridge, and stage fright. It can also control superstition – the feeling that something awful is about to happen. It is also very useful for digestive problems, such as diarrhea and vomiting, particularly if brought on by nerves; and headaches which begin slowly and are caused by overeating sweet foods. It also helps other conditions such as asthma, colic in babies, epilepsy, warts, and sore throats. During labor, it can help bring relief when bearing down.

Which type of person?

🌿 look fraught and prematurely old, with hollowed features, and an accumulation of wrinkles

🌿 do work where quick thinking, rapid responses, and a good memory are necessary, such as acting, lecturing, or executive positions in business

🌿 outwardly exuberant and happy, inwardly suffer from wild emotions, leading them to laugh, cry, or lose their tempers easily

🌿 when worried and agitated, fret about what may go wrong in the future, even becoming irrational

🌿 may break out in sudden nervous sweats

🌿 prefer salty foods, dislike cold food, and crave sweetness, though this causes stomach upset

🌿 children look older than their years; may be sick through apprehension at the thought of school, and dislike airless rooms; overindulge in sweet or salty foods, leading to diarrhea

🌿 breast-fed babies will suffer diarrhea and colic if the mother eats sweet food

BELOW *The source of this remedy is the mineral silver nitrate, tested by Hahnemann to the 15th potency and proved further by Dr. J.O. Müller.*

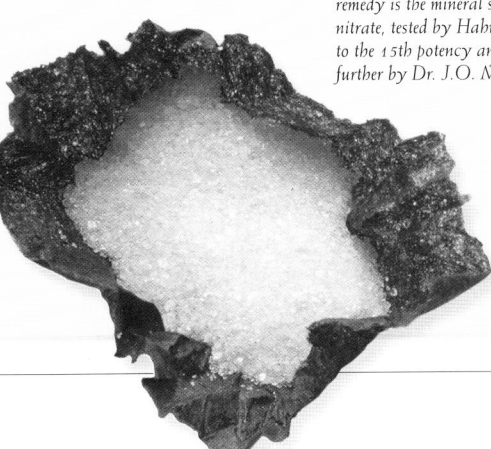

Arnica montana, leopard's bane,
mountain tobacco, sneezewort

ARNICA

Arnica has been used for its healing properties for centuries. It grows in the mountain regions of Europe and Siberia. In folk remedies it was used for aches and bruises, and in conventional medicine for rheumatism, gout, and dysentery. Homeopathically, the remedy was first "proved" by Hahnemann. The whole fresh plant is used when in flower, externally as a cream for sprains and bruises, and internally for shock, often after the patient has suffered an injury.

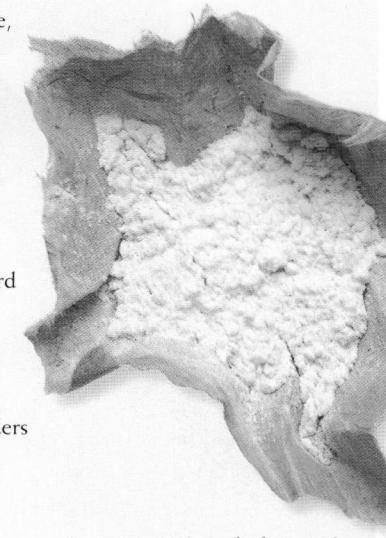

CAUTION

DO NOT USE ARNICA CREAM ON BROKEN SKIN.

ABOVE *The flowers and rootstock of mountain arnica or leopard's bane, Arnica montana, have long been used in folk medicine.*

DATA FILE

Relieves

- bruises, sprains, pain
- shock from injury
- emotional shock, for instance after bereavement

Uses

Arnica is an effective first-aid treatment for sprains, strains, and bruising. Internally, it can help control bleeding

and stimulates the healing of damaged tissue. It is also useful for shock, after either an injury or emotional trauma. It can be used for long-term joint and muscle complaints such as osteoarthritis. Internal treatment can aid external conditions such as eczema and boils.

Which type of person?

- morose, morbidly imaginative
- when ill deny there is a problem, refusing to see a doctor, and preferring to be left alone

SYMPTOMS

MENTAL

- hypochondria
- fear of being touched due to pain
- nightmares
- find it hard to concentrate because easily distracted
- impatient, indifferent, and restless, even in bed
- obstinate

PHYSICAL

- the head feels hot, the body cold
- severe fever
- broken capillaries
- sprained joints
- eczema

Symptoms improve during movement and lying down with the head lower than the feet, and worsen after prolonged movement or rest, under light pressure, in heat.

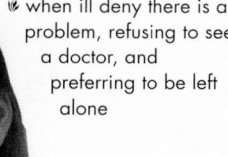

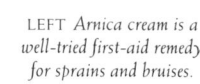

LEFT *Arnica cream is a well-tried first-aid remedy for sprains and bruises.*

Arsenicum album, arsenic trioxide

ARS. ALB.

Arsenic has long been known as a useful poison for those intent on murder! These days, arsenic poisoning is more likely to be the result of accidental ingestion, for instance of agricultural pesticides. In large doses, swallowing arsenic leads to severe stomach upset, vomiting, convulsions, diarrhea, and, if not treated, death. In the past, small doses were given to treat syphilis, anthrax, and to improve stamina. Arsenic is contained in the mineral arsenopyrite, found in countries such as England, Canada, Germany, Norway, and Sweden. It is made up of metallic crystals which cannot be destroyed. In homeopathy, a minute compound of arsenic is used, which works beneficially on the sensitive lining of the digestive tract and respiratory system. Arsenic was first "proved" by Hahnemann.

SYMPTOMS

MENTAL

- fear being alone, burgled, dying
- anxiety leads to restlessness and irritability and a need to do everything meticulously
- possessive, hoard
- sensitive to touch, smell, cold

PHYSICAL

- digestive disorders
- headaches
- dizziness
- vomiting
- asthma which is triggered by anxiety
- fluid retention, diarrhea
- cracked lips, mouth ulcers

Symptoms improve with movement, in warmth, when lying down with the head propped up, and are worse on the right side, in the cold, after cold food and drink.

ABOVE *An oxide of arsenic, the powder known as white arsenic, is the source of this remedy.*

DATA FILE

Relieves

- digestive disorders
- fears and anxiety
- regular, painful headaches
- problems associated with burning pain

Uses

Ars. alb. is given to those suffering from fear – fear of going out alone, fear of the dark, fear of failure, and so on – which is caused by underlying feelings of insecurity. It is also useful for problems of the digestive system, such as indigestion, diarrhea, food poisoning, and excessive eating, such as overconsumption of fruit or ice cream, and drinking too much alcohol. Also, for a range of conditions which particularly sting or burn, such as mouth ulcers, sore lips, eye inflammation, vomiting, burning pains in the rectum. Asthma, fatigue, and fluid retention, especially around the ankles, can also be helped.

Which type of person?

- elegant, even dapper, everything in place
- attentive to detail, plan for every contingency as a way of covering up insecurity and lack of confidence
- strong ideas, making them intolerant of others; want everything to be done perfectly their way
- constant planning does nothing to relieve restlessness and worries, so fret about own health and the health of their family
- children are tidy, restless, and have a wild imagination
- prefer warm foods which are fatty, sweet, or sour; warm drinks, alcohol

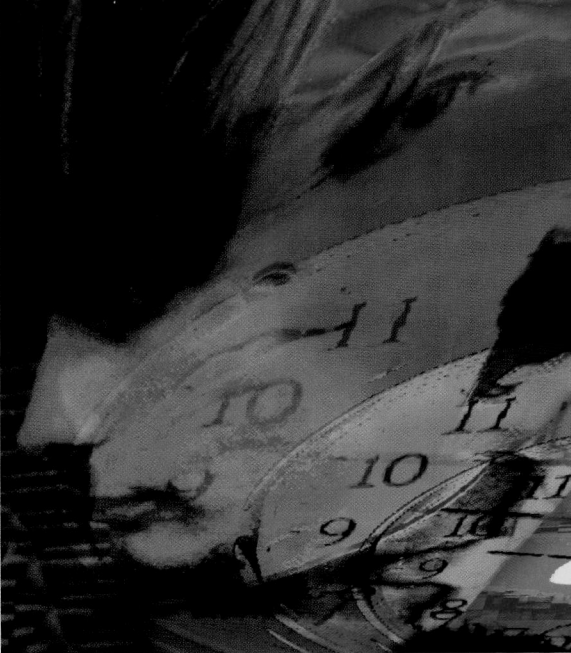

ABOVE *Fear of going out alone, fear of the dark, fear of failure, and so on – caused by underlying feelings of insecurity – are specific problems that can respond to Ars. alb.*

Atropa belladonna, deadly nightshade

BELLADONNA

It was thought during the Middle Ages that deadly nightshade was used in witchcraft. In Italian "bella donna" means beautiful woman, and Italian women used it in eye drops to enlarge their pupils to make themselves more attractive. In conventional medicine, the plant's alkaloid properties of atropine, hyoscamine, and scopolamine are used to treat spasms and nausea. It is grown throughout Europe, and in homeopathy the fresh leaves and flowers are used. Hahnemann first "proved" the remedy in the year 1799.

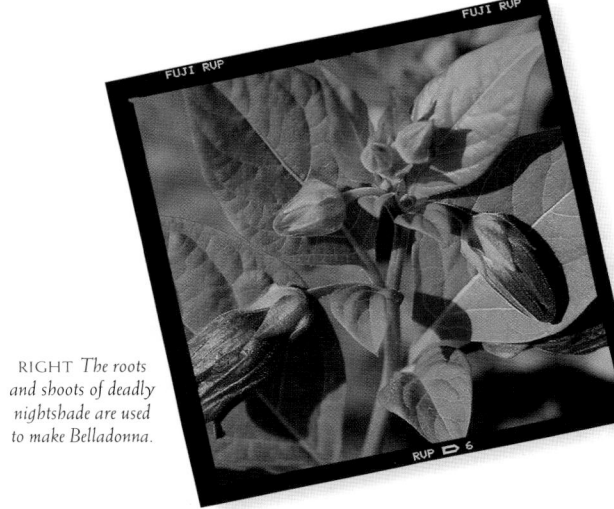

RIGHT *The roots and shoots of deadly nightshade are used to make Belladonna.*

SYMPTOMS

MENTAL

- restless
- excitable behavior
- wild imagination, even hallucinations, nightmares
- fear when approached

PHYSICAL

- very sensitive to light, touch, and movement
- throbbing headaches
- earache, especially on the right side of the head
- hot, dry face, bright red tongue

Symptoms improve in warmth, when standing up, with warm compresses, and worsen when cool, on the right side, at night, with movement, noise, light, pressure.

DATA FILE

Relieves

- sudden, violent complaints, with flushing and throbbing, due to increased circulation
- ailments which include sensitivity to light, noise, pressure, touch
- fever, with staring eyes, dilated pupils

Uses

Commonly used for complaints with sudden onset, inflamed infections, such as fever, tonsillitis, flu, earache – particularly on the right side. Helps severe, pounding headaches jarred by eye movement; boils; labor pain; sore breasts from breast-feeding; fits; cystitis; teething babies.

Which type of person?

- fit, healthy, normally strong in mind and body
- lively and entertaining when well
- agitated, restless, stubborn, and maybe violent when ill
- extremely sensitive to light, touch, movement, and noise

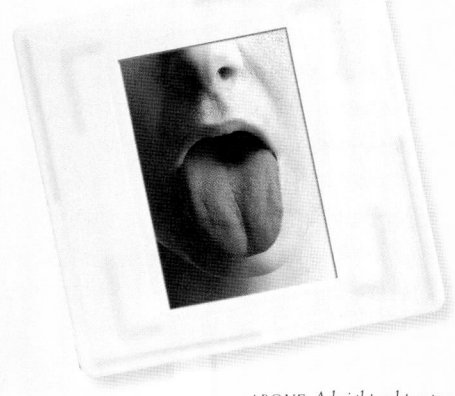

ABOVE *A bright red tongue can indicate the need for the Belladonna remedy, especially if the face is hot and dry.*

Aurum metallicum, gold

AURUM MET.

In the 12th century, gold was used by Arab physicians to treat heart conditions. In the early 20th century, it was used in diagnosing syphilis and treating tuberculosis, and today is used for treating cancer and rheumatoid arthritis. It is found in Canada, the U.S., South Africa, and Australia. Homeopathically, it is given to treat a range of clinical complaints, such as heart disease and depression.

DATA FILE

Relieves

- depression
- ailments accompanied by sensitivity to touch, taste, smell, noise
- vascular complaints

Uses

Useful for mental conditions such as depression and suicidal tendencies. Also for ailments where an increase in blood circulation leads to congestion in the head, as in pulsating headaches, or other organs. Symptoms of heart disease, such as chest pain and breathlessness, can also be helped. Liver problems and sinusitis can be relieved.

Which type of person?

- workaholics who set themselves high goals
- deep sense of duty
- sensitive to the opinions of others as never feel they have achieved as much as they should
- feelings of failure can lead to depression, and even suicidal thoughts

SYMPTOMS

MENTAL

- depression, even suicidal leanings
- explosive behavior if contradicted

PHYSICAL

- red flushes when angry
- blood congestion in organs, such as liver and heart
- inflammation of testes in young boys

Symptoms improve in fresh air and when walking, after washing in cold water and resting, and worsen after mental exertion, when emotionally upset, and at night.

BELOW *Aurum. met. is derived from the precious metal, gold, and is used by homeopaths for a variety of complaints.*

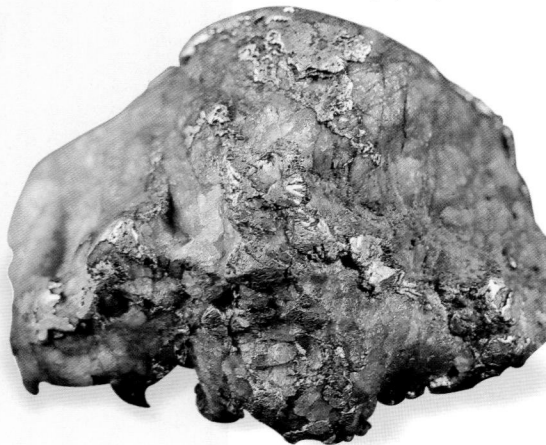

Baptisia tinctoria, wild indigo, horsefly weed, rattlebush

BAPTISIA

Wild indigo is a perennial plant which is native to the U.S. and Canada. Poisonous if ingested in high doses, causing gastrointestinal problems, its medicinal properties were first discovered by Native Americans, who also used it as the basis for indigo dye. It is also used in herbal medicine as a cooling agent, and as an antiseptic and an antibacterial treatment. Homeopathically, the fresh root is used. The remedy was originally "proved" using only seven volunteers, the results being published in the *North American Journal of Homeopathy* in 1857 and 1859.

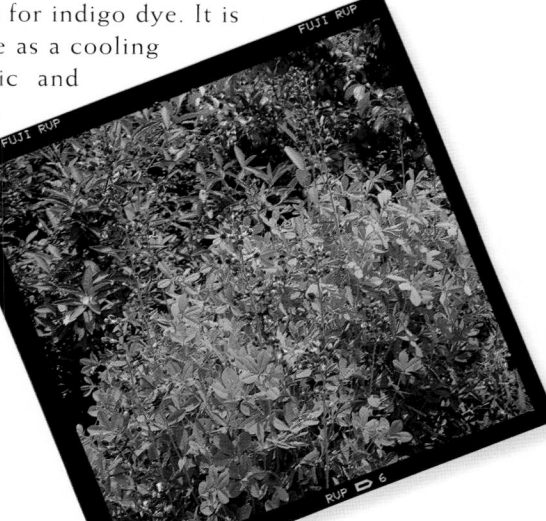

BELOW *The native American plant wild indigo, used to make blue dye, is the source of Baptisia. The plant root is the source of the remedy.*

CAUTION

A PATIENT NEEDING BAPTISIA IS USUALLY SEVERELY ILL AND WILL NEED PROFESSIONAL MEDICAL CARE.

DATA FILE

Relieves

- toxic and septic conditions
- acute feverish illness

Uses

This remedy is mainly used for complaints which have quickly deteriorated into a serious condition, such as acute flu and typhoid fever. Symptoms treated include a rambling mind; restlessness; severe aches and tenderness; prostration and falling asleep mid-sentence; inability to sleep because of delirious mind; foul-smelling breath and stools; dry, coated tongue; mouth ulcers; and persistent ear infections.

Which type of person?

- no particular type, but will be very ill, with puffy face and a drugged look

SYMPTOMS

MENTAL

- restlessness
- confused, wandering mind and talk
- fear of poisoning from food

PHYSICAL

- unable to move around to make themselves more comfortable
- ulcers of the mouth and throat
- foul breath
- coated tongue
- gum sores
- breathing difficulties

Symptoms improve with walking in fresh air and worsen in humidity.

Baryta carbonica, barium carbonate, witherite

BARYTA CARB.

The source of barium carbonate, a poisonous alkaline soluble salt, is barite and witherite, found in the earth's crust in the U.S. and parts of Europe. When heated, it glows and is a useful tool in radiology. Witherite obtains its name from the man who first discovered it in 1783, William Withering. It was given medicinally to treat glandular swellings and tuberculosis. Homeopathically, it was first "proved" by Hahnemann, and the remedy is used mainly for children and the elderly.

ABOVE *Barium carbonate, used in some rat poisons, is the source for Baryta carbonica, one of the remedies proved by Hahnemann.*

DATA FILE

Relieves
- enlarged glands
- headaches
- slow development

Uses
This is a particularly useful remedy for children, adults who have immature tendencies as if going through a second childhood, and the elderly. Children who are shy, are late in walking and talking, are slow to develop physically. Those who are slow intellectually, physically, and emotionally respond well. As they are susceptible to infection, they suffer recurrent problems such as sore throats. The elderly, suffering from senile dementia or a stroke, also respond well.

Which type of person?
- tend to be overweight
- dry, lined skin
- mentally dull, may be mentally challenged

- forgetful, with a short attention span
- children are timid and slow developers
- like cold food

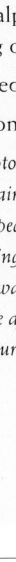

RIGHT *Children, especially those who are shy or slow to develop, are often responsive to Baryta carb.*

SYMPTOMS

MENTAL
- fear of strangers, minor things, things that may happen
- memory loss
- tendency to dwell on past problems
- confusion
- lack of self-confidence
- odd sensations such as cobwebs on face or as if inhaling smoke

PHYSICAL
- recurrent sore throats, accompanied by enlarged glands
- palpitations when lying on the left side
- frequent urination
- constipation

Symptoms improve in the open air, when warmly wrapped, and worsen when thinking about problems, after washing, when lying on the affected side, with exposure to cold or damp.

Bryonia alba, common bryony, white bryony, wild hops

BRYONIA

The Greek physician Hippocrates was one of the first physicians to use bryony, in the 5th century B.C.E. The Romans also used it to treat paralysis, gout, hysteria, and epilepsy. The plant has a deadly, bitter root which, if eaten, can kill within hours. The homeopathic remedy, in which the fresh root is first pounded to a pulp, was one of the first treatments to be "proved" by Hahnemann, in 1834.

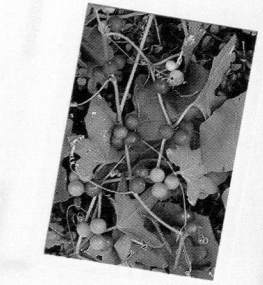

ABOVE *The twining bryony plant yields Bryonia, one of the earliest remedies to be "proved," and still one of the most frequently used.*

DATA FILE

Relieves
- acute complaints with slow onset, painful with movement, thirst
- ailments accompanied by dryness of the mouth, lips, eyes, chest

Uses
Often used for coughs, colds, headaches, and flu which develop slowly and are accompanied by dryness, for instance in the throat, and great thirst. The condition worsens with movement. Also useful for joint inflammation such as rheumatism and osteoarthritis; chest and abdominal inflammation; pleurisy; pneumonia; constipation; mastitis.

Which type of person?
- fear poverty, so materialistic
- worry about financial security, even if well-off; anxious, irritable if security is threatened
- plod, but straightforward, reliable
- meticulous, critical
- usually have dark hair and complexion

SYMPTOMS

MENTAL
- reluctant to speak or to move
- irritable, heavy-headed
- want things, but do not know what, then refuse it when offered
- fears of not getting better, even of dying
- worry about finances and job

PHYSICAL
- excessive sweating
- dryness, constricted throat, thirst
- stabbing headaches
- heavy eyelids
- cravings

Symptoms improve after rest, when pressure is applied, and worsen with movement.

Calcarea carbonica, calcium carbonate

CALC. CARB.

The source of this remedy is the mother-of-pearl in oyster shells. Mother-of-pearl was commonly used for its beauty to adorn combs and the backs of hairbrushes. In homeopathy it also has wide-ranging uses, but is most often used for problems relating to the teeth and bones. It is particularly good for broken bones which are slow to heal, backache, and joint pain.

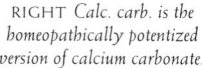

RIGHT *Calc. carb. is the homeopathically potentized version of calcium carbonate.*

SYMPTOMS

MENTAL

- fear of poverty, illness, and death
- swing from being productive at work to lazy
- fear of the dark, ghosts
- dislike small spaces, thunderstorms, mice
- discuss every detail of each illness to the irritation of others

PHYSICAL

- sensitive to cold
- often tired and anxious
- excessive, sour-smelling sweat, even after light exertion
- constipated, but feel better for it

Symptoms improve when lying on the affected side, late morning, and in dry weather, and worsen with sweating, after exertion, in the damp and cold, on waking, and before menstruation.

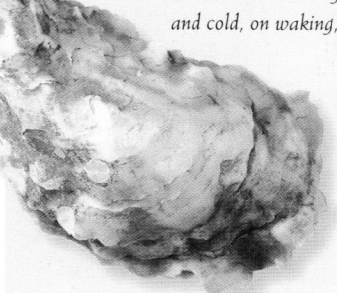

LEFT *Oyster shells are the usual source of Calc. carb., which has an affinity for bone and joint problems, and people who like oysters.*

DATA FILE

Relieves

- aches and pains in the bones and joints
- slow development of teeth and bones
- excessive sweating
- fears, anxieties

Uses

Used to treat bones and joints which are slow to develop, or slow to heal after injury. Also relieves complaints which may be due to this, such as backache. Also helps slow-growing teeth and pain during teething. Eye infections characterized by redness, particularly in the right eye, and ear infections accompanied by unpleasant-smelling discharge are also treated. Right-sided headaches, premenstrual tension, heavy menstruation, the menopause, thrush, eczema, and digestive problems can also be helped by Calc. carb.

Which type of person?

- shy, quiet, sensitive
- seem withdrawn, but are more afraid of making a fool of themselves
- when well, happy and work hard; when ill, slightly depressed and need constant reassurance
- although generally healthy, tend to be overweight, leading to sloth
- prefer sweet, sour, and starchy foods, cold drinks, oysters, and dislike coffee and milk; suffer unusual cravings, chalk, for instance

Calcarea phosphorica, calcium phosphate

CALC. PHOS.

Calcium phosphate is a mineral salt which is the main constituent, along with collagen, of bones and teeth. A natural version is the mineral apatite. For homeopathic use, it is prepared chemically from dilute phosphoric acid and calcium hydroxide, which form fine particles of calcium phosphate. These are then filtered and dried. Calcium phosphate is also used in making porcelain and glass, and as plant food. The remedy is also used as a tissue salt, to treat complaints affecting the bones and teeth.

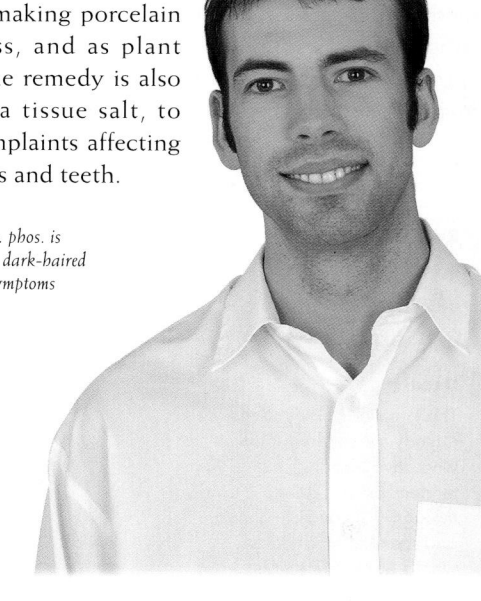

RIGHT *Calc. phos. is suited to thin, dark-haired people with symptoms of fatigue.*

SYMPTOMS

MENTAL

- restless, dislike routine
- need constant stimulation
- hate getting up in the morning

PHYSICAL

- growing pains
- slow-healing fractures
- cravings
- weak digestion

Symptoms improve in dry, warm weather, and worsen in cold, damp weather, when worrying, after excessive sexual activity or other overexertion.

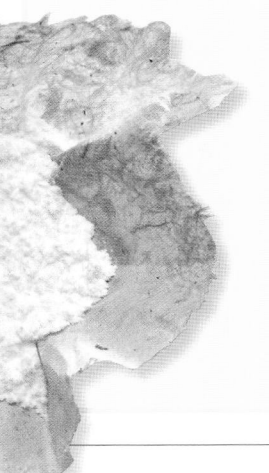

BELOW *This remedy is prepared from phosphate of lime. Calcium phosphate occurs in animal and human bones as well as rocks.*

Calendula officinalis, marigold

CALENDULA

The common, or pot, marigold is a hardy annual bush which grows in southern Europe. It should not be confused with the African marigold, *tagetes*, which is toxic. Calendula has bright orange or yellow daisy-like flowers and narrow pale green leaves, and it grows to a height of about 2ft. (70cm.). The plant has been used for centuries for its healing properties. It is a popular herbal medicine, and is used for its anti-inflammatory and antimicrobial qualities in conditions ranging from skin complaints to cancer. It is a common first-aid treatment for cuts, grazes, and scalds in both herbal and homeopathic medicine. Homeopathically, the fresh leaves and flowers of the plant are used to make the remedy, and a cream for external use.

SYMPTOMS

MENTAL

- none in particular, although patient may be irritable and frightened

PHYSICAL

- cuts, grazes, scalds
- perineal tears
- bleeding after tooth extraction

Symptoms improve when lying still or walking, and worsen in damp, cloudy weather; in draughts, and after eating.

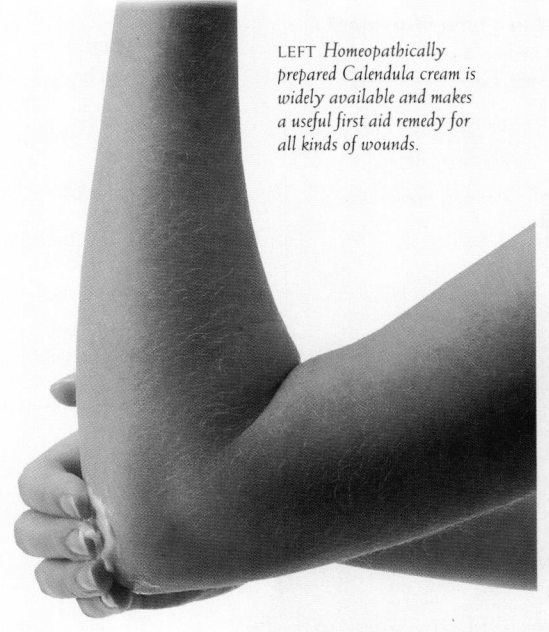

LEFT *Homeopathically prepared Calendula cream is widely available and makes a useful first aid remedy for all kinds of wounds.*

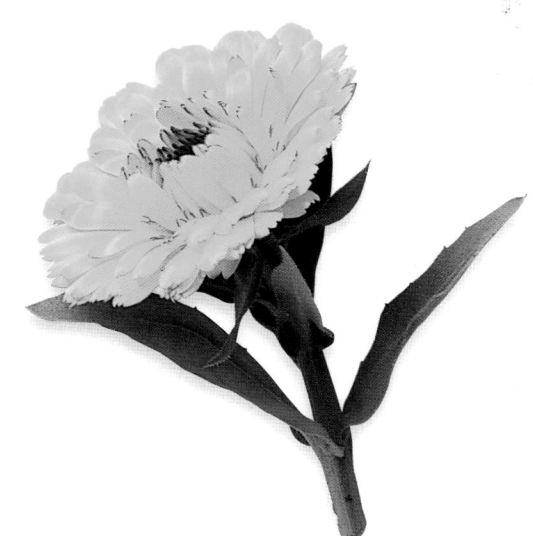

ABOVE *The leaves and flowers of calendula or pot marigold have been used for centuries by herbalists. They also provide the basis for homeopathic preparations.*

CAUTION

ENSURE CUTS ARE CLEAN BEFORE USE SO THAT RAPID HEALING DOES NOT CLOSE IN DIRT OR GERMS. DO NOT USE FOR PUNCTURE WOUNDS OR DEEP CUTS AS RAPID HEALING MAY SEAL THE INFECTION INSIDE THE WOUND.

THERAPY CONNECTIONS

MARIGOLD

- Herbalism   *p.117*
- Aromatherapy *p.148*

Cantharis vesicatoria, Lytta vesicatoria,
Spanish fly, blister beetle

CANTHARIS

Spanish fly is in fact a bright green beetle which is native to southern Europe and western Asia. It emits a fast-acting irritant, cantharidin, causing blistering, hence its other common name. In the past, it was used as an aphrodisiac, causing sexual frenzy in some cases, and medicinally was used to treat a variety of ailments from warts to rheumatism. It was first "proved" by Hahnemann, and the remedy is made up from the whole beetle, dried, and then powdered. Homeopathically, it is used to treat complaints characterized by a burning sensation.

ABOVE *The Spanish fly or blister beetle is the source for Cantharis.*

BELOW *Conditions involving stinging or burning, especially in irritable people who tend to behave violently, can be helped by Cantharis.*

SYMPTOMS

MENTAL
- irritability
- feels excessive sexual desire
- violent tendencies

PHYSICAL
- thirst, but no wish to drink
- loss of appetite
- burning sensation in the stomach
- sweating, and palpitations
- rapidly worsening infections

Symptoms improve in the warmth, with massage, after flatulence or burping, and at night, and worsen with movement, after drinking coffee or cold water, and in the afternoon.

DATA FILE

Relieves
- conditions accompanied by stinging or a burning sensation
- rapidly spreading infection
- stings, burns

Uses
Ailments characterized by burning or stinging, particularly urinary tract infections such as cystitis, frequent but painful urination, insect bites, burns and scalds, infections, burning abdominal pains, and stinging diarrhea. Also for infections which spread rapidly, or conditions which quickly deteriorate. Other conditions which respond well include great thirst without a desire to drink because of breathlessness; pus-filled eruptions on hands; burning throat; burning soles of the feet; loss of appetite. Mental problems such as rage, agitation leading to violence, excessive sexual desire, and severe anxiety can be relieved by Cantharis.

Which type of person?
- have a head full of ideas, but are confused
- maniacal tendencies
- explosive anger
- strong sexual urges

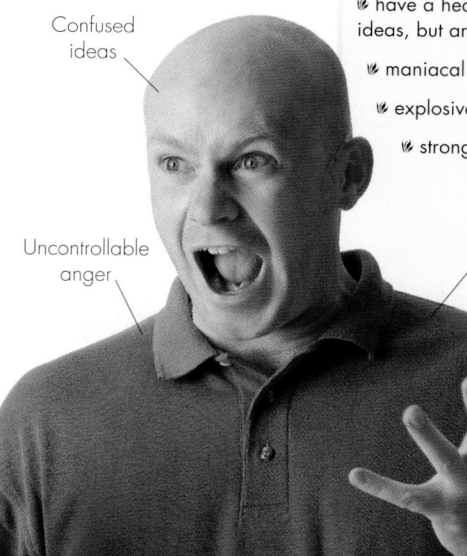

Confused ideas

Uncontrollable anger

Violent tendencies

Carbo vegitabilis, charcoal

CARB. VEG.

Charcoal is wood that has been burnt without air, forming a hard carbon. It has been used as a fuel, in explosives, for smelting, and as an absorbent. In the past, it was used medicinally for its deodorizing and disinfecting qualities, for septic conditions, and flatulence. Today, it is still used to treat the latter in conventional medicine. In homeopathy, charcoal from beech, poplar, and silver birch trees grown in the northern hemisphere is used, and the remedy was first "proved" by Hahnemann.

ABOVE *Charcoal, itself a classic remedy for certain types of digestive problems, is the source of Carb. veg. Beech wood is normally used.*

SYMPTOMS

MENTAL
- never quite feel well following an ailment
- lack mental energy
- fear of the supernatural

PHYSICAL
- burping, regurgitating food
- flatulence
- headaches, especially prevalent in the morning and after eating too much
- clammy hands
- indigestion
- poor circulation

Symptoms improve in cold, fresh air, and are relieved after burping, and worsen in warm, wet air; after fatty, milky foods and wine, and when lying down.

DATA FILE

Relieves
- lack of vitality; fatigue
- cold, clamminess externally, heat internally, associated with shock
- excess mucus from digestive system
- poor circulation

Uses
Used to aid recovery after an illness, when there is exhaustion and weakness, and for shock that may follow an operation which leaves the patient with cold, pale skin, but feeling hot inside. Also treats poor circulation, when the face, hands, or feet are cold and turn bluish; and bleeding varicose veins. Useful for digestive problems, such as indigestion and flatulence; asthma; whooping cough.

Which type of person?
- complain of never quite recovering after an illness
- prefer day to darkness
- fixed ideas
- mentally and physically tired and sluggish
- erratic memory

Causticum hahnemanni, potassium hydrate

CAUSTICUM

This remedy was invented and "proved" by Samuel Hahnemann himself and is unique to homeopathy. It is made chemically from quicklime (calcium oxide) and potassium bisulfate. He found that it caused a burning taste in the back of the mouth and an acerbic sensation. It is used for a set of symptoms known as the Causticum cough (*see Data File below*) and for various neuromuscular conditions.

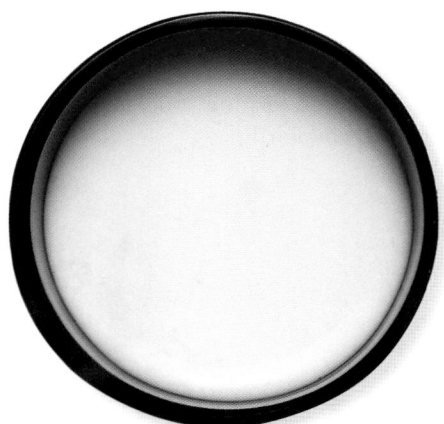

ABOVE *Quicklime (calcium oxide), which becomes slaked lime when combined with water, is used in the preparation of Causticum.*

MENTAL

🐾 fear animals, darkness, ghosts, strangers, death

🐾 can be very critical of others

🐾 empathize with the suffering of others

🐾 despair of recovering from illness

PHYSICAL

🐾 chilly

🐾 prone to warts

🐾 symptoms tend to come on slowly

🐾 tearing, bursting pain in joints, muscles, and bones

🐾 paralytic problems

🐾 contractions of the muscles and tendons

Symptoms improve in warm, damp weather, after cold drinks and washing, and worsen in dry, cold winds, with movement.

Cephaelis ipecacuanha, ipecacuanha

IPECAC.

Ipecacuanha is a small, perennial shrub grown in the tropical rainforests of South and Central America. The first recorded medicinal use – for treating vomiting – was around 1600, by a Portuguese friar in Brazil. It was brought to Europe some 70 years later, where it was used as an anti-dysentery drug in France, as well as for a variety of ailments. It is still used in conventional medicine to induce vomiting in cases of drug overdoses or poisoning, and as an expectorant. Homeopathically, the root is used to treat nausea and vomiting. It is collected when the plant is in flower and then dried.

DATA FILE

Relieves

🍃 persistent nausea

🍃 breathing difficulties

Uses

Commonly used for nausea and vomiting, and accompanying sweats and clamminess. Also good for stomach complaints

accompanied by salivating, lack of thirst, weak pulse, and fainting; conditions causing breathing difficulties, such as asthma and coughing; coughing and vomiting at the same time; persistent nausea.

Which type of person?

🍃 no particular type

BELOW *Ipecac. is obtained from the dried root of the ipecacuanha plant that grows in South and Central America. The plant has a long history of medicinal use.*

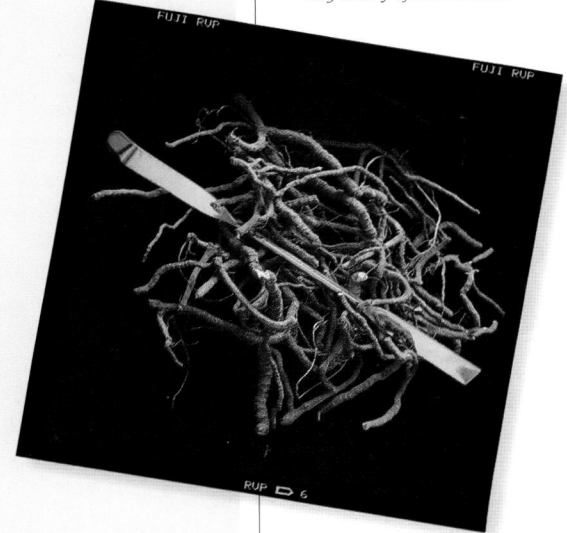

FUJI RUP
FUJI RUP
RUP ▷ 6

DATA FILE

Relieves

🍃 Causticum cough

🍃 progressive weakness leading to paralysis

🍃 burning, bursting pain

Uses

Symptoms of the Causticum cough include a raw, tickly throat with dry cough; burning in the throat; hard, racking cough; chest filled with mucus which is difficult to cough up; incontinence with each cough, and coughing which is worse on breathing out. Also helps neuromuscular problems such as weakness; stiffness; neuralgia; tearing pains in the joints, muscles, and bones; cramps, particularly affecting the vocal cords,

bladder, larynx, or the right side of the face. Other conditions alleviated include dizziness when bending forward; heartburn in pregnancy; burning rheumatic pain; roaring sounds in the ears; nasal soreness; and tender scars and injury sites.

Which type of person?

🍃 dark hair and eyes, with sallow skin

🍃 often mentally and physically exhausted

🍃 narrow-minded

🍃 hypersensitive, weepy

🍃 dislike the smell of food and feel worse after drinking coffee

MENTAL

🐾 contemptuous

🐾 anxiety, including fear of death

🐾 morose

PHYSICAL

🐾 breathing difficulties

🐾 constant nausea

🐾 fainting, cold or hot sweats, clamminess

🐾 bleeding

🐾 weak pulse

Symptoms improve in fresh air, and worsen in warmth, in winter, when moving or lying down, and when under stress or embarrassed.

China officinalis, Cinchona succirubra, Peruvian bark, cinchona bark, Jesuits' bark

CHINA

The China remedy is made from Peruvian bark – grown in the tropical rainforests of South America, in India, and southeast Asia – which is stripped and dried. Quinine, an extract of the bark, was the first substance to be tested and "proven" by Hahnemann, in 1790. He used quinine on himself, noting that large doses caused similar symptoms to malaria, while small doses acted as an antidote. Quinine is still used in conventional medicine today as part of the treatment for malaria. Homeopathically, the dried bark of China is used for exhaustion.

DATA FILE

Relieves

❧ nervous exhaustion after incapacitating illness

❧ weakness after vomiting, diarrhea, or sweating, as a result of loss of body fluids

Uses

Aids recovery from nervous exhaustion after debilitating illness and as a result of loss of fluids from vomiting, diarrhea, or sweating. Also for digestive conditions such as gastroenteritis, flatulence, and gall bladder problems; mental upsets such as lack of concentration, indifference, and outbursts that are out of character; also neuralgia, dizziness, tired and twitchy muscles, tinnitus, hemorrhages.

Which type of person?

❧ sensitive

❧ intense

❧ artistic

❧ idealistic

❧ their own intensity is tiring, making them lazy, depressed, sometimes violent

❧ find it difficult to express themselves to others so do so through their creativity

❧ prefer talking about meaningful issues, not trivia

❧ imaginative mind, fantasize about heroic deeds

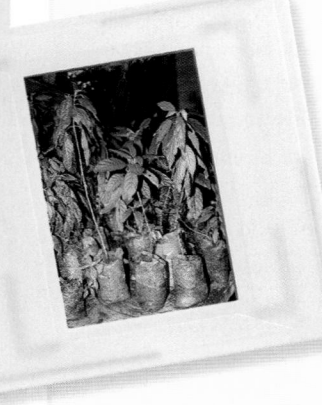

ABOVE *People who are imaginative and artistic, especially if they are exhausted, weakened, or mentally tired out, may be helped by China.*

LEFT *The remedy is obtained from the bark of China officinalis, which also yields quinine.*

SYMPTOMS

MENTAL

❧ emotionally fragile

❧ difficulty in expressing feelings

❧ lacks concentration

❧ nervous exhaustion

PHYSICAL

❧ headaches, dizziness

❧ convulsions

❧ weak muscles

❧ sallow skin

❧ indigestion, flatulence, a feeling that food is stuck behind the breastbone

Symptoms improve in the warmth, when firm pressure is applied to the affected area, and after sleeping, and worsen in the cold or draughts, in the fall.

Cimicifuga racemosa, Actaea racemosa, Black cohosh, bugbane, black snakeroot, rattleroot

CIMIC.

Grown in the U.S. and Canada, the Native Americans used the rhizome or underground stem of this plant to cure rattlesnake bites, giving it one of its common names, rattleroot, and for rheumatism and gynecological problems. It has also been used for menstrual and labor pain as well as being chewed as a sedative to help with depression. Brewed in a tea which was then sprinkled around a room, it was said to prevent the presence of evil spirits. Homeopathically, it was "proved" in the U.S.. The fresh black root is commonly used for treating problems arising during pregnancy and childbirth.

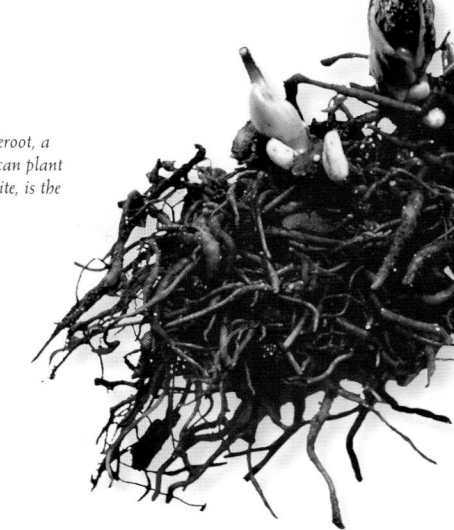

RIGHT *Black snakeroot, a native North American plant once used for snakebite, is the source for Cimic.*

SYMPTOMS

MENTAL

❧ emotional and highly strung

❧ sigh repeatedly when sad

❧ strong fears, such as insanity and death, particularly when menopausal

PHYSICAL

❧ cramps and backache when premenstrual

❧ nausea and vomiting in pregnancy

❧ depression after childbirth

❧ faints and flushes during menopause

Symptoms improve when warm, in fresh air, when pressure is applied, and with gentle movement, but worsen in cold, damp, draughty conditions, with alcohol or excitement.

DATA FILE

Relieves

☙ menstrual symptoms

☙ nausea, vomiting in pregnancy

☙ head, neck aches

☙ woefulness

☙ conditions accompanied by chills

Uses

Cimic. works well on the nerves and muscles of the uterus, making it useful for menstrual problems such as back cramps and headaches; early miscarriage; pregnancy complaints, such as pain in the uterus, difficulty in

sleeping, nausea, and vomiting; and postnatal depression and menopausal problems, such as hot flushes. The upheaval in emotions associated with these problems, such as anxiety and irritability, can also be relieved.

Which type of person?

☙ mainly women

☙ often extrovert, talkative, and excitable

☙ when sad become depressed, often sigh

☙ experience strong, intense emotions

☙ fear death

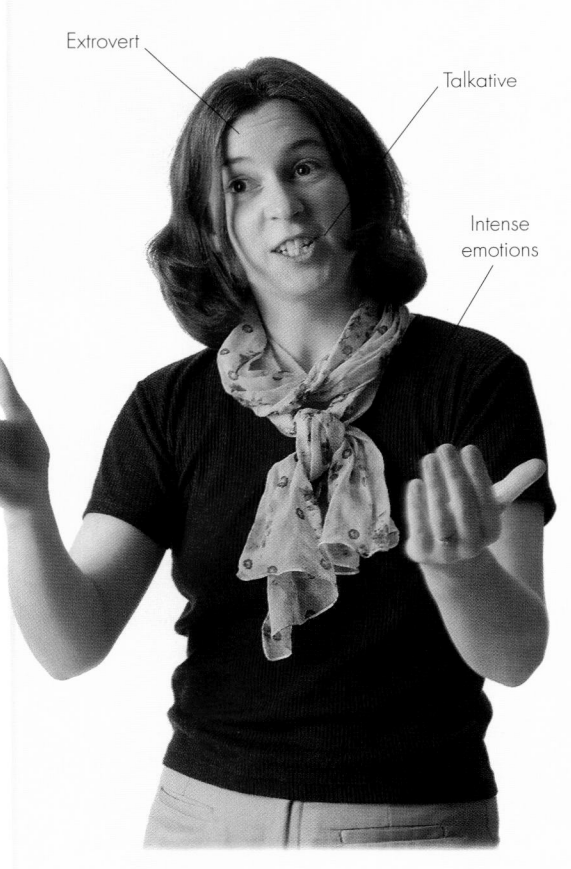

Extrovert

Talkative

Intense emotions

ABOVE *This remedy is well-suited to many female complaints, and can be helpful for women who appear restless and highly strung.*

Cucumis colocynthis, bitter apple, bitter cucumber

COLOCYNTHIS

Colocynthis, or Coloc., comes from a gourd, *Cucumis colocynthis*. In the past, the bitter apple, as it is also known, was used by Arab and ancient Greek physicians as a purgative (with radical results), in order to induce abortion, and to treat derangement, lethargy, and dropsy. The seeds alone are harmless, but when the whole fruit is eaten, it causes bowel inflammation and cramping pains, due to the release of a resin called colocynthin. Homeopathically, the fruit – which grows in hot, arid conditions – is dried and powdered, without the seeds. It was first used in 1834, and is given as treatment for digestive complaints and colic.

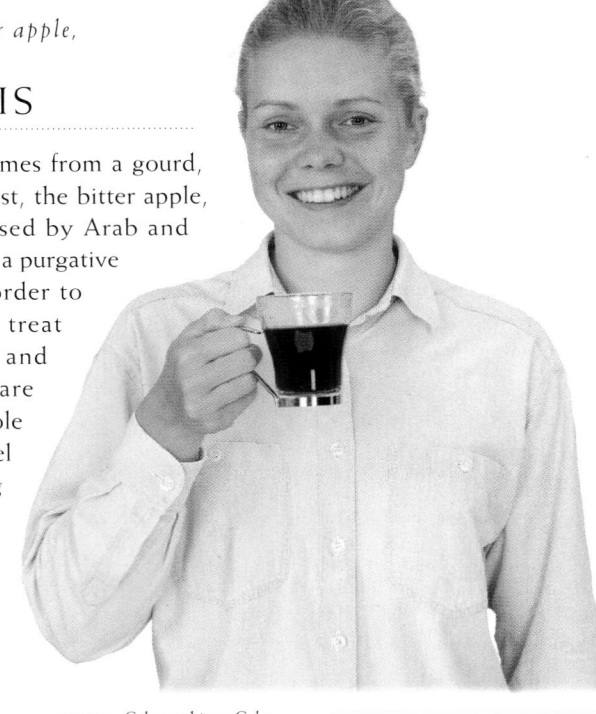

ABOVE *Colocynthis or Coloc. is often found suitable for people who are fair-haired and fair-skinned, when their symptoms are related to anger.*

SYMPTOMS

MENTAL

☙ upset if contradicted, especially if feel humiliated

☙ keen for justice to be done

PHYSICAL

☙ digestive problems

☙ neuralgia and headaches

☙ abdominal pain

Symptoms improve in the warmth, after flatulence, or drinking coffee, but worsen after eating, when indignant or angry, and in damp, cold weather.

BELOW *The leaves of the bitter cucumber (also called bitter apple), whose fruit is the source of Coloc.*

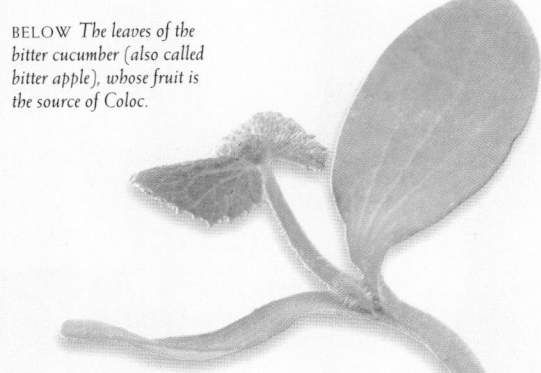

DATA FILE

Relieves

☙ digestive complaints

☙ neuralgia, headaches, and stomach pains brought on by anger

Uses

Mainly used to treat symptoms brought on by anger, particularly suppressed anger, such as neuralgia and abdominal pain; stomach pain, facial neuralgia, and headaches respond well, as does nerve pain in the ovaries or kidneys; gout, sciatica, and rheumatism symptoms can also be helped.

Which type of person?

☙ tend to be fair-haired and fair-skinned

☙ reserved

☙ have a strong sense of right and wrong

☙ dislike being contradicted

☙ suffer physical effects when angry or indignant

Coffea arabica, Coffea cruda, coffee

COFFEA

Coffee is native to Arabia and Ethiopia, and is thought to have been first drunk in Persia. Now grown in Central America and the West Indies, it has been used widely for medicinal purposes as a diuretic, painkiller, and to ease indigestion. It is also a well-known stimulant. Homeopathically, coffea is made from the raw berries of the coffee tree, and was first "proved" by Hahnemann himself and a handful of volunteers. It is mainly used to treat those who are excitable and mentally overstimulated.

SYMPTOMS

MENTAL

- irritable
- heightened senses
- mind buzzing with ideas
- anxiety leading to restlessness
- insomnia
- guilt

PHYSICAL

- trembling limbs
- toothache
- headaches
- palpitations
- hypersensitive skin

ABOVE *Raw coffee beans are the source of Coffea. Coffee has been used for a variety of medicinal purposes as well as in the production of caffeine.*

Symptoms improve in the warmth, after lying down, and when holding cold water in the mouth. They worsen with extreme emotions such as anger, with touch, smell, or noise, and during cold, windy weather.

RIGHT *Coffea can be useful after a failed relationship or other trauma; it helps with palpitations caused by anger, and irritability.*

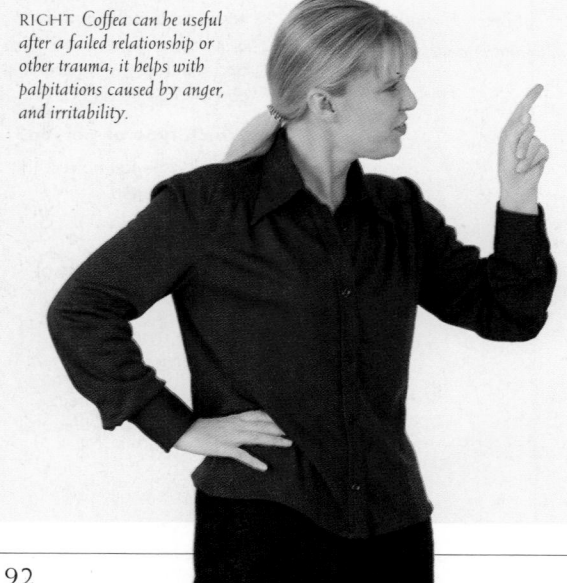

DATA FILE

Relieves

- excitability
- mental overstimulation
- sleeplessness

Uses

Commonly used to treat excessive mental activity when the mind seems to be buzzing; where the person is very excitable and hypersensitive, for instance with toothache or labor pain; when all the senses are acutely affected, making any noise, smell, or touch seem unbearable; headaches which are so severe it feels like a nail is being driven into the skull; palpitations when excited or angry; and for acute premenstrual symptoms.

Which type of person?

- tall, lean, with a tendency to stoop
- dark complexion
- symptoms may appear after a failed relationship, and with exhaustion or after a trauma
- on a high, but will then descend into despair
- tend to "burn out"

Cuprum mettalicum, copper

CUPRUM MET.

Copper, a red-gold metal, is often found in many tools and weapons. In the past, coppersmiths often suffered toxic poisoning due to working with the metal, falling ill with complaints such as coughs, malnutrition, colicky pain, and sometimes even paralysis and death. In the days when alcohol was often made secretly in home distilleries, poisoning occurred from the copper tubing. Small amounts were also used medicinally to help heal wounds. Homeopathically, it was first "proved" in 1834, and is used to treat respiratory problems and various complaints of the nervous system.

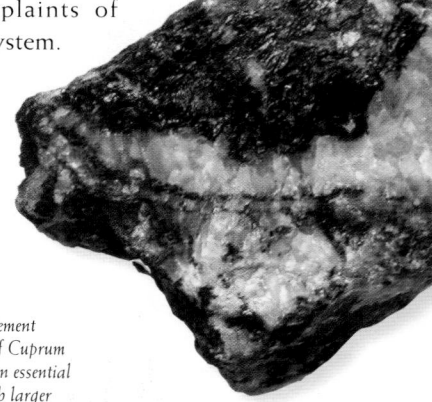

RIGHT *The metal element copper is the source of Cuprum met. Copper itself is an essential trace element although larger amounts are toxic.*

SYMPTOMS

MENTAL

- hide deep emotions
- suppression of feelings leads to physical problems
- cry, becoming morose

PHYSICAL

- twitches, jerks, convulsions
- erratic breathing
- pale color, sometimes turning blue

Symptoms improve after sweating and cold drinks, and worsen if emotions are being suppressed, in the heat, when touched, and after vomiting.

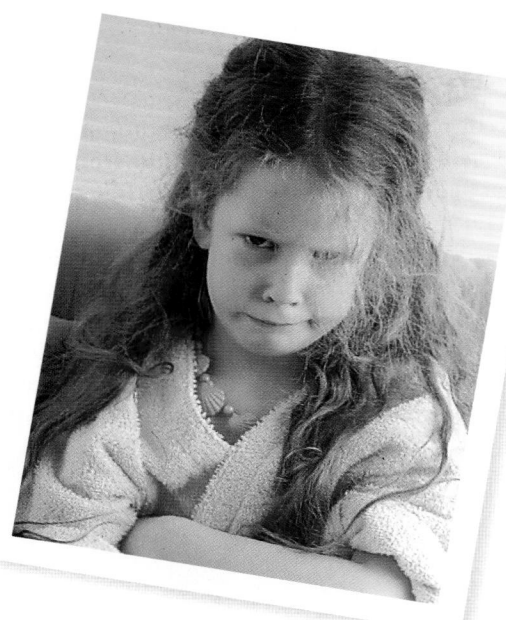

ABOVE *Cuprum met. can be a useful remedy for problems in children who have a destructive mentality, and when angry, hold their breath.*

DATA FILE

Relieves

ᴥ muscular spasm, cramp

ᴥ breathing problems

ᴥ tiredness associated with mental exhaustion

Uses

Problems of the nervous system are commonly treated. Tics, twitches – particularly those that start in a minor way and spread more deeply – and convulsions can be helped. Epilepsy responds well. Tiredness brought on after much mental activity can be treated, as can respiratory problems when breathing seems to be intermittent, such as with asthma.

Which type of person?

ᴥ intensely emotional, but suppress feelings, so may appear reserved

ᴥ serious, self-critical

ᴥ swing from being headstrong to submissive

ᴥ children tend to hold their breath when angry until they go blue, have a destructive mentality, and need their own space; teenagers tend to suppress sexual urges

---

Drosera rotundifolia, sundew, moor grass, red rot, youthwort

DROSERA

The sundew is a carnivorous plant which grows widely in the heaths and boggy areas of Europe, South America, the U.S., China, and India. Insects are attracted by the long, red hairs on the leaves of the plant. Glands on the surface of the leaves then secrete a fluid which traps and breaks down the insect, digesting it. The juice of the plant is caustic, affecting the respiratory system, and when eaten by sheep, leads to a harsh, spasmodic cough. It was used in the Middle Ages to treat the plague, and 16th-century physicians used it for tuberculosis. Homeopathically, it was "proved" by Hahnemann, and the whole fresh plant is used, mainly to treat coughs.

DATA FILE

Relieves

ᴥ severe, spasmodic hollow-sounding cough

ᴥ breathing difficulties

ᴥ retching or the vomiting of mucus

ᴥ growing pains

Uses

Complaints such as whooping cough, characterized by a violent, spasmodic, hollow-sounding cough, triggered by a tickling sensation in the throat. The cough worsens after midnight, and at the acute stage is accompanied by retching and vomiting, cold sweats, and nose-bleeds, after which the patient becomes talkative. Also helps the uncomfortable tingling sensation associated with growing pains, stiffness, and a hoarse voice.

Which type of person?

ᴥ restless, obstinate when ill

ᴥ unable to concentrate

ᴥ dislike being left alone

ᴥ fear of ghosts

ᴥ worry about being given bad news

RIGHT *Children who find it hard to settle, especially when ill, may be cured of coughs by this remedy.*

LEFT *Drosera rotundifolia, the round-leaved sundew plant that is used to produce Drosera.*

MENTAL

ᴥ feel persecuted

ᴥ difficulty in concentrating

ᴥ unable to settle, and become stubborn

PHYSICAL

ᴥ barking cough

ᴥ tingling in leg bones

Symptoms improve when walking, in fresh air, with pressure, when sitting up, and when quiet. They worsen after midnight, after cold food and drinking, when lying down, and if the bed is too warm.

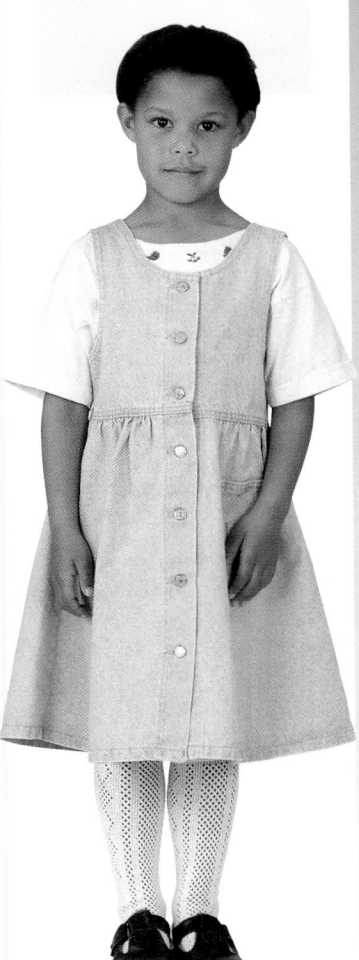

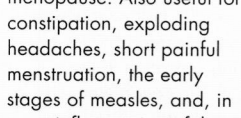
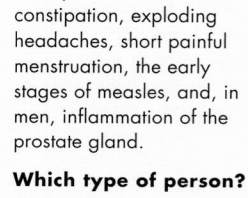
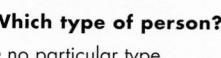
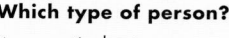

Euphrasia officinalis, Euphrasia stricta, eyebright
EUPHRASIA

Grown in Europe and America, eyebright – as its name suggests – has been used for centuries to treat eye problems. It is believed the name comes from one of the Three Graces, Euphrosyne, who was known for her gladness and joy. First mentioned as an eye treatment in 1305, it was used in later centuries as an infusion for eyes, and in the 19th century was also used as a treatment for coughs, headaches, and earaches. It is commonly used in herbal medicine. Homeopathically, the whole fresh plant is used when in flower to make a remedy for sore, irritated eyes and eye injuries.

ABOVE *The flowering plant* Euphrasia officinalis *or eyebright is used by herbalists as well as in homeopathy.*

DATA FILE

Relieves

🌿 stinging, watery discharge from the eyes

🌿 inflammation or injury to the eyes

🌿 running eyes associated with hay fever

Uses

Any eye irritation or inflammation, such as conjunctivitis, inflammation of the eyelid or iris, small blisters on the cornea. Also for dimmed vision; dislike of bright lights; watery, irritated eyes associated with hay fever sufferers, but accompanied by only bland nasal discharge; colds accompanied by flushed face and runny catarrh; eye injuries; dry

eyes associated with the menopause. Also useful for constipation, exploding headaches, short painful menstruation, the early stages of measles, and, in men, inflammation of the prostate gland.

Which type of person?

🌿 no particular type

SYMPTOMS

MENTAL

🌿 none in particular

PHYSICAL

🌿 stinging discharge from the eyes

🌿 watering eyes

🌿 an intolerance of bright light

🌿 hot cheeks

🌿 bursting headaches

Symptoms improve after lying down in a darkened room and with drinking coffee, and worsen in bright light, in the evening, in enclosed spaces, and during warm, windy weather.

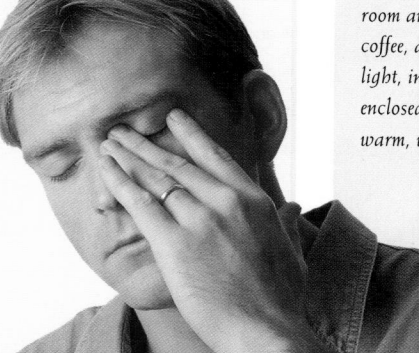

RIGHT *Euphrasia has an affinity for the eyes and is mainly used for eye problems, but it is also used to treat other illnesses.*

Ferrum phosphoricum, iron phosphate
FERR. PHOS.

The Ferr. phos. remedy is made from iron phosphate, which is a chemical combination of iron sulfate, sodium phosphate, and sodium acetate. It is one of the 12 biochemical tissue salts developed by the German physician Wilhelm Schussler between 1872 and 1898. Schussler believed many complaints were the result of a deficiency of minerals, and that by replacing these minerals, or tissue salts, health could be restored. Schussler found Ferr. phos. particularly useful in the early stages of inflammation, and the homeopathic remedy is used for similar purposes.

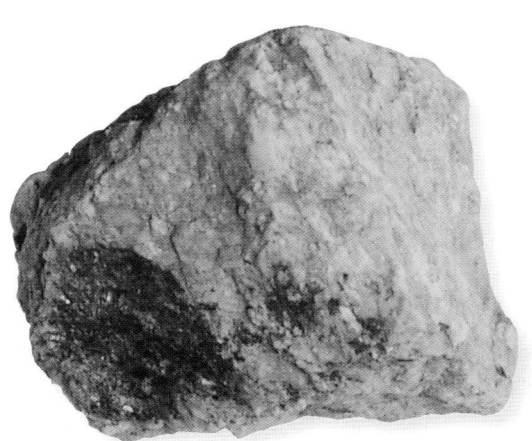

ABOVE *The mineral salt ferrous phosphate, from which Ferr. phos. is prepared, is a compound of iron, the white magnetic metal derived from iron ores.*

SYMPTOMS

MENTAL

🌿 none in particular

PHYSICAL

🌿 headaches and head colds

🌿 dry, hacking cough, laryngitis, hoarseness

🌿 shooting rheumatic pains

🌿 facial flushing and rapid pulse

🌿 chills starting in the early afternoon

Symptoms improve with gentle exercise and cold compresses, and worsen in the heat, with movement, when touched, lying on the right side, between 4 A.M. and 6 A.M., when suppressing sweating.

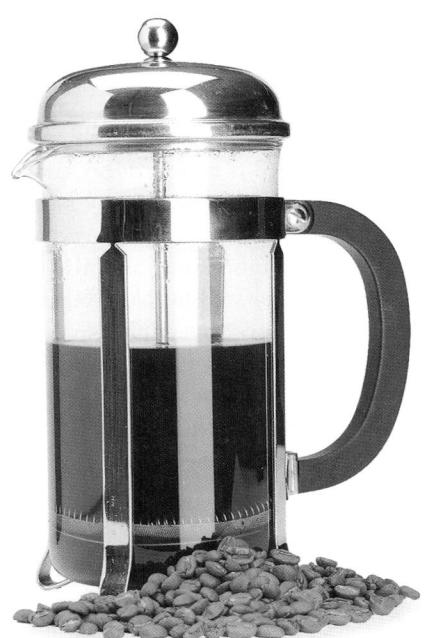

ABOVE *A craving for coffee may indicate Ferrum phosphoricum as an appropriate remedy.*

DATA FILE

Relieves

☙ early stages of inflammation or infection

☙ coughs and colds which come on slowly

Uses

First stages of inflammation or infection, when more blood is flowing to the affected areas, causing congestion, and before the onset of other symptoms. Also slow-starting colds accompanied by nosebleeds and fevers, with hacking cough; headaches which are helped by cool water; rheumatic pain; gastritis including vomiting undigested food; indigestion with sour-tasting burps; hemorrhages; in women, intermittent, painful menstruation; stress incontinence; first stages of dysentery with bloody stools.

Which type of person?

☙ pale, anemic-looking

☙ full of ideas

☙ susceptible to sudden facial flushes

☙ complaining but good-natured

☙ dislike milk, meat, crave coffee

☙ tend to suffer respiratory and gastrointestinal complaints

Gelsemium sempervirens, yellow jasmine, Carolina jasmine, false jasmine

GELSEMIUM

This climbing plant, with its fragrant yellow flowers, is native to the southern states of the U.S. and, despite being attractive to look at, is poisonous if eaten. Ingesting large quantities will affect the respiratory system and movement, leading to shaking, inflammation, and paralysis. Historically, its medicinal uses were first noted when a farmer in Mississippi in the 1840s accidentally ate the plant's root and found his fever was cured. It was used as a treatment for fevers in herbalism before being "proven" in homeopathy.

ABOVE *Gelsemium is produced from the poisonous false jasmine Gelsemium sempervirens, also known as Carolina jasmine.*

SYMPTOMS

MENTAL

☙ fears and phobias, accompanied by trembling and need to urinate

☙ fears such as the dentist, falling or throwing oneself from a height

☙ dull and lethargic

☙ nervous and feel inadequate

PHYSICAL

☙ headaches causing tightness

☙ faintness

☙ facial flushing

☙ visual disturbances

☙ muscle pain

☙ trembling

Symptoms improve after urinating and perspiring, after alcohol or stimulants, and when bending forward. They worsen after physical exertion, in heat, humidity, damp, or fog, with excitement, worry, or stress about symptoms.

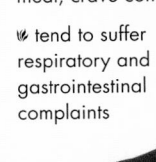

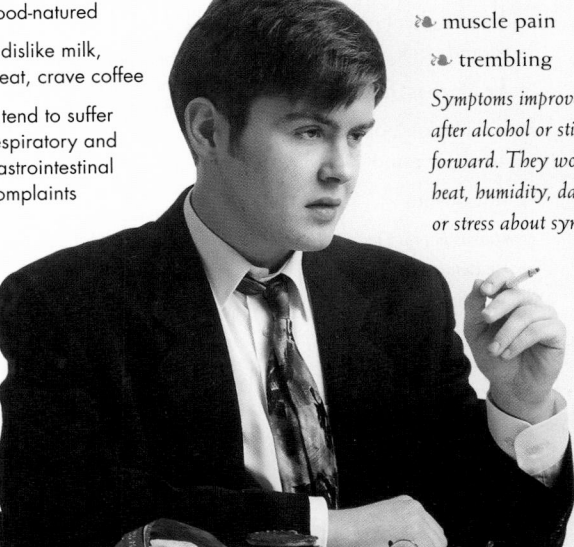

LEFT *People who are heavy smokers may respond to Gelsemium, especially if their symptoms are worse for smoking.*

DATA FILE

Relieves

☙ complaints of the nervous system

☙ fears and phobias

☙ colds, flu

☙ visual disturbances

Uses

Conditions which affect the nervous system respond well, such as problems of the nerves and muscles. Headaches which worsen with movement or light; muscle pain which accompanies fever; nervous disorders such as multiple sclerosis; nerve inflammation; right eye pain; heavy, drooping eyelids; inflamed tonsils and summer colds can all be helped. Also fevers, including flushing; an unpleasant taste in the mouth; twitchy muscles, and chills. It can help alleviate fears and shock accompanied by shaking or trembling. Visual disturbances and blurred vision can also be treated.

Which type of person?

☙ dull and heavy-looking, often with a blue tinge to the skin

☙ intelligence is often below average

☙ heavy smokers

☙ cowardly

☙ mentally weak

Glonoinum, nitroglycerine, glyceryl trinitrate
GLON.

Nitroglycerine, a thick, clear, toxic liquid, was discovered by the Italian chemist A. Sobrero in the mid-19th century. Two decades later, Swedish scientist Alfred Nobel used it as the explosive component in dynamite. In conventional medicine it is used to treat heart disease. Homeopathically, the remedy is made from glycerine, nitric and sulfuric acid. In Victorian times, typesetters and printers who worked under the powerful heat of incandescent gas lamps used it to treat the severe headaches they suffered. The remedy is mainly used for blood and circulation conditions.

ABOVE *Glonoinum (also known as Glonoin) is based on nitroglycerine, which is produced from glycerine with nitric and sulfuric acid.*

DATA FILE

Relieves
- heatstroke
- headaches
- hot flushes

Uses

This is a useful remedy for heatstroke, when an increase in blood circulation flows to the head, causing flushes of heat and a painful bursting sensation in the head. It is also good for headaches and migraine when the head feels very hot and blood vessels seem to be expanding, the patient feels like vomiting, and pressure on the head is unbearable; dizziness; for headaches which are aggravated by heat or cold; and for the cessation of menstruation and the hot flushes often associated with the menopause.

Which type of person?
- no particular type

SYMPTOMS

MENTAL
- quick and violent
- expansive
- strong emotions
- confused
- lacks sense of direction in life

PHYSICAL
- violent symptoms
- bursting feeling in head and neck
- headaches, migraine
- circulation not particularly good
- hot flushes

Symptoms improve in fresh air, and worsen in the heat, if in direct sunlight, with any movement of the head.

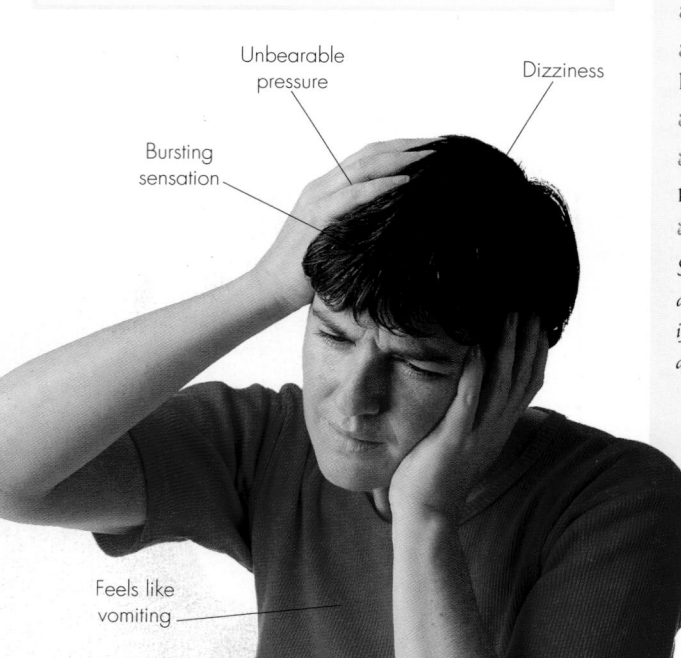

Unbearable pressure

Dizziness

Bursting sensation

Feels like vomiting

LEFT *Nitroglycerine is a characteristically unstable explosive and treats the same kind of symptoms.*

Graphites, graphite, plumbago, black lead
GRAPH.

Graphite is a mineral found in marble, granite, and crystalline rocks, and is mined in Sri Lanka, Canada, the U.S., and Mexico. It is a mixture of carbon, iron, and silica, and is contained in products such as batteries, polishes, lubricants, and also pencils – its name comes from the Greek *graphein*, meaning to write. It was first "proved" by Hahnemann when he discovered that workmen were using black lead to heal cold sores. Homeopathically, graphite is ground to a powder to make the remedy, and is used to treat skin complaints and metabolic imbalances.

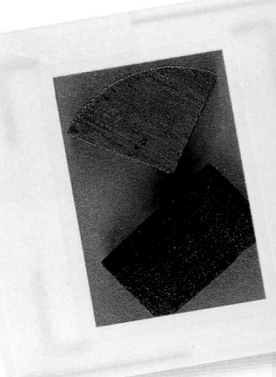

RIGHT *The remedy Graphite is obtained from the powdered natural mineral.*

DATA FILE

Relieves
- skin problems, nail malformation, and obesity, which have been triggered by metabolic imbalances
- menstrual problems
- stomach ulcers
- problems on the left side of the body

Uses

Commonly used for skin problems such as eczema, where the skin cracks in places such as the palms of the hands, behind the knees and ears, and a thick discharge oozes out. Skin complaints which have been triggered by a metabolic imbalance, such as psoriasis, where the skin becomes dry and cracked, and nail malformation; cuts and grazes that refuse to heal and become septic; inflamed, itchy scars, and obesity can be treated. Conditions that develop on the soft mucous membranes, for instance in the mouth or stomach, such as cold sores and ulcers can also be helped. Other conditions, such as hair loss, cramps in hands and feet, catarrh, swollen glands, and sweating after nosebleeds are responsive.

Which type of person?
- dark-haired, coarse-featured, with pale, dry skin
- overweight, even obese
- only able to concentrate for short periods
- moody, apprehensive, indecisive, slow reactions
- prefer sour and acidic cold drinks, dislike seafood, sweet and salty things
- grumpy on waking and become more irritable throughout the day
- prefer outdoor, manual employment
- children tend to be plump and pale-looking; pessimistic and anxious; prone to car sickness; and tend to have little stamina

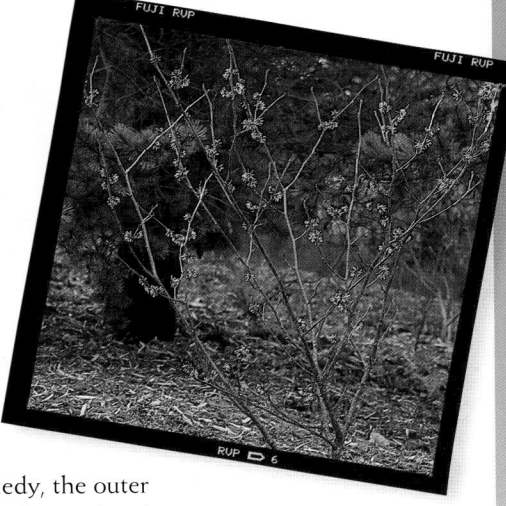

SYMPTOMS

MENTAL

- fear of thunderstorms, insanity, death
- anxiety as do not feel mentally alert
- easily startled
- tend to be morose and occasionally depressed

PHYSICAL

- dry, rough skin
- flaky and crusted scalp
- easily flushed
- no stamina
- headaches if a meal is missed
- ulcers or cold sores
- problems tend to occur on left side

Symptoms improve in warm, fresh air, after eating or sleeping, and in the dark. They worsen in cold, damp air, in the morning and evening, during menstruation, after eating sweet food or seafood, and if the skin problems are suppressed, for instance with steroids.

BELOW *Fear of thunderstorms may be one of a number of symptoms that indicate Glycerine as an appropriate remedy.*

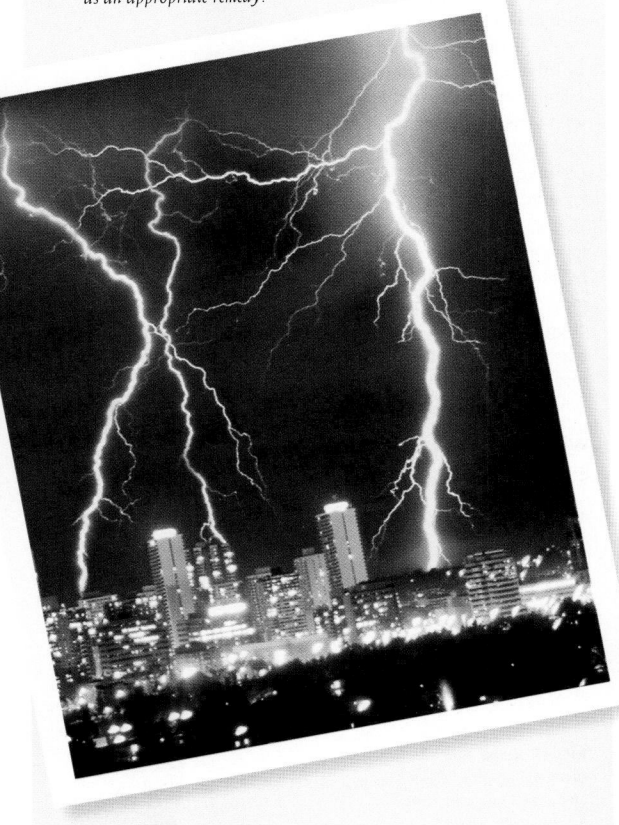

Hamamelis virginiana, witch hazel, snapping hazelnut, spotted alder

HAMAMELIS

Grown in parts of Canada, the U.S., and Europe, witch hazel, which can come from a number of trees or shrubs in the *hamamelis* family, has historically been used for its astringent qualities. In conventional medicine, it has been used for treating minor cuts, burns, rashes, and insect bites. In the homeopathic remedy, the outer skin of the root and bark of the twigs are chopped and pounded to a pulp. The remedy was first "proved" in 1850 by Dr. Hering, an American follower of Hahnemann, and is commonly used to treat piles and varicose veins by improving circulation.

ABOVE *Hamamelis or witch hazel, the plant whose roots and bark are used for the Hamamelis remedy. The plant has long been used in herbal medicine.*

SYMPTOMS

MENTAL

- depression, wanting to be left alone
- restlessness and irritability
- demand respect
- big ideas

PHYSICAL

- piles, varicose veins
- painful bruising
- bloodshot eyes
- headaches, relieved by nosebleeds
- in women, inflammation of the ovaries or uterus
- heavy menstrual bleeding, pain at the time of ovulation

Symptoms improve in fresh air and after thinking about the problem, talking, or reading, and worsen in warm, damp air, and with pressure or movement.

DATA FILE

Relieves

- varicose veins, piles
- nosebleeds
- bruises
- depression

Uses

Primarily used to treat problems associated with bleeding, such as varicose veins and piles (hemorrhoids), which occur when the veins become weakened and swollen with blood; also when the fragile blood vessels in the nose rupture, causing nosebleeds; bruises and soreness due to injury; bloodshot eyes; phlegm dotted with blood after coughing. It is also used for heavy bleeding during menstruation and pain during ovulation, as well as being given to treat bouts of depression.

Which type of person?

- no particular type

THERAPY CONNECTIONS

WITCH HAZEL

- Traditional Home and Folk Remedies   *p.91*
- Herbalism   *p.123*

BELOW *Hamamelis is most often used to treat problems that involve bleeding, such as nosebleeds and bruising.*

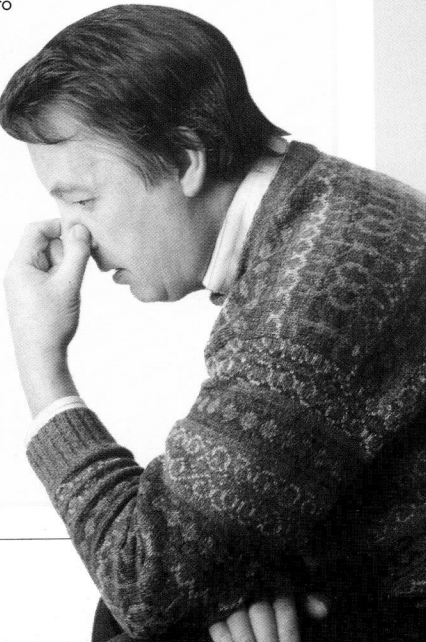

*Hepar sulfuris calcareum,
calcium sulfide*

HEP. SULF.

Historically, calcium sulfide was used to treat a number of complaints such as rheumatism, gout, and itching. In conventional medicine it is used for skin conditions such as acne and boils. It was first "proved" by Hahnemann in 1794 and was used to counter the effects of mercury, which was often used to treat illnesses at that time. Homeopathically, the remedy, made from heating the calcareous inner layer of oyster shells with flowers of sulfur, is used to treat skin infections and ailments accompanied by a discharge.

ABOVE *Flowers of sulfur are used in the preparation of Hep. sulf., mixed in equal parts with powdered oyster shells.*

SYMPTOMS

MENTAL

- anxious and irritable
- tendency to be depressed
- sluggish
- sensitive to touch, pain, cold air, noise

PHYSICAL

- sour-smelling secretions – sweat, urine, stools
- skin moist and sensitive
- low pain threshold
- seeping ailments: ulcers, cold sores, acne, boils
- coughs, colds, sore throats, flu

Symptoms improve in warmth, after applying warm compresses, and after eating, and worsen in the morning, in the cold, when touching or lying on the affected parts.

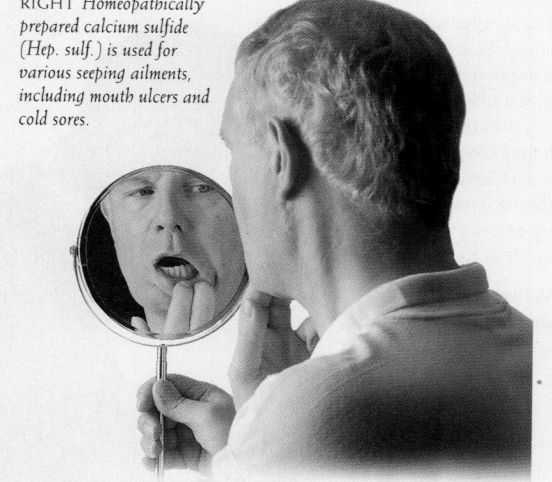

RIGHT *Homeopathically prepared calcium sulfide (Hep. sulf.) is used for various seeping ailments, including mouth ulcers and cold sores.*

DATA FILE

Relieves

- pus-producing infections
- skin infections
- conditions accompanied by sensitivity to touch

Uses

Commonly treats infections in which there is discharge, such as conjunctivitis, sinusitis, cold sores, and mouth ulcers, as well as general infections such as earache, tonsillitis, phlegm-filled chests, and flu. Also used for infections to aid in expelling pus, such as for acne where the spots are sensitive to touch. Other conditions which it can be used to help include colds accompanied by a tickly cough, and dry, hoarse coughs accompanied by a lot of phlegm.

Which type of person?

- tend to be flabby or are quite overweight
- pale-looking
- lethargic and listless
- have exaggerated likes and dislikes
- anxious and frequently bad-tempered
- fail to think things through properly
- easily offended

---

*Hyoscyamus niger, henbane, black henbane,
hog's bean, stinking Roger*

HYOSCYAMUS

It is believed the Romans first brought this poisonous plant to Europe, although it is also grown in parts of the U.S., Canada, and Asia, thriving on rubbish heaps and cemeteries. In conventional medicine it was used as a painkiller, sedative, and anticonvulsant, and the drug hyoscine is currently given as an antispasmodic. Homeopathically, it was first "proved" by Hahnemann. The remedy is made by extracting juice from the whole fresh plant (which is of the same botanical family as Belladonna) when in flower. It is a useful remedy for the elderly due to its gentle approach.

DATA FILE

Relieves

- emotional problems
- twitches
- dry coughs

Uses

Used when emotions, such as jealousy or paranoia, seem to have taken over, and the sufferer feels that he or she is being watched or poisoned. The patient will be either silent or very talkative, with violent outbursts and foul language. Physical conditions are characterized by confusion and passive stupor, with the patient mumbling and weak; twitching and trembling may occur. Dry, spasmodic coughs that are accompanied by twitching and jerking, and helped by sitting up, also respond.

Which type of person?

- lack of self-expression
- suspicious
- may hallucinate
- urge to count things

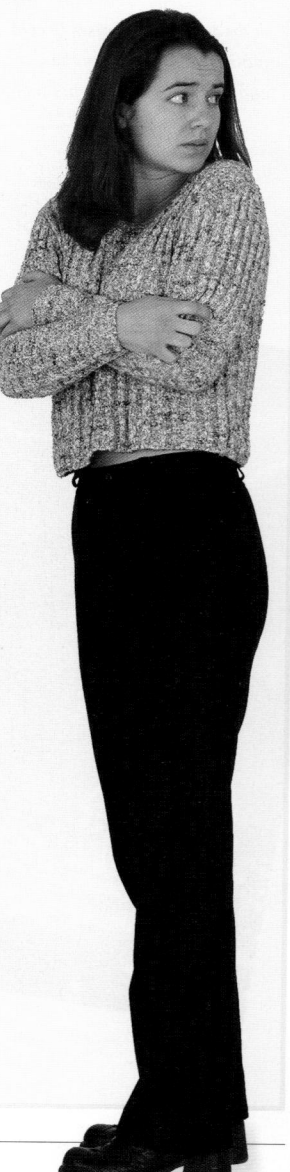

RIGHT *People with emotional problems verging on paranoia may be helped by this gentle remedy.*

SYMPTOMS

MENTAL

- talkative, even obscene
- want to expose body
- may laugh at anything
- fear of animals
- ritual behavior

PHYSICAL

- agitation
- muscle tremors, involuntary jerking
- cough
- sensitive skin
- urge to urinate, although little and infrequent flow

Symptoms improve when bending or sitting up, and worsen after emotional upset, when touched, after food, when lying down, and in the evening.

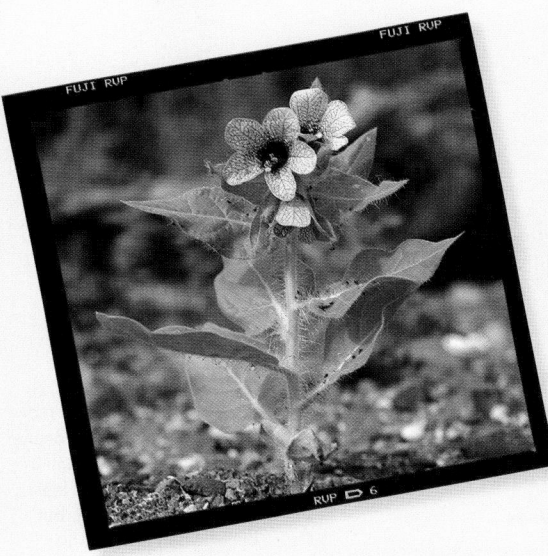

ABOVE *Black henbane, from the same family as Belladonna, is the source for the Hyoscyamus remedy.*

Hypericum perforatum, St. John's wort

HYPERICUM

The St. John's wort shrub is native to Asia and Europe, but is now grown worldwide. Its glandular leaves and yellow flowers secrete a blood-red juice, which led it to be used for cuts and wounds in the past. Its name comes from John the Baptist, and the black marks on the leaves were said to be a symbol of his beheading at the insistence of Herod's daughter, Salome. It is commonly used in herbal medicine, where, as in homeopathy, it is valued for its antidepressant action. In homeopathy, the whole fresh plant is used when in flower, and it is most often given to treat nerve pain following injury, due to its effective action on the central nervous system. Hypericum was "proved" by Dr. G. F. Mueller.

SYMPTOMS

MENTAL

- depression
- sleepiness

PHYSICAL

- neuralgia
- concussion
- toothache
- severe shooting pains that travel upward
- cravings for hot drinks, wine

Symptoms improve when the head is tilted backward, but worsen in warm, stuffy rooms; in damp, cold, or foggy weather; when touched, or when the affected part is exposed.

DATA FILE

Relieves

- nerve pain after injury
- head injuries
- shooting pains

Uses

Hypericum works well on any area affected by nerve pain and injury, but particularly on injuries to parts of the body where there are many nerve endings, such as the spine, head, fingers, toes, and lips. It can also help concussion, neuralgia, back pain, pain that shoots upward, pain after dentistry, small wounds such as bites or splinters, nausea, asthma which worsens in fog, painful piles, and rectal nerve pain. In women, headaches associated with late menstruation can also be alleviated.

Which type of person?

- no particular type

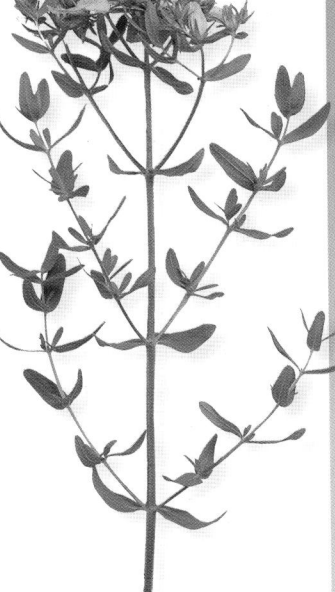

ABOVE *St. John's wort. All parts of the fresh, flowering plant are used to make the Hypericum remedy.*

THERAPY CONNECTIONS

ST. JOHN'S WORT

| Ayurveda | p.40 |
| Herbalism | p.124 |

BELOW *Hypericum can be used as a firstaid remedy for all kinds of injury, including concussion.*

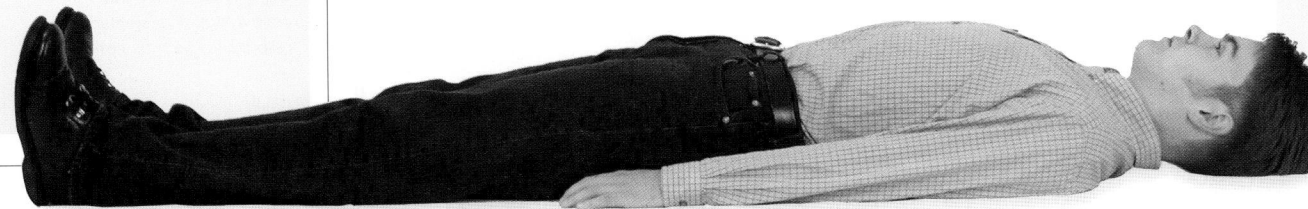

Ignatia amara, Strychnos ignatii, St. Ignatius' bean

IGNATIA

The Ignatia amara tree is found in the Philippines, Indonesia, and China. Its seeds have been used for centuries for healing, and native Filipinos wore them as amulets to ward off disease. The Spanish Jesuits brought the seeds to Europe in the 17th century, naming the tree after the Catholic priest Ignatius Loyola, who founded the Society of Jesus. In conventional medicine, they were used to treat cholera and epilepsy. Homeopathically, the seeds are separated from their pod and powdered. The remedy is used to treat emotional upsets, such as shock and grief, as the strychnine acts on the central nervous system.

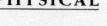

RIGHT *Ignatia amara is made from the fruits of Strychnos ignatii; also known as St. Ignatius' bean.*

DATA FILE

Relieves

- emotional traumas
- bereavement
- depression
- headaches
- changeable ailments

Uses

Ignatia is commonly used to treat shock, anger, and grief characterized by changes of mood, insomnia, and hysteria. All emotional upsets – mild depression, love traumas, self-pity, tearfulness, nervous headaches, fainting, sweating, choking, or a tickly cough – can be alleviated. Contradictory symptoms, for instance a sore throat which feels better after eating solids, are helped. In women, lack of menstruation, or uterine spasm during menstruation, constipation, piles, and shooting pain in a prolapsed rectum are all relieved.

Which type of person?

- mainly thin, dark-haired women
- tired, look strained
- emotionally sensitive, artistic, nervous disposition
- unpredictable
- high expectations
- prefer sour food, dairy products, bread, coffee; dislike fruit, sweet food, and also alcohol
- children tend to be bright, excitable, highly strung; do not cope well with stress, becoming angry and scared. Suffer nervous headaches; are prone to nervous coughing

RIGHT *This remedy can help those in nervous or emotional states, perhaps caused by bereavement or the breakdown of a relationship.*

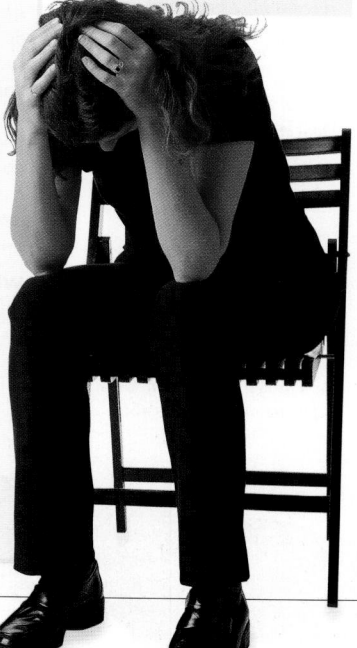

SYMPTOMS

MENTAL

- fears emotional hurt
- dislikes losing control, enclosed spaces, crowds
- difficulty in expressing emotions
- often contradictory
- sensitive to pain
- moody, laughs and cries at the same time

PHYSICAL

- yawns or sighs a lot
- intense headaches, spasmodic cough
- faints in small spaces
- food cravings, constipation

Symptoms improve after eating, urinating, with firm pressure, or lying on the affected side, with heat. They worsen in the cold, when touched, after emotional upset, when taking coffee or smoking, when exposed to strong odors.

Kali bichromicum, potassium dichromate, potassium bichromate

KALI BICH.

Potassium dichromate is an orange-red crystalline substance which has caustic and corrosive effects. It is used in a variety of manufacturing processes such as color dyeing, photography, calico printing, and as a bleaching agent. The homeopathic remedy was first "proved" in 1844, and is commonly given to treat ailments affecting the mucous membranes which lead to mucus and discharge, for example in the nose, throat, stomach, and vagina.

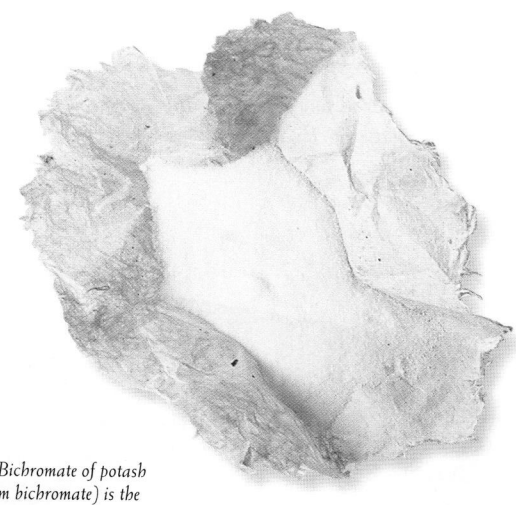

ABOVE *Bichromate of potash (potassium bichromate) is the source of the Kali bich. remedy.*

DATA FILE

Relieves

- all forms of mucus or discharge
- pain that moves about

Uses

This remedy is useful for any condition which affects the mucous membranes, leading to a stringy, yellow, or white discharge. It can help alleviate problems such as sinusitis; glue ear; coughs and colds accompanied by catarrh, where the affected areas feel congested and under pressure. Vomiting where the cause is a digestive disorder and yellow mucus is ejected can also be helped, as can rheumatic pain in joints when the pain tends to move about and becomes worse in hot weather. Migraines which begin at night, feel worse when bending, but better when pressure is applied to the base of the nose also respond well.

Which type of person?

- down-to-earth, straightforward
- high morals
- self-absorbed
- conservative
- like routine, pay attention to detail
- prefer orderliness

SYMPTOMS

MENTAL

- preoccupied with details
- dislike hot weather

PHYSICAL

- chilly and sensitive to cold when ill
- discharge from nose, throat, stomach, vagina
- catarrhal coughs
- heavy colds and blocked ears
- migraines

Symptoms improve in the warmth, after eating, vomiting, or moving. They worsen in cold, wet weather, after drinking, and on waking, between 3 A.M. and 5 A.M., in summer heat, and when feeling cold.

BELOW *A person needing this remedy tends to be chilly, feeling particularly cold in the neck area, and repeatedly suffering from catarrh and fits of coughing.*

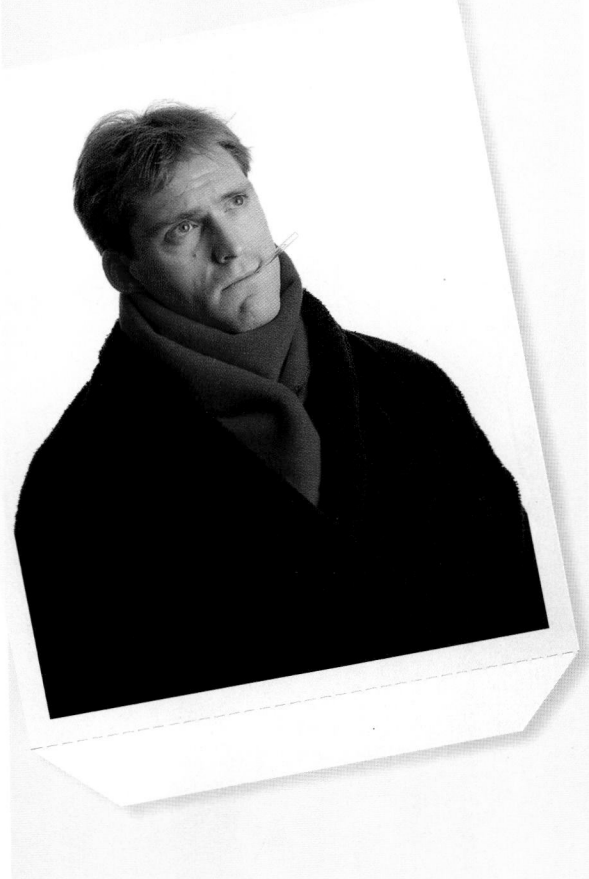

Kali phosphoricum, potassium phosphate, phosphate of potash

KALI PHOS.

Potassium is found naturally in almost all foods and is an essential part of our diet. We need it to maintain healthy function of the brain and nerve cells. In conventional medicine it is given when levels of phosphorus are low, for instance after gastroenteritis or for those who need to be fed intravenously. Kali phos. is also one of the 12 tissue salts identified by the German physician Wilhelm Schussler. Homeopathically, it is prepared by adding dilute phosphoric acid to a solution of potassium carbonate (also known as potash), and is used to treat conditions affecting the nervous system, and for exhaustion.

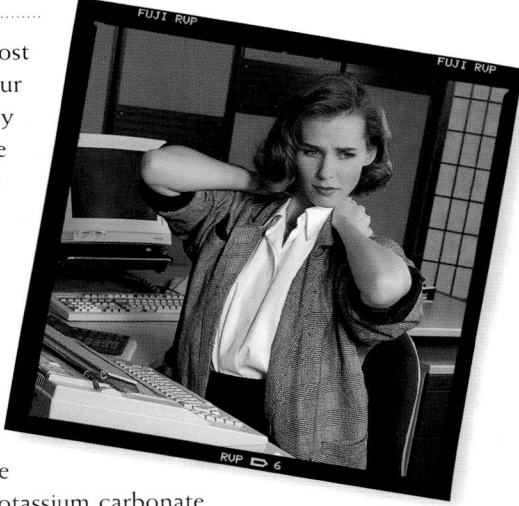

BELOW *Kali phos. types are easily worn down by stress and overwork.*

SYMPTOMS

MENTAL

- worry
- stressed out
- easily upset on hearing sad news

PHYSICAL

- easily exhausted by hard work
- sensitive to disturbances and cold
- suffer a discharge from the bladder, vagina, or the lungs
- muscular weakness

Symptoms improve in the warmth, after eating or gentle movement, and in cloudy weather. They worsen in cold, dry conditions, in winter, after cold drinks, after physical exertion or talking, and when exposed to noise.

DATA FILE

Relieves

- physical and mental exhaustion
- disorders of the nervous system

Uses

Used to treat mental and physical exhaustion, particularly when the nerves become so frayed the patient is on edge, and sensitive to any disturbance or distraction. Sufferers wish to be left alone and become introverted. Conditions such as sensitivity to cold, pus or yellow vaginal discharge, discharge from the lungs or in the stools, muscle fatigue, unwelcome early morning awakening, and chronic fatigue syndrome can all be alleviated.

Which type of person?

- conservative but outgoing
- clear-sighted
- easily upset by bad or distressing news
- stress and overwork tire them out easily

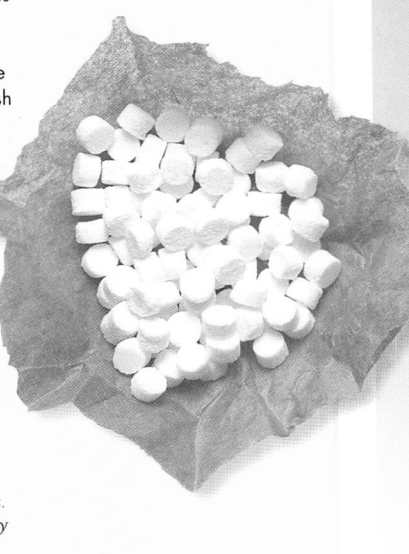

ABOVE RIGHT *The Kali phos. remedy is chemically prepared by adding phosphoric acid to potassium carbonate.*

Ledum palustre, wild rosemary, marsh tea

LEDUM

It is the fine, woolly hairs on the underside of the rosemary plant which give it its Greek name, *ledos*, meaning woolly robe. Wild rosemary has been used for its antiseptic qualities for centuries, and was used more than 700 years ago by the Finns to deter vermin. In the U.S. colonies it was first used in 1773 as a substitute for tea when the tea taxes were introduced. It grows in Ireland, Scandinavia, the U.S., and Canada. Homeopathically, Ledum is made from the whole fresh plant in flower, which is dried and powdered.

RIGHT Ledum
palustre *is the plant
known as wild rosemary,
marsh tea or Labrador tea.
The whole fresh plant or
dried twigs may be used.*

THERAPY CONNECTIONS

ROSEMARY

◐ Herbalism   *p.127*

◐ Aromatherapy *p.168*

DATA FILE

Relieves

🌿 cuts, grazes, stings

🌿 pain that moves about

🌿 prevents wounds becoming infected

Uses

Ledum is a useful first-aid remedy and helps prevent infection in cuts and wounds. Complaints that need immediate treatment – such as stings, cuts, grazes, eye injuries, and puncture wounds – respond well, and Ledum is effective if there is accompanying bruising and the area becomes painful, swollen, and puffy. It can also help to alleviate rheumatic pain which starts in the feet and moves up; painful or injured joints which may look pale or bluish; and where the affected part feels cold to the touch, but the person feels hot inside.

Which type of person?

🌿 no particular type

SYMPTOMS

MENTAL

🐛 timid, but impatient

🐛 morose and want to be left alone

🐛 get extremely angry

🐛 hate others

PHYSICAL

🐛 stiff joints

🐛 puffy, bluish skin

🐛 night sweats

🐛 black eyes

*Symptoms improve when cold
compresses are applied to the
affected part, and if the area is
left uncovered, and worsen if
warm, touched, when
in bed, and at night.*

RIGHT *Ledum is especially
useful for puncture wounds,
such as from an animal's
claws or teeth.*

RIGHT *The Ledum
plant was widely used
in infusions, and in the 18th
century it was imported to be
sold as a substitute for tea in
the U.S.*

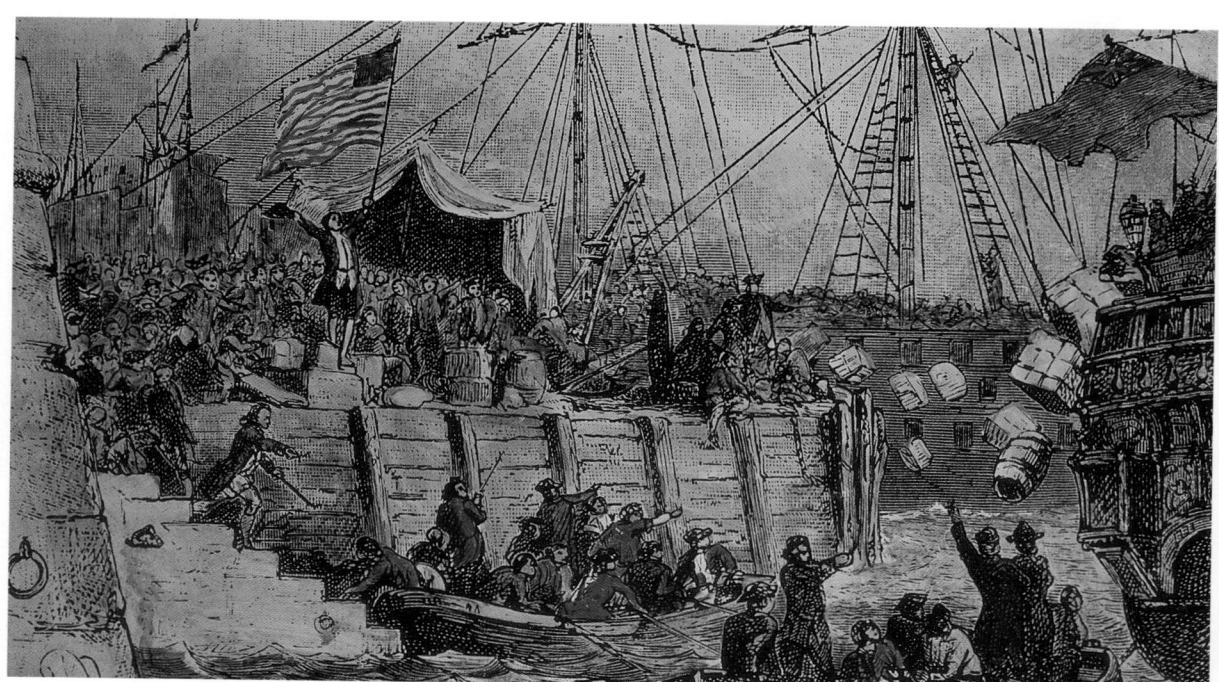

Lycopodium clavatum, club moss, wolf's claw,
stagshorn moss, running pine

LYCOPODIUM

This plant has long been used to treat stomach complaints and urinary disorders, and is grown in the mountains and forests of the northern hemisphere. Historically, Arab physicians used it to disperse kidney stones, while 300 years ago its yellow pollen was used to treat urine retention and gout. It flares up when exposed to naked flame and in the past was used in fireworks. It is also water resistant and was used to coat pills to prevent them from gluing together. Lycopodium was first "proved" by Hahnemann, and for homeopathic use the pollen dust is shaken out of the spikes of the fresh plant.

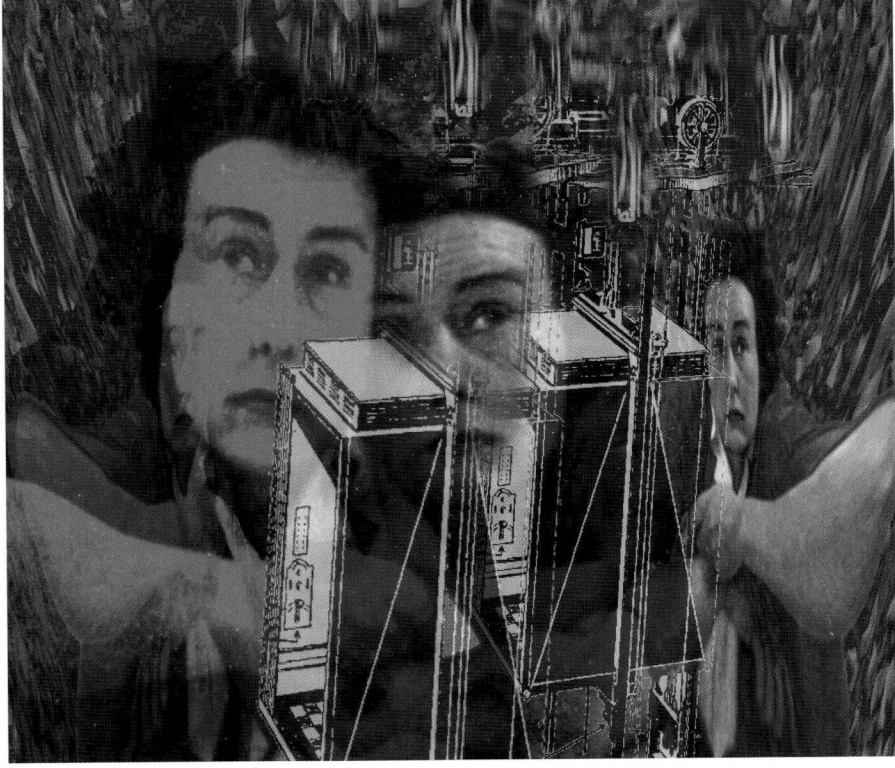

RIGHT *Lycopodium types fear being trapped in enclosed spaces, like elevators.*

SYMPTOMS

MENTAL

- fear of being alone, enclosed spaces, crowds, death
- hatred of the thought of failure
- dislike of the dark
- intolerance of weakness in others and illness
- sexual promiscuity

PHYSICAL

- weakness on right side of body
- sensitive areas include the digestive organs, brain, lungs, skin, liver, kidneys, and bladder
- fatigue

Symptoms improve when in cool, fresh air, when wearing loose clothing, after hot food and drink, and at night. They are worse on the right side, in stuffy rooms, when wearing tight clothing, after overeating or not eating, between 4 A.M. and 8 A.M., and between 4 P.M. and 8 P.M.

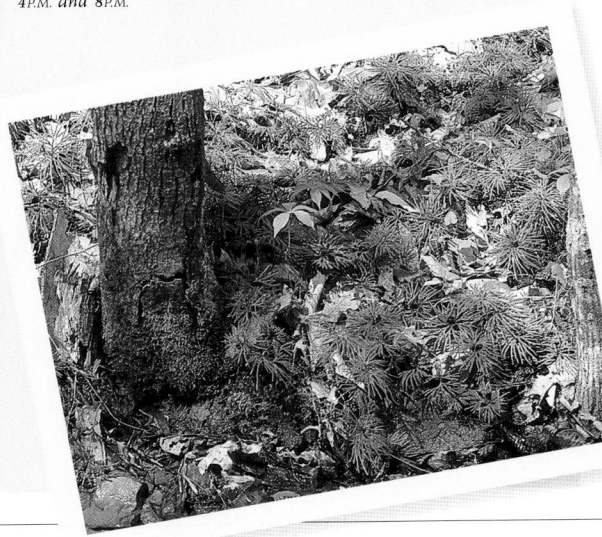

LEFT Lycopodium clavatum
*is a moss which is found growing
on mountain pastures and heaths.*

DATA FILE

Relieves

- stomach disorders
- digestive conditions
- complaints of the bladder and kidney
- problems on the right side
- in men, enlarged prostate, inability to have an erection
- emotional problems and anxiety caused by insecurity

Uses

This remedy is commonly used to treat digestive complaints, such as vomiting, indigestion, distended abdomen with flatulence, constipation, bleeding piles, and hunger which turns to discomfort after eating. Other problems that can be alleviated include swelling in the ankles, feet, or hands (edema); burst blood vessels in the eye; chronic catarrh; psoriasis on the hands; and pneumonia. Most problems tend to occur on the right side of the body, and are accompanied by cravings for sweet food. In men, the remedy is helpful for an enlarged prostate; urine which has a reddish tinge and contains a sandy sediment due to kidney stones; increased libido, but without the ability to achieve or sustain an erection.

Which type of person?

- distinguished appearance
- tall and lean in physique, but not physically strong
- deep facial frown lines, may also be prematurely bald or gray
- detached and poised
- hold important positions, e.g. diplomat or lawyer
- deep insecurity leads to gross exaggerations
- dislike change and having to face challenges
- enjoy company but avoid commitment
- prefer shellfish, sweet food, hot food and drink, cabbage, and onions
- children tend to be thin and sallow, are shy and lack confidence, prefer reading to outdoor activities, have a slightly distended abdomen, and although well behaved at school, are bossy at home

BELOW *People who benefit from Lycopodium may have a liking for shellfish, although they also like sweet food.*

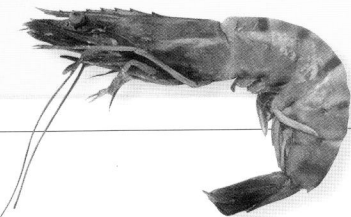

*Magnesia phosphorica, magnesium
phosphate, phosphate of magnesia*

MAG. PHOS.

Magnesium phosphate is one of the homeopathically prepared tissue salts introduced by the German physician Wilhelm Schussler at the end of the 19th century. He believed a deficiency of a mineral salt such as Mag. phos., could lead to disease. In the case of Mag. phos., he found deficiency caused problems associated with muscular nerve endings and tissue. The homeopathic remedy is made chemically from magnesium sulfate and sodium phosphate, and has an antispasmodic effect. Magnesium phosphate is also found naturally in grain cereals like wheat and oats.

ABOVE *Magnesium
phosphate occurs
naturally in grain cereals.*

*Matricaria recutita, German chamomile,
wild chamomile*

CHAMOMILLA

Hippocrates was one of the first physicians to understand the medicinal benefits of chamomile. It is extensively used in herbal medicine to treat conditions such as asthma and eczema, and during childbirth to strengthen the uterus. Chamomile tea is a popular, soothing herbal drink. The plant is a member of the daisy family, and the aromatic flowers can be found all over Europe and America. Homeopathically, the juice is extracted from the whole fresh plant when it is in flower in the late spring, and the remedy is given for those who are sensitive and have a low pain threshold, and is particularly good for children.

SYMPTOMS

MENTAL

- impulsive
- dislike mental effort
- may stammer
- forgetful

PHYSICAL

- complain of coldness in the spine
- headaches
- dizziness
- jerky movements
- pain on right side of body

Symptoms improve in the warmth, with pressure, hot compresses, and bending double, and are worse on the right side, when cool, when touched, and at night.

DATA FILE

Relieves

- cramps
- neuralgia
- pains on the right side

Uses

A useful remedy for any type of cramp from infant colic and abdominal cramp, to menstrual pains and writer's cramp, with the sufferer doubled up in pain.

Abdominal cramps are sharp and intense, with the pain jumping from one part to another, and may improve when bending, with heat, and hard pressure, and worsen in the cold, draughts, and at night. Certain types of headache and neuralgia can also be helped – when the head throbs, the face is flushed, and pain suddenly comes and goes – which improve in the warmth and if the head is bound, but worsen in the cold and draughts, and at night. Pains tend to be on the right side of the body.

Which type of person?

- thin, weak
- sensitive, artistic
- intellectual, intense
- restless and nervous

LEFT *Use of hands and fingers over a long period, whether in writing, playing a musical instrument, or using computer equipment, can cause the kind of cramps for which Mag. phos. is useful.*

DATA FILE

Relieves

- low pain tolerance
- nervous afflictions
- children's ailments

Uses

Chamomilla works well for those who are sensitive to pain and are unable to deal with their discomfort, being impatient, rude, and angry when ill. Often the reaction seems disproportionate to the amount of pain being felt. Even slight pain may cause sweats and fainting in women and children. Children particularly benefit from the remedy. Teething newborns, who are feverish and want to be held all the time, can be soothed; earache when the child is unable to sit still due to the pain and may scream, and toothache which makes one cheek red and hot can also be alleviated. Other conditions treated include heavy, painful menstruation, tinnitus, heartburn, and slimy green diarrhea.

Which type of person?

- low pain tolerance
- whining
- impatient
- never satisfied

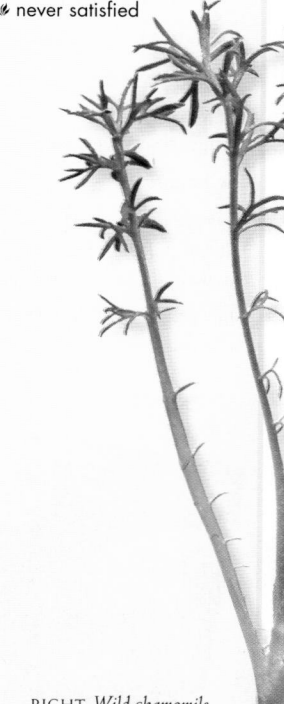

RIGHT *Wild chamomile
is the source for Chamomilla.
In herbalism and homeopathy
alike it is widely used in
treating children.*

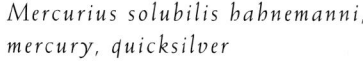

SYMPTOMS

MENTAL

- angry, irritable
- spiteful
- sensitive to people and surroundings
- cries in sleep

PHYSICAL

- restless
- teething
- earache
- toothache

Symptoms improve in the warmth, in wet weather, for not eating, and if carried (children). They worsen in heat, fresh air, cold winds, when angry, and after drinking coffee.

Mercurius solubilis hahnemanni, mercury, quicksilver

MERC. SOL.

In Roman times Mercury was known as the messenger of the gods. In recent centuries the substance has been used for various medicinal purposes. Although it is toxic and if given in too large a dose causes salivation and vomiting, it was once used in small amounts to treat conditions such as syphilis and to encourage secretions. Mercury is usually found in cinnabar, a mineral which forms near hot springs and volcanoes. A silvery-white liquid metal, it is dissolved in dilute nitric acid, forming particles which are dried and powdered for homeopathic use. Although there are many *Mercurius* remedies, Merc. sol. is mainly used to treat conditions associated with foul-smelling secretions.

SYMPTOMS

MENTAL

- restlessness, anxiety
- worry about family becoming ill
- fear of insanity, death
- dislike of thunderstorms
- explosive anger, even murderous feelings if upset

PHYSICAL

- any complaint which is characterized by a strong-smelling discharge
- burning secretions
- eye complaints
- skin conditions
- aching joints
- weak areas include lining of the stomach and respiratory system, skin, bones and joints, blood, mouth and throat, liver

Symptoms improve in temperate weather and after rest, and worsen in changeable weather, when lying on the right side, if too hot in bed, when sweating, and at night.

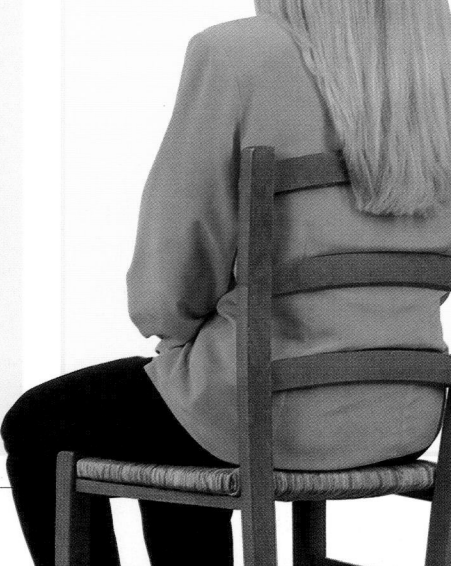

ABOVE *Metallic mercury or quicksilver is the source of Merc. sol. or Mercurius.*

RIGHT *The remedy can be used for children who are outwardly precocious but inwardly quite timid.*

Relieves

- complaints accompanied by strong-smelling secretions
- conditions affecting the mouth and throat
- offensive sweating

Uses

Conditions characterized by a smelly discharge are helped by this remedy, including chronic conjunctivitis, pus secretions from the ears, watery catarrh, nasal cold sores, glutinous saliva which stains the pillow during sleep, throat ulcers which make swallowing painful, phlegmy cough which is worse in the warmth and at night, drenching sweats, pus-filled skin eruptions, sores, and, in women, excessive vaginal discharge and green-looking stools flecked with blood. In the mouth and throat, gingivitis, thrush, bad breath, loose teeth in infected gums, swollen tonsils, and ulcers can be helped. Other symptoms which can be alleviated are foul-smelling sweat which chills the skin as it dries, and oily sweats which make other symptoms worse; stinging, watery eyes and swollen lids due to conjunctivitis; burning nasal secretions; and blisters and scalp lesions.

Which type of person?

- fair-haired, with smooth, clear skin
- outwardly detached, yet sensitive to criticism
- inner sense of haste
- insecure, cautious, and suspicious of others
- dislike being contradicted and may react badly
- strong emotional undercurrents
- when ill, become slow, uncomprehending, forgetful, and lack will-power
- prefer cold drinks, lemons, bread and butter, dislike sweet food, alcohol (except beer), meat, salt
- children tend to appear very grown up, flirty, and precocious, but inwardly are cautious and easily upset; may also be shy and introverted with a tendency to stammer; prone to problems with ears, nose, and throat

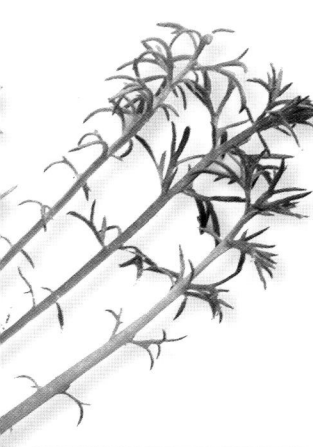

THERAPY CONNECTIONS

CHAMOMILE

- Herbalism   *p.119*
- Aromatherapy   *p.150*

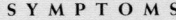
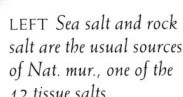

Natrum muriaticum, rock salt, sodium chloride, halite

NAT. MUR.

Salt has long been a valuable commodity. In the past, it was used instead of money for trading purposes and was given as payment to soldiers for services, hence the word salary, which comes from the Latin *salarium*. Many people add salt to food for flavor, but in fact we get more than enough salt, or sodium chloride, naturally from what we eat.

In conventional medicine salt is used in the form of saline solution, for instance, during surgery to replace fluids. Homeopathically, the Nat. mur. remedy is made from rock salt which is formed through the evaporation of salty water, leaving a crusty crystalline solid. The remedy is used to treat a number of conditions resulting from emotional problems and ailments characterized by a discharge. It is also one of the 12 tissue salts identified by Dr. Wilhelm Schussler.

ABOVE *People who may be helped by this remedy will either strongly like or strongly dislike table salt.*

LEFT *Sea salt and rock salt are the usual sources of Nat. mur., one of the 12 tissue salts.*

SYMPTOMS

MENTAL

- impatient, easily upset when judged
- mildly depressed on waking
- fear enclosed spaces, crowds, business failure, insanity, death
- worry about losing self-control, and being hurt in the emotional sense
- dislike the dark, being late, thunderstorms

PHYSICAL

- lower lip often has a center crack
- headaches
- conditions accompanied by discharge
- constipation
- feel the cold but dislike heat

Symptoms improve with fresh air, after sweating, and avoiding food. They worsen in the cold, hot weather, sea air, between 9A.M. and 11A.M., after overexertion, if fussed over.

DATA FILE

Relieves

- anxiety and depression from suppressed emotions
- conditions accompanied by secretions or discharge
- skin complaints
- in women, irregular or absent menstruation
- headaches

Uses

Nat. mur. works well for emotional problems, such as distress, restlessness, and depression, which tend to occur because of the suppression of other emotions, such as fear and grief. Conditions characterized by secretions or discharge, such as colds, catarrh, vaginismus, mouth ulcers, nasal boils, acne, cold sores, and other skin complaints such as hangnails, warts, and a cracked lower lip are alleviated. In women, it helps with erratic menstruation; menstruation which has stopped due to stress, shock, or grief; malaise or swollen ankles before and after menstruation; and a dry or sore vagina. Headaches respond well – those caused by trauma or exercise, explosive headaches, blinding migraines, headaches which feel like the head is being hammered, and are worse between 10A.M. and 11A.M., and those that start on the left side.

Which type of person?

- mainly women
- usually have a square or pear-shaped figure
- sandy or dark hair
- greasy, pale, pasty skin
- watery, red-rimmed eyes
- civilized, sensitive
- when hurt, become quiet and introverted
- enjoy the company of others, but tend to be alone
- prefer sour food and beer, like but cannot tolerate starchy food and milk, dislike chicken and also coffee
- love or loathe salty food
- children tend to be slow walkers and talkers, small for their age, flush and sweat easily, are responsible and diligent, but timid and easily upset, although dislike fuss; prone to headaches and hangnails

SYMPTOMS

MENTAL

- sometimes have suicidal thoughts
- more depressed in the morning
- brood
- sensitive, sometimes cry on hearing music
- sad

PHYSICAL

- prone to asthma brought on by damp
- tend to have profuse discharges of yellow-green mucus
- chest complaints
- triggered by damp

Symptoms improve in fresh air, dry atmosphere, and after changing position, and worsen in the morning, late evening, when lying on the back or left side, when listening to music, and in damp weather.

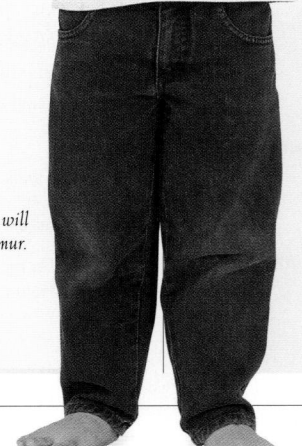

RIGHT *A timid, oversensitive child will benefit from Nat. mur.*

Natrum sulfuricum, sodium sulfate,
Glauber's salt, sal mirabile

NAT. SULF.

Sodium sulfate, a white crystalline compound, is found naturally in spa waters, salt water lakes, and in mineral water. It is also known as Glauber's salt. Sodium sulfate is used in the manufacture of paper, detergents, and glass. It is naturally present in the body and helps to maintain water balance. Homeopathically, it was "proved" by Hahnemann's followers, Nenning and Shieler. It is one of the 12 tissue salts identified by Dr. Wilhelm Schussler.

DATA FILE

Relieves

- chest problems
- emotional changes after head injury
- headaches

Uses

Used to treat chest problems such as asthma, bronchitis, colds, and flu, where there is a build-up of thick yellowish catarrh, which comes from the nose; emotional trauma after an accident in which the head is injured, leading to depression and suicidal thoughts or other emotional changes; headaches which have a vice-like grip at the back of the head and behind the forehead. Other conditions treated include dry mouth, with the tongue having a dirty coating; biliousness; thirst and frequent urination, leading to an inability to deal with damp conditions and sharp liver pains.

Which type of person?

- flabby
- prefer cool weather, dislike damp and humidity
- materialistic
- sometimes sensitive and artistic
- restless
- serious, responsible
- discontented

BELOW *Glauber's salt or sodium sulfate is the source of this remedy; it occurs naturally as the mineral, threnardite.*

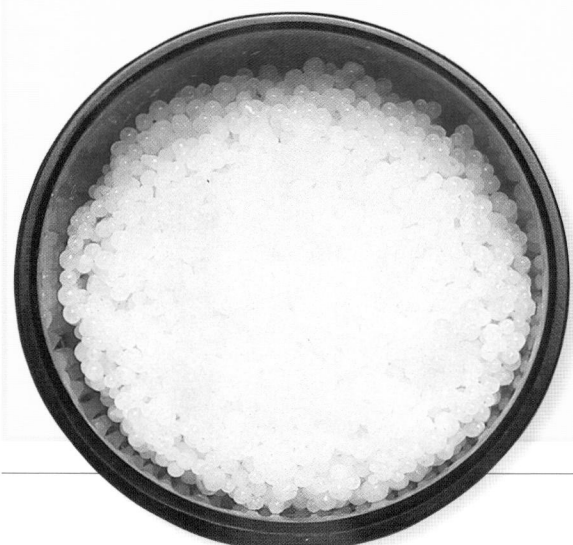

Papaver somniferum, opium poppy

OPIUM

The opium poppy has grayish-green leaves and flowers which range from white to various shades of red. It is grown in Indo-China, India, Turkey, and Iran. Opium is a well-known painkiller and tranquilizer, and an addictive narcotic drug. The unripe seed capsules contain alkaloids such as codeine and morphine, derivatives of which are used in conventional medicine as analgesics and hypnotics. The homeopathic remedy is made from the dried milky juice excreted by the seed capsules.

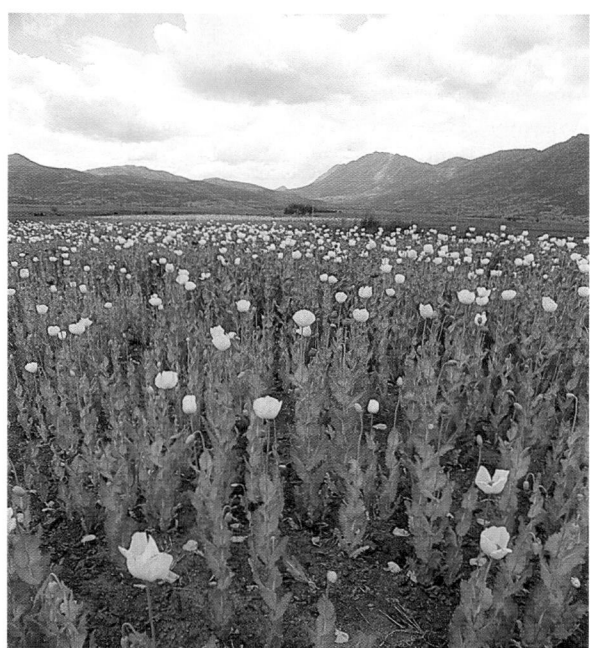

LEFT *A field of opium poppies, whose unripe seeds yield the addictive drug and are also the source of the Opium remedy.*

BELOW *The person needing Opium may want sleep but is unable to, or may actually be sleepy.*

DATA FILE

Relieves

- apathy after shock
- excitability after shock

Uses

Commonly used as a treatment after a shock, such as bereavement, when the patient may be either listless and indifferent to what is going on, or overexcited, even appearing delirious, and unable to sleep; also the patient may not be aware of pain, is very sleepy, but has no recollection of dreams once awake, and perspires easily. It is also given for slow workings of the bowel and urinary system, which can lead to constipation and water retention. Stroke victims also respond well.

Which type of person?

- no particular type

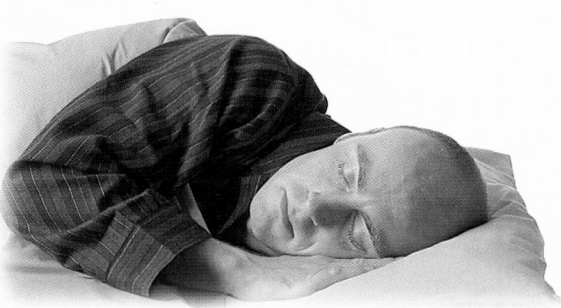

MENTAL

- apathetic
- uncomprehending
- overexcited
- may be delirious
- panicky
- in shock
- frightened

PHYSICAL

- loss of appetite
- constipation
- infrequent urination
- stroke
- irregular breathing
- sweaty skin

Symptoms improve in cool surroundings and with movement, and worsen in the warmth, in heat, during and after sleep.

Phosphorus, phosphorus

PHOS.

The name phosphorus comes from the Greek, meaning "light-bringing." It is a yellowish-white nonmetallic element which occurs in phosphates and living matter. Because of its flammable properties, white phosphate, a toxic substance, was used to make matches and fireworks, but this was replaced by the nontoxic red phosphorus. Because of the ease with which it ignites, phosphorus is kept submerged in water. Our bodies need phosphorus for the healthy functioning of our teeth, bones, bodily fluids, and DNA. In conventional medicine it has been used to treat conditions as diverse as measles and malaria. As a homeopathic treatment, it is mainly given to those suffering from anxiety and digestive disorders.

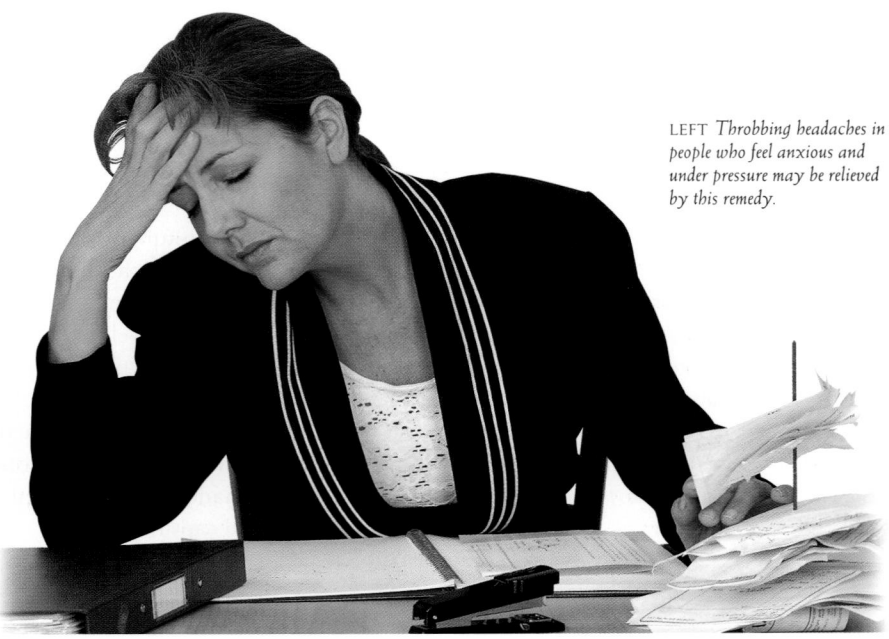

LEFT *Throbbing headaches in people who feel anxious and under pressure may be relieved by this remedy.*

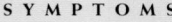

LEFT *The source of the Phosphorus remedy is phosphorus obtained from bone ash.*

SYMPTOMS

MENTAL

- mentally alert
- nervous under pressure
- tend to bottle things up
- indifferent to family and friends when ill
- fear illness and death

PHYSICAL

- weak areas include digestive organs, circulation, nervous system, the left side of the body, liver
- bleeding, such as nosebleeds
- respiratory problems
- headaches

Symptoms improve in fresh air, after sleeping, when touched, and when lying on the right side. They worsen in the morning and evening, after mental or physical exertion, after hot food or drink, when lying on the left side, and in thunderstorms.

DATA FILE

Relieves

- anxieties, fears
- digestive complaints
- circulatory conditions and those causing bleeding
- respiratory problems

Uses

Phosphorus is used to treat symptoms such as exhaustion, insomnia, nerves which are caused by underlying stress, anxiety, and fears, for instance due to exam pressure, overwork, or fear of dying. Other problems that can be helped include digestive problems such as nausea and vomiting due to coughing, stress, or food poisoning, cravings for certain foods, and pressure in the stomach; poor circulation, such as cold or overheated fingers and toes; excessive bleeding, such as bleeding gums, nosebleeds, and heavy menstrual bleeding; respiratory problems such as acute bronchitis or asthma, difficulty in breathing, tight chest, pneumonia, dry tickly coughs, and red-tinged phlegm. Other conditions which can be alleviated include headaches which are worse in heat but

improve after a cold compress or eating; dry skin; sensitive red eyes; perspiring under stress; fever with alternate sweating and shivering; cramps; unresolved sexual problems.

Which type of person?

- well proportioned, tall, and lean
- fine or dark hair, with reddish tinge
- pale skin, blush easily
- intelligent, outgoing, an eye for clothes, often artistic
- open and affectionate
- enthusiastic, but only in short spurts
- tend to offer more than can deliver
- imagination needs constant stimulation

- tend to crumble when subjected to pressure
- crave attention, particularly when ill
- prefer spicy, salty, sweet foods, carbonated drinks, cheese, and wine, and dislike fruit, fish, and tomatoes
- children tend to be tall for their age, smooth-featured, but blush easily; prefer company but become restless and nervous; perceptive, artistic, and affectionate. They dislike doing homework, the dark, and thunderstorms

BELOW *The Phos. patient often has a preference for spicy foods such as curry.*

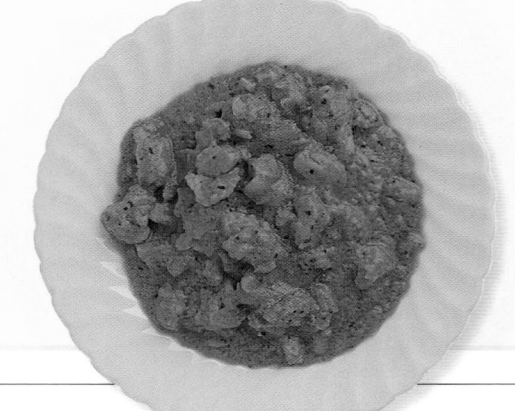

Pulsatilla nigricans, Anemone pratensis,
pasque flower, paschal flower, meadow anemone,
wind flower

PULSATILLA

The pasque flower is distinguishable from other members of the *Pulsatilla* family by its beautiful, deep-purple flowers. It is found growing in central and northern Europe, Russia, and western Asia. The name passe-fleur was given by the French in the 16th century, meaning "flower that excels." It took its later name, pasque or paschal flower, meaning Easter flower, because it usually blooms at that time. It has long been used medicinally for a number of ailments such as ulcers, tooth decay, and cataracts. In homeopathy, the whole fresh plant in flower is used to make the remedy, and it is given for a number of conditions, such as digestive disorders, depression, and gynecological problems.

SYMPTOMS

MENTAL

- avoid confronting people
- depressed
- self-conscious
- cry easily
- fear being alone, the dark, insanity, death
- lack of strength of character

PHYSICAL

- ailments characterized by discharge
- gynecological conditions
- digestive problems
- bad taste in mouth, dry mouth
- aching joints

Symptoms improve in fresh air, with gentle movement, and with sympathy, and worsen in the heat, on eating rich foods, after lengthy standing, when lying on the left side, and in the evening.

DATA FILE

Relieves

- digestive disorders
- gynecological conditions
- emotional traumas
- conditions accompanied by excessive discharge

Uses

Pulsatilla can help relieve a number of digestive problems, such as rich food causing lack of sleep, a stomach which is tight on waking in the morning and which reacts badly to rich or fatty food, particularly pork, heaviness under the breastbone after eating, cravings for sweet foods, and a rumbling stomach. In women it can be used to treat lack of or late menstruation, particularly if due to shock or illness, thick, stinging discharge, and menopausal problems, all of which tend to be accompanied by crying and depression. Moodiness, depression, and fear of being alone can also be treated. Ailments

ABOVE LEFT *The spring-flowering pasque flower, source of Pulsatilla, is also used by herbalists.*

characterized by excessive discharge or secretions, such as conjunctivitis, catarrh with yellow phlegm, sinusitis, and a runny nose, can also be helped. Other troublesome conditions which respond well include headaches above the eyes, backache, rheumatism, varicose veins, corneal ulcers, loose coughs, palpitations, bedwetting.

Which type of person?

- usually women
- fair skin and fair hair, with blue eyes
- blush easily
- tend to be plump
- good-natured, kind, popular, easily influenced by, and depend on, others
- lack assertiveness, and avoid confrontation
- led by emotions rather than head
- relate to those in distress, including animals

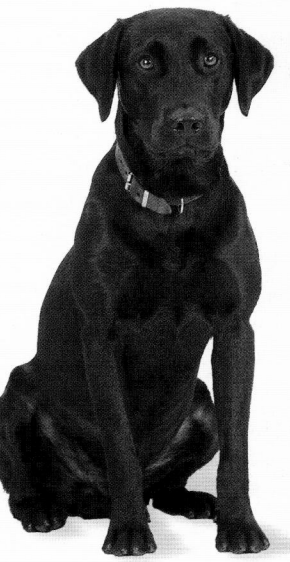

BELOW *The Pulsatilla type is likely to relate well to those in distress, including animals.*

- prefer sweet food, cold food and drink, dislike spicy food, pork, butter, fruit
- children tend to be either small and fair with delicate features, easygoing, affectionate yet shy, blushing easily; or darker-haired, small, listless, needing reassurance and attention, but slow in returning it. Both types are scared of the dark, dislike weather changes, particularly the cold, which can trigger ailments, and are prone to colds

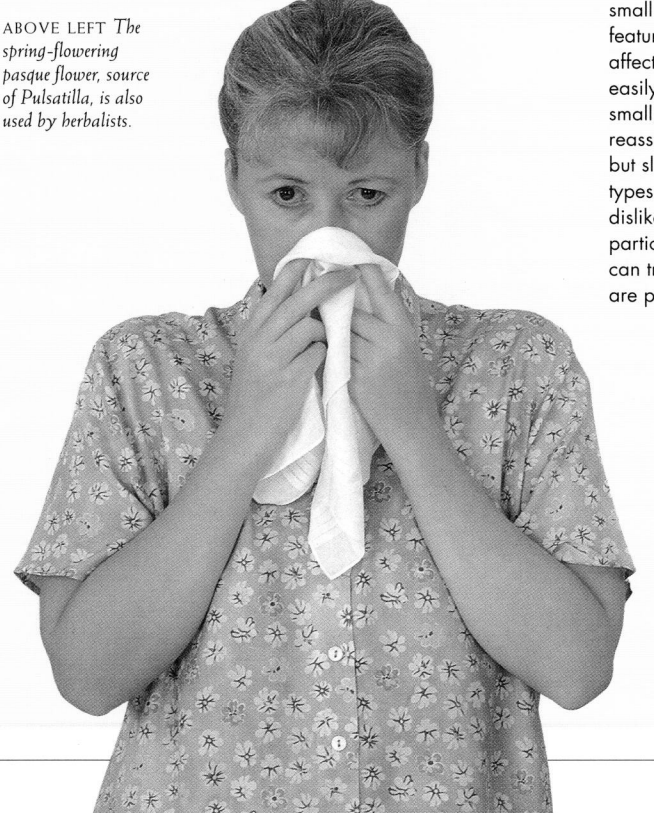

LEFT *Shifting symptoms, changeability and moodiness, with runny eyes and nose, may well indicate Pulsatilla.*

Ruta graveolens, rue, bitter herb, herb of grace

RUTA GRAV.

In the Middle Ages rue was used to ward off the plague. In the 16th and 17th centuries it was scattered over courtroom floors to prevent the spread of typhus, or jail fever, which was carried by the lice which thrived in the squalid jail conditions. It has also been used to treat croup, colic, headaches, and coughs, and was given as an antidote to mushroom poisoning. The homeopathic remedy is made from the juice of the whole plant, which is picked before it flowers. It is given mainly for bruising and restlessness.

DATA FILE

Relieves

- bruises, strained ligaments
- restlessness
- eye strain

Uses

The treatment of bruised bones and tendon injuries, aching bones, deep aching pain, rheumatism, sciatica which is worse when lying down, and the restlessness which goes with having to be still. Also good for eyestrain, when the eyes feel hot and sore from overuse or reading small print, and accompanying headaches. Other conditions treated include infection after tooth extraction; weak chest with breathing difficulties; prolapsed rectum; constipation with stools that are either large and difficult to pass or loose, containing blood and mucus.

Which type of person?

- no particular type

SYMPTOMS

MENTAL

- contradict, criticize others
- depressed when ill
- restless
- anxious, troubled
- dissatisfied with self and with others

PHYSICAL

- painful, aching limbs
- bruises
- headaches due to eyestrain

Symptoms improve with movement and worsen in the cold and damp, when resting or lying down.

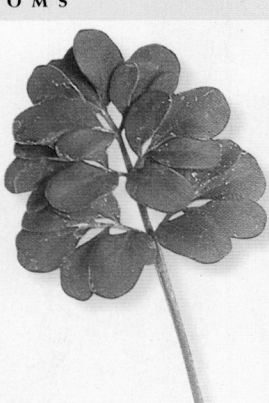

ABOVE *and* TOP *The leaves of rue (the herb* Ruta graveolens)*, the plant used as the source of Ruta. grav.*

Rhus toxicodendron, Rhus radicans, poison ivy, poison oak

RHUS TOX.

Rhus tox. is made from both poison ivy, and a variety of it, poison oak, both of which are native to the U.S. and Canada. Brushing against the leaves can cause a severe skin reaction, as well as headache, swollen glands, and fever, as they contain a poisonous sap. In homeopathy, poison ivy was first "proved" by Hahnemann. The fresh leaves of the plant are collected before it flowers, when the poison is most potent, and pounded to a pulp. The remedy is used for skin conditions and rheumatic pain.

DATA FILE

Relieves

- joint and muscle pain, and general stiffness
- red, itchy skin eruptions

Uses

It can be used to treat skin complaints characterized by red, itchy, puffy areas which feel like they are burning and which tend to form a scaly surface, such as eczema, herpes, diaper rash, and raised patches of skin where there is a clear demarcation line between the affected and unaffected part. Muscle and joint pain, such as that associated with rheumatism, osteoarthritis, cramps, restless legs, stiffness in the lower back, numbness in arms and legs, and strains can also be alleviated. Other complaints, such as headaches, dizziness, fever, stitch pains made worse by cold and damp, and abdominal pain, can also be relieved. In women, early, heavy, or prolonged menstrual bleeding and accompanying abdominal pain can be treated.

ABOVE *Infants with eczema or diaper rash can benefit from Rhus tox. treatment.*

Which type of person?

- lively, extrovert
- diligent workers
- restless
- cry for no reason
- anxious at night
- like milk, always thirsty

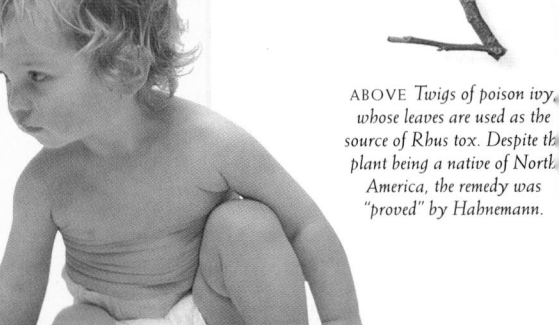

ABOVE *Twigs of poison ivy, whose leaves are used as the source of Rhus tox. Despite the plant being a native of North America, the remedy was "proved" by Hahnemann.*

SYMPTOMS

MENTAL

- fear being poisoned
- anxious at night
- depressed and may contemplate suicide
- may act compulsively

PHYSICAL

- headaches after being cold or damp
- eyes are inflamed after being wet
- backache
- blistering skin

Symptoms improve in the warmth, with movement or after changing position, and after stretching. They worsen during cold, wet weather, with rest, when lying on the back or on the right side, and at night.

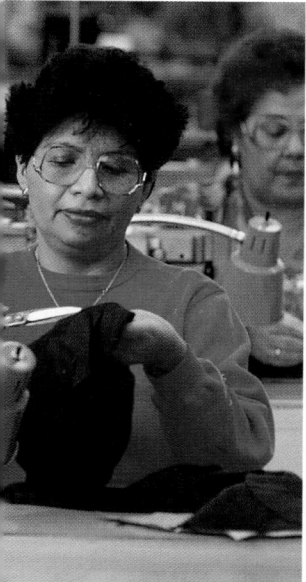

BELOW *The Rhus tox. remedy is suited to people who are diligent workers and has a wide range of applications.*

Silicea terra, quartz, silica, flint, rock crystal

SIL.

Silica, the main constituent of rock, is prepared from silicon dioxide, found in flint, quartz, and sandstone. Plants absorb it through their stems and in humans it is essential for the growth of bones, teeth, hair, and nails, and for the maintenance of connective tissue. In homeopathy, it is useful for problems of the digestive and nervous systems, bone and skin conditions, and for its ability to promote the expulsion of foreign bodies such as thorns and splinters. It is also one of the 12 tissue salts identified by Dr. Wilhelm Schussler.

SYMPTOMS

MENTAL

- fear of failure, exertion, sharp objects
- timidity, lack of self-confidence
- worry about future events
- fear of commitment because of being hurt

PHYSICAL

- feet often sweaty
- chills
- slow healing
- discharges
- cracked lips, brittle nails

Symptoms improve in heat and when wrapped up, and worsen in draughts, cold, and damp, when lying on the left side, after washing, by suppressing sweat, and in the morning.

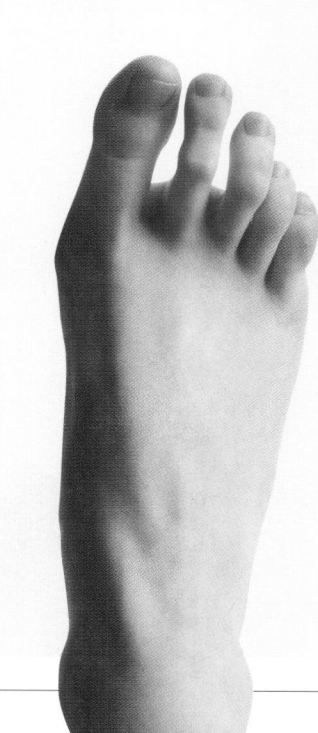

BELOW *Sweaty feet and problems that result from getting the feet wet can indicate the need for Sil.*

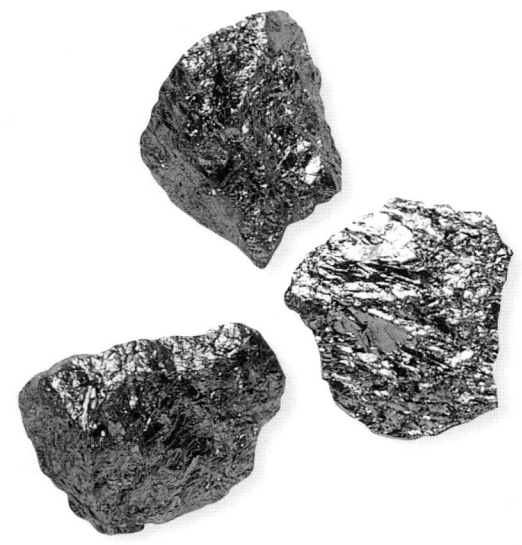

ABOVE *The crystalline form of the element silicon, the source of the homeopathic remedy and tissue salt, Silicea.*

DATA FILE

Relieves

- conditions caused by low immunity due to being malnourished
- bone and skin conditions
- assists in the expulsion of foreign bodies

Uses

Silica is good for complaints which have occurred as a result of low immunity due to lack of nourishment, such as colds, ear infections, catarrh. It can also be used to treat skin and bone conditions, such as acne, weak nails, slow growth, or fontanels which are slow to close in babies, slow-healing fractures; to assist in expelling splinters, glass shards, or thorns from body tissue; and to alleviate problems associated with the nervous system, such as colic and migraines. Other problems alleviated include catarrh with thick, yellow discharge, enlarged lymph nodes, offensive sweat, headaches which start at the back of the head and move over the forehead, glue ear, and restless sleep.

Which type of person?

- slim, small-boned, with lank hair
- neat appearance but prone to cracked lips, and brittle, uneven nails
- appear fragile and lack stamina, but are tenacious
- lack self-confidence, but are strong-willed
- often tired
- worry about new challenges, but take them on anyway
- prefer cold food and dislike milk, meat, cheese, warm food
- children tend to be neat, small, but with large sweaty heads, feel the cold easily, are shy but strong-willed, and conscientious but lacking in confidence

Sepia officinalis, cuttlefish

SEPIA

Historically, cuttlefish ink has been used medicinally to treat conditions such as kidney stones, hair loss, and gonorrhea. It is also used as a pigment in paint, which is where Hahnemann first came across it. He noticed that an artist he was treating for apathy and depression often sucked his brushes, which had been dipped in sepia paint. He published his findings in 1834 after "proving" the remedy. Today, sepia is most commonly taken by women, and is used to treat complaints such as menstrual problems and hormonal imbalances.

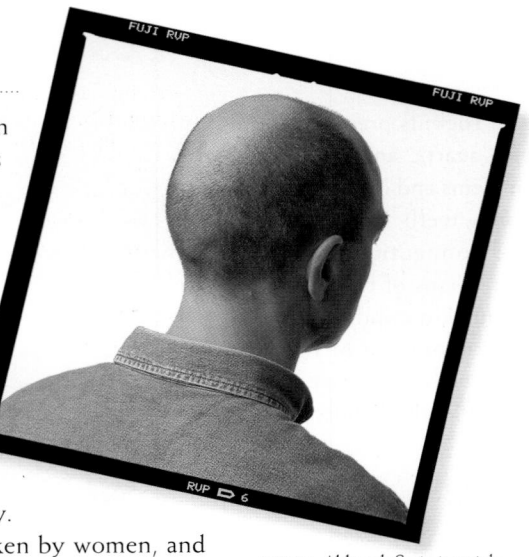

ABOVE *Although Sepia is mainly a women's remedy it is sometimes used for hair loss in either sex.*

SYMPTOMS

MENTAL

- fear poverty, being alone, insanity
- irritable with family, but good in company
- bottle up anger
- find it hard to conceal thoughts

PHYSICAL

- sudden weeping
- easily chilled
- dragging sensation in abdomen
- burning or throbbing pains

Symptoms improve after food, exertion, especially dancing, sleep, and in the warmth, and are worse on the left side, after physical and mental exertion, in the early morning and evening, in thundery weather, and if near tobacco.

DATA FILE

Relieves

- menstrual problems
- conditions associated with hormonal imbalance
- complaints accompanied by exhaustion

Uses

Useful for women who feel "dragged down," both physically and emotionally. Useful for complaints relating to the vagina, ovaries, and uterus, such as heavy or painful menstruation, PMS, menopausal hot flushes, thrush, conditions associated with pregnancy, and the feeling of a sagging abdomen, where the woman feels the need to cross her legs. Pain during sex, aversion to sex, or exhaustion afterward can also be treated. Also, any situation where the woman is feeling emotionally and physically tired, and lacking in energy. Also useful for headaches with nausea, hair loss, dizziness, offensive sweating, indigestion, skin discoloration, and circulatory problems.

Which type of person?

- mainly women
- tall, slim, dark hair and eyes, yellowish facial skin pigmentation
- dignified and attractive
- detached yet emotional
- martyr
- love dancing
- have strong opinions, hating to be contradicted
- resentful of responsibilities
- either career women who appear tough yet are vulnerable, or wives and mothers whose own needs are not met
- prefer sour and sweet foods, alcohol, and dislike milk and pork
- children tend to be sallow, sweaty-skinned, and tire easily; sensitive to weather; moody and negative, dislike parties and being left alone; tendency to constipation

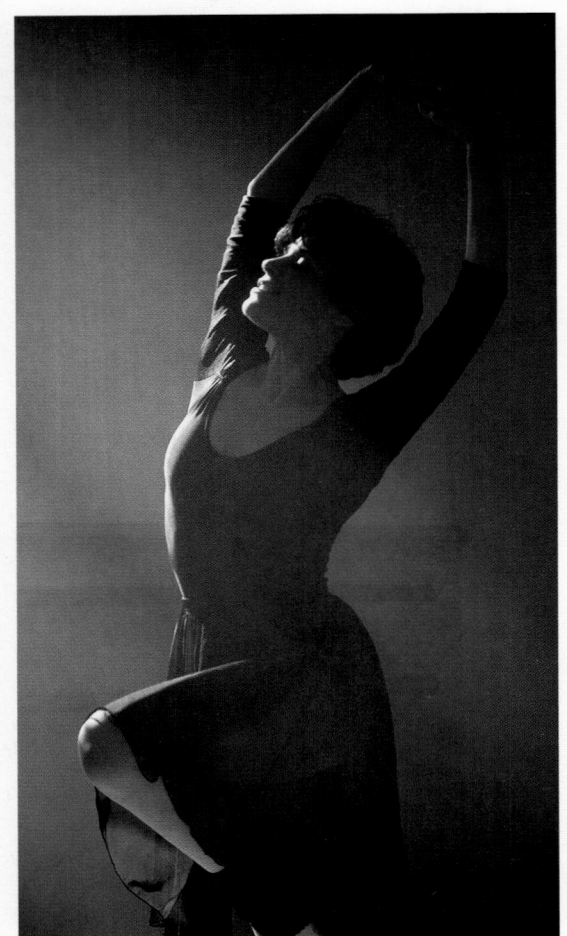

LEFT *A love of dancing may characterize the person who would benefit from treatment with Sepia.*

LEFT *The cuttlefish is the source of sepia used to color ink, and to make the Sepia remedy.*

Spongia tosta, sponge
SPONGIA

Sponge was first treasured for its medicinal properties more than 600 years ago, when it was used as a treatment for goiter, the swelling of the thyroid gland, which is brought on by a deficiency of iodine. Although it was not known then, sponge contains useful amounts of iodine and bromine. Homeopathically, the remedy was first "proved" by Hahnemann, and appears in the sixth volume of his *Materia Medica Pura*. The remedy is made by toasting and powdering the sponge, which is harvested from the waters of the Mediterranean.

LEFT *Sea sponges, source of the remedy Spongia, were first used medicinally hundreds of years ago.*

RIGHT *Those who will benefit from Spongia usually find that their symptoms are soothed by warm drinks.*

DATA FILE

Relieves

- croup
- coughs
- laryngitis

Uses

This remedy works particularly well for children's croup, characterized by sneezing and a hoarse, dry barking cough, with the patient waking in alarm with the feeling of suffocation, later followed by thick mucus which is difficult to bring up. Associated symptoms of coughs, such as hoarseness, dryness of the larynx from a cold, headaches which are worse when lying down, but improve when sitting up, bronchitis, dry mucous membranes, and feelings of heaviness and exhaustion are also alleviated. Laryngitis, where the throat is raw and dry, and feels like it is burning, responds well. Sponge is also good if chest conditions or tuberculosis tend to run in the family.

Which type of person?

- light-haired, blue-eyed
- lean
- dried-up appearance

SYMPTOMS

MENTAL

- anxiety
- fear of suffocation, and death
- waking from sleep, feeling frightened

PHYSICAL

- congestion of the chest or heart region
- coughs
- palpitations
- laryngitis

Symptoms improve with warm food and drink, and when sitting up. They worsen when talking, swallowing, consuming sweet food or cold drinks, moving, touching the affected area, lying with the head lower than the feet, and around midnight.

Solanum dulcamara, woody nightshade, bittersweet
DULCAMARA

Woody nightshade has been used since Roman times as a remedy to help those suffering from conditions such as asthma, catarrh, rheumatism, and pneumonia resulting from the effects of cold and wet. It is also extensively used in herbal medicine, where it is known as bittersweet, for conditions such as eczema, psoriasis, and ulcers. The remedy, first "proved" by Hahnemann, is made from the green shoots and leaves of the flowering plant, and is given for complaints resulting from exposure to wet weather and temperature changes.

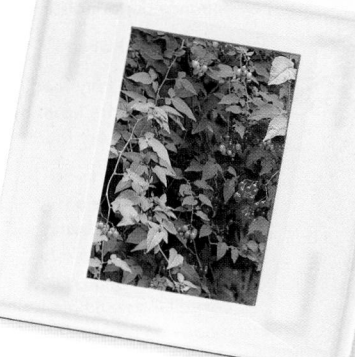

RIGHT *The green shoots and leaves of woody nightshade* (Solanum dulcamara), *a relative of Belladonna, are used to make Dulcamara.*

DATA FILE

Relieves

- conditions which are triggered by or worsen with temperature changes

Uses

Any condition which is brought on by exposure to cold, wet weather, weather changes, for instance from warm to cold or from cooling down too quickly after sweating, can be alleviated. Patients tend to be worse in the fall and in damp, cold weather. Other problems brought on by weather conditions and helped by the remedy include diarrhea triggered by hot days and cold nights; back and neck pains from the damp; fevers due to exposure to the cold while the body is hot; congested eyes; ulcers; sore throat; frequent urination if chilled; and catarrhal, or dry, hoarse coughs. Skin conditions such as urticaria, crusty facial eruptions, fleshy or flat warts, and ringworm.

Which type of person?

- strong-minded, domineering personality
- possessive
- restless, confused
- keen to keep on the move
- eager for something, indifferent when get it

SYMPTOMS

MENTAL

- none in particular

PHYSICAL

- susceptible to cold and weather changes, leading to ailments such as conjunctivitis and diarrhea
- prone to colds
- hungry, but do not want food
- drowsy during the day, restless at night

Symptoms improve in the warmth and with movement, and worsen in the cold and damp, after sweating and then rapidly cooling down, in temperature extremes, and with lack of movement.

Strychnos nux vomica, poison nut, Quaker buttons

NUX VOMICA

The poison nut plant, native to Indonesia, contains strychnine, which is extracted from the seeds. In the past, it was a useful poison for murder. Medicinally, in small amounts, it can help relieve digestive problems, but large doses cause muscular spasm and death from respiratory failure. Strychnine was used during the Middle Ages to help treat sufferers of the plague. Homeopathically, it was first "proved" by Hahnemann. To make the remedy, which is mainly used for oversensitivity and digestive problems, the seeds are extracted from the soft, gelatinous pulp of the fruit and are then dried.

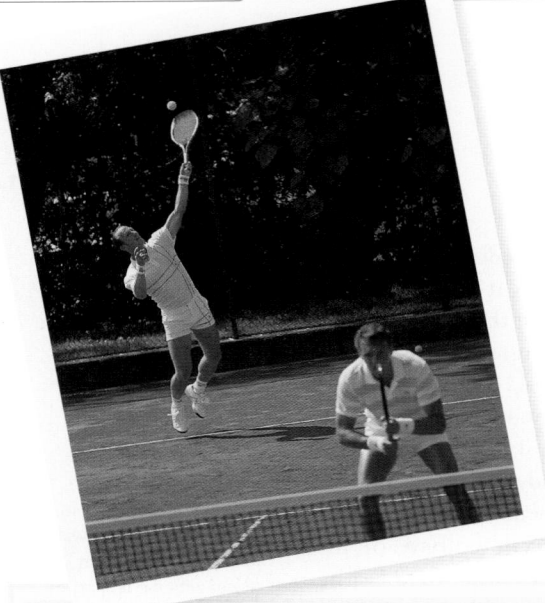

SYMPTOMS

MENTAL

- fear insects, failure, crowds, death
- quarrelsome
- critical of others
- fastidious
- prone to hypochondria

PHYSICAL

- chills
- sensitive to light, smell, noise
- upset by overindulgence in food, alcohol, coffee
- aching, bursting, burning pains

Symptoms improve when lying down and after sleep, in warmth and humidity, in the evening, after washing, and with pressure. They worsen in cold, windy weather, in the morning, in open air or under the sun, two hours after food, and after mental exhaustion.

ABOVE RIGHT *Men, particularly those who are competitive or aggressive, may be Nux vomica types.*

RIGHT *The remedy is derived from the poison nut plant, Strychnos nux vomica, from which strychnine is obtained.*

DATA FILE

Relieves

- digestive upsets
- oversensitivity
- chills

Uses

Commonly used to treat emotional problems such as irritability and oversensitivity, it works well for those who bottle up their anger, who are never satisfied, are prone to arguments, dislike having to depend on others, and prefer being left alone. Also used for digestive conditions, such as nausea, vomiting, diarrhea, indigestion, constipation, and piles, which may be brought on by overindulgence in certain foods, or due to suppressing the emotions, or from mental overwork. Other problems it can alleviate include flu, retching coughs, colds with a blocked nose at night and runny nose during the day, chills, headaches which are worse after mental exertion; in women, erratic, early, or heavy menstrual bleeding, morning sickness, constant urination, and labor pain.

Which type of person?

- mainly men
- hypersensitive
- strained-looking, lined face, sallow skin
- criticize, but cannot take criticism from others
- competitive, enjoy meeting challenges
- verbally and mentally alert, with quick wit
- intolerant of others, and easily angered
- may use stimulants to enhance performance
- disgruntled when ill
- prefer rich, fatty food, and like, but are upset by, alcohol and spicy foods
- children tend to be hyperactive and easily irritated, dislike being contradicted; prone to tantrums; diligent and competitive, but hate losing; moody on awakening; prone to stomach aches

SYMPTOMS

MENTAL

- selfishness, egotism
- argumentativeness, aggressiveness
- fear of ghosts, height, failure
- lethargic depression
- full of bright ideas which fade away

PHYSICAL

- burning, itching sensations
- inflammation of affected part
- offensive odors
- thirstiness
- weak areas include left side of the body, circulation, digestive organs, and skin

Symptoms improve when lying on the right side, in warm, dry, fresh air, after physical activity, and worsen in stuffy atmospheres, in the morning, particularly around 11 A.M., and at night, in the damp and cold, and after washing.

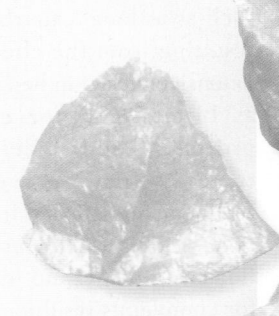

RIGHT *Sulfur, which has many medical and other uses, is the source of the Sulfur remedy.*

Sulfur, brimstone, flowers of sulfur

SULFUR

Sulfur is a mineral which is found in rock forms beside hot springs and in volcanic craters. It has been used medicinally for many centuries – in the 16th century flowers of sulfur was used to fumigate rooms where infection had been present. It was also used as a purgative and to treat rheumatism. Children used to be given brimstone and treacle to encourage bowel function. It has also been used in conventional medicine to treat skin problems such as acne. Homeopathically, it was first "proved" by Hahnemann. A fine, yellow powder is extracted from the mineral. The remedy treats digestive and skin disorders.

DATA FILE

Relieves

- inflamed, itchy skin conditions
- digestive complaints
- offensive odor
- women's conditions
- conditions other remedies do not seem to be helping

Uses

Sulfur can be used to soothe hot, red, itchy skin associated with problems such as eczema and diaper rash, digestive complaints such as vomiting and diarrhea which occur in the morning, indigestion which is made worse by drinking milk, and hunger pangs. It can also treat offensive odors, such as foul-smelling sweat or discharge; premenstrual symptoms such as irritability and headaches; and menopausal symptoms, such as flushing and dizzy spells. It is also useful when another remedy has not worked as hoped or if the picture remedy is not clear. Other problems, such as lack of

energy, restless sleep, depression, fever, burning pains and eruptions, congestion, and back pain, can be helped.

Which type of person?

- either round and red-faced or lanky with bad posture
- dry, flaky skin, dull hair, unclean-looking
- selfish, self-centered, and egocentric, but can be giving and good-natured
- full of ideas, but unable to carry them out, because of a lack of will-power
- fuss over minor details
- quickly angered, but just as quickly calm down
- sensitive to smell
- prefer sweet, fatty, spicy, and sour foods, alcohol, stimulants, and dislike milk, hot drinks, and eggs
- children tend to be either well built, with thick hair and a rosy complexion, or thin and pale with dry skin; both types eat well, look disheveled, are happy when stimulated, take care of their possessions, and are difficult to get to bed

---

Tarentula hispanica, Lycosa tarentula, Spanish spider, wolf spider

TARENTULA

Tarentula gets its name from the Italian town of Taranto (Latin name *Tarentum*), where the wolf spider is commonly found. It was given the name wolf spider because of the way it chases after its prey rather than lying in wait on a web. The European wolf spider does not harm humans, unlike the bite of the poisonous South American tarantula, which was said to cause maniacal behavior, twitching, and the feeling of suffocating. The homeopathic remedy is made from the whole live spider and is used to treat restless, frantic behavior.

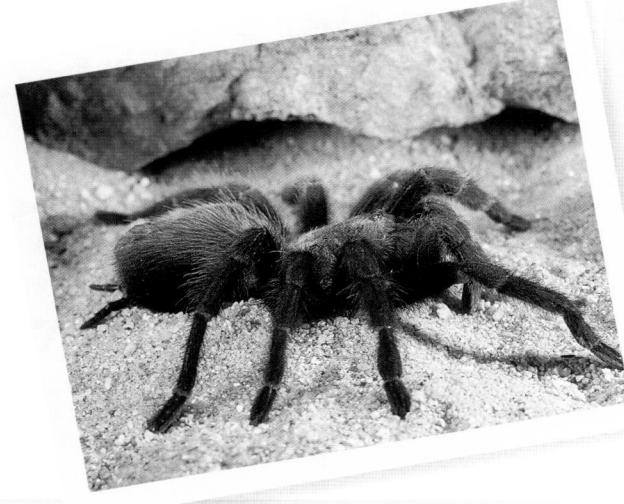

DATA FILE

Relieves

- mental and physical restlessness
- mood swings
- heart complaints
- in women, ovarian disease, genital sensitivity

Uses

It can be used to treat nervous disorders, such as mental and physical agitation, twitchy, restless legs, numbness, extreme mood swings, and impatience. Angina and heart disease also respond well. In women, sensitivity of the genitalia, which become itchy, heavy menstrual

bleeding, and ovarian disease which feels worse on the left side of the body can be alleviated.

Which type of person?

- hyperactive, behave destructively
- extremely impatient
- manipulative
- suffer vertigo
- workaholic

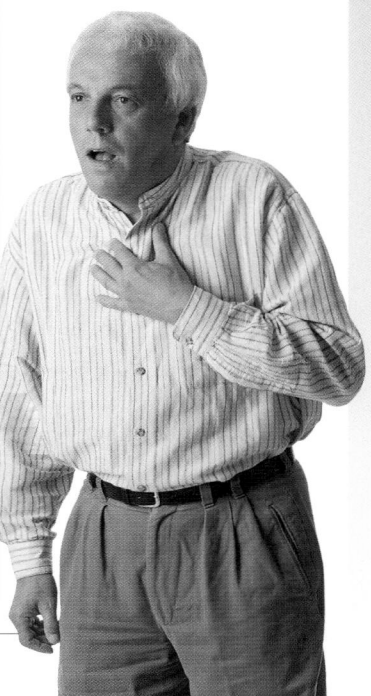

LEFT *The European wolf spider is the source of Tarentula. The whole spider is used in this preparation.*

RIGHT *Choking and feelings of suffocation caused by heart problems can be helped by this remedy.*

Thuja occidentalis, arbor vitae,
white cedar, tree of life

THUJA

The name thuja comes from the Greek word *thero*, meaning to sacrifice or fumigate. In pagan sacrifices, the tree was burnt when victims were executed. The evergreen tree is grown in Canada and the U.S., and Native Americans used its twigs and leaves to treat rheumatism, gout, and malaria. In homeopathy, the scented leaves and twigs are pounded to a pulp to make both the remedy and a cream that is especially useful for rheumatic pain.

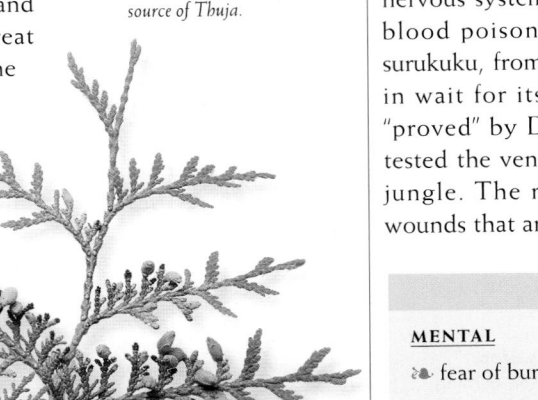

ABOVE *and* BELOW
Leaves of Thuja occidentalis, a member of the extensive Cupressus family, which is the source of Thuja.

DATA FILE

Relieves

- inflamed, swollen joints
- skin complaints
- genitourinary infections

Uses

Thuja can be used for joints that have become swollen and inflamed, as in rheumatism; for skin complaints, particularly warts, and for pale, greasy skin which sweats when exposed; urinary infections; headaches brought on by stress or fatigue; yellow-green catarrh; foul-smelling perspiration; tooth decay; weak nails; in women, for uterine or vaginal infections, early or scant menstruation, and loss of appetite in the morning; gurgling bowels.

Which type of person?

- greasy, pale skin
- take little interest in physical appearance
- sensitive, weep easily
- prefer tea and dislike meat, potatoes, fat
- children are small, with a slim build, and are slow

SYMPTOMS

MENTAL

- paranoia that others are taking advantage
- anxiety
- fear of strangers
- odd fixations

PHYSICAL

- headaches
- warts
- weak nails
- urinary conditions
- catarrh

Symptoms improve when warm in bed and with movement, and worsen in the cold and damp, at night, and on the left side of the body.

Trigonocephalus lachesis,
Lachesis muta, bushmaster snake, surukuku

LACHESIS

The South American bushmaster snake is extremely poisonous – one bite into a vein can cause immediate death – as the venom affects the heart and central nervous system. A lesser bite will cause bleeding and blood poisoning. The snake gets its other name, surukuku, from the humming sound it makes as it lies in wait for its prey. Homeopathically, it was first "proved" by Dr. Constantine Hering in 1837, who tested the venom on himself while in the Amazonian jungle. The remedy uses fresh venom, and treats wounds that are slow to heal or that bleed profusely.

SYMPTOMS

MENTAL

- fear of burglars, poisoning, water, suffocating, death
- disgruntled on waking
- strong ideas and philosophies
- suspicious of people
- jealous
- suffer nightmares
- prone to post-menopausal depression
- short-tempered

PHYSICAL

- blueness around skin problems
- bloating
- restlessness
- oversensitivity to touch and noise
- weak areas include the left side of the body, circulation, nervous system, and female reproductive organs

Symptoms improve after discharges, such as menstruation, nosebleeds, or bowel movements, in fresh air, and after a cold drink, and are worse on the left side, with sleep, when touched, with motion, in heat, and after hot drinks.

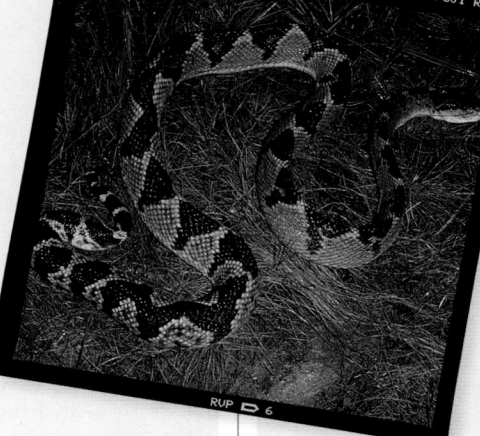

LEFT *The deadly bushmaster snake, native of the Amazonian jungle, is the source of Lachesis.*

DATA FILE

Relieves

- premenstrual and menopausal complaints
- circulatory and vascular problems
- left-sided complaints
- slow-healing wounds

Uses

Helpful for premenstrual problems such as erratic pain relieved by blood flow, and problems associated with the menopause, such as hot flushes and dizziness. It works well for any problems connected with blood flow and circulation, such as varicose veins, irregular pulse, angina, and palpitations. Problems which occur on the left side, for example earache, headaches, and sore throats, can be alleviated; wounds that are not healing well, such as bleeding piles, ulcers, and cuts are helped. Other conditions include nervous disorders such as fainting and petit mal epileptic attacks; blue wounds; purplish, bloated face; fever; sweats; any pulsations or throbbing; waking up with a sensation of choking; and glands which are swollen.

Which type of person?

- tend to be redheaded, freckled, pale-skinned
- puffy or bloated-looking
- egocentric, with no regard for others

- intuitive, creative, aspiring
- selfish, devious, jealous
- dislike commitment, blow hot and cold with partners
- dislike being restricted
- strong ideologists
- may be gloomy and quiet
- creativity is short-lived
- prefer sour and starchy foods and alcohol, and cannot tolerate hot drinks and wheat
- children tend to be hyperactive and difficult to control, prone to jealousy, possessive of friends, but may hurt them with their poisonous tongue

RIGHT *Urtica cream is available to alleviate rashes and stinging, smarting or burning skin conditions.*

Urtica urens, stinging nettle

URTICA

The stinging nettle, a common weed found in many countries, has been used for centuries for its medicinal properties. The Greek physician Dioscorides used it as a purgative and detoxification. It is commonly used in herbal medicine for conditions such as piles, nosebleeds, stomach conditions, and as a tea. The 16th-century herbalist John Gerard used it as an antidote to poison. The small plant is covered in soft, spiny hairs which secrete a sap that causes itching and inflammation if touched. In homeopathy, it was first "proved" by Hahnemann and is used to treat conditions which are accompanied by stinging or burning. Urtica can be used externally in the form of a cream, as well as taken internally.

ABOVE *Allergic reactions, to stings or to eating foods such as strawberries, can be helped by this remedy.*

THERAPY CONNECTIONS

NETTLE

Herbalism   *p.137*

DATA FILE

Relieves

- stinging, burning conditions of the skin
- rheumatic pain
- neuralgia

Uses

Used both as an internal remedy and externally as a cream, Urtica is useful for skin conditions, particularly if the skin is stinging or has the sensation of burning. It is good for rashes where the skin is blotchy and blistered, such as urticaria (hives) and bee stings, or when there is an allergic reaction, for instance after eating strawberries. Other conditions which it can be used to alleviate include rheumatism, neuralgia, neuritis, gout, excess uric acid, and, in women, vulval itching and painful breasts when the milk flow is blocked.

Which type of person?

- no particular type

BELOW *The common stinging nettle is the source of Urtica, also known as Urtica urens and Urt. u.*

SYMPTOMS

MENTAL

- none in particular

PHYSICAL

- stinging, burning skin
- rheumatic pain
- cystitis
- gout

Symptoms improve after massaging the affected area and when lying down, and worsen in cold, damp air, if touched, and with water.

FLOWER REMEDIES

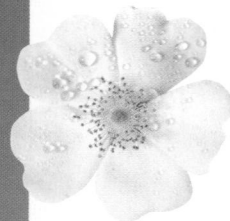

Flower essences, or flower remedies, as they are more commonly known, are used therapeutically to harmonize the body, mind, and the spirit. The essences are said to contain the life force of the flowers used to make them. Thousands of essences are available in health food stores, and they work "vibrationally" on a mental and emotional level, to relieve negative feelings, encourage the healing process, and to balance the energy in the body.

ABOVE *Flower remedies draw on the vibrational power of flowers like wild rose.*

Flower remedies are ideal for home use, being simple to make and use. They are prepared in water and preserved with alcohol. Historically, flower water and the morning dew collected from flower petals were thought to be imbued with magical properties. That flower remedies work is indisputable; but no one knows how, so there is still an element of magic associated with their use – even today, when our understanding of vibrational medicine is growing.

Flower remedies are so simple that they are often dismissed as a placebo. They do not work in any biochemical way, and because no physical part of the plant remains in the remedy, its properties and actions cannot be detected or analyzed as if it were a drug or herbal preparation. Therapists believe the remedies contain the energy, or imprint, of the plant from which it was made and work in a way that is similar to homeopathic remedies. In this way a remedy is believed to provide the stimulus needed to kick-start your own healing mechanism.

DR. BACH

Until recently, the name Dr. Edward Bach was almost synonymous with flower remedies. His set of 38 remedies became the inspiration for the worldwide development of remedies. They are still the cornerstone of flower remedy therapy and easily available. While working in the London Homeopathic Hospital, just after the First World War, he noticed that people with similar attitudes often had similar complaints. He concluded that, independently of other factors, mood and a negative attitude predisposed people toward ill health, and that illness was a manifestation of a deeper disharmony or an indication that the personality was in conflict. Between 1928 and 1932 he identified seven main negative states and found the first 12 of the flower remedies he needed to address them. Over the subsequent few years, he dedicated himself to finding natural remedies from the countryside, and at his death had made 38 separate remedies. His successors at his house in Oxfordshire, Mount Vernon, continue to make his remedies today, and they are sold under the name Bach Flower Remedies.

OTHER REMEDIES

The Bach Flower Remedies are made from the trees and flowers Dr. Bach saw on his travels, which are native to England, with the exceptions of Olive and Vine. In the last 20 years, remedies from the U.S. and Australia have been made. Sometimes they are called flower essences (do not confuse them with essential oils), but they are said to work in the same way as the original flower remedies. They address the emotional self, unlocking repressions, liberating negativity, and encouraging positive well-being.

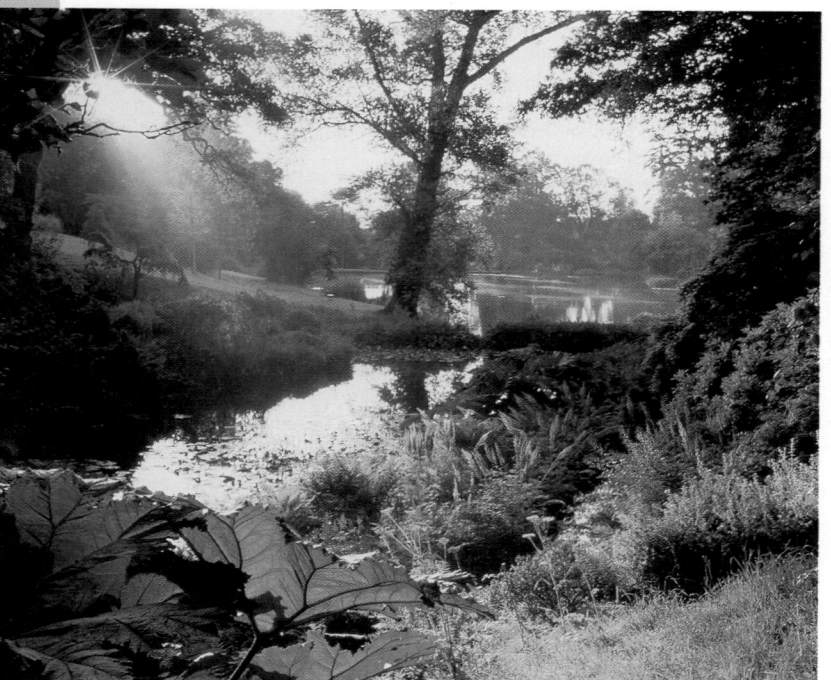

LEFT *Dr. Edward Bach, the originator of the Bach Flower Remedies, sought his ingredients in the English countryside and tested them all on himself.*

THE FUTURE
The world is more complex than it was in 1920, more is demanded, and people have to delve deeper to find the reserves to cope. Human nature has not changed, however, so the same 38 remedies Dr. Bach found still form a complete system that can address all human emotions. Nevertheless, many people have started to make new essences, and remedies are available now from all corners of the world.

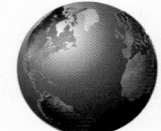

UNITED KINGDOM
It was in the U.K. that Dr. Edward Bach first identified and began to harness the healing power of flowers.

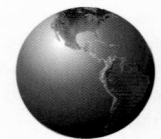

UNITED STATES
American flower essence makers have developed remedies according to the needs of late 20th-century society.

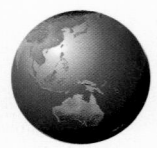

AUSTRALIA
Flower essence makers in Australia have used the natural fauna of their own country to create Australian Bush remedies.

THE BACH FLOWER REMEDIES: A QUICK GUIDE

NEGATIVITY CONTRIBUTES TO ILL HEALTH

Negative emotions depress the mind and immune system, repress activity, and contribute to ill health. All are rooted in one or more of the following, which are headings under which Dr. Bach grouped his 38 remedies:

- fear
- uncertainty
- insufficient interest in present circumstances
- loneliness
- oversensitivity to influences and ideas
- despondency or despair
- over-care for the welfare of others

By learning the healing capacity of peace, hope, joy, faith, certainty, wisdom, and love it is possible to develop a positive outlook and a sense of well-being.

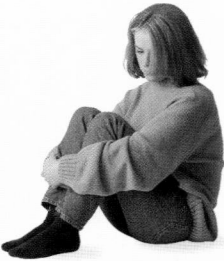

ABOVE *Negative emotions have a detrimental effect on the health.*

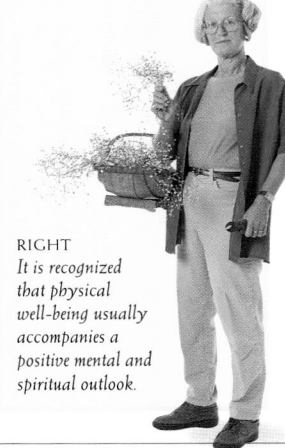

RIGHT *It is recognized that physical well-being usually accompanies a positive mental and spiritual outlook.*

- **AGRIMONY** For those who hide their feelings behind humor and put on a brave face.

- **ASPEN** For fear of the unknown; vague, unsettling fears which cannot be explained.

- **BEECH** For the perfectionist who tends to be intolerant of other people's methods and experience.

- **CENTAURY** For those who find it impossible to say no to the demands of others and thus exhaust themselves by doing too much.

- **CERATO** For those who lack confidence in themselves and are constantly seeking the advice of others to make up their mind.

- **CHERRY PLUM** For the fear of loosing one's mind, and for irrational thoughts or behavior.

- **CHESTNUT BUD** For those who find it hard to learn from life and keep making the same mistakes.

- **CHICORY** For the self-obsessed, mothering type who is overprotective and possessive.

- **CLEMATIS** For the absent-minded daydreamer who needs to be awake and focus the mind on the here and now.

- **CRAB APPLE** For those who feel unclean or polluted on any level, either physically, emotionally, or spiritually; Crab Apple is for those who feel they need purification.

- **ELM** For those who suffer temporary feelings of inadequacy brought on by all the responsibilities they have taken on.

- **GENTIAN** For despondency, and for those who are easily discouraged by a setback in life.

- **GORSE** For those who suffer feelings of hopelessness and despair, and who are stuck in a negative pattern; pessimism.

- **HEATHER** For those who like to be listened to when they talk constantly about themselves; for poor listeners and those who are self-obsessed.

- **HOLLY** For those who suffer dissipating bouts of hatred, jealousy, envy, and suspicion.

- **HONEYSUCKLE** For those who suffer from nostalgia or who dwell on the events of the past instead of living in the present.

- **HORNBEAM** For those who are stuck in a rut and feel tired, so that work which used to be fulfiling is now tiresome.

- **IMPATIENS** For impatience and irritability; Impatiens helps those for whom life is always a rush and who are too busy to slow down.

- **LARCH** For those who feel worthless and are suffering from lack of confidence or low self-esteem.

- **MIMULUS** For the fear of known things; for the strength to face everyday fears and all fears which can be named.

- **MUSTARD** For depression without cause, those who feel they are under a dark gloomy cloud for no apparent reason.

- **OAK** For the fighter who never gives in and is exhausting himself or herself by being too persistent in the same old fight.

- **OLIVE** For those who are exhausted on all levels, fatigued, and drained of further optimism and spirit after a long struggle or effort.

- **PINE** For those who suffer self-reproach and guilt; for those who say sorry even when things are not their fault.

- **RED CHESTNUT** For those who are overanxious about the welfare of family or friends; for those who fear that something awful may happen to their loved ones.

- **ROCK ROSE** For those who feel helpless and experience extreme terror or panic, when there may or may not be a reason but the feeling is real.

- **ROCK WATER** For perfectionists who are hard on themselves and demand perfection in all things.

- **SCLERANTHUS** For those who suffer from indecision and who cannot make up their mind.

- **STAR OF BETHLEHEM** For shocks of all kinds, accidents, bad news, sudden startling noise, and trauma.

- **SWEET CHESTNUT** For utter despair and hopelessness; for when there seems no way out.

- **VERVAIN** For enthusiasts and those with a strong sense of justice; those who never rest in their pursuit of an aim.

- **VINE** For the over-strong and dominating leader who may tend toward tyranny; for bullying.

- **WALNUT** For change; for breaking links so that life may develop without hindrance.

- **WATER VIOLET** For people who are aloof, self-reliant, and self-contained; to relax the reserved and enable sharing.

- **WHITE CHESTNUT** For tiresome mental chatter and the overactive mind, full of persistent and unwanted patterns of thought.

- **WILD OAT** For those who need help in deciding on the path and purpose of their life.

- **WILD ROSE** For those who drift through life resigned to accept any eventuality; for fatalists and people too apathetic to try.

- **WILLOW** For those who feel they have been treated unfairly; for resentment and self-pity.

USING FLOWER REMEDIES

Flower remedies are simple and effective, and they can be used:

- ❀ to support in times of crisis.
- ❀ to treat the emotional outlook produced by illness.
- ❀ to address a particular recurring emotional or behavioral pattern.
- ❀ to give strength during a temporary emotional setback.
- ❀ as a preventive remedy when things start to go out of balance.

Remedies act swiftly for passing moods and there should be an improvement very quickly, although it may take months to start to change a long-standing pattern.

The flower remedies or essences bought in a store are sold in stock bottles. They can be used straight from the bottle, but it is better to make a personal remedy mix. Sometimes a single flower remedy is needed, but in most cases two or more are combined.

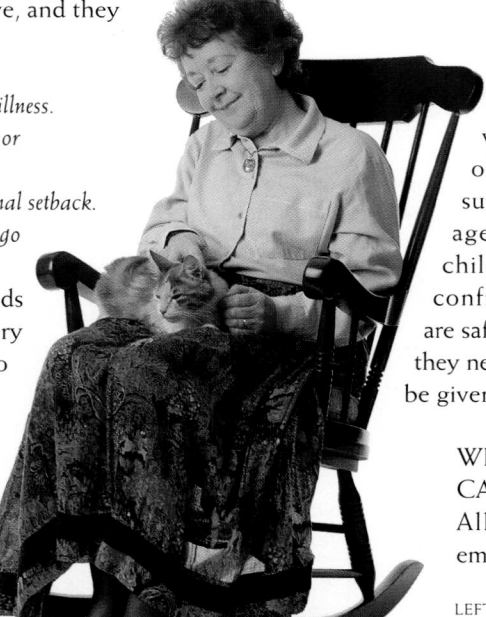

LEFT *Many claim that animals as well as people can be helped by flower remedies.*

ARE THEY SAFE?

The remedies are not addictive or dangerous, nor do they interfere with any other form of treatment. They are suitable for people of all ages. Pregnant women and children can take them with confidence. Flower remedies are safe for young babies, should they need them, and they can also be given to animals and plants.

WHICH PROBLEMS CAN THEY HELP?

All types of mental or emotional problems.

USING THE REMEDIES

Successful treatment depends on accurate diagnosis. Get to know the different essences available and then aim to match the remedies to the individual character.

FOR YOURSELF If you find it hard to decide on a remedy, make a note of the one you think you need and then ask yourself the same questions you would ask anyone for whom you were prescribing:

- ✵ How do you feel?
- ✵ Why are you feeling like that?
- ✵ How do the symptoms affect you?
- ✵ What could have caused the problem?

FOR CHILDREN Children show their nature in their behavior and play. Try to match the behavior of the child to the remedy:

- ✵ Is the child always active like Vervain?
- ✵ Timid and shy like Mimulus?
- ✵ Gentle and obedient like Centaury?
- ✵ Bossy like Vine?
- ✵ Or sulky like Willow?

FOR ANIMALS You need to know the animal's nature and note how differently it behaves when ill. For example, a dog which looks sorry for itself needs Willow; an aggressive one needs Holly or Vine; and cats often need Water Violet for their pride and independence. Add 4 drops to a small animal's drinking water, and 10 drops for large animals such as horses and cows. Add more drops whenever the water is replaced.

TO MAKE A PERSONAL REMEDY

✣ You'll need:

– 1fl.oz. (30ml.) amber glass dropper bottle
– 1fl.oz. (30ml.) spring water; or 1 teaspoon (5ml.) brandy and 5 teaspoons (25ml.) spring water

✣ Decide on the remedies which are most applicable. Usually between one and six is enough. If you think you need several, simplify to a maximum of seven covering immediate issues, and check again in a few weeks.

✣ Put 2 drops of each remedy into a clean 1fl.oz. (30ml.) amber glass dropper bottle. This is the standard amount, but read the label, as occasionally some of the newer essences suggest you use 4 or 7 drops.

✣ If the remedies are to be used within a week, fill the bottle with clean spring water.

✣ If the remedies are to be taken for a prolonged period, add 1 teaspoonful (5ml.) of brandy to the bottle and then fill with spring water.

✣ Label the bottle with your name and the date.

✣ Give the remedy a title or a few words to remind you of the purpose. Would an affirmation be useful?

✣ Take as directed (*see below*).

✣ Keep remedies, like other medicines, out of the reach of children.

To use

✣ The standard dose is 4 drops, on or under the tongue, 4 times a day.

✣ At times of crisis, 2 drops from the stock bottle can be put into a glass of water (or, in an emergency, any drink) and sipped as needed.

✣ If for any reason it is impossible to take anything by mouth, put the drops on the skin or in washing water.

BELOW *Flower essences are usually added to water; up to six kinds are mixed.*

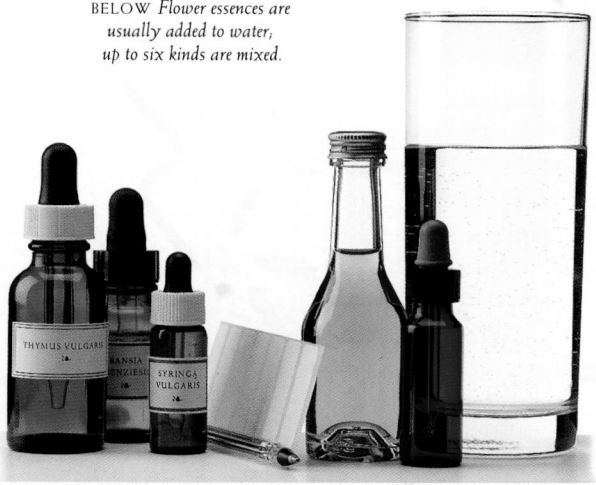

CHILDREN

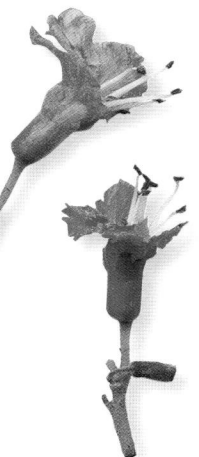

ABOVE *The flowers of Red Chestnut are a good remedy for parents who are over-anxious about their family's welfare.*

❋ Flower remedies are ideal for children. Treat them as soon as you notice that something is "not quite right."

❋ Physical symptoms must be professionally treated. Consult a physician if in doubt.

❋ Listen and do not trivialize children's emotional lives. Be calm and methodical. Notice the mood or address a previously known pattern. Give the remedy for a day or two, then reassess. Moods in children may change rapidly.

❋ If worried about a child (or other family member) take Red Chestnut, Rescue Remedy, or any other remedy which seems relevant, to settle yourself before deciding on treatment.

❋ If the child is of breast-feeding age, give the remedy to the mother. It may also be put in the bath: for example, use Impatiens to treat the hot and restless frustration of a teething baby.

❋ Support the parents. If home nursing, give Mimulus to minimize known fears. Give Rescue Remedy and Walnut if the child is hospitalized. Other remedies may be applicable.

❋ Treat the parents. Their emotional problems (even if suppressed) may be the root of a child's distress.

ATTITUDE AND AFFIRMATIONS

Flower remedies should not be taken without thought and due care.

Ask these questions:
❧ Why is it needed?
❧ What do I expect?
There should be a clear reason for taking a herb or remedy and a positive treatment aim or goal.

Some people recommend the use of affirmations, suggesting that an appropriate affirmation is written down several times a day for a week while taking the remedy. An example of a positive affirmation for the Clematis daydreamer would be: "I am awake (or becoming awake) and open to the experience of here and now."

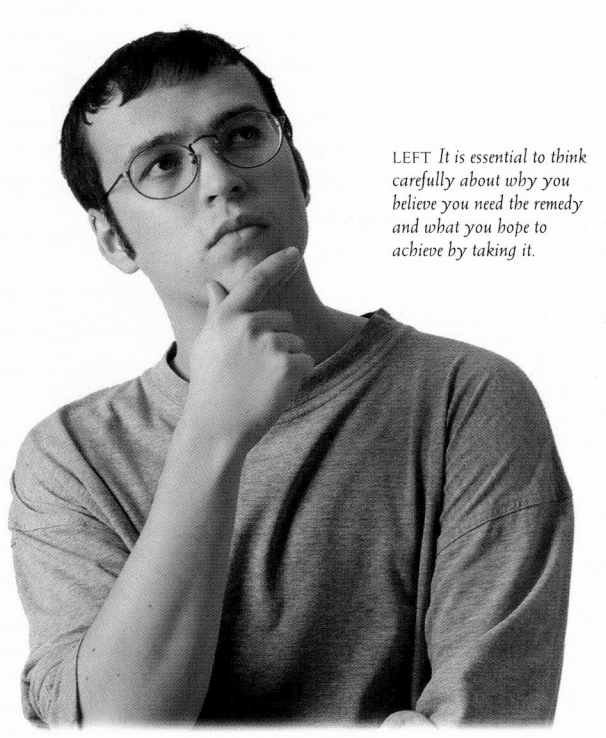

LEFT *It is essential to think carefully about why you believe you need the remedy and what you hope to achieve by taking it.*

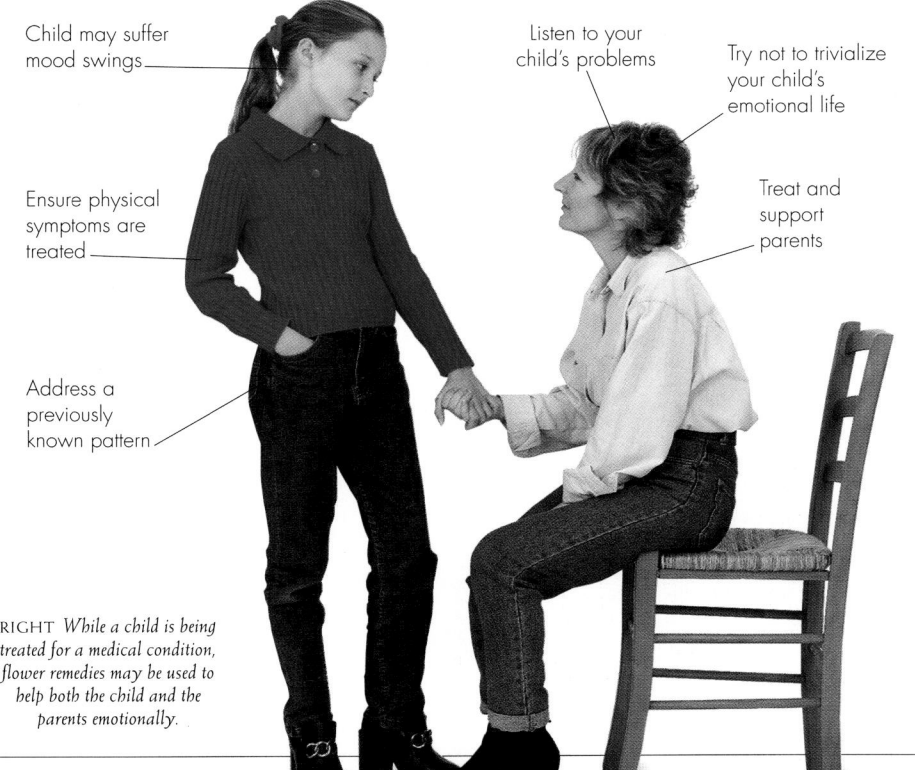

Child may suffer mood swings

Listen to your child's problems

Try not to trivialize your child's emotional life

Ensure physical symptoms are treated

Treat and support parents

Address a previously known pattern

RIGHT *While a child is being treated for a medical condition, flower remedies may be used to help both the child and the parents emotionally.*

REMEDIES AND ALCOHOL

Flower remedies and essences are preserved in alcohol. The amount of alcohol in a personal remedy made solely with water is minute, but it is enough to upset those who are alcohol intolerant or recovering from alcoholism. Always check the status of those to whom you give a remedy. Thoughtlessness can do untold damage.

It is possible to remove the alcohol by putting the diluted drops of remedy in a boiling hot drink – the steam will evaporate the alcohol. Leave the remedy to cool before taking. Sip throughout the day.

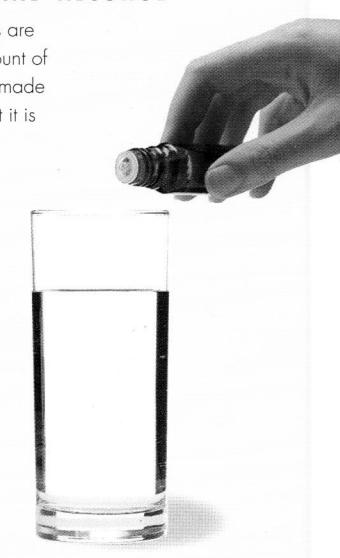

ABOVE *The remedies can be taken in hot or cold water as the patient prefers.*

MAKING THE REMEDIES

HOW TO MAKE FLOWER REMEDIES

Flower remedies are simple to make, and rewarding and effective to use. Remedies are made in two ways: the sun method and the boiling method.

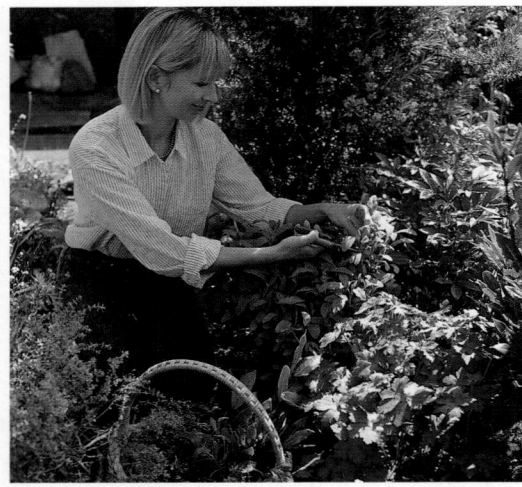

ABOVE *Whichever method you are using, collect your materials on a fine day, preferably before noon.*

Whatever the method there are a few basic rules:

CORRECT IDENTIFICATION Find the plant and site well before the day of picking. Make sure that it is legal to pick it or that you have the landowner's permission.

PREPARATION Collect essentials. Absolute cleanliness is essential. Wash your hands and rinse them several times. Utensils can be cleaned by boiling in spring or rain water for 20 minutes and then allowing them to drain dry. Wrap them in a clean cloth to keep them ready for a suitable day.

THE RIGHT DAY For sun method remedies, choose a warm, sunny day with no clouds. For boiling method remedies any bright, sunny day is good.

ON THE DAY Pick with respect. Remember that you are making a remedy and what the remedy is designed to treat. Pick flowers that you are drawn to. Pick from all sides of the plant, from the top and bottom branches of trees, or from a wide area with meadow plants. Work quickly so there is only a little time between picking the flowers and putting them into the water to make the remedy. If you need to carry the flowers, cover your palm with a large leaf (preferably from the plant being picked) to prevent the heat and oils from the hand contaminating the blossoms. Use a twig to stir and remove the flowers.

LABELING When you have finished, label and date your remedy clearly. Keep it in a cool, dark place, away from direct sunlight.

Pick when the flowers are coming into full bloom. This will depend on the climate and the type of season, but the following can serve as a general guide:

❖ **EARLY SPRING:** oak, gorse, olive, vine.
❖ **LATE SPRING:** white chestnut, water violet.
❖ **SUMMER:** rock water, mimulus, agrimony, rock rose, centaury.
❖ **LATE SUMMER:** scleranthus, wild oat, impatiens, chicory, vervain, clematis, heather.
❖ **FALL:** cerato, gentian.

A 3fl.oz. (100ml.) bottle of mother tincture will last the average family many years. The recipe can make more, up to six bottles. If you wish to make more for family or friends, prepare more bottles. Each 3fl.oz. (100ml.) should contain 1½fl.oz. (50ml.) of brandy and be made up as outlined below:

❖ You'll need:
 bottle of spring or mineral water
 plain glass bowl
 3fl.oz. (100ml.) amber bottle(s)
 1½fl.oz. (50ml.) brandy
 natural and unbleached filter paper
 pen and label

❖ Decide beforehand on the plants, where to pick from, and where to place the bowl, then wait for a suitable sunny day.

THE SUN METHOD

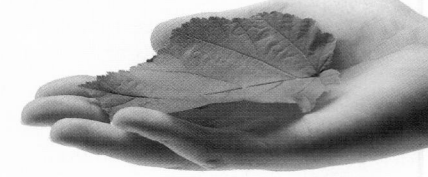

ABOVE *Use a leaf, ideally of the plant being picked, to protect the flowers from the heat of your hand.*

The bowl should be placed in a clear open place, as close to the plants as possible, but away from shadows and possible contamination.

❖ The best time of the day for harvesting the plants is between 9 A.M. and midday. The flowers are dry from the dew, but not yet exhausted by the sun.
❖ Pick the flowers and put in the water as quickly as possible.
❖ Float the flowers on the water until the whole surface is covered. Use a twig or leaf to arrange them, not your fingers.
❖ Leave the bowl out in the open where it will receive direct sunshine for three hours.
❖ After 3 hours, remove the flowers with a twig and filter the liquid.
❖ Pour 1½fl.oz. (50ml.) of the water into the bottle with the brandy. Shake and label with the name, "flower essence mother tincture," and date. This mother tincture will be used to prepare stock bottles and it will keep for many years. To prepare a stock bottle, put 2 drops of mother tincture into a 1fl.oz. (30ml.) dropper bottle, and top up with brandy. Then, from the stock bottle, use 2 drops to make up the treatment bottle as already described.

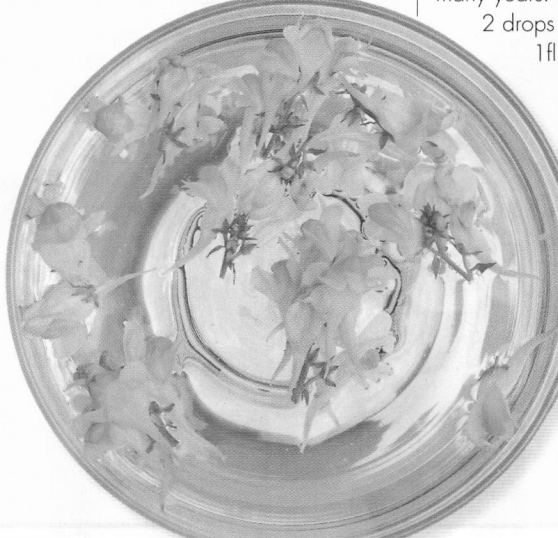

LEFT *Leave the flowers floating on the surface of the water in the sun.*

THE BOILING METHOD

The boiling method is mainly used for the flowers of trees. In any case, more than just the flower are picked – in addition, it is necessary to collect twigs that have a few leaves on them.

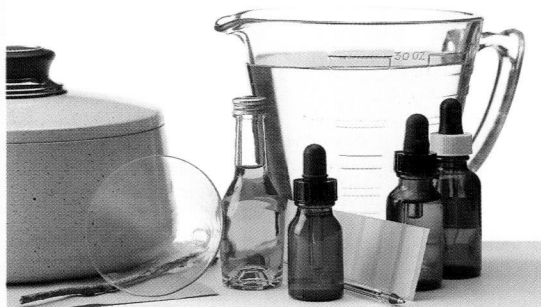

ABOVE *The equipment needed for the boiling method, which is used for the flowers of trees.*

Pick when the flowers are at their best:
* EARLY SPRING: cherry plum.
* SPRING: elm, aspen.
* LATE SPRING: beech, chestnut bud, hornbeam, larch, walnut, and Star of Bethlehem.
* LATE SPRING: holly, crab apple, willow.
* EARLY SUMMER: red chestnut, pine, mustard.
* SUMMER: honeysuckle, sweet chestnut, wild rose.

Again, cleanliness is vital to avoid contamination. Sterilize utensils.
* You'll need:
  6pt. (3l.) saucepan with lid (use an enamel, glass, or stainless steel pan; avoid copper, aluminum, and Teflon-coated pans)
  a glass measuring jug
  2pt. (1l.) of cold water (rain water or mineral water)
  3fl.oz. (100ml.) amber glass bottle(s) (up to six)
  1½fl.oz. (50ml.) of brandy
  natural and unbleached filter paper
  pen and label

* Decide on the plants beforehand; prepare and clean the utensils. If you are going to boil the remedy outside, check your camping stove and equipment. Wait for the perfect day.
* Take everything into the field between 9A.M. and 11A.M. on a sunny day.
* Touch as little as possible. Pick twigs or flowers until the saucepan is three-quarters full; put on the lid and take to the heat source as quickly as possible.
* When the pan is on the heat source, cover the flowers and twigs with the cold water and bring to the boil.
* Once it has reached boiling point, simmer for a half-hour. Use a twig from the tree to push the twigs under the water.
* After a half-hour, remove the pan from the heat, put the lid on it, and stand it outside to cool.
* When cool, remove the twigs, then carefully filter the water into the jug.
* Put 1½fl.oz. (50ml.) of the flower water into the 3fl.oz. (100ml.) bottle(s) with the brandy. Label with the name, "flower essence mother tincture," and date.
  This is the mother tincture from which a stock bottle is made. It will keep for many years, and is used to make up personal remedies as previously described.

SEEING A PROFESSIONAL

Flower remedies were created to be so simple to use that people could treat themselves. However, many practitioners of other disciplines – such as herbalism, homeopathy, and aromatherapy – use flower remedies to complement their own remedies, and a few flower essence therapists use the remedies exclusively.

Most therapists have their own ways of working. But every consultation should begin with an interview between you and the therapist. This can last from as little as 15 minutes to over an hour. During this time the therapist will explain the system to you if you do not already know how it works. He or she will ask why you have come to see a therapist and will listen while you talk about yourself and your worries. The therapist will observe your posture and appearance, and will listen to the tone of your voice and the way you say things, as these can be as revealing as what you say. While you chat, the therapist may take notes and ask questions to work out, by a process of elimination, which remedies would be best for you. He or she might ask questions about your fears, how you feel about your children or other family members, or how easily you give up when something you attempt does not work out. It is not enough for the therapist to know that you have a problem at home or at work.

At the end of the consultation the therapist will help you select the remedies. The number of remedies prescribed depends on the individual, but it is unlikely to be more than six, and will often be much fewer. Most people feel at least a little better at the end of the consultation because they have been able to talk through their problems.

The Dr. Edward Bach Foundation maintains an international register of qualified practitioners in the Bach Flower Remedies. A list of practitioners may be obtained from the Bach Center (*see page 489*).

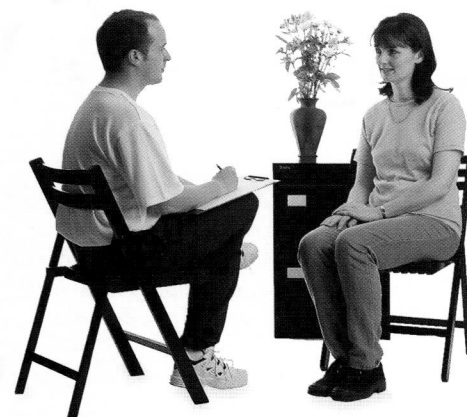

ABOVE *Talking through your problems is part of the consultation process.*

FLOWER ESSENCES

Aesculus carnea
RED CHESTNUT

This essence is extracted from the pink-flowered chestnut tree, which is frequently grown for ornamental decoration in parks.

DATA FILE

Use

❦ Red Chestnut is for those who suffer fear and anxiety for others. They may have forsaken worrying about themselves, but project their fear onto their loved ones. They often anticipate that some unfortunate accident or illness (the worst scenario) will befall friends and relations, and ceaselessly worry. This inappropriate fear limits the social interactions of both the sufferer and his or her loved ones. Red Chestnut helps us realize that the anxiety is a projection of personal fear. It brings the calm necessary to be sensitive to the real problems and concerns of our loved ones, and to give empathetic support.

Method

❦ The boiling method *(see page 223)*

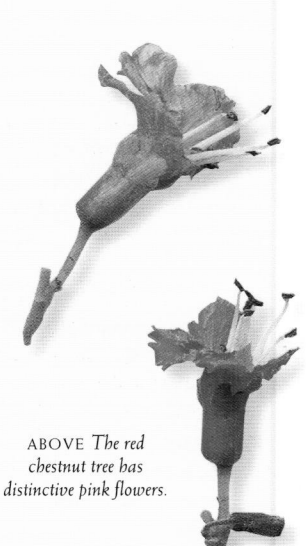

ABOVE *The red chestnut tree has distinctive pink flowers.*

PROFILE

🙠 GOAL – Sensitivity to others 🙠 **People who need Red Chestnut fear that something awful may happen to their loved ones.** 🙠 They experience unnecessary fear, over-worry, even hypochondria on another person's behalf. 🙠 **Red Chestnut encourages calm and rationality, a response based on sensitivity to others, to replace the projected fear.**

Aesculus hippocastanum
WHITE CHESTNUT

The common horse chestnut tree has distinctive, upright clusters of white flowers and divided spatulate leaves.

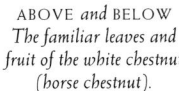

ABOVE *and* BELOW *The familiar leaves and fruit of the white chestnut (horse chestnut).*

DATA FILE

Use

When the mind is full of unwanted thoughts, ideas, or persistent and worrying mental arguments – overactive and exhausting mental chatter going round and round in a never-ending circle.

Method

❦ The sun method *(see page 222)*

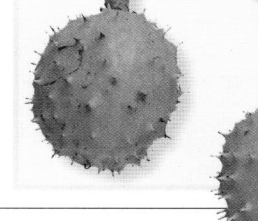

PROFILE

🙠 GOAL – Clear mind; clarity 🙠 **For people who suffer from constant mental chatter, persistent thoughts, and worries.** 🙠 **For sleeplessness due to worry.** 🙠 **White Chestnut switches off unwanted thoughts so that it is possible to find peace and mental clarity.** 🙠 Other remedies might be needed to address the root cause.

Aesculus hippocastanum
CHESTNUT BUD

The white chestnut tree is used to make two remedies: White Chestnut and Chestnut Bud. The large leaf buds, called "sticky buds," are picked when they are just about to open to make this particular essence.

DATA FILE

Use

For those who make the same mistake over and over again, and who are thus slow to learn from experience. Chestnut Bud is for people who find themselves stuck in the same repeating pattern, who regretfully do not seem able to learn the lessons of past experience, events, and relationships.

Method

❦ The boiling method *(see page 223)*

PROFILE

🙠 GOAL – Vision 🙠 **The person who needs Chestnut Bud may suffer poor health, chronic conditions may continually "flare up," or they may suffer from preventable illness.** 🙠 If the same pattern is continually repeated they are stuck in the energy of that moment. 🙠 **Chestnut Bud helps focus the mind and enable us to see our path with greater objectivity.**

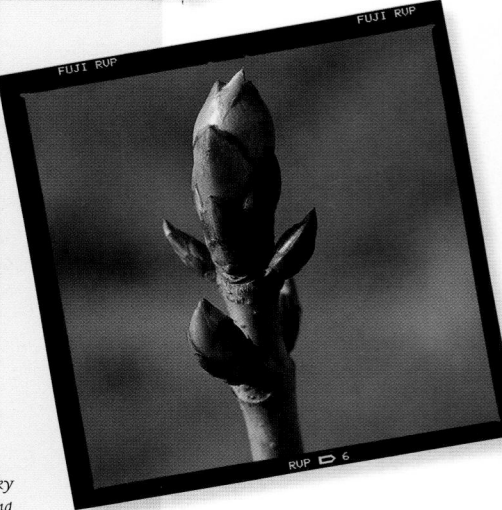

RIGHT *The leaves of the white chestnut or horse chestnut grow from the "sticky buds" produced in early spring.*

Agrimonia eupatoria
AGRIMONY

A wild plant with small yellow flowers on tapering spikes like church spires, sometimes known as "church steeples." The seed vessels are covered in hooked hairs and cling to animals coming into contact with them.

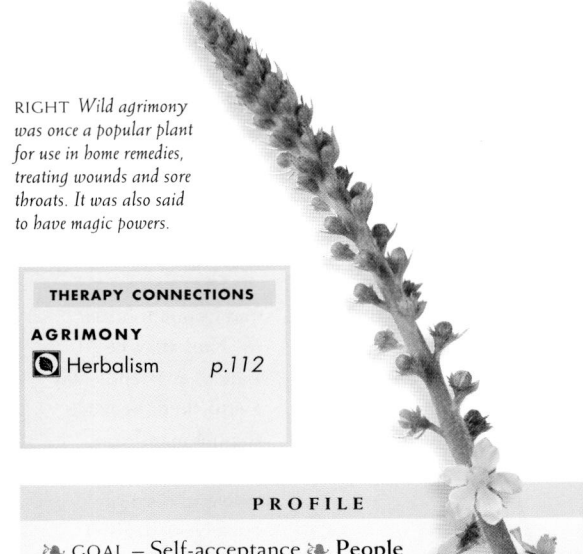

RIGHT *Wild agrimony was once a popular plant for use in home remedies, treating wounds and sore throats. It was also said to have magic powers.*

THERAPY CONNECTIONS

AGRIMONY

🜂 Herbalism   *p.112*

PROFILE

🍃 GOAL – Self-acceptance 🍃 **People who need Agrimony will put on a brave face of cheerfulness. Laughter hides things as well as being distracting; other distractions may be drink, drugs, or dangerous or thrill-seeking hobbies or occupations.** 🍃 They may be restless sleepers or unable to sleep without help. 🍃 **Agrimony helps us to love ourselves as we are, and to put aside the mask. It helps us cope with the difficult sides of our nature and use humor appropriately.**

DATA FILE

Use

For those who hide their problems and inner selves behind a cheerful face, masking real feelings of unhappiness and unworthiness. They are the life and soul of a party, and will make jokes, perhaps even inappropriately. The person who needs Agrimony finds it hard to deal with the darker, less pleasant parts of life and extreme emotions. They are reluctant to burden others and dread arguments, pursuing peace at all costs. This can lead to an inner anguish that is often masked by alcohol or drugs.

Method

🌿 The sun method *(see page 222)*

Anigozanthos manglesii
KANGAROO PAW

This large Australian perennial is one of the first plants to recolonize after bush fires. It is so named because the flowers at the end of the long stems resemble a kangaroo's front paw.

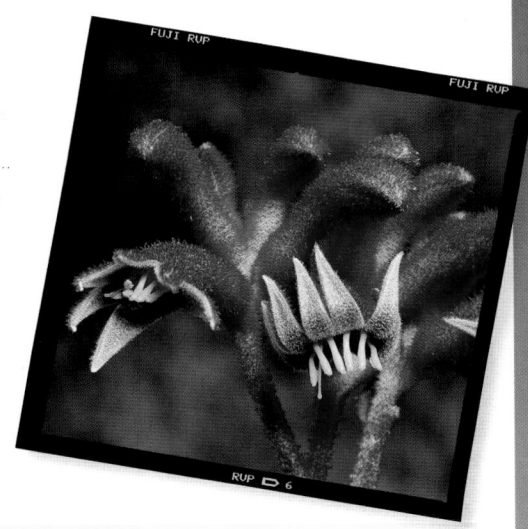

RIGHT *The flowers of kangaroo paw are a more recent addition to the list of available remedies.*

PROFILE

🍃 GOAL – Kindness and sensitivity
🍃 **For people who are inexperienced, socially inept, or embarrassed.**
🍃 Associated symptoms include clumsiness, nervousness, stuttering or stammering; blushing and embarrassment; shyness and timidity.
🍃 **Kangaroo Paw encourages sensitivity and empathy, and gives us the courage to just be, to accept, and be kind to ourselves and others. It allows us to experience true two-way communication.**

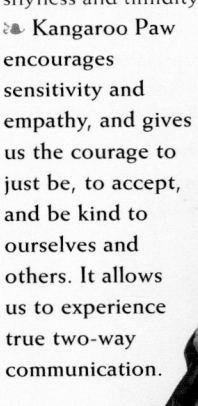

RIGHT *People who feel nervous and ill-at-ease with others can be helped to relax with Kangaroo Paw.*

DATA FILE

Use

For people who have poor social skills, and difficulties relating to and communicating with others, who are so self-conscious and self-aware that they feel "out of place" at work, at meetings, gatherings, or parties. This may be noticed by others and become a joke. Interactions feel like competitions, and they find it impossible to find the space to think before acting, or to be aware of other people's feelings. Kangaroo Paw makes it possible for them to relax and get in tune with themselves and others, and to become aware of their surroundings. It encourages sensitive and appropriate social interaction.

Method

🌿 The sun method *(see page 222)*; pick the whole cluster (or paw) of flowers

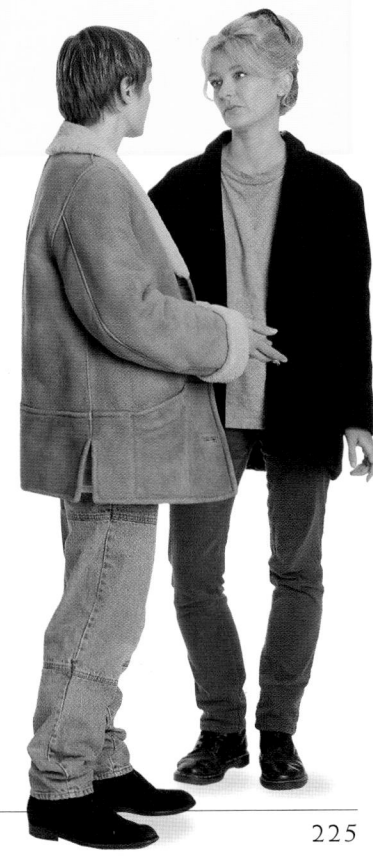

Bromus ramosus
WILD OAT

An elegant woodland grass, wild oat stands between 2 and 5 feet (½–1½m.) high. The common name is hairy or wood brome grass, because of the soft, hairy leaves.

PROFILE

🌿 GOAL – Meaningful purpose, a positive direction 🌿 **Wild Oat is for uncertainty and frustration with current activities, when a person has the desire to find a purpose, yet is aimless, drifting from one job or relationship to another.** 🌿 Wild Oat helps us listen to our calling, find our true vocation, and gives the strength of character to act on this.

DATA FILE

Use

Wild Oat is for capable people who have ambition to do something meaningful in their lives but have not yet found their true calling. They may have several choices or directions they could follow and may be working hard on a given path, but fundamentally they are dissatisfied and frustrated. Somewhere deep down they know that they have not found their vocation in life, and are emotionally or spiritually unsatisfied. Wild Oat helps to tune the heart to what will bring true meaning and purpose. It helps us to make choices, sometimes difficult, which unite all aspirations. It also helps us to balance the needs of spirituality and making a living.

Method

🌸 The sun method *(see page 222)*

THERAPY CONNECTIONS

WILD OATS
🔘 Herbalism   *p.117*

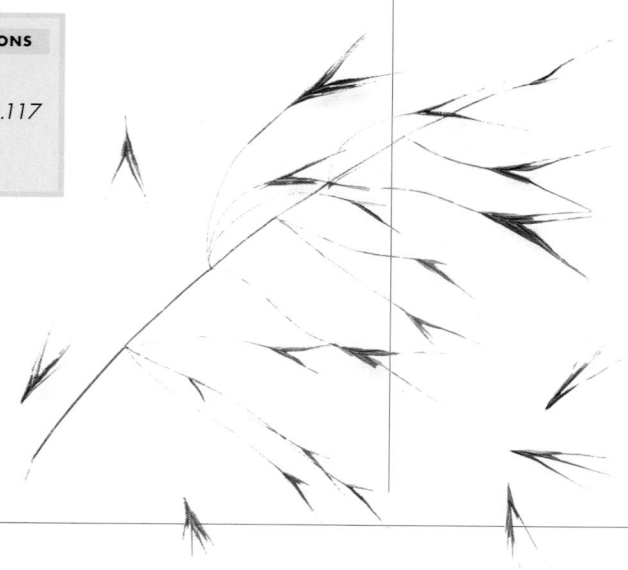

RIGHT *Wild oat is a hairy woodland grass, not to be confused with the common wild oat of open pastures.*

Calluna vulgaris
HEATHER

This common plant is often found in Alpine areas, on heaths, and waste ground. *Calluna* prefers acid soil. According to variety, flowers are produced from summer to fall.

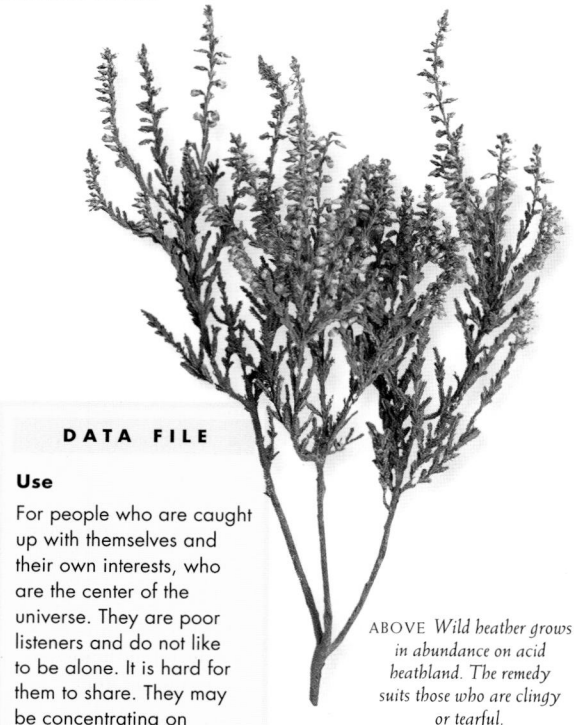

DATA FILE

Use

For people who are caught up with themselves and their own interests, who are the center of the universe. They are poor listeners and do not like to be alone. It is hard for them to share. They may be concentrating on fulfiling personal needs in order to avoid loneliness.

Method

🌸 The sun method *(see page 222)*

ABOVE *Wild heather grows in abundance on acid heathland. The remedy suits those who are clingy or tearful.*

BELOW *People who need Heather often become isolated from others because they are self-obsessed or demanding.*

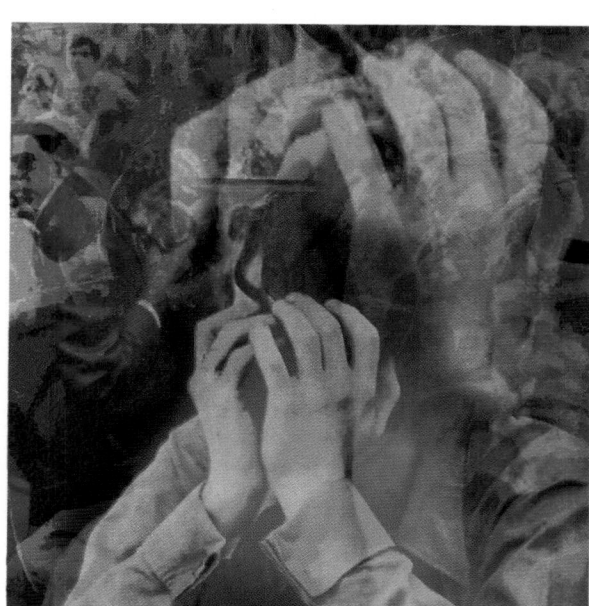

PROFILE

🌿 GOAL – Love with space to share; to listen: A useful affirmation might be: "I am listening and letting the love of the world nourish my heart." 🌿 **People who need Heather can be self-centered and self-obsessed. They may intrude into other people's personal space, cling, or be aggressively talkative.** 🌿 They can be weepy and hypochondriac. 🌿 **They may be lonely, as friends may avoid them because they demand too much.** 🌿 We should love and nurture ourselves. Heather helps us to look after ourselves without being obsessed with our own personal needs. It gives us the space to listen to others, and experience genuine love and companionship.

Carpinus betulus
HORNBEAM

A medium-sized, deciduous tree common in woods. It grows well in a sunny or lightly shaded position, and its leaves turn a rich yellow-orange in the fall.

DATA FILE

Use

Hornbeam is for those who feel that they do not possess enough strength to fulfill the responsibilities of daily life, for the "Monday morning blues." This feeling often comes from boredom or some basic dissatisfaction with the work they are doing. These people might feel that they are in the wrong job, or in some way not fully expressing their creative potential.

Hornbeam restores confidence and optimism, and helps us find the satisfaction in the mundane "nine-to-five" aspects of our lives.

Method

☙ The boiling method *(see page 223)*

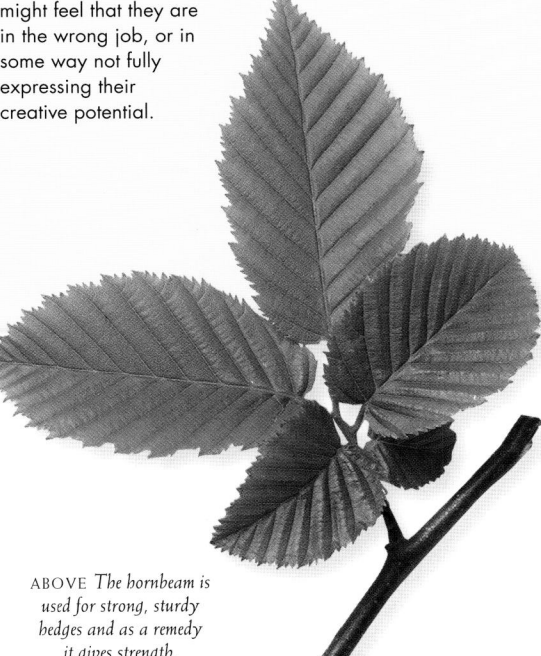

ABOVE *The hornbeam is used for strong, sturdy hedges and as a remedy it gives strength.*

PROFILE

☙ GOAL – Strength to carry out daily tasks
☙ **People who need Hornbeam feel exhausted at the thought of working. They may feel stuck in a rut.**
☙ Procrastination is a common avoidance stratagem.
☙ **Hornbeam is usually for a temporary feeling. If the weakness is a regular occurrence, the person may be exhausting himself or herself in the wrong direction, and other remedies may be needed.**

Castanea sativa
SWEET CHESTNUT

This chestnut tree produces edible fruits after its creamy flowers. The tree grows to 100ft. (30m.) and is deciduous.

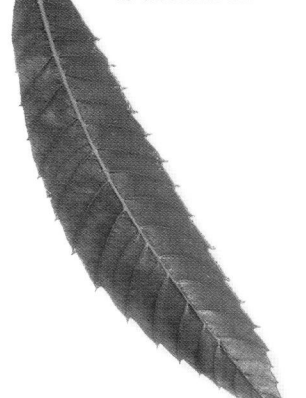

ABOVE *A leaflet and fruit of the edible chestnut tree, a remedy for anguish.*

PROFILE

☙ GOAL – Transformation; to widen the boundaries
☙ **Hornbeam is for the feeling Dr. Bach called the "dark night of the soul," when it feels that annihilation is all that will be left.**
☙ Associated symptoms may include sleep disturbance, hopelessness, and perhaps hidden despair.

DATA FILE

Use

Sweet Chestnut is for those moments when anguish is so great as to seem unbearable, when people feel that they have "come to the end of their tether," reached their limit, and are being stretched beyond endurance. When this happens things have to change. Sweet Chestnut helps to bring out hidden reserves, opening boundaries and expanding limits, which gives people the strength to grow.

Method

☙ The boiling method *(see page 223)*

Centaurium erythraea
CENTAURY

A small pink flower of chalky soil. It is named after a centaur in Greek mythology, who used it to cure himself from a poisoned arrow wound.

DATA FILE

Use

Centaury is for people who have an excessive desire to please and a willingness to serve. They can be taken for granted and exploited. Their will to help others is so strong that it undermines their individuality and they find it hard to say "no." They can become servants rather than helpers, and end up doing more than their fair share. This leads to frustration and a loss of self-confidence, appreciation, and expression. Their life becomes one of drudgery or self-martyrdom.

Method

☙ The sun method *(see page 222)*

PROFILE

☙ GOAL – Service, in the widest sense
☙ **People who need Centaury lack will-power; they may be tired and exhausted. Inner frustration and anger may sap their inner strength.**
☙ The "weaker" partner in a co-dependent relationship may benefit from Centaury. ☙ **Centaury helps balance the desire to serve by strengthening our will power and appreciation of ourselves. It helps us make a choice, to say "yes" or "no" from the heart.**

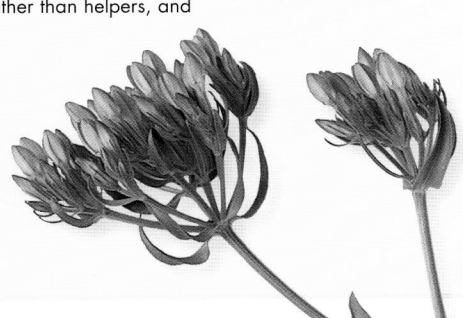

LEFT *The flowers of centaury, a plant which grows more readily in the wild than in cultivation.*

Ceratostigma willmottiana
CERATO

A small shrub with bright blue flowers which is often grown in gardens. It originally came from China and the Himalayas. Cerato is the only Bach Flower Remedy to be made from a cultivated plant.

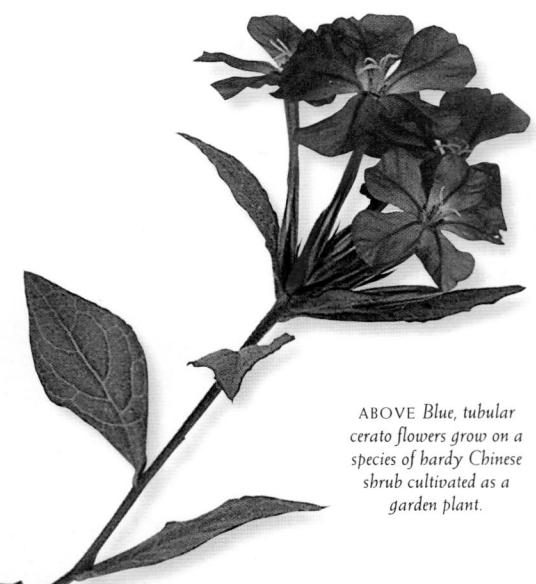

ABOVE *Blue, tubular cerato flowers grow on a species of hardy Chinese shrub cultivated as a garden plant.*

PROFILE

🍃 GOAL – Inner confidence; to trust intuition
🍃 People who need Cerato may appear weak-willed and silly. They lack constancy, and may imitate others or become an ever-changing "fashion victim."
🍃 They may join cults or take up fads. 🍃 Cerato helps us to listen to advice from within, restores confidence, and strengthens our trust in ourselves to follow our path even if it runs contrary to the expectations of others.

DATA FILE

Use
Cerato is for lack of trust in our own abilities and judgment. People who need Cerato are intelligent and curious, but they lack confidence in themselves, distrust their own intuition, and constantly seek the advice and approval of other people.

They like to be seen to be doing the "right thing."

Method
🌿 The sun method *(see page 222)*

Chicorium intybus
CHICORY

A wayside plant with bright blue flowers. It is cultivated as a vegetable and blanched as a bitter plant to add to salads. The flowers close in the afternoon and open again in the morning.

PROFILE

🍃 GOAL – Love, free-flowing and without strings
🍃 Those who need Chicory may be possessive and selfish. They may be fussy, nagging, and manipulative. They may be prone to illness if not "loved," or to hypochondria. 🍃 Chicory helps us to see love as a universal force, to give love selflessly and freely so that it may freely return to us.

DATA FILE

Use
Chicory is for those who see love as a transaction incurring duty, and as a method of control. They give love in order to receive it. Chicory types love and care publicly, even melodramatically, building up a stock of good works which they expect to be reciprocated, but love still does not flow their way.

Method
🌿 The sun method *(see page 222)*

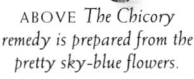

ABOVE *The Chicory remedy is prepared from the pretty sky-blue flowers.*

BELOW *Chicory helps people to be selfless in love, which makes for more satisfying relationships.*

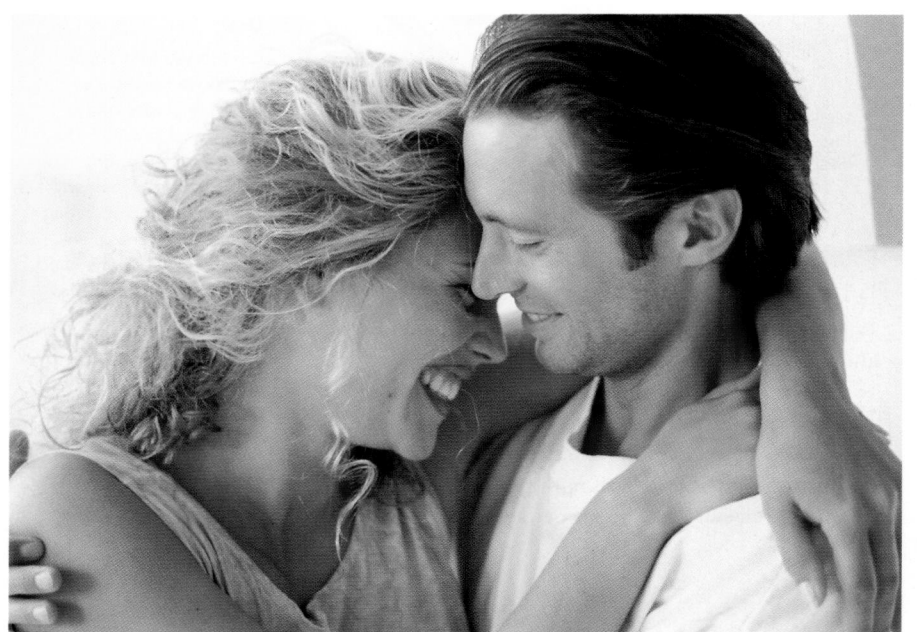

Clematis vitalba

CLEMATIS

The wild clematis is a rambling, perennial climber of woods and country hedges. Its common name is travelers' joy, and it bursts forth with a mass of beautiful flowers.

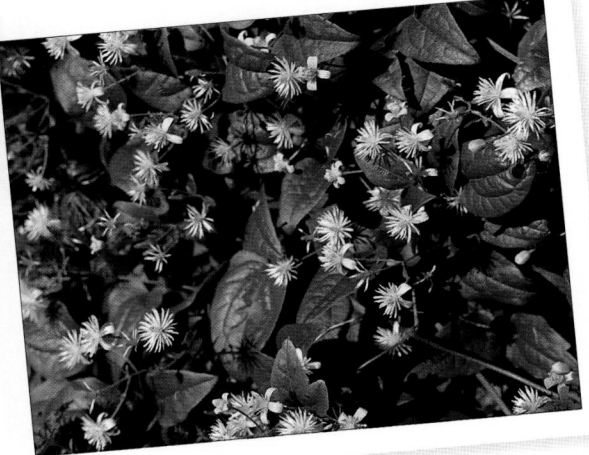

ABOVE *Wild clematis, travelers' joy or old man's beard is a poisonous plant and must be used carefully.*

DATA FILE

Use

For those who are dreamy and not fully awake. Sometimes they daydream or fantasize about a utopian future. Clematis people prefer to live in the mind or the spirit, rather than deal with contemporary issues and the mundane functions of everyday life. They tend to be airy and impractical individuals, drifting off into their own ideas, the typical "mad professor." They sometimes lead a sedentary life, are pale, and lack vitality and ambition. They are sensitive and sometimes need lots of sleep.

Method

The sun method (*see page 222*)

GOAL— Being awake and grounded in the body and in the present People who need Clematis are dreamy, absent-minded, and lack interest in the present. They sometimes have a poor will to live. They may forget to eat, experience faintness and tiredness. If children resort to daydreaming as an escape, Clematis may be useful, although the child should be questioned to find the underlying cause.

GOAL— Mental balance and clarity; to read or speak clearly People who need Bush Fuchsia may be nervous and stammer. Although intelligent, they are slow to learn. They may avoid situations which highlight this, or become shy. They have difficulties with determining left and right, up and down. Bush Fuchsia is specific for children with dyslexia or learning difficulties. Bush Fuchsia aids concentration and confidence. It is also useful when we are "stuck" in one mode of thinking, releasing energy to rebalance the mind.

Epacris longiflora

BUSH FUCHSIA

A low, straggly shrub, bush fuschia flowers throughout the year with bright red, elongated, bell-like flowers hanging in a row from the stem. The leaves are small and heart-shaped. The plant needs full sun.

DATA FILE

Use

Bush Fuchsia is used to balance the hemispheres of the brain so that the rational left side and creative right side can be expressed with confidence. It is useful for all problems with learning difficulties, or translating marks from the page (words, symbols, music) into physical action. It boosts confidence when performing or speaking in public. Dyslexia and other learning disabilities, if not understood and addressed, can seriously affect self-worth and hinder the development of social skills.

Method

The sun method (*see page 222*)

BELOW *The long, hanging flowers of bush fuchsia adorn the shrub throughout the summer months.*

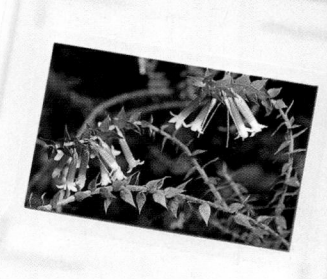

Fagus sylvatica

BEECH

The common beech tree grows to a majestic 100ft. (30m.), with a spread of 80ft. (25m.). The leaves take on rich yellow and orange hues in the fall.

DATA FILE

Use

Beech is for those who are being over-critical and intolerant, and according to Dr Bach, "for those who need to see beauty in all that surrounds them." Beech types have their own "way" and are very proud that they can cope. They think problems can be solved in their way, and are intolerant of those who cannot do this. They do not understand that everyone has different strengths and experiences. They think "cannot" means "will not," and therefore become irritable and short-tempered with others. They may also feel unappreciated.

Method

The boiling method (*see page 223*)

GOAL – Tolerance and empathy People who need Beech may be lonely and isolated. Lack of understanding leads to narrow views and behavior. Beech fills hearts with empathy and opens eyes to see beauty without judgment. It shows that we are individuals, with different ways of dealing with the world.

LEFT *The leaves and twigs of the common beech tree produce a remedy that can help those who are intolerant.*

Gentianella amarella
GENTIAN

Gentianella amerella flowers from late summer onward, with rich blue, violet to purple flowers. It likes dry, well-drained conditions, and sandy or chalky soils.

PROFILE

🍃 GOAL – Courage to accept what is; encouragement to face the future positively 🍃 Gentian helps us to put setbacks and disappointments into perspective, and to once again display a positive attitude.

DATA FILE

Use

For despondency and mild depression due to circumstances. Gentian people are easily discouraged. When everything is going well they are happy, but they can be easily disheartened, and can slip back into a negative outlook. Doubt and lack of faith are important elements. Gentian restores the courage to recognize that life is not a competition and that there is no failure when trying our best.

Method

🌿 The sun method *(see page 222)*

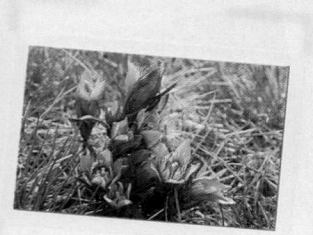

LEFT *The twisted purple flowers of this* Gentianella *species are similar to those of the honeysuckle.*

Grevillea buxifolia
GRAY SPIDER FLOWER

A common Australian evergreen, this shrub flowers for most of the year. It prefers acid soil and full sun.

DATA FILE

Use

Aspen and Mimulus are both for fear, but Gray Spider Flower is for extreme and intense feelings of terror, a blind panic which is immobilizing. The fear may be known or unknown, and it is associated with physical symptoms of inner terror which freeze the mind and body, and prevent thoughts moving forward. Gray Spider Flower frees the body and the mind to move, bringing faith that the terror will pass.

Method

🌿 The sun method *(see page 222)*; pick the whole flower head at the end of the branch

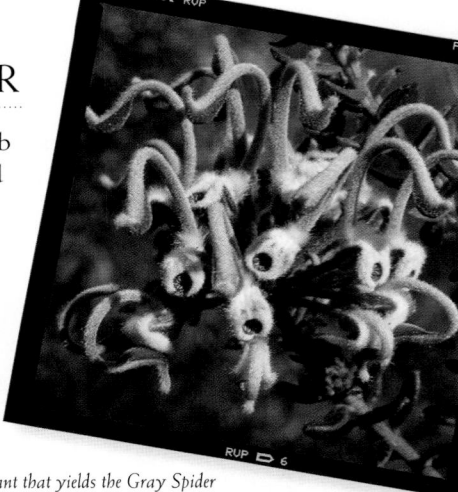

ABOVE *The plant that yields the Gray Spider Flower remedy is a tender evergreen that can be grown in sheltered areas outdoors in milder regions.*

PROFILE

🍃 GOAL – Faith 🍃 **For extreme, immobilizing terror of day or night; nightmares, disturbed sleep, or fear of sleep.** 🍃 For shivering, pallor, palpitations, depression, and feelings of being psychically drained and exhausted. 🍃 **Gray Spider Flower brings lightness, courage, and faith, the certainty that we are loved by the world.** 🍃 It is ideal for children terrorized by bad dreams. 🍃 **Take with Fringed Violet Flower for protection from fear of the supernatural and of psychic attack.**

Gossypium sturtianum
STURT DESERT ROSE

Sturt desert rose is a small shrub with mauve, hibiscus-like flowers which likes dry, stony ground. The flower remedy is good for feelings of worthlessness.

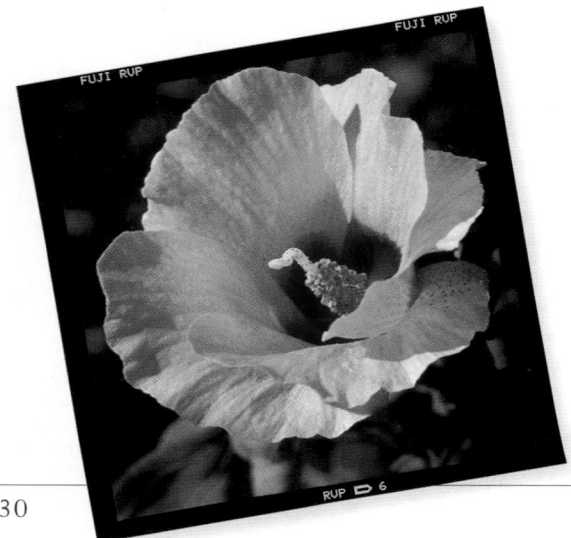

LEFT *Sturt desert rose is a delicate-looking, sun-loving plant that thrives in poor, dry soil and is a tough survivor.*

DATA FILE

Use

People who need Sturt Desert Rose are always apologizing for themselves and their actions. They blame themselves for everything, for things they should or should not have done, and feel guilt and remorse. They may have an acute sense of obligation and duty which is hard (or impossible) to live up to. Guilt and shame are both disabling emotions. Sturt Desert Rose enables self-acceptance, the understanding that we do what we can and must take responsibility (not blame) for the consequences. It enables reconciliation, allowing us to accept, forgive, and move on to pastures new.

Method

🌿 The sun method *(see page 222)*

PROFILE

🍃 GOAL– Self-acceptance, conciliation, communication true to self 🍃 For guilt, regret, remorse. People who need Sturt Desert Rose feel useless. They have low self-esteem and a sense of shame. They are characterized by self-criticism. 🍃 Associated symptoms include anxiety dreams, depression, especially of old hidden guilt. 🍃 Sturt Desert Rose facilitates self-acceptance, allowing forgiveness and healing.

Helianthemum nummularium
ROCK ROSE

A low-growing, yellow-flowered plant found on chalky or gravely soils. Some varieties of rock rose are cultivated in rock gardens, but these are not suitable for use as flower remedies.

DATA FILE

Use

Rock Rose is one of the main ingredients of Rescue Remedy. It is to be taken in all cases of extreme fear, terror, panic, urgency, or danger. Rock Rose gives the courage to face life and death, frees the mind to act, bringing faith that the terror or panic will soon pass.

Method

🌿 The sun method *(see page 222)*

ABOVE The rock rose thrives in a dry, stony, sunny spot and bears an endless succession of short-lived, fragile flowers.

BELOW Rock Rose is for people who suffer from extremes of panic or helplessness.

PROFILE

🌿 GOAL– Personal courage 🌿 **The person who needs Rock Rose experiences feelings of helplessness, terror, and blind panic.** 🌿 Fear may cause palpitations, heart jitters, or panic attacks. 🌿 **Rock Rose should be given for any perceived threat to the person, their self-image, or personal integrity.**

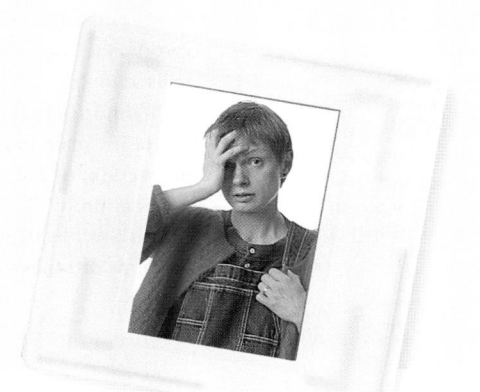

DATA FILE

Use

People who need Hibbertia love ideas and pursue knowledge at all costs. They may repress or deny their body and its needs, or have a rigid or dogmatic lifestyle. They continually read, attend lectures, courses, and workshops to improve themselves and gain status. They want to "know it all." They look deep within books, but never around at their surroundings. Their head is in the air and they are ungrounded. The search is ultimately unsatisfactory; knowledge grows from within and they must find themselves before they can change.

Method

🌿 The sun method *(see page 222)*

ABOVE RIGHT With its bright yellow flowers and its preference for open spaces, Hibbertia encourages openness and confidence.

RIGHT Hibbertia is a good remedy for studious young people who may neglect the physical side of themselves.

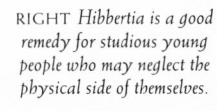

Hibbertia pedunculata
HIBBERTIA

A low, trailing plant of the open bush. The large, bright, and gleaming yellow flowers bloom in spring. It is frost-tender. The flower essence is good for those with a love of learning.

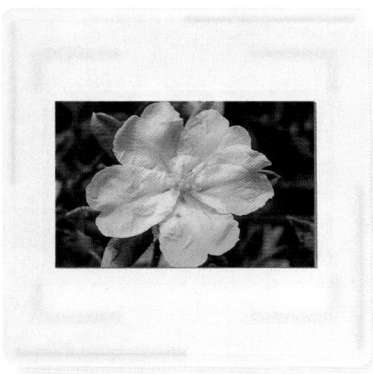

PROFILE

🌿 GOAL – Wisdom 🌿 **For those who are intelligent, the "constant student," characterized by continual pursuit of knowledge for self-improvement or status, and love of "hidden knowledge." Such people may be fanatical or cult followers.**
🌿 They may be neglectful of their body, or suffer sedentary and stress-related illnesses, indigestion, skin rashes, wasting or stiffness of muscles and joints.
🌿 **Hibbertia encourages confidence and contentment. It links external knowledge with personal observations and physical needs, producing wisdom.**

Hottonia palustris
WATER VIOLET

This is a delicate perennial plant with pale violet flowers and feathery leaves which is often found in ditches, as it grows submerged in water. The flowers appear above the water in summer.

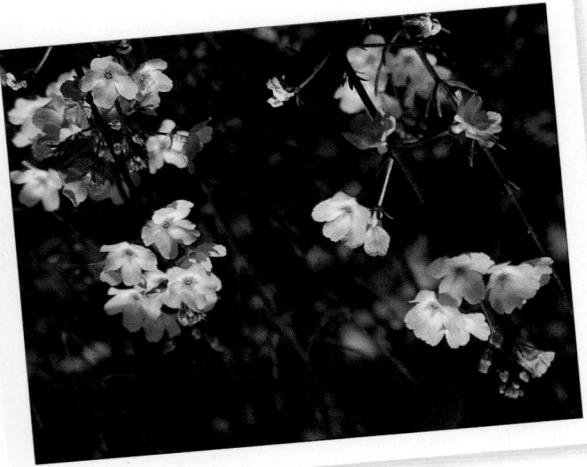

ABOVE *Water violets grow under water, and issue forth a delicate foam of lilac-colored flowers in early spring.*

DATA FILE

Use

Water Violet is for self-reliant people with an aloof, "live-and-let-live" attitude. They are quiet and spend much time alone, keeping others at a distance. When ill they keep to themselves and do not wish to be any "trouble" to those around them. They find it hard to share. In their isolation they may feel special, or chosen, a sensation which can distort their sense of belonging and self-worth. Water Violet gives the confidence to share – the strengths and weaknesses, the ups and downs, all of life's rich tapestry.

Method

☙ The sun method *(see page 222)*

PROFILE

☙ GOAL – Communication; sharing ☙ **The person needing Water Violet is reserved and self-contained. This can be seen as standoffish aloofness and pride, and thus lead to loneliness.** ☙ **He or she may be solitary yet proud.** ☙ **Water Violet allows us to acknowledge the inner self as a starting point from which to expand, communicate with the world, and share from the heart.**

Ilex aquifolium
HOLLY

Holly is a common evergreen tree, with spiky leaves and red berries. It is a powerful symbol of winter and is used in Christmas decorations. To produce berries on a female plant, a male plant needs to be grown nearby.

BELOW *The holly is not noted for its flowers, but these have an unmistakable and pervasive scent.*

DATA FILE

Use

Holly is for those who are attacked by feelings of hatred, envy, jealousy, suspicion, and revenge. The person who needs Holly has intense negative feelings. They also have other intense emotions, but they are too frightened to express these fully. The free flow of emotion and love is then blocked or expressed unclearly. This leads to tension, unclear communication, frustration, anger, and emotional outbursts.

Method

☙ The boiling method *(see page 223)*

PROFILE

☙ GOAL – Unconditional expression of affection and love. A useful affirmation might be: "I am opening my heart to express my love." ☙ **The negative emotions of the person who needs Holly may be spiteful and nagging, with intense feeling and outbursts of temper. They may be suspicious or mildly paranoid.** ☙ **Useful for the "no!" negative states and temper tantrums of two-year-olds.** ☙ **Holly allows us to recognize that these feelings are the negative expression of our caring interaction with others. It gives us the strength to open our hearts to the full flow of love.**

Juglans regia
WALNUT

A large, handsome, deciduous tree which is easily recognized by its popular edible nuts, walnut grows to about 50ft. (15m.) tall and is wide-spreading.

DATA FILE

Use

Walnut is for people who need to find constancy and protection from outside forces, those who need to move on and break links and old patterns with people and things. Walnut frees the person from interference, and gives protection so that it is possible to break inappropriate ties and pursue personal freedom. Walnut is useful for people on the brink of some major decision or change, for example children leaving home, the menopause, marriage, or having babies.

LEFT *The walnut fruit resembles the human brain and the remedy from the flowers is thought to strengthen and protect the mind.*

Method

☙ The boiling method *(see page 223)*

PROFILE

☙ GOAL – Protection, sanctuary ☙ **Walnut is useful at any of the milestones of life: puberty, marriage, leaving home, change of job or country, etc.** ☙ **People who have moved on but find old habits persistent can take Walnut to break links with the past.** ☙ **Walnut is also useful for temporary distraction, or for domination by enthusiasm, or strong opinions of others.**

Impatiens glandulifera
IMPATIENS

A tall annual with large mauve flowers and exploding seed pods, Impatiens is common in damp places. It is sometimes called "touch me not," as the tightly coiled seed pods are apt to explode at the slightest touch.

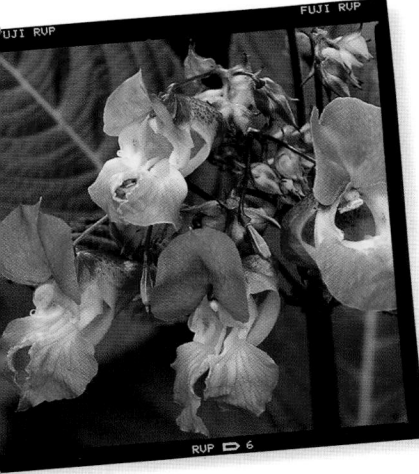

LEFT *Impatiens grows on the banks of streams and ditches, and its flowers nod gently in the breeze.*

🌿 GOAL– Patience 🌿 **Impatiens is for impatience and irritability at slowness, the desire to do everything quickly.** 🌿 People who need Impatiens may fidget, find it hard to sit still, and therefore suffer from indigestion and nervous tension. 🌿 **People who have learnt the lesson of Impatiens have patience, they are capable and decisive, knowing how to get things done and turn the pace of life to advantage.**

DATA FILE

Use

For those who are quick in thought and action, and who are always on the go. They know their mind and want things to be done at speed. They become irritable at hindrance, hesitation, and delay, and impatiently blame others. They can alienate people by being brusque and unsympathetic, speaking their mind quickly and without thought. They refuse to slow down even when illness overtakes them. They are truly in the "rat race." Impatiens restores acceptance of the natural pace of life, rather than fighting against it.

Method

🌷 The sun method (see page 222)

Larix decidua
LARCH

Larch is a tall conifer with needle-like leaves that are shed in the fall. Male and female flowers appear on the same tree in spring. It can grow to 100ft. (30m.) high, and the cones are small and erect.

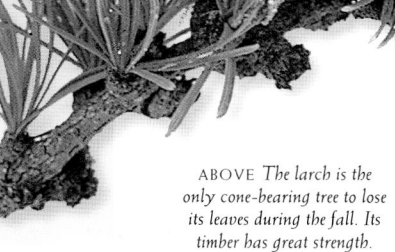

WALNUT

✋ Traditional Home and Folk Remedies *p.92*

🌿 GOAL– Confidence 🌿 **Larch can be used for any lack of confidence and self-esteem, for passivity and fear of trying, and for poor self-image and feelings of inferiority.** 🌿 It is suitable for children starting a new school, and who feel they will not be as clever as the other children and so fear failure. 🌿 **Feelings of worthlessness may hide deeper problems or a pattern of abuse. Other remedies may also be useful.** 🌿 Larch strengthens confidence, and helps us appreciate our real worth and value our personal contribution to the planet.

ABOVE *The larch is the only cone-bearing tree to lose its leaves during the fall. Its timber has great strength.*

Fear of trying

Lack of confidence

Poor self-image

Feels worthless

DATA FILE

Use

Larch is for those who lack confidence in themselves and fear failure, those who feel that they are not as capable as those around them. At times, lack of confidence may completely immobilize them and prevent them from even trying. They do not think that they are capable, or worthy of success. Feelings of total uselessness also can lead to great unhappiness, despair, and isolation. Larch increases confidence and strengthens personal will.

Method

🌷 The boiling method (see page 223)

LEFT *The Larch remedy can help bring confidence and self-esteem, especially in teenage years.*

Lonicera caprifolium
HONEYSUCKLE

Lonicera caprifolium is a strongly scented climber found in woods. The fragrance is sweet and long-lasting. The flowers are tubular and form a spreading head.

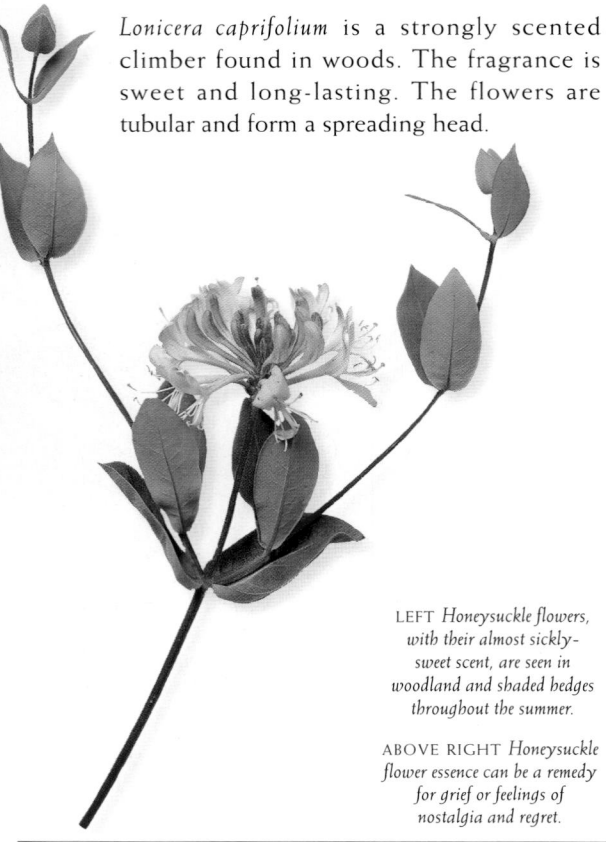

LEFT *Honeysuckle flowers, with their almost sickly-sweet scent, are seen in woodland and shaded hedges throughout the summer.*

ABOVE RIGHT *Honeysuckle flower essence can be a remedy for grief or feelings of nostalgia and regret.*

DATA FILE

Use

Honeysuckle is for those who dwell too much on memories of the past, on the "good old days," and who do not expect to experience such happiness and companionship again. The past seems rosy and familiar; the future seems dark, bleak, forbidding, and unknown. For nostalgia, a faraway sense of regret or loss, often tinged with pessimism. Nostalgia may be a temporary sensation, a fleeting regret, or it may be a pattern which prevents further joy and expression. Honeysuckle is appropriate for both.

Method

❦ The boiling method *(see page 223)*

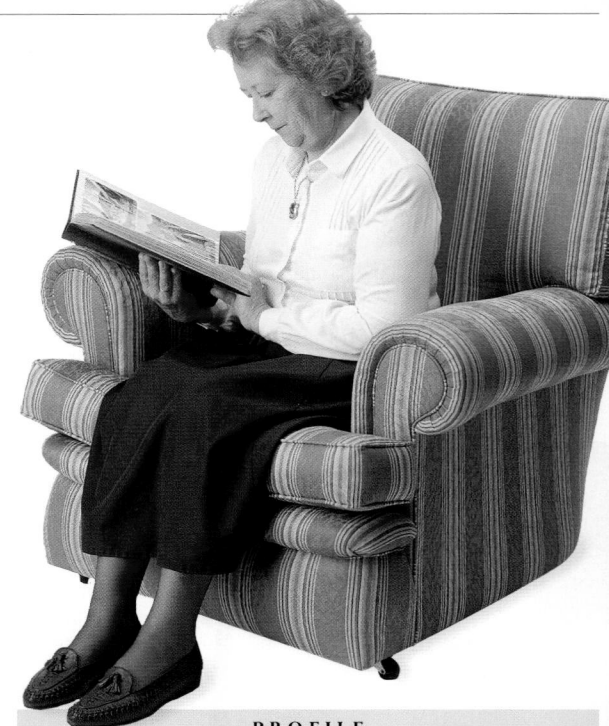

PROFILE

❧ GOAL – To be completely "here" ❧ **A useful affirmation might be "I am here and now, growing from my past into a positive future."** ❧ Honeysuckle is for people who are not grounded in the present, who (for many reasons) are stuck in the past. ❧ **It is for homesickness or regrets.** ❧ It is also useful for grief and bereavement where these cause the person to dwell on the past. ❧ **Honeysuckle integrates past experiences and gives strength to face new challenges.**

Malus sylvestris
CRAB APPLE

The fruits yielded by this plant are small, yellow, and very acid. It grows in hedges and on waste ground. The crab apples make a piquant preserve. *Malus* provides a good show of color in the fall.

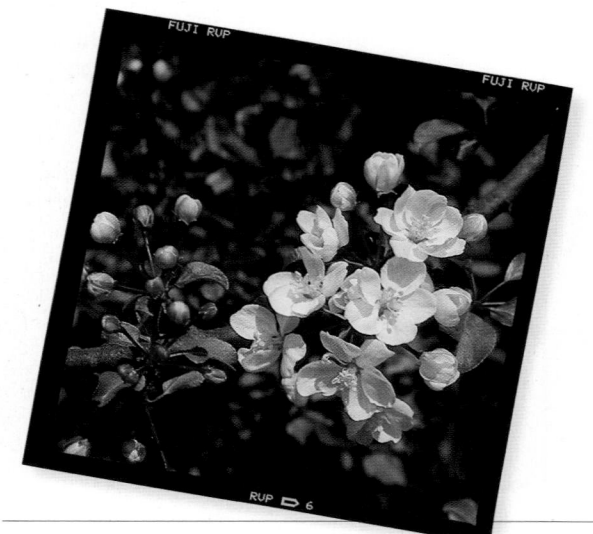

LEFT *The blossoms of the crab apple produce a fresh but bitter fruit that is also used to make country jellies and wines.*

PROFILE

❧ GOAL – Cleaning and purification ❧ **Crab Apple is for people who feel unclean on any level. They may feel self-disgust or self-loathing and may hurt, punish, cut, or otherwise abuse themselves. They may have phobias or rituals around purity or cleanliness.** ❧ Crab Apple is also useful for spots and rashes on the face, so that they can be faced and the self accepted. ❧ **This remedy is a cleanser on all levels: physical, emotional, and spiritual.** ❧ It is also used to cleanse the body and spirit after contact with anything contagious or which feels unclean. ❧ **It may be added to baths or to skin creams.**

DATA FILE

Use

Crab Apple is a bitter acid fruit, useful for those who feel self-condemnation and disgust, in need of cleaning or detoxification. This may be a temporary feeling brought on by shame or remorse, or guilt over some act of which they are ashamed, or thoughts which are felt to be unclean. Crab Apple is also useful to encourage acceptance of spots or physical blemishes, and for a deep phobia or cleanliness fetish. It cleanses both the mind and body.

Method

❦ The boiling method *(see page 223)*

Mimulus guttatus
MIMULUS

A pretty, water-loving plant common in damp places, Mimulus has rich yellow flowers in midsummer that resemble the snapdragon. It grows to 2ft. (60cm.)

DATA FILE

Use

Mimulus is for fear which can be identified, of known or worldly things. (Aspen is also for fear, but for unknown fears.) Mimulus should be taken for the everyday fears of pain, accidents, poverty, being alone, and misfortune. These understandable fears dominate responses, either prodding people into hasty action or freezing them into inaction. They are easily identified and faced, but underneath they are fed by insecurity and a negative attitude toward past experience. Mimulus is also for shy, timid people who tend to avoid social occasions and large crowds of people.

Method

☙ The sun method
(see page 222)

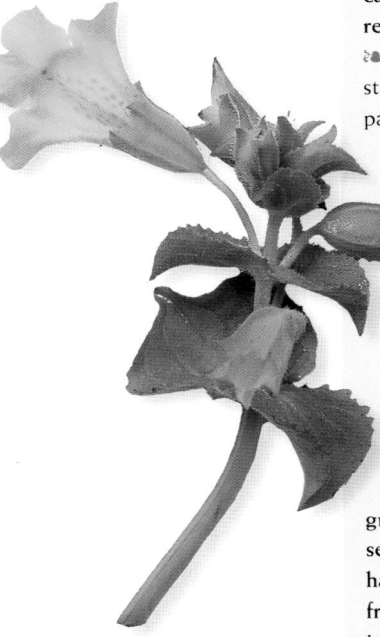

ABOVE *The mimulus or monkey plant is a bog plant, in need of shade and cool, damp conditions.*

PROFILE

☙ GOAL – Freedom; freedom from fear
☙ **For any fear which can be named. A trivial fear or phobia, if it can be named, will respond to Mimulus.**
☙ Fear can lead to stammering, palpitations, indigestion, sleeplessness, and troubled dreams.
☙ **Mimulus liberates us from fear and helps us to understand the rhythms and balances of everyday life, to grow beyond the limits set by fear, and to have the courage and freedom to respond in appropriate ways.**

Ornithogalum umbellatum
STAR OF BETHLEHEM

The delicate flowers of this wild lily are like six-pointed stars and bloom in late spring. *Ornithogalum umbellatum* is a spring-flowering bulb.

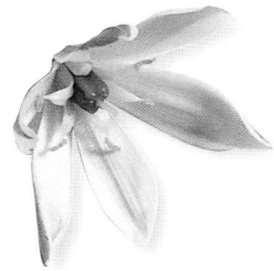

ABOVE *Star of Bethlehem grows wild in Asia and North Africa, and as far north as the U.K.*

PROFILE

☙ GOAL – Peace and comfort ☙ **For shock, and its physical and emotional effects.**
☙ Long-repressed shock or trauma may lead to psychosomatic symptoms.
☙ **Star of Bethlehem neutralizes the effects of shock, so that the body and mind can again find equilibrium and comfort.**

DATA FILE

Use

Star of Bethlehem is used in Rescue Remedy to ameliorate the effects of shock – the shock of bad news, of loss, of an accident, even of being born. People "jump" with shock; waves ripple outward through the body, affecting every cell and tissue. Time is needed for everything to settle, to be comfortable in the body, but sometimes the trauma may be so extreme, or the shock unrealized or repressed, that the effects continue to resonate years later. Star of Bethlehem neutralizes the effects so that the body is able to harmonize.

Method

☙ The boiling method
(see page 223)

Olea europea
OLIVE

Olive is a small evergreen common in southern Europe. The fruits yield olive oil.

PROFILE

☙ GOAL – Renewal and regeneration ☙ **For all exhaustion, physical, and mental tiredness after some effort or struggle.** ☙ Exhaustion can be so profound that life loses its interest and spark.
☙ **Olive helps restore vitality by helping people to relax and take a more balanced attitude toward life, making sure they allow themselves "quality" time for unwinding, rest, and spiritual renewal.**

DATA FILE

Use

For extreme fatigue of mind, body, or spirit after effort. People in need of Olive feel totally exhausted in every way. They feel that life is hard and without pleasure, that they have no more strength, and at times hardly know how they manage to keep going. They burn the candle at both ends, and become too tired even to think. They may depend on others for help.

Olive helps people relax and switch off, so that the simple things of life – a warm bath, a walk in the sunshine, watching children, or sharing with friends – can refresh the spirit.

Method

☙ The sun method
(see page 222)

RIGHT *Olive oil has been used to soothe and heal for thousands of years, and the Olive remedy heals the spirit.*

THERAPY CONNECTIONS

OLIVE
✋ Traditional Home and Folk Remedies p.95

APPLE
✋ Traditional Home and Folk Remedies p.94

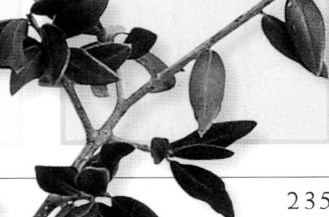

Pinus sylvestris
PINE

The Scotch pine is an evergreen tree often depicted in painting and song as the "lonesome pine." It has blue-green leaves and gray or reddish cones.

DATA FILE

Use

Pine is a very specific remedy for those who blame themselves and are suffering from self-reproach. Even when successful they are never content, and always feel that they could have done better. They blame themselves even when the fault is someone else's.

Method

🌿 The boiling method *(see page 223)*

ABOVE *The Scotch pine is a native of Europe and Asia that can grow to a great age.*

PROFILE

🌿 GOAL – Appropriate response; responsibility 🌿 **For self-reproach and guilt, frequently groundless.** 🌿 People who need Pine may carry the blame for the actions of others, and may apologize frequently and often needlessly. 🌿 **Pine helps us understand that "responsibility" is the ability to respond. If we respond honestly and freely there is no need for blame and we can move on.**

Prunus cerasus
CHERRY PLUM

A small tree with red or yellow fruit, cherry plum is often grown as hedging and windbreaks. It flowers from early spring, with delicate pale pink flowers.

PROFILE

🌿 GOAL – Release; to let go of fear and to regain control of the emotions 🌿 **People who need Cherry Plum may feel desperate, and fear they may hurt themselves and others. They may have bouts of hysteria.** 🌿 Cherry Plum is useful for uncontrolled tantrums in children, when they are frightened by their own loss of temper. 🌿 **Cherry Plum restores control and trust of the mind and emotions.**

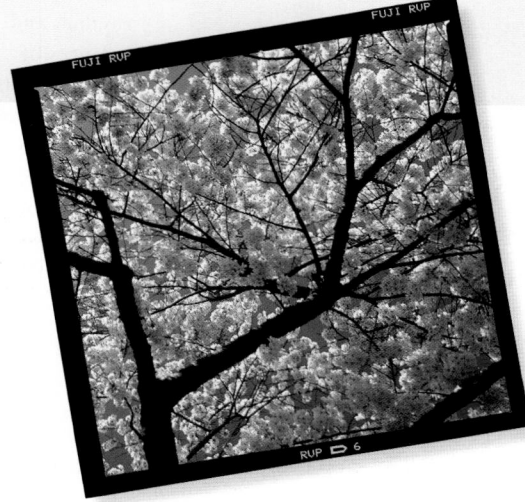

LEFT *The wild cherry plum is in flower almost before the arrival of spring. Flowering twigs are used for the remedy.*

DATA FILE

Use

Cherry Plum is for the fear of letting go or of losing control. The fearful thoughts may be of a suicidal, compulsive, or destructive nature. This mental pain and turmoil may happen during a period of great emotional or physical change, when the person is worn and stressed. Dr. Bach says it is "for fear of the mind being overstrained, of reason giving way, of doing fearful and dreaded things, not wished and known wrong, yet there comes the thought and impulse to do them."

Method

🌿 The boiling method *(see page 223)*

Populus tremula
ASPEN

Aspen is a slender, silver-barked, deciduous tree. It grows to 30ft. (10m.), its almost circular leaves trembling in the slightest breeze.

THERAPY CONNECTIONS

PINE

◉ Aromatherapy *p.166*

PROFILE

🌿 GOAL – Courage to face the unknown 🌿 **The person who needs Aspen may feel frightened, a sense of dread, and that something awful may happen. This may be extreme enough to affect appetite, produce palpitations, and interrupt sleep patterns, bringing nightmares.** 🌿 Aspen is suitable for the fears and nightmares of children where they cannot describe what they are frightened of. 🌿 **Aspen brings reassurance that there is nothing to fear. It helps us to face the unknown with courage and trust.**

LEFT *Aspen is a type of poplar with gray-green leaves that flutter in the breeze. It also has cottony catkins.*

DATA FILE

Use

Dr. Bach says it is for "vague fear, for which there is no explanation or reason." The fear can be so deep that it is too frightening to express, and the sufferer feels burdened by doom, and inexplicable terror.

Method

🌿 The boiling method *(see page 223)*

Ptilotus atripicfolius
MULLA MULLA

A small plant from desert regions, mulla mulla responds to the weather, and sends out clusters of pink, long-lasting flowers when conditions are favorable. All but one of the many species of *Ptilotus* are exclusive to Australia.

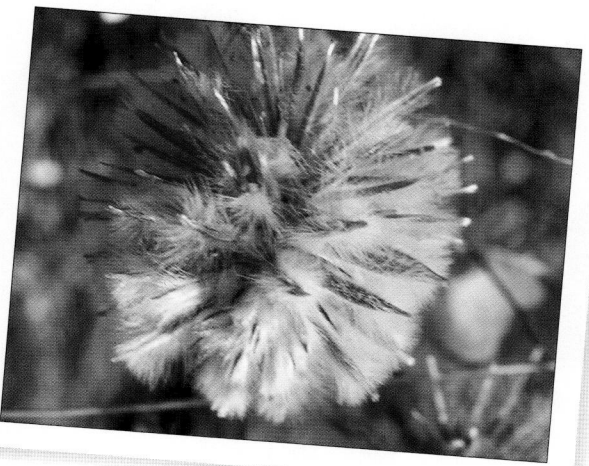

ABOVE *Like many desert plants, mulla mulla has stunning flowers which seem to symbolize hope and life.*

DATA FILE

Use

For those suffering the effects of fire, heat, or radiation. In reality and symbolically, fire is profoundly powerful. In most traditions fire was a gift from the gods and had to be used with wisdom. Do we understand fire and use it wisely? Burning fossil fuels adds to the greenhouse effect and to the depletion of the ozone layer. Mulla Mulla helps the body recover from damage and protects it from harmful rays.

Method

🌿 The sun method *(see page 222)*

PROFILE

🐚 GOAL – Rejuvenation 🐚 People who need Mulla Mulla may have obvious burns, sunburn, or hot rashes. They may be suffering exhaustion from heat, or from working in over-hot conditions, or a hot climate. 🐚 Mulla Mulla helps them to be comfortable with the inner and outer manifestations of fire.
🐚 Mulla Mulla also protects from the damaging effects of heat, for example in laser treatment.

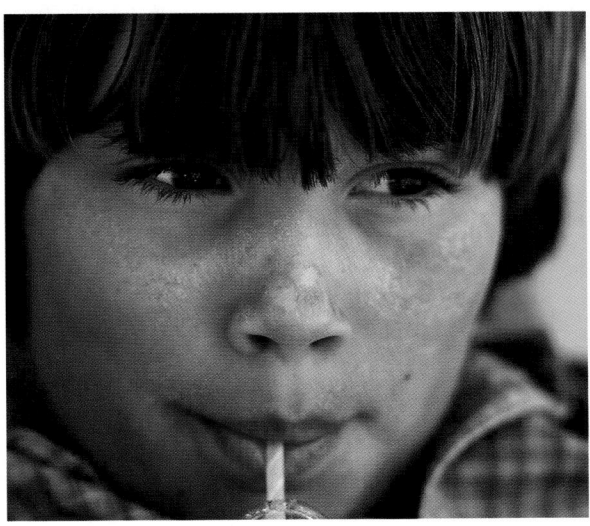

RIGHT *Mulla Mulla can help cool the effects of burns or heat exhaustion and over-exposure to the sun.*

Quercus robur
OAK

Quercus robur is the common oak. Most people recognize the acorns, but the flowers are less familiar. Male and female flowers are borne on the same tree and appear from April onward.

RIGHT *Oak leaves and flowers both appear toward the end of spring.*

DATA FILE

Use

Oak people are strong and brave fighters. They struggle through events and physical illnesses even when there is no hope, never thinking of surrender. Their strength may sometimes be inappropriate, and they can exhaust themselves by pushing blindly on in one narrow direction. Strength is a virtue, but it is pointless pushing against an immovable object. Oak helps us surrender, step back, look around, and consider different answers.

Method

🌿 The sun method *(see page 222)*; pick the small, female catkins only

PROFILE

🐚 GOAL – Adaptability and flexibility 🐚 Oak is for those who struggle on, never giving up. 🐚 People who need Oak may overwork, and drive themselves relentlessly.
🐚 They can be obstinate, and, unless they rest or find another strategy, may exhaust themselves and break down.
🐚 Oak restores the true inner strength, which is flexible and adaptable.

Ricinocarpus pinifolius
WEDDING BUSH

Ricinocarpus pinifolius is a small bush with abundant, six-petaled white flowers. Male and female flowers grow on the same bush. The flowers were traditionally used for wedding decorations, giving the bush its name.

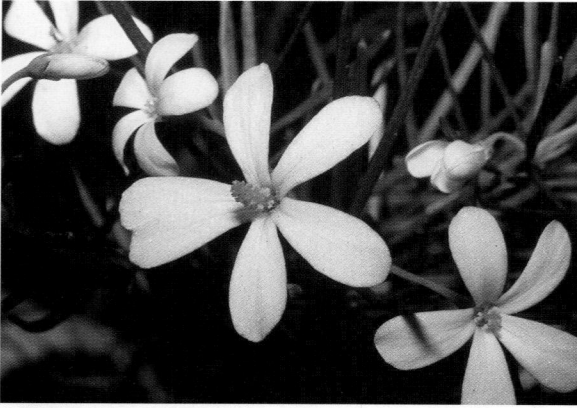

DATA FILE

Use

Wedding Bush is like the glue which holds people together through thick and thin. It is for those who doubt their ability to commit or accept the responsibility of deep caring; for those with a pattern of starting but not finishing, moving on, and running away from the self in all aspects of life; for those who are an "emotional rolling stone." They may be in love with love (or the newness of love) and move from one affair to another, or they may have one job after another. Commitment is not just about long-term endurance; it is an attitude of mind involving self-worth. Wedding Bush reminds us of the privilege of being, and of our commitment to life.

Method

❧ The sun method *(see page 222)*; pick both male and female flowers

ABOVE *Just as the flowers of Wedding Bush make bridal bouquets, so the remedy keeps a sense of dedication alive.*

BELOW *Wedding Bush can help to bring a feeling of confidence to a relationship and an ability to see things through.*

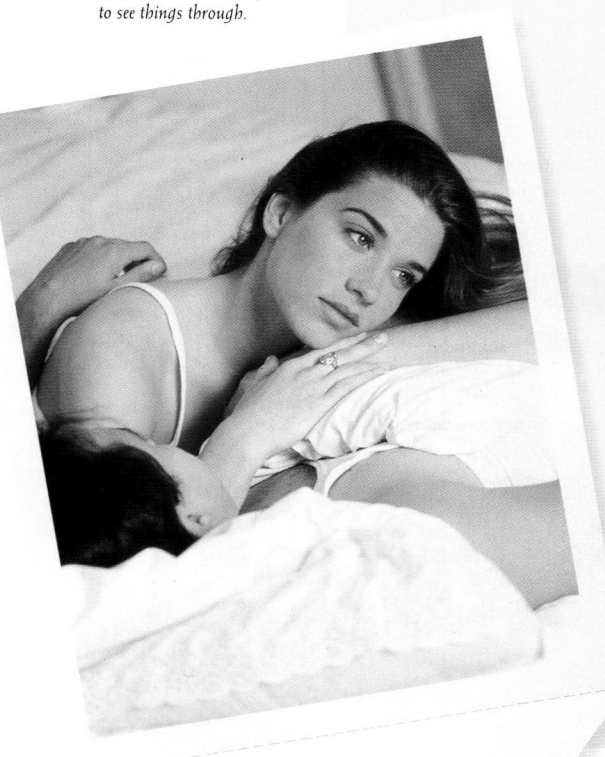

PROFILE

❧ GOAL – Commitment and dedication ❧ **For those who find commitment difficult and suffer indecision and procrastination.** ❧ For those with a pattern of starting but not finishing. ❧ **Wedding Bush encourages the confidence to commit, to feel the comfort rather than the burden of responsibility, to make a long-term dedication to life and its purpose.** ❧ Wedding Bush can also help us to carry through short-term jobs or commitments to a satisfying conclusion.

Rosa canina
WILD ROSE

The common wild rose, *Rosa canina* can be seen rambling over country hedges. The flowers appear in early summer, and vary in color from almost white to deep pink. The fruit, or rosehip, is a striking scarlet.

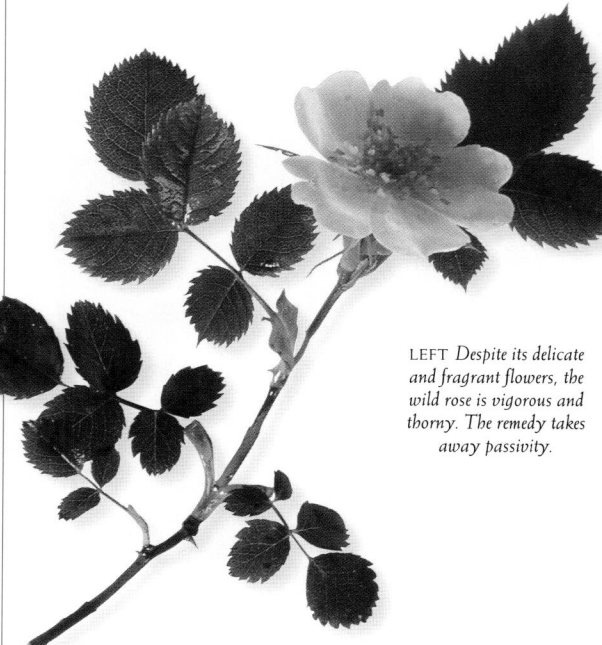

LEFT *Despite its delicate and fragrant flowers, the wild rose is vigorous and thorny. The remedy takes away passivity.*

DATA FILE

Use

Dr. Bach recommends Wild Rose for those who have become resigned to all that happens, for the fatalist. This person glides through life passively, taking it as it is, without motivation or expectation. He or she is apathetic about change and asks, "What is the use?". Such a person has given away his or her power and interest in life. Wild Rose stimulates this interest and an appreciation of life's color and joy. The remedy encourages action, and a purposeful pleasure in being and doing.

Method

❧ The boiling method *(see page 223)*

PROFILE

❧ GOAL – Interest in life; participation and action ❧ **People who need Wild Rose are fatalistic, resigned to events, and apathetic about change.** ❧ Wild Rose helps us to interact with all aspects of life and make an impact by creating our own unique and dynamic reality.

Salix alba var. vitellina
WILLOW

The willow is an attractive tree with thin, bright yellow twigs and long, narrow leaves. It is also known as the golden osier. The tree is often cut back hard to encourage the growth of strong, young shoots.

PROFILE

GOAL – Maturity and natural balance **People who need Willow may be sulky and selfish, embittered with self-pity, and ungrateful for help.** They may experience psychosomatic illness, and tearfulness. **Willow helps us see that we create our own reality by focusing on different elements of our life. It encourages a more positive and mature attitude.** Willow may also be taken for a brief temporary embitterment.

LEFT *Tall and graceful, with slender, silvery leaves, the willow is a water lover with supple, flexible branches.*

DATA FILE

Use

Willow is for people who find the bad things that happen to them hard to accept and are embittered. They take problems personally, and feel life has become a personal trial to endure, without hope or happiness. They blame the world when things go wrong. "It's not fair," they say, like a two-year-old child. Willow helps them see that with this self-pitying outlook they are creating their own oppression by continual negative thoughts.

Method

The boiling method *(see page 223)*

Scleranthus annuus
SCLERANTHUS

Scleranthus is a small, bushy, spreading plant with green flowers which grows to 4in. (10cm.) on sandy soils and in cornfields. The green flowers have no petals and grow at the forks and end of the stems.

DATA FILE

Use

For those who are unable to decide and who suffer much from hesitation and uncertainty. For confusion. People who need Scleranthus tend to be quiet and are not inclined to discuss their options with others. They need to learn to decide for themselves; it is important that they do so, but they cannot. Scleranthus gives the stability to listen to the inner self, and integrate the emotional and intellectual extremes (which sometimes seem contradictory) into balanced and sustained action.

Method

The sun method *(see page 222)*

RIGHT *This branching annual plant has tiny green flowers from early spring to late summer.*

PROFILE

GOAL – Stability and balance **For people who are unable to decide between two things.** They are uncertain, indecisive, vacillate, and subject to erratic mood swings. Scleranthus brings harmony, stability, and balance, allowing us to act decisively.

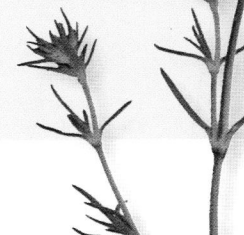

Synapse arvensis
MUSTARD

The common wild mustard found growing in hedges and on waste ground has large yellow flowers that appear in early summer. This annual plant grows to about 2ft. (60cm.) and self-seeds readily.

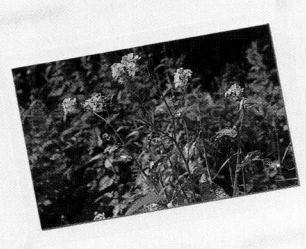

ABOVE *The mustard used for this remedy is the yellow-flowered wild field mustard, also known as charlock.*

DATA FILE

Use

Mustard is used for dark clouds of gloom or deep, black depression that seems to come from nowhere. It is for the feeling of being under a cloud which blocks out the warming rays and optimism of the sun. It may lift just as suddenly as it arrived. While a person is under the dark cloud, it is hard for him or her to muster any feeling of happiness or hope. All clouds pass and Mustard restores hope and a sense of pleasure in living.

Method

The boiling method *(see page 223)*

PROFILE

GOAL – Hope and hopefulness **Mustard is for depression with no known cause, and for melancholia.** It is for people whose thoughts turn inward and whose life lacks light and pleasure. **Although these bouts of depression seem to come from nowhere, there may be a deeply hidden reason. If it happens frequently, look for a cause; if there is a physiological or psychological root, seek professional assistance.** Mustard lightens our mood, giving us the faith and hope to carry on.

THERAPY CONNECTIONS
ROSE
Aromatherapy *p.168*
MUSTARD
Traditional Home and Folk Remedies *p.98*
Ayurveda *p.30*
WILLOW
Herbalism *p.129*

Telopea speciosissima
WARATAH

Waratah is the Aboriginal word for beautiful. It is a shrub with magnificent red flowers packed together into a globe measuring 5in. (12cm.) across. It is a very striking plant.

PROFILE

🌿 GOAL – To have the courage to be courageous
🌿 **Waratah should be taken in times of crisis, emotional or physical. People who need it may feel unable to go on, trapped in a dark night of despair, even suicidal.** 🌿 Physical signs may be exhaustion, interrupted or prolonged sleep, loss of the ability or interest to care for oneself. 🌿 **Waratah reunites all aspects of the personality.** 🌿 It also helps maintain personal integrity for coping with everyday challenges.

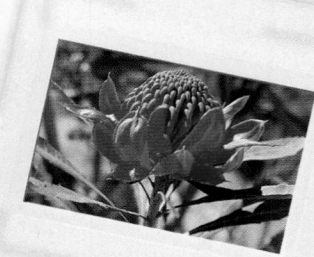

DATA FILE

Use

Waratah is a very powerful and fast-acting remedy. It should be taken for despair, deep distress, and any emotional or physical crisis. The image of the globe of the flowers reflects how the remedy of Waratah brings everything in the personality together: strength, old and forgotten skills and lessons, trust, and love. It gives us the faith and confidence to hold our head up in all weathers, to stand erect and just be ourselves – blooming, obvious, and beautiful.

Method

🌾 The sun method *(see page 222)*

LEFT *With its stunning, globe-shaped flowers Waratah is a powerful remedy, bringing strength and confidence.*

Tetratheca ericifolia
BLACK-EYED SUSAN

This small scrubby plant of the Australian woodland is called "black-eyed" as the drooping, bell-like flowers have a core of black pollen-covered stamens surrounded by four mauve petals.

PROFILE

🌿 GOAL – The "stand and stare" remedy; inner peace
🌿 **People who need Black-eyed Susan are always "on the go." They hate waiting or delay, as they rush to accomplish things quickly.** 🌿 Accompanying physical symptoms are irritability, poor digestion, restless sleep, and general tension and stress. They may also have nervous rashes. 🌿 **Black-eyed Susan releases stress and helps us slow down and find the inner peace to "stand and stare,"** as in the lines of the poem, "What is this life if full of care/ We have no time to stand and stare."

DATA FILE

Use

Black-eyed Susan is for people who are always rushing and striving, for the workaholic who does not have time for himself or herself or the people around, and is expending all his or her energy at a fast rate. The flowers' petals protect the black center, so the remedy helps us turn inward, slow down, and pay attention to our inner rhythm.

Method

🌾 The sun method *(see page 222)*

LEFT *Just as this plant's petals draw attention to the dark centers of the flowers, so the remedy can help people to focus on their inner core.*

Ulex europaeus
GORSE

Gorse is a bushy shrub with pea-like yellow flowers, which is abundant on poor, stony soils and heaths. It is almost leafless, but its green, spiny stems give it an evergreen appearance.

DATA FILE

Use

Gorse is for strong feelings of hopelessness and despair. People who need Gorse may seek help in order to please others, but underneath feel that nothing more can be done for them. They have lost the will to strive, perhaps in response to a life event, an accident, a medical diagnosis, or to a long-standing illness or fear. They are caught up in negativity, unwilling to try new avenues, and unwilling to hope. Gorse gives them the courage to try, building renewed hope, and giving the will to continue the fight toward recovery.

Method

🌾 The sun method *(see page 222)*

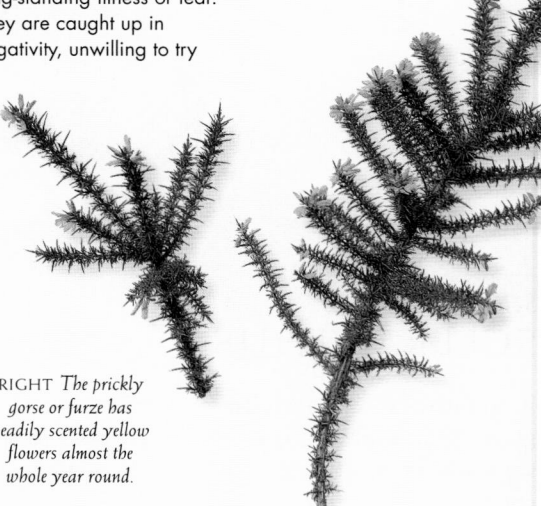

RIGHT *The prickly gorse or furze has headily scented yellow flowers almost the whole year round.*

PROFILE

🌿 GOAL – Anything is possible; positive possibilities
🌿 **Gorse is for hopelessness and despair when the person has decided to give up.** 🌿 Gorse can help give people the heart to stay with a course of treatment. It is useful when a long period of retraining is necessary, for example after a stroke, loss of limbs, or a major accident, when the person feels that there is no use in trying. 🌿 **Gorse helps open a door to possibilities, encourages an objective attitude, and strengthens the heart to face them.**

Ulmus procera
ELM

The magnificent English elm, once common in hedgerows and fields, is now sadly rare due to Dutch elm disease. It grows to a towering 120ft. (35m.) and spreads to 50ft. (15m.).

DATA FILE

Use

Elm is for temporary feelings of inadequacy. People who benefit from Elm do good work and are proud of themselves and their calling. They hope to do something important, and to be of service and benefit to all of humanity. They seek and aim for perfection. When this goal seems unattainable they can become overwhelmed. Elm is for brief faltering moments of despair and lack of confidence, when the task seems too much. Elm restores faith in ability, so that we do not strive for unattainable perfection, but instead appreciate the worth of our own actions.

Method

🌿 The boiling method *(see page 223)*

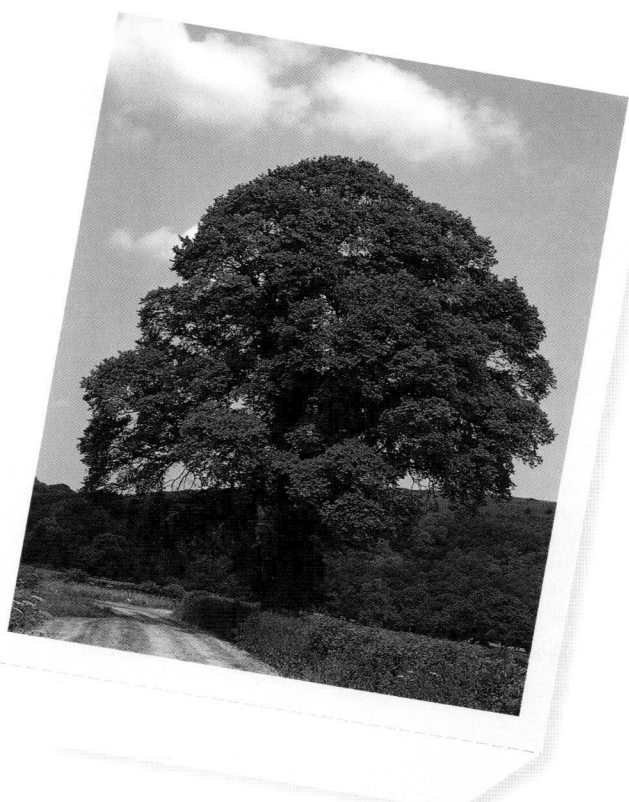

ABOVE *The English elm has clusters of small green flowers with long purple-pink stamens that appear before the leaves open.*

PROFILE

🌿 GOAL – Restores confidence. 🌿 People who need Elm are usually confident and capable, but are temporarily over-whelmed with the scope, weight, and burden of their work. They may be tired or feel exhausted, which can lead to mild depression. 🌿 Elm gives the strength to balance responsibilities with the practical needs of everyday reality and carry on. 🌿 *(See also* Larch.*)*

THERAPY CONNECTIONS

VERVAIN

🔘 Herbalism   *p.138*

Verbena officinalis
VERVAIN

A common wayside perennial found in meadows, on the roadside, and in dry, sunny places, vervain bears many small, unscented lilac flowers.

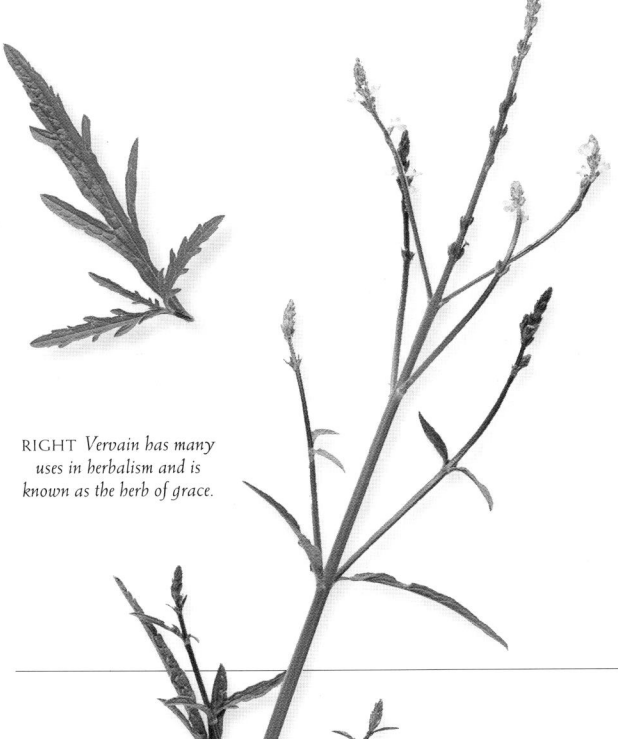

RIGHT *Vervain has many uses in herbalism and is known as the herb of grace.*

DATA FILE

Use

Vervain people have fixed ideas and principles. They are strong-willed and rarely change their views; they think they are right and obstinately maintain a stance, or fight on when others would have conceded. They are great doers and wish to convert all those around them. They strive with mental energy and will power, but the effort of trying to persuade others is extremely stressful, even exhausting. Vervain brings calm and the ability to relax a little and see the other point of view.

Method

🌿 The sun method *(see page 222)*

PROFILE

🌿 GOAL – Will; to relax and hear the will of the world 🌿 People who need Vervain are those whose activity is self-driven, often with overcommitment. 🌿 They may be overworked and experience stress-related illnesses, including anxiety, indigestion, insomnia, and sleep disorders. 🌿 Vervain brings calm and a space for reflection. It relieves stress and helps to bring the personal will into harmony with the world.

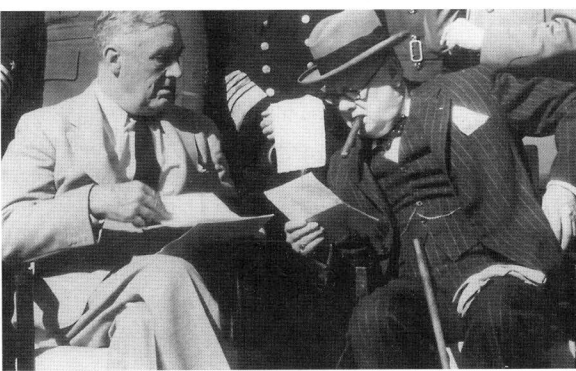

ABOVE *Vervain can be an aid to people who have to face stress and challenges.*

241

Vitis vinifera
VINE

The grapevine is a thick-trunked shrub which climbs by means of tendrils. The flower clusters are small and green, and give way to the well-known fruit – green or purple berries.

DATA FILE

Use

Vine is for capable, confident, and successful people; for those who would be "king" (or "queen"). They believe they know best and that others would be happier if they followed. They can bully and dominate, disempowering others, and gaining authority at the expense of their confidence. Even in illness, from the sickbed, they can be ruthless and dominating, ordering their carers around. Vine encourages equality, and the respect each of us, as a fellow human being, is due.

Method

❦ The sun method *(see page 222)*

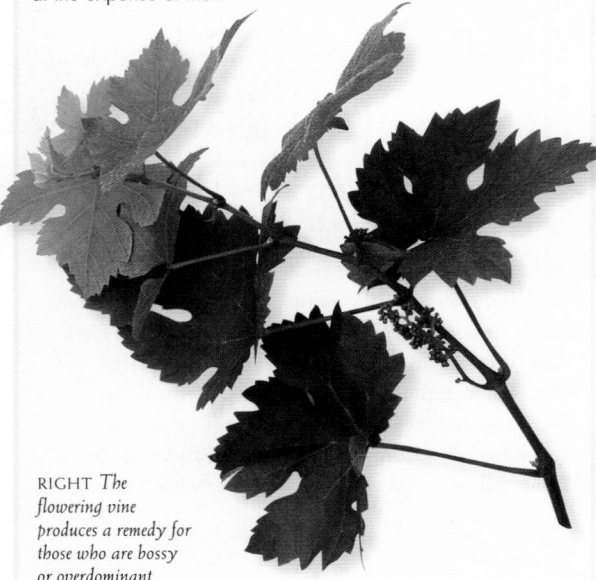

RIGHT *The flowering vine produces a remedy for those who are bossy or overdominant.*

PROFILE

❧ GOAL – Power and natural authority; leadership by consent not through fear ❧ **Those who need Vine are dominating and bullying.** ❧ They can be cruel and callous through thoughtlessness. ❧ **They may also experience stress-related illnesses.** ❧ Vine allows us to stand back and let others express themselves, to respect the absolute authority of each person over their own inner life, and to acknowledge their personal choices.

Wahlenbergia spp.
BLUEBELL

This is a small perennial bluebell that is native to Australia. The small, blue, bell-like flowers appear in spring. *Wahlenbergia* thrives best in partial shade, and prefers a well-drained soil.

DATA FILE

Use

Bluebell is a remedy for the heart – it opens the heart to the flow of the universe. The heart may be closed through hurt, fear, or loneliness. People who need Bluebell are emotionally closed and fearful. They fear that love will run out and they will be left with nothing. They may be possessive and greedy, with objects representing love.

Method

❦ The sun method *(see page 222)*

BELOW *Bluebell remedy helps to conquer greed and possessiveness, and brings a will to love and share.*

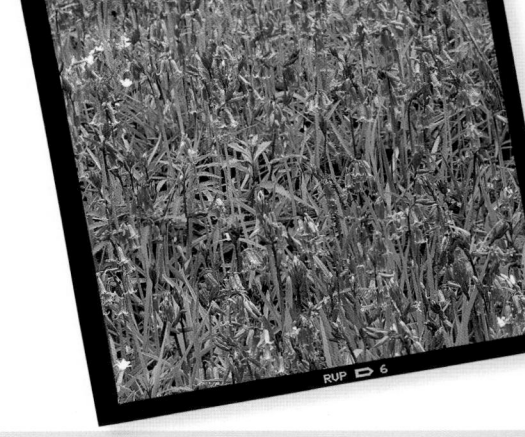

BELOW *A patch of wild Australian bluebells makes a breathtaking sight in spring.*

PROFILE

❧ GOAL – Wholehearted abundance of love; sharing ❧ **People who need Bluebell are emotionally closed, and find it hard to share without keeping mental tally of all emotional transactions.** ❧ They are possessive, greedy, and possibly house-proud. Children will not share. ❧ **They may also have congestive and containing symptoms such as indigestion, cramps, constipation, or hemorrhoids.** ❧ Bluebell helps us own ourselves. The heart is like the magic wine flask in the fairy story; it never runs out. Each morning it is refilled to overflowing abundance.

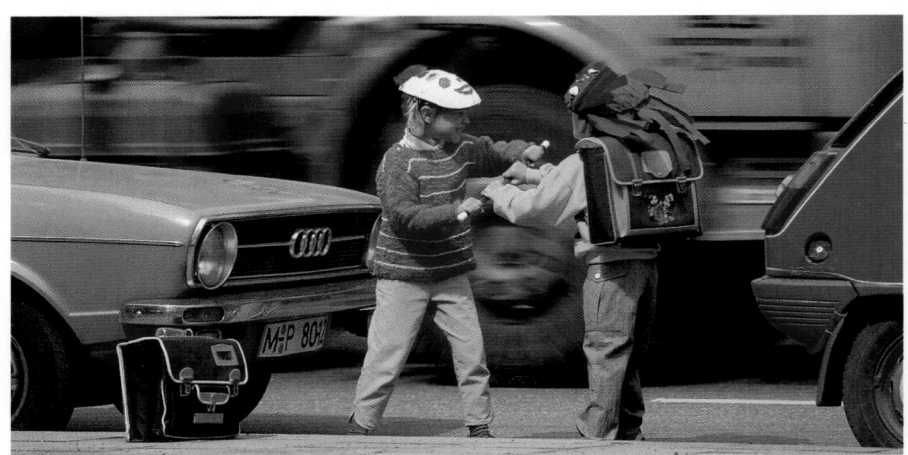

Wisteria sinensis
WISTERIA

Wisteria is a large, woody vine, originally from China. The flowers come before the leaves in spring, and hang in large drooping plumes of pale lilac and mauve. This climber can grow to 100ft. (30m.).

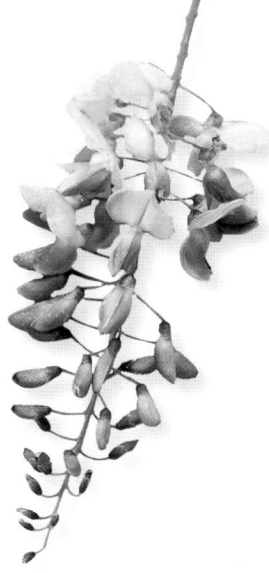

RIGHT *The soft gray racemes of wisteria have a gentle perfume which is found to be very soothing.*

DATA FILE

Use

In Western culture, sex and gender issues are sometimes seen as a matter of power and control. The term "war of the sexes" expresses this. Rape and sexual abuse frequently confirm this role and attitude to power. Wisteria helps people to overcome the inhibitions, blocks, and emotional conflicts produced by this dualistic attitude. It can help them to transcend the roles and to be comfortable with their sexuality. Wisteria can enable them to be open, express themselves, and experience the intimate power and passivity of the orgasm.

Method

🌢 The sun method *(see page 222)*

PROFILE

🌢 GOAL – To be comfortable with own sexuality; intimacy and trust 🌢 **Women who need Wisteria may be frigid, cold, have a touch taboo, or not enjoy sex. They cannot "lose control" or give themselves.** 🌢 Men who need Wisteria may be equally fearful and "role-bound," being macho or a "New Man," when they should let go and be themselves. 🌢 **Associated symptoms may be genital herpes, warts, or pelvic congestion linked to a pattern or history of abuse, as well as very painful menstruation. If there is a history of abuse (in either sex), give other appropriate remedies.** 🌢 Wisteria helps us experience intimacy and mutual trust.

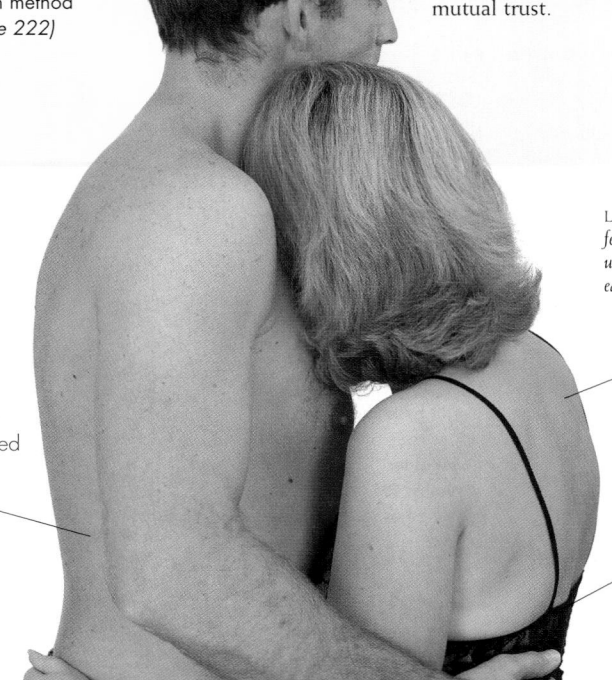

LEFT *Both partners may feel trapped in a role and unable to behave toward each other with true feeling.*

Man trapped by macho image

Woman may feel frigid

Cannot let go

ROCK WATER

Water taken from a natural well or spring, preferably one with a traditional reputation for healing. There are many half-forgotten springs and wells. The water should be open and free-flowing. Choose a well or spring which is open to the air and sunshine, and is as natural as possible. Do not use water from a well dedicated to a saint, or within a church or shrine.

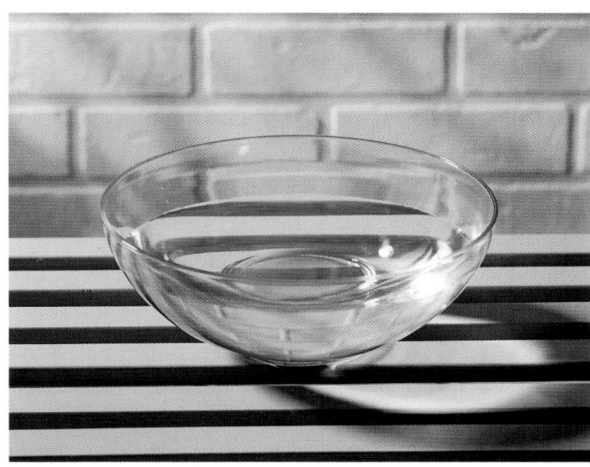

ABOVE *Pure, clear water, filtered by rock can encourage the spirit to flow.*

PROFILE

🌢 GOAL – Harmony and discipline
🌢 People who need Rock Water may be rigid, narrow-minded, and very strict with themselves, to the point of self-denial.
🌢 They are perfectionists with exaggerated ideals, but unlike Vervain people they do not try to convert others. They are content to make themselves perfect.
🌢 Rock Water encourages flexibility in reaching goals which harmonize with the natural order of the world.

DATA FILE

Use

Rock Water is for people who are very strict with themselves and unforgiving – like the rock. They practise self-discipline and deny themselves anything which might distract them from their goal. They have high ideals and are hard on themselves. True self-discipline does not involve denial. Denial is only necessary when the person is not acting from the heart and has a narrow view of his or her goal. Rock Water gives the flexibility of water, a pure spring flowing toward the sea.

Method

🌢 The sun method *(see page 222)*

RESCUE REMEDY

Rescue Remedy can be bought as a liquid or as a cream. It is made from equal amounts of the five following essences:

* CHERRY PLUM – *for feelings of desperation*
* ROCK ROSE – *to ease terror, fear, or panic*
* IMPATIENS – *to soothe irritability and agitation*
* CLEMATIS – *to counteract the tendency to drift away from the present*
* STAR OF BETHLEHEM – *to address the mental and physical symptoms of shock*

Together, these flower essences make a safe mental sanctuary in which to recover. Carry Rescue Remedy with you for all emergencies.

CLEMATIS

STAR OF BETHLEHEM

IMPATIENS

CHERRY PLUM

ROCK ROSE

ABOVE *The five flowers whose essences are used to make up the Bach Flower Rescue Remedy.*

DATA FILE

Use

Rescue Remedy rebalances the body after any emotional or physical upset. It should be taken when a person feels in need of rescue, is unsettled, or is not quite in step with himself or herself. This may be after a shock, an accident, an argument, a trying event like a divorce or separation, or any circumstance which has demanded supreme nervous effort. Rescue must take place before salvage and restoration.

Rescue Remedy speeds healing after surgery.

Use Rescue Remedy cream after sunburn, cuts, bruises, or damage from accidents.

Rescue Remedy can be added to any skin wash, douche, or compress if some element of rescue is needed. This method is also useful if nothing is allowed by mouth.

Rescue Remedy can also be given before a trying event, examination, court appearance, operation, hospital test, etc., to minimize the trauma. It is for all emergencies; always carry a small bottle with you.

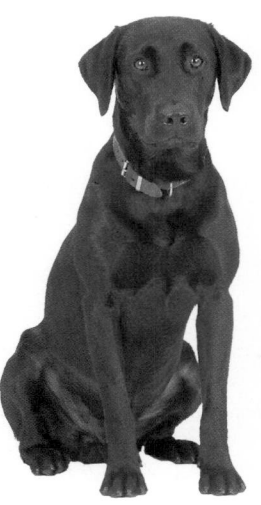

ABOVE *Even frightened or traumatized animals respond to treatment with Rescue Remedy.*

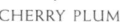

244

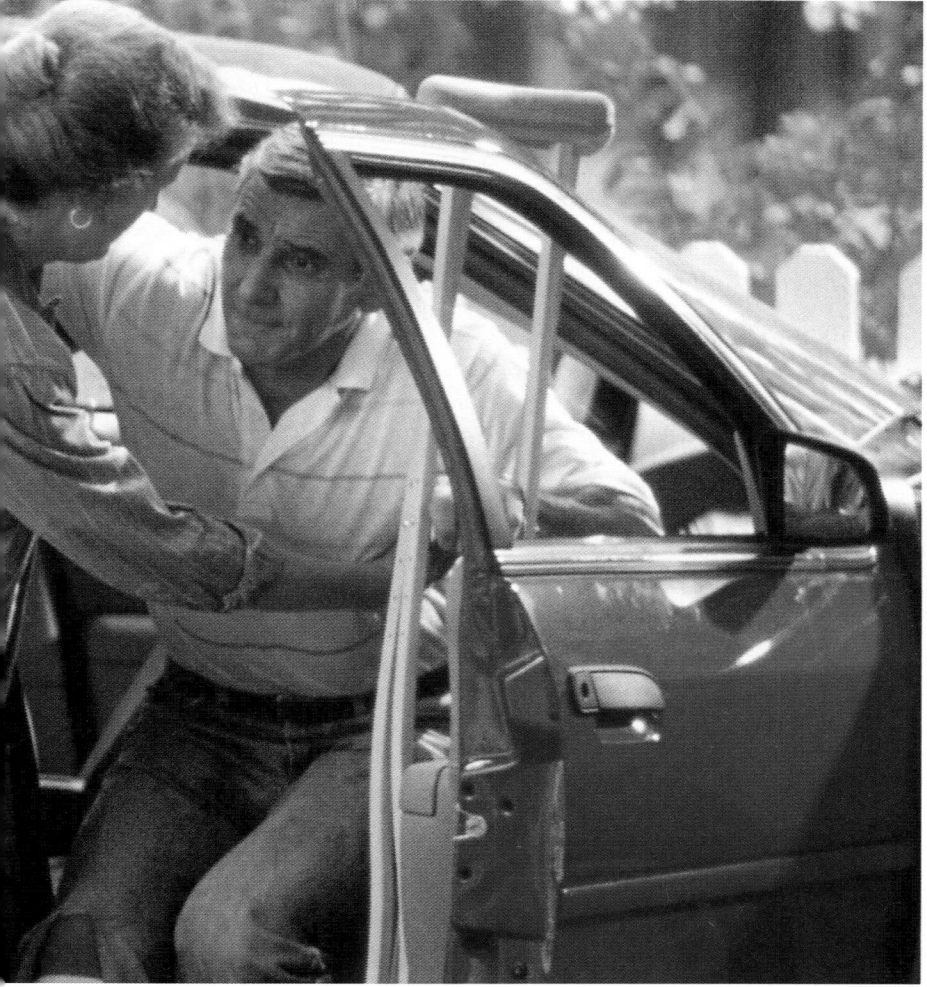

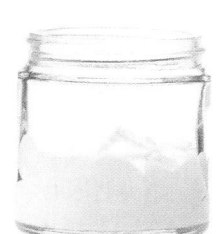

LEFT *Rescue Remedy can have a calming, stabilizing effect after an event such as a car crash.*

LEFT *A few drops of Rescue Remedy can be mixed into skin cream for external use.*

RECIPE

Home-made Rescue Remedy

🌿 🌿 🌿 🌿

Make a treatment bottle of Rescue Remedy by adding 2 drops of each constituent Bach Flower Remedy to a 1fl. oz. (30ml.) bottle of brandy.

A cream can be made at home by adding 4 drops of stock Rescue Remedy to a favorite skin cream or neutral base, then adding 2 drops of Crab Apple.

PROFILE

🌿 GOAL– Rescue or salvation 🌿 **Rescue Remedy is the only Bach Flower Remedy that is usually taken neat, straight from the stock bottle. Put 4 drops directly onto or under the tongue. Repeat dosage as often as needed.** 🌿 Put 4 drops into a glass of water and sip throughout the day until you feel more settled. 🌿 **Rescue Remedy is ideal for children and animals, and can be dropped into food or drinking water. A startled infant or baby can be reassured by putting 4 drops into the evening bath.** 🌿 It can be given to plants and seedlings with success. 🌿 **It is never too late to take Rescue Remedy. It will help overcome old and unspoken trauma if these are still upsetting you. But it is not a panacea, so once the immediate emotional crisis has calmed, look at the other remedies with a view to creating your own personal combination.**

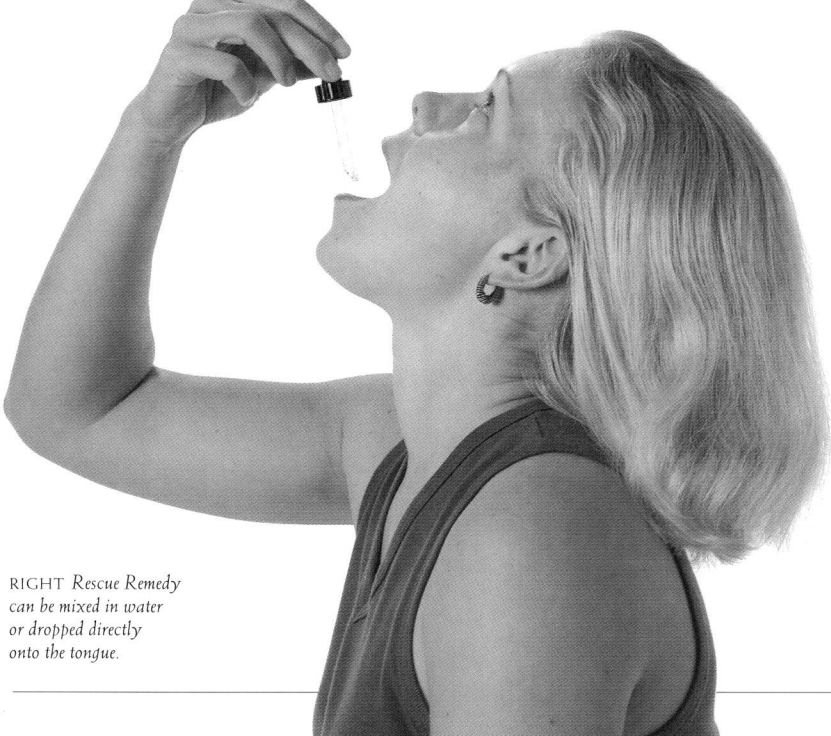

RIGHT *Rescue Remedy can be mixed in water or dropped directly onto the tongue.*

VITAMINS AND MINERALS

Our understanding of vitamins and minerals — and other micronutrients, compounds, and elements — and their role in our body has improved dramatically over the last decades. We now know that "micronutrition" — or the vitamins, minerals, and other health-giving components of our food, such as amino acids, fiber, enzymes, and lipids — is crucial to life, and that by manipulating our nutritional intake, we can not only ensure good health and address ailments, but prevent illness and some of the degenerative effects of aging. Exciting new discoveries related to the nutrient components of our food mean that more than half of us are now taking supplementation in one form or another, convinced that diet itself — bearing in mind the stresses on our body and the polluted world in which we live — is inadequate to supply us with our nutritional needs.

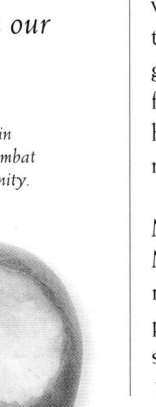

ABOVE *More than 50 percent of the U.K. population now take some form of dietary supplement.*

BELOW *Apples contain vitamin C, which helps combat infection and boost immunity.*

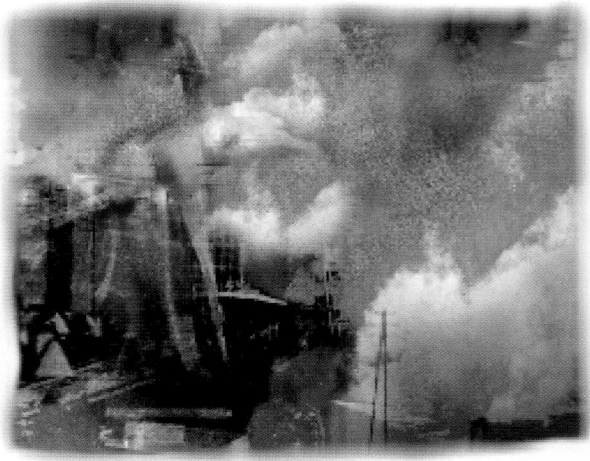

ABOVE *Pollutants in the atmosphere have a harmful effect on our health, making it even more important that we supplement our diet with vitamins and minerals.*

VITAMINS

Vitamins are a group of unrelated organic nutrients which are essential to regulate the chemical processes that go on in the body — such as releasing the energy from food, maintaining strong bones, and controlling our hormonal activity. Ideally, vitamins are present in roughly the same quantity in various foods.

MINERALS

Minerals are inorganic chemical elements, which are necessary for many biochemical and physiological processes that go on in our bodies. Inorganic substances that are required in amounts greater than 100mg. per day are called minerals; those required in

A HISTORY OF NUTRITION

PREHISTORY

From the very earliest days of civilization, nutrition has formed the backbone of healthcare. Obtaining and eating food consumed most of early humans' time, and food and herbs were our first medicine, used to treat a large number of conditions ranging from wounds and insect bites to infection. It became clear that food had powerful healing effects, and that a varied diet, rich in natural ingredients, was a prerequisite for good health. From that time, diet became a fundamental part of most therapies, and an integral element in almost all of the others.

18TH CENTURY

In the 18th century, English sailors were given lime or lemon juice in order to prevent scurvy, a disease caused by lack of vitamin C, which occurred as a result of long periods of time away at sea without fresh fruit or vegetables.

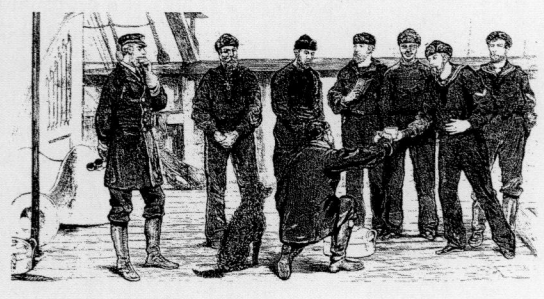

LEFT *From the 18th century English sailors ate limes as a protection against scurvy.*

19TH CENTURY

In the late 19th century, naturopaths drew attention to the use of food and its nutritional elements as medicine, a concept that was not new, but which had not been acknowledged as a therapy in its own right until that time. Naturopaths used nutrition and fasting to cleanse the body, and to encourage its ability to heal itself. As knowledge about food, its make-up, and the effects it has on our body became greater with the development of biochemistry, the first nutritional specialists undertook to treat specific ailments and symptoms with the components of food.

ABOVE *Since the 19th century, the nutritional components of food have been used as medicine.*

amounts less than 100mg. per day are called trace elements. Minerals are not necessarily present in foods – the quality of the soil and the geological conditions of the area in which they were grown play an important part in determining the mineral content of foods. Even a balanced diet may be lacking in essential minerals or trace elements because of the soil in which the various foodstuffs were grown.

There is evidence that "sub-clinical" deficiencies – in other words, a deficiency which is not extensive enough to be life-threatening or to produce large-scale symptoms – may be the cause of certain forms of cancer, heart disease, weight and skin problems, and a host of other health conditions.

AMINO ACIDS

An amino acid is any compound that contains an amino group and an acidic function. There are 20 amino acids necessary for the synthesis of proteins, which are essential for life. These 20 amino acids form the building blocks of all proteins and are involved in important biological processes, such as the formation of neurotransmitters in the brain. There are eight essential amino acids, which are:

- *phenylalanine*
- *valine*
- *threonine*
- *tryptophan*
- *isoleucine*
- *methionine*
- *lysine*
- *leucine*

The remaining 12 are called "nonessential," which means that they can usually be made by the body from other substances. In some conditions, however, nonessential amino acids are necessary, for example in cases of extreme illness or a very poor diet.

LIPIDS AND DERIVATIVES

Lipids are commonly called "fats," and while many fats are now known to be unhealthy, there are many that are essential to body processes and actually work to prevent the effects of "unhealthy" fats in our bodies. Many lipids and their derivatives are used to unclog arteries, work to retard the effects of aging, and to discourage heart disease and the build-up of cholesterol.

OTHER SUPPLEMENTS

There are a number of other food supplements that do not fall strictly within the definitions of vitamins, minerals, lipids, and amino acids. These include various elements that either have healing properties or are now known to be crucial to health.

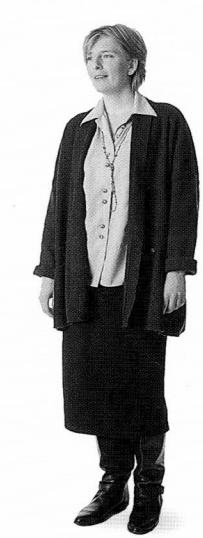

NUTRITION TODAY

Nutrition has changed from a mainly physician-led dietary therapy, also called clinical nutrition, to a more profound theory of health based on treating the patient as a whole (holistic health), and looking for deficiencies that may be causing illness, which are specific to each individual.

RIGHT *Many nutritionists now treat their patients holistically as a "whole being" composed of body, mind, and soul.*

20TH CENTURY

By the middle of the 20th century, scientists had put together a profile of proteins, carbohydrates, and fats, as well as vitamins and minerals, which were essential to life and to health. More than 40 nutrients were uncovered, including 13 vitamins. It was discovered that minerals were needed for body functions, and a new understanding of the body and its biochemistry fed the growing interest in the subject. In the 1960s, physicians began to treat patients with special diets and supplements, prescribed according to individual symptoms, problems, and needs, but while conventional medical physicians still discussed nutrition in terms of basic food groups, nutritionists were prescribing vitamins in megadoses.

ABOVE AND RIGHT *Conventional medical practioners discuss nutrition in terms of food groups, while nutritionists tend to prescribe vitamins.*

Other elements and compounds were soon identified as necessary to human life, and we are now able to purchase and take substances like amino acids; bee pollen; lipids, such as evening primrose oil and cod liver oil; and seaweeds, acidophilus (healthy bacteria), and dietary enzymes.

WHAT DO VITAMINS, MINERALS, AND OTHER ELEMENTS DO IN OUR BODIES?

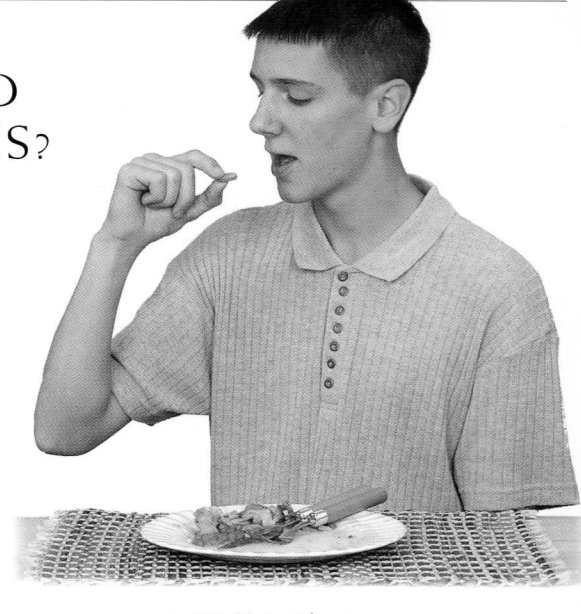

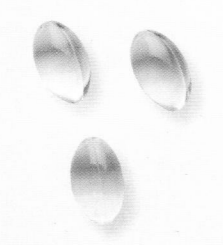

ABOVE *In some cases vitamin and mineral supplements should only be taken on the advice of a registered nutritionist.*

Vitamins, minerals, and other elements work together within the body to ensure that all processes can be carried out. When even one element is missing, the body becomes unbalanced and unable to work at its optimum level.

WHEN SHOULD SUPPLEMENTS BE TAKEN?

☙ The best time for taking most supplements is after meals, on a full stomach, although some vitamins and minerals work best on an empty stomach. Read the label on any supplement you plan to take to find out the best time to take it.

☙ Time-release formulas need to be taken with food, as their nutrients are slowly released over a number of hours. If there is not enough food to slow their passage through the body, they can pass the sites where they are normally absorbed before they have had a chance to release their nutrients.

☙ Take supplements evenly throughout the day for best effect.

WHEN TO SEE A PRACTITIONER

Most supplements can be taken safely without input from a nutritionist, but if you suffer from chronic health problems, or a specific ailment, it is best to seek expert advice. Amino acids and other elements should only be taken with the advice of a professional. A nutritionist will make sure that you are taking a balanced combination of nutrients that will work together to make you healthy. Remember that everyone's needs are different, based on overall health, diet, whether or not you smoke or drink, are pregnant, and other influences. It is sensible to ensure that you receive advice that is tailored specifically to your individual needs.

RIGHT *If you suffer from chronic health problems, consider visiting a nutritionist for expert advice.*

ABOVE *Most supplements are best taken on a full stomach, but read the label on the packet for precise information.*

CHILDREN

Children need far lower doses than adults, and a healthy, organic diet should offer a large proportion of their nutritional needs. A good vitamin and mineral supplement will provide anything extra that is required, but if you feel your child needs further supplements, see a practitioner. If you are buying products yourself, read the label to ensure that the product is safe for children, and follow the advice carefully.

PREGNANCY

A growing baby puts heavy demands on your body when you are pregnant, and it is more important than ever to ensure that you have a good diet. Research has now proved that we need extra folic acid and iron during pregnancy, and a good multivitamin and mineral supplement is often suggested. Do not take vitamin A supplements while pregnant (*see page 252*).

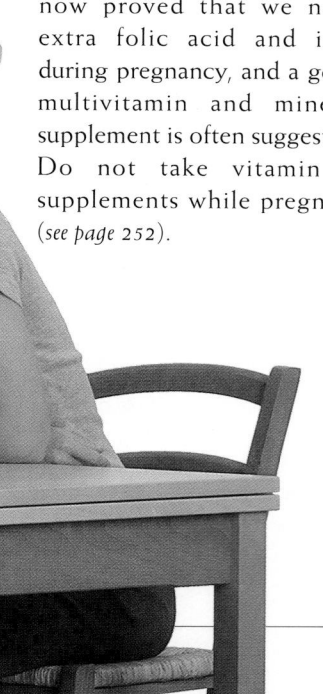

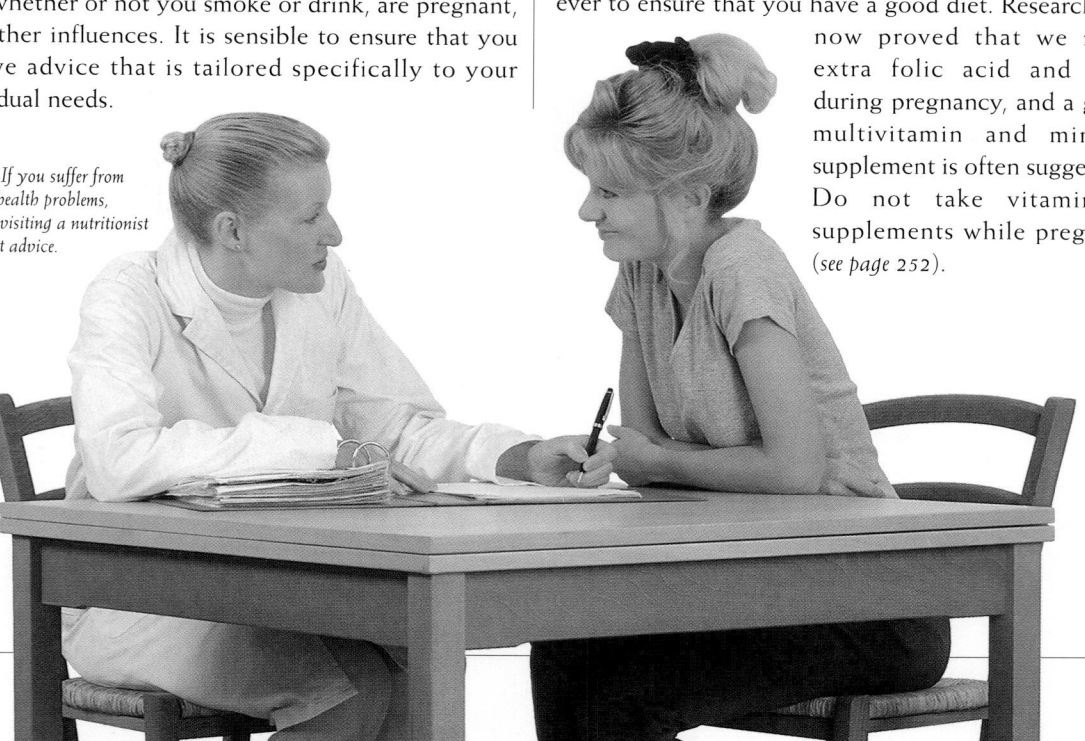

A HEALTHY DIET

Our diet should be made up of complex carbohydrates (5–9 portions per day), fruits and vegetables (4–9 portions), proteins (3–5 portions), and fat (under 30g. per day is recommended for a healthy diet). But eating the right foods doesn't necessarily mean that you are getting enough nutrients. Refining and processing foods takes out much of the nutritional value, and pesticides and other agents used in the growing process place extra demands on our bodies. Before our food ever reaches the grocery store it may be nutritionally deficient. Therefore, take extra steps to preserve the nutritional content of your food whenever possible:

- Eat the skins of vegetables.
- Don't cut, wash, or soak fruit and vegetables until you are ready to eat them. Exposing their cut surfaces to air destroys many nutrients.
- Eat brown, unpolished rice and whole grains.
- Choose fresh fruit and vegetables first, but remember that nutritional value decreases with age. Frozen is a better option if you aren't going to eat the food immediately.
- Eat raw whenever possible; if cooking, use as little water as possible.
- If you do boil fruit or vegetables, use the water remaining after cooking in your sauces or gravy.
- Eat organic food whenever possible. It may be more expensive, but you can be sure that the food you are eating has not been processed, and has been grown without the use of pesticides and other chemicals.

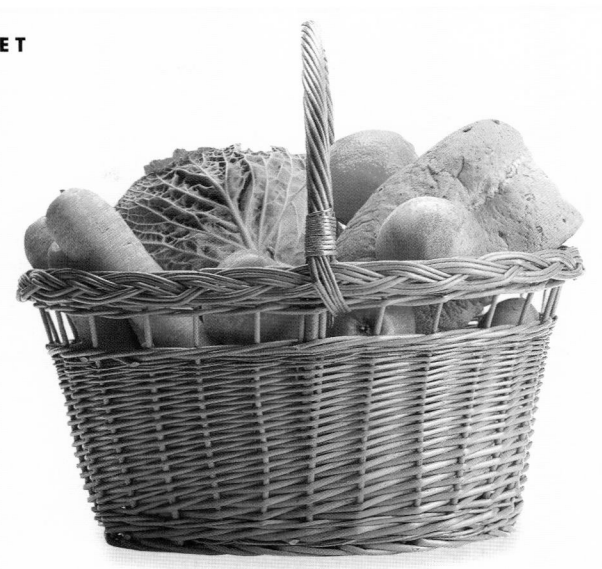

BELOW Choose your daily dietary requirements from different groups of food – complex carbohydrates, fruit and vegetables, and fats and proteins.

ABOVE By the time our food reaches the grocery store it may have lost many of its valuable nutrients. Try to choose organic fruit and vegetables.

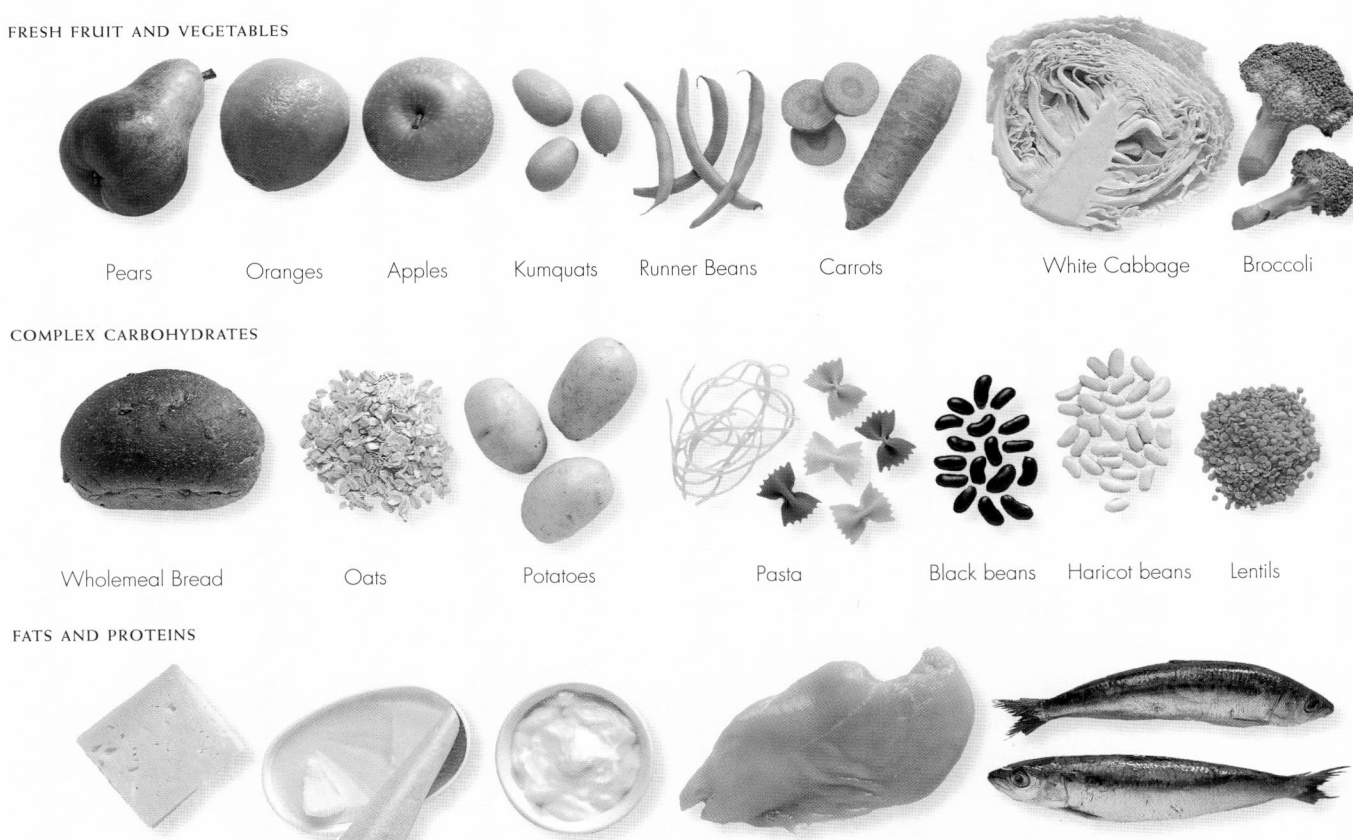

FRESH FRUIT AND VEGETABLES

Pears   Oranges   Apples   Kumquats   Runner Beans   Carrots   White Cabbage   Broccoli

COMPLEX CARBOHYDRATES

Wholemeal Bread   Oats   Potatoes   Pasta   Black beans   Haricot beans   Lentils

FATS AND PROTEINS

Cheese   Vegetable Spread   Yogurt   Chicken   Fish

SUPPLEMENT FORMS

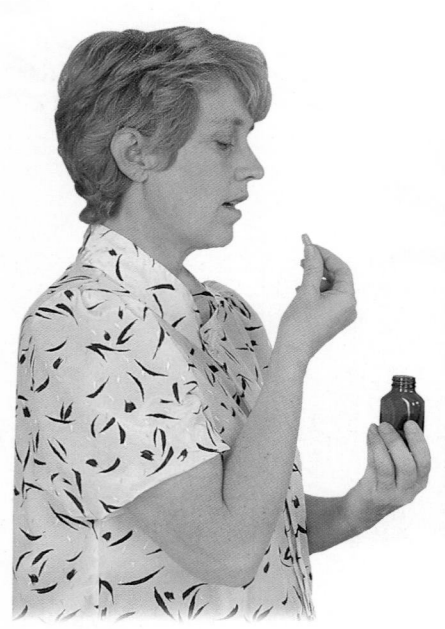

Most supplements come in a variety of forms, to allow for individual needs. They are also prepared with different quantities of the active ingredients, so read the label carefully to ensure that you are getting the correct quantity for your needs.

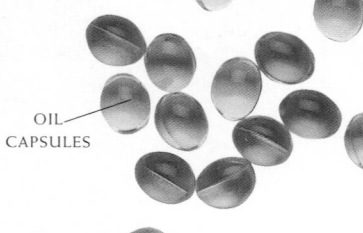

OIL
CAPSULES

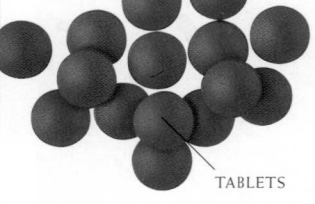

TABLETS

POWDER
CAPSULES

ABOVE Some supplements come in a variety of forms, allowing the individual to choose between powders, capsules, liquids, or tablets.

WHICH SUPPLEMENT?

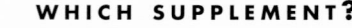
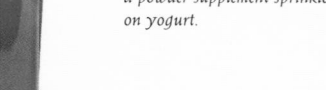

- **POWDERS** Many supplements come in powder form, which will usually provide you with extra potency, with no binders or additives. This is useful for people with allergies, or those who find it difficult to swallow a tablet. Powders are particularly useful for children – sprinkle a little powder in their breakfast juice, or stir it into some yogurt or dessert.

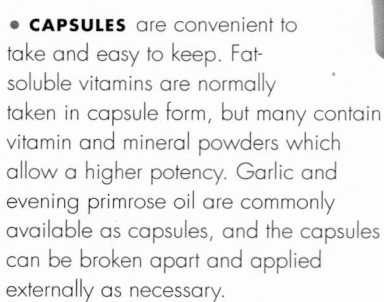

LEFT If you find it too hard to swallow tablets, try taking a powder supplement sprinkled on yogurt.

- **CAPSULES** are convenient to take and easy to keep. Fat-soluble vitamins are normally taken in capsule form, but many contain vitamin and mineral powders which allow a higher potency. Garlic and evening primrose oil are commonly available as capsules, and the capsules can be broken apart and applied externally as necessary.

- **LIQUIDS** are appropriate for people who have difficulty swallowing tablets or capsules. Many children's formulas come in liquid form for easy administration. Liquids can be mixed with food or stirred into drinks. Liquid supplements can also be applied externally.

- **TABLETS** Many supplements come in tablet form and these are the most practical for many people because they can be easily stored and they will keep for a long time. Check the label to see what is added to your tablets in the form of binders or fillers, which are added to preserve or bulk out the active ingredient.

RIGHT Liquid formulas can be added to fruit juices, making them a popular form of supplement for children.

Reading the Label

Supplements work in different ways, and you will need to understand some of the key words that appear on the labels in order to choose which are most suitable for you.

Chelated is a term which appears on mineral supplements, and it means that the mineral is combined with amino acids to make assimilation more efficient. Most nutritionists recommend taking chelated minerals because they are 3 to 5 times more effective.

Time-release formulas are created with a process that allows them to be released into the body over an 8–10-hour period. These are particularly useful for water-soluble vitamins (*see pages 253–56*), any excess of which is excreted within 2 or 3 hours of taking the supplement. Time-release formulas are reputed to provide stable blood levels during the day and night.

ANTIOXIDANTS

Much of the cell damage that occurs in disease is caused by highly destructive chemical groups known as free radicals. These are the products of oxidation, a process which occurs naturally in our body as we breathe. Today, because of the other elements in the air, there are more free radicals than ever. In small quantities free radicals can fight bacteria and viruses; in larger quantities they encourage the aging process and cause damage to our cells.

Fortunately, these can be combated by antioxidants – the ACE vitamins (vitamin A in the form of beta carotene, vitamin C, and vitamin E), the minerals selenium and zinc, and to a lesser extent manganese and copper. Antioxidants protect other substances from oxidation. Many trials have shown that additional antioxidant vitamins – such as 2,000mg. of C and 400mg. of E daily – can significantly reduce the incidence of heart attacks, strokes, cataracts, and other diseases, and slow down the process of aging.

BELOW *Antioxidants, such as the ACE vitamins and zinc, can help combat cell damage caused by free radicals.*

BETA-CAROTENE

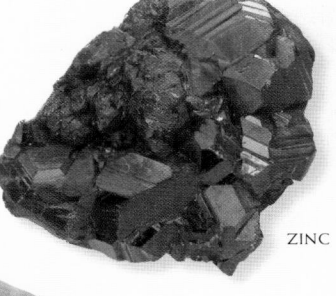

ZINC

WHICH PROBLEMS CAN VITAMINS, MINERALS, AND OTHER SUPPLEMENTS HELP?

The use of nutrition for health, or nutritional therapy, can help with almost anything, since food is the basic fuel of all the chemical processes which take place in the body. Therefore, almost all ill health can have a basis in nutritional elements which are missing or insubstantial within the diet. Great success has been achieved treating conditions like rheumatism and arthritis, high blood pressure, fatigue, constipation and other digestive disorders, the healing and recuperation processes following injury or surgery, skin problems, and many psychological and behavioral problems. Neuralgia, osteoporosis, PMS, post-natal illness, pregnancy problems, reduced immunities, stress, and viruses may respond to dietary treatment. In effect, however, all the systems in the body will be improved by a healthy diet. In a fit state you are much more likely to fight off infection and deal efficiently with any health problems or injury.

Governments around the world have provided guidelines for how much of each vitamin or mineral we need in our diets. These are called RDAs (recommended daily allowance) or RDIs (recommended daily intake) and they apply to healthy individuals with a good, balanced diet. These levels are an "adequate" intake, and do not reflect new thinking on nutrition for optimal health and longevity. In other words, they are not therapeutic levels and they do not take into account the varying needs of the population. People with illnesses, a stressful lifestyle, or who are on medication, or eat a highly refined diet may need much more than the RDA.

RDA AND SUPPLEMENTS

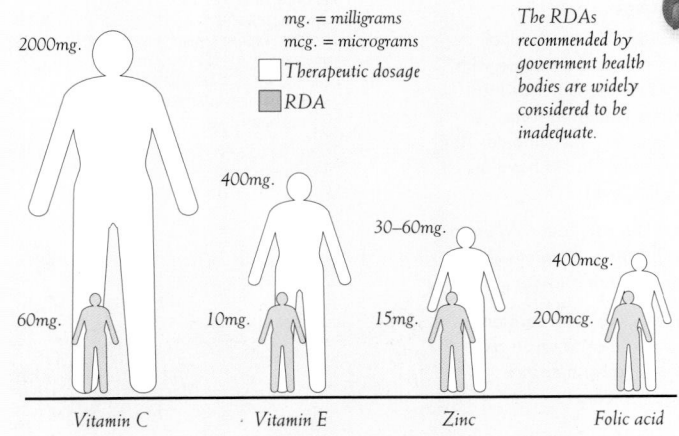

mg. = milligrams
mcg. = micrograms
☐ Therapeutic dosage
▨ RDA

2000mg.
60mg.
Vitamin C

400mg.
10mg.
Vitamin E

30–60mg.
15mg.
Zinc

400mcg.
200mcg.
Folic acid

The RDAs recommended by government health bodies are widely considered to be inadequate.

ABOVE *Conditions such as rheumatism respond to dietary change, combined with vitamin and mineral supplements.*

VITAMIN A

U.S. RDA 3mg. E.U. RDA 800mcg.

Vitamin A is a fat-soluble vitamin that comes in two forms: retinol, which is found in animal products such as liver, eggs, butter, and cod liver oil; and beta-carotene, which our body converts into vitamin A when we need more. Beta-carotene is found in any brightly-colored fruits and vegetables.

Vitamin A was for many years called a "miracle" vitamin because of its effect on the immune system and growth. It is necessary for healthy skin and eyes, and allows us to see in the dark. Beta-carotene is an antioxidant (*see page 251*), and it has anti-carcinogenic properties.

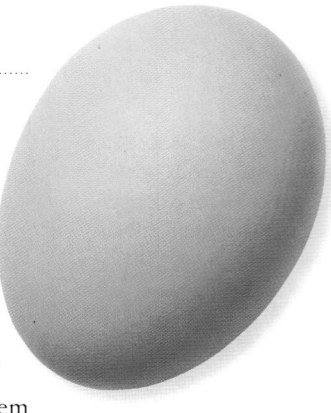

ABOVE *Retinol, one form of vitamin A, can be found in animal products such as eggs.*

ABOVE *Vitamin A is necessary for good vision and helps prevent night blindness.*

BELOW LEFT *Carrots are a good source of beta-carotene, which our body converts into vitamin A when necessary.*

DATA FILE

Properties

❦ Anticarcinogenic.

❦ Prevents and treats skin disorders and aging of skin.

❦ Improves vision and prevents night blindness.

❦ Improves the body's ability to heal.

❦ Promotes the growth of strong bones, hair, teeth, skin, and gums.

❦ May help in the treatment of hyperthyroidism.

Best Sources

Vitamin A: cod liver oil, liver, kidney, eggs, and dairy produce.

Beta-carotene: carrots, tomatoes, watercress, broccoli, spinach, cantaloupe, apricots.

Dosage

❦ The RDA is very much a minimum, and people with special needs (following illness, suffering from infections, with diabetes, for example) should have a higher level.

❦ Taken as vitamin A, up to 6,000mcg. is permissible if you are not pregnant.

❦ Taken as beta-carotene, 15mg. can be taken as a preventative measure against illness.

CAUTION

VITAMIN A AS RETINOL IS TOXIC AND SHOULD NOT BE TAKEN AT ALL AS A SUPPLEMENT BY PREGNANT WOMEN, AS IT CAN CAUSE BIRTH DEFECTS IN THE UNBORN CHILD.

B1 (THIAMINE)

U.S. RDA 1.2–1.5mg. E.U. RDA 1.4mg.

Thiamine is involved in all key metabolic processes in the nervous system, the heart, the blood cells, and the muscles. It is useful in the treatment of nervous disorders, and can protect against imbalances caused by alcoholism.

There are more cases of vitamin B1 deficiency than of any other nutritional element – this has been said to be due to a growth in alcoholism. Thiamine is found in all plant and animal foods, but good sources are whole grains, brown rice, seafood, and pulses.

DATA FILE

Properties

❦ Protects against imbalances caused by alcohol consumption.

❦ B1 may be useful in treating heart disease.

❦ May be beneficial in the treatment of neurological disease (particularly when caused by B1 deficiency).

❦ May help to treat anemia.

❦ May improve people's mental agility.

❦ May help to control diabetes which has been linked to deficiency.

❦ Useful in the treatment of herpes and infections.

❦ Helps to convert sugar to energy, in the muscles and the bones.

Best Sources

Pork, milk, eggs, whole grains, organ meats, brown rice, barley, seafood.

Dosage

❦ Heavy drinkers, smokers, pregnant women, or those taking the pill should increase normal dosage to up to 100–300mg. per day.

❦ Increase intake in stressful conditions. Will be most effective as part of a good B-complex supplement.

CAUTION

THIAMINE IS NONTOXIC, BUT IT IS RECOMMENDED THAT YOU DO NOT TAKE MORE THAN 400MG. DAILY.

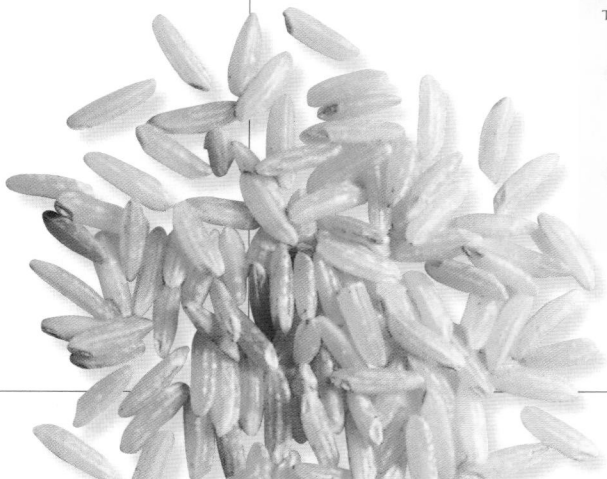

LEFT *Brown rice can help protect against imbalances caused by alcohol as it contains thiamine.*

B2 (RIBOFLAVIN)

U.S. RDA 1.7mg. E.U. RDA 1.6mg.

Riboflavin is a water-soluble member of the B-complex family of vitamins. It is crucial to the production of body energy and has antioxidant qualities. Riboflavin is not stored in any significant amount in the body, and deficiency is common.

Riboflavin is necessary for healthy skin, hair, and nails. Because it is destroyed by sunlight, it is recommended that you keep foods containing this vitamin in a dark, cool place. In particular, milk loses its riboflavin content after only two hours' exposure to sun.

BELOW *Dairy products, such as cheese, are one of the best sources of riboflavin. Intake should be increased during pregnancy and breast-feeding.*

CAUTION

RIBOFLAVIN IS NONTOXIC IN MOST DOSES, BUT IT IS RECOMMENDED THAT YOU DO NOT TAKE IN EXCESS OF 400MG. PER DAY UNLESS SUPERVISED BY A REGISTERED PRACTITIONER.

ABOVE *Avocado is a rich source of many vitamins, including niacin.*

DATA FILE

Properties

ᴗ Works with enzymes to metabolize fats, protein, and carbohydrates.

ᴗ Aids vision.

ᴗ Promotes healthy skin, hair, and nails.

ᴗ Promotes healthy growth and reproductive function.

ᴗ Boosts athletic performance.

ᴗ Protects against cancer.

ᴗ Protects against anemia.

Best Sources

Milk, eggs, cheese, fortified breads and cereals, green leafy vegetables, fish.

Dosage

ᴗ Pregnancy, breast-feeding, taking the pill, and heavy drinking all call for an increased intake.

ᴗ Take as part of a B-complex supplement, and increase dosage in stressful situations. 100–300mg. per day is commonly suggested.

B3 (NIACIN)

U.S. RDA 13–18mg. adults, 5–6mg. infants, 9–13mg. children under ten. E.U. RDA 15–18mg.

Niacin is one of the water-soluble B-complex vitamins, and it is essential for the synthesis of sex hormones and a healthy nervous system. Niacin may also be valuable in helping to prevent and treat schizophrenia, and in acting as a detoxicant, ridding the body of toxins, pollutants, and drugs.

Niacin takes the form of nicotinic acid and nicotinamide, and is a fairly recent addition to the family of B-complex vitamins, named as a vitamin only in 1937. Niacin has been shown to lower blood cholesterol and other body fats, and is useful in the prevention of heart disease. It may help to prevent diabetes.

CAUTION

IN HIGH DOSES, NIACIN MAY CAUSE DEPRESSION, LIVER MALFUNCTION, FLUSHING, AND HEADACHES.

AVOID DOSES LARGER THAN ABOUT 120MG. UNLESS YOU ARE UNDER THE SUPERVISION OF A REGISTERED PRACTITIONER.

DATA FILE

Properties

ᴗ Prevents and treats schizophrenia.

ᴗ Aids in cell respiration.

ᴗ Produces energy from sugar, fat, and protein.

ᴗ Maintains clear, healthy skin, nerves, tongue, and good digestion.

ᴗ May lower cholesterol and therefore protect against heart disease.

ᴗ Believed to be antioxidant.

ᴗ May help prevent migraine headaches.

ᴗ Reduces blood pressure.

ᴗ May alleviate arthritis.

Best Sources

Meat, fish, wholegrain cereals, eggs, milk, cheese.

Dosage

ᴗ Large doses may be used therapeutically, but should be taken under the supervision of a physician or health practitioner.

ᴗ Doses of 20–100mg. of niacin, taken daily, may be beneficial. Best taken as part of a B-complex supplement.

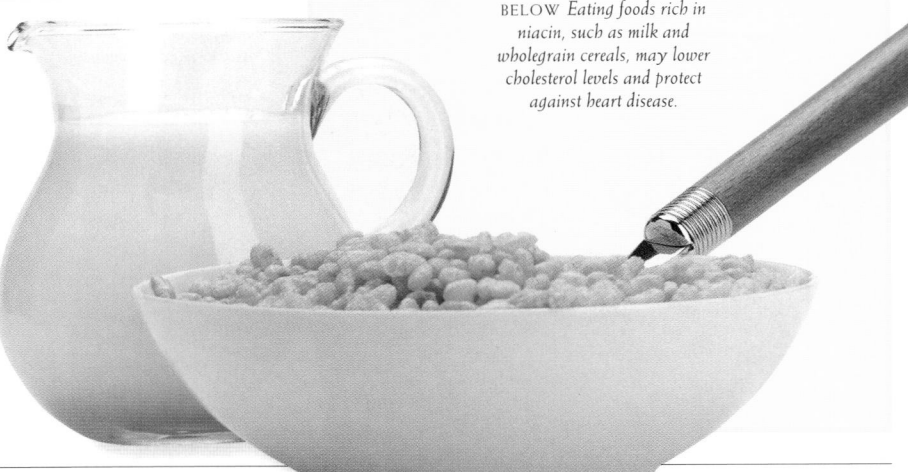

BELOW *Eating foods rich in niacin, such as milk and wholegrain cereals, may lower cholesterol levels and protect against heart disease.*

B5 (PANTOTHENIC ACID)

U.S. RDA 10mg. E.U. RDA 6mg.

Pantothenic acid is a water-soluble member of the B-complex family of vitamins that helps maintain normal growth and the health of the nervous system. Pantothenic acid has become a popular supplement over the past decade for its ability to boost energy levels and improve immune response.

There is also evidence that pantothenic acid can lower cholesterol and protect against heart disease. Pantothenic acid is useful in reducing the effects of stress on the body, and is needed to convert choline into acetylcholine, which is necessary for brain functioning.

ABOVE *Pantothenic acid is an ideal supplement to take to boost the immune system.*

CAUTION

NO KNOWN TOXICITY, ALTHOUGH DOSES OF OVER 300MG. PER DAY SHOULD BE SUPERVISED BY A PRACTITIONER.

SOME PEOPLE REPORT STOMACH UPSETS AT DOSES HIGHER THAN 10G.

DATA FILE

Properties

- B5 encourages the healing of wounds.

- Helps the body in the production of energy.

- Reduces stress levels.

- Controls the metabolism of fat.

- Encourages functioning of the immune system.

- Prevents fatigue.

- Lowers cholesterol levels and so protects against heart disease.

- Prevents arthritis, and also treats it.

- May prevent hair loss and graying of hair.

Best Sources

Yeast, organ meats, eggs, brown rice, wholegrain cereals, molasses.

Dosage

- Best taken in B-complex formulas, up to 300mg. per day for therapeutic use.

- The normal dosage, which should help to prevent disease, is about 100mg. per day.

LEFT *An adequate intake of vitamin B5 will help to keep your hair in good condition.*

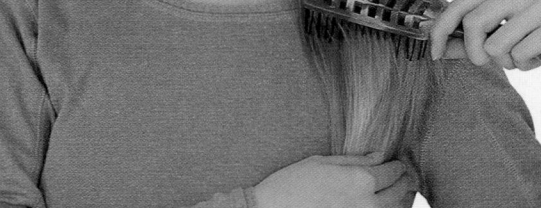

B6 (PYRIDOXINE)

U.S. RDA 2mg. E.U. RDA 1.6–2mg.

Pyridoxine is a water-soluble B-complex vitamin which is necessary for the production of antibodies and white blood cells. B6 is necessary for the absorption of vitamin B12. B6 is required for the functioning of more than 60 enzymes in the body and also for protein synthesis.

Of all the B vitamins, B6 is the most important for a healthy immune system, and it is thought to protect the body against some cancers. B6 is widely used for relieving the symptoms of PMS and menopause, and may cure some forms of infertility. This vitamin is also used to prevent skin inflammation, and maintain healthy teeth and gums.

DATA FILE

Properties

- Boosts immunity.

- Helps to control diabetes.

- B6 assimilates proteins and fats.

- Helps prevent skin and nervous disorders.

- Alleviates nausea.

- Treats symptoms of PMS and menopause.

- Reduces muscle cramps and spasms.

- Acts as a natural diuretic.

- Protects against cancer.

Best Sources

Meat, fish, milk, eggs, wholegrain cereals, fresh vegetables.

Dosage

- Should always be taken as part of a B-complex supplement, and in equal amounts with B1 and B2.

- Time-release formulas are best because it lasts for only eight hours in the body.

CAUTION

VITAMIN B6 IS TOXIC IN HIGH DOSES, CAUSING SERIOUS NERVE DAMAGE WHEN TAKEN AT QUANTITIES OF MORE THAN 2G. PER DAY.

SOME PEOPLE REPORT SIDE-EFFECTS WITH DOSES AS LOW AS 100MG.

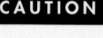

ABOVE *Vegetables like cabbage are one of the best sources of B6 and will help protect against cancer.*

B9 (FOLIC ACID)

U.S. RDA 400mcg. E.U. RDA 200–360mcg.

Folic acid is a water-soluble vitamin that forms part of the B-complex family. It is also known as vitamin Bc or vitamin B9. Low levels of folic acid may lead to anemia. Folic acid is essential for the division of body cells, and it is also necessary for the utilization of sugar and amino acids.

Recent findings indicate that folic acid can prevent some types of cancer and birth defects, and it is helpful in the treatment of heart disease. Most folic acid deficiency is the result of a poor diet, because it is abundant in foods such as leafy green vegetables, yeast, and liver. Taken from just before conception, and particularly in the first trimester of pregnancy, folic acid can help to prevent spina bifida.

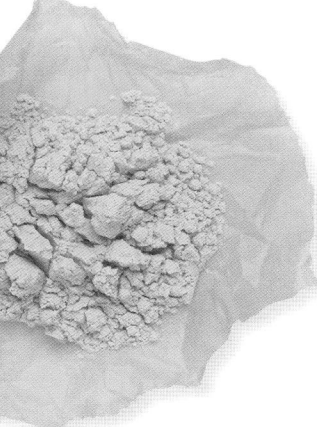

ABOVE Folic acid is part of the B-complex family. It helps prevent some types of cancer.

RIGHT Recent scientific studies have shown that folic acid can help prevent birth defects such as spina bifida if taken prior to conception and during the first trimester.

CAUTION

FOLIC ACID IS TOXIC IN LARGE DOSES AND CAN CAUSE SEVERE NEUROLOGICAL PROBLEMS.

HIGH DOSES MAY CAUSE INSOMNIA AND INTERFERE WITH THE ABSORPTION OF ZINC IN THE BODY.

DATA FILE

Properties

- Improves lactation.
- May protect against cancer.
- Improves skin condition.
- Natural analgesic.
- Increases appetite in debilitated patients.
- Needed for metabolism of RNA and DNA.
- Helps form blood.
- Builds up babies' resistance to infection.
- Essential for transmission of genetic code.
- Prevents spina bifida.

Best Sources

Green leafy vegetables, wheat germ, nuts, eggs, bananas, oranges, and organ meats.

Dosage

- There are many people at risk of deficiency, including heavy drinkers, pregnant women, the elderly, and those on low-fat diets. Supplementation at 400–800mcg. is recommended for those at risk.
- It is best taken with a good multivitamin and mineral supplement.

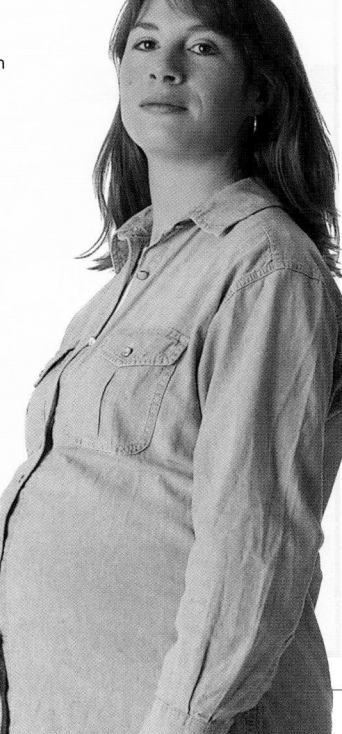

B12 (COBALAMIN)

U.S. RDA 3mcg. E.U. RDA 2mcg.

Cobalamin is a water-soluble member of the B-complex vitamin family, and it is the only vitamin that contains essential minerals. B12 is essential for the healthy metabolism of nerve tissue, and deficiencies can cause brain damage and neurological disorders. Vitamin B12 was once considered to be a "wonder drug" and was given by injection to rejuvenate. B12 may also reduce the risk of cancer and the severity of allergies, as well as boosting energy levels. Low levels of this vitamin result in anemia.

ABOVE LEFT A deficiency of B12 can result in anemia.

DATA FILE

Properties

- Needed for maintenance of the nervous system.
- Improves memory and concentration.
- Required to utilize fats, carbohydrates, and proteins.
- Increases energy.
- Promotes healthy growth in children.
- May protect against cancer.
- Protects against allergens and toxic elements.

Best Sources

Liver, beef, pork, eggs, cheese, fish, milk.

Dosage

- Dosages of 5–50mcg. should be adequate for most people; higher dosages should be supervised.
- Best taken as part of a B-complex supplement.

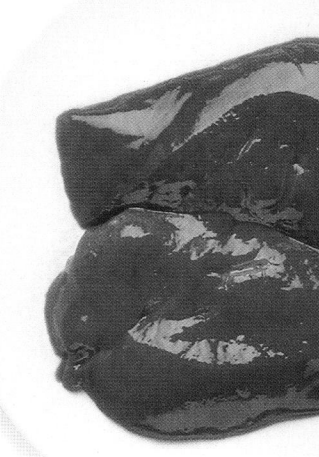

ABOVE B12, necessary for proper maintenance of the nervous system, can be found in liver.

CAUTION

ALTHOUGH VITAMIN B12 IS NOT CONSIDERED TO BE TOXIC, IT IS RECOMMENDED THAT YOU DO NOT TAKE MORE THAN 200MG. DAILY UNLESS YOU ARE UNDER THE SUPERVISION OF A REGISTERED PRACTITIONER.

Vitamin C

U.S. RDA 60mg. E.U. RDA 60mg.

Vitamin C is water soluble, which means that it is not stored by the body and we need to ensure that we get adequate amounts in our daily diet. More people take vitamin C than any other supplement, and yet studies show that a large percentage of the population have deficiencies.

Vitamin C is also known as ascorbic acid, and it is one of the most versatile of the vitamins we need to sustain life. It is one of the antioxidant vitamins (see page 251) and is believed to boost immunity, and to fight cancer and infection.

DATA FILE

Properties

🍃 Reduces cholesterol and helps prevent heart disease.

🍃 Speeds up the healing of wounds.

🍃 Maintains healthy bones, teeth, and sex organs.

🍃 Acts as a natural antihistamine.

🍃 May help to overcome male infertility.

🍃 Fights cancer.

🍃 Boosts immunity and reduces the duration of colds and other viruses.

🍃 Helps maintenance of good vision.

🍃 Antioxidant.

Best Sources

Rosehips, blackcurrants, broccoli, citrus fruits, all fresh fruits and vegetables.

Dosage

🍃 At least 60mg. per day is necessary for health, but more is required by smokers (25mg. is depleted with every cigarette), and people who are under stress, taking antibiotics, suffering from an infection, drink heavily, as well as after an accident or injury.

🍃 Daily dosages of up to 1,500mg. per day appear to be safe, but take this in three doses, preferably with meals, and use a time-release formula.

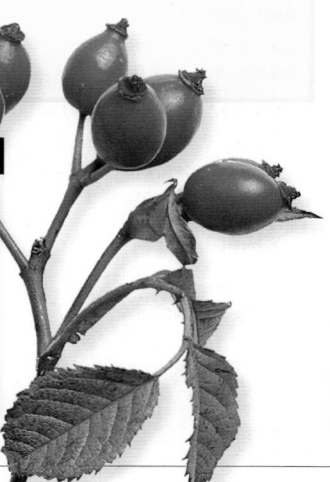

BELOW *Rosehips are a good source of this important vitamin.*

ABOVE *Citrus fruits like oranges are rich in vitamin C.*

CAUTION

VITAMIN C MAY CAUSE KIDNEY STONES AND GOUT IN SOME INDIVIDUALS.

—◆—

SOME PEOPLE SUFFER FROM DIARRHEA AND CRAMPS AT HIGH DOSAGES, ALTHOUGH THE VITAMIN IS CONSIDERED TO BE NONTOXIC AT EVEN VERY HIGH LEVELS.

DATA FILE

Properties

🍃 Protects against osteoporosis.

🍃 May help in the treatment of psoriasis.

🍃 Boosts immune system.

🍃 May be useful in the treatment of cancer.

🍃 Protects against cancer.

🍃 Necessary for strong teeth and bones.

Best Sources

Animal produce, such as milk, eggs, oily fish, butter, cheese, cod liver oil.

Dosage

🍃 Supplementation between 5–10mcg. is suggested for those at risk of deficiency.

CAUTION

VITAMIN D IS THE MOST TOXIC OF ALL THE VITAMINS, CAUSING NAUSEA, VOMITING, HEADACHE, AND DEPRESSION, AMONG OTHER PROBLEMS.

—◆—

DO NOT TAKE IN EXCESS OF 10MCG. DAILY.

BELOW *Animal foods, such as oily fish, contain vitamin D – although sunlight, not food, is this vitamin's best source.*

Vitamin D

U.S. RDA 10mcg. E.U. RDA 5mcg.

Vitamin D is a fat-soluble vitamin that is found in foods of animal origin and is known as the "sunshine" vitamin. Vitamin D can be produced in the skin from the energy of the sun, and it is not found in rich supply in any food.

Vitamin D is important for calcium and phosphorus absorption, and helps to regulate calcium metabolism. Recent research suggests that it could have a role in protecting against some cancers and infectious diseases. Deficiency is caused by inadequate exposure to sunlight, and low consumption of foods containing vitamin D.

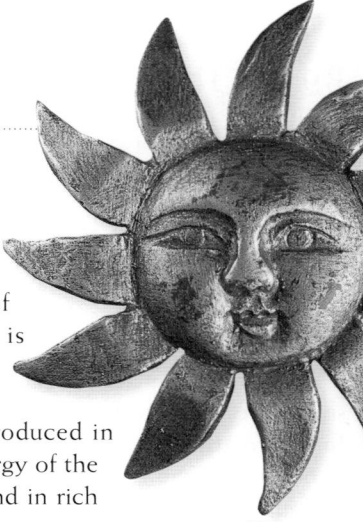

ABOVE *The human body will manufacture vitamin D itself if the skin is exposed to sunlight.*

BELOW *It has been shown that smoking seriously hampers the body's ability to absorb vitamins.*

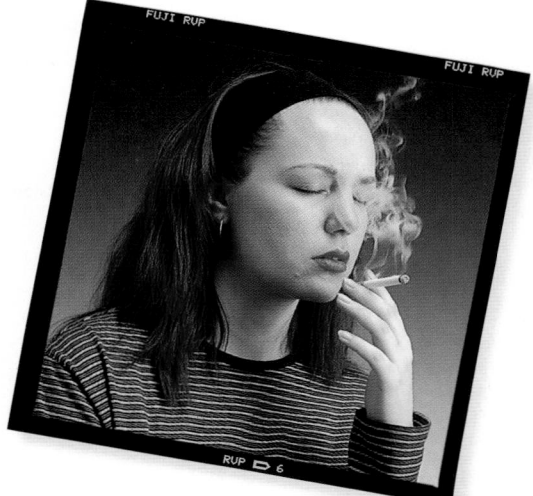

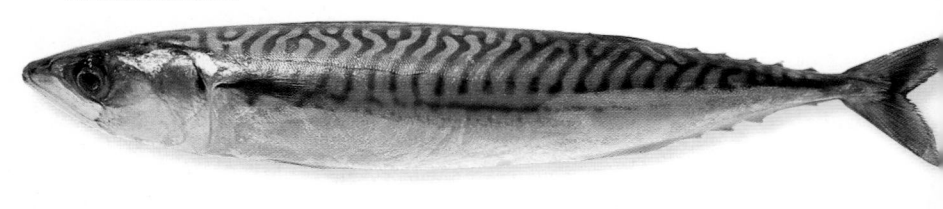

Vitamin E

U.S. RDA 20mg. E.U. RDA 10mg.

Vitamin E is fat soluble and one of the key antioxidant vitamins (*see page 251*). Its key function is as an anticoagulant, but its role in boosting the immune system and protecting against cardiovascular disease is becoming increasingly clear.

Apart from its crucial antioxidant value, vitamin E is important for the production of energy and the maintenance of health at every level. Unlike most fat-soluble vitamins, vitamin E is stored in the body for only a short period of time, and up to 75 percent of a daily dose is excreted in the feces.

DATA FILE

Properties

☙ Antioxidant, so helps to slow the process of aging.

☙ Protects against neurological disorders.

☙ Boosts immunity.

☙ Protects against cardiovascular disease.

☙ Alleviates fatigue.

☙ Accelerates healing, particularly of burns.

☙ Reduces the various symptoms of PMS.

☙ Treats skin problems and baldness.

☙ Helps prevent miscarriage.

☙ Acts as a natural diuretic.

☙ Prevents formation of thickened scars.

Best Sources

Wheatgerm (fresh), soybeans, vegetable oils, broccoli, leafy green vegetables, whole grains, peanuts, eggs.

Dosage

☙ Available in many forms (the dry form is best for people with skin problems or oil intolerance).

☙ Daily dosage may be from 250–280mg., but you may be advised to take higher doses in some cases.

BELOW LEFT *One of the main antioxidant vitamins, vitamin E can be found in vegetable oils.*

BIOTIN (VITAMIN H)

U.S. RDA 300mcg. E.U. RDA 0.15mg.

Biotin is not a true vitamin, but it works with B-complex vitamins and is often called vitamin H, or co-enzyme R. Biotin is water soluble and is found in many common foods. It is essential for breaking down and metabolizing fats in the body.

Biotin is depleted in the body by alcohol, cooking or refining food, antibiotics, and when taken with raw egg whites, which contain avidin, a protein that prevents biotin absorption. Biotin works more effectively with vitamins B2, B6, B3, and A.

DATA FILE

Properties

☙ Prevents the hair from turning gray.

☙ Eases various muscular aches and pains.

☙ Treats eczema, dermatitis, and other skin conditions.

☙ Helps to prevent baldness.

Best Sources

Nuts, fruits, beef liver, egg yolks, milk, kidneys, unpolished rice, and brewer's yeast.

Dosage

☙ Biotin is normally included in most readily-available B-complex supplements.

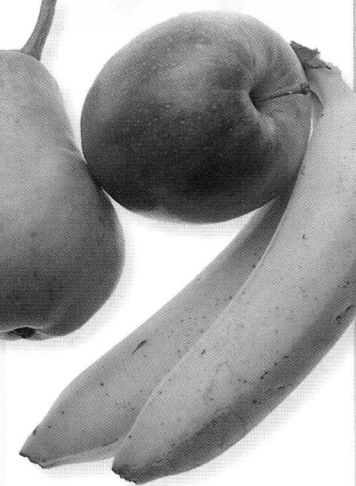

ABOVE *Found in fruits, biotin is essential for energy release from fats.*

Vitamin K

U.S. RDA none. E.U. RDA none.

The K vitamins are fat soluble, and are necessary for normal blood clotting. They are often used to treat the toxic effects of anticoagulant drops, such as Warfarin, and in people who have a poor ability to absorb fats.

Vitamin K occurs naturally in foods as vitamin K1, and is produced by intestinal bacteria as vitamin K2. Synthetic vitamin K is known as K3. Vitamin K1 injections are routinely given to newborn babies to prevent hemorrhage, but since a recent scare linked the vitamin with childhood leukemia it is now more often given as oral drops.

DATA FILE

Properties

☙ Controls blood clotting.

Best Sources

Cauliflower, spinach, peas, wholegrain cereals.

Dosage

☙ We need an estimated 500–1,000mcg. of vitamin K from our diet per day.

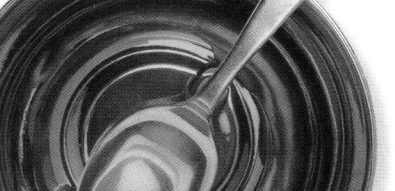

LEFT *Vitamin K, found in cauliflower, spinach, peas, and whole grains, is essential for normal blood clotting.*

VITAMIN B BORON

U.S. RDA none. E.U. RDA none.

Boron is a trace mineral found in most plants, and it is essential for human health. Recent research has reported that boron added to the diet of post-menopausal women prevents calcium loss and bone demineralization – a revolutionary discovery for sufferers of osteoporosis.

It is also claimed that boron will raise testosterone levels and build muscle in men, and boron is therefore often used by athletes and bodybuilders. Boron is found in most fruit and vegetables, and does not appear in meat and meat products. Boron supplements are usually taken in the form of sodium borate.

DATA FILE

Properties

❧ Assists in the external treatment of bacterial and fungal infections.

❧ Helps to lower the incidence of arthritis.

❧ Prevents osteoporosis.

❧ Used to build muscles.

Best Sources

Root vegetables (such as potatoes, parsnips, and carrots) grown in soil that is rich in boron.

Dosage

❧ No RDA, but it is suggested that 3mg. should be taken daily to prevent osteoporosis.

CAUTION

BORON CAN BE TOXIC, WITH SYMPTOMS INCLUDING A RED RASH, VOMITING, DIARRHEA, REDUCED CIRCULATION, SHOCK, AND THEN COMA.

A FATAL DOSE IS 15–20G., 3–6G. IN CHILDREN. SYMPTOMS APPEAR AT ABOUT 100MG.

RIGHT *Bodybuilders and athletes take boron supplements to help build their muscles.*

LEFT *Most fruits contain boron, which helps prevent osteoporosis.*

Ca CALCIUM

U.S. RDA 800–1,200mg. E.U. RDA 800mg.

Calcium is an important mineral, and recent research shows that we get only about one-third of what we need for good health. Calcium is essential for human life – it makes up bones and teeth, and is crucial in the process of conducting messages along nerves. It ensures that our muscles contract, and that our hearts beat, and it is extremely important in the maintenance of the immune system, among other things.

There are many groups at risk of calcium deficiency – in particular the elderly – and because it is so important to body processes our bodies take what they need from our bones, which causes them to become thin and brittle. It is used therapeutically for allergies, depression, panic attacks, insomnia, and hyperactivity, and extra should be taken during pregnancy and while breast-feeding.

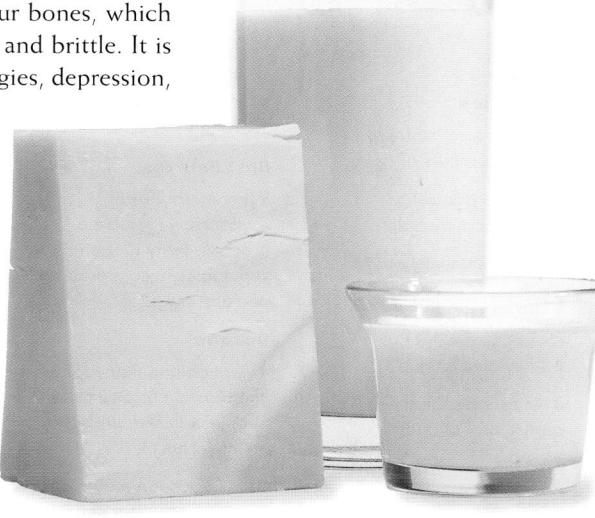

RIGHT *All dairy products are rich in calcium, essential for healthy bones and teeth.*

CAUTION

DOSES OVER 2,000MG. PER DAY MAY CAUSE HYPERCALCEMIA (CALCIUM DEPOSITS IN THE KIDNEYS), BUT SINCE EXCESS CALCIUM IS EXCRETED, IT IS UNLIKELY TO OCCUR UNLESS YOU ARE ALSO TAKING EXCESS QUANTITIES OF VITAMIN D.

DATA FILE

Properties

❧ Prevents osteoporosis, and helps to treat the condition once symptoms manifest.

❧ Prevents cancer.

❧ Useful in the treatment of high blood pressure.

❧ Prevents heart disease.

❧ Useful in treating arthritis.

❧ Helps to keep skin healthy.

❧ Alleviates leg cramps.

❧ Encourages regular beating of the heart.

❧ Soothes insomnia.

❧ Helps the body to metabolize iron.

❧ Necessary for nerve-impulse transmission and muscular function.

Best Sources

Milk, cheese, dairy produce, leafy green vegetables, hard tap water, salmon, tinned fish, eggs, beans, nuts, tofu.

Dosage

❧ Experts recommend that calcium be taken in a good multivitamin and mineral supplement, although extra doses may be given up to 1,000mg. per day.

❧ More calcium is needed by women after the menopause, and while pregnant or breast-feeding.

Co COBALT

U.S. RDA none.
E.U. RDA none

Cobalt is an essential trace mineral. It is a constituent of vitamin B12. The amount of cobalt in the body is dependent on the amount of cobalt in the soil, and therefore in the food we eat. Most of us are not deficient in cobalt, although deficiency is much more common in vegetarians.

DATA FILE

Properties
Cobalt is able, with vitamin B12, to:

- Prevent pernicious anemia.
- Help in the production of red blood cells.
- Aid in the synthesis of DNA and choline.
- Encourage a healthy nervous system.
- Reduce blood pressure.
- Maintain myelin, the fatty sheath protecting the nerves.

Best Sources
Fresh leafy green vegetables, meat, liver, milk, oysters, clams.

Dosage
- Cobalt is rarely found in supplement form, but forms part of a good multivitamin and mineral supplement with the B-complex vitamins.
- An intake of 8mcg. daily appears to be adequate.
- Used therapeutically, side-effects occur at regular doses above 30mg. – hypothyroidism, goiter, and heart failure.

Cu COPPER

U.S. RDA 1.5–3mg. E.U. RDA 1.2mg.

Copper is an essential trace mineral, and is necessary for respiration – iron and copper are required for oxygen to be synthesized in red blood cells. Copper is also important for the production of collagen, which is responsible for the health of our bones, cartilage, and skin. Copper is also one of the antioxidant minerals (*see page 251*), which protect against free-radical damage. Arthritis sufferers report that copper bracelets reduce pain and inflammation associated with the condition, probably because traces of the mineral are absorbed by the skin and enter the bloodstream.

DATA FILE

Properties
- May prevent cancer.
- Protects against cardiovascular disease.
- Useful mineral in the treatment of arthritis.
- Boosts the immune system.
- Acts as an antioxidant.

Best Sources
Animal livers, shellfish, nuts, fruit, oysters, kidneys, and legumes.

Dosage
- Copper appears in good multivitamin and mineral supplements, and can be taken alone up to 3mg. daily.

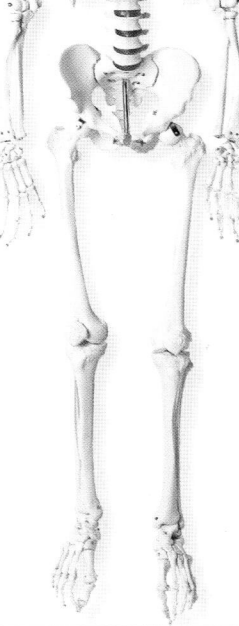

ABOVE RIGHT *Copper is important for collagen production, essential for healthy bones.*

Cr CHROMIUM

U.S. RDA none. E.U. RDA none.

Chromium is a trace mineral that was discovered in the body in the 1950s. It is an important regulator of blood sugar, and has been used successfully in the control and treatment of diabetes. It is involved in the metabolism of carbohydrates and fats, and is used in the production of insulin in the body.

High levels of sugars in the diet cause chromium to be excreted through the kidneys, so it is important to get enough in your diet if you eat sugary foods. The incidence of diabetes and heart disease decreases with increased levels of chromium in the body.

DATA FILE

Properties
- Aids in the control and production of insulin.
- Aids in the metabolism of carbohydrates and fats.
- Controls levels of cholesterol in the blood.
- Stimulates the synthesis of proteins in the body.
- Increases general resistance to infection.
- Suppresses hunger pains.

Best Sources
Wholegrain cereals, meat, cheese, brewer's yeast, molasses, egg yolk.

Dosage
- There is no RDA, but it is suggested that 25mcg. per day is adequate.
- If necessary, supplements of up to 200mcg. per day can be taken.

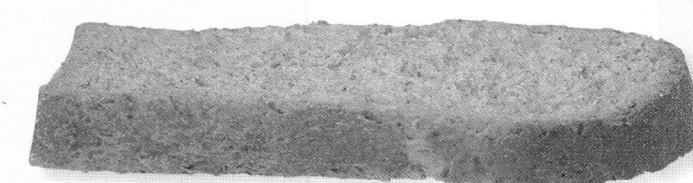

RIGHT *Eat wholegrain bread to ensure an adequate intake of chromium.*

F FLUORINE

U.S. RDA 1mg. fluoride, 3.6mg. sodium fluoride.
E.U. RDA none.

Fluorine is a trace mineral found naturally in soil, water, plants, and animal tissues. Its electrically charged form is "fluoride," which is how we usually refer to it. Although it has not yet been officially recognized as an essential nutrient, studies show that it is important in many processes, and may play a major role in the prevention of many 20th-century killers, like heart disease.

The major source of fluorine is drinking water, which is sometimes fluoridated, or has enough naturally occurring fluoride to make fluoridation unnecessary. Fluoride supplements should always be taken with calcium.

DATA FILE

Properties

≈ Fluorine protects against dental caries.

≈ Protects against, and also treats, osteoporosis.

≈ It may help to prevent heart disease.

≈ May help to prevent calcification of organs and musculoskeletal structures.

Best Sources

Seafood, animal meat, fluoridated drinking water, and tea.

Dosage

≈ The major source is drinking water, and typical daily intake is 1–2mg.

≈ Tablets and drops are available from pharmacies, but should be limited to 1mg. daily in adults, and 0.25–0.5mg. for children.

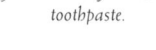

ABOVE *Fluoride can be found in many makes of toothpaste.*

CAUTION

AN EXCESS OF FLUORIDE CAUSES FLUOROSIS, CHARACTERIZED BY IRREGULAR PATCHES ON TOOTH ENAMEL, AND DEPRESSES THE APPETITE. EVENTUALLY THE SPINE CALCIFIES. FLUOROSIS IS RARE AND OCCURS AT LEVELS FAR ABOVE 10MG. PER DAY.

DO NOT SUPPLEMENT FLUORIDE WITHOUT THE ADVICE OF YOUR DENTIST.

LEFT *Fluoride in drinking water and dental products helps to prevent dental cavities.*

Fe IRON

U.S. RDA 10–18mg., pregnant women 30mg.
E.U. RDA 14mg.

Iron is a trace mineral which is essential for human health. Iron-deficiency anemia, which is the condition most commonly associated with deficiency, was described by Egyptian physicists as long ago as 1500 B.C.E. Today, 10 percent of all women in the Western world suffer from iron-deficiency anemia.

We now know that iron is present in our bodies as hemoglobin, which is the red pigment of blood. Iron is required for muscle protein and is stored in the liver, spleen, bone marrow, and muscles. Efficient absorption of iron is highest in childhood, and reduces as we age. Our bodies need vitamin C in order to assimilate iron in an effective fashion.

CAUTION

EXCESS IRON CAN CAUSE CONSTIPATION, DIARRHEA, AND, RARELY, IN HIGH DOSES, DEATH.

BE VERY CAUTIOUS WHEN GIVING CHILDREN IRON SUPPLEMENTS – EVEN DOSES AS LITTLE AS 3G. CAN CAUSE DEATH.

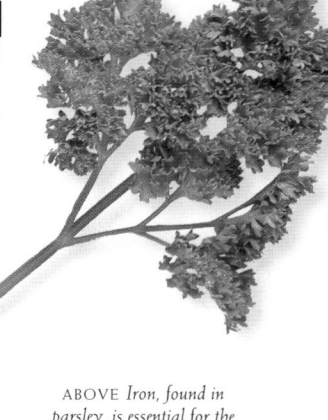

ABOVE *Iron, found in parsley, is essential for the formation of red blood cells.*

DATA FILE

Properties

≈ Improves physical performance.

≈ Anti-carcinogenic.

≈ Prevents learning problems in children.

≈ Prevents and cures iron-deficiency anemia.

≈ Improves immunity.

≈ Boosts energy levels.

≈ Encourages restful sleep and maintains energy levels.

Best Sources

Shellfish, brewer's yeast, wheat bran, offal, cocoa powder, dried fruit, cereals.

Dosage

≈ Pregnant, breast-feeding, and menstruating women, infants, children, athletes, and vegetarians may require increased levels of iron. Your general physician will prescribe iron supplements if they are necessary.

≈ Maximum dosage is around 15mg. daily, unless under medical supervision.

Ge GERMANIUM

U.S. RDA none. E.U. RDA none.

Germanium is a mineral which is abundant in the surface of the earth. Almost all foods commonly eaten contain some germanium. Some conditions have been reported to respond favorably to germanium given at therapeutic doses, including arthritis, angina, stroke, Raynaud's disease, burns, and pain associated with cancer.

Germanium is believed to function by boosting the action of oxygen in generating energy. Because it maintains an equilibrium within the body, germanium is said to reduce high blood pressure, lower cholesterol levels, and generally to exert a good effect on the immune system. Germanium is now considered to be one of the antioxidant minerals (*see page 251*).

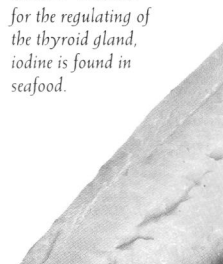

ABOVE *Although it is a useful mineral in the treatment of cancer, it is recommended that germanium supplement should only be taken with medical supervision.*

BELOW *The mineral germanium is found in almost all commonly eaten foods, including garlic.*

CAUTION

GERMANIUM IS SAFE UP TO QUITE A HIGH LEVEL, ALTHOUGH SKIN ERUPTIONS AND DIARRHEA HAVE BEEN REPORTED IN SOME PATIENTS TAKING THERAPEUTIC DOSES. ONLY USE THE SUPPLEMENT UNDER THE SUPERVISION OF A PHYSICIAN OR NUTRITIONIST.

DATA FILE

Properties

๛ Maintains the homeostasis in the body, and therefore may reduce high blood pressure and cholesterol levels.

๛ Germanium boosts the immune system.

๛ May be analgesic.

๛ May have antiviral, antibacterial, and antitumor activity.

๛ Useful as part of a cancer treatment program.

๛ Helps chronic Epstein-Barr virus syndrome.

๛ Useful in the treatment of HIV/AIDS.

Best Sources

Bran, wholewheat flour, vegetables, seeds, meats, dairy products.

Dosage

๛ Germanium supplementation is not recommended without a physician's supervision.

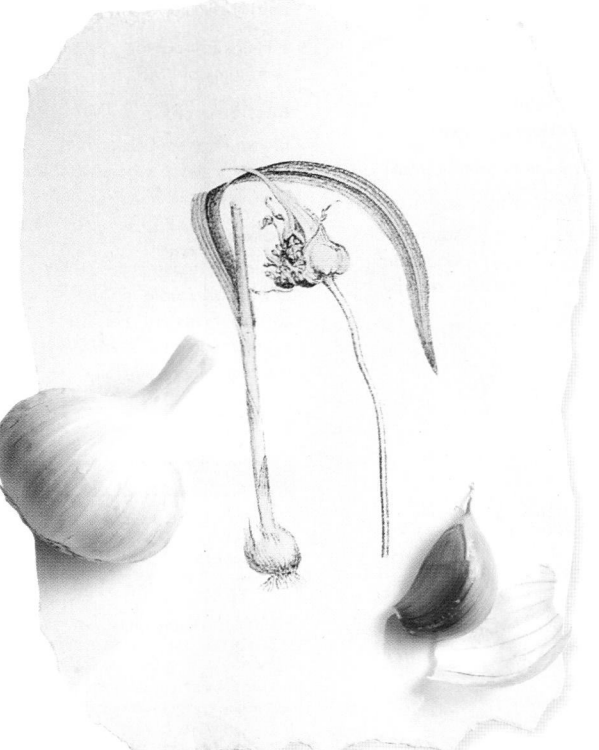

I IODINE

U.S. RDA 80–150mcg. E.U. RDA 150mcg.

Iodine is a mineral, which was first discovered in 1812 in kelp. Iodine was extracted and given its name because of its violet color. It occurs naturally and is a crucial constituent of the thyroid hormones, which monitor our energy levels.

Iodine deficiency is one of the key world health problems, and at least 200 million people suffer from conditions linked to inadequate iodine in the diet. Lack of iodine can cause goiter, underactive thyroid, cretinism, and can eventually lead to myxedema.

CAUTION

IODINE IS TOXIC IN HIGH DOSES AND MAY AGGRAVATE OR CAUSE ACNE. LARGE DOSES MAY INTERFERE WITH HORMONE ACTIVITY.

CRUCIFEROUS FOODS LIKE CABBAGE, BRUSSELS SPROUTS, CAULIFLOWER, AND BROCCOLI CONTAIN SUBSTANCES WHICH CAN CAUSE HYPOTHYROIDISM BY ANTAGONIZING IODINE. ANYONE WHO EATS LARGE QUANTITIES OF THESE VEGETABLES SHOULD CONSIDER AN IODINE SUPPLEMENT.

BELOW *Essential for the regulating of the thyroid gland, iodine is found in seafood.*

DATA FILE

Properties

๛ Determines the level of metabolism and energy in the body.

๛ Relieves the pain of fibrocystic breasts.

๛ Protects against the toxic effects of exposure to radioactive materials.

๛ Prevents goiter.

๛ Prevents thyroid disorders.

๛ Loosens mucus in the respiratory tract.

๛ Natural antiseptic.

Best Sources

Seafood and seaweed. Most table salt is fortified with iodine.

Dosage

๛ Iodine is best taken as potassium iodide.

๛ Take under the supervision of your physician or nutritionist.

๛ 150mcg. RDA iodine is adequate.

K POTASSIUM

U.S. RDA 3,500mg. E.U. RDA 3,500mg.

Potassium is one of the most important minerals in our body, working with sodium and chloride to form "electrolytes," the essential body salts that make up our body fluids. Potassium is crucial in order for the body to function. It plays a role in nerve conduction, the beating of the heart, energy production, the synthesis of nucleic acids and proteins, and the contraction of muscles.

Sweating can cause a loss of potassium, as do chronic diarrhea and diuretics. People taking certain drugs, including corticosteroids, high-dose penicillin, and laxatives, may suffer from potassium deficiency. Symptoms of this can include vomiting, abdominal distension, muscular weakness, loss of appetite, low blood pressure, and intense thirst.

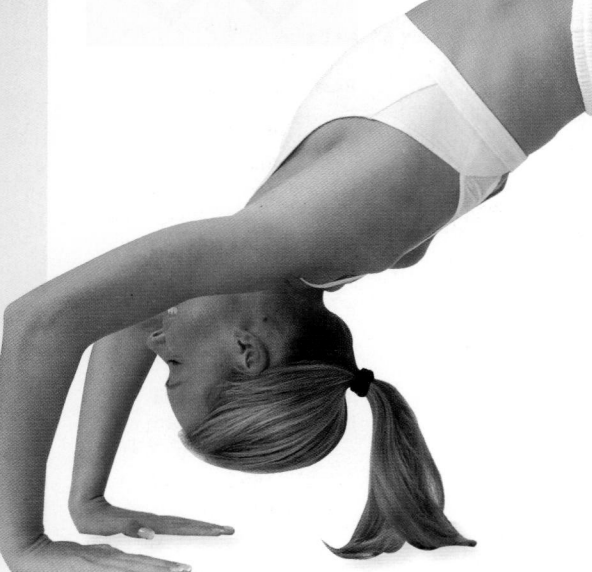

ABOVE *Dried fruits are a rich source of potassium, one of the most important minerals in our body.*

CAUTION

IN EXCESS (DOSES ABOVE 3,500MG.), POTASSIUM MAY CAUSE MUSCULAR WEAKNESS AND MENTAL APATHY, EVENTUALLY STOPPING THE HEART.

BELOW *To achieve athletic excellence, ensure that you have the recommended daily intake of potassium.*

DATA FILE

Properties

- Activates enzymes which control energy production.
- Prevents and treats high blood pressure.
- May help to protect against stroke.
- Improves athletic performance.
- May help treat and prevent cancer.
- Maintains water balance within cells.
- Stabilizes the internal structure of cells.
- Acts with sodium to conduct nerve impulses.

Best Sources

Fresh fruit and vegetables, particularly bananas.

Dosage

- Eat more fresh fruit and vegetables to increase potassium intake. Diuretic users and those in a hot climate may need up to 1.5g. in supplementary potassium daily.
- Take with zinc and magnesium for best effect.

ABOVE *Increase your intake of wholewheat bread to prevent magnesium deficiency.*

Mg MAGNESIUM

U.S. RDA 300–400mg. E.U. RDA 300mg.

Magnesium is a mineral that is absolutely essential for every biochemical process taking place in our bodies, including metabolism and the synthesis of nucleic acids and protein.

Magnesium deficiency is very common, particularly in the elderly, heavy drinkers, pregnant women, and regular, strenuous exercisers, and it has been proved that even a very slight deficiency can cause a disruption of the heartbeat. Other symptoms of magnesium deficiency include weakness, fatigue, vertigo, nervousness, muscle cramps, and hyper-activity in children.

DATA FILE

Properties

- Magnesium is necessary for many body functions, including energy production and cell replication.
- Essential for transmission of nerve impulses.
- Helps to prevent kidney stones and gallstones.
- Useful in the treatment of prostate problems.
- Repairs and maintains body cells.
- Required for hormonal activity.
- Required for most body processes, including production of energy.
- Useful in the treatment of high blood pressure.
- Protects against cardiovascular disease.
- Helps to treat the symptoms of PMS.

Best Sources

Brown rice, soybeans, nuts, brewer's yeast, whole wheat flour, legumes.

Dosage

- Dietary intake is thought to be inadequate in the average Western diet; supplements of 200–400mg. are recommended daily.

CAUTION

MAGNESIUM IS TOXIC TO PEOPLE WITH RENAL PROBLEMS OR ATRIOVENTRICULAR BLOCKS.
◄◆►
HIGH DOSES ARE BELIEVED TO CAUSE FLUSHING OF THE SKIN, THIRST, LOW BLOOD PRESSURE, AND LOSS OF REFLEXES IN SOME PEOPLE, ALTHOUGH THIS IS RARE.

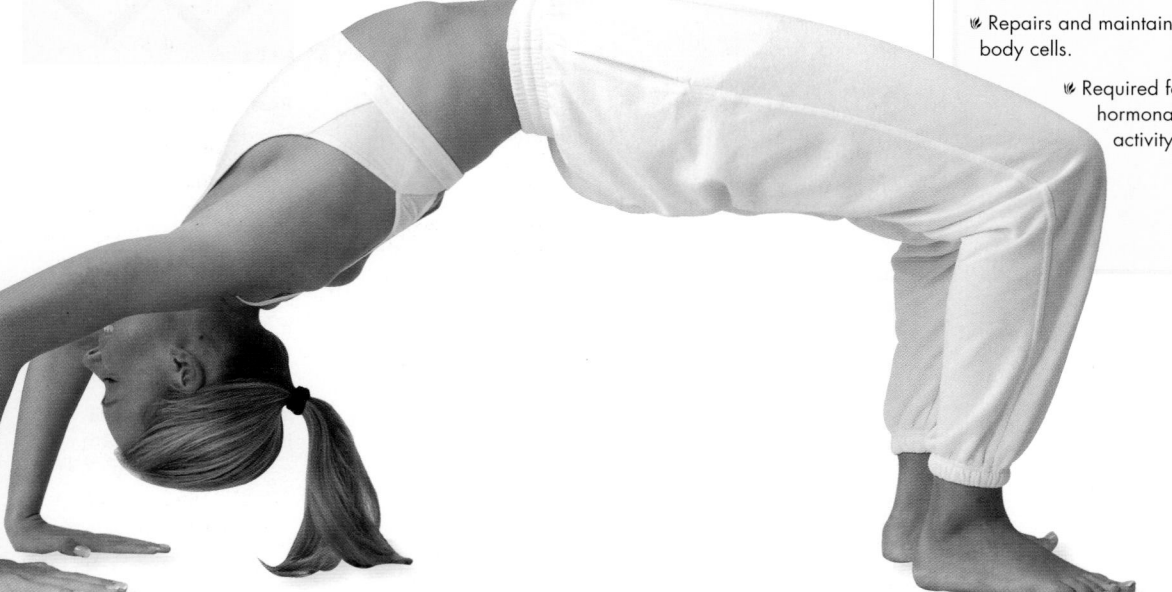

Mn MANGANESE

U.S. RDA 2.5–7mg. E.U. RDA none.

Manganese is an essential trace element that is necessary for the normal functioning of the brain, and effective in the treatment of many nervous disorders, including Alzheimer's disease and schizophrenia. Deficiency is usually related to a poor diet – particularly one where there is a high intake of foods that are processed and refined.

Our understanding of manganese is still incomplete, but it may prove to be one of the most important nutrients in human pathology. It appears likely that manganese is one of the antioxidant minerals (*see page 251*). There is some evidence that diseases such as diabetes, heart disease, and schizophrenia are linked to manganese deficiency.

DATA FILE

Properties

𝄞 Manganese maintains the healthy functioning of the nervous system.

𝄞 Necessary for female sex hormones.

𝄞 Necessary for the synthesis of the structural proteins of body cells.

𝄞 Necessary for normal bone structure.

𝄞 Important in the formation of thyroxin in the thyroid gland.

𝄞 Necessary for the functioning of the brain.

𝄞 Used in the treatment of some nervous disorders.

𝄞 Necessary for metabolism of glucose.

Best Sources

Cereals, tea, green leaf vegetables, wholewheat bread, pulses, nuts.

Dosage

𝄞 2–5 mg. is adequate, but doses up to 10mg. are thought to be safe.

CAUTION

TOXIC LEVELS ARE USUALLY QUITE RARE, BUT SYMPTOMS OF EXCESS MANGANESE MAY INCLUDE LETHARGY, INVOLUNTARY MOVEMENTS, POSTURE PROBLEMS, AND COMA.

BELOW LEFT *The trace element manganese, which can be found in pulses, is used in the treatment of some nervous disorders.*

Mo MOLYBDENUM

U.S. RDA 150–500mcg. E.U. RDA none.

Molybdenum is an essential trace element, and a vital part of the enzyme which is responsible for the utilization of iron in our bodies. Molybdenum may also be an antioxidant, and recent research indicates that it is necessary for optimum health.

Molybdenum can help to prevent anemia and is known to promote a feeling of well-being. A deficiency may result in dental caries, sexual impotence in men, and cancer of the gullet. Deficiency is usually the result of eating foods from molybdenum-deficient soils, or a diet that is high in refined and processed foods.

CAUTION

MOLYBDENUM IS TOXIC IN DOSES HIGHER THAN 10–15MG., WHICH CAUSE GOUT (A BUILD-UP OF URIC ACID AROUND THE JOINTS).

DATA FILE

Properties

𝄞 For utilization of iron, fats, carbohydrates; excretion of uric acid.

𝄞 Prevents impotence.

𝄞 Protects against cancer, anemia, dental caries.

Best Sources

Wheat, canned beans, wheat germ, liver, pulses, whole grains, offal, eggs.

Dosage

𝄞 Optimal intake is not decided; 0.075–0.25mg. per day is adequate, and experts suggest 50–100mcg. per day as a preventive measure. Toxic in doses higher than 10-15mg., causing gout.

LEFT *Wheat is a good source of molybdenum. An adequate intake protects against cancer, anemia, and dental caries.*

P PHOSPHORUS

U.S. RDA 800–1,200mg. E.U. RDA 800mg.

Phosphorus is a mineral that is essential to the structure and function of the body. It is present in the body as phosphates, and in this form aids the process of bone mineralization and helps to create the structure of the bone.

Phosphorus is also essential for communication between cells, and for energy production. Phosphorus appears in many foods and deficiency is rare. Because of its role in strengthening our bones, we should eat twice as much calcium as phosphorus.

CAUTION

PHOSPHORUS CAN BE TOXIC AT DOSAGES OR INTAKE ABOVE 200MG. PER DAY, IN SOME CASES CAUSING DIARRHEA, THE CALCIFICATION OF ORGANS AND SOFT TISSUES, AND MAKING THE BODY UNABLE TO ABSORB IRON, CALCIUM, MAGNESIUM, AND ZINC.

DATA FILE

Properties

𝄞 Forms bones and teeth.

𝄞 Produces energy.

𝄞 Cofactor for many enzymes and activates B-complex vitamins.

𝄞 Increases endurance, and fights fatigue.

𝄞 Forms RNA and DNA.

Best Sources

Yeast, dried milk and milk products, wheat germ, hard cheeses, canned fish, nuts, cereals, eggs.

Dosage

𝄞 Phosphorus deficiency usually accompanies deficiency in potassium, magnesium, and zinc, so take a supplement containing all four.

𝄞 Take under medical supervision only.

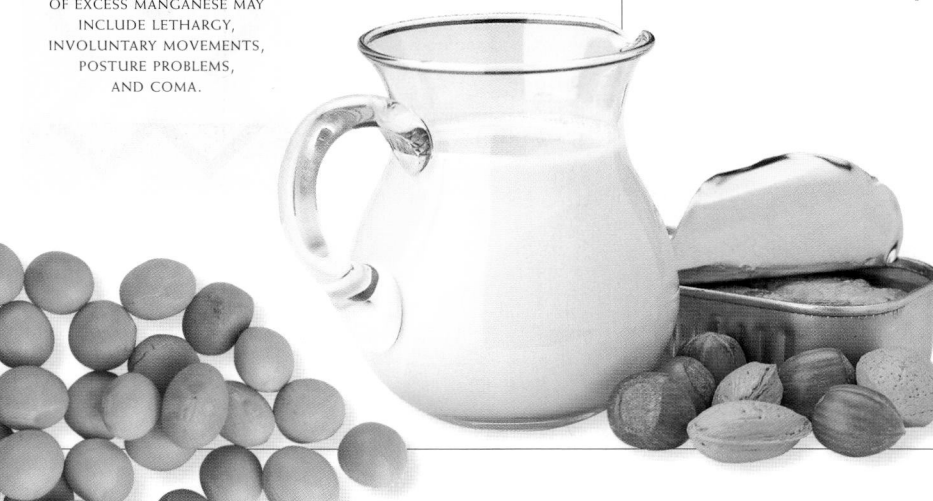

LEFT *Phosphorus, found in milk products, canned fish, and nuts, is essential for maintaining body functions.*

Se SELENIUM

U.S. RDA 50–100mcg.
E.U. RDA 10–75mcg.

Selenium is an essential trace element that has recently been recognized as one of the most important nutrients in our diet. It is an antioxidant (*see page 251*) and is vitally important in human metabolism. Selenium has been proved to provide protection against a number of cancers, and other diseases.

Selenium is necessary for the body's manufacture of proteins, and helps the liver to function efficiently. It also forms part of the male sperm, which means that deficiency can be linked to infertility in men. Other symptoms of deficiency include reduced immune activity, hair loss, and chest pains.

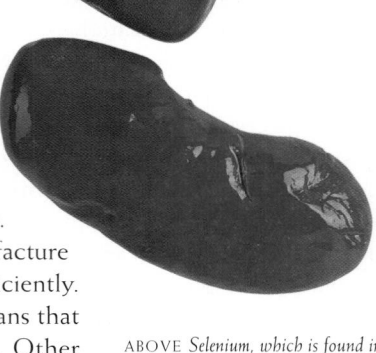

ABOVE *Selenium, which is found in kidneys is one of the most important nutrients in our diet. It helps the liver to function effectively.*

DATA FILE

Properties

❧ Maintains healthy eyes and eyesight.

❧ Maintains good skin and healthy hair.

❧ Stimulates immune system.

❧ Prevents many cancers.

❧ Improves liver function.

❧ Protects against heart and circulatory diseases.

❧ May work to impede the aging process.

❧ Can detoxify alcohol, many drugs, smoking, and some fats.

❧ Increases male potency and sex drive.

❧ Useful addition to the treatment of arthritis.

❧ Alleviates hot flushes and symptoms of menopause.

❧ Helps treat dandruff.

Best Sources

Selenium is found in wheat germ, bran, tuna fish, onions, tomatoes, broccoli, kidneys and whole wheat bread.

Dosage

❧ There is no RDA, but it has been suggested that men take 75mcg. of supplementary selenium and women take 60mcg.

❧ Selenium supplementation should be taken with 9–120mcg. of vitamin E to ensure that selenium works most efficiently.

❧ Dosages of 400–1,000mcg. have been used for immune stimulation, and for anticarcinogenic effects, but it is recommended that 50–200mcg. should be adequate to experience benefits.

CAUTION

SELENIUM CAN BE TOXIC IN VERY SMALL DOSES.

SYMPTOMS OF EXCESS INCLUDE BLACKENED FINGERNAILS AND A GARLIC-LIKE ODOR ON THE BREATH AND SKIN.

TAKE NO MORE THAN 500MCG. DAILY UNLESS SUPERVISED BY A REGISTERED PRACTITIONER.

RIGHT *Take vitamin E with selenium supplementation to ensure maximum benefit.*

Si SILICON

U.S. RDA none. E.U. RDA none.

Silicon is a trace element which is only just starting to be understood. It has been proved to be essential to animals, and it is thought that it is crucial to human life as well. Scientists believe that silicon plays some part in the make-up of our connective tissues, bones, skin, and fingernails.

Silicon is also known to play a role in preventing osteoporosis, by assisting the utilization of calcium within the bones. It also improves the strength of hair and nails by improving the production of keratin and collagen. Silicon is available as a supplement in the form of silicon dioxide. Silicea is a homeopathic remedy for disorders of the bones, joints, and skin.

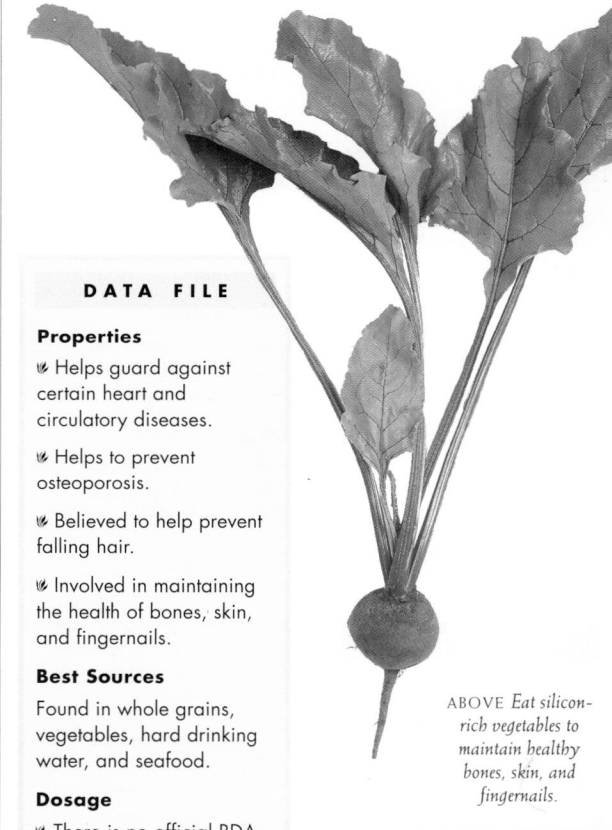

DATA FILE

Properties

❧ Helps guard against certain heart and circulatory diseases.

❧ Helps to prevent osteoporosis.

❧ Believed to help prevent falling hair.

❧ Involved in maintaining the health of bones, skin, and fingernails.

Best Sources

Found in whole grains, vegetables, hard drinking water, and seafood.

Dosage

❧ There is no official RDA, but we need 20–30mg. each day. Most of us get about 200mg. in our diet.

ABOVE *Eat silicon-rich vegetables to maintain healthy bones, skin, and fingernails.*

CAUTION

EXCESS SILICON CAN CAUSE KIDNEY STONES, BUT ONLY AT VERY HIGH DOSES.

V VANADIUM

U.S. RDA none. E.U. RDA none.

Vanadium is a trace mineral that has only recently been proved necessary for human life. At the turn of the 20th century, French physicians believed that vanadium was a miracle cure for a variety of illnesses, but it proved to be toxic at the levels they were prescribing, and it became less popular.

Today, it is believed that elevated levels of vanadium may cause manic depression, which is perhaps a clue to a little-understood disease. Normal doses are thought to reduce appetite, and to reduce blood fat and cholesterol levels.

DATA FILE

Properties
- Reduces high blood sugar by mimicking the effect of insulin on the cells.
- Prevents dental caries.
- Aids in the production of red blood cells.
- Encourages normal tissue growth and fat metabolism.
- Slows down cholesterol formation in blood vessels.
- Prevents heart disease and heart attacks.

Best Sources
Found in fish, parsley, radishes, strawberries, lettuce, and cucumber.

Dosage
- Vanadium supplements are not available, although some newer multivitamin and mineral supplements may contain low levels of it.

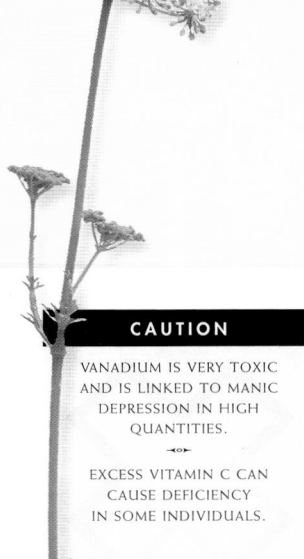

BELOW *Present in parsley, vanadium is essential for human life – although high levels may cause manic depression.*

CAUTION

VANADIUM IS VERY TOXIC AND IS LINKED TO MANIC DEPRESSION IN HIGH QUANTITIES.

EXCESS VITAMIN C CAN CAUSE DEFICIENCY IN SOME INDIVIDUALS.

Zn ZINC

U.S. RDA 15mg. E.U. RDA 15mg.

Zinc is one of the most important trace elements in our diet, and it is required for more than 200 enzyme activities within the body. It is the principal protector of the immune system, and is crucial for regulating our genetic information. Zinc is also vital for the structure and function of cell membranes.

Zinc is an antioxidant (*see page 251*) and can help to detoxify the body. A zinc deficiency can cause growth failure, infertility, impotence, and, in some cases, an impaired sense of taste. Eczema is commonly linked to zinc deficiency, and new research points to the fact that postnatal illness may be attributable to insufficient zinc in the diet. A weakened immune system and a poor ability to heal may also indicate deficiency.

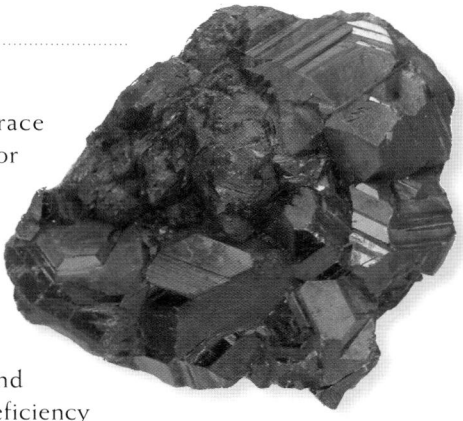

ABOVE *A vital trace element in our diet, zinc is needed for over 200 enzyme functions in the human body.*

DATA FILE

Properties
- Boosts the immune system.
- Prevents cancer.
- Prevents and treats colds.
- Maintains senses of taste, smell, and sight.
- May help to prevent age-related degenerative effects.
- Prevents hair loss.
- Treats acne and various other skin problems.
- Useful in treatment of rheumatoid arthritis.
- Prevents blindness associated with aging.
- Increases male potency and sex drive.
- Used to treat infertility.

Best Sources
Offal, meat, mushrooms, oysters, eggs, wholegrain products, brewer's yeast.

Dosage
- Take 15–30mg. daily, and increase copper and selenium intake if taking more zinc.

CAUTION

VERY HIGH DOSES (ABOVE 150MG. PER DAY) MAY CAUSE SOME NAUSEA, VOMITING, AND DIARRHEA.

THERAPY CONNECTIONS

SILICON
Homeopathy *p.211*

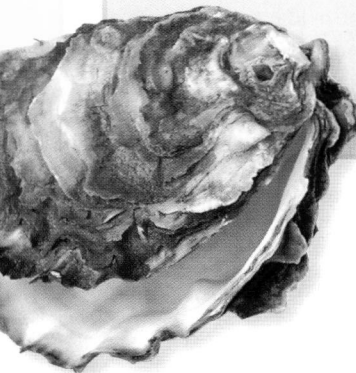

ABOVE AND LEFT *Shellfish such as oysters contain high levels of zinc. This mineral helps boost the immune system and is necessary for healthy growth and development.*

AMINO ACIDS

L-ARGININE

L-arginine is one of the most important and most useful of the amino acids, with a significant role to play in the function of the muscles, growth, and healing, helping to regulate and support key components of the immune system. It is also extremely important for male fertility.

For adults, L-arginine is a nonessential amino acid, which means that it is capable of being synthesized in the body and it is therefore not essential that we get additional amounts in our daily diet. For children, however, L-arginine is essential.

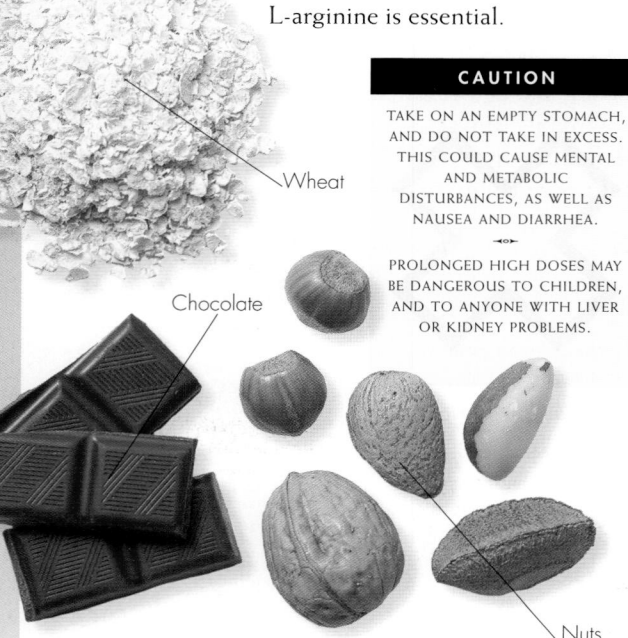

Wheat

Chocolate

Nuts

DATA FILE

Properties

❧ Boosts immunity.

❧ Inhibits the growth of a number of tumors.

❧ Builds muscle and burns fat, by stimulating the pituitary glands to increase growth hormone secretion.

❧ Helps to promote the healing of burns and other wounds.

❧ Helps to protect the liver and to detoxify harmful substances.

❧ Increases sperm count in men with a low count.

Best Sources

Raw cereals, chocolate, and nuts.

Dosage

The optimal intake is unknown, but doses up to 1.5g. appear to be safe. Take L-arginine with lysine, which inhibits herpes attacks in carriers.

LEFT *Found in chocolate, nuts, and cereals, L-arginine is one of the most important amino acids and is essential for young children.*

L-ASPARTIC ACID

L-aspartic acid is a nonessential amino acid which has been used for many years in the treatment of chronic fatigue. Studies confirm the efficiency of this amino acid in raising energy levels, and in helping to overcome the side-effects of drug withdrawal.

DATA FILE

Properties

❧ Disposes of ammonia, helping to protect the central nervous system.

❧ Helps treat fatigue.

❧ May improve stamina and endurance.

Dosage

❧ Supplements are available in 250–500mg. tablets; take 3 times daily with juice or water.

BELOW *L-aspartic acid has long been used to treat chronic fatigue.*

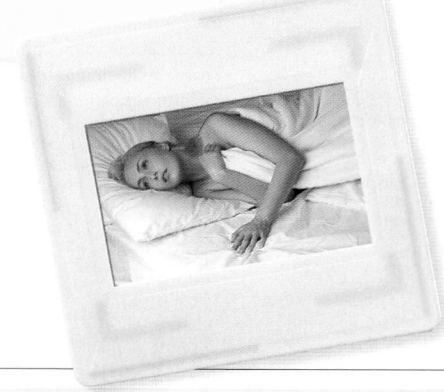

L-CYSTEINE

Cysteine contains sulfur, which is said to work as an antioxidant, protecting and preserving the cells in the body. It is also believed to protect the body against pollutants, but much work has still to be done to understand the effects of this amino acid.

BELOW *Eggs, meat, and dairy products all contain cysteine, which helps protect the body against free radicals.*

Meat

Yogurt

Eggs

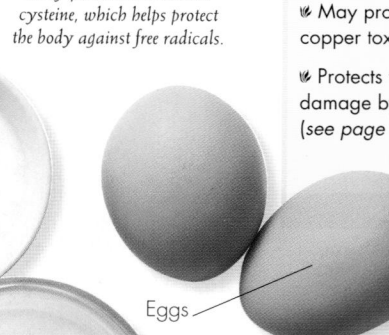

DATA FILE

Properties

❧ May protect against copper toxicity.

❧ Protects the body against damage by free radicals (*see page 251*).

❧ May help to reverse damage done by smoking and alcohol abuse.

❧ Offers protection against X-rays and nuclear radiation.

❧ May help to treat arthritis.

❧ Helps to repair DNA, thereby preventing the effects of aging.

Best Sources

Eggs, meat, dairy products, some cereals.

Dosage

❧ Take with vitamin C for best effect (three times as much vitamin C as L-cysteine). Doses up to 1g. are considered to be safe, but consult your physician first.

L-GLUTAMINE

L-glutamine is a derivative of glutamic acid, which is believed to help reduce cravings for alcohol. Studies are inconclusive as to the real benefits of taking this amino acid, and it is recommended that you do not take more than 1g. daily unless you are supervised by your physician.

DATA FILE

Properties

❦ Believed to help reduce craving for alcohol.

❦ May help to speed the healing of peptic ulcers.

❦ May help to counter attacks of depression.

❦ May energize the mind.

❦ May help to treat and prevent colitis.

Dosage

Up to 1g. daily is believed to be safe, but supplement only under the supervision of your physician.

L-HISTADINE

L-histadine is one of the lesser-known amino acids, and its role in our bodies is not yet fully understood. Research is ongoing into the possible effects of histadine supplementation.

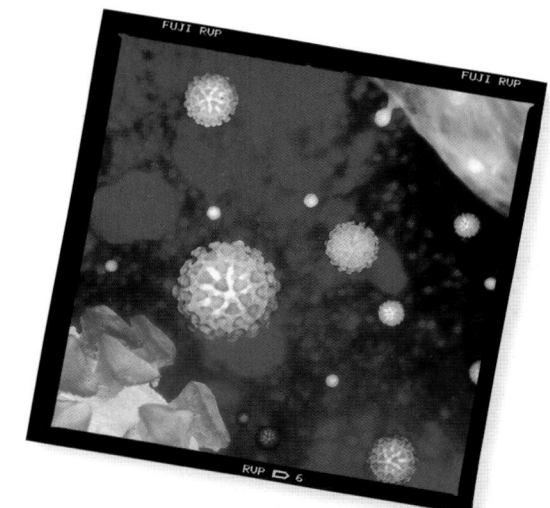

DATA FILE

Properties

❦ Used in the treatment of arthritis sufferers, who have an abnormally low level of this amino acid in their blood.

❦ May boost the activity of suppressor T-cells, which could be useful in the fight against HIV/AIDS and auto-immune conditions.

Dosage

Do not take more than 150mg. daily unless supervised by your physician.

LEFT *Research suggests that L-histadine may boost T-cell activity, which could make it important in HIV/AIDS treatment.*

GLYCINE

Glycine is considered to be the simplest of the amino acids, with a variety of properties which are still being studied by scientists.

CAUTION

IT IS RECOMMENDED THAT YOU DO NOT TAKE THIS AMINO ACID AS A SUPPLEMENT UNLESS SUPERVISED BY YOUR PHYSICIAN.

DATA FILE

Properties

❦ May help to treat low pituitary gland function.

❦ May be used in the treatment of spastic movement – particularly in patients suffering from multiple sclerosis.

❦ May help treat progressive muscular dystrophy.

❦ Used in the treatment of hypoglycemia, since it stimulates the release of glucagon, which mobilizes glycogen, which can then be released into the bloodstream as glucose.

Dosage

❦ Doses below 1g. are thought to be safe, but research is ongoing.

L-LYSINE

L-lysine is an essential amino acid, which means that it is necessary for life. It is needed for growth, tissue repair, and for the production of antibodies, hormones, and enzymes. Lysine should be obtained from eating foods such as fish, milk, cheese, and eggs, although it is possible to purchase lysine supplements.

CAUTION

NOT SUITABLE FOR CHILDREN.

DATA FILE

Properties

❦ Inhibits herpes – high doses are now believed to be effective in reducing the recurrence of outbreaks.

❦ May assist in building muscle mass.

❦ Helps to prevent fertility problems.

❦ Improves concentration.

Best Sources

Found in fish, milk, lima beans, meat, cheese, yeast, eggs, all proteins.

Dosage

❦ Up to 500mg. daily is believed to be safe.

❦ Some experts recommend 1,000mg. daily at mealtimes.

❦ It is usually advised that amino acids are taken on an empty stomach, with some juice or water.

❦ Take L-lysine with an equal quantity of arginine if an increase in muscle mass is the desired goal.

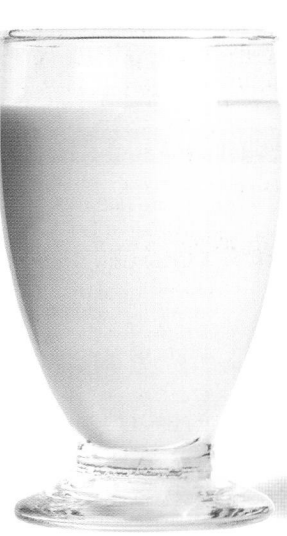

RIGHT *Milk is an ideal source of lysine, an essential amino acid that aids concentration and helps prevent fertility problems.*

L-METHIONINE

Methionine is a sulfur-containing amino acid that is very important in numerous processes in the body. Research shows that it may help to prevent clogging of the arteries by eliminating fatty substances.

BELOW Eating methionine-rich foods, such as fish, milk, liver, and eggs, may help the body eliminate fatty substances in the blood.

Eggs

Yogurt

Fish

Liver

DL-PHENYLALANINE (DLPA)

DLPA is a form of the amino acid phenylalanine created from equal parts of D (synthetic) phenylalanine and L (natural) phenylalanine. DLPA has a unique role of activating and producing endorphins, which are the body's natural painkillers. Many people who do not respond to conventional painkillers respond successfully to DLPA, and its painkilling action increases over time. Do not confuse DLPA with L-phenylalanine.

L-PHENYLALANINE

L-phenylalanine is an essential amino acid that is necessary for a number of biochemical processes, including the synthesis of neurotransmitters in the brain. It is said to promote sexual arousal and to release hormones that help to control appetite.

Almonds

Peanuts

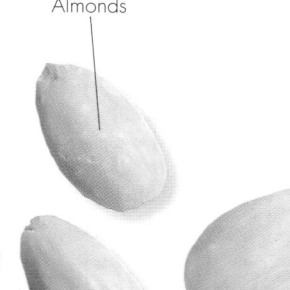

LEFT Present in almonds, peanuts, soybeans, and sesame seeds, L-phenylalanine is said to control the appetite and alleviate depression.

Soybeans

Sesame seeds

L-TRYPTOPHAN

This essential amino acid is used by the brain, along with several vitamins and minerals, to produce serotonin, a neurotransmitter. Serotonin, which regulates and induces sleep, is also said to reduce sensitivity to pain. It was one of the first amino acids to be produced for sale as a supplement, and it is useful as a natural sleeping aid.

DATA FILE

Properties

❧ May help to encourage sleep and to prevent jet lag.

❧ Reduces sensitivity to pain.

❧ Lessens a craving for alcohol.

❧ Natural antidepressant, and may help to reduce anxiety and panic attacks.

Best Sources

Cottage cheese, milk, meat, fish, turkey, bananas, protein sources.

Dosage

❧ Used to prevent panic attacks and depression,

L-tryptophan should be taken between meals with juice or water (no proteins).

❧ To help induce sleep, take 500mg. along with vitamin B6, niacinamide, and magnesium an hour or so before bedtime.

CAUTION

THERE IS SOME EVIDENCE THAT IT MAY CAUSE LIVER PROBLEMS IN HIGH DOSES, AND ALTHOUGH STUDIES VARY, IT IS NOW BELIEVED THAT IT CAN BE TOXIC IN VERY HIGH DOSES. TAKE ONLY ON THE ADVICE OF YOUR PHYSICIAN.

L-TYROSINE

L-tyrosine is not an essential amino acid, which means that it is synthesized in the body. Tyrosine is involved with important neurotransmitters in the brain, and it is said to energize and help to relieve the effects of stress.

DATA FILE

Properties

❧ Helps to relieve stress, and encourages alertness and fewer physical symptoms of tension and stress.

❧ May act as an antidepressant.

❧ May be used to treat the emotional symptoms of PMS.

❧ May help to aid in the treatment of addiction to and withdrawal from cocaine and other addictive drugs.

Dosage

❧ Take with juice or water on an empty stomach (do not take with proteins, such as milk).

❧ Some experts suggest that it is more effective when taken in conjunction with up to 25mg. of vitamin B6.

CAUTION

DO NOT TAKE TYROSINE IF YOU SUFFER FROM MIGRAINE HEADACHES, OR IF YOU TAKE MAOI ANTIDEPRESSANTS.

PEOPLE SUFFERING FROM HIGH BLOOD PRESSURE OR SKIN CANCER SHOULD NOT TAKE SUPPLEMENTARY TYROSINE WITHOUT THE APPROVAL OF A PHYSICIAN.

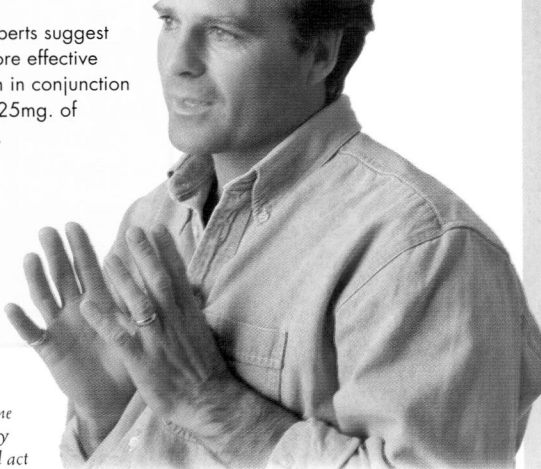

RIGHT *Tyrosine supplements may alleviate stress and act as an antidepressant.*

LIPIDS AND DERIVATIVES

FISH OILS

Fish oils contain two long-chain fatty acids called eicosopentaenoic acid (EPA) and docosahexaenoic acid (DHA) that affect the synthesis of prostaglandins, which have a regulatory effect on the body. There are numerous claims for fish oils, which are now believed to improve overall health and treat many health conditions.

CAUTION

FISH OILS MAY BE HARMFUL IN DIABETICS, CAUSING INCREASES IN BLOOD SUGAR AND A DECLINE IN INSULIN SECRETION.

DATA FILE

Properties

❧ May be useful in the treatment of kidney disease, and can counteract the effects of some immuno-suppressive drugs.

❧ May help to prevent cancer, in particular the onset of breast cancer.

❧ Stops progression of arthritis symptoms.

❧ May help to protect against high blood pressure.

❧ Helps to prevent cardiovascular disease.

❧ May help to prevent and treat psoriasis.

Best Sources

Fish, in particular herring, salmon, tuna, cod, prawns.

Dosage

❧ People suffering from arthritis or psoriasis can take up to 4g. daily, but for most people it is more appropriate to increase your intake of fish and seafood in order to achieve the benefits of the fish oils in their natural form.

❧ The maximum suggested dosage for supplements, taken without the supervision of your physician, is 900mg. per day.

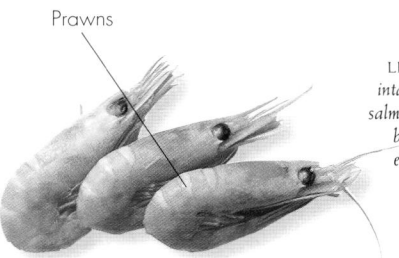

Prawns

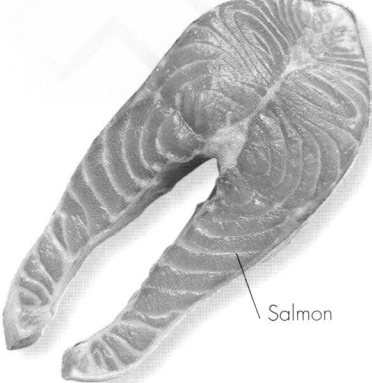

LEFT *Increase your intake of fish, such as salmon and prawns, to benefit from health-enhancing fish oils.*

Salmon

EVENING PRIMROSE *(GLA)*

Native Americans were the first to recognize the potential of evening primrose oil as a healer, and they decocted (boiled) the seeds to make a liquid for healing wounds. Evening primrose oil is a rich source of gamma-linoleic acid, which is better known as GLA. The body makes GLA from essential fatty acids (EFAs). EFAs have numerous functions in the body, one of which is to manufacture hormone-like substances called "prostaglandins," which have very important effects on the body, such as toning blood vessels, balancing our water levels, and improving the action of the digestive system, and brain functioning. Prostaglandins also have a beneficial effect on the immune system.

BELOW *Evening primrose oil will help to keep your skin from becoming dehydrated.*

DATA FILE

Properties

• Reduces scaling and redness, prevents itching, and encourages healing in cases of eczema. Also used in the treatment of psoriasis.

• Discourages dry skin, and ensures that the cellular membranes that make up the skin are stable and strong. There is some evidence that the oil retards the aging process.

• Evening primrose oil may help to prevent MS, and appears to be particularly useful for children suffering from the condition.

• May help in cases of liver damage caused by alcohol (cirrhosis of the liver), hyperactivity in children, and cystic fibrosis.

• May have a stimulating effect on the body, encouraging it to convert fat into energy, which would make it an excellent treatment for obesity.

• Hormonal imbalances, perhaps causing conditions like PMS, and symptoms of the menopause may be eased by evening primrose oil, reducing symptoms of bloating, water retention, irritability, and depression.

• Reduces the inflammation of rheumatoid arthritis.

• Evening primrose may have an immunosuppressive effect on the body.

Dosage

• Evening primrose oil is most often taken in the form of capsules, but it is also available as an oil (sometimes flavored), and it can be applied to the skin to treat skin conditions.

• Take 500mg. each day for two months, and then for the 10 days preceding menstruation if you suffer from PMS. During the menopause, 2,000–4,000mg. should be taken daily for four weeks, and then 500–1,000mg. daily thereafter.

• For asthma, take two 500mg. tablets three times daily for three to four months; then one tablet three times daily. If you are taking steroids, this treatment will not work because steroids interfere with evening primrose oil's action.

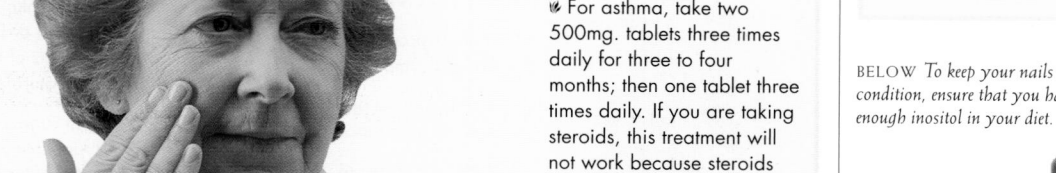

INOSITOL

Inositol is not a true vitamin, as it can be synthesized by the body, but it forms part of the B-complex family of vitamins, and is present in cereals and vegetables as phytic acid. There is a high concentration in the brain, stomach, spleen, liver, and heart.

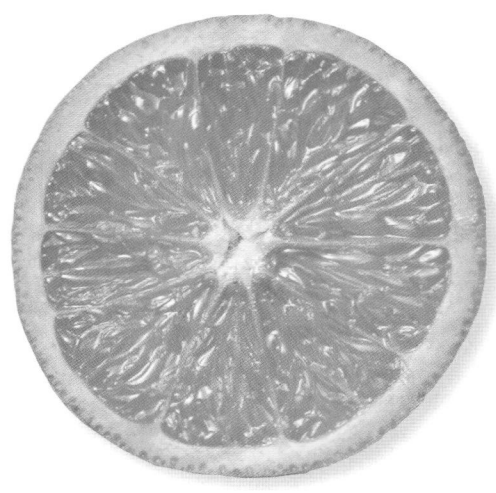

ABOVE *Citrus fruits are a valuable source of inositol, part of the B-complex vitamin family.*

DATA FILE

Properties

• Helps to dissolve fat.

• May help to prevent anxiety and tension.

• Ensures healthy hair and strong nails.

• Controls levels of cholesterol in the blood.

• Helps to encourage natural sleep.

• May help to treat schizophrenia and other nervous disorders.

Best Sources

Lethicin, liver, wheat germ, brown rice, citrus fruits, nuts, and cereals.

Dosage

• Natural sources are best, but if you are prescribed supplements, take in the form of myo-inositol to a maximum of 1,000mg. daily.

BELOW *To keep your nails in good condition, ensure that you have enough inositol in your diet.*

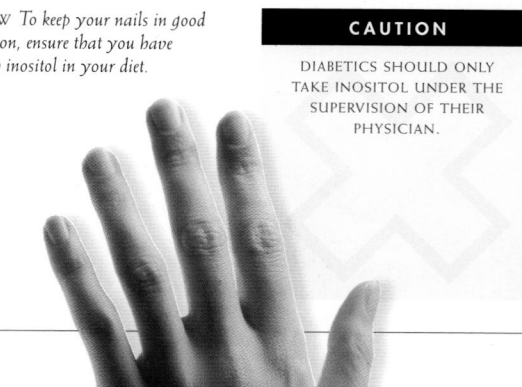

LECITHIN

Lecithin has for some time been a popular supplement, used for a variety of health conditions. It is comprised of choline, inositol, fatty acids, and phosphorus, and is available as a liquid or as dry granules. It is widely used in foods to maintain consistency, and is probably one of the few nutritious food additives.

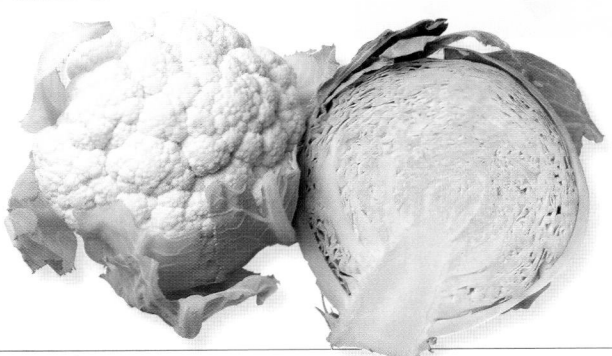

RIGHT *Increase your intake of lecithin-rich foods, such as cauliflower and cabbages to treat a wide variety of ailments.*

DATA FILE

Properties

๕ Protects against cardiovascular disease.

๕ Helps to reduce high blood pressure.

๕ Used to treat memory loss and conditions of the nervous system such as dementia and Alzheimer's.

๕ May help in the treatment of mental disorders such as manic depression.

๕ Lecithin has some action against viruses.

๕ May prevent and also treat gallstones.

๕ May help to treat viral hepatitis, repairing the membranes of the liver cells.

Best Sources

Found in egg yolks, soybeans, liver, meats, fish, cauliflower, and cabbage.

Dosage

๕ Doses of up to 1g. daily are acceptable, but see your physician to discuss your individual needs.

๕ Lecithin appears in a wide range of foods, and it is probably best to increase your intake of these rather than supplementing.

OTHER SUPPLEMENTS

ACIDOPHILUS

Acidophilus (also known as *lactobacillus acidophilus*) is a source of friendly intestinal bacteria (flora). Healthy bacteria play an important role in our bodies, and unless they are continually supplied with some form of lactic acid or lactose (such as acidophilus) they can die, causing a host of health problems. Many physicians and health practitioners recommend taking acidophilus alongside oral antibiotics which can cause diarrhea, destroy the healthy flora of the intestines, and lead to fungal infections. Acidophilus may also help to ensure vaginal health.

DATA FILE

Properties

๕ Keeps the intestines clean.

๕ Prevents yeast infections of the vagina.

๕ Aids the absorption of nutrients in food.

๕ Can eliminate bad breath (which has been caused by intestinal putrefaction).

๕ Can relieve and prevent constipation and flatulence.

๕ Can aid the treatment of acne and other skin troubles.

๕ Maintains intestinal health.

Best Sources

Natural, unflavored, "live" yogurt, sometimes known as "bio yogurt."

Dosage

๕ Acidophilus is not toxic and can be taken daily, with food, in unlimited amounts.

BEE AND FLOWER POLLEN

In flowering plants the pollen-producing spores are located in the stamens of flowers. Flower pollen is said to be purer than bee pollen. Bee pollen is found in the hives themselves. It is rich in protein and amino acids, and forms, with honey, the basic diet of all the bees in the hive, except for the queen (*see royal jelly, page 276*). Pollen has been used as medicine around the world for thousands of years.

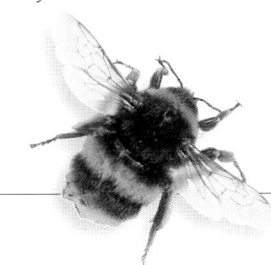

LEFT *Bee pollen is found in the hives of bees but it also present in small amounts in unpasteurized honey.*

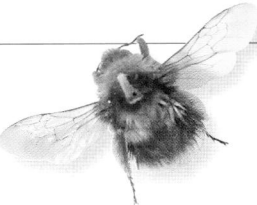

DATA FILE

Properties

๕ Rich in both amino acids and protein.

๕ Helps to suppress appetite and cravings.

๕ May help to improve skin problems and retard the aging process.

๕ May help to treat problems of the prostate.

๕ Energizes the body.

๕ Regulates the bowels.

๕ May boost immunity and diminish allergies.

Best Sources

Unpasteurized honey contains small amounts of bee pollen.

Dosage

๕ 400mg. doses, taken daily, appear to be safe.

๕ Take pollen with food.

BIOFLAVONOIDS

Bioflavonoids were originally called vitamin P, and are also known as flavones. They accompany vitamin C in natural foods, and are responsible for the color in the leaves, flowers, and stems of food plants. Their primary job in the body is to protect the capillaries, to keep them strong, and to prevent bleeding. Bioflavonoids are also anti-inflammatory. Many of the medicinally active substances contained in herbs are bioflavonoids.

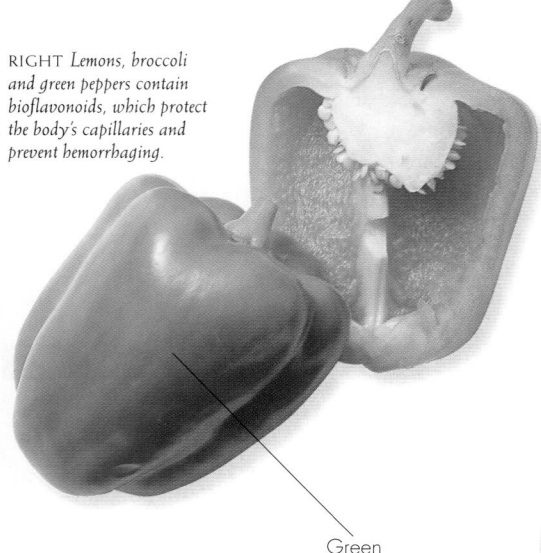

RIGHT *Lemons, broccoli and green peppers contain bioflavonoids, which protect the body's capillaries and prevent hemorrhaging.*

Green peppers

Lemons

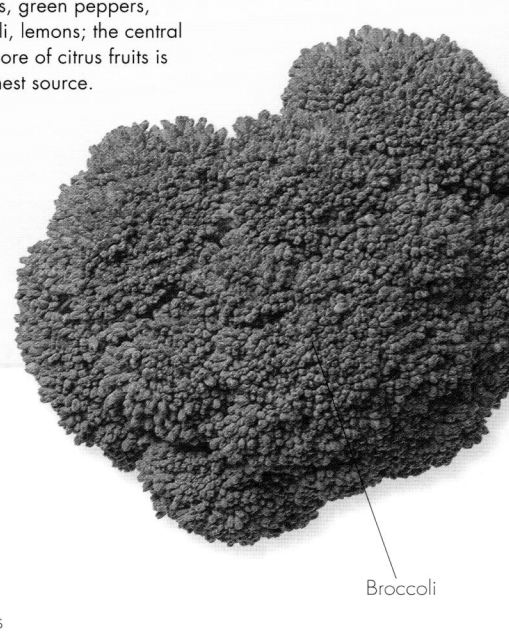

Broccoli

DATA FILE

Properties

❦ Reduce bruising in susceptible individuals.

❦ Protect capillaries.

❦ Protect against cerebral and other hemorrhaging.

❦ Reduce bleeding during menstruation.

❦ Antioxidant (*see page 251*), and encourage the antioxidant qualities of vitamin C.

❦ Antiviral activity.

❦ Anti-inflammatory.

❦ Antiallergy.

❦ May help to cure colds.

Best Sources

Citrus fruits, apricots, cherries, green peppers, broccoli, lemons; the central white core of citrus fruits is the richest source.

Dosage

❦ Bioflavonoids are not toxic, and should be taken together with vitamin C for best effect.

BREWER'S YEAST

Brewer's yeast is the same type of yeast that is used in the brewing process, and is quite different from the yeast that causes thrush. It is a rich source of B-vitamins and amino acids, as well as some minerals, in particular chromium and selenium. It also contains naturally occurring nucleic acids (DNA and RNA), which are said to enhance the immune system, among other things.

CAUTION

BREWER'S YEAST IS NOT TOXIC AND CAN BE TAKEN DAILY WITHOUT ANY SIDE-EFFECTS.

—◦—

SOME EXPERTS SUGGEST THAT IT MAY CAUSE YEAST INFECTIONS AND CHRONIC FATIGUE SYNDROME, BUT THIS HAS LARGELY BEEN DISCLAIMED.

RIGHT *Brewer's yeast, which comes in powder or tablet form, contains B-vitamins and amino acids, as well as some minerals.*

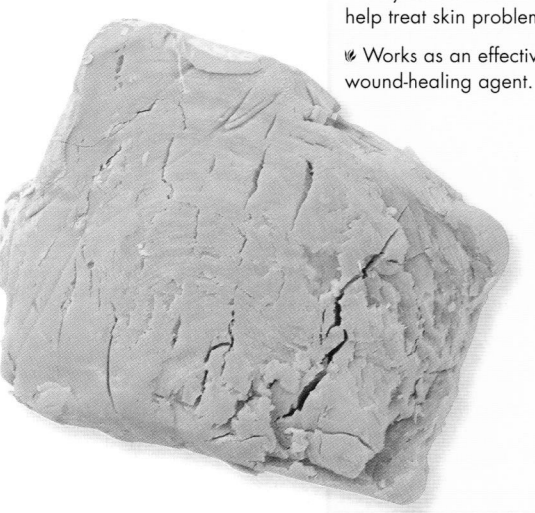

DATA FILE

Properties

❦ May reduce wrinkling and help treat skin problems.

❦ Works as an effective wound-healing agent.

❦ Encourages the healing of burns.

❦ Rich source of B-vitamins, which can help to relieve stress and nervous disorders.

❦ Encourages the activity of the immune system.

❦ Increases energy.

❦ Used externally, to detoxify skin.

Dosage

❦ Brewer's yeast comes in tablets, or as a powder that can be sprinkled on food or drink.

CHARCOAL

Charcoal is a porous, solid product obtained when materials such as cellulose, wood, peat, bituminous coal, or bone are partially burned in the absence of air. Charcoal has always been popular for dealing with flatulence, bloating, and irritable bowel syndrome, by soaking up gas. Charcoal can also be useful in the long-term management of kidney patients.

DATA FILE

Properties

- Reduces cholesterol in the blood.

- Reduces the risk of atherosclerosis.

- Absorbs gas and so acts as an antacid.

- Binds with cholesterol, toxins, and waste in the intestine, which has a cleansing effect.

Dosage

- Charcoal is available in tablet, powder, and capsule form.

- High doses (more than 50g. per day) should be supplemented with a well-balanced vitamin and mineral supplement.

CAUTION

ACTIVATED CHARCOAL CAN BIND WITH AND INACTIVATE SOME THERAPEUTIC DRUGS AND SUPPLEMENTAL NUTRIENTS, AND SHOULD BE TAKEN AT LEAST ONE HOUR BEFORE OR AFTER DRUGS OR SUPPLEMENTS ARE TAKEN.

IF YOU ARE ON PRESCRIPTION DRUGS, TAKE CHARCOAL ONLY WITH YOUR PHYSICIAN'S ADVICE.

BELOW *Charcoal is good for kidney problems, but only take it on your physician's advice.*

CO-ENZYME Q10

Co-enzyme Q10 is a vitamin-like substance found in all cells of the body. It is biologically important, since it forms part of the system across which electrons flow in the cells during the process of energy production. When there is a Q10 deficiency, the cell cannot function effectively, and the rate at which the muscle cells work is adversely affected.

DATA FILE

Properties

- Enhances immunity.

- Improves the heart-muscle metabolism.

- May help to prevent coronary inefficiency and heart failure.

- Anti-aging.

- Necessary for healthy functioning of the nervous system and the brain cells.

Best Sources

Meat (it is also made within the body).

Dosage

- 10mg., taken 3 times a day, has a therapeutic effect within the body.

CAUTION

CO-ENZYME Q10 IS FAT SOLUBLE, AND THEREFORE MAY BE TOXIC IN HIGH DOSES.

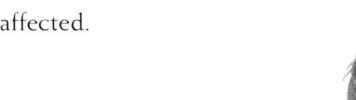

BELOW *Co-enzyme Q10 is an important substance for the efficient functioning of muscle cells.*

DHEA

Dehydroepiandrosterone (DHEA) is a hormone which we produce in our adrenal glands, and which also occurs naturally in the Mexican wild yam (potato). DHEA was for many years considered to be a cure-all, and indeed research has proved that it has invaluable therapeutic benefits, particularly in the prevention and treatment of cancer, but it is still very much under investigation and its many qualities have yet to be proven. It should be taken only if you have a known deficiency (less than 130mg/dl. in women and less than 180mg/dl. in men).

CAUTION

MANY SUPPLEMENTS THAT HAVE BEEN ANALYZED HAVE NO DHEA IN THEM, SO EXERCISE CAUTION WHEN CHOOSING A SUPPLEMENT.

DATA FILE

Properties

- Anticancer effects.

- Inhibits weight gain.

- May extend life span.

- DHEA is thought to have anti-aging effects.

- Works to reduce stress.

- Improves immunity.

Best Source

Mexican wild yam.

Dosage

- There is still some debate as to whether or not oral DHEA has any effect within the body, as in some studies it appears to be destroyed by the liver before it reaches the necessary tissues.

- See a registered practitioner for advice on supplementation.

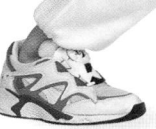

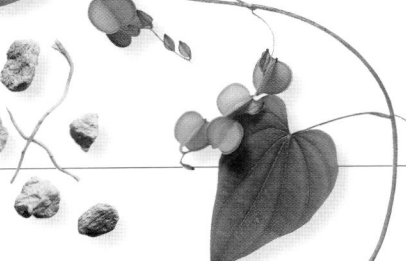

RIGHT *Mexican wild yam is the chief source of DHEA.*

DIETARY FIBER

Dietary fiber, also known as bulk and roughage, is an essential element in the diet, even though it provides no nutrients. It consists of plant cellulose and other indigestible materials in foods, along with pectin and gum. The chewing it requires stimulates saliva flow, and the bulk it adds in the stomach and intestines during digestion provides more time for absorption of nutrients. A diet with sufficient fiber produces softer, bulkier stools, and helps to promote bowel regularity and avoid constipation and disorders such as diverticulosis.

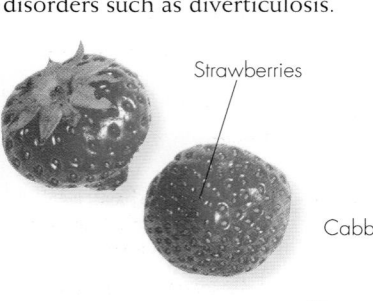
Strawberries

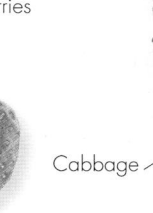

Cabbage

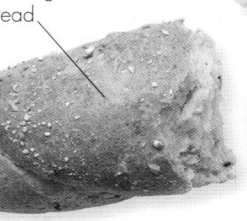
Wholegrain bread

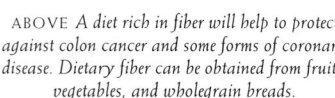
Nuts

ABOVE *A diet rich in fiber will help to protect against colon cancer and some forms of coronary disease. Dietary fiber can be obtained from fruits, vegetables, and wholegrain breads.*

DATA FILE

Properties

☙ Reduces the production of cholesterol in the body.

☙ May protect against some coronary heart diseases.

☙ Helps to control diabetes.

☙ Helps to control weight.

☙ Can be used to treat certain intestinal disorders such as diverticulosis.

☙ Protects against cancers of the colon.

Best Sources

Fruit and vegetables, wholegrain breads and cereals, products made from nuts and legumes.

Dosage

☙ An intake of 20–60g. per day is ideal, and can be taken in the form of food, or as "soluble fiber," which is less likely to cause loose bowel movements.

GLANDULARS

Glandulars are concentrates of the hormonal glands, and have, over the past decade, been hailed as a wonder drug. Evidence does not, however, support these claims and many experts now discourage their use. The premise is that failing or aging glands can be rejuvenated by supplementation.

DATA FILE

Properties

☙ May improve sexual performance and libido.

☙ May help to build muscle.

☙ May help to control the spread of cancer.

☙ May help to treat hypoglycemia.

☙ May be used in the treatment of asthma.

Dosage

☙ Consult a registered practitioner before taking any glandulars.

☙ Do not take them at night, as they will cause insomnia.

BELOW *Inhalers are most often used to treat asthma but glandulars have been said to help - only take them under medical supervision.*

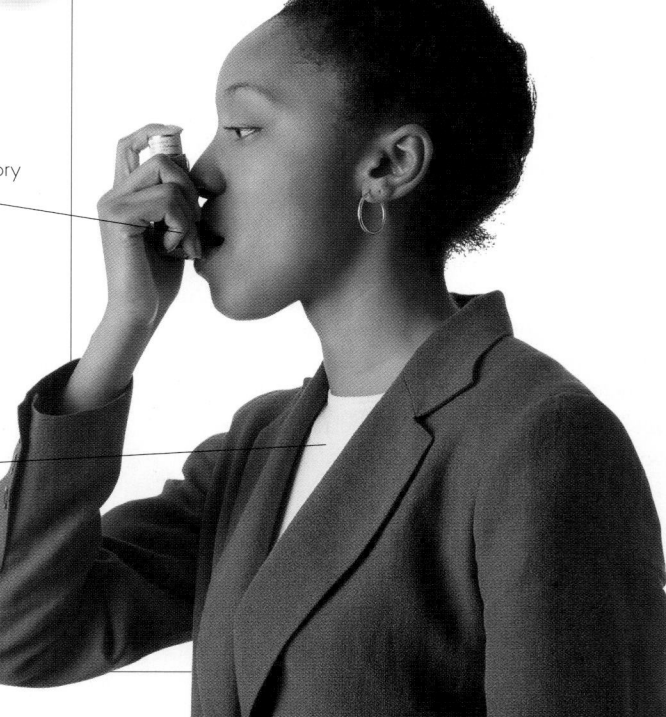
Respiratory inhaler

Chest tightness

PABA

Para-aminobenzoic acid (PABA) is often grouped with the B-vitamins, and although it is water soluble, it is stored in the tissues and can be toxic at high doses. Freckles can sometimes be minimized by the use of sunscreen lotions containing para-aminobenzoic acid (PABA). PABA can be synthesized in the body, helps to form folic acid, and is important in the efficient utilization of protein.

CAUTION

HIGH DOSES CAN CAUSE NAUSEA, FEVER, SKIN RASH, AND DIARRHEA.

PABA MAY PROVE TOXIC TO THE LIVER IN HIGH DOSES.

DO NOT TAKE PABA IF YOU ARE USING ANY SULFONAMIDE ANTIBIOTICS.

ABOVE *Many sunscreens contain PABA as it helps shield the skin from harmful ultraviolet rays.*

DATA FILE

Properties

💧 Used for the treatment of Peyronie's disease.

💧 Shields the skin from the damage of ultraviolet rays.

💧 May rejuvenate skin.

💧 May help in the treatment of arthritis.

💧 May restore color to graying or white hair.

💧 Reduces the pain of burns (used externally).

💧 Keeps skin healthy and smooth, and helps to delay wrinkles (used externally).

💧 PABA is used in the treatment of eczema.

Best Sources

Liver, brewer's yeast, kidney, whole grains, rice, bran, and molasses.

Dosage

💧 Available in 30–1,000mg. strengths, and should be taken three times daily for best effect.

💧 Experts suggest that you do not take more than 30mg. daily because of side-effects (*see Caution*).

💧 Best taken in a good multivitamin supplement.

💧 Ointments are available for external use, and PABA is included in many sunscreen preparations.

PANGAMIC ACID

Also called vitamin B15, pangamic acid is not a vitamin in the strictest sense of the word, but it is a good antioxidant and some studies show promising results. Pangamic acid is water soluble, and it works much like vitamin E. It stimulates the carriage of oxygen to the blood from the lungs, and from the blood to the muscles and vital organs of the body. It also acts to detoxify poisons and free radicals, and to stimulate the "anti-stress" hormones.

CAUTION

THE FDA (FOOD AND DRUG ADMINISTRATION) IN THE U.S. HAS ATTEMPTED TO BAN THE SALE OF PANGAMIC ACID AS AN UNSAFE FOOD ADDITIVE, AND, APART FROM RUSSIAN STUDIES, THERE HAS BEEN LITTLE TO PROVE THE BENEFITS OF THE SUPPLEMENT. ONE STUDY SUGGESTS THAT IT MAY BE CARCINOGENIC.

DATA FILE

Properties

💧 Extends the lifespan of cells in the body.

💧 Helps to reduce a craving for alcohol.

💧 Encourages the body to deal efficiently with stress.

💧 Protects against pollution and cirrhosis of the liver.

💧 Helps synthesize protein.

💧 Helps angina and asthma.

💧 Lowers cholesterol levels.

Best Sources

Brewer's yeast, brown rice, whole grains, pumpkin seeds, sesame seeds.

Dosage

💧 Available in 50mg. capsules, and should be taken after the day's largest meal to avoid toxicity.

💧 Do not take more than 50mg. daily, and only supplement with the approval of your physician or registered practitioner.

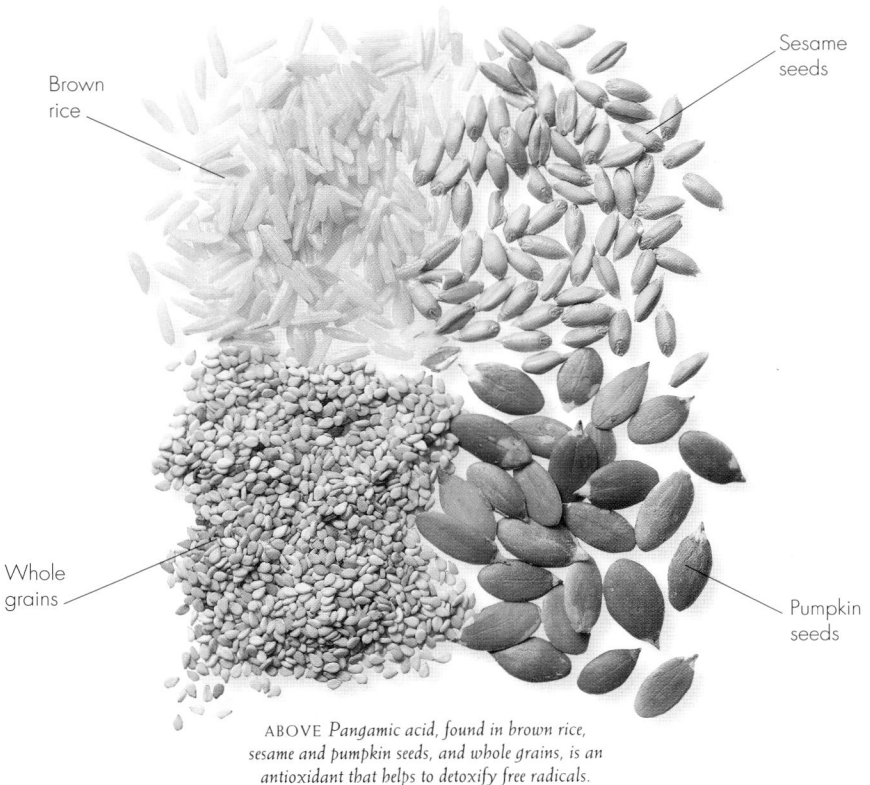

Brown rice

Sesame seeds

Whole grains

Pumpkin seeds

ABOVE *Pangamic acid, found in brown rice, sesame and pumpkin seeds, and whole grains, is an antioxidant that helps to detoxify free radicals.*

PROPOLIS

Propolis is a sticky material collected by bees from buds or tree bark and used to seal the inside of the hive. It is a mixture of wax, resin, balsam oil, and pollen. It is said to act as an antibiotic and bactericide, and may be used to help wounds to heal. Propolis is rich in bioflavonoids.

CAUTION

BECAUSE THIS PRODUCT CONTAINS POLLEN, IT MAY CAUSE AN ALLERGIC REACTION IN SUSCEPTIBLE INDIVIDUALS.

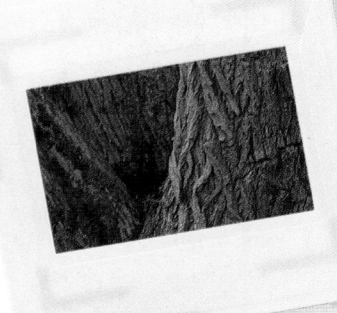

RIGHT *Propolis, which is a mixture of wax, resin, balsam oil, and pollen, is a sticky substance found on tree bark.*

DATA FILE

Properties

- Enhances immunity.
- Helps wounds to heal.
- Boosts energy.
- A natural anesthetic.
- Reduces cholesterol levels in the blood.
- Helps to reduce incidence and duration of colds.
- Natural antibiotic.

Dosage

- Propolis is available in tablet and liquid form, and does not appear to have any toxic levels.
- See your practitioner for details of suitable dosage.

ROYAL JELLY

Royal jelly has been used for centuries for its health-giving and rejuvenating properties, and it is rich in vitamins, amino acids, and minerals. It is also the prime source of fatty acid, which is said to increase alertness and act as a natural tranquilizer (when necessary). Royal jelly is secreted by the salivary glands of the worker bees to feed and stimulate the growth and development of the queen bee.

DATA FILE

Properties

- Antibacterial.
- May prevent the development of leukemia.
- Has a yeast-inhibiting function, preventing conditions such as thrush and athlete's foot.
- Contains the male sex hormone testosterone, which may increase libido.
- Used to treat subfertility.

- May be useful in the treatment of ME and MD (muscular dystrophy).
- Helps to reduce allergies.
- Boosts the body's resistance to the harmful side-effects of chemotherapy and radiotherapy.
- Controls cholesterol levels.
- Boosts the immune system.
- Royal jelly is used in the treatment of skin problems, including eczema, psoriasis, and acne.

- Combined with pantothenic acid, royal jelly provides relief from the symptoms of arthritis.

Dosage

- Most tablets contain 100–500mg. of royal jelly.
- Optimum dosage is about 150mg. per day.
- Fresh is better, although more expensive.

SEAWEEDS

Seaweeds are not plants, but part of the Protista kingdom. They are better known as "algae," and there are four main types. Seaweeds appear in many foods, medicines, and cosmetics, and have been used therapeutically for thousands of years. Rich in iodine, they are used in the treatment of goiter.

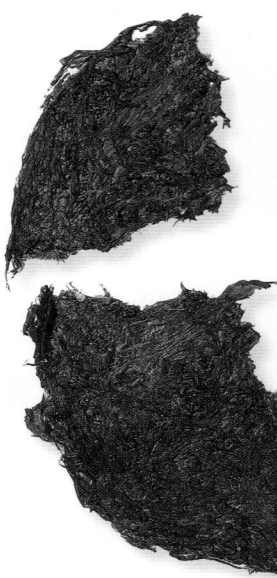

BELOW *Seaweeds are an excellent source of protein, and should be included in your diet. They are also the richest natural source of iodine.*

ABOVE *Seaweeds have been used in different cultures as a healing remedy and in cosmetics for centuries.*

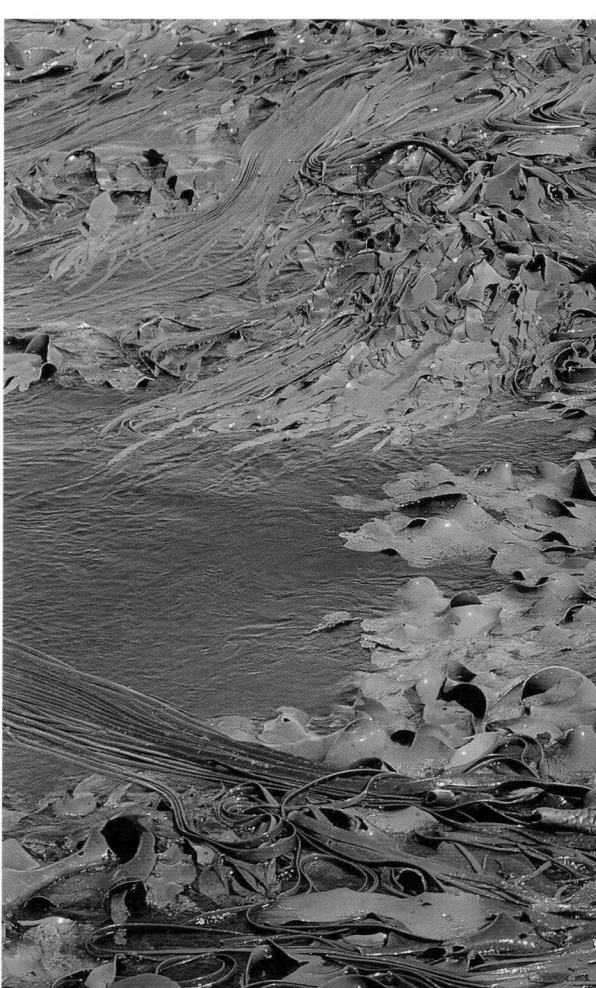

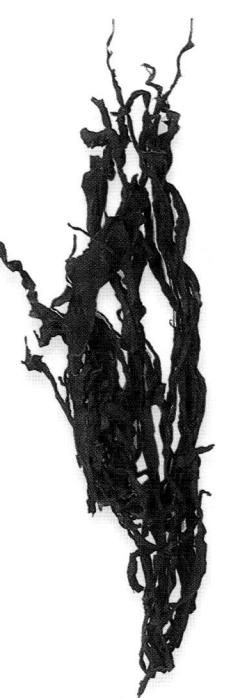

DATA FILE

Properties

✦ Antiviral activity.

✦ May prevent cancer.

✦ Used in the prevention and treatment of goiter.

✦ May help to reduce the effects of carcinogen, as well as radioactive material.

✦ Helps to counter the side-effects of radiotherapy and chemotherapy treatment.

✦ Natural antacid.

✦ Used in the treatment of intestinal disorders.

✦ Used in the treatment of exudative wounds.

Best Sources

Take seaweeds in their natural form, available from health food stores and many grocery stores (particularly oriental food stores).

Dosage

✦ There is no recommended dosage – consult a registered practitioner.

SPIRULINA

Spirulina are blue-green bacteria or algae, which are rich in GLA (gamma-linoleic acid, *see page* 270) and a wide variety of nutrients, including beta-carotene, inositol, calcium, vitamin E, magnesium, and phosphorus. In ancient times, spirulina was used as a staple food by the Aztecs of Mexico. It is now marketed in health food stores as a high-protein food supplement.

LEFT *Spirulina food supplements will help to keep your skin healthy and free of blemishes.*

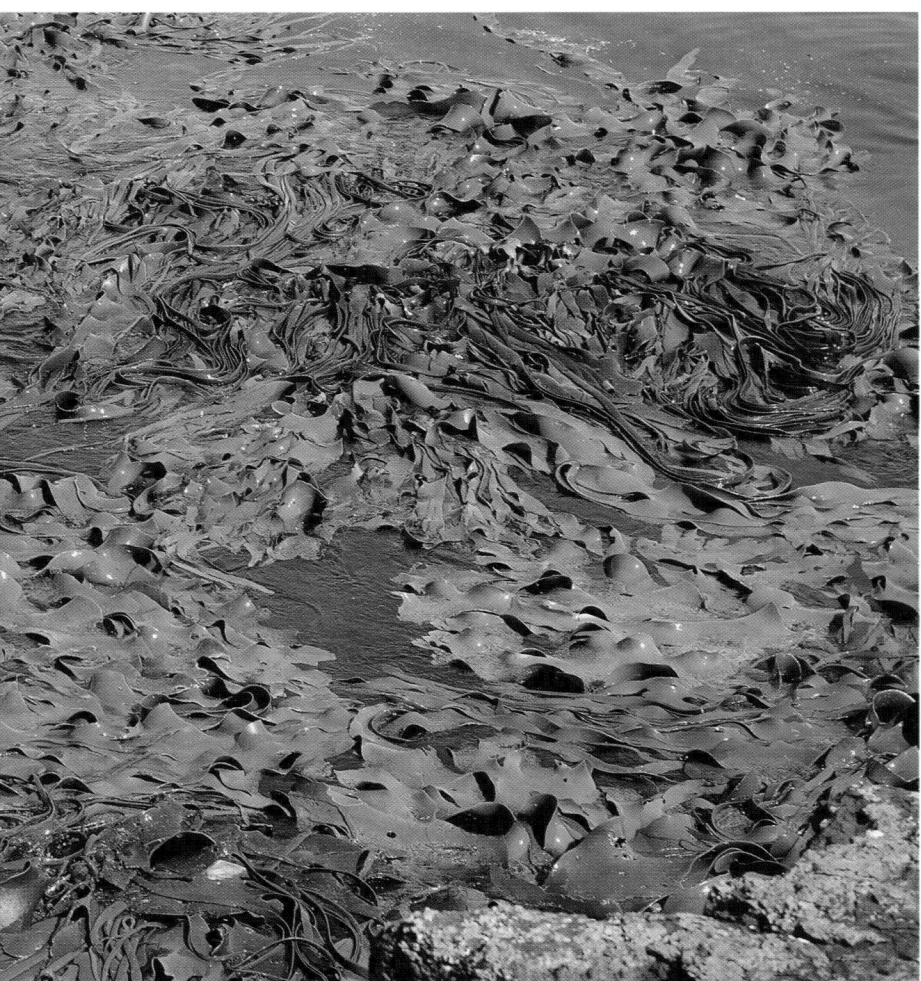

DATA FILE

Properties

✦ Rich in nutrients and high in protein (particularly useful for vegetarians).

✦ May suppress appetite.

✦ Maintains skin health and treats skin disorders.

✦ May contribute to healthy functioning of the intestines.

✦ General tonic properties.

✦ May be rejuvenating.

✦ Many spirulina have anti-cancer properties.

Best Sources

Fresh or freeze-dried spirulina.

Dosage

✦ There is no recommended dosage for spirulina – consult a registered practitioner.

LEFT *Spirulina algae contain protein and are also rich in nutrients.*

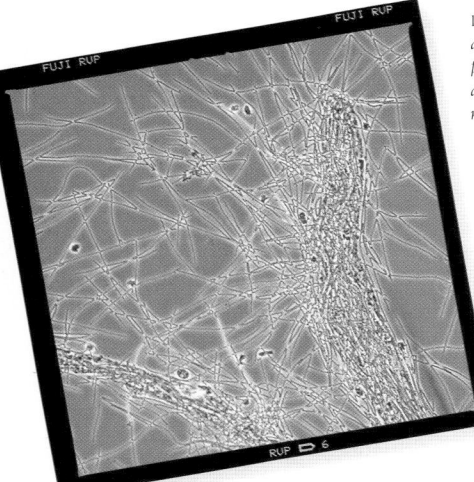

TREATING
COMMON AILMENTS

DISORDERS OF THE MIND AND EMOTIONS

Addictions

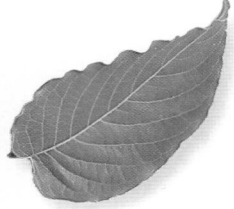

ABOVE *Add ylang ylang oil to the bath for its antidepressant qualities.*

An addiction is an overwhelming craving for or dependence on a substance, usually a drug, alcohol, or nicotine. The addiction may be limited to mental dependence, but it can become physiological if the way in which the body functions has changed through prolonged use of a substance. In such cases the addict will experience physical "withdrawal" symptoms without the substance in question.

SYMPTOMS

• *loss of control over use of the drug or other substance* • *mood swings and irrational behavior* • *in drug addiction: — sore or red eyes with dilated or constricted pupils — irregular breathing — trembling hands — itchy or runny nose — nausea* • *drug withdrawal symptoms may include craving, depression, restlessness, yawning, sweating, abdominal pain, vomiting, diarrhea, loss of appetite, and suffering from gooseflesh*

DATA FILE

• Drugs with potential for misuse are narcotics, including morphine, opium, heroin, and methadone; depressants such as alcohol, barbiturates, and sedatives; stimulants such as cocaine and amphetamines; hallucinogenic drugs; and marijuana.

• Nicotine and caffeine can also be abused, and anabolic steroids and human growth hormone are often misused by athletes and bodybuilders seeking to increase muscle mass.

• True physical addiction is known to occur with the narcotics and depressants; psychological dependence, with or without physical symptoms, can develop from using many other prescription drugs, such as tranquilizers.

• Studies show that 50–80 percent of all alcoholics have a close relative who is an alcoholic. Some researchers therefore suggest that some alcoholics have an inherited physical predisposition to alcohol addiction.

• Alcoholism and alcohol abuse in the U.S. cost an estimated $98 billion and take 100,000 lives per year, according to the National Institute on Alcohol Abuse and Alcoholism.

• One-half of all traffic fatalities and one-third of all traffic injuries are related to the abuse of alcohol.

• One-third of all suicides and one-third of all mental health disorders are estimated to be associated with serious alcohol abuse.

• The relaxation smokers feel is because tobacco contains nicotine, an addictive alkaloid. A number of diseases have been directly linked to smoking, and in the U.S. alone tobacco use kills about 420,000 smokers each year.

• Every day about 3,500 Americans successfully quit smoking.

CAUTION

ADDICTIONS TO PHYSICAL SUBSTANCES SHOULD ALWAYS BE TREATED BY A REGISTERED PRACTITIONER.

DO NOT DISCONTINUE ANY PRESCRIPTION DRUGS UNLESS YOU ARE UNDER SUPERVISION.

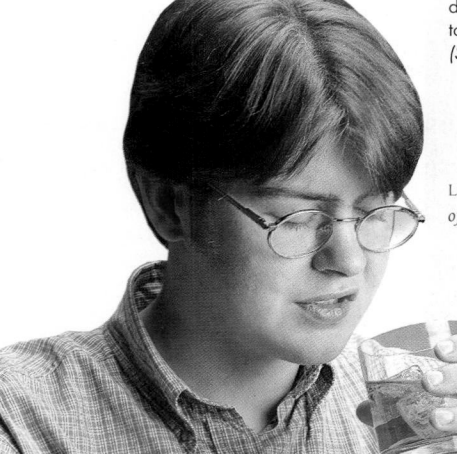

LEFT *Alcohol causes a third of all mental disorders.*

TREATMENT

AYURVEDA
• This has proved very successful in treating addictions of all types, which it sees as fundamental imbalance within the body. Treatment will be tailored to your specific constitution and personal characteristics. *(See page 20.)*

CHINESE HERBALISM
• For alcoholism, heat would be cleared from the Lung and Liver, with watermelon or kudzu vine to detoxify Blood.
• Treatment would be specific for various other types of addiction.
• Strong green tea is used to cool the liver.

HERBALISM
• Oats will calm you down and help to strengthen your willpower. *(See page 117.)*
• Other herbs to calm the nervous system and reduce symptoms when you wish to withdraw from your addiction include skullcap and valerian. Drink daily as a tea. *(See pages 131 and 136.)*
• Cramp bark helps nervous tension and jitters. *(See page 138.)*

AROMATHERAPY
• Antidepressant oils include chamomile, clary sage, and ylang ylang. Use in the bath, and in a vaporizer by your bedside. A few drops on your clothing during the day will allow the effect to be maintained. *(See pages 146–71.)*

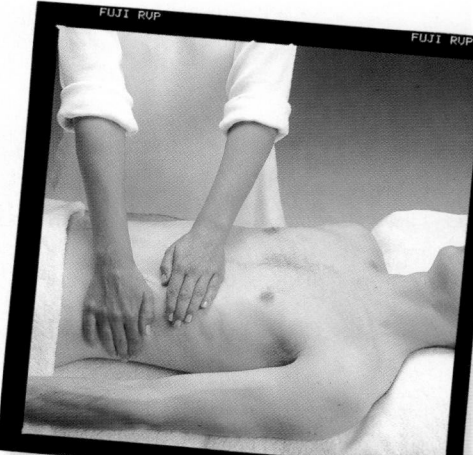

ABOVE *An aromatherapy massage encourages a positive attitude.*

• Massage with aromatherapy oil is extremely rewarding and a positive treatment. Try detoxifying oils such as juniper. *(See page 160.)*
• Aromatherapists suggest changing the oils used at regular intervals; although it is almost impossible to become physically addicted to an essential oil, you may come to regard it as a prop. *(See pages 146–71.)*
• Bergamot seems to be extremely useful in cases of food addiction. *(See page 153.)*

HOMEOPATHY
Homeopathic treatment would be constitutional, or tailored to your individual needs. Some useful addiction treatments are:
• Nux vomica, which helps to overcome a craving for smoking. *(See page 214.)*
• Kali phos., which strengthens the nervous system and may make it easier for a person to give up an addiction. *(See page 201.)*
• Arsenicum, for great anxiety, restlessness and fear of being alone. *(See page 182.)*

• Absinthium, when you feel depressed, disoriented, and dizzy.

FLOWER ESSENCES
• Crab Apple, for anyone who needs purification. *(See page 234.)*
• Gorse, when you are stuck in a negative pattern. *(See page 240.)*
• Mustard, for depression for no apparent reason. *(See page 239.)*
• Olive is particularly good for the recovery period. *(See page 235.)*

VITAMINS AND MINERALS
Treatment would ensure that there are no small nutritional deficiencies making you crave certain substances, and that deficiencies caused by addictions (such as vitamin B in alcoholics) are righted. Some amino acids may be used to create a specific physical effect, or act as a natural tranquilizer, which may help. Alcoholics are often deficient in GLA (gamma-linolenic acid), and it is recommended that you take evening primrose (a rich source) to help prevent mood swings. *(See page 270.)*

Obsessions and Compulsions

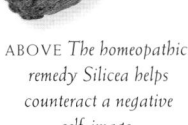

ABOVE *The homeopathic remedy Silicea helps counteract a negative self-image.*

An obsession is a persistent, recurring thought or idea, while a compulsion is an overwhelming drive to perform a particular act. When a person becomes dominated by these intrusions, despite knowing that they are irrational, he or she is said to be suffering from an obsessive-compulsive disorder. This may take the form of a hand-washing ritual, for example, or repeated checking that doors and windows are locked. The problem is often triggered by a stressful life event, but can also be due to subtle brain damage (usually the result of illnesses affecting the brain), especially when due to encephalitis. Obsessive-compulsive disorder is rare, although minor obsessional symptoms probably occur in about 15 percent of the population. At least two-thirds of all people who have obsessive-compulsive disorder respond well to therapy. Symptoms may recur under stress but can usually be controlled.

SYMPTOMS

- *fear of contamination*
- *dermatitis caused by repeated washing*
- *inefficiency caused by repeated and meticulous checking*
- *aggressive thoughts and behavior*
- *possible depression*

RIGHT *An irrational fear of germs and contamination may culminate in repeated, excessive hand washing.*

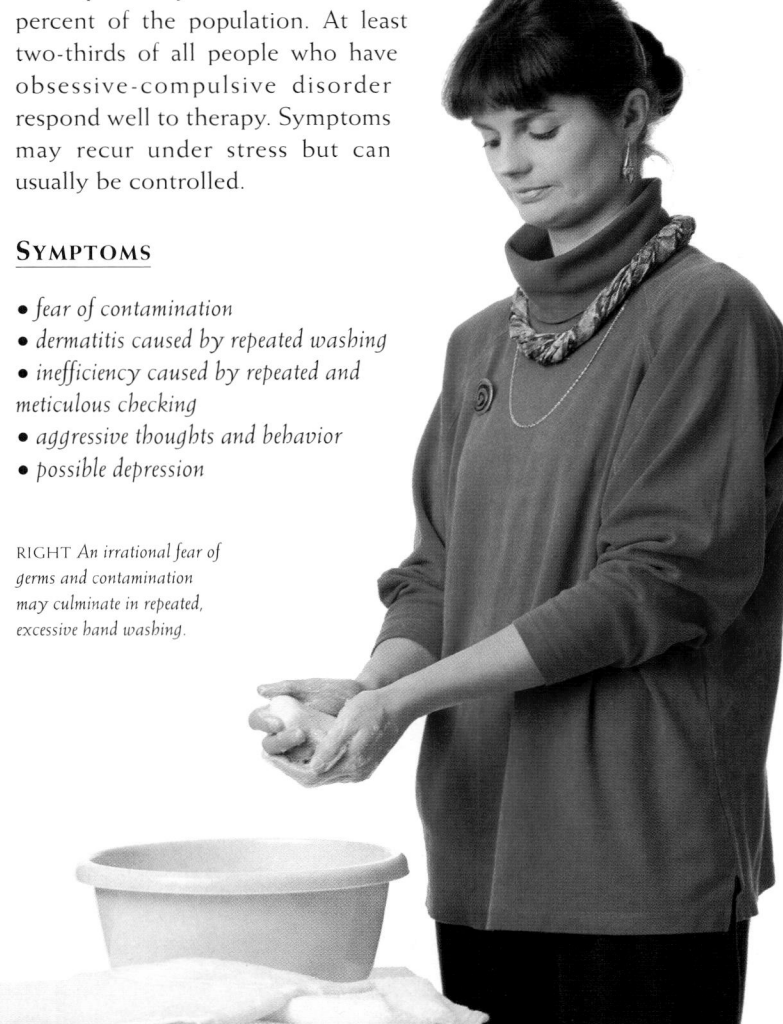

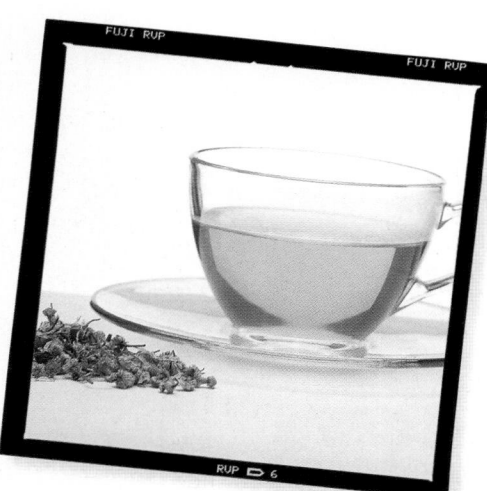

RIGHT *Certain herbs have beneficial effects on the nervous system. Take them in the form of an infusion.*

HERBALISM
• Drink certain infused herbs which act on the nervous system, including hops, valerian, vervain, chamomile, and passiflora. Taken on a regular basis, these herbs may help to ease tension and restrict various behavioral problems. *(See pages 119, 136, and 138.)*

AROMATHERAPY
• Relaxing oils, such as Roman chamomile or marjoram may help to achieve balance. Use regularly in the bath or on a burner in your room. *(See pages 150 and 165.)*
• Ylang ylang and clary sage may also help. *(See pages 169 and 148.)*

HOMEOPATHY
• Aurum is useful for feelings of worthlessness and overwhelming thoughts of death and dying. *(See page 184.)*
• Silicea for unshakable feelings of inadequacy, and an overwhelming urge to count small objects. *(See page 211.)*
• Take Anacardium when you feel that your mind is not your own and is being controlled by an external force. *(See page 179.)*

FLOWER ESSENCES
• Cherry Plum, for the fear of losing your mind, and to deal with irrational thoughts or behavior. *(See page 236.)*
• Crab Apple, for those who feel unclean or polluted on any level. *(See page 234.)*
• Vervain, for those who are strong-willed and need space for reflection. *(See page 241.)*
• White Chestnut, for an overactive mind, full of unwanted patterns of thought. *(See page 224.)*

RIGHT *The flower remedy Cherry Plum helps quell illogical behavior patterns.*

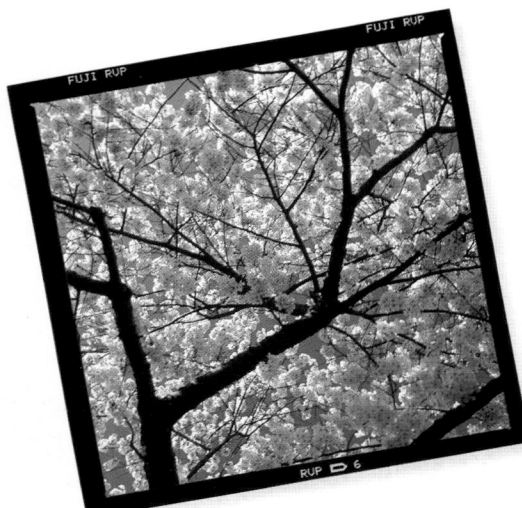

Phobias

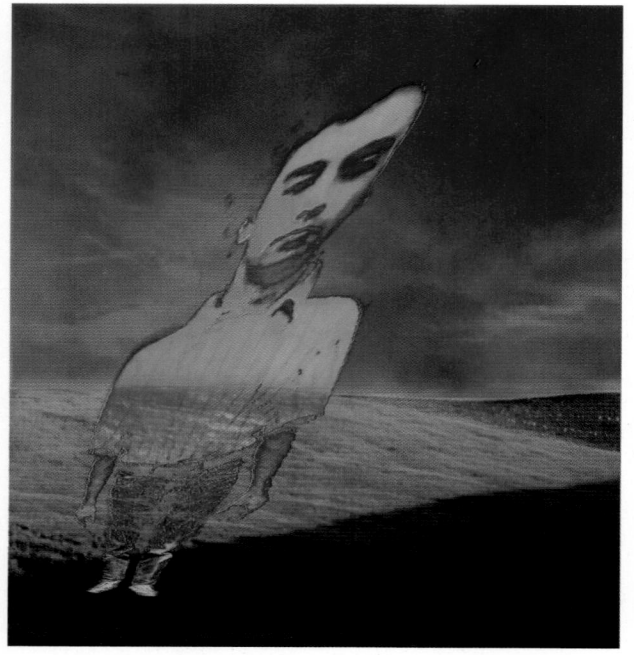

A phobia is an irrational fear which the sufferer finds impossible to overcome. Some of the most common fears are claustrophobia (fear of enclosed spaces), agoraphobia (fear of open spaces), and acrophobia (fear of heights). A phobia can, however, relate to just about any object, person, or situation, and is probably caused by a subconscious reflex to avoid repeating an unpleasant experience. For the sufferer it may cause little more than mild embarrassment, or it may be totally debilitating and disruptive to everyday life. An estimated 10 percent of people in the U.K., and slightly more in the U.S., suffer from phobias of some description. Recent research indicates that most sufferers can cure themselves.

LEFT Jasmine essential oil has a scent which calms an agitated mind.

SYMPTOMS

- rapid pulse • profuse sweating
- high blood pressure • trembling • nausea

TREATMENT

ABOVE Phobias range from the manageable to the totally incapacitating.

AYURVEDA
• Lemon or lime may be suggested for dizziness, and individual treatment would be prescribed according to your specific needs. *(See page 20.)*

CHINESE HERBALISM
• A herbalist may suggest cooling herbs, and Gui Pi Wan, which addresses emotional problems.

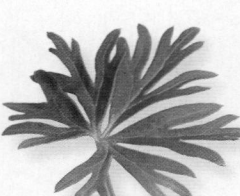

ABOVE Aconite is a homeopathic remedy for agoraphobia.

• Ginseng, Chinese angelica and senega root may also be useful. *(See pages 56, 67, 70.)*

HERBALISM
• Valerian tea can help to reduce tension. Drink an infusion as required. *(See page 136.)*

AROMATHERAPY
Essential oils can be very useful in the treatment of phobias. The effect of certain smells can help to release tension and induce a feeling of calm. Some of the best oils to try are: bergamot, chamomile, clary sage, geranium, jasmine, juniper, lavender, marjoram, melissa, and ylang ylang, which are sedative. They can be used in the bath, in massage with a light carrier oil (such as sweet almond), or in a vaporizer. Carry a

bottle of diluted oils with you – perhaps in a small sprayer – and apply them to the temples or pulse points in times of fear. *(See page 140.)*

HOMEOPATHY
There are dozens of homeopathic remedies which can be used to treat phobias, but they will be prescribed constitutionally, that is, the treatment would be tailored to your exact needs. Some to try may be:
• Arg. nit., for fear of heights. *(See page 181.)*
• Phosphorus, for fear of the dark. *(See page 208.)*
• Gelsemium, for fear of performing in public, when you feel weak at the knees. *(See page 195.)*
• Aconite, for agoraphobia, when you are terrified of dying or collapsing if you go out. *(See page 178.)*
• Arnica, for fears that are brought on by an accident. *(See page 182.)*
• Sulfur, when you need help and no other remedy seems to be indicated. *(See page 215.)*

FLOWER ESSENCES
Treatment would be based on your individual state of mind, but some of the following may help:
• Mimulus, for the everyday fears of known things, spiders, being late for work, flying, and being ill. *(See page 235.)*
• Aspen is for unknown fears, the vague and dark fears which hover and play on the imagination. *(See page 236.)*
• Rock Rose should be added when the fear is turning into terror and perhaps even panic. *(See page 231.)*
• Cherry Plum is for the fear that everything will fall apart. *(See page 236.)*
• Red Chestnut is for fear for another's safety. *(See page 224.)*
• The most important Bach Flower Remedy for fear, anxiety, and phobias, Rescue Remedy, is made up of five essences, Cherry Plum, Rock Rose, Impatiens, Clematis, and Star of Bethlehem.

It works to treat fear, loneliness, despondency, and loss of focus. It rebalances the sufferer after an emotional upset and is particularly useful in panic attacks. Apply a few drops of the remedy to your tongue or pulse points. *(See page 244.)*

VITAMINS AND MINERALS
Vitamin B-complex and C are important for nerve functioning. Ensure that you eat regular meals, since low blood sugar can exacerbate the problem.

BELOW Use an atomizer to apply your favorite essential oil at stressful moments.

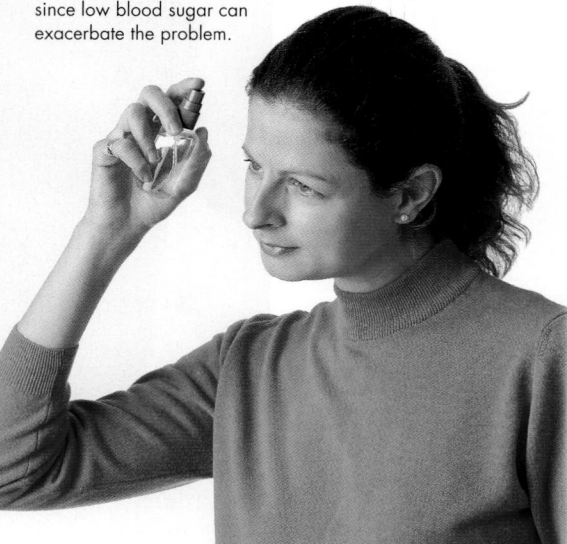

Depression

Depression is a prolonged feeling of unhappiness and despondency, often magnified by a major life event such as bereavement, divorce, or retirement. Many women experience depression after childbirth. Clinical depression is a genuine illness which overwhelms the sufferer so that he or she feels a hopelessness, dejection, and fear out of all proportion to any cause. Someone who is depressed may contemplate or attempt suicide.

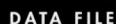

ABOVE *Chamomile essential oil has antidepressant qualities.*

SYMPTOMS

- *slow speech* • *poor concentration* • *confusion and irritability* • *self-accusation and loss of self-esteem*
- *insomnia and early-morning waking*
- *a feeling of emptiness and despair*
- *loss of appetite*
- *loss of sexual drive*

DATA FILE

- Major depressions occur in 10–20 percent of the world's population in the course of a lifetime.

- Women are more often affected than men, by a 2:1 ratio.

- Relatives of patients with major depressive illnesses seem to be at some higher risk of becoming depressed, and about 2 percent of the population may have a chronic disorder known as a depressive personality.

- Unipolar depression consists of episodes that can recur several times in a person's life.

- Manic depression, or bipolar disorder, is a severe mental disorder involving manic episodes (characterized by an abnormally elevated or irritable mood, grandiosity, sleeplessness, extravagance, and a tendency toward irrational judgment) that are usually accompanied by episodes of depression (possibly including lethargy, a sense of worthlessness, lack of concentration, and guilt). Manic depression occurs in males and females equally, and is found more frequently in close relatives of people with the disorder.

- More than 8 billion people in the U.S. consult their general physician about treatment for depression.

- Up to 50 percent of people who suffer have a hereditary tendency.

- Seasonal affective disorder (SAD) is thought to be caused by a deficiency of corticotropin-releasing hormone.

- Cases of SAD are on the increase, and are thought to be partly due to increased stress levels.

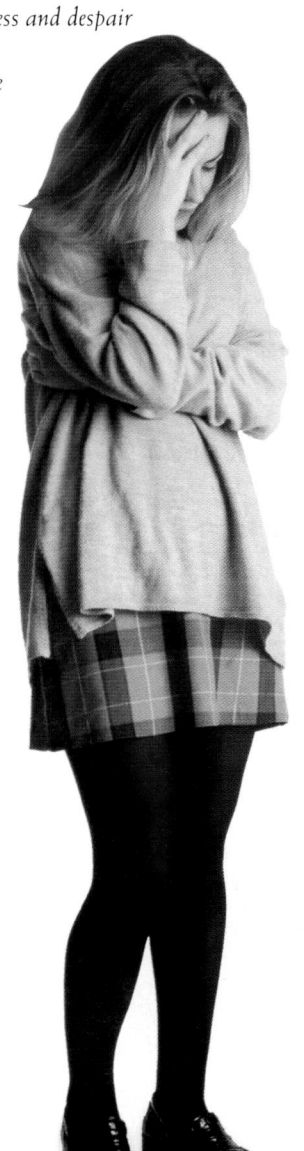

TREATMENT

AYURVEDA
- Detoxification treatment would be followed by specific oral medication to balance the three doshas. Treatment is always individual. *(See page 20.)*

CHINESE HERBALISM
- Depression is believed to be caused by stagnation of the Liver qi, and may be treated with angelica, peony root, licorice, and thorowax root. *(See pages 56, 64, 67.)*

HERBALISM
- The best antidepressant and nervine (with a specific action for nerves) herbs include: balm, borage, limeflower, oats, rosemary, and vervain. These can be taken as herbal teas, added to the bath, or taken as tablets, or in tincture form (herbs suspended in alcohol). *(See page 104.)*

AROMATHERAPY
- There are a number of antidepressant oils, which can be used in the bath, in a vaporizer, on a light bulb and in massage. They include: neroli, jasmine, geranium, melissa, and rose.
- Ylang ylang, lavender, clary sage, and chamomile are sedative and antidepressant.

LEFT *Depression affects more women than men.*

HOMEOPATHY
It will be necessary to see a homeopath to receive treatment that is suited to you, and which addresses the cause of your depression. Specific remedies include:
- Aurum, for feelings of worthlessness, suicidal feelings, and self-disgust. *(See page 184.)*
- Pulsatilla, for bursting into tears at the smallest hurt. *(See page 209.)*
- Arsenicum, if you feel chilly, tired, restless, and obsessively tidy. *(See page 182.)*
- Ignatia, if depression has an external cause, such as bereavement. *(See page 200.)*

FLOWER ESSENCES
- Cherry Plum, for "fear of the mind being over strained, of doing dreaded things," and of being violent to oneself or others. *(See page 236.)*
- Agrimony, for deeply held emotional tensions which are hidden from others. *(See page 225.)*
- Gorse helps to combat feelings of hopelessness. *(See page 240.)*
- Gentian will help to improve a mild depression and despondency caused by a setback. *(See page 230.)*
- Mustard is for blacker and deeper feelings when there is no apparent cause. *(See page 239.)*

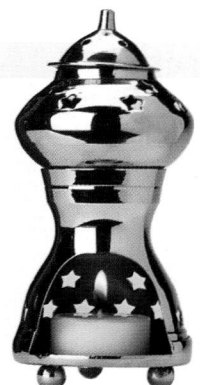

ABOVE *A vaporizer heats an essential oil to release its therapeutic qualities.*

- Sweet Chestnut should be taken if you feel anguished and stretched beyond endurance. *(See page 227.)*

VITAMINS AND MINERALS
Depression which occurs just before menstruation (PMS) may be caused by a vitamin B6 deficiency; post-natal depression may be caused by a deficiency of vitamin B12, and folic acid. Nutritional supplements and allergy tests may be suggested by a practitioner. Ensure you have an adequate intake of vitamin C. Some therapists may recommend supplementing the amino acid tryptophan. *(See page 246.)*

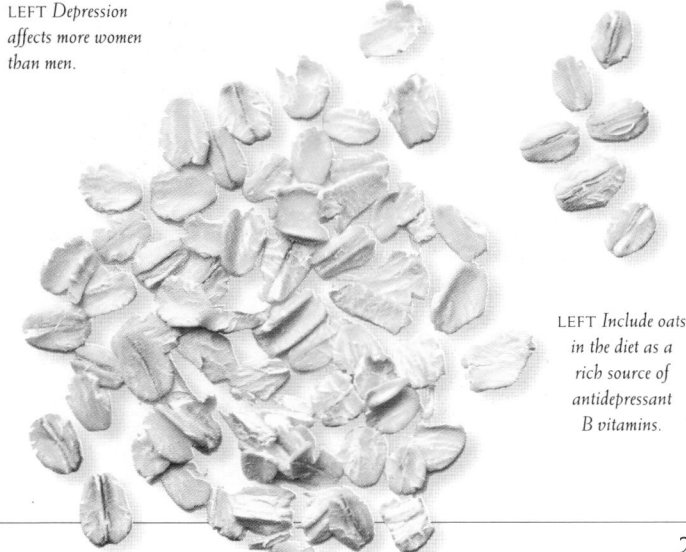

LEFT *Include oats in the diet as a rich source of antidepressant B vitamins.*

Stress

Each individual is able to cope with a different amount of stress in life, and while some seem to draw on endless reserves to keep going, others succumb. A certain amount of stress provides stimulation, but prolonged stress can cause mental and physical damage.

Most of us think of tense situations and worries as being the cause of stress. In reality, stresses are wide-ranging. They include environmental stresses, such as pollution, noise, housing problems, cold, or overheating; physical stresses, such as illnesses, injuries, an inadequate diet; and mental stresses, such as relationship problems, financial strains, bereavement; and job difficulties. All these factors affect the body, causing it to make a series of rapid physiological changes, called "adaptive responses," to deal with threatening or demanding situations.

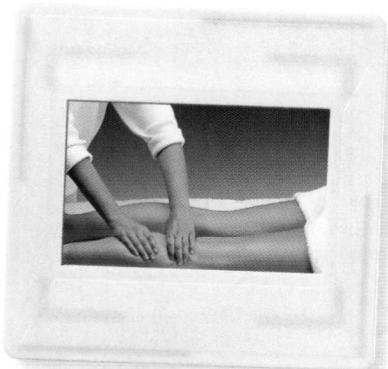

ABOVE *Human touch is very comforting and can be utilized in massage.*

In the first stage of stress, hormones are poured into the bloodstream. The pulse quickens, the lungs take in more oxygen to fuel the muscles, blood sugar increases to supply added energy, digestion slows, and perspiration increases. In the second stage of stress, the body begins to repair the damage caused by the first stage. If the stressful situation is resolved, the stress symptoms vanish. If the situation continues, however, exhaustion sets in, and the body's energy gives out. This stage may continue until vital organs are affected, and then disease or even death can result.

SYMPTOMS

• *the increase in hormones such as adrenaline, noradrenaline, and corticosteroids in response to stress may cause the following: increased breathing and heart rate – nausea – tense muscles* • *in the long term it is thought that stress can lead to: insomnia – depression – high blood pressure – hair loss – allergies – ulcers – heart disease – digestive disorders – menstrual problems – palpitations – impotence and premature ejaculation*

DATA FILE

• Psychological stress results from perceived or anticipated threats. The stress may be acute, as in response to immediate danger, or chronic, as when an individual is experiencing an unhappy life situation. In either case, the body mechanisms are similar.

• Chronic physical illness is almost always accompanied by significant psychological effects.

• Long-lasting psychological stress, in turn, often leads to debilitating changes.

• Medical scientists divide people's behavior into two types, depending on their reactions to stress. People with type-A behavior react to stress with aggressiveness, competitiveness, and self-imposed pressure to get things done. Type-A behavior has been linked to increased rates of heart attack and other diseases. People with type-B behavior may be equally serious in their intentions, but are more patient, easygoing, and relaxed.

• Stress is a major factor in diseases whose physical symptoms are induced or aggravated by mental or emotional problems.

• Stress-related disorders comprise 50–80 percent of all illnesses, though stress may not be the only cause.

TREATMENT

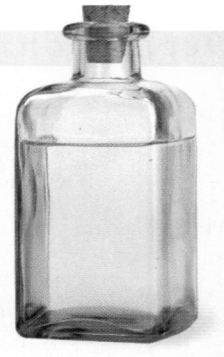

ABOVE *A massage blend which includes rosemary essential oil strengthens the adrenal system.*

AYURVEDA
• An Ayurvedic practitioner would prescribe supportive herbs, and use a balancing treatment specific to your needs. *(See page 20.)*

CHINESE HERBALISM
• Chinese medicine takes the view that it is not stress that causes illness, but how we deal with it. Herbs would be prescribed according to your specific needs, in order to support you throughout stressful periods, and tonify. *(See page 51.)*
• Treatment may be aimed particularly at the Kidneys, which have become exhausted through overwork, and to support the Blood and qi, which need to circulate harmoniously in the body. *(See page 50.)*

TRADITIONAL FOLK AND HOME REMEDIES
• Pumpkin seeds, which contain high quantities of zinc, iron and calcium, as well as B vitamins and proteins, which are necessary for brain function, will help you to deal with the effects of stress.
• Oats are vital for a healthy nervous system. In periods of stress, start the day with oatmeal, which will help to keep you calm, and prevent depression and general debility. *(See page 84.)*

HERBALISM
• Herbs that encourage relaxation and act as a tonic to the nervous system include balm, lavender, chamomile, passiflora and oats. These can be drunk as an infusion – as often as necessary when in a stressful situation. *(See pages 117 and 119.)*
• Ginseng is an excellent "adaptogenic" herb, which means that it lifts you when you are tired and relaxes you when you are stressed. It also works on the immune system and energizes. Some therapists recommend a daily dose at stressful times. *(See page 126.)*

AROMATHERAPY
• Essential oils are excellent for stress reduction because many of them work on the nervous system and the brain to relax and soothe. *(See pages 146–71.)*
• Other oils are uplifting, which can be invaluable in times of serious stress. *(See pages 146–71.)*
• Massage with aromatherapy oils is very comforting – particularly the physical element of touch – and a few drops of essential oil in the bath can offer an opportunity to "wash away" the problems of the day while experiencing the benefits of the oil. Suitable oils include basil, chamomile, geranium, lavender, neroli, and rose. *(See pages 146–71.)*
• Oils which strengthen the adrenal system, which is weakened by stress, include rosemary, ginger, and lemongrass. *(See pages 146–71.)*

VITAMINS AND MINERALS
Eating a good, balanced diet will make your body stronger and able to cope more efficiently with stress. B vitamins are often depleted by stress, so ensure that you are getting enough in your diet, or take a good supplement. There is some evidence that bee and flower pollen, available in tablets or in grains, can boost immunity and energize the body. Do not eat this if you are allergic to honey or bee stings. An amino acid called L-Tyrosine appears to energize and relieve stress, and studies show that people taking this supplement react better to stressful situations, staying more alert, less anxious, more efficient, and have fewer complaints about physical discomforts. Vitamin C is a great stress reliever, and boosts immunity, making you fitter and more healthy. *(See page 256.)*

LEFT *A healthy, balanced diet shores up the body against stress.*

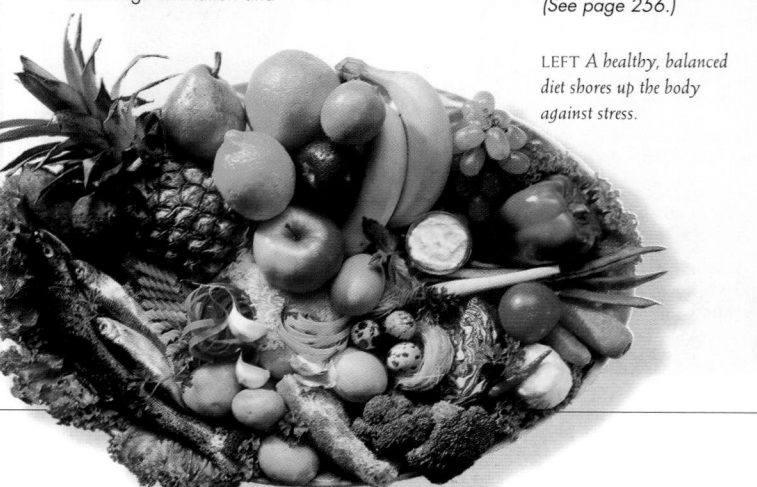

Anxiety

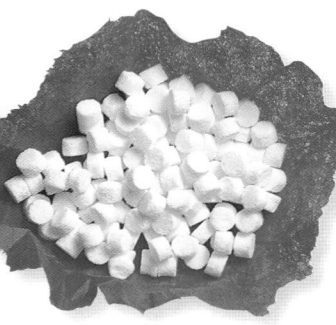

ABOVE *The homeopathic remedy Calcarea balances calcium levels in the body.*

Anxiety is a state of fear or apprehension in the face of threat or danger. It is a natural, healthy response since it allows the body to prepare itself (through adrenaline) to cope with the danger. Anxiety can, however, take a person over – a condition known as anxiety neurosis – and the person is then said to be in an anxiety state. This may be chronic anxiety, with a constant feeling of worry, associated with depression, or an acute anxiety attack, when the sufferer will be suddenly overwhelmed by fear and feelings of dread.

DATA FILE

• When we are faced with a frightening or threatening situation, our body goes into a "fight or flight" response, when adrenaline pours into the system and the body prepares itself for action. When no action follows, and nervous energy is not discharged, there is physiological confusion – otherwise known as a panic attack. Symptoms may include dizziness, visual disturbance, clammy hands, racing heart, dry mouth, and overbreathing.

• Up to 70 percent of people who have panic attacks end up seeing as many as ten physicians before being correctly diagnosed.

• Anxiety appears to affect twice as many women as men.

• Evidence exists that some people may be biochemically vulnerable to panic attacks.

• The National Center for Health Statistics reports that drugs for anxiety disorders are among the 20 drugs most frequently prescribed.

• In the U.K., a report by the Royal College of Psychiatrists stated that more than 9 million Britons will suffer from abnormal anxiety and fears at some point in their lives.

• Anxiety is an element of many psychological disorders, including phobias, panic attacks, obsessive-compulsive disorders, and post-traumatic stress disorder.

SYMPTOMS

• *dry mouth* • *sweaty palms* • *rapid pulse and palpitations* • *in anxiety neurosis: – breathlessness – headaches, general weakness, and fatigue – feeling of tightness in the chest – high blood pressure – abdominal pain and diarrhea – insomnia – loss of appetite*

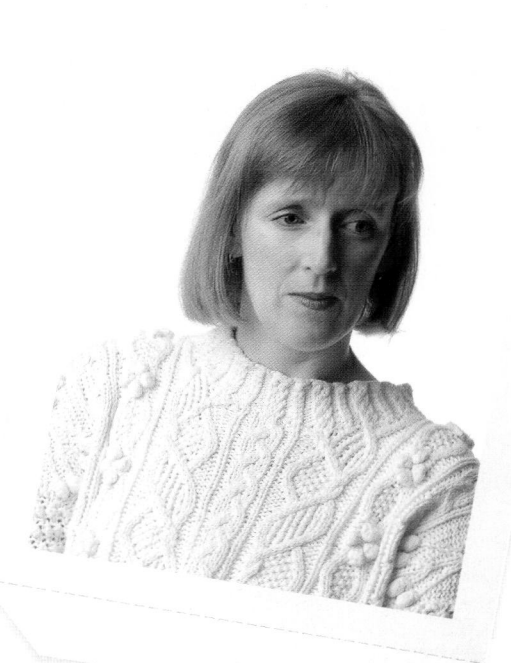

RIGHT *A persistent state of anxiety can sap energy and so self-perpetuate.*

AYURVEDA
• An Ayurvedic medical practitioner would balance the tri-doshas, and use panchakarma for balancing the vátha. *(See page 20.)*

CHINESE HERBALISM
• A Chinese herbalist might suggest ginseng, Chinese angelica, and white peony root with thorowax root for relaxation. Treatment would be designed to strengthen the Spleen and enliven Liver qi. *(See pages 56 and 67.)*

TRADITIONAL FOLK AND HOME REMEDIES
• Oats contain thiamin and pantothenic acid, which act as gentle nerve tonics *(See page 84.)*

HERBALISM
• Herbal remedies would be used to calm the nervous system and to generally relax you.
• Skullcap and valerian are useful herbs, blended together for best effect. Drink this as a tea three times daily while suffering anxiety symptoms. *(See pages 131 and 136.)*

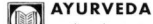

ABOVE *Make an infusion with 1-2 teaspoonsful of dried skullcap and boiling water.*

• Lady's slipper and lime blossom may also work to ease anxiety and tension. *(See page 134.)*

AROMATHERAPY
• A relaxing blend of essential oils of lavender, geranium, and bergamot in sweet almond oil or peach kernel oil may be used in the bath at times at great stress and anxiety. *(See pags 146–71.)*

HOMEOPATHY
Constitutional treatment will be appropriate for chronic conditions, and there are a number of remedies which will prove useful for relieving acute attacks. These include:
• Aconite, for dispelling a sudden panic attack. *(See page 178.)*
• Arsenicum may be useful if you feel insecure, restless, tired, and tend to fight anxiety by being obsessively tidy or really well organized. *(See page 182.)*
• Nat. mur. may be useful if you have a tendency to dwell on morbid topics and generally hate fuss. *(See page 206.)*

• Calcarea, if you fear for your sanity, forget things, and feel the cold. *(See page 186.)*
• Ignatia, if your anxiety follows the loss of a loved one or a specific, distressing event. *(See page 200.)*

FLOWER ESSENCES
• Remedies are prescribed according to the personal characteristics of the sufferer, and the cause and the nature of the anxiety.
• Try Elm for anxiety accompanying a feeling of being unable to cope, or Red Chestnut for anxiety over the welfare of others. *(See pages 241 and 224.)*
• Aspen, for anxiety for no apparent reason. *(See page 236.)*
• Rescue Remedy or Emergency Essence are useful during attacks. *(See page 244.)*

VITAMINS AND MINERALS
Increase your intake of B vitamins, which work on the nervous system, and avoid caffeine in any form. *(See pages 252–5.)*

Insecurity

Insecurity is a feeling that affects everybody at one time or another. It can be triggered by physical, social, financial, or emotional factors, and can often induce anxiety and its associated symptoms. Whatever the initial cause, when a person feels insecure that person's entire perception of his or her own competence and self-worth are thrown into question. Chronic insecurity, which can manifest itself as depression, shyness, lack of confidence, or an inability to form stable relationships, has less to do with external events than with unrealistic expectations and a poor self-image.

SYMPTOMS

- *dry mouth* • *sweaty palms*
- *rapid pulse and palpitations*
- *in anxiety neurosis:*
breathlessness – headaches, general weakness, and fatigue – feeling of tightness in the chest – high blood pressure – abdominal pain and diarrhea – insomnia – loss of appetite

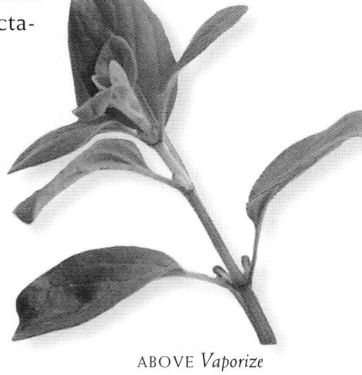

ABOVE *Vaporize marjoram oil to cheer yourself up.*

TREATMENT

CHINESE HERBALISM
- Try herbs which work to balance the nervous system, including fleeceflower stem, poria, and wild jujube seeds. *(See pages 71 and 75.)*

HERBALISM
- Uplifting herbs such as rosemary, lavender, ginseng, damiana, or valerian. They can be drunk as infusions 3 times daily. *(See pages 125, 127, 135, and 136.)*

AROMATHERAPY
- Jasmine lifts the spirits and improves mental outlook – add a few drops to a vaporizer or your bath (not at bedtime). *(See page 161.)*
- Marjoram and thyme are cheering and can boost self-image. *(See pages 165 and 170.)*

HOMEOPATHY
- Aconite, for insecurity brought on by a traumatic experience. *(See page 178.)*
- Ignatia, for insecurity stemming from a particular cause, for example a bereavement. *(See page 200.)*
- Pulsatilla, if you feel tearful, worse for heat, and longing for company. *(See page 209.)*

FLOWER ESSENCES
- Mimulus is appropriate for fear and of known things, timidity and shyness. *(See page 235.)*
- Crab apple, for poor self-image. *(See page 234.)*
- Elm, for those who are usually confident but are experiencing a temporary crisis of confidence because they are overwhelmed by responsibility. *(See page 241.)*

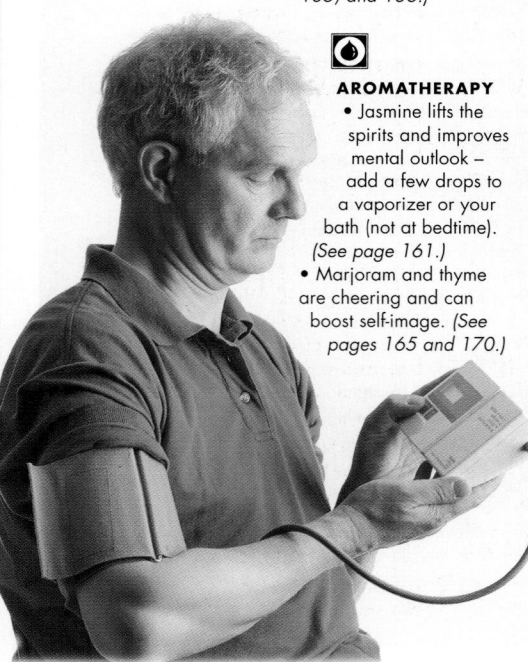

LEFT *Feelings of insecurity may trigger a rise in blood pressure.*

Memory Loss

A total or partial loss of memory is known as amnesia. It occurs as a result of either physical or mental disease (such as senile dementia), or physical trauma (such as a blow to the head or a fractured skull). The latter may induce a state of retrograde amnesia where the sufferer has no memory of the events immediately before the injury as well as those after. The period of amnesia in such cases is usually in proportion to the severity of the injury. Amnesia is caused by damage to, or disease of, brain regions concerned with memory function, and can also occur in some forms of psychiatric illness in which there is no apparent physical damage to the brain. Amnesia can very often be a complication of alcoholism, and can result from depression, anxiety, stress, poor nutrition, inadequate sleep, or lack of stimulation.

ABOVE *Sunflower oil and eggs contain lecithin, which enhances functioning of the brain.*

TREATMENT

CHINESE HERBALISM
- Herbs to aid memory include fleeceflower root and black ginger seed. *(See page 71.)*
- Memory loss caused by stress or fatigue may be treated with Chinese wolfberry. *(See page 66.)* *(See also Anxiety, page 241.)*

HERBALISM
- Ginseng powder can act as a memory aid and general stimulant. *(See page 126.)*
- Add a small amount of gotu kola to your food or drink for several days, to revive your memory.
- Rosemary is said to comfort the brain and refresh the memory, and sage is also useful. *(See page 127.)*

HOMEOPATHY
Treatment would be constitutional, but the following may be of use:
- Anacardium when you are absent-minded because of an inner conflict. *(See page 179.)*
- Sulfur, for difficulty remembering words and names. *(See page 215.)*
- Calcarea, for wandering attention, particularly in the elderly. *(See page 186.)*
- Ignatia, for memory loss caused by a traumatic event or bereavement. *(See page 200.)*

FLOWER ESSENCES
- Star of Bethlehem, when memory is affected by an accident, bad news, or trauma. *(See page 235.)*

VITAMINS AND MINERALS
Your diet should be rich in B vitamins and protein, for amino acids are necessary for the brain to function efficiently. An amino acid supplement (containing all 22 acids) may be useful. Acetylcholine, which is formed in the body from lecithin, may help. Increase your intake of lecithin (found in sunflower oil and eggs) or take it as a supplement. *(See page 271.)*

Insomnia

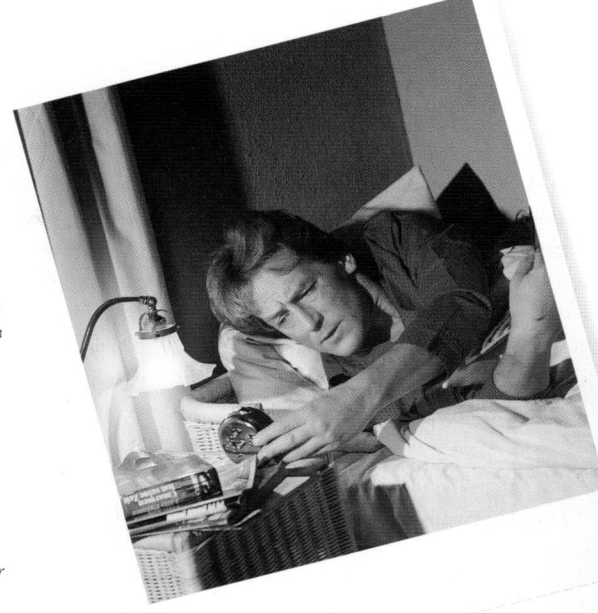

A common complaint, insomnia is the inability to sleep or the disturbance of normal sleep patterns. It is difficult to qualify, because everyone has different sleep requirements, and sleeplessness is, in fact, a natural feature of aging. Insomnia is often caused by worry, emotional stress, and exhaustion. Other causes include pain; excess caffeine, alcohol and drugs; food allergy; or sleeping in a stuffy room. Insomnia can also be a symptom of depression.

RIGHT *To achieve a peaceful sleep, rest on a pillow containing dried lavender.*

SYMPTOMS

• *overactive mind causing difficulty in falling asleep*
• *nervousness and restlessness* • *nightmares once asleep*
• *irritability* • *mood swings involving hysterical behavior*
• *a fear of bedtime may eventually develop*

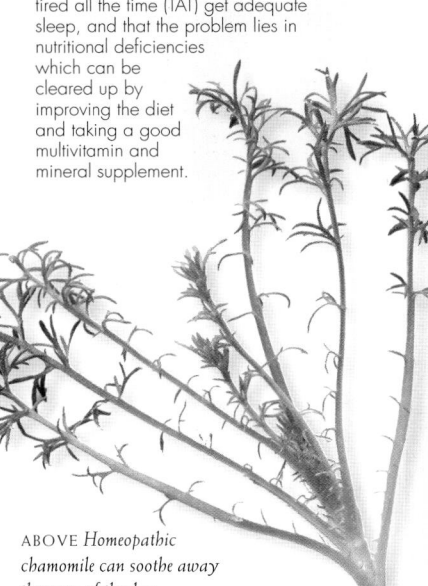

ABOVE *Homeopathic chamomile can soothe away the cares of the day.*

TREATMENT

AYURVEDA
• Specific herbs to treat insomnia may include henbane, which is sedative.

CHINESE HERBALISM
• Useful herbs include hoelen, fleeceflower stem, and wild jujube. *(See pages 71 and 75.)*
• The herbalist may suggest that you sleep on a gypsum pillow.

TRADITIONAL FOLK AND HOME REMEDIES
• A hot foot-bath before bed helps relaxation by drawing blood away from the head. Add a little mustard powder to the water to increase the effect. *(See page 98.)*
• Lettuce is said to encourage sleep. Eat a large leaf about half an hour before bedtime.

HERBALISM
• A warm bath with a an infusion of chamomile, catnip, lavender, or limeflowers may be recommended. *(See pages 119 and 134.)*
• A cup of warm herb tea just before bed will soothe and help you to relax. Try chamomile, catnip, lemon balm, and limeflowers. *(See pages 119 and 134.)*
• Make a lavender pillow and place it under your usual pillow.

AROMATHERAPY
• A few drops of chamomile oil, clary sage, or lavender can be added to the bath. *(See pages 146–71.)*
• Try a gentle massage just before bedtime, with a few drops of chamomile, lavender, rose, or neroli blended into a light carrier oil. *(See pages 146–71.)*
• Place a few drops of lavender oil on your bedroom light bulb, just before bed, or place a few drops on a handkerchief and tie it to the bed. *(See page 161.)*

HOMEOPATHY
Remedies can be taken an hour before going to bed, for up to 14 days. Repeat the dose if you wake in the night and cannot get back to sleep. Insomnia is usually treated "constitutionally," so you may need to consult a registered homeopath for treatment. The following remedies may be helpful:
• Coffea, when your mind is overactive, and you are unable to switch off. *(See page 192.)*
• Nux vomica, when your sleeplessness is exacerbated by food or alcohol; you wake around 3 or 4A.M., then fall asleep just as it is time to get up; and consequently are irritable during the day. *(See page 214.)*
• Pulsatilla, when you are restless in the early hours of sleep, feeling uncomfortable, hot and then cold, are not thirsty and sleep with your arms above your head. *(See page 209.)*
• Arnica, when the bed feels too hard, and you are overtired, fidgety, and dream of being chased by animals. *(See page 182.)*
• Lycopodium, when your mind is active at bedtime, going over and over work done that day; you dream a lot, talk and laugh in your sleep, and then wake up at around 4A.M. *(See page 203.)*
• Arsenicum, for when you tend to wake between midnight and 2A.M., feeling restless, worried, and apprehensive. *(See page 182.)*
• Rhus tox., when you cannot sleep, are irritable, restless, and feel a need to walk about; especially if in pain. *(See page 210.)*
• Aurum, when you have dreams about dying, hunger, or problems at work, and consequently become depressed. *(See page 184.)*
• Aconite, when sleep problems are worse after shock or trauma; there is restlessness, nightmares, and fear of dying. *(See page 178.)*
• Chamomilla, when you are feeling irritable bedtime. *(See page 204.)*

FLOWER ESSENCES
• Worrying thoughts and mental arguments might respond to White Chestnut. *(See page 224.)*
• Indecision can be treated with Scleranthus. *(See page 239.)*
• Stress, strain, frustration, and inability to relax might respond to Vervain or Rock Water, Vine, Elm, Beech, or Impatiens could apply. *(See pages 229, 233, 241, 242, and 243.)*

VITAMINS AND MINERALS
Increase your intake of vitamins B, C, folic acid, zinc and calcium. Try a calcium supplement just before bedtime. *(See page 258.)*

DISORDERS OF THE BRAIN AND NERVES

MS (Multiple Sclerosis)

Multiple sclerosis is a chronic disease of the nervous system in which the protective sheaths that cover the nerves become inflamed and scarred, resulting in loss of nerve function. The initial attack is usually followed by recovery, but sufferers inevitably experience a cycle of remission (sometimes for years) and relapse with steadily increasing neurological damage and disability. The degree of improvement after each attack decreases and the physical disability is usually progressive. Eventually there may also be intellectual impairment. The cause of MS is unknown.

DATA FILE

• MS is not an inherited disease, but a predisposition may run in families.

• The cause remains unknown, but some researchers propose that it is an auto-immune disorder; others believe a viral infection may trigger the disease.

• MS is more common in temperate climates and is relatively rare in Asia and Africa, lending credibility to the theory that it might be related to diet or climate.

• U.S. cases are usually diagnosed from age 20 to 40.

• In most cases, MS follows a course of repeated remissions, with the symptoms returning with increased severity, over a period of years.

• Because of lack of persistent symptoms, many MS patients go for a number of years before being correctly diagnosed.

• The average life expectancy after onset is over 30 years, although some patients die within a few years of onset and others survive more than 50 years.

SYMPTOMS

• *limb weakness* • *visual deterioration, particularly in the center of the visual field* • *double vision* • *loss of sensation* • *staggering* • *impaired speech* • *facial paralysis*

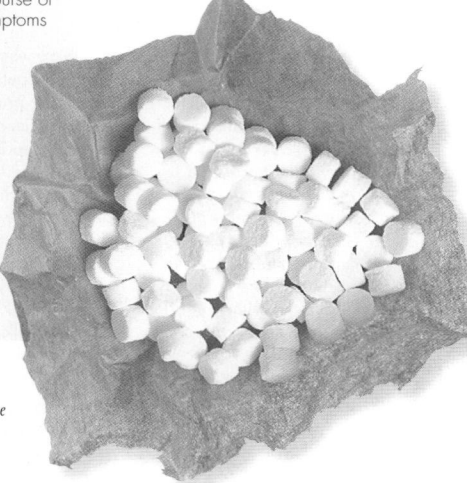

RIGHT *Potassium phosphate is the source for the homeopathic remedy Kali phosphoricum.*

TREATMENT

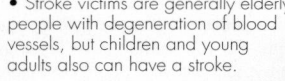

HOMEOPATHY
Treatment is constitutional, but the following remedies may be useful while you are waiting for treatment:
• Tarantula, when movements of the hands, feet, and tongue are jerky. *(See page 215.)*
• Agaricus, for sharp, shooting pains, and weakness with shaking.
• Phosphorus, for exaggerated reflexes and a tendency to fainting. *(See page 208.)*
• Kali phos., for weakness in the back and legs, made worse by exercise, which causes overwhelming fatigue, pain, and even paralysis. *(See page 201.)*

FLOWER ESSENCES
• Rescue Remedy or Emergency Essence may help to ease the symptoms and control shaking and anxiety. *(See page 244.)*

VITAMINS AND MINERALS
• Eat plenty of foods that contain gamma-linoleic acid, which is found in sunflower and safflower oil, as well as evening primrose products. *(See page 270.)*
• Get plenty of vitamins B3, B6, B12, folic acid, C and E, and the minerals zinc and magnesium. *(See pages 253–57, 264 and 265.)*

Stroke

A stroke (cerebrovascular accident, or CVA) results from an interruption of the blood supply to any part of the brain. This may be caused by bleeding into or around the brain (cerebral hemorrhage), a clot which blocks an already damaged artery (cerebral thrombosis), or a small clot elsewhere in the bloodstream that eventually causes obstruction in an artery to the brain (cerebral embolism). Smoking, diabetes, high blood pressure, and atherosclerosis are all risk factors.

DATA FILE

• The effects of a stroke vary according to its cause and the part of the brain affected. The most serious (and often fatal) cause is cerebral hemorrhage, the first sign of which is a severe headache followed by: paralysis down one side of the body – loss of vision to one side – fixed turning of the eyes to one side – possibly a seizure.

• The effects of cerebral thrombosis or embolism are similar to the above, but less serious, and recovery often follows.

• In the U.S. stroke is the third-ranking cause of death after heart disease and cancer, and about one-fourth of the neurologic patients in nursing homes are stroke victims.

• The death rate has declined by nearly 50 per cent since the late 1960s; in the early 1990s about 150,000 Americans of the 450,000 each year who suffered a new stroke died as a result.

• Stroke victims are generally elderly people with degeneration of blood vessels, but children and young adults also can have a stroke.

• More men than women are afflicted by a stroke.

• More people of African descent have strokes than any other race.

• Prior history of stroke increases the chance that you will have a repeat.

• Women using oral contraceptives are at greater risk of a stroke.

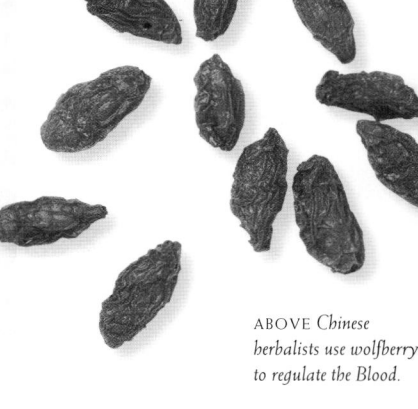

ABOVE *Chinese herbalists use wolfberry to regulate the Blood.*

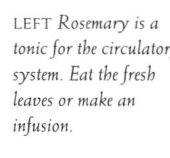

LEFT *Rosemary is a tonic for the circulatory system. Eat the fresh leaves or make an infusion.*

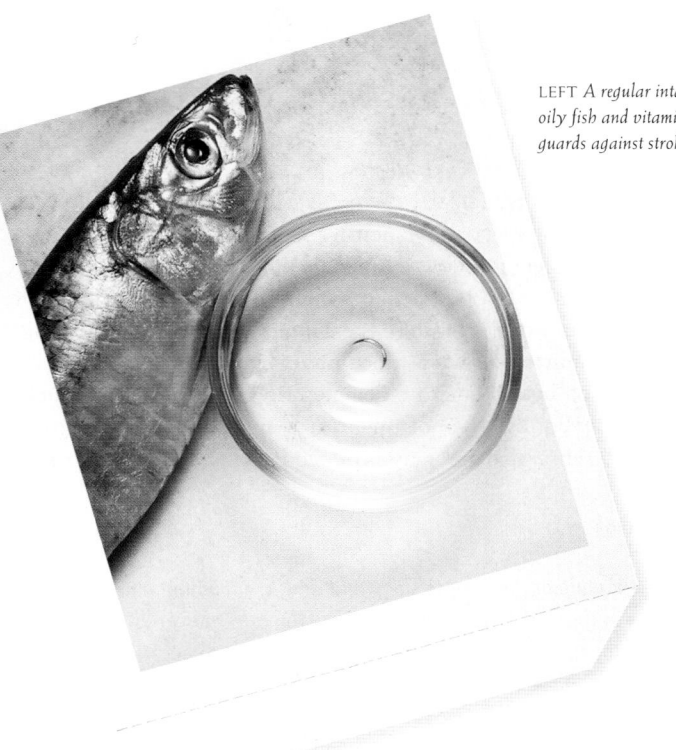

LEFT *A regular intake of oily fish and vitamin E guards against stroke.*

Meningitis

The epidemic disease called cerebrospinal meningitis is caused by the meningococcus bacterium, an organism that inhabits the nose of healthy human carriers but sometimes infects the blood and cerebrospinal fluid. The most common cause of bacterial meningitis is *Haemophilus influenzae* type b. Meningitis may result from head injuries and infections involving the eyes, ears, and nose; it can also be a complication of systemic disorders such as pneumonia and syphilis, both of which reach the brain via the bloodstream. Diagnosis is often made by lumbar puncture (spinal tap). A vaccine against *Haemophilus influenzae* type b was licensed for use in 1985. Children and immune-suppressed people are most susceptible.

CAUTION

MENINGITIS CAN LEAD TO SERIOUS BRAIN DAMAGE, BLINDNESS, DEAFNESS, OR EVEN DEATH. URGENT MEDICAL ATTENTION IS REQUIRED IF MENINGITIS IS SUSPECTED.

SYMPTOMS

• *viral meningitis: headache, worse on bending – fever – nausea and vomiting – stiff neck – in severe cases there may also be muscle weakness, paralysis, impaired speech, double vision, and epileptic fits* • *bacterial (meningococcal) meningitis: any/all of the above – a rash of red spots on the trunk of the body – drowsiness and eventually coma – convulsions and a characteristic high-pitched cry in babies and infants – in infants the fontanel on the top of the head may bulge and feel more tense than usual*

RIGHT *The homeopathic remedy Belladonna can be taken for meningitis until a physician arrives.*

TREATMENT

HOMEOPATHY Constitutional treatment from an experienced homeopath can aid recovery after a stroke. Changes in diet, exercise, and lifestyle will be recommended. There are also specific remedies which can be used while waiting for medical attention. These include:
• Belladonna, when the face is hot and flushed, with staring eyes. *(See page 183.)*
• Opium, when there is unconsciousness, and a blue face, and the patient is breathing heavily. *(See page 207.)*
• Nux mosch., for the first signs of an attack, often brought on by overindulgence.
• Aconite, for fear and panic. *(See page 178.)* Following an attack:
• Aconite, immediately afterward and for the next 4 weeks. *(See page 178.)*
• Baryta, when there is physical and mental weakness after an attack, particularly in the elderly. *(See page 185.)*

• Aurum, for depression. *(See page 184.)*
• Gelsemium, when there is numbness, trembling, pain at the back of the head, and an inability to speak. *(See page 195.)*
• Lachesis for slow speech. *(See page 216.)*

FLOWER ESSENCES
• These remedies could play a part in helping to promote a more positive frame of mind in sufferers who are frightened, depressed, or affected by other negative attitudes.

VITAMINS AND MINERALS
• Prevention is easier than cure, and a good intake of oily fish and vitamin E with a wholefood diet is the best prevention against the small blood clots in the brain which are the cause of strokes. *(See page 257.)*
• Nutritional therapists use the herb ginkgo biloba after a stroke to improve the circulation in the brain and help to prevent further strokes.

HERBALISM
• Yarrow is recommended to improve circulation and tone the blood vessels. Drink an infusion 3 times daily. *(See page 112.)*
• Rosemary is useful and can be drunk or eaten fresh as soon as possible to improve the health of the circulatory system. *(See page 127.)*

CHINESE HERBALISM
• A Chinese herbalist is likely to offer herbs to regulate the Blood condition, such as peony bark and wolfberry. *(See pages 66 and 67.)*

AYURVEDA
• Ayurveda is a very popular method for rehabilitation of paralysis – special panchakarma therapy for vátha. *(See page 20.)*

TREATMENT

CHINESE HERBALISM
• A registered practitioner could treat this condition with herbal laxatives and anti-inflammatories, but treatment should be alongside conventional medical treatment.
• Herbs to boost the immune system following infection include ginseng. Treatment would address Deficient Blood and qi. Peony root and mulberry might be appropriate. *(See page 67.)*

HOMEOPATHY Emergency remedies, to be taken every 10 minutes, until help arrives include:
• Arnica, for symptoms which arise after a head injury. *(See page 182.)*
• Aconite, for restlessness, fear and great thirst. *(See page 178.)*
• Bryonia, which treats a severe headache made worse by eye movement. *(See page 185.)*

• Belladonna, for staring eyes, delirium, and fever. *(See page 183.)*

FLOWER ESSENCES
• Take Rescue Remedy or Emergency Essence (apply to the temples or moisten the lips if the sufferer is not conscious) to calm and encourage the healing process. *(See page 244.)*

Encephalitis

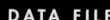

Encephalitis is an inflammation of the brain tissue, usually caused by infection, but occasionally by poisoning. Primary encephalitis is caused by direct infection with viruses, which include herpes simplex, herpes zoster, or mosquito- and tick-borne viruses. Secondary encephalitis usually occurs as a complication of a viral infection such as mumps, measles, rubella, or chickenpox. The causative infection may enter the brain via the bloodstream. Many other infections involve only the surface membranes (*see Meningitis, page 289*), whereas others affect both meninges and brain, and cause meningoencephalitis. Encephalitis can be fatal within hours of onset, although many people make a full recovery even from serious attacks.

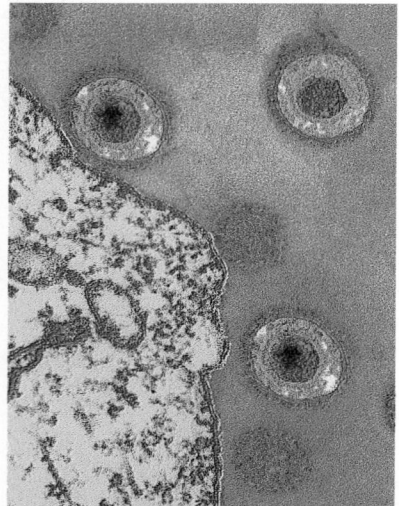

SYMPTOMS

• in mild cases the symptoms are similar to those of other viral infections: fever – headache – loss of appetite – lethargy and drowsiness • in more severe cases sufferers may experience: double vision – mental confusion and impaired speech – stiff neck and back – epileptic fits – coma

LEFT *The chicken pox virus. Encephalitis may occur as a complication after infection by this virus.*

TREATMENT

HERBALISM
• Echinacea is antiviral, and can be taken alongside orthodox treatment, in order to boost the immune system and treat the infection. *(See page 120.)*
• Eat plenty of fresh garlic following the illness to speed recovery and treat the immune system. *(See page 113.)*
• Drink chamomile, catnip, or skullcap when you feel uncomfortable or restless. *(See pages 119 and 131.)*

AROMATHERAPY
• Essential oils of chamomile, lavender, peppermint, or tea tree can be dropped on a cold compress and used to bathe the forehead to soothe and encourage healing. *(See pages 146–71.)*

HOMEOPATHY
This condition is very serious and must be dealt with by a conventional doctor and treated as a medical emergency. While waiting for help, the following remedies may help:

• Belladonna, for a flushed face, delirium, and staring eyes. *(See page 183.)*
• Nux mosch., for drowsiness – especially in infants.
• Gelsemium, for dizziness, a tight band around the forehead, and weakness with trembling. *(See page 195.)*

VITAMINS AND MINERALS
• Take plenty of extra vitamin C and zinc, which will boost the immune system. *(See pages 256 and 265.)*

Parkinson's Disease

Parkinson's is a progressive disease in which degeneration of the nervous system, particularly the nerve cells in the brain, causes loss of control over voluntary movement. The damage is irreversible and the exact cause as yet unknown. It occurs most commonly among the elderly, and affects men more than women. Parkinson's involves the central gray matter of the brain (basal ganglia), resulting in deficiency of a neurotransmitter known as dopamine. The common form of this disease is caused by a premature degeneration of certain basal nuclei. Many centrally acting psychotropic drugs, manganese, other toxins, and anoxic cerebral damage may produce Parkinsonian syndromes.

SYMPTOMS

• difficulty in walking, tending to stoop and shuffle • involuntary head movements • stiffness of facial muscles, resulting in a fixed expression • stiffness of tongue muscles, causing impaired speech and dribbling • worsening of the tremor, making it impossible to write, use cutlery or drink from a cup • eventually there may be senile dementia

BELOW *Include foods rich in vitamin C, such as capsicum, in your diet to help the nervous system.*

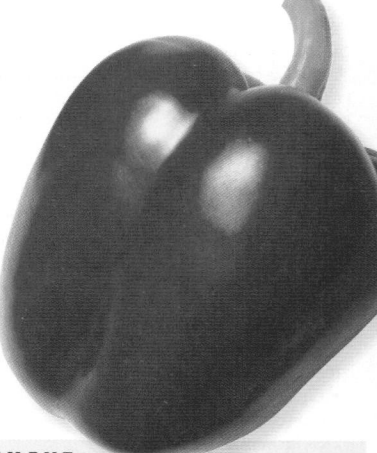

DATA FILE

• Onset of the disease is between the ages of 40 and 70.

• It can be induced by certain chemicals, such as one known as MPTP – a by-product of the street drug MPPP, a Demerol analogue – suggesting that Parkinsonism might be environmental in origin.

• Parkinson's affects a half-million people annually in the U.S.

TREATMENT

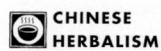

CHINESE HERBALISM
• The cause is believed to be Deficient Blood and Kidney Yang, and the following herbs might be useful: gastrodia tuber, peony root, peony buds, and wolfberry root. *(See pages 62, 66 and 67.)*

HERBALISM
• Herbs which work to boost the nervous system and brain function include ginseng, wild oats, which are calming and strengthening, astragalus and Chinese

angelica, which also works to boost the immune system. *(See pages 115–7, and 126.)*

HOMEOPATHY
Treatment will be constitutional, under the supervision of an experienced homeopath. Specific remedies which are useful when symptoms are bad include:
• Hyoscyamus, for restless, twitching motions, and rude, suspicious, and jealous behavior. *(See page 198.)*
• Mercurius, for a sweet taste in the mouth,

trembling hands, drooling, and sensitivity to heat and cold. *(See page 205.)*
• Gelsemium, for trembling and weakness affecting the tongue and eyes; and for a staggering gait. *(See page 195.)*
• Rhus tox., when there is stiffness and cramping made worse by damp and inactivity. *(See page 210.)*

VITAMINS AND MINERALS
• Take extra vitamin B6 and C to aid nervous function.
(See pages 254 and 256.)

Epilepsy

Epilepsy is an indication of an abnormality in brain function. Generalized epilepsy (grand mal and petit mal) is the most common form and is caused by a great electrical discharge across the surface of the brain on both sides. Partial-seizure epilepsy (simple and complex) is confined to a localized area of the brain – often, but not always, the temporal lobe. The symptoms vary according to which area of the brain is affected.

ABOVE *Avoid certain aromatherapy oils, such as fennel.*

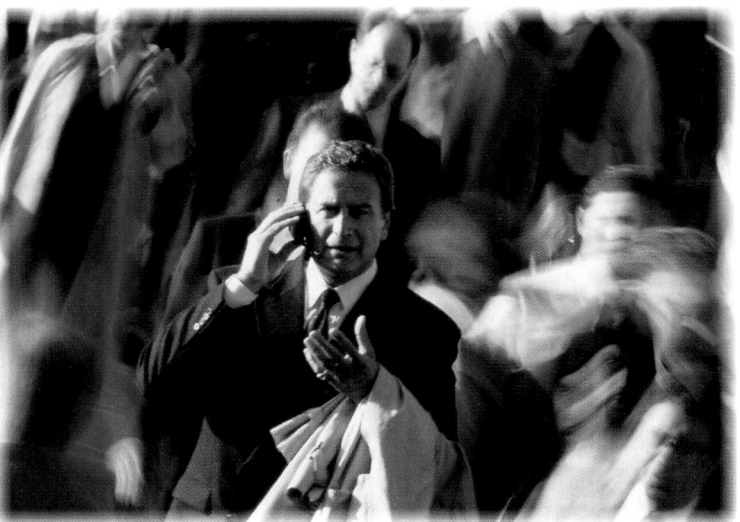

ABOVE *One percent of the U.S. population suffers from some form of epilepsy.*

SYMPTOMS

• *grand mal: seizure may begin with a shout – loss of consciousness – foaming at the mouth – loss of bladder and bowel control – rhythmic contraction of all the body's muscles – the sufferer may end the seizure in a deep sleep* • *petit mal (particularly common among children): momentary loss of consciousness – possibly jerky contractions of facial and finger muscles* • *simple partial seizure – hallucinations of smell, vision, or taste – twitching movements* • *complex partial seizure – as for simple partial seizure but with a feeling of fear and anger, and a period of unresponsiveness – the sufferer may behave in a robot-like way, and can be violent if interfered with*

DATA FILE

• 1 in 100 people in the U.S. suffer from epilepsy.

• In 70 percent of cases the cause is unknown; genetic susceptibility may be a factor.

• In 75 percent of cases, epilepsy begins during the sufferer's childhood.

• When drugs fail to control seizures, surgery to remove the affected portion of the brain or to interrupt the pathways of seizure spread may be considered.

• For children who do not respond to other treatment, the ketogenic diet – high in fat, very low in carbohydrates – may be an option.

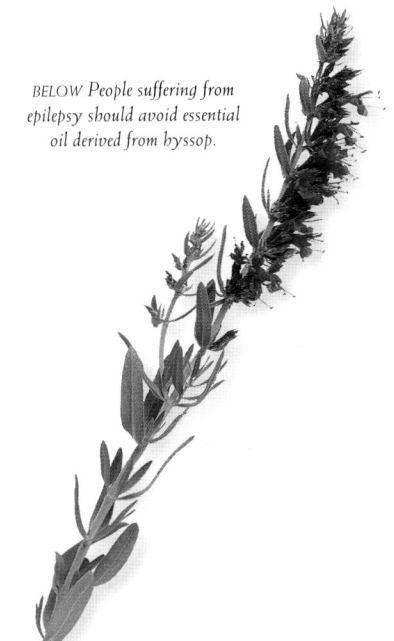

BELOW *People suffering from epilepsy should avoid essential oil derived from hyssop.*

TREATMENT

CHINESE HERBALISM
• The source of the problem is believed to be excess Heart mucus, internal Damp and stagnant qi or Blood. Sweet flag root and the juice of the young bamboo can prevent attacks in some cases.

HERBALISM
• Herbs to relax the central nervous system, including vervain and valerian, may be useful in reducing the frequency and severity of attacks. *(See pages 136 and 138.)*

AROMATHERAPY
• Studies show that extremely small doses of rosemary might be helpful in treating epilepsy, but this must only be done under the supervision of an aromatherapist with a medical qualification. *(See page 168.)*

• There are a number of oils to avoid if you have epilepsy, and these include sage, fennel, hyssop, and wormwood. *(See pages 146–71.)*

HOMEOPATHY
Remedies should be given as soon as the fit wears off.
• Chamomilla, for an attack brought on by an outburst of anger, characterized by one red cheek and greenish stools. *(See page 204.)*
• Ignatia, for a fit brought on by emotional upset. *(See page 200.)*
• Zinc, for fits brought on through illness, with fidgety, restless movements of the limbs and a bad temper.
• Aconite, for fits brought on by fright or fever. *(See page 178.)*
• Belladonna, when symptoms are made worse by jolting, and the sufferer is red-faced and staring. *(See page 183.)*

FLOWER ESSENCES
• Take a few drops of Emergency Essence or Rescue Remedy if you feel an attack coming on. This will calm you and may well abort an attack. *(See page 244.)*

VITAMINS AND MINERALS
• Extra vitamin B5, magnesium, calcium and zinc may help to prevent attacks. *(See pages 245, 258, 262, and 265.)*
• Vitamin D and B6 deficiency can prompt attacks. *(See pages 254 and 256.)*
• The amino acid taurine has been shown to control seizures.

Guillain-Barré Syndrome

Guillain-Barré syndrome is a specific type of neuropathy, or disruption of the nerves of the body. It is a serious disorder in which widespread inflammation of the nerves, caused by an immune problem, prevents normal nerve conduction. No cause is known, but an infectious agent, probably viral, is suspected. The disease often occurs one to three weeks after a mild gastrointestinal or respiratory infection. There has also been a noticeable incidence of the disease in certain recently inoculated patients. A vaccine used to combat the 1976–77 swine flu epidemic was implicated in several cases of Guillain-Barré syndrome.

ABOVE *Supplement your diet with a daily multivitamin and mineral tablet, to assist the nervous system.*

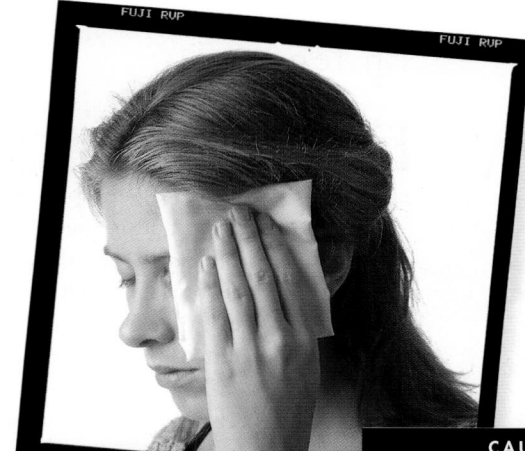

LEFT *A few drops of melissa oil on a cold compress, applied to the temples, will help.*

SYMPTOMS

• *back pain* • *tingling in the limbs and muscular weakness* • *paralysis rapidly follows and may include the facial and respiratory muscles*

CAUTION

IF THE SUFFERER HAS ANY TROUBLE BREATHING, RING FOR AN AMBULANCE IMMEDIATELY.

TREATMENT

HERBALISM
• Valerian root calms the nervous system and helps to encourage healing. *(See page 136.)*
• Herbs to boost the immune system include ginseng and echinacea, and they can be taken as a tincture or in tablet form. *(See pages 120 and 139.)*
• Vervain and skullcap will support an ailing nervous system and help you to cope better. *(See pages 131 and 138.)*
• Oats are considered to be food for the nervous system, and are a general tonic. *(See page 117.)*

AROMATHERAPY
• The following oils are nervine, which means that they strengthen the nervous system, and they can be used alongside conventional drugs: chamomile, lavender, marjoram, melissa, and rosemary. Apply a few drops to a cold compress and hold over the temples. *(See pages 146–71.)*

HOMEOPATHY
Treatment must be constitutional, but specific remedies may help in the interim:
• Thuja, if symptoms begin after vaccination and the patient has no trouble breathing. *(See page 216.)*
• Aconite, if symptoms begin after a viral infection and there is no trouble breathing. *(See page 178.)*

VITAMINS AND MINERALS
• Increase your intake of B vitamins, which aid the health of the nervous system. *(See pages 252–5.)*
• Nutritional deficiencies can disrupt the normal function of the nervous system, and extra vitamin E, along with most of the minerals and trace elements, including calcium, magnesium, zinc and manganese, are vital to normal brain function. Take a good vitamin and mineral supplement daily. *(See page 248.)*

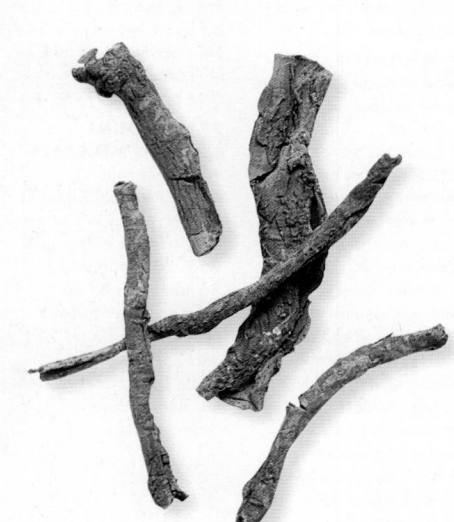

ABOVE *Ginseng is a good general tonic but should not be taken continuously for a long period. Make a decoction, or purchase ready-made tablets or other remedies.*

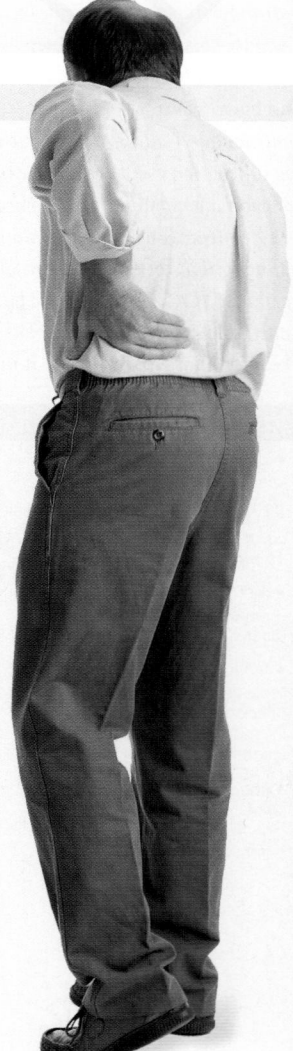

RIGHT *Back pain and muscular weakness can be a symptom of Guillain-Barré syndrome.*

Shingles

Shingles is an extremely painful disease caused by the herpes zoster virus (which is also the chicken pox virus). Following an attack of chickenpox the virus remains dormant in the body. Many years later a drop in the efficiency of the immune system may cause reactivation of the virus, this time in the form of shingles, causing acute inflammation in the ganglia near the spinal cord.

DATA FILE

- Occurs most often in people over the age of 50 and may be activated through surgery or X-ray therapy to the spinal cord and its roots.

- In younger people, it is often associated with a weakening of the immune system.

- The pain, which can be disabling, may continue for a few months after the blisters heal.

- Shingles strikes 850,000 Americans each year.

SYMPTOMS

- *the first sign of shingles is sensitivity in the area to be affected, then pain* • *fever* • *sickness* • *a rash of small blisters develops on the fourth or fifth day; these turn yellow within a few days, form scabs, then drop off, sometimes leaving scars* • *in some cases there may be persistent pain for months or years (post-herpetic pain)*

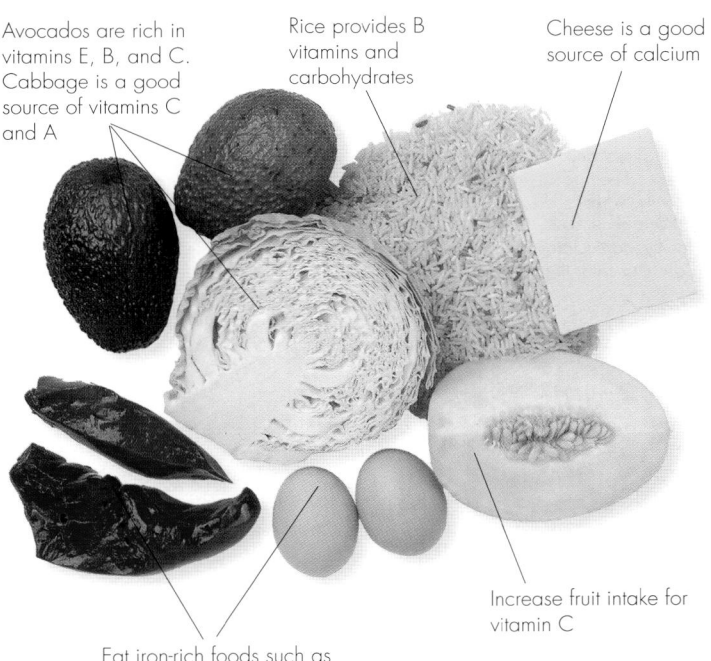

Avocados are rich in vitamins E, B, and C. Cabbage is a good source of vitamins C and A

Rice provides B vitamins and carbohydrates

Cheese is a good source of calcium

Increase fruit intake for vitamin C

Eat iron-rich foods such as liver and eggs

CAUTION

SHINGLES OF THE FACE MAY AFFECT THE EYES AND SHOULD RECEIVE APPROPRIATE SPECIALIST MEDICAL ATTENTION.

ABOVE *It is important to eat a balanced, nutritious diet, especially if it is suspected that a weakened immune system has caused shingles.*

TREATMENT

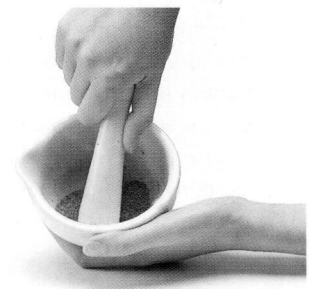
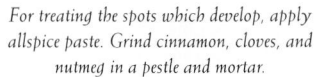

For treating the spots which develop, apply allspice paste. Grind cinnamon, cloves, and nutmeg in a pestle and mortar.

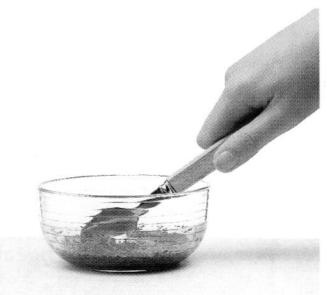

Add water to make a thick paste. Apply to spots to numb the pain. (You can also buy allspice as a pre-ground powder.)

HERBALISM
- Make an infusion of the following nervine herbs and drink three times daily: oats, skullcap, St. John's wort, and vervain. *(See pages 117, 124, 131, and 138.)*
- Diluted tinctures or cold infusion of marigold, plantain, and St. John's wort can be used to bathe the affected area. *(See pages 117, 124, 126.)*

AROMATHERAPY
- Essential oils can combine analgesics with antiviral properties, and can be applied as a compress, added to the bath, or massaged into the skin. Try combining two or more of bergamot, chamomile, geranium, eucalyptus, melissa, lavender, and tea tree. *(See pages 146–71.)*
- Dab the sores with lemon or geranium oil diluted in a little water. *(See pages 154 and 165.)*

CHINESE HERBALISM
- Treatment would address gall bladder heat and damp. Useful herbs include gentian and Oriental wormwood.

TRADITIONAL HOME AND FOLK REMEDIES
- Grind allspice and make a paste, then apply to the spots to relieve pain.
- Celery juice or celery tea can alleviate the pain and help to tone up the nervous system.
- Apply bruised juniper berries to the spots for effective pain relief.
- Fresh lemon can be cut and applied to the affected areas to relieve the pain. *(See page 87.)*

HOMEOPATHY
The following remedies can be taken every two hours for up to ten doses:
- Arsenicum, for burning pains which are worse between midnight and 2 A.M., accompanied by skin eruptions and feeling restless, chilly, and anxious. *(See page 182.)*
- Lachesis, when the left side of the body is affected by swelling. *(See page 216.)*

- Rhus tox., for red, blistered, and itching skin which is improved with movement and warmth. *(See page 210.)*
- Fanunculus, for nerve pains and itching which are made worse by movement and eating.
- Sponge the blisters with a blend of Hypericum and Calendula tinctures, added to a little hot water. *(See pages 187 and 199.)*

VITAMINS AND MINERALS
- Eat plenty of foods that are rich in the B-complex vitamins, to aid nervous health. *(See pages 252–5.)*
- Increase your intake of vitamin C, and take a supplement of 1g. up to 4 times daily. *(See page 256.)*
- Supplementation with Vitamin E is now known to reduce the long-term symptoms associated with shingles. Take up to 1mg. daily, broken into 3 doses, with food. *(See page 257.)*
- Vitamin E oil, applied directly to the sores, will encourage healing. *(See page 257.)*
- An attack of shingles is a sign of general debility, and any of the treatments suggested for stress *(see page 284)* will help to tone up the system.

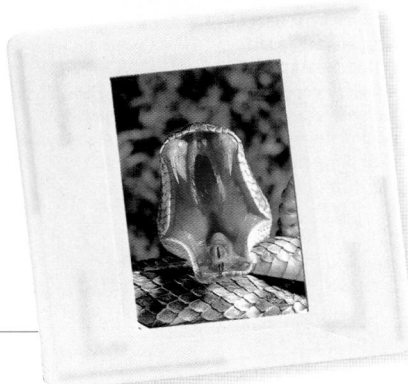

RIGHT *The homeopathic remedy Lachesis is made from the venom of the bushmaster snake.*

Neuralgia

Neuralgia is the term used to describe any pain originating in a nerve. If there is damage at any point along the route of a nerve, pain will then be referred to the area served by the affected nerve. Infection causing inflammation in a nerve can also cause neuralgia. The pain may be intermittent or continuous. Neuralgia has different causes, which give rise to certain specific types of neuralgic pain – trigeminal neuralgia, sciatica, post-herpetic neuralgia, and glossopharyngeal neuralgia.

DATA FILE

Specific types of neuralgia include:

• trigeminal neuralgia, in which the facial nerve is affected, causing severe one-sided facial pain.

• sciatica, in which spinal nerves are trapped between vertebrae, causing pain of varying severity in the back, sometimes extending down to the foot.

• Post-herpetic neuralgia, which causes a burning pain at the site of a previous attack of shingles.

• Glossopharyngeal neuralgia, in which pain is felt in the ear, the throat, and at the back of the tongue.

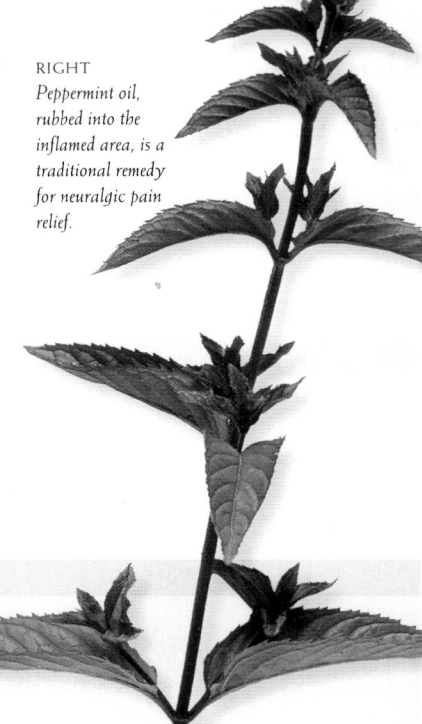

RIGHT *Peppermint oil, rubbed into the inflamed area, is a traditional remedy for neuralgic pain relief.*

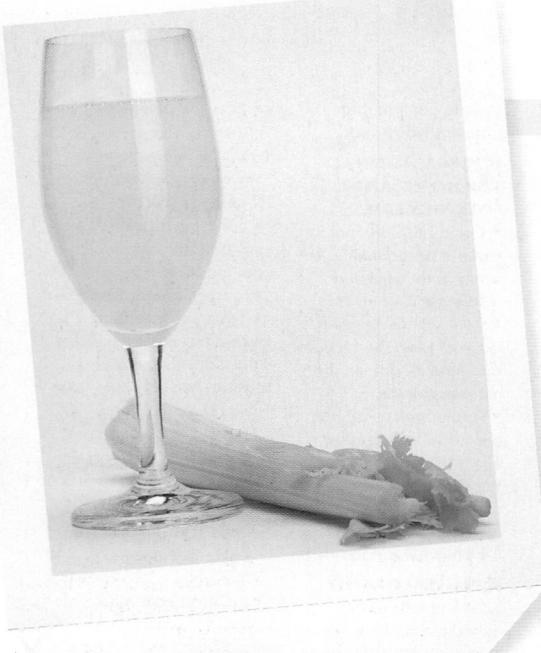

ABOVE *Celery juice relieves neuralgic pain. Make it by liquidizing fresh celery.*

TREATMENT

• Warm chamomile compresses applied to the affected area will ease inflammation and pain.
• Rub lemons on the affected area for pain relief. *(See page 87.)*
• Rub peppermint oil into the affected area.
• Clove oil can be used where pain is experienced inside the mouth. *(See page 90.)*

AROMATHERAPY
• Massage essential oil of eucalyptus, lavender, or chamomile into the affected area, or add the infused herbs to the bath. *(See pages 146–71.)*
• A compress of rosemary essential oil will improve the circulation in that area, which will encourage healing. *(See page 168.)*
• Blend one drop of mustard and pepper oils in some grapeseed oil, and massage into the affected area. *(See pages 146–71.)*

HOMEOPATHY
Treatment should be constitutional, and supervised by an experienced homeopath. Some of the following remedies may be helpful:

• Arsenicum, for an attack brought on by dry cold. You feel chilly, tired, restless, and have burning pains. *(See page 182.)*
• Lachesis, for pain that is worse after sleep. *(See page 216.)*
• Mag. phos., for pain that is relieved by applying heat and pressure. *(See page 204.)*
• Aconite, when symptoms come on suddenly, particularly after exposure to cold; the body feels congested and numb. *(See page 178.)*
• Colocynthis, for a neuralgia attack brought on by cold or damp, and which feels better for heat. *(See page 191.)*

VITAMINS AND MINERALS
• Vitamins B1, B2, and biotin help nerve health. *(See pages 252, 253, and 257.)*
• Take both extra vitamin E and chromium. *(See pages 257 and 259.)*

CHINESE HERBALISM
• Treatment would be aimed at addressing Wind, Damp and Heat which may have entered the meridians and are causing the illness. *(See page 50.)*
• Gentian and oriental wormwood may be useful.

TRADITIONAL HOME AND FOLK REMEDIES
• Celery juice or celery tea will help to ease the pain of neuralgia. *(See page 83.)*

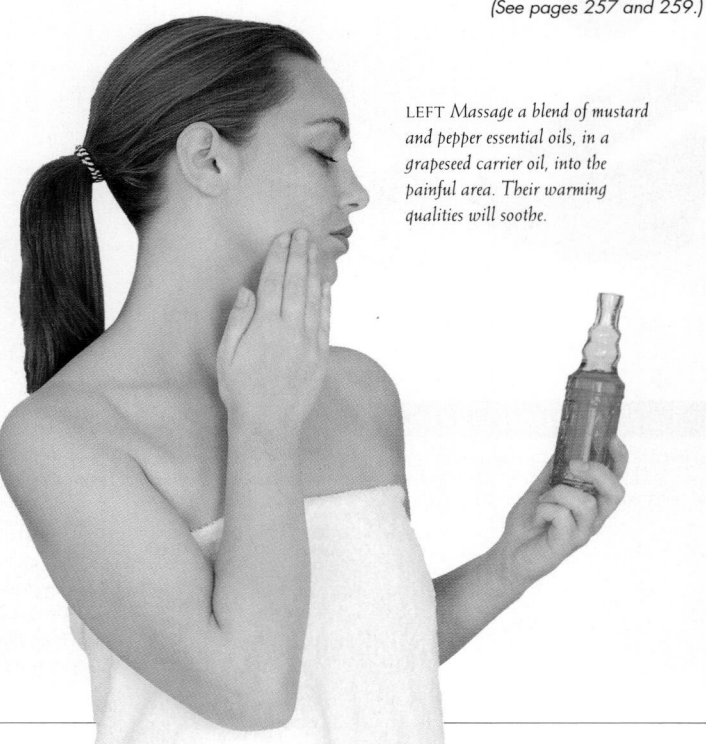

LEFT *Massage a blend of mustard and pepper essential oils, in a grapeseed carrier oil, into the painful area. Their warming qualities will soothe.*

Migraine

The classic feature of a migraine is a throbbing headache, usually on one side of the head only. This is caused by the narrowing and dilating of the blood vessels in a part of one side of the brain. An attack may last for up to two days. There are two main types of migraine, common and the comparatively rare classical. Migraine can be hereditary, and may be triggered by many factors, including stress, hormonal changes (around menopause, menstruation, and occasionally pregnancy), oral contraceptives, and food that contains tyramine, an amino acid which affects the blood vessels. Foods rich in tyramine include bananas, cheese, chocolate, eggs, oranges, spinach, tomatoes, and wine. Other triggers include changes or extremes in temperature, lighting, or noise level. Migraine occurs in about 10 percent of the population, and is more common in women. Children may suffer from migraine, but this often manifests itself as an abdominal pain rather than a headache.

ABOVE *Eating a couple of feverfew leaves daily may stave off an attack of migraine.*

SYMPTOMS

• *common migraine: slowly developing severe headache, lasting from a few hours to two days — made worse by the smallest movement or noise — nausea and sometimes vomiting.* • *classical migraine: headache preceded by an aura which generally takes the form a visual disturbance — this may consist of temporary loss of vision, focusing problems, blind spots, and flashing lights — possible speech problems — occasional weakness or temporary paralysis of the limbs or extremities — nausea and vomiting — sensitivity to light*

DATA FILE

• Some 16–18 million Americans suffer from migraine. Studies suggest that people who feel compelled to excel are especially susceptible to migraine.

• About 60 percent of all migraine sufferers are women, and most patients first develop symptoms between the ages of 10 and 30.

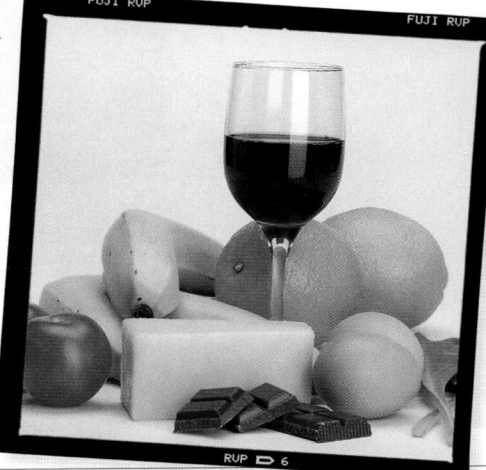

RIGHT *These foods contain tyramine, an amino acid which may trigger a migraine in some people.*

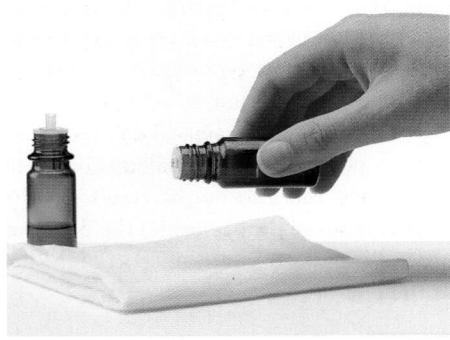

LEFT *Make a cool compress with a few drops each of lavender and peppermint essential oils on a damp cloth.*

AYURVEDA
• Treatment would be aimed at Ayurvedic oral formulas, and panchakarma shirovirechana. *(See page 20.)*
• Vilwadi lehya, an Ayurvedic product, can help with nausea.

CHINESE HERBALISM
• The cause is believed to be excess Liver qi stagnation, weakness in the stomach, and an imbalance of stomach and liver. Useful herbs include cassia tora and chrysanthemum.

HERBALISM
• Feverfew is an effective remedy for reducing the frequency of migraine. Take 2 or 3 small leaves between a little fresh bread, daily. Feverfew tablets are also available. *(See page 133.)*
• The following herbs can be infused for treating a mild attack of neuralgia: balm, meadowsweet, rosemary, and skullcap. *(See pages 121, 127, and 131.)*
• Apply a warm compress with Jamaican dogwood to the temples and forehead during an attack.

AROMATHERAPY
• Peppermint and lavender oils, applied to a cool compress, will help to relieve symptoms. *(See pages 161 and 164.)*
• Inhalations, baths, or massage of melissa, rosemary, or sweet marjoram can relieve the pain and shorten the duration of attacks. Used regularly, these methods can be preventive. *(See pages 146–71.)*
• A dab of lavender oil at the base of the nostrils can be used at the first signs of an attack. *(See page 161.)*

HOMEOPATHY
Treatment is constitutional, but the following remedies may be helpful in the event of an attack:
• Pulsatilla, for headache which is worse in the evening or during menstruation, and aggravated by rich, fatty foods; also for tearfulness. *(See page 209.)*
• Thuja, for a left-sided headache with the sensation of a nail being drilled into the skull. *(See page 216.)*

• Silicea, for pain that begins in the back of the head, settling above an eye. This is alleviated by wrapping the head. *(See page 211.)*
• Lycopodium, for pain that is worse on the right side of the body, painful temples and dizziness. *(See page 203.)*
• Nat. mur., for headache which is blinding and throbs, and which is worsened by warmth and movement, and where the attack is preceded by numbness around the mouth and nose. *(See page 206.)*

VITAMINS AND MINERALS
• Take extra vitamins B5, C, and E, and also evening primrose oil. *(See pages 254, 256, 257, and 270.)*
• Add fresh root ginger to food.

RIGHT *Nat. mur. homeopathic remedy is common salt.*

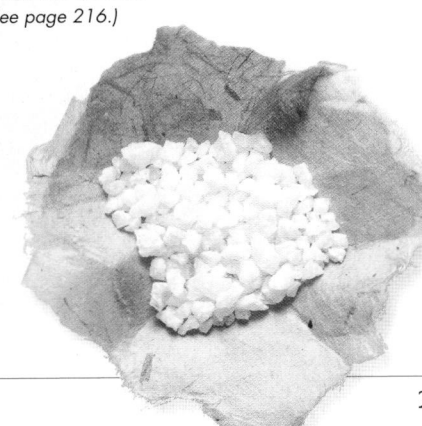

Headache

Headaches are an extremely common complaint, and for the most part are due to muscular tension in the head, neck, or shoulders, or to congestion of the blood vessels supplying blood to the brain and muscles. In some cases a headache may be a symptom of a more serious underlying disorder, but often headaches are caused by stress, tiredness, poor posture, caffeine, alcohol, drugs, food allergy, eyestrain, sinusitis, or low blood sugar. They can also be the result of a head injury. There are many different types of headache and the degree and intensity of pain vary accordingly. It may occur in any part of the head, usually worsening towards the end of the day.

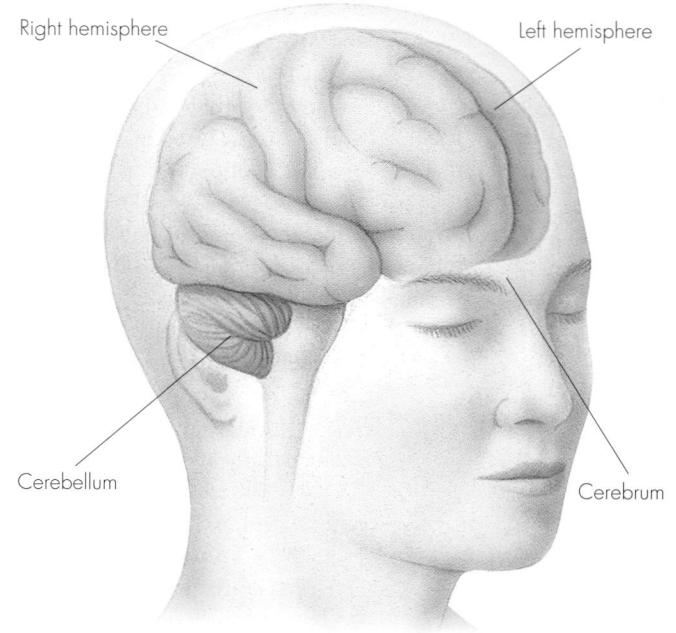

Right hemisphere

Left hemisphere

Cerebellum

Cerebrum

ABOVE *Headaches are very occasionally an indication of a serious disorder, such as a brain tumor.*

CAUTION

HEADACHES WITH ASSOCIATED FEATURES SUCH AS DOUBLE VISION, PROJECTILE VOMITING, WEAKNESS, PARALYSIS, VERTIGO, OR ONE-SIDED DEAFNESS REQUIRE URGENT MEDICAL ATTENTION.

SYMPTOMS

• sensation of a tight band around the head • a feeling of pressure at the top of the head • bursting or throbbing sensation • eye and neck pain • dizziness

DATA FILE

• In the U.S., up to 50 million people every year seek medical advice about their headaches.

• $0.5 billion is spent on headache remedies annually.

• Almost 90 percent of all people seeking medical help for headaches suffer from tension-type headaches.

• Cluster headaches produce short, severe attacks of pain centered over one eye. They are so called because they occur in clusters, many times a day, for several months. Spontaneous remissions often take place, but the pain usually returns some months or years later.

• Cluster headaches are suffered most often by males.

• Researchers suspect that cluster headaches may be caused by a disorder in histamine metabolism, since they are usually accompanied by allergy symptoms such as tearing, nasal congestion, and a runny nose.

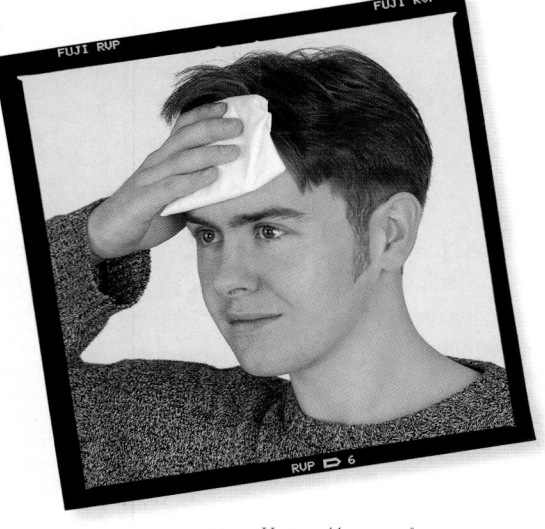

ABOVE *Heat 3 tablespoons of mustard oil, pour on to a cloth, and apply to the forehead to ease throbbing.*

RIGHT *The Chinese trust ginger to relieve headaches. Chew a small piece of fresh root.*

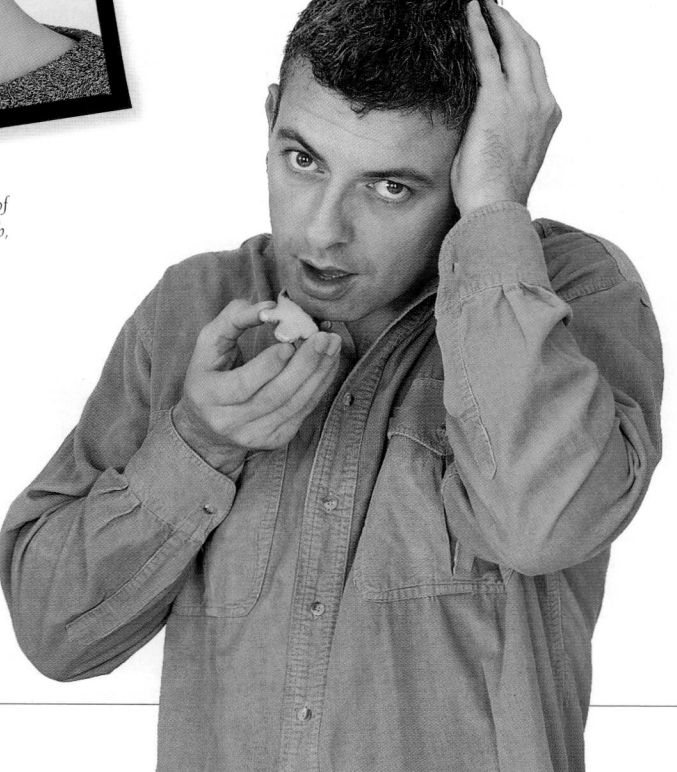

TREATMENT

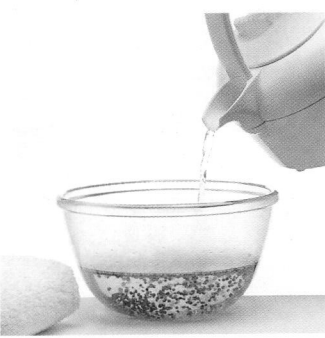

An Ayurvedic treatment for sinus-related headaches is the steam inhalation of coriander seeds. Put the coriander seeds into a small bowl.

Pour on some boiling water, drape a towel over your head and the bowl, and inhale the steam. Coriander's active ingredient is a volatile oil.

🏠 HOMEOPATHY
Most headaches would be dealt with constitutionally, that is, the treatment would be tailored to your individual needs. Other remedies to try include:
• Ignatia, for headaches caused by emotional stress. (See page 200.)
• Nux vomica, for headaches caused by overindulgence or stress. (See page 214.)
• Cimicifuga may be useful for pain caused by nervous muscular tension in the shoulders and neck. (See page 190.)
• Nux vomica or Pulsatilla are both useful in many cases of migraine. (See pages 209 and 214.)
• Aconite, for a sudden headache which feels worse for cold and is characterized by a tight band around the head. (See page 178.)
• Apis, for stinging, stabbing or burning headaches; when the body feels tender and sore. (See page 180.)
• Belladonna, for throbbing, drumming headaches with a flushed face. (See page 183.)
• Bryonia, for sharp, stabbing pain when the eyes are moved. (See page 185.)
• Hypericum, for a bursting, aching headache with a sensitive scalp. (See page 199.)
• Ruta, for a pressing headache caused by fatigue, and made worse by reading. (See page 210.)

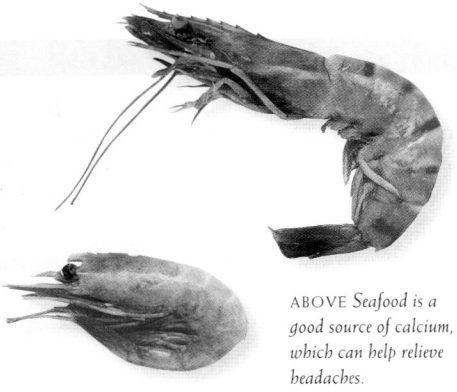

ABOVE Seafood is a good source of calcium, which can help relieve headaches.

💊 VITAMINS AND MINERALS
• Frequent headaches could be a signal that you are low on some important vitamins and minerals. Low levels of niacin and vitamin B6 can cause headaches, for example, and all the B vitamins are needed to help combat stress and avoid tension headaches. Protein-rich foods such as chicken, fish, beans and peas, milk, cheese, nuts, and peanut butter are all good dietary sources of both niacin and vitamin B6. (See page 253 and 254.)
• The minerals calcium and magnesium work together to help prevent headaches, especially

those related to a woman's menstrual cycle. Good sources of calcium are dairy products, tofu, dark green leafy vegetables such as kale or broccoli, and beans and peas. Magnesium is found in dark green leafy vegetables, nuts, bananas, wheat germ, seafood, and beans and peas. (See page 258 and 262.)
• If you can't eat some of these foods because they are headache triggers for you, taking a good daily multivitamin with minerals should provide enough of all the nutrients you need to help prevent headaches.

📖 AYURVEDA
• For headaches, heat 3 tablespoons of mustard oil, soak a cloth in the solution and apply to the forehead as required. (See page 30.)
• Coriander seeds, steeped for several minutes in boiling water, can be inhaled under a towel to relieve sinus-related headaches. (See page 35.)
• Asna vilwadi thaila is an oil, for external use, which relieves headaches.

🍵 CHINESE HERBALISM
• Traditional Chinese herbal medicine recommends ginger for headaches. Eat a small piece of fresh ginger root or make ginger tea from the fresh root or tea bags. If you prefer, mix a large pinch of powdered ginger into a glass of cool water and drink it, or try powdered ginger in capsules, available from health food stores.
• Ginseng is another favorite Chinese herbal remedy for headaches. (See page 67.)

✋ TRADITIONAL HOME AND FOLK REMEDIES
• A ginger foot bath may ease the pain and warm the body.
• Chamomile tea soothes headache symptoms.
• A mustard foot bath is a traditional headache remedy. (See page 98.)
• A few grains of cayenne pepper, added to tea, ease a headache. (See page 86.)
• Fresh garlic bulbs, eaten in a salad, will clear headaches which have a feeling of congestion. (See page 82.)
• Parsley and peppermint teas will clear the head.

🌿 HERBALISM
• Sitting down with a relaxing cup of mild herbal tea is often good for a tension headache. Good choices are peppermint, spearmint, chamomile, rose hip, meadowsweet, or lemon balm. (See pages 119, 121, and 125.)
• Valerian root tea can also be helpful, but it may induce sleep – use it with caution. (See page 136.)
• Researchers are studying the benefits of the herb feverfew for treating chronic headaches and migraines.

The leaves of this plant contain a substance that relaxes the blood vessels in your brain. Studies suggest that patients who eat a few fresh feverfew leaves or take an extract of the leaves every day have fewer and less severe migraines; the herb has no unpleasant side-effects. (See page 133.)

💧 AROMATHERAPY
• The relaxing qualities of lavender oil make it a good treatment for a tension headache. This essential oil is very gentle, so you can massage a few drops of neat oil into your temples and the base of your neck. (See page 161.)
• Try mixing a drop or two of peppermint oil in a bowl of hot water and inhaling the steam, then lie down with a warm compress soaked in sweet marjoram oil on your forehead. (See pages 164 and 165.)
• Place a few drops of lavender oil at the base of your nostrils for almost instant pain relief. (See page 161.)
• Try taking a bath with relaxing oils such as chamomile or ylang ylang to soothe and relieve pain. (See pages 146–71.)

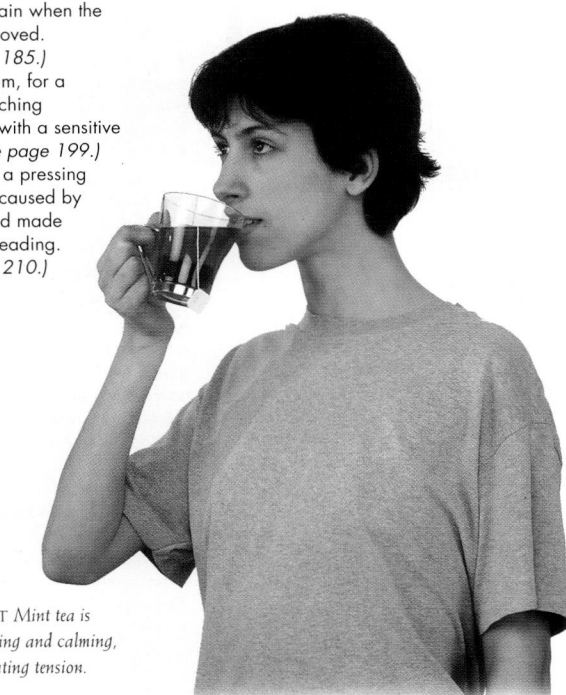

RIGHT Mint tea is refreshing and calming, dissipating tension.

Fainting

Fainting (or a vasovagal attack) is a brief loss of consciousness, usually brought on by strong emotion, shock, distress, or pain, and is most likely to occur in warm, crowded places. It is caused by a temporary shortage of blood supply to the brain, and there is also a slowing of the heart rate. A fainting episode acts, in fact, as a type of safety mechanism in that the fall restores the blood supply to the brain by gravity.

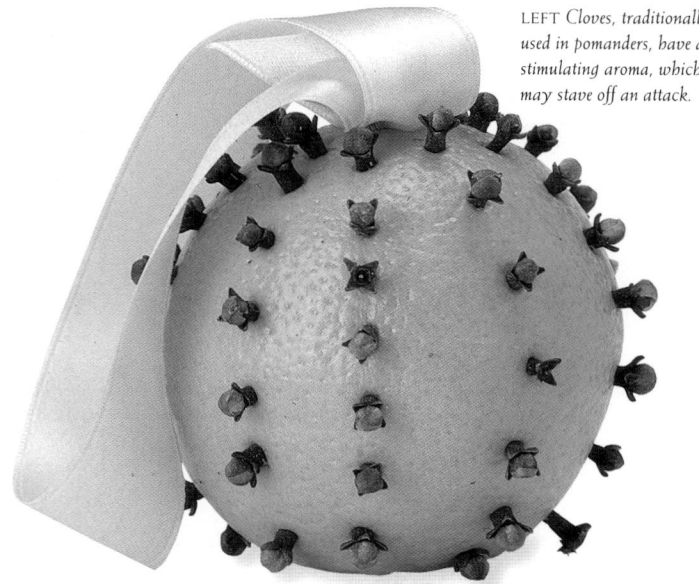

LEFT *Cloves, traditionally used in pomanders, have a stimulating aroma, which may stave off an attack.*

SYMPTOMS

The characteristic loss of consciousness may be preceded by:
• *yawning* • *sweating* • *nausea*
• *deep, rapid breathing and a weak pulse* • *impaired vision* • *ringing in the ears* • *weakness and confusion*

DATA FILE

• Fainting often occurs as a result of a vasovagal attack, in which overstimulation of the vagus nerve causes slowing of the heartbeat and a fall in blood pressure – which reduces the flow of blood to the brain. These attacks are commonly caused by pain, stress, shock, fear, or in a room with little oxygen. Other causes include prolonged coughing, straining to defecate or urinate, or blowing an instrument.

• Fainting may also result from postural hypotension (see page 299), which may occur when a person stands still for a long time, or suddenly stands up. This is common in the elderly, in sufferers of diabetes, and people taking high blood pressure medication or vasodilator drugs.

TREATMENT

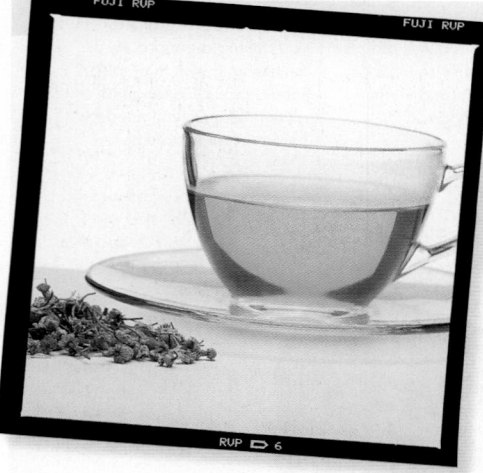

ABOVE *An infusion of ginger, cinnamon, and peppermint prevents fainting.*

AYURVEDA
The following Ayurvedic preparations will help to cure the condition: Aswagandharishta, an oral tonic; Chandanadi thaila, an external oil; Kalyanaka ghritha, oral ghee. *(See page 20.)*

CHINESE HERBALISM
• Fresh ginger, cinnamon twigs, and peppermint would be useful, taken internally as an infusion or decoction, as required. *(See page 54.)*

TRADITIONAL HOME AND FOLK REMEDIES
• Eat fresh or grated apple when you start to feel faint; it is both restorative and calming. *(See page 94.)*

• Chew dried cloves, which are stimulating and can improve circulation. *(See page 90.)*

HERBALISM
• Small sips of ginger tea, or root ginger chewed, will help to restore, and prevent an attack. *(See page 139.)*
• Rosemary is stimulating, and taken regularly can prevent fainting spells. *(See page 127.)*
• A hot drink of honey and peppermint will help to prevent loss of consciousness. Drink when you first start to feel faint. *(See page 125.)*

AROMATHERAPY
• Hold a tissue with a few drops of peppermint or neroli oil, which can help when you feel faint or are in a state of shock. *(See pages 152 and 164.)*
• A few drops of rosemary oil, massaged into the temples, prevents loss of consciousness. *(See page 168.)*

HOMEOPATHY
Constitutional treatment is necessary if the condition is chronic, but specific remedies which can be taken every 5 minutes after or immediately before fainting (when the sensation of fainting begins) include:
• Veratrum, for fainting caused by anger.
• Coffea, for fainting brought on by excitement. *(See page 192.)*
• Ignatia, for fainting caused by an emotional shock or trauma. *(See page 200.)*

• Aconite, for fainting caused by fright and characterized by tension and pale, clammy skin. *(See page 178.)*
• Cocculus, for fainting caused by lack of sleep.
• Gelsemium, when you feel weak and shaky. *(See page 195.)*

FLOWER ESSENCES
• Rescue Remedy or Emergency Essence placed on the tongue or temples may help to prevent fainting. If you are prone to fainting, carry a bottle at all times and take at the first signs of weakness. *(See page 244.)*
• Clematis can be taken for the "far away" feeling that comes before an attack, to bring the mind back to present reality. *(See page 229.)*

LEFT *Crunch an apple when feelings of faintness threaten to overwhelm.*

Dizziness

Dizziness is the sensation that everything around the sufferer is spinning, or that the brain is moving within the skull. In severe cases the sufferer may lose his or her balance and fall to the ground. Dizziness can be caused by a fault in the inner ear's balancing mechanism, or it may be due to a neurological disturbance. It can also be brought on by travel sickness, hyperventilation, anxiety, alcohol, drugs, and standing up suddenly from a sitting or lying position (postural hypotension). Postural hypotension is more common in the elderly and in people taking antihypertensive (high blood pressure) drugs.

SYMPTOMS

- *spinning sensation* • *nausea* • *vomiting* • *pallor*
- *cold sweats*

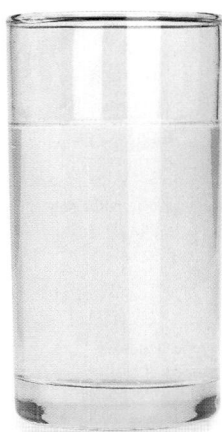

ABOVE *Ayurveda recommends drinking soda water with the juice of a lime or lemon.*

TREATMENT

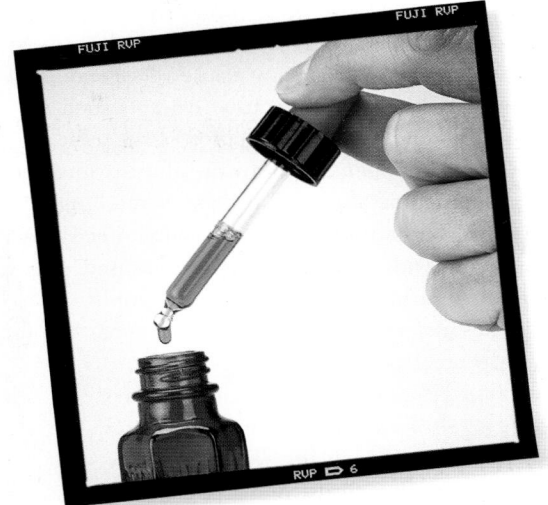

ABOVE *Rescue Remedy, made up of five flower essences, calms the patient and restores equilibrium.*

CAUTION

SEVERE OR PROLONGED DIZZINESS SHOULD BE REPORTED TO YOUR PHYSICIAN.

BELOW *Ginger tea's stimulant qualities help to fend off an attack of dizziness.*

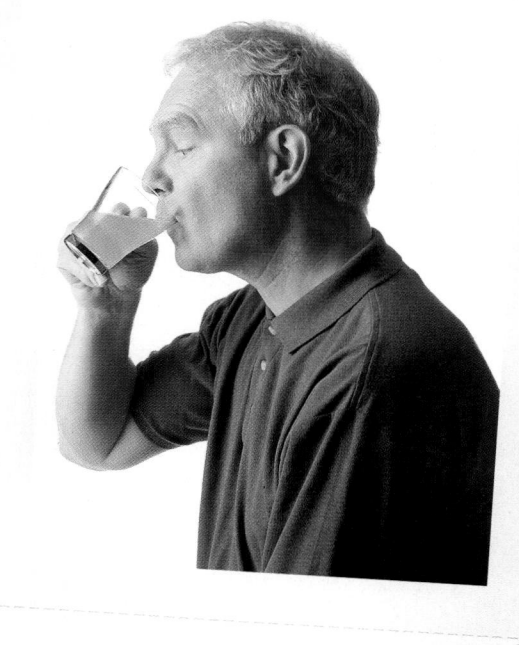

AYURVEDA
- Add the juice of a lime or lemon to half a glass of soda water and sip in small doses.

CHINESE HERBALISM
- Fresh ginger, cinnamon, and peppermint may help. *(See page 59.)*
- Mulberry can be used to nourish the blood.

HERBALISM
- Small sips of fresh ginger tea, made with root ginger, will help to ease the symptoms. *(See page 139.)*
- Teas of rock rose flowers or wild rose flowers, with a little honey, will be helpful.

HOMEOPATHY
- Gelsemium, for dizziness accompanied by a fit of trembling. *(See page 195.)*
- Nux vom., for when symptoms are made worse by flickering lights.
- Calcarea, when symptoms become worse after looking up. *(See page 186.)*
- Borax, for symptoms made worse by downward motion.
- Conium, when you feel worse lying down.

FLOWER ESSENCES
- If dizziness is associated with panic, stress, or anxiety, Emergency Essence or Rescue Remedy will be calming and restorative; take as required. *(See page 244.)*

VITAMINS AND MINERALS
- Take vitamins B2 and B3, and extra salt if you are sweating a great deal. *(See page 253.)*

RIGHT *Peel fresh ginger thinly, to preserve the richest active properties which lie just under the skin.*

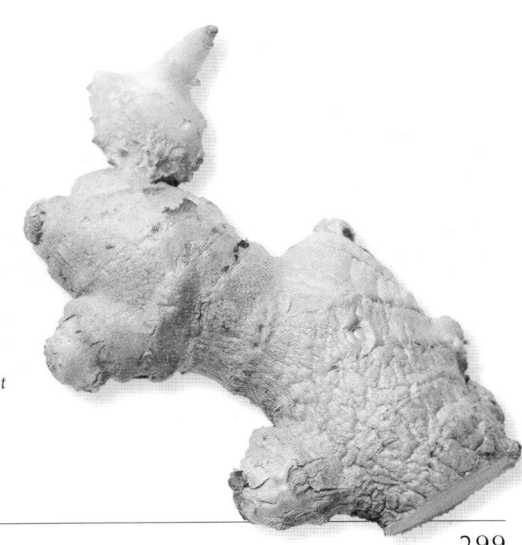

SKIN AND HAIR PROBLEMS

Dermatitis

Dermatitis is a very loose term (often used inter-changeably with eczema) used to describe an inflammation of the skin from any cause. Exogenous dermatitis is caused by external factors (irritants such as washing powder), and tends to occur around infected wounds or ulcers. Endogenous forms are due to internal problems, including metabolic disorders. Scratching always aggravates dermatitis and may also cause infection. Types of dermatitis include: diaper rash, caused by the ammonia in urine; atopic dermatitis, complicated by allergies such as hay fever; infantile eczema; seborrheic dermatitis (see Dandruff, page 306); dermatitis artefacta, caused by unnecessary scratching (it is self-inflicted and usually indicates an underlying emotional problem). The symptoms of dermatitis vary in severity and appearance according to the cause.

SYMPTOMS

• *redness and blistering* • *swelling, weeping, and crusting of skin* • *itching with a strong impulse to scratch* • *burning sensation*

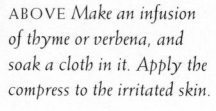

ABOVE *Make an infusion of thyme or verbena, and soak a cloth in it. Apply the compress to the irritated skin.*

DATA FILE

• Skin-contact dermatitis includes primary irritant dermatitis, allergic dermatitis, and photochemical dermatitis.

• Primary irritant dermatitis is the most common type and is caused by the direct toxicity of certain chemicals that come in contact with the skin.

• Allergic dermatitis involves the immune mechanism and requires prior sensitization of an individual to agents such as cosmetics, chemicals, plants, drugs, or costume jewelry.

• Photochemical dermatitis occurs when an individual with photosensitizing chemicals on his or her skin is exposed to light.

• Atopic dermatitis, or eczema, is a chronic inflammation that appears to run in families with a history of asthma and hay fever.

• Dermatitis can occur in single episodes, or may be chronic. Up to 90 percent of the U.S. population will suffer from dermatitis during their lifetime.

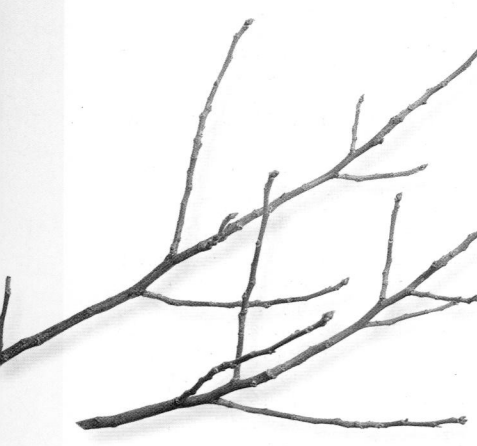

ABOVE *Rhus tox. is a homeopathic remedy for dermatitis which has erupted into blisters.*

CHINESE HERBALISM
• Dittany bark and puncture vine fruit may help with itching.

TRADITIONAL HOME AND FOLK REMEDIES
• For dermatitis on the hands, rub them with the cold wet coffee grounds left after you have brewed a pot of coffee, to soothe.

HERBALISM
• Apply compresses of verbena or thyme tea to the area to soothe and cool. (See page 135.)

AROMATHERAPY
• Dilute and massage a few drops of aspic, cedarwood, niaouli, or chamomile into the affected area to ease itching. (See pages 146–71.)
• For contact dermatitis, calendula or chamomile oil. (See pages 148 and 150.)

HOMEOPATHY
• Sulfur, for when the skin feels as if it is burning, and becomes red, hot, and itchy. (See page 215.)
• Graphites, when the skin appears infected. (See page 196.)
• Petroleum, when there are deep cracks with a watery discharge.

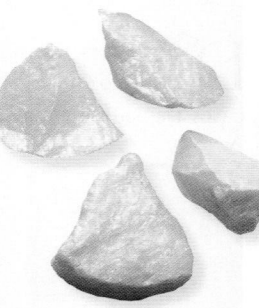

ABOVE *Homeopaths may prescribe Sulfur for a feeling of burning.*

• Urtica urens, for a nettle rash-type itchiness. (See page 217.)
• Rhus tox., for blisters that are worse at night and improve with warmth. (See page 210.)

FLOWER ESSENCES
• Crab Apple is the cleansing remedy. It works well when added to water for washing and baths. (See page 234.)
• Impatiens is very useful for people whose rashes are associated with feelings of irritability and impatience. Take internally or mix into a neutral cream. (See page 233.)
• Rescue Remedy, taken internally or used externally in a cream or wash, is useful for treating most skin problems. (See page 244.)

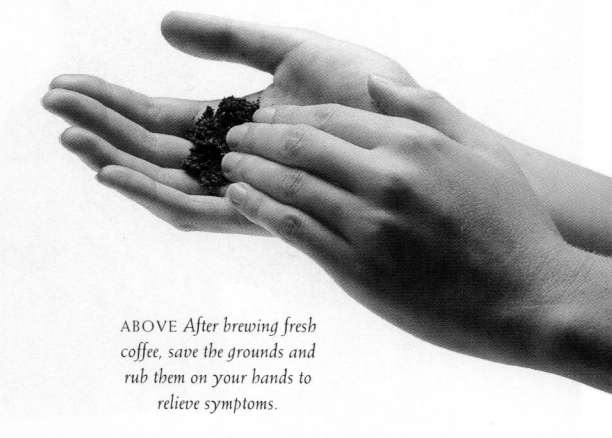

ABOVE *After brewing fresh coffee, save the grounds and rub them on your hands to relieve symptoms.*

Eczema

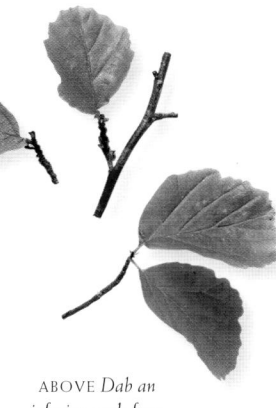

ABOVE *Dab an infusion made from witch hazel on the affected skin.*

Eczema (also called dermatitis) is an inflammation of the skin that causes itching and redness. It is a feature of many different skin disorders arising from many different causes. It can also be hereditary. Eczema is only infectious if it becomes secondarily infected. Types of eczema include: contact eczema (caused by allergens such as plants, metals, detergents, and chemical irritants); atopic eczema (associated with allergies such as hay fever); pomphylox eczema (triggered by emotional stress); and varicose eczema (occurring in the region of varicose veins).

SYMPTOMS

• *red, scaly, cracked patches of skin, particularly on the hands, ears, feet, and legs* • *burning and itching with a strong urge to scratch, possibly leading to infection, particularly in children* • *small fluid-filled blisters which may burst to form sores*

BELOW *Sometimes eczema is brought on by stress. Massage helps to relax the sufferer.*

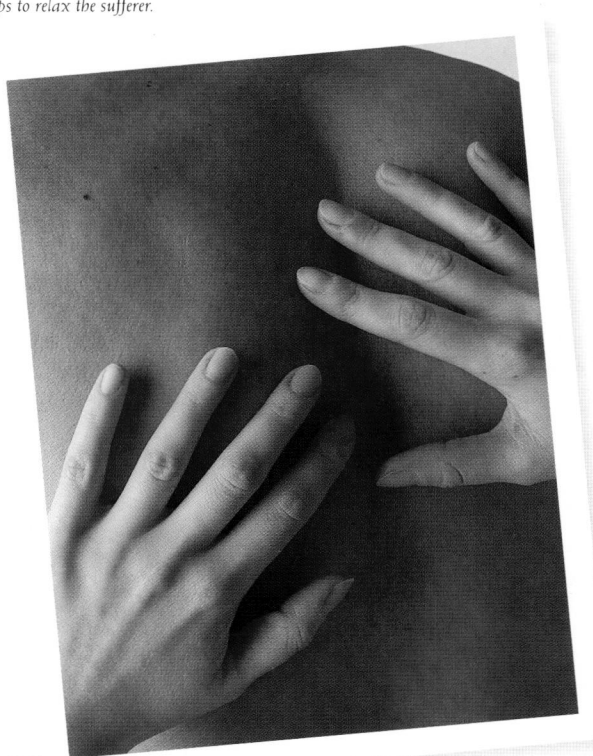

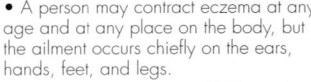

DATA FILE

• A person may contract eczema at any age and at any place on the body, but the ailment occurs chiefly on the ears, hands, feet, and legs.

• In infants, eczema is often caused by allergy to certain proteins in wheat, milk, and eggs.

• Emotional problems and severe mental stress are suspected of causing eczema in adults.

• Often, a family history of eczema exists, implying that heredity is also involved in some way.

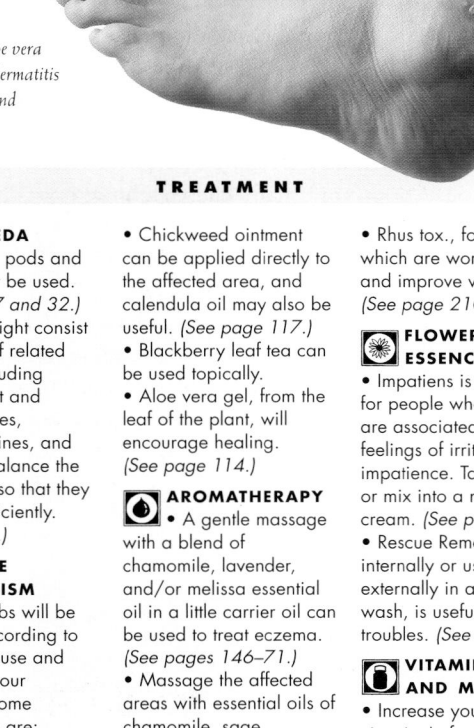

RIGHT *Smooth aloe vera gel into patches of dermatitis to relieve itchiness and aid healing.*

TREATMENT

AYURVEDA
• Cassia pods and aloe vera may be used. *(See pages 27 and 32.)*
• Treatment might consist of a number of related therapies, including herbalism, diet and lifestyle changes, cleansing routines, and treatment to balance the body systems so that they work more efficiently. *(See page 20.)*

CHINESE HERBALISM
• Chinese herbs will be prescribed according to the specific cause and symptoms of your eczema, but some possible herbs are: wormwood, peony root, and Chinese gentian. *(See page 67.)*
• Dittany bark and puncture vine fruit may help with itching

TRADITIONAL HOME AND FOLK REMEDIES
• An oatmeal bath will soothe irritation and reduce annoying itching. *(See page 84.)*
• Bathe sore patches with an infusion of witch hazel diluted in some warm water. *(See page 91.)*

HERBALISM
• Try drinking an infusion of burdock, chamomile, heartsease, marigold, and red clover, all of which are anti-inflammatory herbs. *(See pages 115, 117, and 119.)*

• Chickweed ointment can be applied directly to the affected area, and calendula oil may also be useful. *(See page 117.)*
• Blackberry leaf tea can be used topically.
• Aloe vera gel, from the leaf of the plant, will encourage healing. *(See page 114.)*

AROMATHERAPY
• A gentle massage with a blend of chamomile, lavender, and/or melissa essential oil in a little carrier oil can be used to treat eczema. *(See pages 146–71.)*
• Massage the affected areas with essential oils of chamomile, sage, geranium, and lavender, all blended together with a little carrier oil. *(See pages 146–71.)*

HOMEOPATHY
Eczema requires constitutional treatment, which means that treatment is tailored to your specific needs. The following remedies may be useful in the meantime:
• Sulfur, when the skin is burning, red, hot, and itchy. *(See page 215.)*
• Graphites, when the skin appears infected. *(See page 196.)*
• Petroleum, when there are deep cracks with a watery discharge.
• Urtica urens, for a nettle rash-type itchiness. *(See page 217.)*

• Rhus tox., for blisters which are worse at night and improve with warmth. *(See page 210.)*

FLOWER ESSENCES
• Impatiens is very useful for people whose rashes are associated with feelings of irritability and impatience. Take internally or mix into a neutral cream. *(See page 233.)*
• Rescue Remedy, taken internally or used externally in a cream or wash, is useful for skin troubles. *(See page 244.)*

VITAMINS AND MINERALS
• Increase your intake of vitamin A, found in liver, eggs, butter, milk, and red and orange vegetables. *(See page 252.)*
• Take a B-complex supplement each day, and make sure your tablet contains good levels of niacin (B3), which is also found naturally in peanuts, meat, fish, and pulses. *(See page 253.)*
• Vitamin C and bioflavonoids (which are often contained in a good vitamin C supplement) act as a natural antihistamine. *(See pages 256 and 272.)*
• Evening primrose oil has been used successfully in the treatment of eczema, reducing itching and encouraging healing. *(See page 270.)*

Psoriasis

Psoriasis is a common skin disorder which may affect any part of the body, but most often the elbows, knees, shins, scalp, and lower back. The characteristic bright pink or red plaques covered with silvery scaling are caused by a thickening of the outer skin layers. Psoriasis tends to run in families and usually begins in adolescence. Cold damp conditions, stress, anxiety, or an acute illness (such as tonsillitis) may all be triggers. There is also an association with arthritis of the fingers or toes. Psoriasis does not usually cause itching, nor is it contagious.

SYMPTOMS

• *pain (rather than itching), with cracks appearing in the dry areas of the hands and feet* • *pustules on the palms of the hands or soles of the feet (pustular psoriasis)* • *glazed but not scaly plaques in moist areas of the body (flexural psoriasis)* • *distortion and pitting of the nails in some cases*

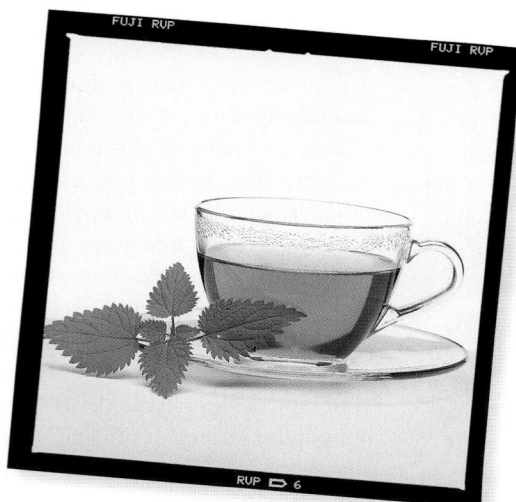

ABOVE *Sip nettle tea as a skin tonic. Nettles contain formic acid.*

TREATMENT

Scalp massage with aromatherapy oil may help

Some exposure to sunlight may be of benefit

Nettle skin cream may improve symptoms

Take a multivitamin and mineral supplement daily

ABOVE *Psoriasis affects many different sites in the body with scaly red patches.*

CHINESE HERBALISM
• Dittany bark and puncture vine fruit may help with itching.

TRADITIONAL HOME AND FOLK REMEDIES
• Take at least 1 tablespoonful of olive oil a day and at least one raw vegetable salad. *(See page 95.)*
• Garlic is cleansing, and may ease the symptoms and prevent attacks. *(See page 82.)*

HERBALISM
• Licorice, for the inflammation of psoriasis. *(See page 122.)*
• Yarrow used twice weekly in bath water has proved beneficial in some cases. *(See page 112.)*
• Nettle tea and products based on nettles may be helpful. *(See page 137.)*

AROMATHERAPY
• Sedative and antidepressant oils such as lavender and chamomile can help to reduce the stress that exacerbates the condition. Use in the bath, massage, and skin creams. *(See pages 150 and 161.)*
• Bergamot essential oil, cajeput, and Roman chamomile can all be used as a beneficial massage oil. They may also be added to a bath, or placed in a vaporizer. *(See pages 146–71.)*

HOMEOPATHY
• Kali ars., for scaly skin aggravated by warmth.
• Arsenicum, for burning, hot areas, and feeling chilly and restless. *(See page 182.)*
• Graphites, for psoriasis that is worse behind the ears and weeping. *(See page 196.)*
• Sulfur, for patches that become worse after a bath and in heat. *(See page 215.)*
• Petroleum, when the condition is worse in winter.

FLOWER ESSENCES
• Impatiens is very useful for people whose rashes are associated with feelings of irritability and impatience. Take internally or mix into a neutral cream. *(See page 233.)*
• Rescue Remedy, taken internally or used externally in a cream or wash, treats most skin troubles. *(See page 244.)*
• Crab Apple is the cleansing remedy. It works well when added to water for washing and baths. *(See page 234.)*

VITAMINS AND MINERALS
• Increase your intake of vitamin A (as beta carotene), vitamin C, vitamin E, selenium, B-complex vitamins as part of a good multivitamin and mineral supplement, and also protein. *(See pages 252–57 and 264.)*

Urticaria

Urticaria is an allergic condition also known as hives or nettle rash. The rash of raised, whitish-yellow areas of skin surrounded by red inflammation is caused by the release of histamine into the tissues in response to triggers which may include heat, cold, sunlight, scabies, bites and stings, contact with plants, food additives, sensitivity to certain foods, and stress or anxiety. Acute urticaria typically develops very quickly, and usually disappears just as quickly; chronic urticaria is more persistent.

SYMPTOMS

• *rash of weals, especially on limbs and trunk* • *intense itching* • *swelling of the tongue and larynx may occur, possibly interfering with breathing* • *a feverish feeling* • *possibly nausea*

LEFT *The leaves of the aloe vera plant produce a gel which soothes a range of skin problems.*

TREATMENT

AYURVEDA
• Aloe vera can be used topically to soothe the rash. *(See page 27.)*

CHINESE HERBALISM
• The source of urticaria is considered to be Heat and Wind when red; and Heat, Cold and Wind for a cold white rash. Treatment may include chizomeotea or ledebouriella. *(See page 64.)*

TRADITIONAL HOME AND FOLK REMEDIES
• Add a few tablespoons of baking soda to the bath to relieve itching. *(See page 100.)*
• An oatmeal bath will soothe the rash. *(See page 84.)*
• Add a cupful of vinegar to the bath water to restore the balance of the skin. *(See page 102.)*

HERBALISM
• An infusion of chickweed and chamomile can be used to bathe the affected area. *(See page 119.)*
• Balm and heartsease can be drunk 3 times daily to soothe and reduce inflammation.
• For urticaria brought on by anxiety and stress, drink an infusion of valerian twice daily. *(See page 136.)*
• Urtica urens cream will soothe and promote healing.

AROMATHERAPY
• A warm bath with essential oil of chamomile or melissa will soothe the skin and help to prevent stress-related attacks. *(See pages 150 and 163.)*

HOMEOPATHY
• Apis, for burning and swelling, particularly of the lips and eyelids. *(See page 180.)*
• Urtica, for a rash that feels like stinging nettles, and is worse when touched or after it has been scratched. *(See page 217.)*
• Nat. mur., for chronic urticaria exacerbated by stress. *(See page 206.)*
• Rhus tox., for burning, itching, and blisters. *(See page 210.)*
• Sulfur, for relief of red, itchy, puffy skin, which is made worse by heat. *(See page 215.)*
• Arsenicum, for symptoms accompanied by restlessness and anxiety. *(See page 182.)*

FLOWER ESSENCES
• Impatiens is very useful for people whose rashes are associated with feelings of irritability and impatience. Take internally or mix into a neutral cream. *(See page 233.)*

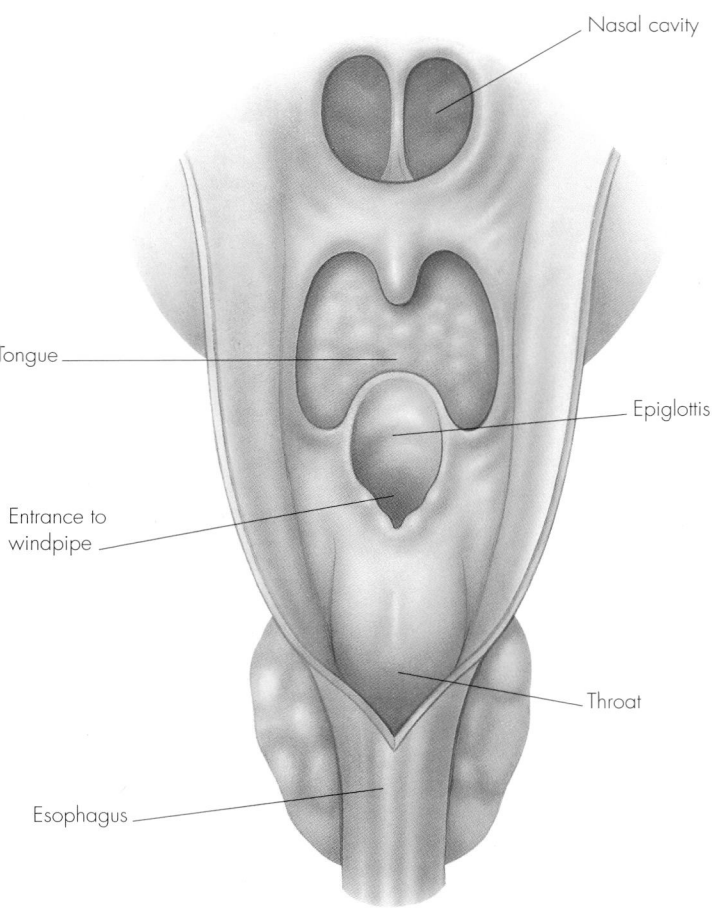

Nasal cavity

Tongue

Epiglottis

Entrance to windpipe

Throat

Esophagus

ABOVE *The larynx. Sometimes urticaria causes the tongue and larynx to swell, which may restrict breathing.*

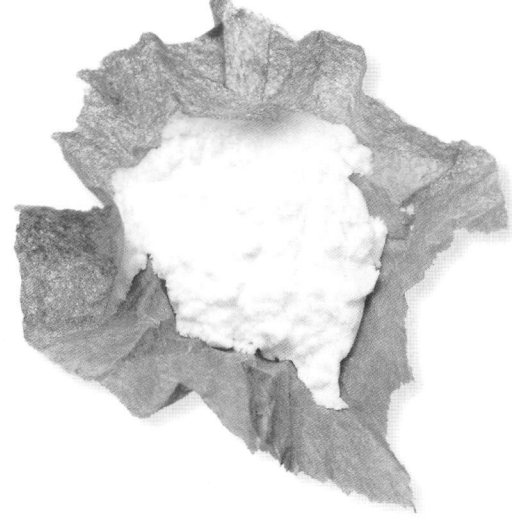

RIGHT *Sprinkle a few tablespoonsful of baking soda into your bathwater to temper the itching.*

Prickly Heat

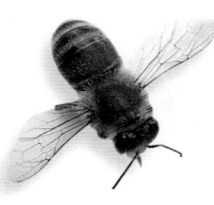

ABOVE *The honey bee is the source of the homeopathic remedy Apis.*

Prickly heat, or heat rash, occurs as a result of sweat duct blockage (probably due to excessive dampness of the skin) in particularly hot and humid weather. It produces a rash of red spots on the face and/or body, which usually disappears within hours of the sufferer moving into the shade, or his or her acclimatization. Occasionally, however, it may develop into patches of eczema. Children, the elderly and the obese are all particularly susceptible.

TREATMENT

HERBALISM
• Chickweed infusions can be made into cool compresses and applied to the affected area. Chickweed ointment can be applied as needed.

AROMATHERAPY
• Add a few drops of lavender and sandalwood oils to a little calendula oil, and massage into the affected area. *(See pages 146–71.)*

HOMEOPATHY
• Apis, taken every 2 hours for up to 10 doses. *(See page 180.)*
• Merc. Sol. can be used as a preventive measure. *(See page 213.)*

FLOWER ESSENCES
• Impatiens is very useful for itching. Take internally or mix into a neutral cream. *(See page 233.)*
• Rescue Remedy, taken internally or applied externally in a cream or wash, helps most skin troubles. *(See page 244.)*

VITAMINS AND MINERALS
• Take plenty of vitamin C, which will help to discourage itching and the rash. *(See page 256.)*

SYMPTOMS

• *a constant prickling or itching sensation*
• *tiny blisters may form in severe cases as a result of salt crystals forming in the sweat gland ducts*

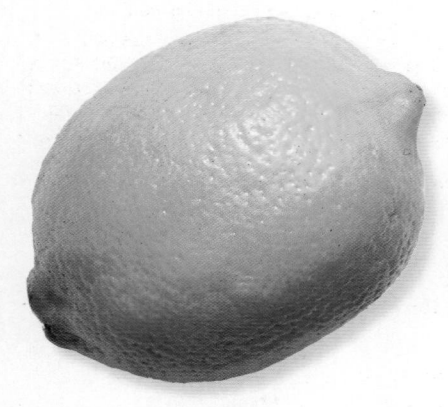

BELOW *Citrus fruit is a good source of vitamin C, needed to alleviate skin problems.*

Perspiration

Perspiration is generally stimulated by heat and is the body's way of regulating temperature. Excessive sweating (or hyperhidrosis) is caused by overactive sweat glands. It may be confined to specific areas such as the palms of the hands, armpits, groin and feet, or it may occur all over the body. When perspiration exceeds the bounds of what is considered normal, it may be due to an overactive thyroid gland, the menopause, prolonged fever, or stress or other psychological factors.

SYMPTOMS

• *an unpleasant body odor may occur if perspiration comes into contact with bacteria on the skin* • *in severe cases the skin in affected areas may become damp and damaged*

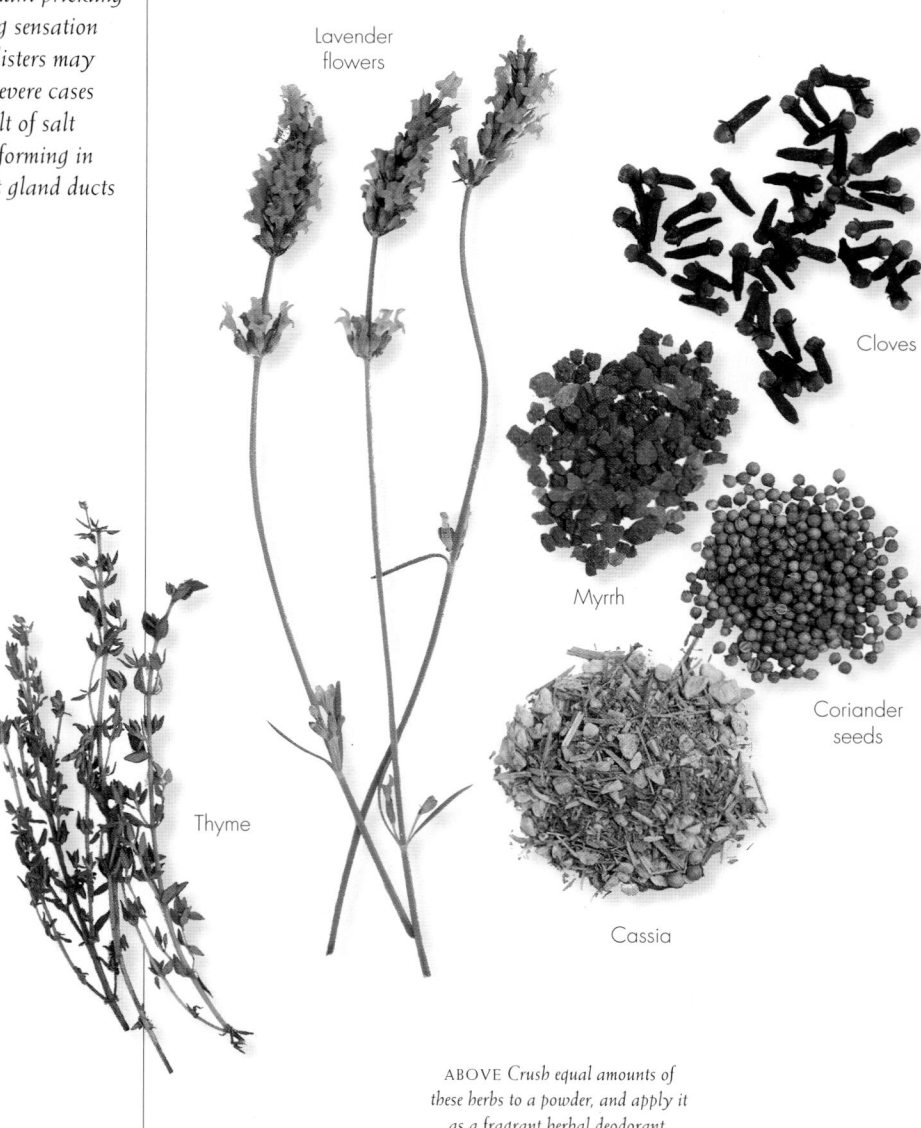

Lavender flowers

Cloves

Myrrh

Coriander seeds

Thyme

Cassia

ABOVE *Crush equal amounts of these herbs to a powder, and apply it as a fragrant herbal deodorant.*

CHINESE HERBALISM
• Excess sweating is thought to be caused by a deficiency of qi or yin. *(See page 49.)*
• For yin deficiency, use gray lily turf root, cork tree bark, and peony. *(See pages 67 and 68.)*
• Try ledebouriella and astragalus for deficient qi. *(See pages 57 and 64.)*

HERBALISM
• Marigold infusion can be drunk to produce a perspiration increase, when necessary. *(See page 117.)*
• A herbal deodorant would include cloves, myrrh, coriander seeds, cassia, lavender flowers, and thyme, in equal amounts and ground into a powder. Use in the bath, or under the arms. This may cause a rash in sensitive people. *(See page 135.)*

AROMATHERAPY
• Cypress oil is astringent and refreshing, and can be massaged into the feet for excess perspiration, or combined with lavender oil in a light massage oil and massaged under the arms. *(See page 156.)*
• Oils with deodorizing properties are bergamot, clary sage, eucalyptus, lavender, neroli,

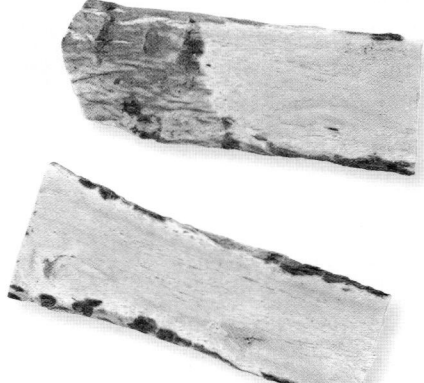

ABOVE *Astragalus. In Chinese medicine, depleted qi causes health problems. Astragalus restores qi.*

petitgrain, and rosewood. *(See pages 146–71.)*
• Detoxifying oils include fennel, garlic, juniper, and rose. *(See pages 146–71.)*
• Basil, chamomile, juniper, peppermint, and tea tree oils promote sweating, if there is a lack of it. *(See pages 146–71.)*

HOMEOPATHY
Constitutional treatment is most appropriate, but the following may help:
• Lycopodium, for smelly perspiration, worse on feet and under arms. *(See page 203.)*

• Mercurius, for smelly sweat. *(See page 205.)*
• Sulfur, for sweating on the head, with morning diarrhea. *(See page 215.)*
• Calcarea, for sour sweat. The sufferer is likely to be overweight, and feels cold and clammy. *(See page 186.)*
• Silicea, for sweaty, smelly feet in a thin person. *(See page 211.)*
• Aethusa, for insufficient perspiration production.

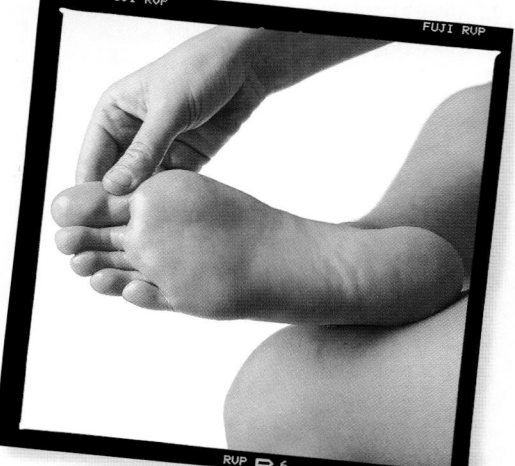

RIGHT *To help stop sweaty feet, rub a little cypress oil into the skin.*

Bruising

(See under Heart, Blood, and Circulation, page 354.)

Sunburn

Sunburn occurs on exposure to bright sunlight and is caused by the effects of ultraviolet light. It is most likely to affect people with pale complexions or those who are unused to being in the sun.

SYMPTOMS

• *redness and extreme soreness in affected areas* • *a sensation of heat in burned areas* • *blistering in severe cases*

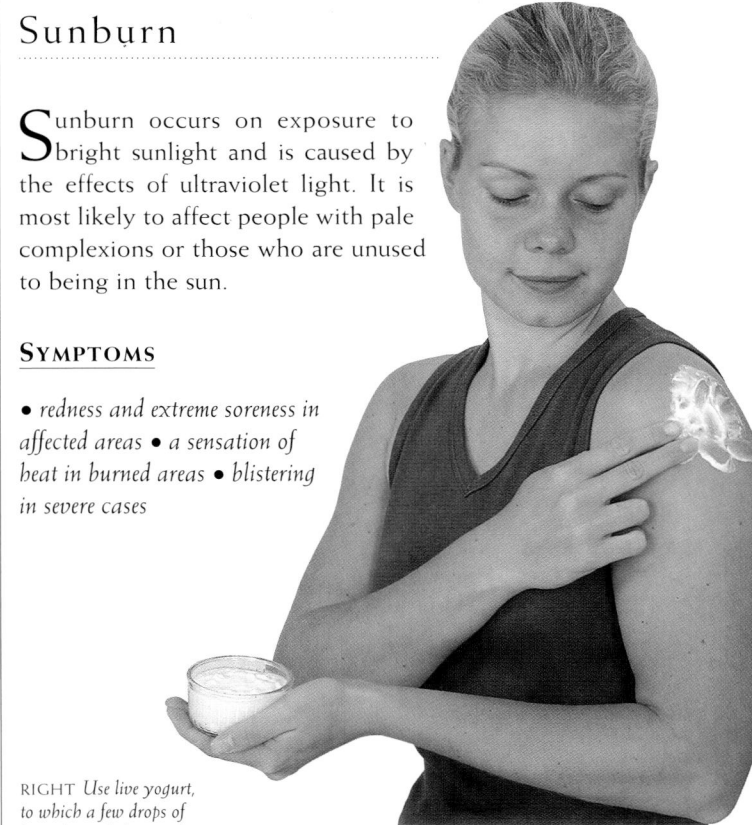

RIGHT *Use live yogurt, to which a few drops of lavender and chamomile oils have been added.*

AYURVEDA
• Aloe vera can be used on burned areas to soothe and to heal. *(See page 27.)*

HERBALISM
• Urtica urens ointment eases the pain and helps to prevent skin damage.

AROMATHERAPY
• Add a few drops of lavender and chamomile oils to a tub of live yogurt, and apply to affected areas to soothe, encourage healing, and reduce inflammation. *(See pages 146–71.)*

HOMEOPATHY
• Merc. Sol. can be used to prevent and treat sunburn. *(See page 213.)*

FLOWER ESSENCES
• Rescue Remedy cream heals damaged tissue and reduces the discomfort. *(See page 244.)*

VITAMINS AND MINERALS
• Rub a little vitamin E oil into the affected area, soon after the burning, to help the healing process and prevent peels and scarring. *(See page 257.)*

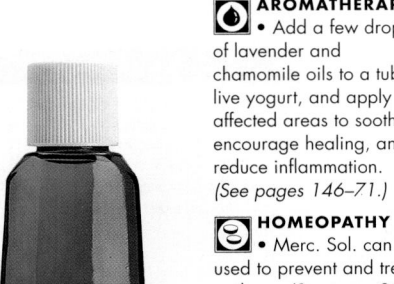

LEFT *Vitamin E oil encourages the sunburned skin to repair itself. Rub it in as an aftersun treatment.*

Warts

A wart is a small, hard growth, usually brown or flesh-colored, on the skin. It may be caused by any one of 30 strains of the human papilloma virus. Warts are highly contagious, but not dangerous, and can occur more frequently when the immune system is compromised.

TREATMENT

TRADITIONAL HOME AND FOLK REMEDIES
• Rub fresh lemon into the wart daily, and keep moist (with a plaster), paring back any hardened skin. (See page 87.)
• Rub fresh garlic into the wart to fight the fungal infection, and eat lots of garlic to boost immunity. (See page 82.)
• Mix castor oil and baking powder into a paste, and apply at night with a plaster, leaving it exposed during the day.

HERBALISM
• Squeeze the fresh sap of a dandelion stalk on to the wart every day

until it disappears. (See page 134.)
• Milkwort can be mashed and applied directly to the wart.

AROMATHERAPY
• Apply a little lemon oil directly to the wart; continue treatment until the wart disappears. (See page 154.)
• When the wart disappears, add a few drops of lavender oil to vitamin E oil and apply to the area for a week, to encourage healing and prevent scarring and further infection. (See page 161.)
• Overall body massage with rosemary, juniper, or geranium will help to

strengthen the immune system. (See pages 146–71.)

HOMEOPATHY
• Thuja, for soft, fleshy warts that ooze and bleed. (See page 216.)
• Causticum, for warts on the face or fingertips, and painful verrucas. (See page 189.)
• Dulcamara, for hard, smooth, fleshy warts on the back of hands. (See page 213.)
• Kali mur., for warts growing on the hands.
• Nat. carb., for weeping warts on the toes.
• Antimonium, for horny warts caused by or associated with a callus. (See page 179.)

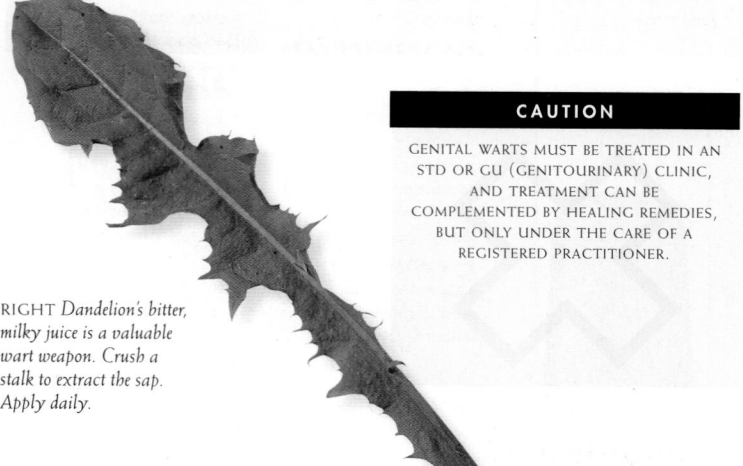

RIGHT *Dandelion's bitter, milky juice is a valuable wart weapon. Crush a stalk to extract the sap. Apply daily.*

Dandruff

Dandruff occurs when the fine cells of the outer layer of skin on the scalp are shed at a faster rate than normal, causing the characteristic flakes of dead skin. This is caused by a disorder of the sebaceous glands. If too little sebum is secreted the hair is dry and dandruff appears as white flakes; if too much sebum is produced the hair is greasy, and the dandruff yellow. The flakes are usually most obvious after brushing or combing the hair, which loosens them. Certain types of seborrheic dermatitis are also responsible for dandruff, which will cause inflammation and itchiness in addition to flaking.

ABOVE *A homeopath may suggest Arsenicum if the scalp is sensitive and feels dry.*

TREATMENT

HERBALISM
• Improve circulation to the scalp. Rosemary is the herb of choice, taken internally as a tea and used as an application. (See page 127.)
• For dry hair, rub rosemary-infused oil into the scalp before washing. (See page 127.)
• For greasy hair, add rosemary vinegar or a few drops of rosemary essential oil to the rinsing water. (See page 127.)
• Take a combination of the herbs burdock, kelp, and heartsease internally to improve the general condition of the scalp. (See pages 115 and 122.)

AROMATHERAPY
• Rosemary, cedarwood, tea tree, or patchouli can be massaged into the scalp, added to unscented shampoos, and used in the final rinse when washing your hair. (See pages 146–71.)
• Dilute lavender oil in a little almond or coconut oil and massage into the scalp to eliminate dandruff. (See pages 146–71.)

HOMEOPATHY
Constitutional treatment may be useful, but the following remedies may help:
• Arsenicum, for a dry, sensitive, hot scalp with bare patches of skin. (See page 182.)

• Nat. mur., for a white crust around the hairline, and greasy hair. (See page 206.)
• Fluoric acid, for flaky scalp and hair loss.
• Graphites, for a moist scalp with smelly crusting. (See page 196.)
• Sulfur, for thick dandruff which is itchier at night. (See page 215.)
• Sepia, for moist, greasy scalp, which is sensitive around the ears. (See page 212.)

VITAMINS AND MINERALS
• Increase your intake of selenium, vitamin E, vitamin C, B-complex vitamins, and zinc. (See pages 252–57, 264, and 265.)

Hair Loss

It is normal to shed about 150 hairs a day, but sometimes this number may be increased by various stresses on the body. Hereditary hair loss is known as alopecia. It affects men far more than women and tends to be a feature of aging, starting with a receding at the temples or forehead, which gradually progresses (though rarely ending in total baldness). Other causes of hair loss include severe illness with high fever, pregnancy and childbirth, shock, stress, damage to the skin (from burns, infection, radiation, chemical injury), skin cancer, chemotherapy, excess of vitamin A, hypothyroidism, and syphilis.

LEFT If you suffer from hair loss try drinking sage tea as it stimulates growth.

RIGHT Male pattern baldness affects over 80 percent of men to some degree.

DATA FILE

• Baldness, or alopecia, is total or partial loss of scalp hair. The condition may be temporary or permanent.

• The most common type of alopecia is pattern baldness, a hereditary trait that is expressed more often in males than in females because it depends on the influence of the male hormone testosterone.

• Pattern baldness in males extends until only a sparse growth of hair remains on the back and sides of the head. Up to 86 percent of men in the U.S. will experience some pattern balding.

• In women, baldness usually extends until only a sparse growth remains across the crown.

• Premature baldness may partly result from an imbalance of sex hormones.

• Sudden temporary hair loss sometimes occurs as a result of typhoid fever, flu, pneumonia, or stress.

• Gradual thinning of the hair may be caused by severe nutritional deficiency, tuberculosis, cancer, and disorders of the thyroid gland or pituitary gland.

• Temporary baldness may also be caused by exposure to nuclear radiation or X-rays, or by the internal use of certain anticancer drugs.

TREATMENT

CHINESE HERBALISM
• Shou Wu Pian nourishes Liver Blood, Kidney qi and jing. It is commonly used in China to keep hair from graying.
• Hair loss is attributed to Deficient Liver and Kidneys, and specific herbs to address this include wolfberry, mulberry, and fleeceflower root. *(See pages 66 and 71.)*

TRADITIONAL HOME AND FOLK REMEDIES
• Sage tea, drunk and applied externally, will stimulate hair growth.
• Nettle tea helps to cleanse the system, and encourages the growth of hair.

HERBALISM
• Improve circulation to the head with daily intake of rosemary tea and shoulder stands. *(See page 127.)*
• Massage the scalp with infused oil of fenugreek or ginger. *(See page 139.)*
• Rinse with nettle vinegar. *(See page 137.)*

AROMATHERAPY
• Lavender, rosemary, sage, cedarwood, patchouli, or ylang ylang can be massaged into the scalp and added to mild unfragranced shampoos. *(See pages 146–71.)*

HOMEOPATHY
• Lycopodium, for hair loss after childbirth. *(See page 203.)*

• Aurum, for hair loss with headaches and boils breaking out on the scalp. *(See page 184.)*
• Phosphoric acid, for hair loss after grief, and with exhaustion.
• Arnica, for hair loss starting after injury. *(See page 182.)*
• Selenium, for painful scalp and loss of body hair along with hair on head.
• Sepia, for hair loss related to the menopause and childbirth. *(See page 212.)*

VITAMINS AND MINERALS
• Increase your intake of vitamin B-complex (high-dosage tablet, twice daily), choline, inositol, calcium, magnesium, vitamins and minerals in a good supplement. *(See pages 252–5, 258, 262, and 270.)*

BELOW Make sage tea by pouring a cup of boiling water on 1-2 teaspoonsful of leaves.

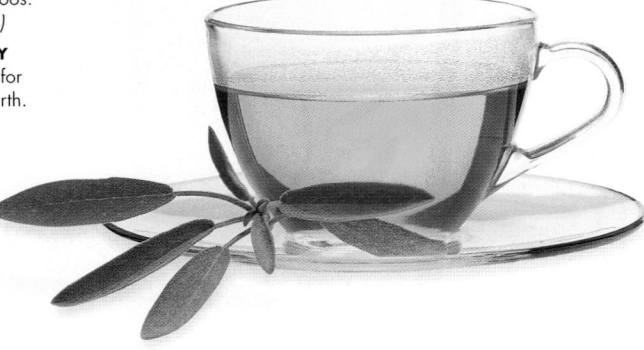

Boils

A boil is a swollen, pus-filled area occurring on the site of an infected hair follicle. The staphylococcus bacterium is usually responsible, but other causes may include eczema, scabies, diabetes, poor personal hygiene, or obesity. A boil begins as a painful red lump, then hardens and forms a yellow head. The most common areas for boils to appear are the back of the neck, the groin, and the armpits. A boil on an eyelash is known as a stye, and where a group of adjacent hair follicles are affected the resultant boil is known as a carbuncle.

SYMPTOMS

• *burning, throbbing sensation in and around the affected area* • *sensitivity to the slightest touch once pus has formed*

TREATMENT

TRADITIONAL HOME AND FOLK REMEDIES
• Apply a warm poultice made with figs or honey to the affected area. *(See pages 90 and 101.)*
• Soak a sterile cloth with hot thyme tea and hold it over the boil for a time.
• A hot cabbage leaf poultice, applied to the area, will help to draw out the infection. *(See page 85.)*
• Eat plenty of garlic if you are prone to boils; garlic is cleansing and

chronic boils indicate that you may have a high level of toxins in your body. *(See page 82.)*

HERBALISM
• Drink infusions of thyme or red clover 3 times daily during attacks. *(See page 135.)*
• Drink echinacea 2 or 3 times daily to boost the immune system and purify the blood. *(See page 120.)*

AROMATHERAPY
• A warm compress with essential oil of chamomile, lemon,

lavender, or thyme will help to bring the boil out. *(See pages 146–71.)*

HOMEOPATHY
• Belladonna, for red, tender, new boils. *(See page 183.)*
• Hep. sulf., for boils that are sensitive and weep easily. This will also bring the boil to a head. *(See page 198.)*
• Gunpowder, for weeping but not painful boils.
• Arsenicum, for burning skin aggravated by heat. *(See page 182.)*

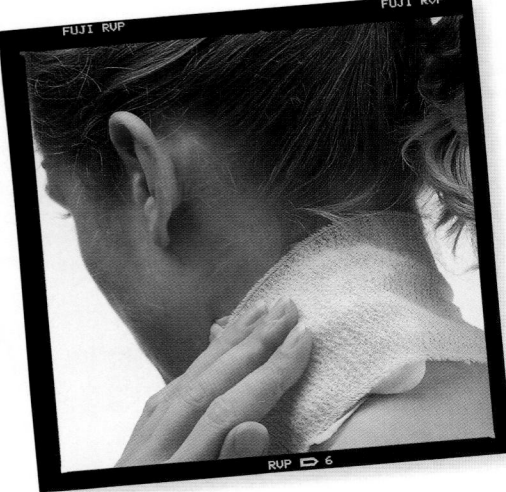

RIGHT *A warm poultice, made with mashed figs, will relieve pain and bring the boil to a head.*

Cold Sores

Cold sores are painful fluid-filled blisters which crust over after bursting. They usually appear on the mouth and around the lips or nose, sometimes in clusters. They are caused by viral infection (herpes simplex). The virus is harbored by most people, most of the time, but is most likely to cause problems when the immune system is compromised, dealing with other viral infections (such as a cold), or when one is run down. Cold sores are highly contagious.

ABOVE *A healthy diet prevents many health problems by keeping the immune system at optimum efficiency.*

CAUTION

COLD SORES ARE INFECTIOUS – WASH HANDS CAREFULLY AFTER APPLYING ANY LOTION, AND USE A PERSONAL TOWEL.

SYMPTOMS

• *pain and soreness from the characteristic crusting blister*
• *cracking and weeping may occur, particularly if sores are in the corners of the mouth*

TREATMENT

HERBALISM
• St. John's wort tincture, applied immediately, should prevent development of a sore. *(See page 124.)*
• Once the cold sore is established, myrrh tincture can be applied sparingly to help dry it up.

AROMATHERAPY
• Bergamot, eucalyptus, and tea tree oils will help to treat the blisters, and should be applied at the first sign of a sore. *(See pages 146–71.)*
• Lavender oil will help to heal blisters that erupt. *(See page 161.)*

HOMEOPATHY
Constitutional treatment is best, but the following remedies may help:

• Nat. mur., for deep cracks in the lower lip, dry mouth, and puffy burning cold sores. *(See page 206.)*
• Rhus tox., for mouth and chin sores, and ulcers at the corner of the mouth. *(See page 210.)*
• Sempervivum, for ulcers in the mouth, and bleeding gums; and when the condition is worse at night.
• Capsicum, for cracks at the corners of the mouth, pale lips, a rash on the chin, blisters on the tongue, and bad breath.

VITAMINS AND MINERALS
Cold sores tend to crop up when you feel run down, so it is important that you eat healthily and ensure that you get plenty of the following nutrients, which boost immunity:

• Wholegrain cereals like brown rice and whole-wheat bread, fruit, pulses (beans and lentils), a few nuts and seeds for their vital oils.
• A daily multivitamin and multimineral preparation – especially one containing high amounts of the antioxidant nutrients – acts to boost immune activity. *(See page 251.)*
• Vitamin C stimulates immunity and is antiviral as well as being anti-fungal. *(See page 256.)*
• Acidophilus will encourage the healthy bacteria in your gut, which will help to fight off infections and infestations. *(See page 271.)*
• Zinc stimulates the immune system, and acts as an antiviral and antifungal agent. *(See page 265.)*

Abscess

An abscess is a pocket of pus which may occur in any bacterially infected area of the body. White blood cells are sent by the body's defense system to attack the bacteria in question and they do so by engulfing them, thereby creating the pus-filled swelling. Dental abscesses (usually around the root of a tooth) are particularly common – and very painful.

SYMPTOMS

• swelling, pain, and discomfort in the affected area • the abscess and surrounding area may feel hot to the touch • fever
• nausea • sweating

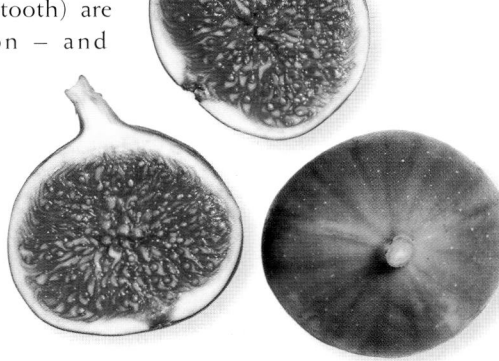
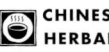

ABOVE and RIGHT
Figs are mentioned in the Bible as a treatment used by Hezekiah.

TREATMENT

AYURVEDA
• Kalanchoe may be useful.

CHINESE HERBALISM
• Treatment would address Heat and Fire poison in the Blood.
• Externally, use peony flowers or rhubarb ointment. *(See pages 67 and 73.)*
• Internally, violet, wild chrysanthemum, dandelion, and golden thread are useful. *(See page 61.)*

TRADITIONAL HOME AND FOLK REMEDIES
• Apply a warm fig or honey poultice to the abscess. *(See pages 90 and 101.)*
• Soak a sterile cloth with hot thyme tea and apply.
• A hot poultice, made with cabbage leaves, will help to draw out infection. *(See page 85.)*

HERBALISM
• Drink infusions of thyme or red clover 3 times daily during attacks. *(See page 135.)*
• Drink echinacea 2 or 3 times daily to boost the immune system and purify the blood. *(See page 120.)*

AROMATHERAPY
• A warm compress with essential oil of chamomile, lemon, lavender, or thyme will help to bring the abscess out. *(See pages 146–71.)*

HOMEOPATHY
• Hep. sulf., for an abscess which is tender, causing sharp pain. *(See page 198.)*
• Belladonna, for early stages, where there is tenderness and throbbing pain. *(See page 183.)*
• Silicea, for a slow-forming abscess, with swelling, which does not appear to come to a head. *(See page 211.)*
• Mercurius, for the early stages, if perspiration is smelly and you are irritable. *(See page 205.)*

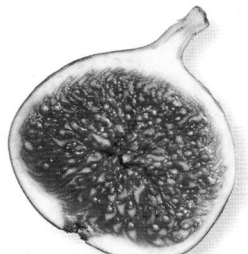

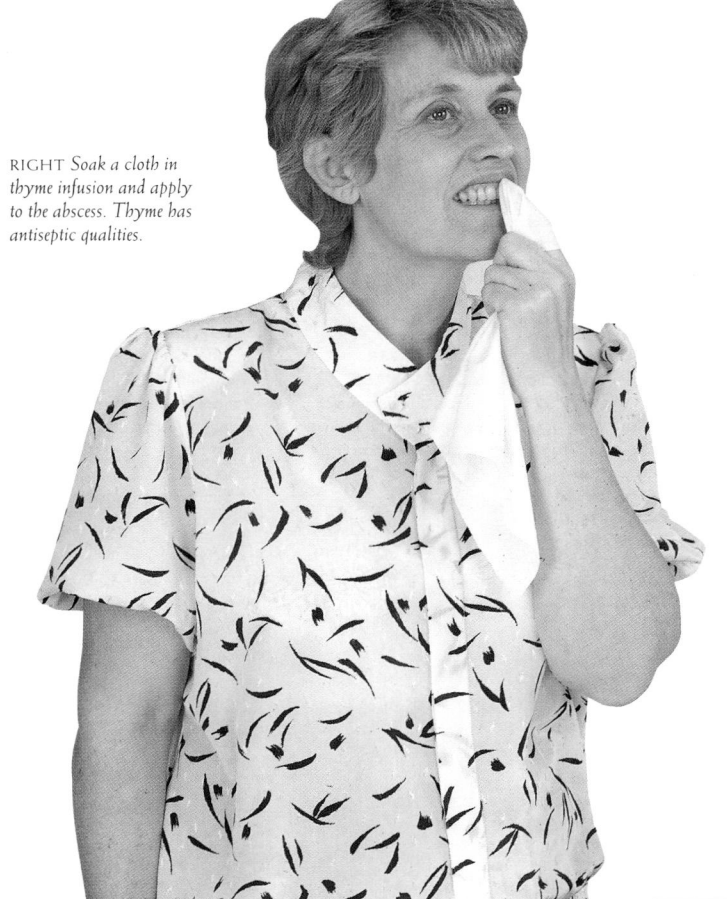

RIGHT *Soak a cloth in thyme infusion and apply to the abscess. Thyme has antiseptic qualities.*

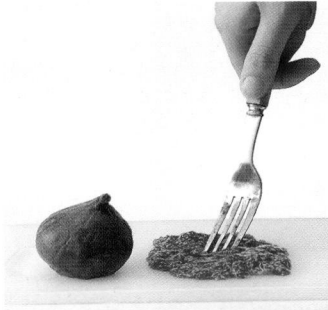

To make a warm fig poultice, you can use either lightly roasted fresh figs, or dried figs. Split the fig and mash up the soft, pulpy interior. This can be warmed by adding a little boiling water.

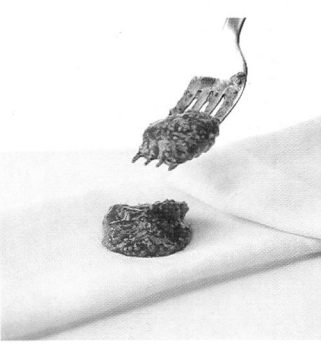

Place the mixture on a clean piece of cloth. Use either linen, gauze or cotton. The whole compress can then be warmed by placing on a hot water bottle. (This is also useful to warm it up again after it cools.) Apply to the skin.

Acne

Acne is a skin disorder most common among adolescents. It is caused by the hormonal changes at puberty, which lead to an increase in the activity of the sebaceous (oil-producing) glands. Sebaceous glands secrete through pores and hair follicles – which are most abundant on the face and scalp – a fatty lubricant known as sebum. Acne occurs when the pores become clogged with sebum. Blackheads – external plugs formed of sebum and dead cells – may be invaded by bacteria, which cause pus-filled inflammations, or pimples. The overlying skin may become stretched to the point of rupture, resulting in lesions and, in prolonged severe cases, eventual scarring. Sweating can aggravate acne, as do some oral contraceptives, lack of sunlight, poor skin hygiene, face creams, cosmetics, and exercise.

SYMPTOMS

• red spots • spots may become inflamed and infected, in which case they are extremely painful

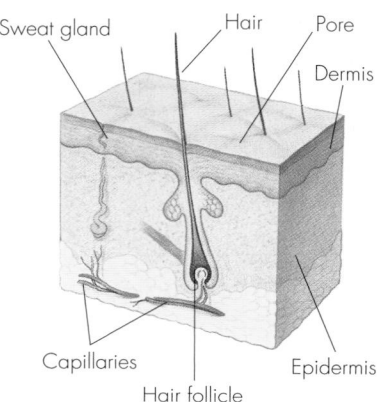

RIGHT *The structure of skin. Spots break out when the pores become blocked with sebum, which is produced to lubricate the skin.*

Sweat gland Hair Pore
Dermis
Capillaries
Hair follicle
Epidermis

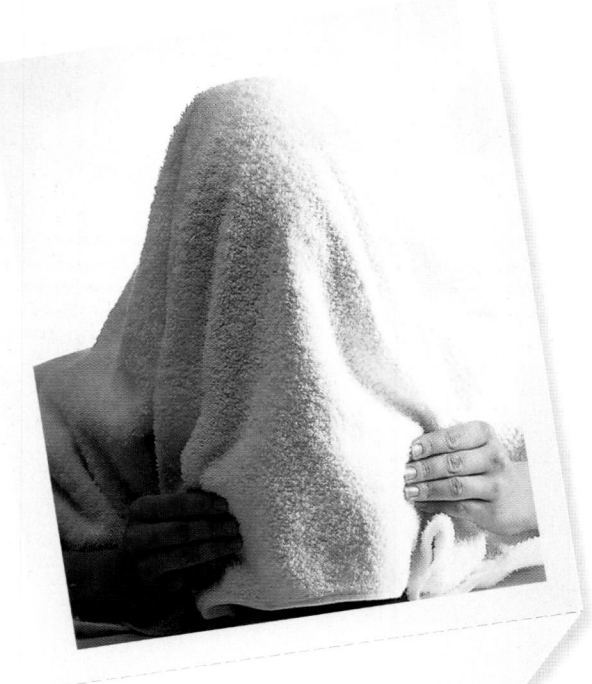

LEFT *Try steaming the face with a herbal infusion. Put chickweed, elderflower, and marigold in a bowl, and pour on boiling water.*

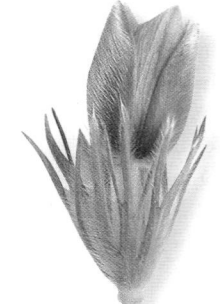

RIGHT *Pulsatilla is often prescribed by homeopaths for complaints starting in adolescence.*

TREATMENT

CHINESE HERBALISM
• Cai Feng Zhen Zhu an Chuang Wan/Margarite acne pills. This is an excellent remedy for acne. It contains Pearl.
• Treatments to clear excess Heat in the Blood and Stomach include chrysanthemum, dandelion, and honeysuckle, with cucumber and watermelon juice applied externally. *(See page 65.)*

HERBALISM
• A facial steam with chickweed, elderflower, and marigold may be useful for soothing and drawing out infection. *(See pages 117 and 130.)*
• Take echinacea, burdock root, cleavers, or yellow dock, sipped 3 times daily as a decoction, to cleanse the system and fight infection. *(See pages 115, 120, and 128.)*
• Massage comfrey ointment into any old spots to reduce scarring. *(See page 132.)*

HOMEOPATHY
Treatment should be constitutional, but the following remedies may help:
• Silicea, when there is scarring. *(See page 211.)*
• Ant. tart., for pus-filled pimples. *(See page 179.)*
• Sulfur, for chronic acne, with rough hard skin, and proneness to diarrhea. *(See page 215.)*
• Kali brom., for itchy spots, accompanied by unpleasant dreams.
• Hep. sulf., for large spots resembling boils. *(See page 198.)*
• Pulsatilla, when the spots are aggravated by rich, fatty foods; and if the sufferer dislikes stuffy rooms and is often tearful. *(See page 209.)*

FLOWER ESSENCES
• Gorse is useful for people who have given up hope of finding a cure. *(See page 240.)*

VITAMINS AND MINERALS
• Try a multivitamin and mineral supplement which is low in iodine. *(See page 261.)*
• Increase intake of vitamin E, vitamin A (as retinol, see Vitamin A, caution, page 252), zinc. *(See pages 252, 257, and 265.)*
• Eliminate processed foods.

Impetigo

Impetigo is a highly contagious skin infection caused by bacteria such as streptococci and staphylococci. Infection may follow a break in the skin or occur secondarily to dermatitis, insect bites, and fungus infections. The skin reddens and small, fluid-filled blisters appear on the surface. The blisters tend to burst, leaving moist, weeping areas underneath. The released fluid dries to leave honey-colored crusts on the skin. The infected area may spread at the edges, or another patch may develop nearby. In severe cases there may be swelling of the lymph nodes in the face or neck, accompanied by fever. Itching is common and scratching can spread the infection. It usually first appears around the mouth and nose, but can spread rapidly if other parts of the body are touched after touching a blister. It can be passed on to others by direct contact or by sharing towels. Impetigo occurs most commonly (although not exclusively) in children, particularly in hot, humid climates. Severe attacks are often attributed to poor standards of personal hygiene.

SYMPTOMS

• *reddening of affected areas* • *small fluid-filled blisters which often burst and weep, then dry out to form a yellow crust* • *itching* • *very rarely, a kidney inflammation or blood poisoning may develop*

TREATMENT

TRADITIONAL HOME AND FOLK REMEDIES
• Dab the area with cider vinegar, as often as possible throughout the day. *(See page 102.)*
• Clean the area with fresh cabbage juice 2 or 3 times daily. *(See page 85.)*
• Honey is a strong antibiotic and can be applied directly to the sores, and taken internally to boost the immune system. *(See page 101.)*

HERBALISM
• Heartsease can be taken internally or used as a wash to treat impetigo; it is both softening and drying, and can soothe the skin.

AROMATHERAPY
• A few drops of tea tree oil, applied neat to the affected area, will encourage healing and prevent the infection from spreading; it also has immuno-stimulant properties to help your body fight infection. *(See page 162.)*

HOMEOPATHY
• Antimonium, for blisters cropping up around the nostrils and mouth. *(See page 179.)*
• Arsenicum, for blisters and feelings of exhaustion and restlessness. *(See page 182.)*
• Croton, for blisters around the scrotum.

VITAMINS AND MINERALS
• Vitamin A is necessary for healthy skin. *(See page 252.)*
• Ensure that you get enough of the B-complex vitamins in your diet. *(See pages 252–5.)*
• Vitamin C will help the body to fight infection. *(See page 256.)*

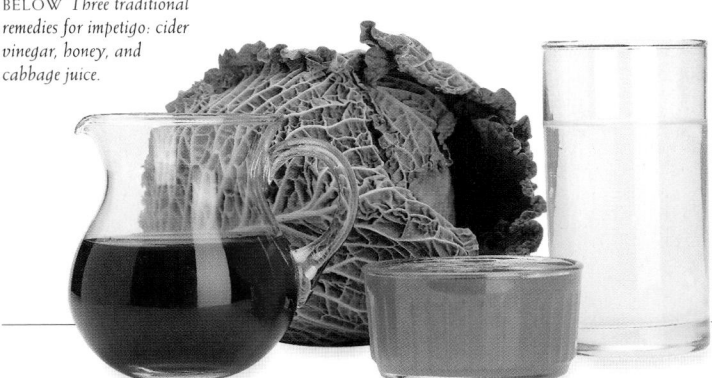

BELOW *Three traditional remedies for impetigo: cider vinegar, honey, and cabbage juice.*

Nail Problems

The nail forms a shield at the end of the fingers and toes. The nail itself is colorless and transparent, but appears pink because of the blood vessels lying under the skin. The end of the nail is white because of air beneath it. The crescent or moon, also called the lunule, located near the root of the nail, appears white because it does not firmly adhere to the connective tissue. The nail plate consists of dead, cornified cells. Nails grow from between 1/500–1/20in. (0.05–1.2mm.) per week. If the nail is lost, it takes approximately seven months to grow out fully.

Fingernails grow faster than toenails, and nails of individual fingers of the same hand grow at different rates. Growth increases during the summer, and is slower in cold climates, and sometimes during illness.

Nails are vulnerable areas and subject to several possible problems *(see Data File)*.

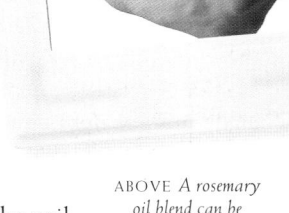

ABOVE *A rosemary oil blend can be massaged into the base of the nails to help improve circulation.*

DATA FILE

• Onycholysis – detachment of the nail from its bed. This may occur as a result of a collection of blood (a hematoma) forming underneath it, most commonly caused by injury. Other possible causes of onycholysis include psoriasis, thyrotoxicosis, and fungus infection. Complete shedding of the nail can lead to a cessation of nail growth.

• Paronychia – an infection of the soft tissue around the nail. It is usually the result of repeated minor injury, causing pain, swelling, and inflammation. Pus may sometimes appear at the nail edge.

• Horizontal ridges – these usually indicate an infection in the skin around the nail.

• Nail thickening – a feature of psoriasis and fungus infection.

• Nail-biting – an anxiety- or boredom-related habit which, in severe cases, may cause damage to the cuticles and even infection.

TREATMENT

CHINESE HERBALISM
• Brittle nails are attributed to the kidneys, and watermelon and nori (seaweed) would be advised.

AROMATHERAPY
• Add a little rosemary oil to a light carrier oil and massage into the base of the finger and toenails to improve circulation to the area. *(See page 168.)*
• Use tea tree oil on the affected area for bacterial or fungal infections. *(See page 162.)*

HOMEOPATHY
• Antimonium, for brittle, horny nails. *(See page 179.)*
• Thuja, for brittle nails with a red base. Also for ingrown toenails. *(See page 216.)*
• Graphites, for thick, deformed, brittle, painful, or crumbling nails. *(See page 196.)*
• Silicea, for deformed nails with white spots. *(See page 211.)*
• Belladonna, for the early stages of infection (yeast or bacterial). *(See page 183.)*

VITAMINS AND MINERALS
• Take zinc, vitamin C, and vitamin B-complex for fungal infections. *(See pages 252–56 and 265.)*
• White spots are often a sign of a deficiency of zinc or vitamin A. *(See pages 252 and 265.)*
• Deformed nails can be caused by deficiency of vitamins A, B-complex, and C, calcium, magnesium, zinc, and essential fatty acids. *(See pages 252–56, 258, 262, and 265.)*
• Iron deficiency can lead to nail problems; increase your iron intake. *(See page 260.)*
• Fungal infections can be improved by eating live yogurt each day, or taking acidophilus supplements. *(See page 271.)*

Edema

Edema is swelling or puffiness of tissues due to fluid retention. It is an obvious physical symptom of a number of disorders including kidney disease, heart failure, and cirrhosis of the liver. Edema may also occur as a result of injury (where the injured blood vessels are made more water-permeable) and changes in hormonal levels (before menstruation, during pregnancy, or through the use of oral contraceptives).

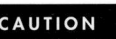

ABOVE *Evening primrose oil contains gamma-linoleic acid, which is a highly unsaturated fatty acid.*

SYMPTOMS

• *edema may be accompanied by weight gain and breathing difficulties*

TREATMENT

AYURVEDA
• Hollyhock is a diuretic, and may help ease the condition.

CHINESE HERBALISM
• The problem is thought to be due to excess water and Kidney Deficiency; useful herbs for treatment include ginseng, water plantain, poria, cinnamon twigs, and ephedra. *(See pages 59, 67, and 71.)*

• Wu Ling San pills tonify the Spleen Yang to move water and resolve edema, particularly edema of the lower abdomen.
• Jin Gui Shen Qi Wan tonifies the Kidney Yang to resolve edema, particularly of the lower legs.
• In practice, the latter two may be applicable in any particular case.

TRADITIONAL HOME AND FOLK REMEDIES
• Evening primrose oil, taken in capsule form daily, can help to prevent water retention.
• Swelling can be relieved by eating plenty of fresh apples. *(See page 94.)*
• Celery is also a good diuretic, and acts on the kidneys to encourage their action. *(See page 83.)*
• Eat fresh grapes to prevent bloating.

HERBALISM
• Yarrow, dandelion, and uva ursi are natural diuretics, and they can be drunk three times daily, as required. *(See page 112.)*

AROMATHERAPY
• Essential oils of rosemary, lavender, and geranium will help to reduce bloating and discourage depression. *(See pages 146–71.)*
• Rub a little cedarwood, fennel, rosemary, or sandalwood oils, blended in a light carrier oil, into the areas most affected, or in a whole body massage to have an overall diuretic effect. *(See pages 146–71.)*

HOMEOPATHY
• Arsenicum, when the feet and ankles are swollen, and you feel restless and chilly. *(See page 182.)*
• Apis, for swelling accompanying inflammation, with stinging pains that become worse in heat. *(See page 180.)*
• Nat. mur., for swelling in hot weather or in hot rooms. *(See page 206.)*

LEFT *Grapes have a cleansing action, and will prevent bloating. They are also rich in vitamin C.*

Scabies

Scabies is an infestation of the skin by the mite *Sarcoptes scabiei*, or itch mite. The mites burrow in the skin to lay eggs, particularly in the sides of the fingers, the elbows, groin, buttocks, nipples, and penis. The newly hatched mites reach adulthood within 14 days, and they, in turn, mate on the skin, thus perpetuating the infestation. Scabies is extremely infectious and can be transmitted by direct or indirect contact.

SYMPTOMS

• *intense itching, particularly at night* • *a rash, which may become infected as a result of scratching*

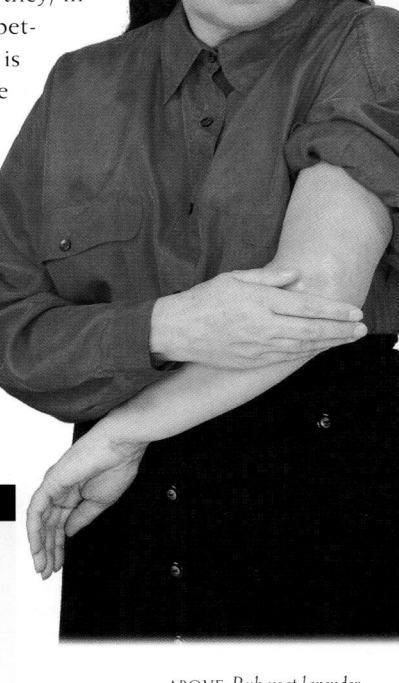

CAUTION

DO NOT GIVE SULFUR TO ANYONE SUFFERING FROM ECZEMA WITHOUT THE SUPERVISION OF A HOMEOPATH.

ABOVE *Rub neat lavender oil into the infestation as an initial measure, to help control the itching.*

TREATMENT

AROMATHERAPY
• Use tea tree or lavender oil on the sores, to heal and prevent itching and inflammation. *(See page 162.)*
• Rub the whole body with neat lavender oil, and then make a solution of lavender, aspic, and juniper in 4 teaspoons of vodka, and use that daily until symptoms improve. *(See page 161.)*

HOMEOPATHY
• Try Sulfur, given every 10 hours for 3 or 4 days, for the infected or anyone who has been in contact with someone infected. *(See page 215.)*

• Psorinum, derived from the scabies mite, may be useful.

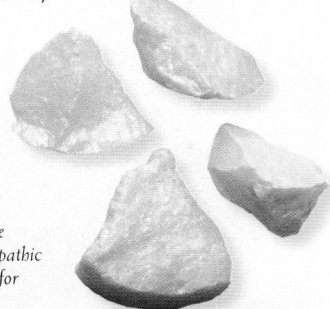

RIGHT *Sulfur is the source for the homeopathic remedy Sulfur, used for skin eruptions.*

Cellulite

Cellulite, believed to be accumulations of fat under the skin, is recognizable by its characteristic orange peel look. The uneven appearance results from the thickened fat cells, fluids, and toxins. It is far more prevalent among women than men, and is thought to have some links with female hormones. Possible triggers are poor circulation, alcohol, refined sugars, and caffeine, which contribute to the build-up of toxins in the body. Cellulite is not generally recognized as a medical condition by many doctors. Persistent, unsightly fat is often a deposit for toxins, either environmental or dietary. Exercise, skin brushing, massage, and eating as many organic and as few processed foods as possible may help.

SYMPTOMS

• *areas of skin with a dimpled orange peel appearance which may be slightly tender* • *these patches occur predominantly on the buttocks, hips, thighs, and upper arms*

CAUTION

DO NOT USE JUNIPER BERRIES IN HERBAL PREPARATIONS IF YOU HAVE DIABETES, FOR THEY LOWER THE BLOOD SUGAR. DO NOT EAT FRESH PARSLEY IN PREGNANCY.

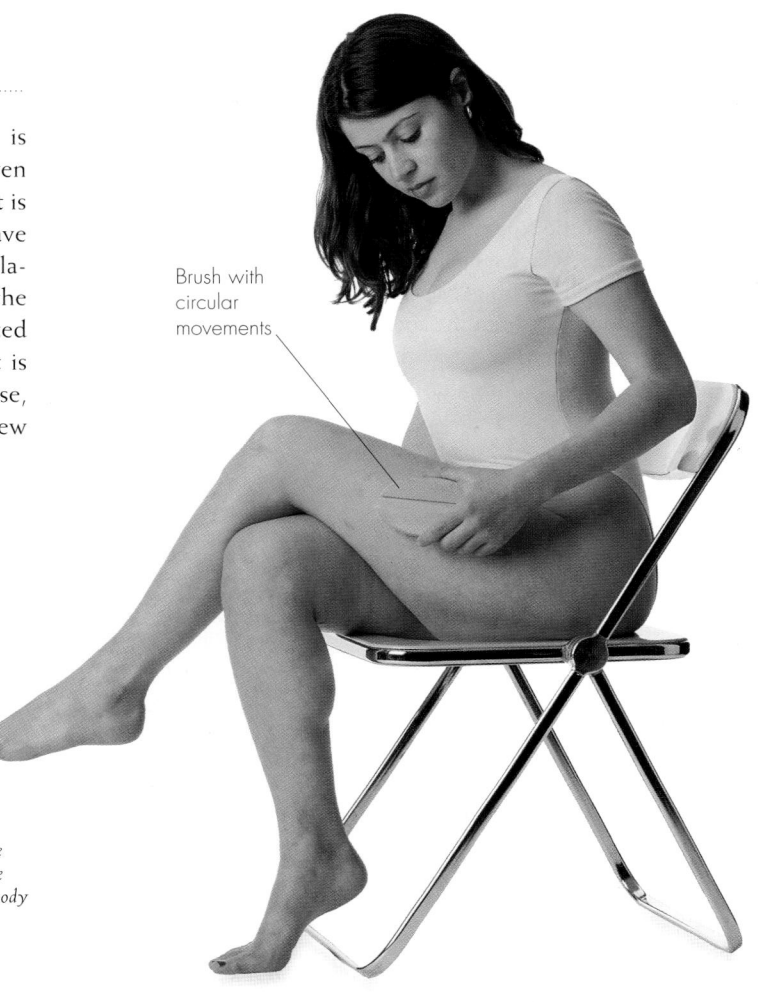

Brush with circular movements

RIGHT *Brushing the skin will stimulate the system and help the body to flush out toxins.*

TREATMENT

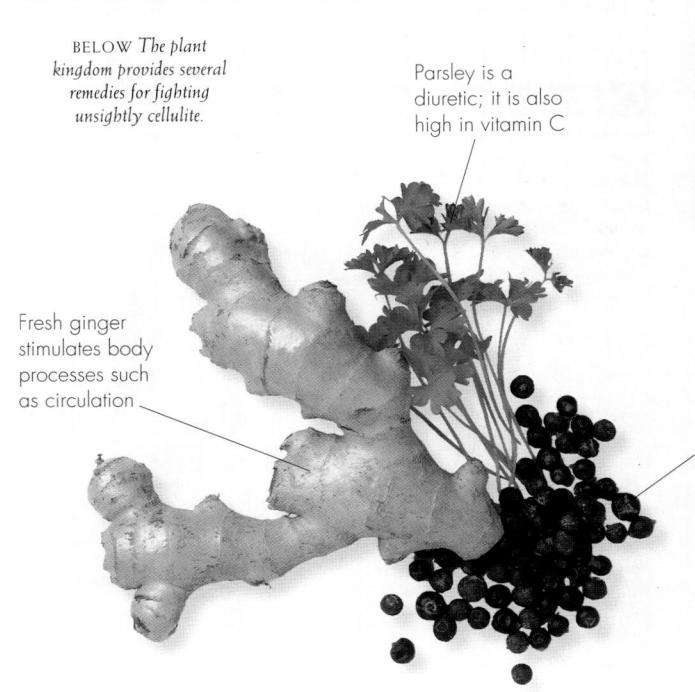

BELOW *The plant kingdom provides several remedies for fighting unsightly cellulite.*

Parsley is a diuretic; it is also high in vitamin C

Fresh ginger stimulates body processes such as circulation

Juniper's volatile oil helps cleanse the system

TRADITIONAL HOME AND FOLK REMEDIES
• Eat fresh parsley, which is a good detoxificant and diuretic.

HERBALISM
• Massage with juniper-infused oil and take a cleansing tea with herbs such as marigold. (See page 117.)

• Fresh ginger improves circulation in the body; drink an infusion, or chew fresh ginger daily to help reduce the condition. (See page 139.)
• Juniper berries are cleansing and detoxifying, and chewing them can help prevent and treat cellulite.

AROMATHERAPY
• A blend of geranium and rosemary or grapefruit, juniper or cypress used in massage and skin lotion, or add to the bath and use a loofa to stimulate the tissues. (See pages 146–71.)

• Rose oil soothes tissues, and affects the liver function, to encourage cleansing. It also strengthen the veins, which helps circulation. Add a little to the bath, or massage some into the area. (See page 168.)

VITAMINS AND MINERALS
• Avoid cigarettes, caffeine, alcohol, and other toxins, which are believed to build up in the body, and drink plenty of fresh water to flush the system.

Corns and Calluses

A callus is a hardened and thickened area of skin occurring as a result of constant friction. The skin cells respond to the friction by reproducing, which results in the characteristic hardening of skin. Calluses generally appear on the fingers and toes, knees, palms of the hands, and soles of the feet. When a callus on a toe joint becomes painful, it is known as a corn. The pain is caused by pressure on nerve endings. Soft corns can appear between the toes. Manual laborers are prone to calluses, which can be permanent, while ill-fitting shoes and high heels can be responsible for calluses on the feet or corns.

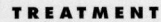

LEFT *Garlic was a traditional antiseptic treatment for dispersing hard swellings.*

TREATMENT

TRADITIONAL HOME AND FOLK REMEDIES
• Corns can be softened and treated by painting them with fresh lemon juice or vinegar. (*See page 87.*)
• Apply compresses of fresh garlic to the area. (*See page 82.*)

AYURVEDA
• Place your feet in a basin with 4 tablespoons of mustard seeds and some boiling water to soothe. (*See page 30.*)

AROMATHERAPY
• Tea tree is a good oil for skin problems, and has mild analgesic and anti-inflammatory properties, which will help to ease the discomfort of corns and calluses. (*See page 162.*)
• Pare the thickening skin away, and apply an emollient cream with rose oil. (*See page 168.*)

HOMEOPATHY
• Antimonium is the most effective remedy. (*See page 179.*)

VITAMINS AND MINERALS
• Increased intake of vitamins A and E can help to encourage the health of the skin. (*See pages 252 and 257.*)

LEFT *Lemon juice contains citric acid and will help soften hard skin.*

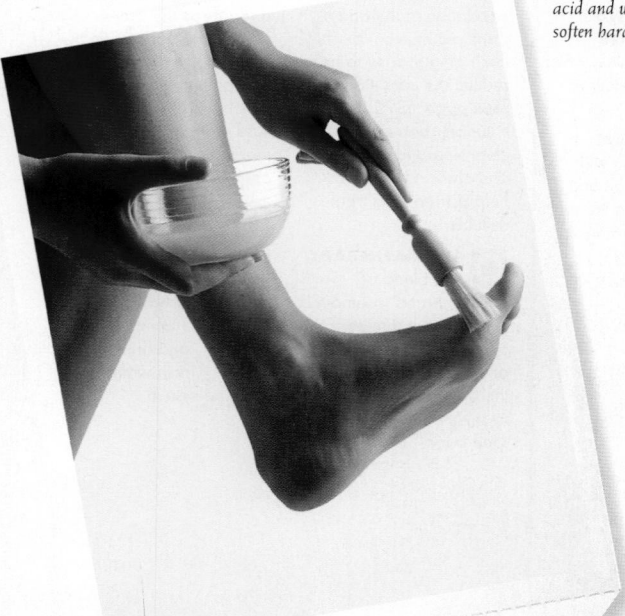

Athlete's Foot

Athlete's foot (or tinea pedis) is a fungal infection which attacks the warm, moist areas between the toes, most commonly between the fourth and fifth toes. It is highly infectious, spreading through close physical contact, notoriously in the changing facilities at public swimming baths. Once acquired, athlete's foot is very persistent. It usually affects people with particularly sweaty feet, and those whose personal hygiene is inadequate.

SYMPTOMS

• *discomfort and itching in the affected area*
• *painful cracks in the skin* • *peeling skin* • *blisters*
• *dry and scaly or damp and blistered skin*
• *unpleasant odor*
• *in severe cases the toenails may crumble*

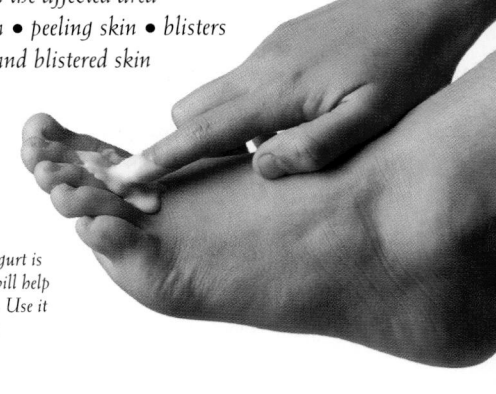

RIGHT *Live yogurt is antifungal, and will help soothe itchy skin. Use it every day.*

TREATMENT

HERBALISM
• Echinacea, marigold, and myrrh tinctures, which are antifungal, can be dabbed on the affected area as often as required. (*See pages 117 and 120*)

AROMATHERAPY
• A foot bath with tea tree oil, eucalyptus, patchouli, myrrh, and/or lavender is effective as all the oils are soothing and antifungal. Also add to unscented skin lotion. (*See pages 146–71.*)

HOMEOPATHY
• Treatment would be constitutional to boost the immune system, but Silicea might be useful. (*See page 211.*)

VITAMINS AND MINERALS
• Take extra vitamin C and zinc, to boost immune activity and help fight infection. (*See pages 256 and 265.*)

• Apply a little live yogurt to the area daily, for its antifungal properties.
• Take acidophilus tablets daily to help restore natural bacteria in the body which help to fight fungal infections. (*See page 271.*)

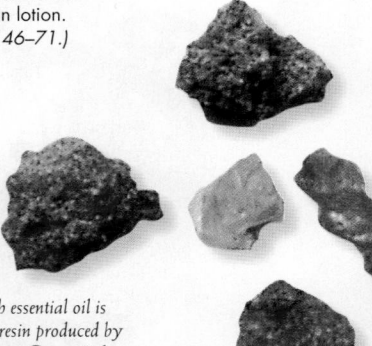

RIGHT *Myrrh essential oil is extracted from resin produced by the trunk of a tree, Commiphora myrrh. It is used to make a soothing and antifungal foot bath.*

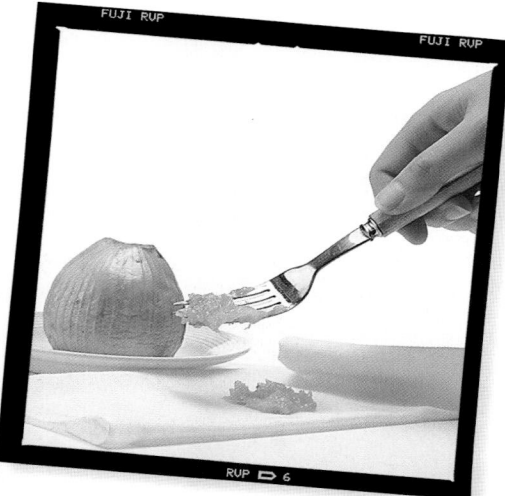

LEFT *Mash a roasted onion and make into a poultice. It will help chilblains to heal.*

Chilblains

A chilblain is a circular, raised, red swelling appearing on the fingers or toes during cold weather. It is caused by the narrowing of small arteries in the cold, which restricts the flow of blood. This leads to tissue damage in the area concerned from shortage of oxygen and glucose fuel, and bacteria may also accumulate there.

SYMPTOMS

• *pain and itching in the area of skin affected* • *swelling and redness*

TREATMENT

CHINESE HERBALISM

• Treatment would be aimed at Deficient Yang qi, and useful herbs include cinnamon twigs, red sage, angelica, dried ginger, and aconite root. *(See pages 56 and 59.)*

TRADITIONAL HOME AND FOLK REMEDIES

• Ginger, taken internally as a tea, or chewed (the root), or externally (in the bath) will warm the body, and both prevent and treat chilblains.

• A roasted onion poultice can be applied to chilblains to draw the heat to the surface and encourage healing. *(See page 82.)*
• A poultice of mustard can be applied to chilblains to warm the area. *(See page 98.)*

HERBALISM

• Nettle tea, and creams and ointments can be applied to the affected area. Drink an infusion of nettle. *(See page 137.)*

• Improve the general circulation of the body by taking rosemary tea with a pinch of cayenne. *(See pages 118 and 127.)*
• Rub a hot oil made with cayenne, pepper or mustard over the chilblain. Do not apply this if the skin is broken; use marigold ointment instead. *(See pages 117 and 118.)*
• When chilblains have caused the skin to break, apply calendula ointment to promote healing. *(See page 117.)*

AROMATHERAPY

• Lemon, lavender, chamomile, cypress, peppermint, or black pepper essential oil can be used in massage, in a bath or foot bath, or dabbed on the affected area. *(See pages 146–71.)*

HOMEOPATHY

• Agaricus, for chilblains that burn and itch and are not relieved by cold compresses.

• Petroleum, for burning, itching chilblains worsened by damp.
• Calcarea, when the chilblains are worse in cold weather, and the patient feels chilly and prone to head sweats. *(See page 186.)*
• Pulsatilla, for chilblains that are most painful when the limbs hang down, and which are worsened by warmth. *(See page 209.)*

VITAMINS AND MINERALS

• Eat plenty of garlic, and brewer's yeast, which will encourage the healthy functioning of the circulatory system.
• Increase your intake of oily fish.
• Vitamins C and E will encourage the healthy functioning of the circulatory system. *(See pages 256 and 257.)*
• Vitamin E oil, applied to burst chilblains, will help prevent scarring and encourage healing. *(See page 257.)*

BELOW *Pay attention to your diet, and aim to include foods supplying beneficial vitamins and minerals.*

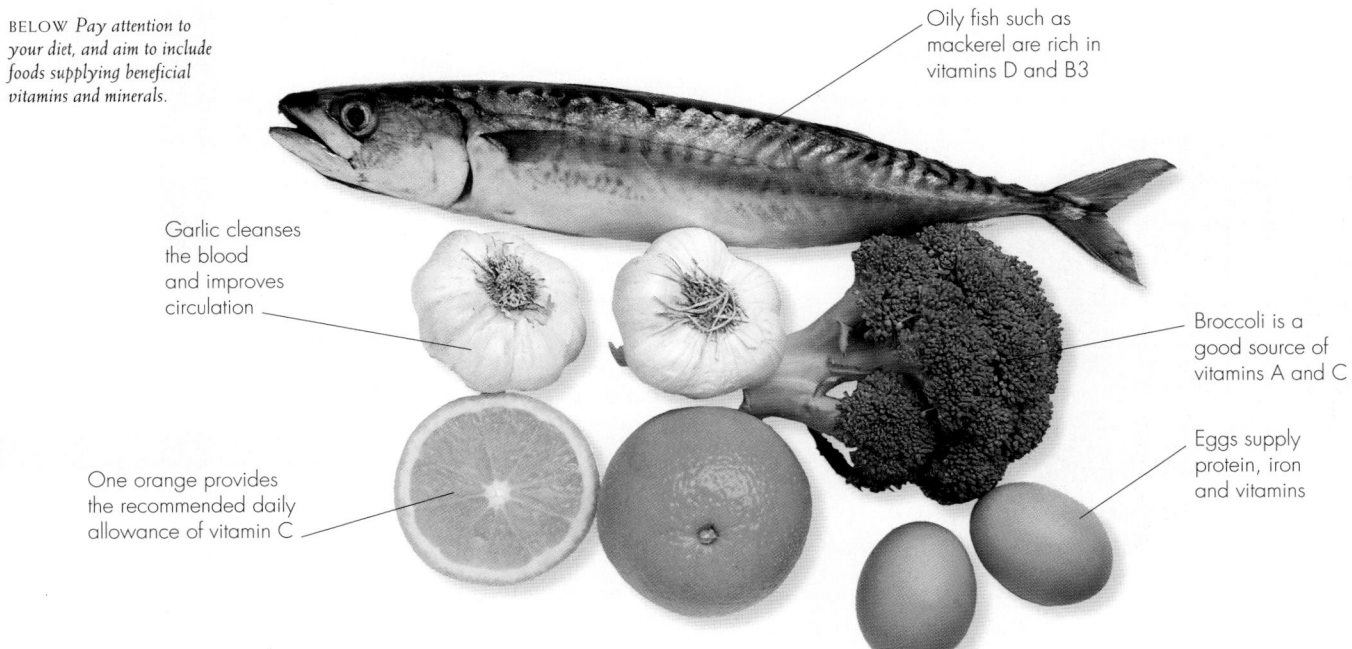

Oily fish such as mackerel are rich in vitamins D and B3

Garlic cleanses the blood and improves circulation

Broccoli is a good source of vitamins A and C

Eggs supply protein, iron and vitamins

One orange provides the recommended daily allowance of vitamin C

EYE PROBLEMS

Glaucoma

Glaucoma results from the pressure of fluid in the eyeball becoming too high. This causes compression and obstruction of the blood vessels which feed the optic nerve, resulting in optic nerve fiber damage and visual disturbances. Untreated, glaucoma leads to blindness, but is usually only found if looked for, say through routine checks. It tends to run in families, and its incidence increases with age.

SYMPTOMS

• *acute glaucoma: painful, red eye, hard and tender to touch, possibly with dilated pupil – misting of vision, then severe visual impairment – nausea and/or vomiting – possibly abdominal pain* • *a warning sign of acute glaucoma may be a sub-acute attack, usually at night. There will be: visual disturbances such as seeing concentric rings around lights – fogginess of vision – dull aching pain in the eye* • *chronic simple glaucoma: slow but progressive loss of peripheral vision which can go unnoticed until the damage is irreversible – loss of central vision follows*

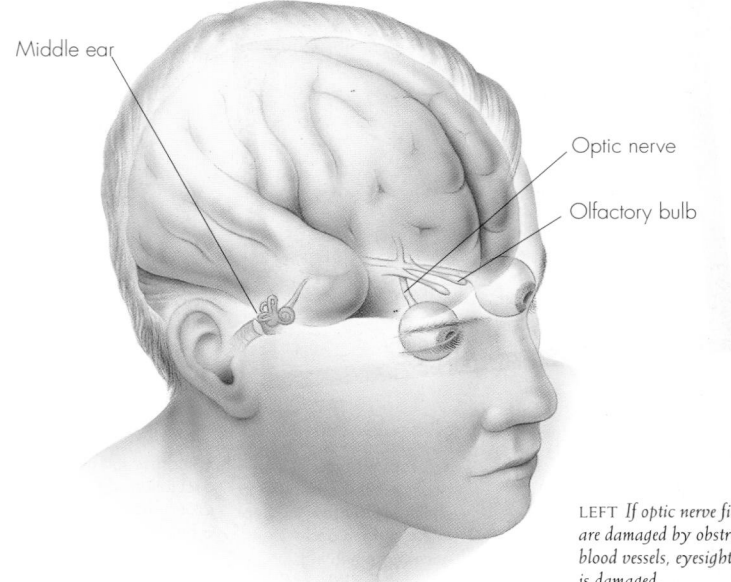

LEFT *If optic nerve fi[be]rs are damaged by obstru[cted] blood vessels, eyesight is damaged.*

TREATMENT

HOMEOPATHY
• Belladonna is the prime remedy, and it can be taken every 15 minutes, for up to 10 or 12 doses, as soon as you experience symptoms. This is suitable for chronic simple glaucoma only. *(See page 183.)*

FLOWER ESSENCES
• When symptoms begin, take Rescue Remedy or Emergency Essence, which will calm you and help you to deal with the pain. *(See page 244.)*

VITAMINS AND MINERALS
• Avoid excessive quantities of protein in your diet, which can exacerbate or contribute to glaucoma.
• Ensure you have an adequate intake of vitamins A, B1, B12, C, and the minerals chromium and zinc, which can contribute to the health of the eyes. *(See pages 252, 255, 256, 259, and 265.)*

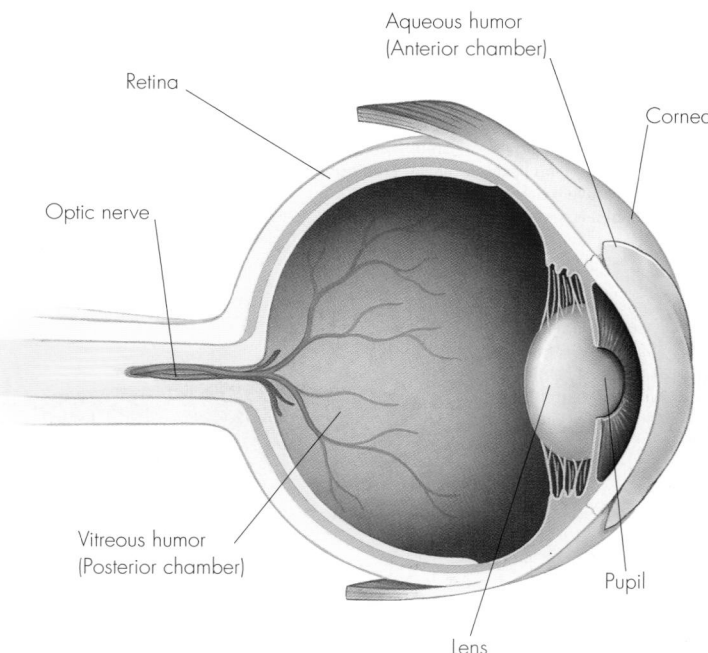

ABOVE *The eyeball is filled with fluid: if its pressure becomes too high, loss of vision ensues.*

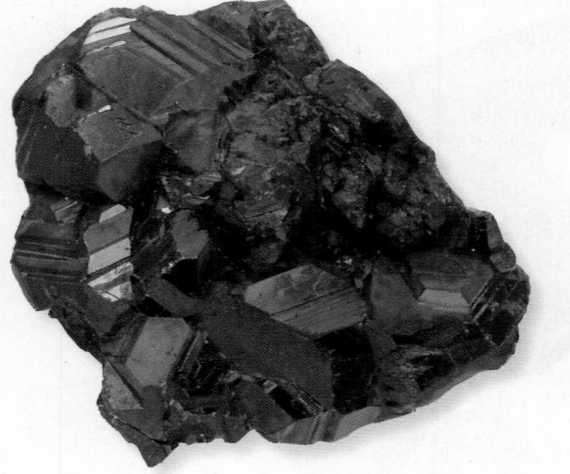

ABOVE *Vital for the protection of cell membranes, zinc can help maintain healthy eyes.*

CAUTION

SYMPTOMS OF ACUTE OR SUB-ACUTE GLAUCOMA REQUIRE URGENT MEDICAL ATTENTION.

Cataract

A cataract is an opacification of the edges of the lens of the eye which has spread inward to reach the part of the lens that is directly behind the pupil. It is caused by a coagulation of the proteins of the lens. Cataracts are often hereditary or a part of aging, but may also be a feature of Down's syndrome, diabetes, nutritional deficiencies, severe skin problems, or long-term use of steroids. Radiation or injury to the eye can also cause cataracts, and they may be present at birth as a result of German measles during pregnancy.

SYMPTOMS

• *loss of image clarity and blurring, with progressively less and less perception of detail; a person with a fully formed cataract may only be able to distinguish the presence of light and the direction from which it is coming* • *a change in the perception of colors* • *scattering of light rays caused by the opacity of the lens, which can make night driving difficult or even dangerous*

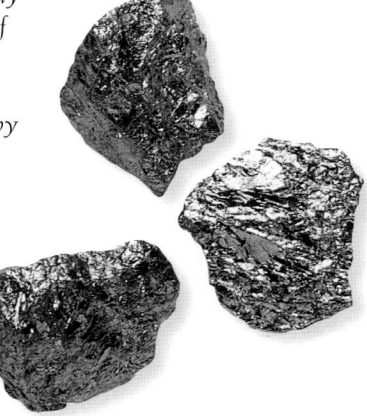

RIGHT *Silicea is prepared from silicon, found in quartz, flint, and sandstone.*

TREATMENT

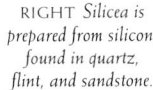 **CHINESE HERBALISM**
• Treatment would address weak Liver and Kidneys resulting from Deficient Blood. Herbal remedies might include wolfberry, chrysanthemum flowers, dendronbrum, rumania.

HOMEOPATHY
See a homeopath for constitutional treatment, or if the following remedies fail to work after about two

months. Specific remedies, which can be taken 3 times daily for up to a week, and then twice daily thereafter include:
• Silicea, if your cataract has begun to affect your sight. *(See page 211.)*
• Phosphorus, for a misting sensation. *(See page 208.)*
• Calcarea, when circular lines are evident on the lens. *(See page 186.)*

VITAMINS AND MINERALS
• Increase your intake of antioxidants, including vitamins A, C, and E, and also selenium, which prevent the growth of cataracts in the eyes. *(See pages 252, 256, 257, and 264.)*
• Bioflavonoids will also help in prevention and treatment, and these can be taken separately or in conjunction with vitamin C. *(See pages 256 and 272.)*

Black Eye

A "black eye" (known medically as a periorbital hematoma) is the result of blood being released from veins in the eyelids and surrounding area into the tissues around the eye. This produces the characteristic blackish-blue bruising. It is usually caused by a blow to the eye. The bruising can last from a few days to a month, and will go through several color changes, usually ending in pale yellow before fading completely.

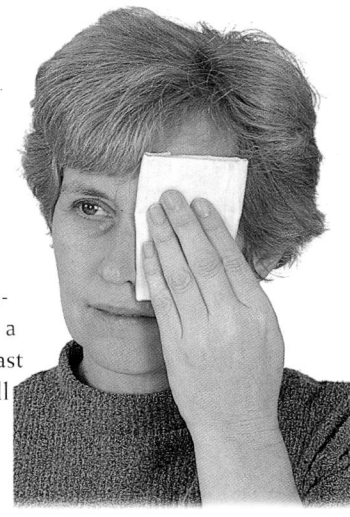

ABOVE *For a black eye, infuse lavender leaves and wrap in a handkerchief.*

SYMPTOMS

• *soreness in and around the eye* • *pain on pressure* • *in severe cases there could be swelling, which may make it difficult to open the eye*

TREATMENT

HERBALISM
• Make an infusion of fresh lavender leaves, and wrap it in a fine handkerchief. Place it on the bruised area when the leaves have cooled.

TRADITIONAL HOME AND FOLK REMEDIES
• Bruise caraway seeds, and heat them with hot, soft bread. Cool slightly and apply to the bruised area.
• A cool witch hazel compress can be applied to the area to encourage healing. *(See page 91.)*
• Place a cold compress on the area, which will reduce swelling and allow

fluid to circulate, which will facilitate healing.

AROMATHERAPY
• A few drops of calendula, lavender, and marjoram oil can be placed on a cool cloth and applied to the bruise. Avoid the eyelids and the corner of the eye. *(See pages 146–71.)*

HOMEOPATHY
• Arnica should be taken as soon as possible after the injury, and continued until the bruising disappears. Follow this with Ledum, which will disperse the swelling. *(See page 182.)*
• Aconite is useful in the initial stages, following

the blow or trauma to the area. *(See page 178.)*

FLOWER ESSENCES
• Use Rescue Remedy or Emergency Essence cream and lightly dab over the affected area to help the healing process. *(See page 244.)*
• Rescue Remedy or Emergency Essence can be taken internally after the trauma to help you cope with pain and encourage healing. *(See page 244.)*

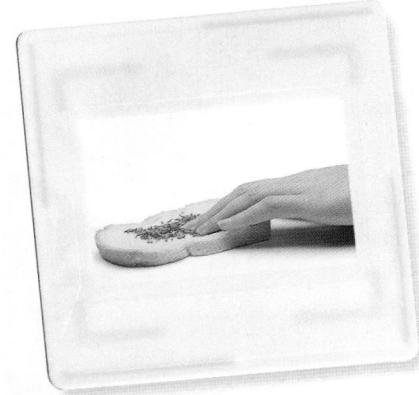

LEFT *Bruise caraway seeds in a pestle and mortar, and spread on soft bread. Heat, and apply to the area.*

Conjunctivitis

Conjunctivitis is an inflammation of the conjunctiva (the mucous membrane that covers the outer layer of the eyeball and lines the eyelids). It is generally caused by either viral or bacterial infection, or by an allergic reaction to substances such as pollen, cosmetics, and solutions used for contact lenses. Either one or both eyes may be affected. Viral conjunctivitis is a common ailment which sometimes occurs in epidemic proportions, spreading rapidly.

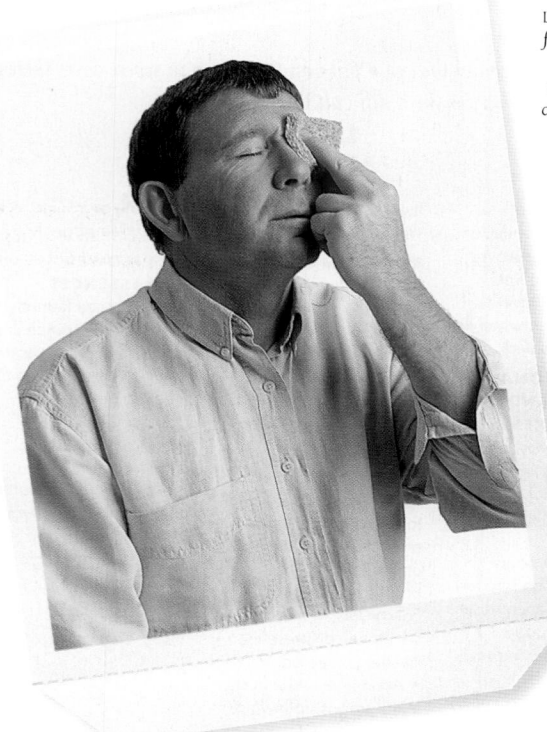

ABOVE *Drink sage infusion to invigorate the immune system.*

LEFT *Cut the crusts from a slice of bread and put it in the refrigerator. When cold, hold to the eye.*

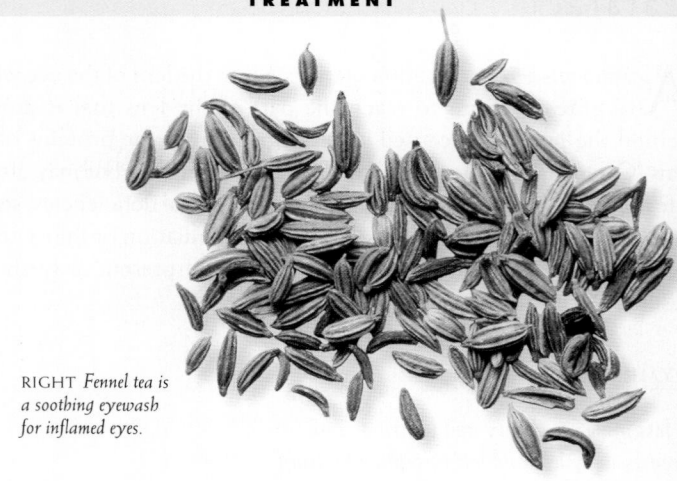

RIGHT *Fennel tea is a soothing eyewash for inflamed eyes.*

SYMPTOMS

• *redness and soreness with irritation, dryness, and grittiness of the eyes* • *possibly slightly blurred vision* • *bacterial conjunctivitis produces a yellow discharge which hardens during sleep, causing stickiness in and around the eye* • *viral conjunctivitis produces only minimal discharge*
• *swollen and puffy eyelids in allergic conjunctivitis, but no discharge*

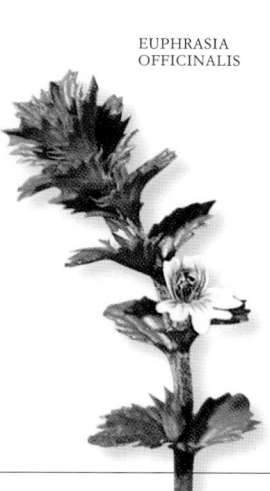

EUPHRASIA
OFFICINALIS

AYURVEDA
• Treatment would consist of panchakarma treatment (detoxification), and nasya, together with inhalations and an eyewash. Treatment would be specific to your needs. *(See page 20.)*

CHINESE HERBALISM
• The source of the problem is believed to be Wind Heat in the Liver meridians, and herbal treatment might include bamboo leaves, violets, and chrysanthemum flowers. Boil these together, strain, and use the cool water to bathe the eyes.

TRADITIONAL HOME AND FOLK REMEDIES
• Apply cold bread to closed eyes to reduce the inflammation of conjunctivitis, and soothe itching. *(See page 101.)*
• Boil fennel seeds to make an eyewash for conjunctivitis and sore, inflamed eyes.

• Honey water can be used to cleanse the eye; it acts to destroy any infection, soothe, and encourage healing. *(See page 101.)*

HERBALISM
• Infusions of the following herbs can be taken internally to ease the condition: echinacea (which boosts the immune system and acts as a natural antibiotic), eyebright, golden seal, sage. *(See pages 120 and 129.)*
• Infusions of chamomile, elderflower, eyebright, and golden seal can be applied externally. A tincture of some of these herbs can also be used to make an eyewash. *(See pages 119 and 130.)*

AROMATHERAPY
• Make a warm compress with a few drops of lavender, chamomile, or rose oil, and apply to the affected area to encourage healing and draw out infection. *(See pages 146–71.)*

HOMEOPATHY
• Euphrasia is suitable for burning, itchy eyes. *(See page 194.)*
• One or two drops of Euphrasia tincture can also be used to bathe the eyes. *(See page 194.)*
• Pulsatilla can be used when there is mucus collecting in the corner of the eyes. *(See page 209.)*
• Hep. sulf. will be useful to draw out infection. *(See page 198.)*

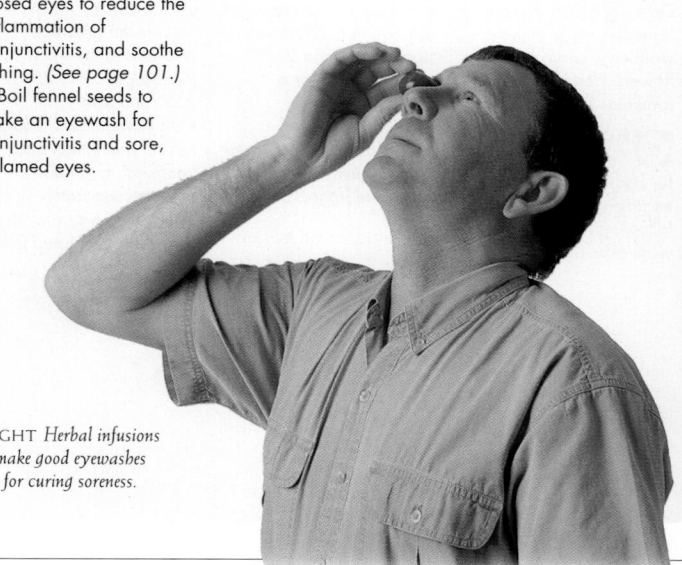

RIGHT *Herbal infusions make good eyewashes for curing soreness.*

Stye

A stye is an abscess occurring around the root of an eyelash, usually caused by staphylococcal bacteria. A collection of pus at the base of the eyelash produces the characteristic small, yellow head. Styes usually last for around seven days, but the infection may spread to adjacent follicles. They tend to occur when general resistance is low.

SYMPTOMS

• *redness, soreness, and swelling* • *pain and sometimes irritation*

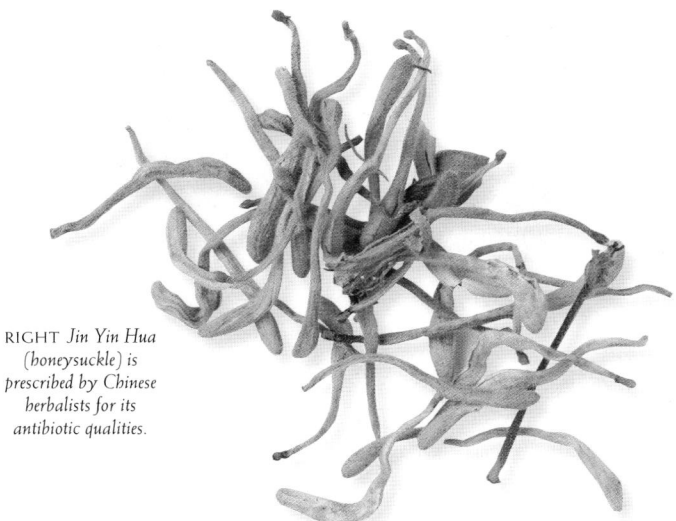

RIGHT *Jin Yin Hua (honeysuckle) is prescribed by Chinese herbalists for its antibiotic qualities.*

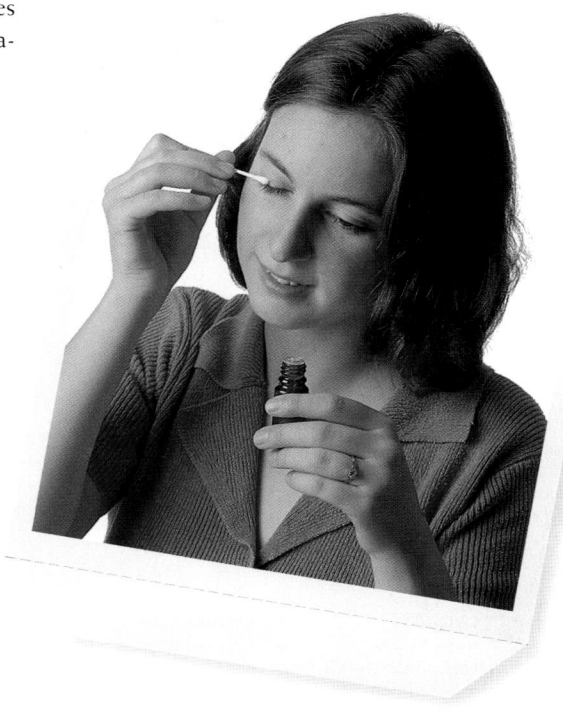

LEFT *Dab a stye with tea tree oil to utilize its bactericidal properties.*

TREATMENT

CHINESE HERBALISM
• Anti-inflammatory herbs, and herbs to detoxify and boost the immune system will be appropriate, including the preparation Jin Yin Hua, which acts as an antibiotic to help fight the bacterial infection. *(See page 65.)*

TRADITIONAL HOME AND FOLK REMEDIES
• A warm bread poultice applied directly to the stye will help bring out the infection. *(See page 101.)*

HERBALISM
• Echinacea and poke root will boost the immune system, which is particularly useful if you suffer from recurrent styes. *(See page 120.)*
• Chamomile or eyebright can help to reduce swelling. *(See page 119.)*
• Marigold tincture can be applied directly to the stye, and taken internally to boost the immune system. *(See page 117.)*

AROMATHERAPY
• A drop of lavender or tea tree oil, on a cotton swab, can be dabbed at the base of the stye. Take care not to let it enter your eyes. *(See pages 146–71.)*

HOMEOPATHY
Recurrent styes should be treated constitutionally, and your homeopath will take steps to improve your overall immune response.
• Pulsatilla, in the first instance. *(See page 209.)*
• If this does not work, try Staphisagria, every hour, for up to 10 doses.

CAUTION
RECURRENT EPISODES OF STYES MAY BE AN INDICATION OF DIABETES AND SHOULD THEREFORE BE INVESTIGATED.

RIGHT *Marigold treats all skin inflammations. Apply tincture to a stye.*

Eyestrain

Eyestrain is used to describe any discomfort or distress related to the eyes or seeing. It is not, however, a medical term. The body's response to visual difficulty is to contract the muscles around the eye, and it is this that may cause the sensation of strain. Prolonged and constant use of a VDU system, intense periods of reading, wearing incorrectly prescribed glasses, and working in bad light can all lead to eyestrain, but these things do not necessarily damage the eyes as is popularly believed.

SYMPTOMS

- *feeling of tightness around the eyes*
- *focusing difficulties* • *recurrent headaches, particularly across the forehead and behind the eyes*

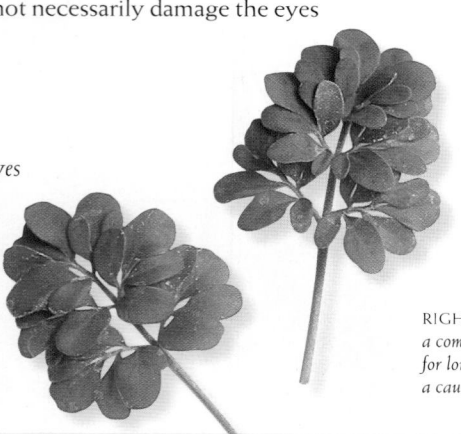

RIGHT *Rue, itself an antispasmodic, is the source of Ruta, a homeopathic remedy sometimes prescribed for eyestrain.*

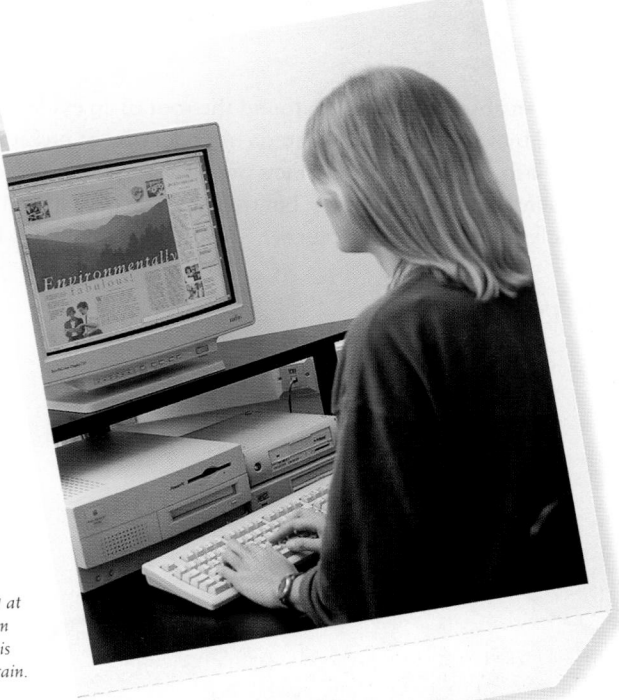

RIGHT *Staring at a computer screen for long periods is a cause of eyestrain.*

TREATMENT

TRADITIONAL FOLK AND HOME REMEDIES
- A slice of cucumber over tired, strained eyes is invigorating and soothing. *(See page 89.)*
- Drink fresh lemon juice, which is restorative. *(See page 87.)*
- Roast an apple and apply the pulp to the eye area to relieve inflamed or tired eyes. *(See page 94.)*
- The ancient Greeks used fresh white cabbage juice, mixed with a small amount of honey, to relieve sore or inflamed eyes. *(See page 85.)*

CHINESE HERBALISM
- Chinese practitioners believe that eye problems may be due to exhausted Blood, and the following herbs may be useful: wolfberry, mulberry, chrysanthemum flowers, and cassia seed. *(See page 66.)*

HERBALISM
- Cool compresses of chickweed, eyebright, or marigold should be placed over the eyes and left for 10–15 minutes. *(See page 117.)*

AROMATHERAPY
- A few drops of fennel oil, on a cool compress laid over the eye area, will soothe puffy, inflamed eyes. *(See page 159.)*
- Add 1 drop of lemon or rose aromatherapy oil to 2 tablespoons of carrier oil, and massage into the temples and the bony areas around the eyes (avoid the immediate eye area). *(See pages 146–71.)*

HOMEOPATHY
- The following remedies can be taken up to 4 times per day for a week. If the symptoms persist, see your homeopath.
- Ruta, when eyes feel strained after reading for long periods; also good for a burning sensation. *(See page 210.)*
- Arnica, for tired eyes resulting from long periods of driving and looking into the distance. *(See page 182.)*

- Nat. mur., when eyes are painful on looking up, down, or sideways. *(See page 206.)*

VITAMINS AND MINERALS
- Vitamin A and vitamin B12 are useful if you suffer from periodic or chronic eyestrain. *(See pages 252 and 255.)*

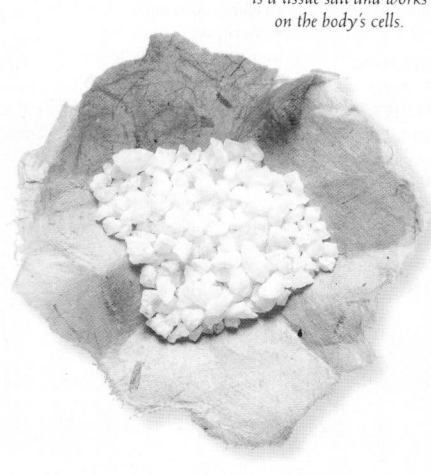

BELOW *Natrum mur. is a tissue salt and works on the body's cells.*

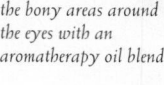

RIGHT *Massage the bony areas around the eyes with an aromatherapy oil blend.*

Squint

A squint (or strabismus) is a condition in which only one eye focuses on an object of interest. In a divergent squint the other eye looks outward, while in a convergent squint it looks inward. A squint in children may be caused by congenital hypermetropia (long-sightedness), or physical defects in the cornea, lens, retina, nerves, and muscles of the eye. Acquired in adulthood, a squint is usually indicative of an underlying disease elsewhere in the body (possibly encephalitis, meningitis, septicemia, syphilis, or various brain disorders).

LEFT Gelsemium remedy, first made in 1862 from the false jasmine plant, may help a squint.

SYMPTOMS

• *in addition to the characteristic squint appearance adults may also experience double vision*

CAUTION

IF YOU BEGIN TO EXPERIENCE DOUBLE VISION, SEE YOUR PHYSICIAN.

TREATMENT

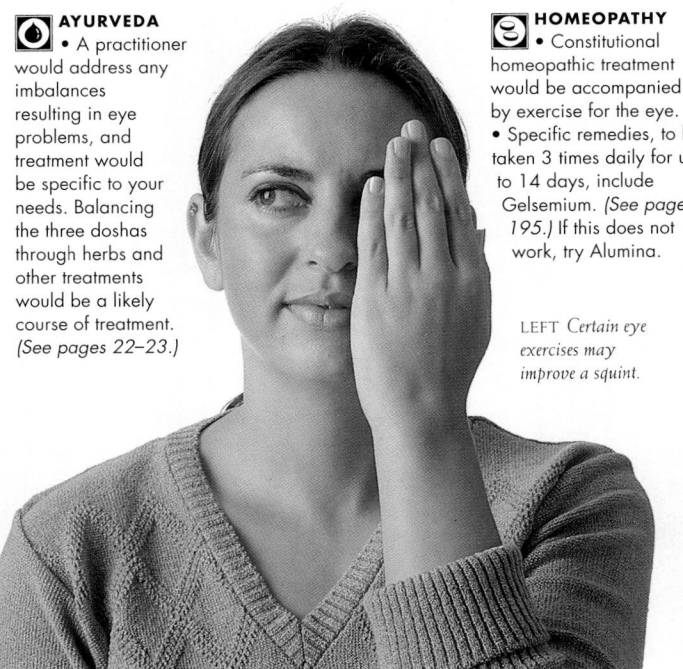

AYURVEDA
• A practitioner would address any imbalances resulting in eye problems, and treatment would be specific to your needs. Balancing the three doshas through herbs and other treatments would be a likely course of treatment. *(See pages 22–23.)*

HOMEOPATHY
• Constitutional homeopathic treatment would be accompanied by exercise for the eye.
• Specific remedies, to be taken 3 times daily for up to 14 days, include Gelsemium. *(See page 195.)* If this does not work, try Alumina.

LEFT Certain eye exercises may improve a squint.

Twitching Eyelids

Twitching (fasciculation) of the eyelids is caused by a brief, involuntary contraction of the flat muscle around the eye. It is a very common phenomenon and is only a cause for concern if it is very persistent, as it may then be an indication of nerve disease. A twitch or tic commonly affecting adults is blepharospasm, in which there is spasmodic closure of one or both eyes. This is usually a feature of psychological disturbance and may be associated with other bodily tics.

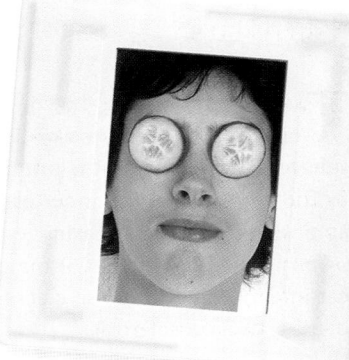

ABOVE Cucumber is cooling and refreshing for irritated eyes.

TREATMENT

TRADITIONAL HOME AND FOLK REMEDIES
• Place a slice of cucumber on the eyes to soothe and reduce irritation. *(See page 89.)*

HERBALISM
• Because most twitches are caused by tension or tiredness, relaxing herbs would be prescribed, including chamomile, lavender, and vervain. Drink as infusions. *(See pages 119 and 138.)*

AROMATHERAPY
• A few drops of lavender or marjoram oil added to the bath will relax and rejuvenate. *(See pages 161 and 165.)*
• Try a few drops of chamomile or rose oil on a cool compress, placed over the eye area, and massage a drop in a light carrier oil into the muscles surrounding the eye area. Avoid the immediate eye area. *(See pages 150 and 168.)*

HOMEOPATHY
• Constitutional treatment would be most appropriate, but the following remedies can be taken every 4 hours for up to 6 doses:
• Pulsatilla, for twitching accompanied by inflammation of the eye. *(See page 209.)*
• Codeinum, for twitching eyelids.

FLOWER ESSENCES
• Vervain is useful for those whose overenthusiasm is putting them under stress. *(See page 241.)*
• Hornbeam, for exhaustion and the feeling of being in a rut. *(See page 227.)*
• Impatiens, for irritability and a rushed lifestyle. *(See page 233.)*

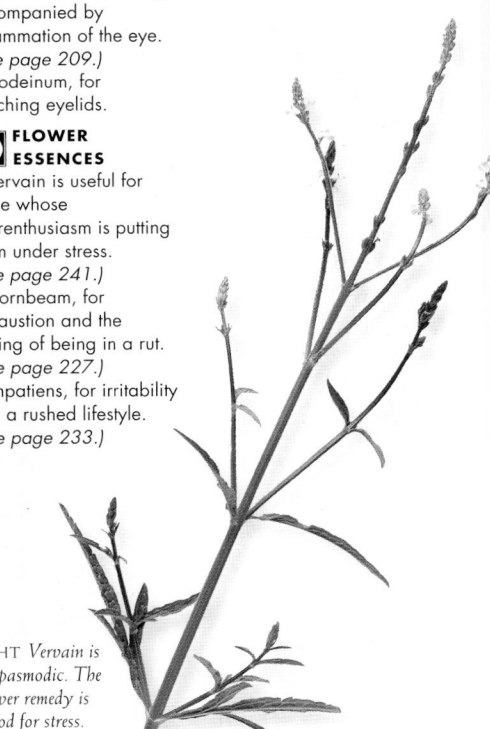

RIGHT Vervain is antispasmodic. The flower remedy is good for stress.

EAR PROBLEMS

Tinnitus

Tinnitus is a hissing, buzzing, whistling, or ringing sound experienced in the ear (one or both). It is usually continuous, but the sufferer's awareness of it is intermittent. Tinnitus is related to damage to the hair cells of the inner ear. Persistent tinnitus is usually associated with a degree of hearing loss, and can be triggered by explosions or prolonged loud noise. It may also be a symptom of colds and flu, ear infections and excessive ear wax, brain or head injuries, Ménière's disease, and otosclerosis.

DATA FILE

• The ringing, roaring, clicking, or hissing sounds heard with tinnitus are actually warning signs of such things as infection, Ménière's disease, and otosclerosis. They may also be caused by hard masses of wax in the ear; a stuffy nose; such drugs as quinine, antibiotics, aspirin, and alcohol; and excessive smoking.

• Sensorineural hearing loss is often accompanied by ear noise, or tinnitus. Because the inner ear has no pain fibers, damage is not accompanied by pain.

• More people lose hearing today than in past years; the average pop concert or stereo headset can impair hearing in less than a half-hour.

• About 30 percent of adults over 65 have hearing loss, and as much as one-third of cases are associated with exposure to loud noise.

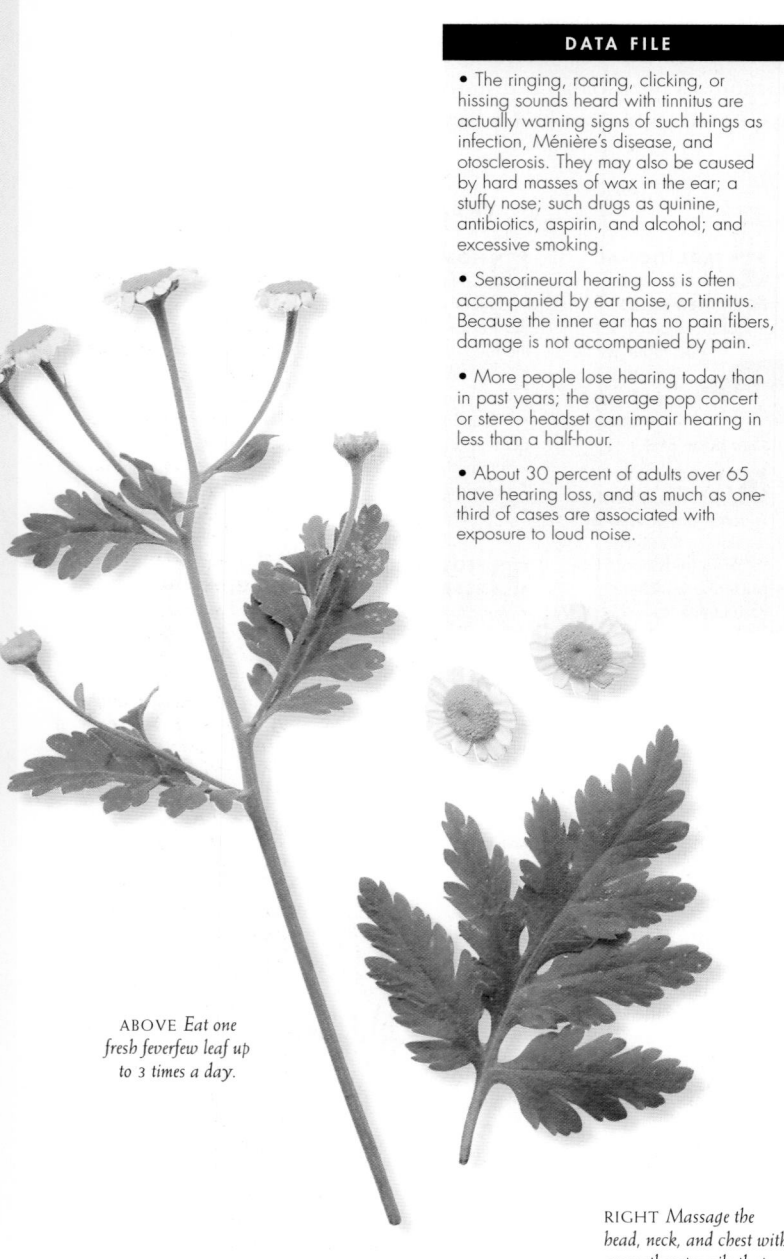

ABOVE *Eat one fresh feverfew leaf up to 3 times a day.*

RIGHT *Massage the head, neck, and chest with aromatherapy oils that increase circulation.*

TREATMENT

CHINESE HERBALISM
• A herbalist might treat a Blood Deficiency, and use the following herbs: Shu di Huang and Tu Su Zi, which are commonly used in the treatment of tinnitus. *(See pages 62 and 73.)*

HERBALISM
• For tinnitus caused by blood congestion or pressure in the head, try black cohosh. Use 10–30 drops of tincture diluted in water, and drink it as often as necessary.
• Feverfew is effective for tinnitus, and taken daily may prevent attacks. *(See page 133.)*
• Tinnitus caused by poor circulation or high blood pressure may respond to treatment with hawthorn. *(See page 119.)*

AROMATHERAPY
• Use oils which increase the circulation, including rosemary, cypress, lemon, and rose. Massage of the head, neck, and chest using these oils may help, as will one or more in a blend heated in a vaporizer or burner. *(See pages 146–71.)*

HOMEOPATHY
• Treatment should be constitutional, but some remedies which may help include:
• Salicylic acid, for roaring in the ears, dizziness, and deafness.
• China sulf., for any buzzing, hissing, or singing sounds in the ears.
• Kali iod., for ringing in the ears and no other obvious symptoms.

VITAMINS AND MINERALS
• Try increasing the following nutrients in your diet: magnesium, potassium, and manganese. Deficiency of these has been linked with tinnitus. *(See pages 262 and 263.)*
• Eat plenty of food rich in vitamins A and C, and bioflavonoids, which are very good for circulation. *(See pages 252 and 256.)*

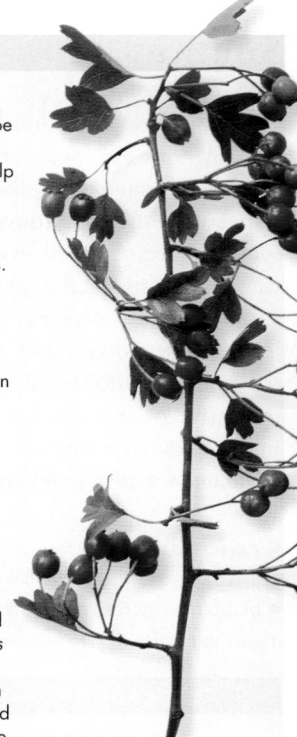

ABOVE *Hawthorn is a tonic for the circulatory system, which may help some cases of tinnitus.*

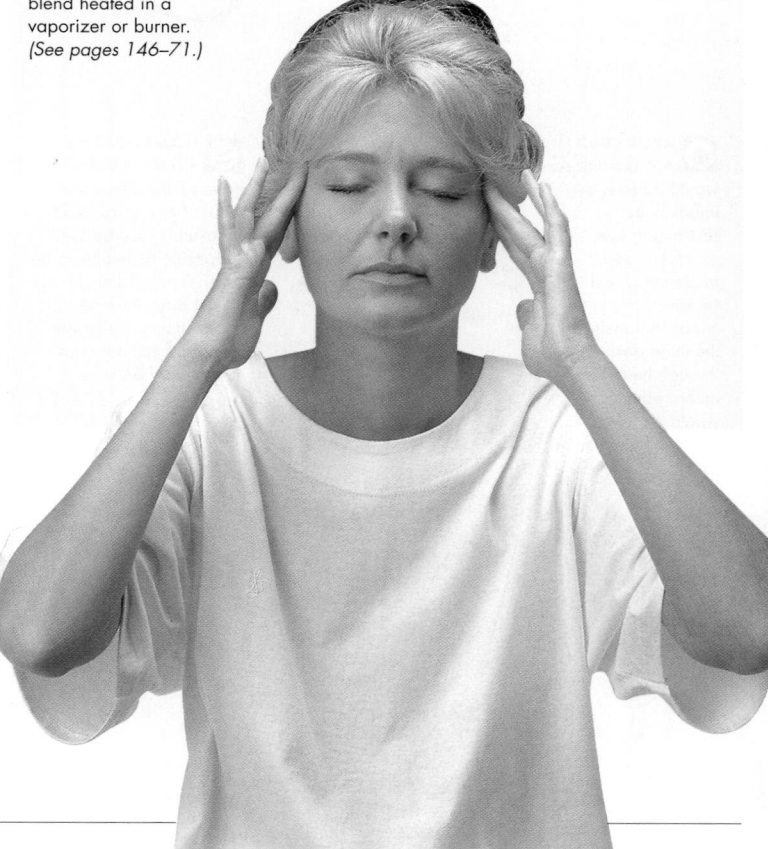

Middle Ear Infection (Otitis Media)

The most common ear infections are middle ear infections (otitis media). The middle ear is located behind the eardrum and connected to the throat by the Eustachian tube. Bacteria may therefore travel to the middle ear from the throat when infections occur there, or they may also enter through a perforation in the eardrum. The eardrum may be perforated, or ruptured, by shattering blasts or sharp objects, as well as by infection. Very loud noises, a change in pressure (such as when flying), and violent sneezing while suffering an ear infection may also, in some cases, cause perforation.

Young children, with shorter and straighter Eustachian tubes than adults, are especially prone to middle ear infections. The tendency is also apparently inherited. Chronic infections may also be associated with allergies, tuberculosis, measles, and other diseases.

ABOVE *Garlic's medicinal properties will help to combat ear infections.*

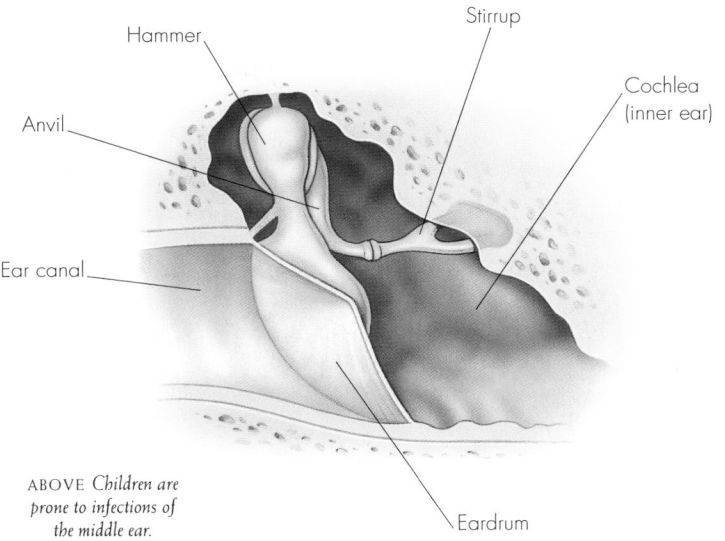

ABOVE *Children are prone to infections of the middle ear.*

SYMPTOMS

• *intense pain* • *fever* • *in severe cases pressure in the middle ear builds up to such an extent that the eardrum perforates in order to release the discharge; this may lead to external ear infection and a degree of temporary or permanent hearing loss*

CAUTION

ALWAYS CONSULT YOUR PHYSICIAN IF THE EAR DRUM "BURSTS" OR PERFORATES, AS IT CAN LEAD TO SERIOUS COMPLICATIONS, INCLUDING DEAFNESS AND, IN SOME CASES, MENINGITIS.

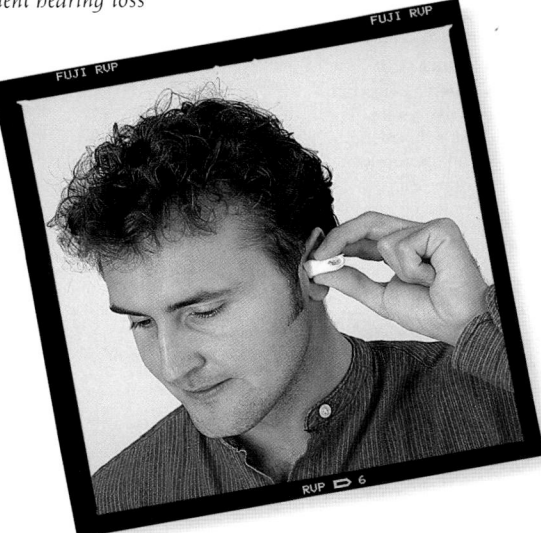

RIGHT *Wrap a piece of garlic in gauze, warm it, and insert gently into the ear canal.*

TREATMENT

AYURVEDA
• Purified and concentrated extracts of garlic might be used to control and treat infection. *(See page 26.)*
• Panchakarma would be appropriate. *(See page 22.)*

TRADITIONAL HOME AND FOLK REMEDIES
• Peel the skin from a bud of garlic, and cut to fit the outside of the ear canal. Wrap in a piece of gauze, heat gently, and insert into the canal. *(See page 82.)*

HERBALISM
• Mullein oil is a traditional herbal treatment. Place a few drops on a cotton ball and gently place in the ear canal. *(See page 137.)*
• Anti-inflammatory and antibacterial herbs include chamomile, echinacea, golden rod, and golden seal, and they can be taken internally or infused and dropped into the ear canal. *(See pages 119 and 120.)*
• Steep yarrow and pour the warm liquid into the ear canal to soothe and reduce infection. *(See page 112.)*

AROMATHERAPY
• Massage a blend of anti-infectious oils around the ear and down the neck. Suitable oils include lavender, chamomile, and tea tree. *(See pages 146–71.)*
• Mix a drop of clove oil in a little grapeseed carrier oil and massage around the neck and ear. *(See pages 146–71.)*

HOMEOPATHY
• Chronic ear infections should be treated constitutionally. Acute attacks may respond to the following, taken every half-hour for up to 10 doses.
• Hep. sulf. may be useful for infection accompanied by sharp pain. *(See page 198.)*
• Belladonna, for a throbbing earache with redness around the ear, accompanied by fever. *(See page 183.)*
• Aconite, for an attack which comes on suddenly, particularly after exposure to cold. *(See page 178.)*
• Pulsatilla, when there is pain, as if the eardrum is being pushed out. *(See page 209.)*

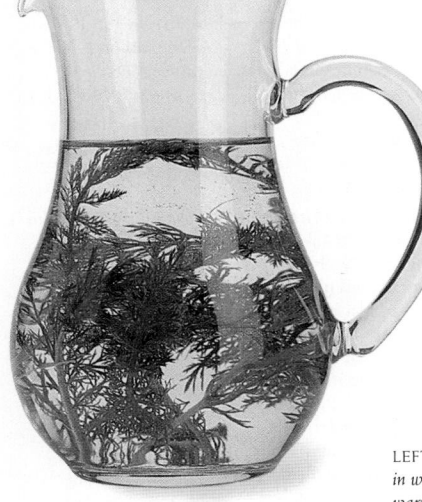

LEFT *Steep yarrow leaves in water, and pour the warm liquid into the ear.*

Outer Ear Infection (Otitis externa)

An inflammation or infection of the outer ear can cause severe pain, possibly a discharge, and impaired hearing. Such symptoms may be due to a number of factors, such as infection by fungi or bacteria, or a foreign body in the ear. Boils or abscesses lead to a build-up of pus which causes severe pain in the ear.

BELOW Regular swimmers may be more likely to suffer outer ear infections, particularly if the water is not clean.

DATA FILE

Reasons for infection include:

• Boils often result from infection by staphylococcus bacteria. Infection often occurs through a break in the skin caused by scratching an itch, or may enter the ear from polluted water. Boils are painful, the ear may swell, and infection may spread to the inner ear.

• Fungus infections are sometimes called "swimmer's ear" because dampness is favorable to fungal growth.

• Damage from constant probing of the ear may lead to bacterial or fungal infection or inflammation.

• An allergic reaction to a foreign body can cause an ear infection.

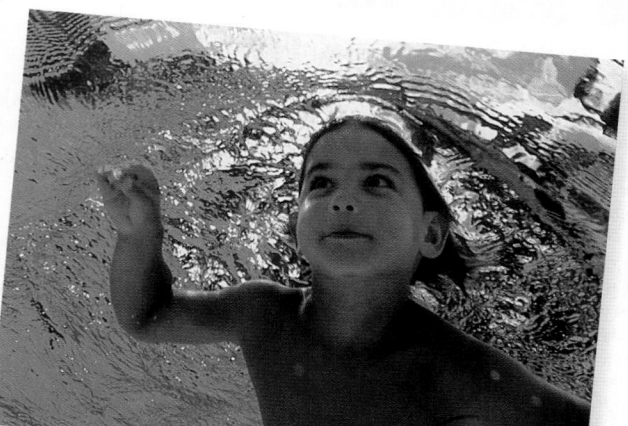

TREATMENT

TRADITIONAL HOME AND FOLK REMEDIES
• A roasted onion can be applied to the outer ear canal (hot) to draw out infection and to ease the pain. *(See page 82.)*
• A bread poultice *(see Earache, page 326)* will reduce inflammation and pain. *(See page 101.)*
• Warm a little garlic oil, saturate a cotton bud, and place in the ear canal to draw out infection. *(See page 82.)*

HERBALISM
• Mullein oil will reduce external pain and encourage healing. St. John's wort oil exerts a similar beneficial effect. *(See pages 124 and 137.)*
• Wash the ear canal with a warm infusion of herbs such as chamomile, elderflower, or golden seal, which are antiseptic. *(See pages 119 and 130.)*

AROMATHERAPY
• Apply a little tea tree oil to the end of a cotton bud and gently swab the outer ear canal, and the ear itself. *(See page 162.)*
• Warm some marjoram oil in grapeseed oil, massage around the ear and dab a few drops into the ear canal. Apply a little more to a cotton ball and insert into the ear and leave overnight. This will reduce pain and encourage healing. *(See pages 146–71.)*

HOMEOPATHY
• Belladonna, for pain and redness. *(See page 183.)*
• Mercurius, when there is a smelly discharge. *(See page 205.)*
• Aconite, for an acute infection characterized by sharp shooting pains. *(See page 178.)*

FLOWER ESSENCES
• Take Rescue Remedy or Emergency Essence to ease symptoms and induce calm. *(See page 244.)*

Labyrinthitis (Otitis interna)

Labyrinthitis (otitis interna) is an inflammation of the part of the inner ear responsible for balance (the labyrinth). A viral infection is usually the cause of labyrinthitis (possibly in the course of mumps or flu), although it may be the result of infection spreading through the bone from middle ear infection. Infection may also reach the inner ear (via the bloodstream) from somewhere else in the body. Less commonly, a bacterial labyrinthitis results from a head injury. In labyrinthitis, inflammation of the fluid-filled chambers (labyrinth) of the inner ear causes disruption of the individual's sense of balance. As well as vertigo, labyrinthitis may cause nausea, vomiting, nystagmus (abnormal, jerky movements of the eyes), tinnitus, and hearing loss.

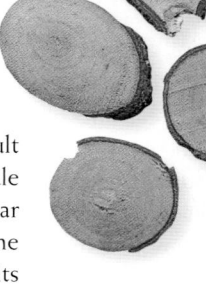

ABOVE The Chinese herbal remedy Gui Zhi, or cinnamon twigs. It is prescribed to counteract episodes of dizziness.

CAUTION

UNTREATED BACTERIAL LABYRINTHITIS MAY LEAD TO PERMANENT DEAFNESS, OR SPREAD TO CAUSE MENINGITIS.

SYMPTOMS

• *a spinning sensation* • *unsteadiness, faintness, and possibly falling* • *nausea and vomiting* • *partial deafness* • *ringing or hissing in the ears (see Tinnitus, page 322)*

TREATMENT

CHINESE HERBALISM
• Fresh ginger, cinnamon twigs, and peppermint will help with the dizziness. *(See page 59.)*
• Mulberry can be taken to nourish the Blood.

HERBALISM
• Treatment to boost the immune system, including echinacea, would be appropriate. *(See page 120.)*

• Ginger root, candied or chewed raw, will help to ease the nausea. *(See page 139.)*
• Try Chinese angelica, which can restore energy, stimulate white blood cells and the formation of antibodies to fight infection. *(See page 115.)*
• Licorice helps recovery, stimulating formation and efficiency of white blood cells and antibodies. *(See page 122.)*

HOMEOPATHY
• Conium, for dizziness which worsens when lying down.
• Belladonna, for a feeling of fullness in the ear, worsened by moving around. *(See page 183.)*
• Nat. mur., for symptoms accompanied by a headache and sometimes by constipation. *(See page 206.)*
• Phosphorus, when dizziness is made worse by looking down. *(See page 208.)*
• Gelsemium, when you feel weak and trembling. *(See page 195.)*
• Calcarea, when an attack of dizziness is made worse by looking up. *(See page 186.)*

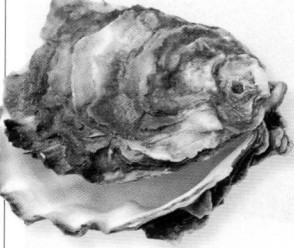

LEFT The European edible oyster is the source for Calcarea carbonica.

Glue Ear

Glue ear is a persistent condition in children in which there is a build-up of sticky fluid in the middle ear. It may be caused by chronic nose or throat infection, but can also be due to allergies or exposure to draughts. It may also be associated with chronically enlarged tonsils and adenoids, causing Eustachian tube obstruction. Glue ear does not cause any pain but does impair normal hearing. This in turn can lead to other problems, such as falling behind in class, since hearing is essential for speech development and learning.

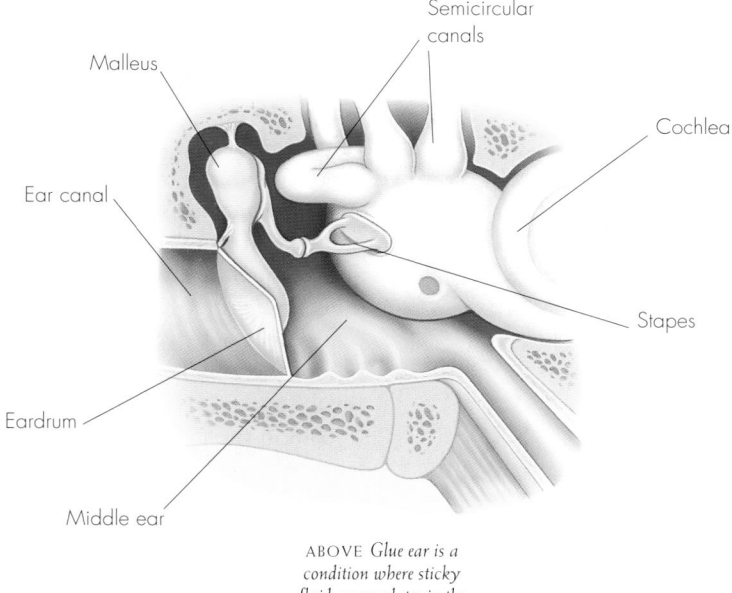

ABOVE *Glue ear is a condition where sticky fluid accumulates in the middle ear.*

CAUTION

SEVERE INATTENTION AMONG CHILDREN UNDER TWO YEARS COULD WELL BE DUE TO PARTIAL DEAFNESS CAUSED BY GLUE EAR. IT IS ESSENTIAL THAT THIS IS INVESTIGATED IN ORDER TO AVOID LONG-TERM SPEECH, COMPREHENSION, AND INTELLECTUAL IMPAIRMENT.

SYMPTOMS

• *hearing impairment*

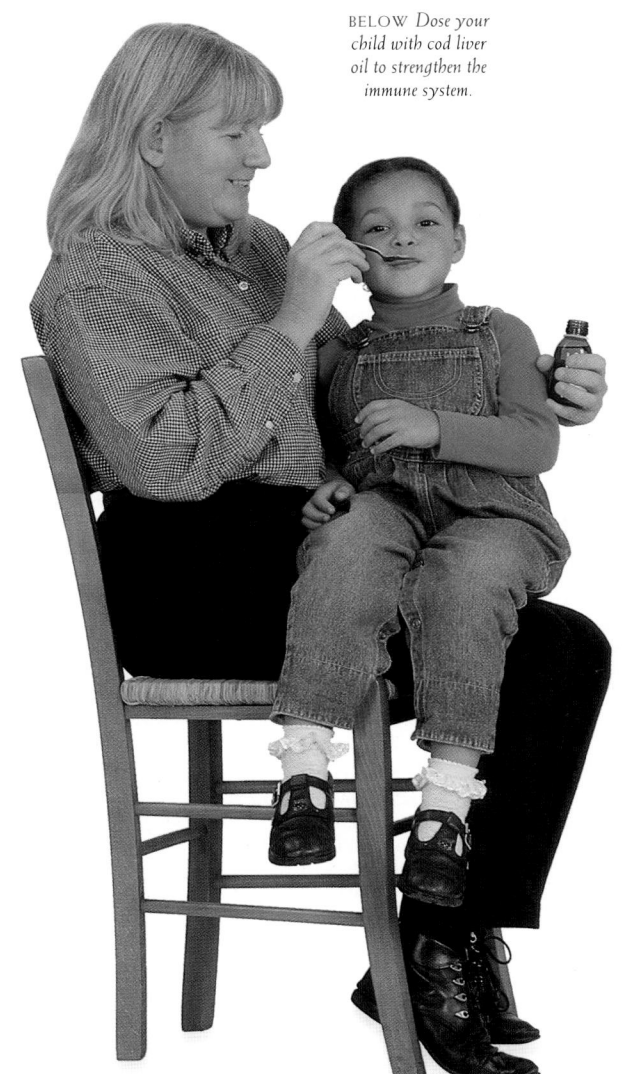

BELOW *Dose your child with cod liver oil to strengthen the immune system.*

TREATMENT

CHINESE HERBALISM
• Herbs to reduce inflammation and mucus (phlegm) would be Sheng di Huang or Chinese senega root/Polygala. *(See pages 70 and 72.)*

TRADITIONAL HOME AND FOLK REMEDIES
• Drink lemon and honey or cider vinegar to clear the mucus and to strengthen the immune system. *(See pages 87, 101, and 102.)*

HERBALISM
• Clean away discharge with a warm infusion of herbs such as chamomile or golden seal, which are antiseptic. *(See page 119.)*
• Herbal remedies to boost the immune system include chamomile, echinacea, peppermint, and wild indigo. *(See pages 120 and 125.)*
• Herbs to help clear the catarrh include elderflowers, euphrasia, golden rod, and hyssop. *(See page 130.)*
• Herbs which are able to reduce catarrh include golden rod, ground ivy, and elderflower. *(See page 130.)*

AROMATHERAPY
• Dilute essential oils of lavender, chamomile, eucalyptus, or rosewood in a light carrier oil. Warm and massage around the ear and neck. *(See pages 146–71.)*

HOMEOPATHY
• Kali mur., when there are cracking sounds in the affected ear, accompanied by swollen glands in the neck.
• Lycopodium, when there is deafness and a roaring sound is experienced in the affected ear. *(See page 203.)*
• Pulsatilla, for a full feeling in the ear, and weepiness. *(See page 209.)*

• Mercurius, when there is thick, smelly discharge. *(See page 205.)*

VITAMINS AND MINERALS
• Chronic infection can be caused by a build-up of catarrh *(see page 329)*. Reduce consumption of dairy produce and any other possible allergens, including wheat.
• Take cod liver oil and vitamin C to give a boost to the immune system. *(See page 256.)*

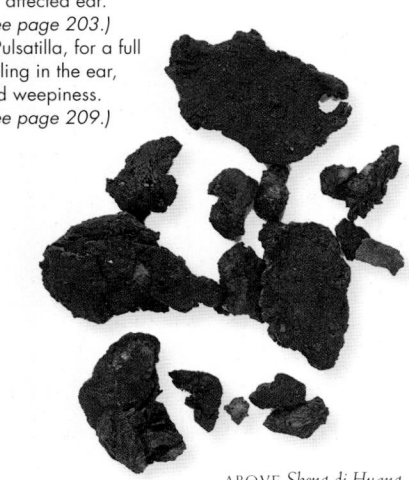

ABOVE *Sheng di Huang. In Chinese medicine this is a cooling herb, prescribed to relieve Heat.*

Earache

Earache is particularly common among children. It is usually (but not always) caused by a change in pressure in the middle ear as a result of a failure in the ear's pressure-equalizing mechanism. The failure occurs when the flow of air to and from the middle ear is impeded by a blockage in the Eustachian tube. The other most frequent causes of earache are acute infection of the middle ear or the ear canal (*see pages 323 and 324*).

Pain in the ear area may be a feature of problems in other nearby parts of the body, such as the teeth, jaw, throat or neck.

DATA FILE

Earache may be a feature of:

• enlarged adenoids causing Eustachian tube blockage

• infection of the middle ear in which the obstruction in the Eustachian tube interferes with fluid drainage

• a boil or infection by viruses, bacteria or fungi in the external ear passage

• teething in babies, and dental decay

• sinusitis

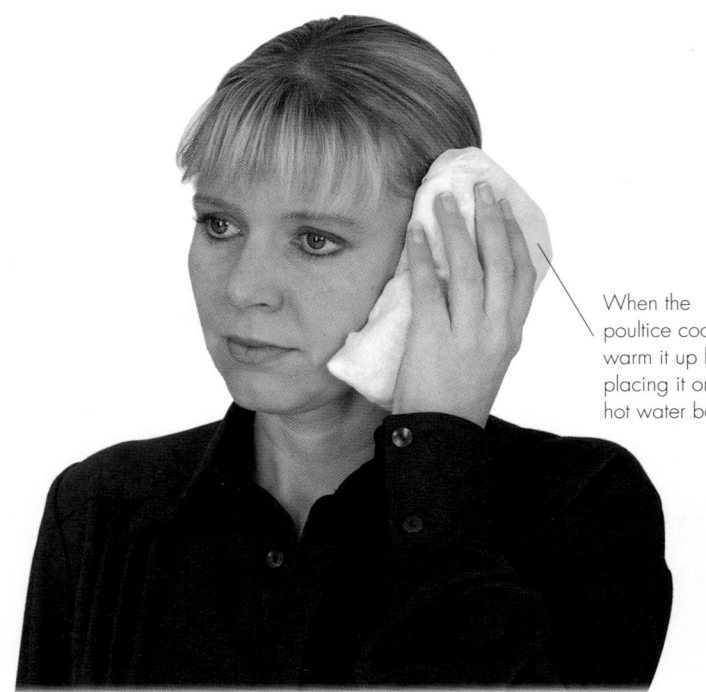

When the poultice cools, warm it up by placing it on a hot water bottle

RIGHT *A warm poultice of ginger or roasted onion will help earache.*

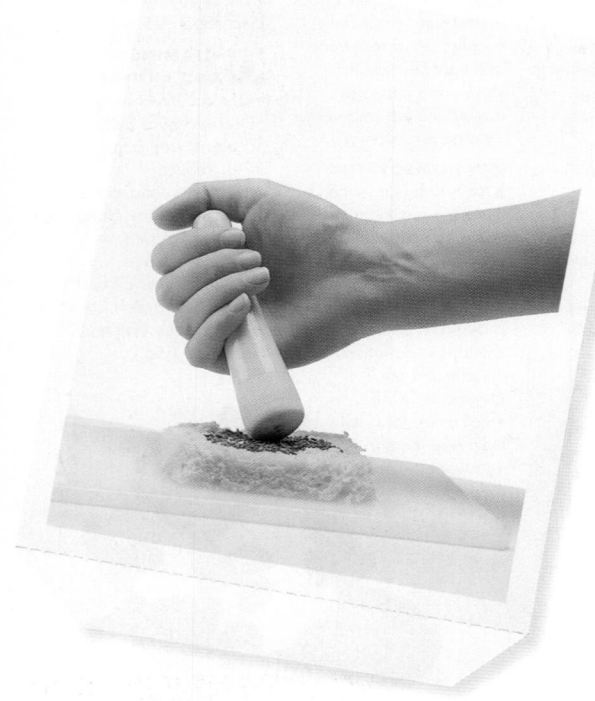

ABOVE *Make a poultice paste by pounding caraway seeds on a slice of bread, and moistening with hot brandy.*

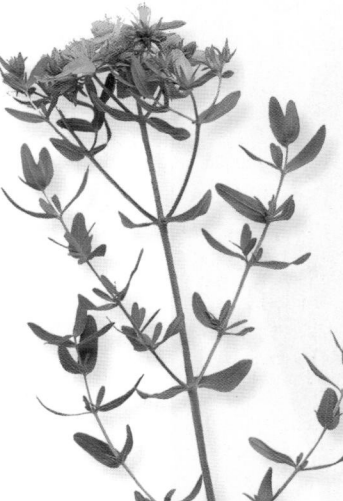

RIGHT *Massage St. John's wort oil into the ear area.*

TREATMENT

TRADITIONAL HOME AND FOLK REMEDIES
• Warm a slice of bread with the crusts removed, and pound it with a handful of bruised caraway seeds. Add some hot brandy to make a paste, and apply as a hot poultice to reduce inflammation of the ear. *(See page 101.)*
• Crush and simmer root ginger and make a poultice to apply to the affected ear.
• Roast an onion, and then apply it hot (take care – test first) to the ear for relief of pain and control of discharge. *(See page 82.)*

HERBALISM
• Apply a little St. John's wort oil to the area, and massage in gently. *(See page 124.)*
• Massage a little warmed olive oil, with a few drops of chamomile or elderflower tincture, around the ear, and use a dropper to insert a little into the affected canal. *(See pages 119 and 130.)*

AROMATHERAPY
• Make a hot compress, to apply directly to the ears and neck to ease the pain, using diluted chamomile, eucalyptus, lavender, or rosewood oils. *(See pages 146–71.)*

HOMEOPATHY
• Chamomilla, for severe pain and need of comfort. *(See page 204.)*
• Pulsatilla, if the pain feels like the eardrum is being pushed out, and you feel weepy. *(See page 209.)*
• Hep. sulf., for throbbing pain made better by a warm compress. *(See page 198.)*
• Belladonna, for throbbing pain that is improved by application of a cold compress. *(See page 183.)*
• Aconite, for an earache that comes on suddenly. *(See page 178.)*

FLOWER ESSENCES
• Emergency Essence or Rescue Remedy can be applied to the temples or taken internally to soothe and reduce any panic. *(See page 244.)*

Ear Wax

Ear wax is a sticky, fatty secretion produced by the glands in the outer ear to protect the eardrum by trapping dust and small objects. Normal soft wax is disposed of naturally by the ear, but hard or dried wax accumulates. An excess of ear wax obstructs the ear canal, and the blockage may be worsened by swimming or bathing since the wax absorbs water.

SYMPTOMS

- *a sensation of fullness or aching in the ear*
- *partial hearing loss caused by inflammation in the ear canal*

TREATMENT

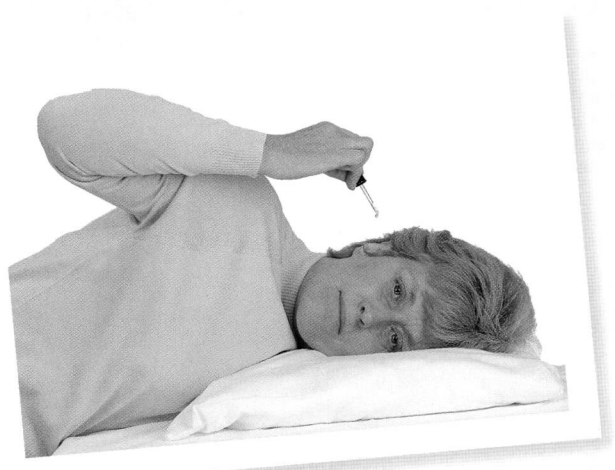

ABOVE *To use an ear dropper, lie with the head on a pillow. This allows the oil to penetrate the ear canal.*

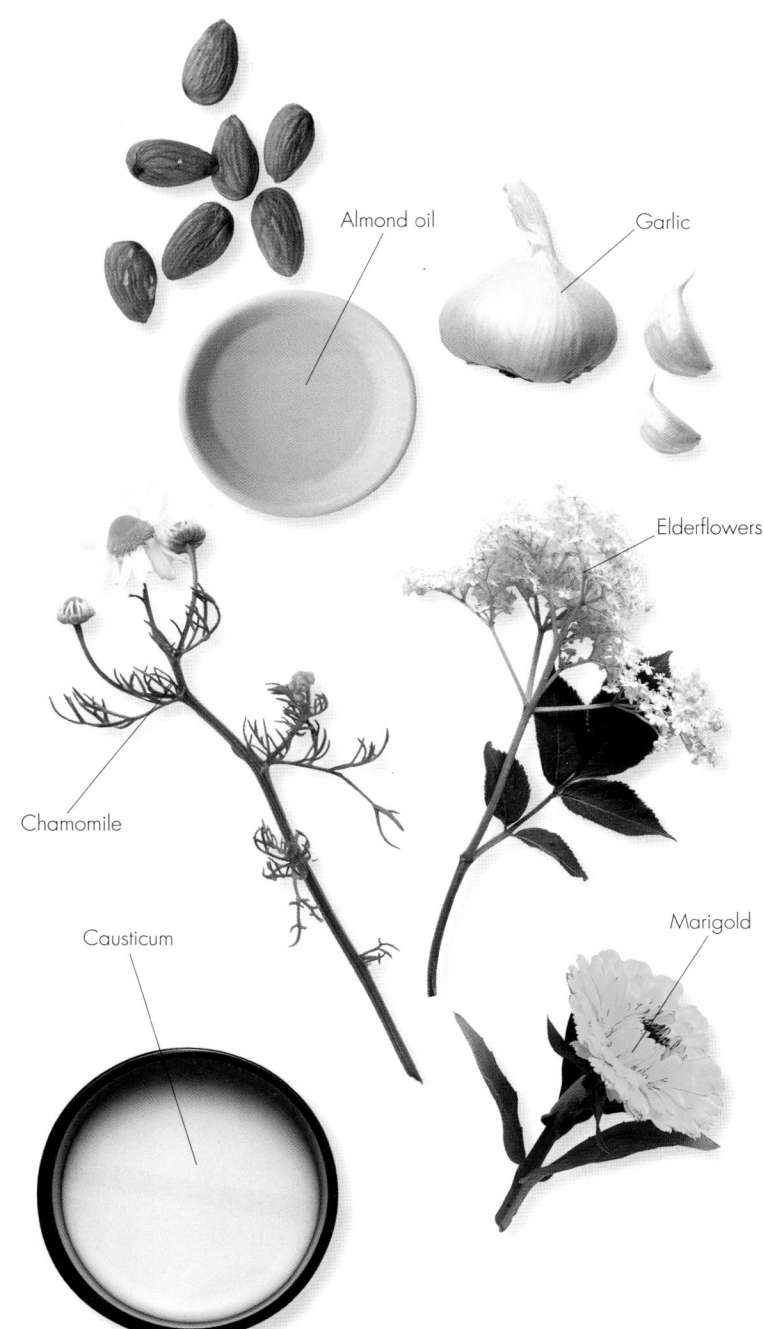

Almond oil · Garlic · Elderflowers · Chamomile · Causticum · Marigold

ABOVE *Sources of treatment in some of the major healing remedies: almonds and their oil (Chinese), garlic (traditional home remedies), elderflower and marigold (herbalism), slaked lime (source of Causticum in homeopathy), chamomile (source of chamomile oil in aromatherapy).*

CHINESE HERBALISM
- Drop a little warmed almond oil into the ear to soften the wax, making it easier to remove.

TRADITIONAL HOME AND FOLK REMEDIES
- A little warmed garlic oil, dropped into the ear, will soften the wax and occasionally dislodge it. (See page 82.)
- Use an ear candle (available from health stores) to heat and draw out excess wax.

HERBALISM
- Make a warm infusion of chamomile, elderflowers, or marigold, or put a few drops of the tincture into some warm water. Using a dropper, place the liquid in the ear canal and stop with a cotton ball. Repeat several nights running until the wax has softened and is absorbed by the cotton. (See pages 117, 119, and 130.)

AROMATHERAPY
- Put a few drops of warm chamomile oil, blended in a light carrier oil, into the ear canal and block gently with a cotton ball. Repeat until wax has softened. (See page 150.)

HOMEOPATHY
- Causticum, when there is a build-up of wax with some related loss of hearing. (See page 189.)

CAUTION
CONSTANT PRODDING OR CLEANING OF THE EAR CAN LEAD TO EXCESSIVE EAR WAX PRODUCTION.

NASAL PROBLEMS

Sinusitis

Sinusitis is an inflammation of the sinuses – the air-filled cavities located in the bones around the nose. When this occurs the lining of the sinuses swells, causing a blockage in the channel that drains them. A build-up of mucus discharge results, creating intense pressure and pain. Sinusitis usually develops as a complication of a viral infection such as a cold, but pollution or tobacco can also be triggers. Severe symptoms should be referred to your physician.

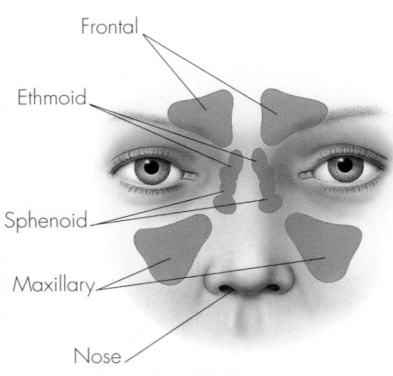

Frontal
Ethmoid
Sphenoid
Maxillary
Nose

ABOVE *The sinus cavities within the skull are lined with mucous membrane. Inflammation of this membrane can be very painful.*

SYMPTOMS

• *nasal congestion with thick, stretchy mucus* • *nosebleeds and sneezing* • *loss of sense of smell* • *headache with a sensation of pressure in and around the head* • *severe pain around the eyes and cheeks (particularly on bending down), sometimes feeling like toothache*

DATA FILE

• More than 50 percent of cases are caused by bacterial infection.

• In one U.S. study, 50 percent of sufferers had an immune-system problem.

• 10 percent of all cases are caused by dental problems.

• The proximity of the paranasal sinuses to the brain makes sinus infections potentially dangerous.

• Inflammation of the sinuses may develop from an allergy or from bacteria introduced through the nasal channels, causing an infection accompanied by pain and tenderness.

• Chronic sinusitis may result from either form or a combination of both.

• Maxillary sinusitis can result from a cold or can be caused by swimming in contaminated water.

• Rarely, extraction of a molar tooth will break the floor of the maxillary sinus, leaving an opening for bacteria to enter and cause infection.

• Frontal and ethmoid sinusitis share symptoms of localized headache, surface tenderness, and, occasionally, swelling of the eyelids.

• Sphenoid sinusitis can cause blurred vision because of the proximity of this sinus to the optic nerves.

TREATMENT

AYURVEDA
• Treatment will involve the elimination of kapha with nasya (inhalation of oils). Herbal treatment may be prescribed, including coriander for sinus problems and related headaches. Detoxification will be appropriate. *(See page 20.)*

CHINESE HERBALISM
• Bi Yan Pian pills are very good for sinusitis, especially with sticky yellow nasal discharge, which is hard to get out.
• A herbal prescription of Cang er Zi San, when there is lots of green nasal discharge, headache and pain.
• Xin Yi San, when there is lots of clear or white nasal discharge, nasal congestion, and pain.

• Peppermint, honeysuckle, tangerine peel, and zanthium fruit may all be useful. *(See pages 59 and 65.)*

TRADITIONAL HOME AND FOLK REMEDIES
• Peppermint is antispasmodic and decongestant. Infuse some fresh or dried leaves in a bowl of boiling water, and inhale the steam.
• Combine the juice of a fresh peeled and pulped horseradish root with the juice of two or three lemons, and take a half-teaspoon between meals. Use for several months until the mucus in the sinus clears. *(See pages 84 and 87.)*

HERBALISM
• Elderflower is excellent for catarrh and sinusitis. Drink an infusion as required to reduce symptoms and encourage healing. *(See page 130.)*

• Drink an infusion of golden seal every two hours during an acute attack.

AROMATHERAPY
• Try steam inhalations of lavender, eucalyptus, and tea tree, which are anticatarrhal and antibacterial. Lavender in particular will act as an anti-inflammatory and ease any painful symptoms. *(See pages 146–71.)*

HOMEOPATHY
• Kali bich. is the main remedy, particularly for thick, sticky mucus that accumulates in the throat, and which is difficult to clear. *(See page 200.)*
• Try Hep. sulf. if Kali bich. does not help. *(See page 198.)*
• Pulsatilla, for sinusitis accompanied by weepiness and pain above the eyes. *(See page 209.)*

VITAMINS AND MINERALS
• Many cases are caused by food allergy or intolerance. See a practitioner if you suspect this is the cause.

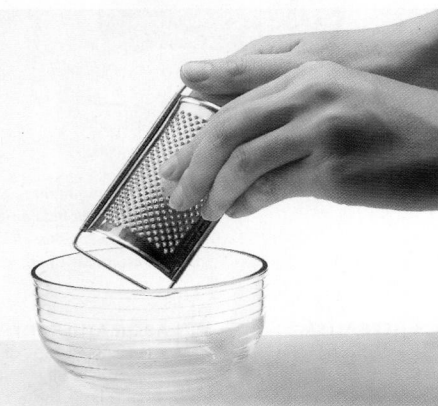

LEFT *Grate a freshly peeled horseradish root to a pulp and combine this with lemon juice. Taken between meals, it will help to clear the sinuses.*

CAUTION

GOLDEN SEAL IS NOT APPROPRIATE FOR PEOPLE WITH HIGH BLOOD PRESSURE, OR FOR PREGNANT WOMEN.

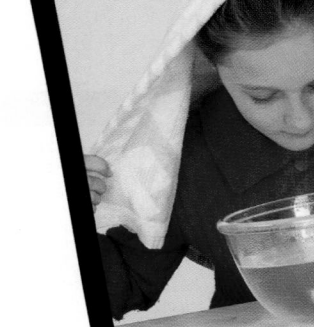

RIGHT *Steam inhalation can quickly bring relief to sinusitis in many cases. There are several herbs and plant oils that can be added to the water.*

Catarrh

Catarrh is the term used to describe the overproduction of thick phlegm by the mucous membranes of the air passages to the lungs, the larynx, the nose, and sinuses. Cells which produce and secrete a watery mucus are present in the mucous membranes, which line the passages, and they are composed of large, thin-walled veins whose blood supply serves to warm incoming air. Inflammation of the membranes as a result of a cold or flu is the usual cause, but other triggers include smoking, inhalation of dust, chronic sinusitis, upper respiratory tract infection, and allergy. A series of colds in close succession may lead to chronic catarrh. Complementary therapists believe that chronic catarrh that is not obviously due to viral or bacterial infection, allergy, chemical irritants, or dry air (all of which irritate or inflame the mucous membranes) is a symptom of general toxicity of the body – catarrh is the body's attempt to rid itself of toxins that are not being adequately dealt with by the liver, or properly excreted by the kidneys, bowels, and skin.

LEFT *In catarrh there is an excess of mucus in the nose and throat, caused by a cold or other illness, or in allergic reactions.*

Nasal cavity

Pharynx

Larynx

SYMPTOMS

- *blocked, possibly painful nose, or excessively runny nose*
- *cough with phlegm* • *earache* • *ulcers may develop on the septum (the bone that separates the nostrils)* • *possibly nosebleeds*

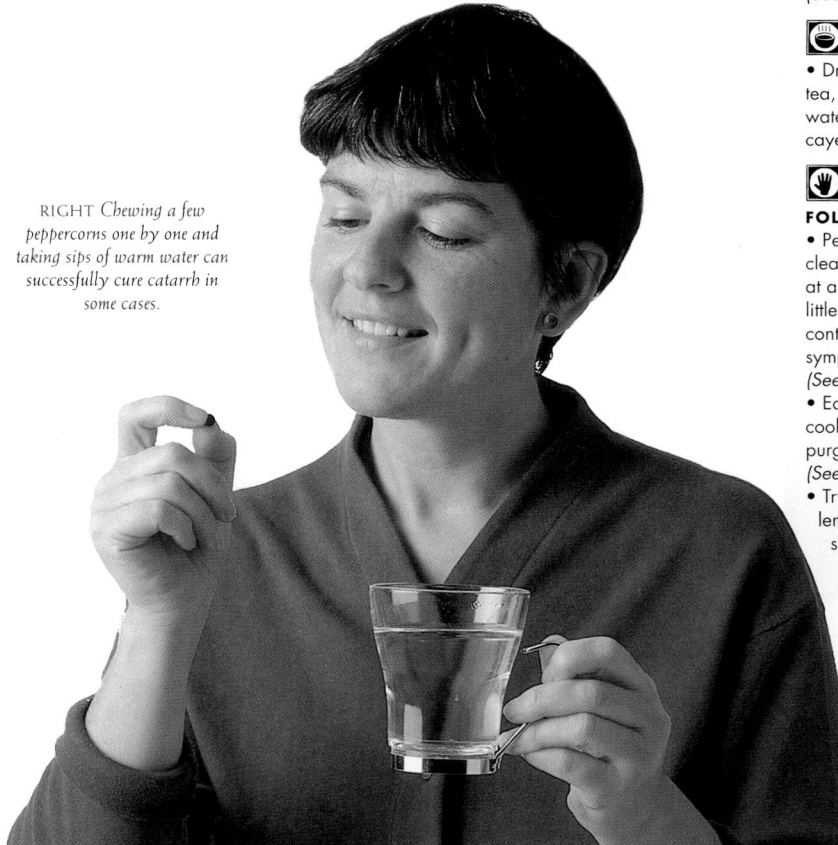

RIGHT *Chewing a few peppercorns one by one and taking sips of warm water can successfully cure catarrh in some cases.*

TREATMENT

AYURVEDA
• Coriander can help to relieve sinus problems and prevent the build-up of catarrh. Brown the seeds and boil them in water with root ginger. Boil until the liquid is reduced and drink (with a little honey) as required. *(See page 35.)*

CHINESE HERBALISM
• Drink ginger or sage tea, and drink onion water with a pinch of cayenne pepper.

TRADITIONAL HOME AND FOLK REMEDIES
• Peppercorns will help to clear catarrh. Chew one at a time, followed by a little hot water, and continue until the symptoms have gone. *(See page 97.)*
• Eating either raw or cooked onions helps to purge stubborn catarrh. *(See page 82.)*
• Try a drop of fresh lemon in each nostril – slightly painful, but enormously powerful! *(See page 87.)*
• Mustard powder can be added to a foot bath to help decongest nasal passages and clear catarrh. *(See page 98.)*

HERBALISM
• Herbs such as golden rod, elderflower, and eyebright are anti-catarrhal and astringent. When catarrh is accompanied by infection, supplement with echinacea and garlic. *(See pages 113, 120, and 130.)*
• Poke root is a good tonic and acts to prevent and reduce catarrh.

AROMATHERAPY
• Thyme and eucalyptus oils may be inhaled to ease symptoms, and it is a good idea to keep niaouli by the bed, as it can help you to sleep. *(See pages 146–71.)*
• Many oils are decongestant and expectorant, including chamomile, hyssop, mint, niaouli, pine, and clary sage. Rub into the chest and temples in a light carrier oil, or place several drops in a bowl of boiling water and inhale. *(See pages 146–71.)*

HOMEOPATHY
Chronic catarrh should be treated constitutionally, but the following remedies may be helpful:
• Arsenicum for thick, yellow discharge which makes the nose and the surrounding area sore. *(See page 182.)*

• Pulsatilla, for yellow or green catarrh that is not painful, accompanied by feelings of weepiness. *(See page 209.)*
• Nat. mur., for catarrh resembling raw egg white, with a dry nose and the loss of taste and smell. *(See page 206.)*
• Calcarea, for yellow and smelly catarrh. *(See page 186.)*
• Sulfur, when there are dry scabs inside the nose, causing bleeding, and when the nose is stuffier indoors than outdoors. *(See page 215.)*

VITAMINS AND MINERALS
• Increase your intake of vitamin C and zinc, which help to reduce symptoms. *(See pages 256 and 265.)*
• If you are prone to chronic catarrh, cut down on intake of dairy produce, which may exacerbate the condition. *(See pages 249.)*
• It may also be caused by over-consumption of sugar and too many refined carbohydrates.
• Ensure that your home is free of dust and avoid smoking.

Hay Fever

Hay fever (also known as allergic rhinitis) is an allergic reaction to airborne irritants such as grass, tree, or flower pollens. These allergens (and others including dust, animal fur, feathers, spores, plants, and chemicals) trigger a reaction which causes swelling of the nasal membrane and the production of the antibodies which release histamine. It is this chemical substance that is responsible for the characteristic allergic symptoms.

SYMPTOMS

- *runny nose, congestion, and sneezing* • *red, itchy eyes*
- *sore throat* • *wheezing, which can develop into asthma*

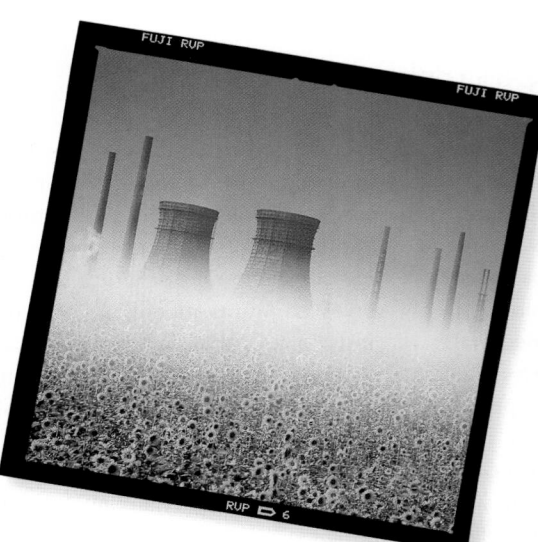

RIGHT *Susceptibility to hay fever will increase near to sources of airborne irritants such as flower pollen and emissions from factory sites and power stations.*

DATA FILE

- The timing of the symptoms will depend on the type of pollen at fault: for tree pollen, grass pollen; and weeds such as nettles, golden rod, and mugwort. In the autumn, spores and mould are likely to cause hay fever.

- At least 22 million Americans suffer from hay fever in some form.

- Most cases involve some dermatitis (in the form of urticaria or hives), and temporary asthma is common during the hay fever seasons in susceptible people.

- German researchers have found that three bananas contain enough magnesium to quell a hay fever attack.

- Babies born in the spring, when more pollen is in the air, are more likely to develop hay fever later in life.

RIGHT *A daily drink of elderflower or yarrow tea can strengthen resistance to airborne allergens.*

TREATMENT

CHINESE HERBALISM
- Bi Yan Pian/Nose inflammation pills, for Wind Cold or Wind Heat to the face; sneezing, itchy eyes, facial congestion and sinus pain, acute and chronic rhinitis, and nasal allergies.
- A herbal prescription of Yu Ping Feng San/Jade screen helps prevent hay fever, and guards against allergies.
- Cang er Zi Tang/ Xanthium powder, for allergic rhinitis with a thickened yellow catarrh or a blocked nose.

TRADITIONAL HOME AND FOLK REMEDIES
- A teaspoon of local honey, before and during the season, helps many people. *(See page 101.)*
- Eat plenty of fresh garlic to boost the immune system, and to act as an anticatarrhal agent. *(See page 82.)*

HERBALISM
- Strengthen resistance with a tea of elderflowers and yarrow for some weeks before the pollen season starts. *(See pages 112 and 130.)*

- Soothe itchy eyes with an elderflower, eyebright, or chamomile compress. Eyebright tea or capsules will relieve symptoms.

AROMATHERAPY
- Chamomile in the bath and in massage will help to ease symptoms. *(See page 150.)*
- Steam or dry inhalations of lavender and/or eucalyptus can help for sneezing and runny nose. Also use in the bath. *(See pages 159 and 161.)*
- Melissa may soothe and calm the allergic reaction. *(See page 163.)*

HOMEOPATHY
Hay fever can be deep-seated and take some time to cure, and treatment should be constitutional. However, there are preventive remedies, including the following:
- Allium, for hay fever where the sufferer has a burning nasal discharge. *(See page 178.)*
- Sabadilla, for hay fever with a sore throat.
- Arsenicum, when there is a constant need to sneeze. *(See page 182.)*

- Euphrasia, when the eyes are itching and red. *(See page 194.)*

FLOWER ESSENCES
- Rescue Remedy or Emergency Essence will help to ease symptoms during an attack, and help to produce a more positive frame of mind. *(See page 244.)*

VITAMINS AND MINERALS
- Vitamin C combined with bioflavonoids will act as a natural antihistamine to control symptoms. *(See pages 256 and 272.)*
- Taking extra pantothenic acid may help to relieve hay fever symptoms. *(See page 254.)*
- Bee pollen can help prevent allergies when taken for several weeks before the hay fever season. *(See page 27.)*
- Royal jelly is also a useful hay fever treatment. *(See page 276.)*

BELOW *Unfortunately, many people can be allergic to their own pets.*

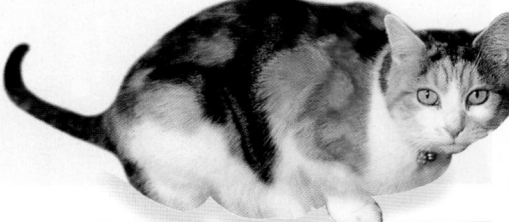

Disturbed Sense of Smell

The olfactory nerves in the nose have many hair-like nerve fibers or smell receptors. When we sniff, a waft of air passes over the receptors, allowing us to identify a smell. Loss of the sense of smell (or "anosmia"), whether temporary or permanent, can be severely debilitating and in some instances dangerous – if it fails to alert us to the presence of gas or smoke, for example. It may occur as a result of head injury in which damage is sustained to the twigs of the olfactory nerve, colds or flu.

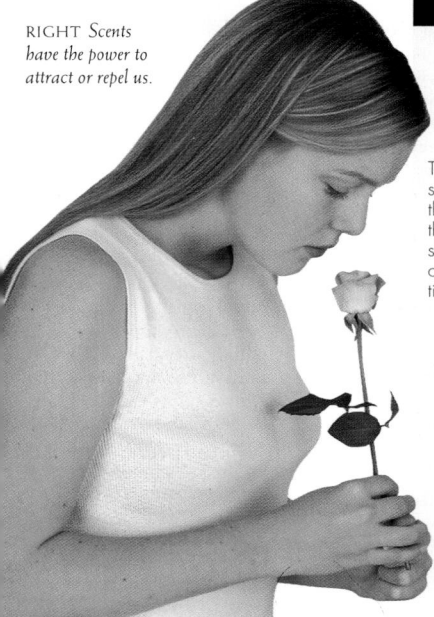

RIGHT *Scents have the power to attract or repel us.*

DATA FILE

Despite the close association, taste and smell are distinct. In the case of taste, chemicals that evoke sweet, sour, bitter, and salty sensations stimulate taste bud receptors located in the throat and on the tongue and palate. This stimulation triggers nerve cells to send signals to the brain stem, located in the base of the brain. Odors register in the brain when airborne chemicals stimulate receptors located on the olfactory epithelium, a small patch of tissue positioned high in the nose.

The olfactory system is vitally important in determining food flavors. During chewing and swallowing, odor-laden air is forced from the rear of the oral cavity to the olfactory receptors, evoking many flavor sensations that people usually associate with taste but which are almost completely dependent on the sense of smell. If you pinch your nose while swallowing food, the flow of air to the olfactory receptors is prevented, resulting in a decrease or elimination of the perception of the food's taste.

TREATMENT

AYURVEDA
• The senses are linked to the elements in Ayurvedic medicine, and any imbalance can be adjusted through balancing treatment. Treatment will be specific to the patient's needs. *(See page 20.)*

HOMEOPATHY
Treatment will be constitutional, but the following remedies may be useful:
• Ignatia, for sensitivity to tobacco smoke. *(See page 200.)*
• Graphites, for sensitivity to flower scents. *(See page 196.)*

• Carbolic acid, when all smells are overpowering.
• Belladonna, for a sudden smell of rotten eggs. *(See page 183.)*

VITAMINS AND MINERALS
• A zinc deficiency can cause problems with your sense of smell – ensure that you have an adequate dietary intake, or take a daily supplement of zinc. *(See page 265.)*

CAUTION

VERY RARELY, CANCER PATIENTS REPORT SPECIFIC SMELL AND TASTE CHANGES. IF YOU SUDDENLY DEVELOP AN ACUTE SENSE OF SMELL, SEE YOUR PHYSICIAN.

Nosebleeds

Nosebleeds are very common, resulting either from persistent probing, an injury, infection of the mucous membrane, or from drying and crusting. Injury or infection which damages the moist lining of the nose can quite easily rupture tiny local blood vessels and cause bleeding; more often, bleeding occurs for no apparent reason. There is some association between nosebleeds and high alcohol intake.

RIGHT *Lavender oil applied on a cotton bud will encourage healing.*

TREATMENT

TRADITIONAL HOME AND FOLK REMEDIES
• Lemon is a natural styptic. Place a drop in the offending nostril, on the end of a cotton bud. *(See page 87.)*

AROMATHERAPY
• A drop of lavender oil, placed in the nostril on a cotton bud, will encourage healing and help to staunch the flow of blood. *(See page 161.)*

HOMEOPATHY
• Aconite, for a sudden nosebleed. *(See page178.)*
• Arnica, for a nosebleed brought on by injury or bruising. *(See page 182.)*

• Phosphorus, for a nosebleed brought on by blowing the nose violently. *(See page 208.)*
• Rhus tox., for nosebleeds after strenuous exercise. *(See page 210.)*
• Lachesis, for nosebleeds occurring in hot weather. *(See page 216.)*

FLOWER ESSENCES
• Rescue Remedy or Emergency Essence will help in cases of emotional distress, and a few drops diluted in water and placed in the nostril may help to encourage the healing process. *(See page 244.)*

CAUTION

NOSEBLEEDS WHICH DO NOT STOP WITHIN A COUPLE OF HOURS SHOULD BE CHECKED BY A PHYSICIAN. DO NOT STEM THE BLEEDING TOO QUICKLY IN THOSE SUFFERING FROM HIGH BLOOD PRESSURE – ALLOW THE BLEEDING TO CONTINUE FOR 10 MINUTES BEFORE TAKING ACTION.

CONTRARY TO POPULAR MYTH, NOSEBLEEDS ARE NOT ALWAYS A SIGN OF HIGH BLOOD PRESSURE, BUT IF YOU ARE OVER 40, OR SUSPECT HIGH BLOOD PRESSURE, SEE YOUR PHYSICIAN.

LEFT *Leaning forward and lightly pinching the sides of the nose can often stem a nosebleed.*

DENTAL PROBLEMS

Gingivitis

Gingivitis is inflammation of the gums. It may sometimes occur as a result of infection or ill-fitting dentures, but most usually it is caused by an accumulation of plaque and impacted food around and under the gums. Left untreated, gingivitis may lead to loosening of the affected tooth (periodontitis) through damage to the membrane securing it. It is a very common problem, particularly during pregnancy. Gingivitis may also result from systemic disorders such as vitamin C deficiency (scurvy) and endocrine disturbances (diabetes mellitus). Prevention and treatment include good oral hygiene and control or correction of local and systemic factors. The incidence of gingivitis appears to increase with age: at 10 years old, 15 percent of the U.S. population suffer; by the age of 50, more than 50 percent have gingivitis. A blood test can now detect gum disease six months before symptoms set in.

✋ TRADITIONAL HOME AND FOLK REMEDIES
• Peach pit tea is useful for mouth infections. Rinse your mouth with the hot tea three times a day.

🌿 HERBALISM
• Depending on the problem, some herbs, such as myrrh, are highly astringent and antiseptic, and may be useful locally. Other treatments may be used internally to increase the patient's resistance.
• Golden seal can make an effective poultice, and will treat any infection.
• Comfrey mouthwash will help to heal mouth abrasions, and reduce swelling and bleeding. *(See page 132.)*

⊘ HOMEOPATHY
Gingivitis may be treated homeopathically. One of the following specific remedies may be taken every 4 hours for up to 3 days:

• Mercurius, when the gums are spongy and the breath smells bad. *(See page 205.)*
• Kreosotum, when the gums are red, inflamed, and swollen, and bleed easily, with the roots of the teeth exposed.
• Nat. mur., when gums bleed easily, there are ulcers and a taste of pus in the mouth, accompanied by sensitive teeth. *(See page 206.)*
• Phosphorus, for gums which bleed easily when touched, gaps between teeth and gums. *(See page 208.)*
• Silicea, for painful, swollen gums, very sensitive to cold, and which bleed easily. *(See page 211.)*
• Abscesses generally seem to respond well to Hep. sulf., Belladonna, Silicea, or Mercurius. *(See pages 183, 198, 205, and 211.)*

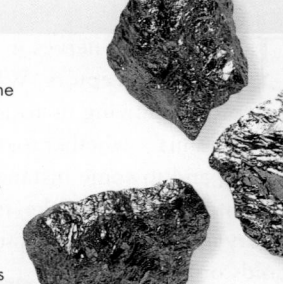

ABOVE *Silica, source of the homeopathic remedy Silicea, which can be an effective treatment.*

💊 VITAMINS AND MINERALS
• Apart from a visit to a dental hygienist, followed by daily brushing and flossing, a healthy diet will promote healthy gums.
• Vitamin C is important for the production of collagen. Most tissues in the body are made from this. *(See page 256.)*
• Co-enzyme Q10 supplements have been found beneficial in some cases of gum disease.

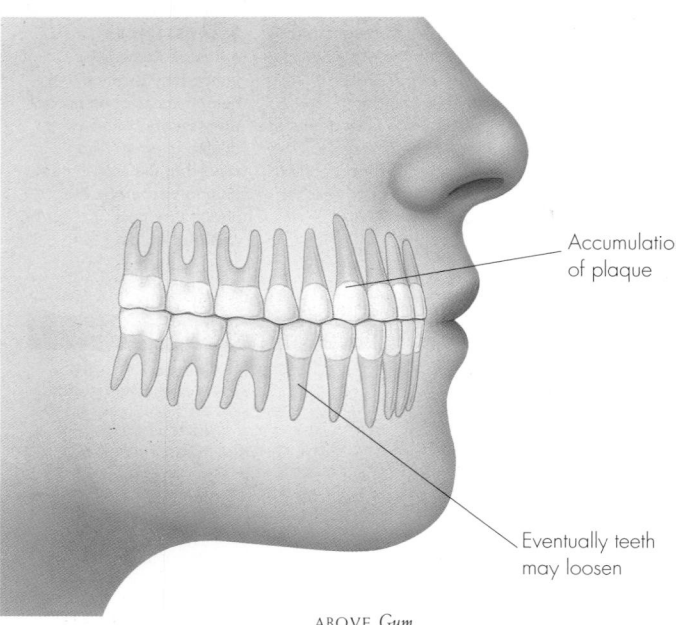

Accumulation of plaque

Eventually teeth may loosen

ABOVE *Gum inflammation can lead to periodontitis if not treated, and this causes the teeth to loosen and fall out.*

SYMPTOMS

• *swollen and tender gums which bleed easily after brushing* • *halitosis (bad breath) if areas of tissue death occur*
• *possibly earache from referred pain*

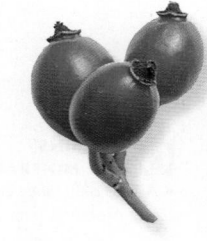

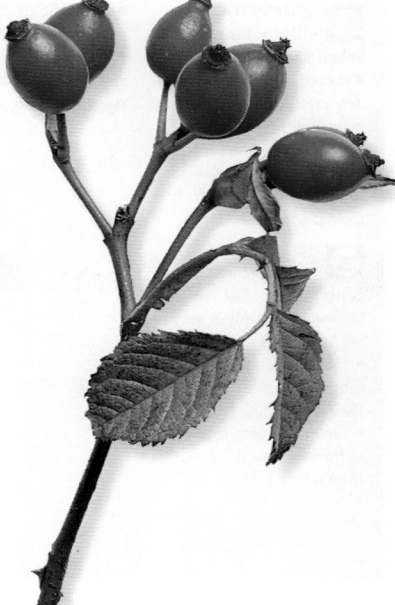

RIGHT AND LEFT *Rosehips and oranges are an excellent source of vitamin C, which is required to maintain healthy gums. Included in the diet they can prevent vitamin C deficiency, one of the factors that can lead to gingivitis.*

Toothache

Aching or pain in a tooth is generally a result of tooth decay (or "caries"). When the hard enamel of the tooth is damaged, this allows infecting organisms to enter the tooth, which results in inflammation and pain. If a tooth is sensitive to heat, cold, or sweet things, or gives pain lasting for more than a few minutes, nerves in the tooth may be inflamed due to advanced decay. If pain is absent, except when you bite, your tooth or filling may be broken. In either case, it is recommended that you see your dentist within 48 hours. Toothache after a filling is not unusual, on contact with cold air or drinks, but if the pain persists and the tooth becomes sensitive to heat as well, a return visit will be necessary.

RIGHT *Cayenne pepper, a temporary remedy for toothache and sore gums.*

TREATMENT

AYURVEDA
• Crush a clove of garlic and apply to the tooth. *(See page 26.)*
• Dip a small cotton ball into cinnamon oil and apply to the affected area. *(See page 34.)*

CHINESE HERBALISM
• Treatment would address Heat in the Stomach, and decayed or damaged teeth.
• Gypsum and ginseng might be used to relieve heat. *(See page 67.)*

HERBALISM
• A herbalist might recommend tinctures of echinacea or myrrh to encourage healing and reduce the risk of infection. *(See page 120.)*
• Cayenne can act as a local anesthetic for painful teeth and gums. *(See page 118.)*
• Fennel may be applied to the cheek in the form of a poultice, which will reduce inflammation and ease symptoms. *(See page 121.)*

AROMATHERAPY
• Peppermint or clove oils can be applied directly to the area to act as a natural analgesic. *(See pages 146–71.)*
• Oil of coriander will reduce inflammation and pain. *(See page 156.)*
• Rub a little lavender oil on to the face and jaw to ease pain and distress. *(See page 161.)*

HOMEOPATHY
• Chamomilla, when there is unbearable pain, made worse by cold air, or warm food and drinks. *(See page 204.)*
• Mercurius, for tender spongy gums which bleed easily, and when there is great thirst and shooting pains. *(See page 205.)*
• Apis, when gums feel tight and swollen, and the toothache burns and stings. *(See page 180.)*

• Staphisagria, for severe toothache made worse by cold air, food, and pressure, and where the cheeks are red and swollen.
• Plantago, for nervy teeth, aggravated by cold air and pressure, but which are better on eating.
• Belladonna, for throbbing pain and a dry mouth. *(See page 187.)*
• Aconite, when pain comes on quickly. *(See page 178.)*
• Arnica, for pain after a filling or an extraction. *(See page 182.)*

FLOWER ESSENCES
• Rescue Remedy or Emergency Essence can be applied to the affected area, and taken internally to reduce pain and encourage healing. *(See page 244.)*

DATA FILE

Dental caries is a bacterially-caused destruction of the enamel and dentine of the tooth. If untreated, it leads to an infection of the dental pulp and an abscess of the apex of the tooth. The bacteria produce both acid and enzymes to break down the tooth. Sweet foods that stick to the tooth increase the activity of the bacteria. Saliva tends to protect against caries, so decreased saliva flow usually increases caries. Tooth shape and hereditary factors also determine susceptibility to the disease.

CAUTION

TOOTHACHE IS AN INDICATION OF AN UNDERLYING PROBLEM, WHICH SHOULD BE INVESTIGATED BY A DENTIST IMMEDIATELY.

Tooth Abscess

In cases of badly neglected decay infection may gain access to the root canal of the affected tooth or teeth. Inflammation of the tissues around the root causes tissue destruction and the collection of pus, forming an abscess. A tooth abscess may spread sideways under the gum to form what is known as a gumboil, which may open, giving relief from pain. Plaque re-forms within 24–48 hours of brushing, so regular brushing is essential to prevent decay. Some research shows that allergy sufferers – whose immune activity is heightened – have fewer cases of tooth decay. Periodontal disease is the second most common infectious ailment in the U.S.

SYMPTOMS

• *intense pain, which may be intermittent, or continuous and throbbing*
• *increased pain on biting or chewing* • *swelling and inflammation of the surrounding gum* • *in severe cases there may be fever*

TREATMENT

TRADITIONAL HOME AND FOLK REMEDIES
• Break the large ridges of a cabbage, heat gently, and apply to the abscessed tooth. *(See page 85.)*
• Split a fig and heat it. Apply to the abscessed tooth. *(See page 90.)*
• Rinse your mouth with apple cider vinegar to reduce inflammation and infection. *(See page 102.)*
• Chew fresh sage leaves or garlic, for antiseptic effect. *(See page 82.)*

HERBALISM
• Comfrey mouthwash or ointment will help to heal and draw out the infection. *(See page 132.)*
• Clove oil will reduce inflammation and ease the pain.
• A hot garlic compress, applied to the area, will help to draw out infection and encourage healing. *(See page 113.)*
• A tincture of myrrh can be used as an antiseptic and healing mouthwash.

AROMATHERAPY
• Dab on some clove oil, or suck a clove, for its analgesic and antiseptic properties.
• Make a gargle containing a few drops of antiseptic oils, such as chamomile, clove, lemongrass, or niaouli. *(See pages 146–71.)*

HOMEOPATHY
• Mercurius, where there is copious saliva and the gums are spongy. *(See page 205.)*
• Gunpowder, for the discharge of pus from boils on the gums.

• Hypericum and Calendula, used in solution as a mouthwash. *(See page 199.)*
• Belladonna, at the first hint of an abscess. *(See page 183.)*
• Hep. sulf., when the abscess is in place. *(See page 198.)*

BELOW *Sulfur, the source for Hep. sulf., which is a homeopathic remedy for toothache with an abscess.*

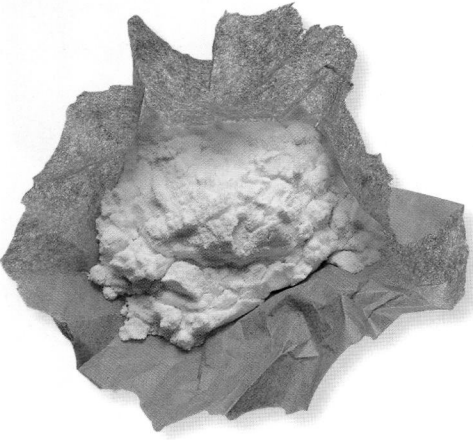

Dental Discomfort (following treatment)

Discomfort following dental treatment is usually caused by injury (perhaps to a nerve) or bruising around the tooth that has been worked on. This may occur immediately after treatment, or pain may follow initial discomfort after an anesthetic has worn off. There may also be some blood loss. Persistent pain following treatment may signal infection.

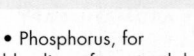

RIGHT *Arnica root, a source of the homeopathic remedy Arnica, which can be used after dental treatment.*

TREATMENT

TRADITIONAL HOME AND FOLK REMEDIES
• Oil of clove or macerated cloves can be applied to the area to prevent infection, reduce the inflammation and prevent discomfort. *(See page 90.)*

HOMEOPATHY
• Arnica should be taken immediately after treatment, every hour for up to 10 doses. *(See page 182.)*
• Ruta, for infections after teeth have been removed. *(See page 210.)*

• Phosphorus, for bleeding after a tooth has been extracted. Take every 10 minutes for 1 hour. *(See page 208.)*
• Hypericum, for pain occurring after treatment. *(See page 199.)*
• Ledum, for pain after an injection. *(See page 202.)*

FLOWER ESSENCES
• Rescue Remedy or Emergency Essence will help to reduce the effects of trauma, and encourage the healing process. *(See page 244.)*

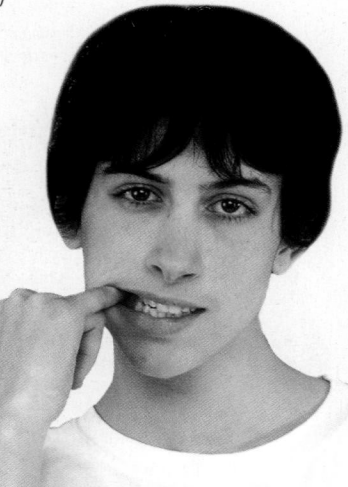

LEFT *Oil of cloves can be gently applied to the painful area inside the mouth.*

Grinding of Teeth

Habitual grinding or clenching of the teeth is known as bruxism. It is usually performed unconsciously, but is audible to others. It is common among children and the elderly, and often occurs during sleep. In severe cases the enamel of the teeth may be worn away. There may be some links with anxiety and with alcohol consumption.

TREATMENT

AYURVEDA
• An Ayurvedic medical practitioner would balance the tri-doshas, and use panchakarma for balancing the vátha. *(See page 22.)*

CHINESE HERBALISM
• A Chinese herbalist might suggest ginseng, Chinese angelica, and white peony root with thorowax root for relaxation. Treatment would be designed to strengthen the Spleen and enliven Liver qi. *(See pages 56 and 67.)*

TRADITIONAL HOME AND FOLK REMEDIES
• Oats contain thiamine and pantothenic acid, which are gentle nerve tonics. *(See page 84.)*

HERBALISM
• Herbal remedies would be used to calm the nervous system and to relax you. Skullcap and valerian are useful herbs, blended together for best effect. Drink this as a tea 3 times daily while suffering the symptoms. *(See pages 131 and 136.)*
• Lady's slipper and limeflowers may ease anxiety and tension that may exacerbate the condition. *(See page 134.)*

AROMATHERAPY
• A relaxing blend of essential oils of lavender, geranium, and bergamot in sweet almond oil or peach kernel oil may be added to the bath to calm nerves and prevent attacks. *(See pages 146–71.)*

HOMEOPATHY
• Constitutional treatment will be appropriate if there are emotional causes, but some of the following remedies may be useful:
• Arsenicum, for grinding of teeth during sleep, especially between midnight and 2 or 3 A.M. *(See page 182.)*
• Zinc, when the gums bleed and teeth become loose.
• Phytolacca, when there is an overwhelming urge to clench the teeth.

FLOWER ESSENCES
• Remedies would be useful if there is an emotional cause underlying the condition. *(See page 244.)*
• Elm, for anxiety accompanying a feeling of being unable to cope. *(See page 241.)*
• Red chestnut, for anxiety over the welfare of others. *(See page 224.)*
• Aspen, for anxiety for no apparent reason. *(See page 236.)*

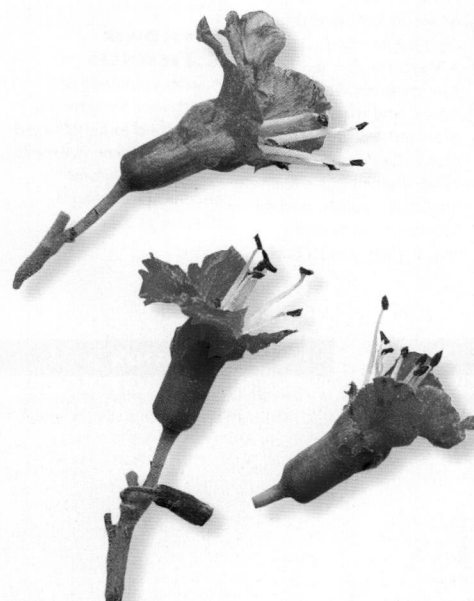

LEFT *Red chestnut is one of the flower essences that may help with the emotional causes of tooth grinding.*

Fear of Dental Treatment

Fear of dental treatment (dental phobia) is an extremely common phenomenon – some studies show that nearly 80 percent of the U.S. population suffer some feelings of fear about dental treatment. Full-scale phobia is one of the most common types of phobia in both the U.K. and the U.S. Sufferers develop intense feelings of anxiety and panic from an association between dentists and pain and discomfort, despite the fact that modern dental technology has eliminated much of the pain of treatment. Both adults and children may be affected (children are particularly vulnerable if they sense that their parents are frightened).

Most modern dentists are aware of the nervousness affecting many people, and may offer home visits or sedation, anesthetics, hypnosis, and other forms of relaxation. Relaxation for Living, in the U.K., has produced a pamphlet called "Don't Dread the Dentist", with tips for overcoming dental phobia. (*See also Phobias, page 282.*)

RIGHT *Aconite leaves, the source for Aconite, a homeopathic remedy for acute fear.*

SYMPTOMS

- *rapid pulse* • *profuse sweating*
- *high blood pressure* • *trembling*
- *nausea*

AYURVEDA
• Lemon or lime may be suggested for dizziness, and individual treatment would be prescribed according to your specific needs. *(See page 20.)*

CHINESE HERBALISM
• A herbalist may prescribe cooling herbs, and Gui Pi Wan, to help with emotional problems.
• Ginseng and Chinese angelica and senega root may also be useful. *(See pages 56, 67 and 70.)*

HERBALISM
• Valerian tea can help to reduce tension. Drink an infusion as required. *(See page 136.)*

AROMATHERAPY
• The effect of certain smells can help to release tension and induce a feeling of calm. Some of the best oils to try are bergamot, chamomile, clary sage, geranium, jasmine, juniper, lavender, marjoram, melissa, and ylang ylang, which are sedative. They can be used in the bath, in massage with a light carrier oil (such as sweet almond), or in a vaporizer. Carry a bottle of diluted oils with you and apply to the temples or pulse points before dental treatment. *(See pages 146–71.)*

HOMEOPATHY
• Aconite, for intense fear. Take before and after treatment. *(See page 178.)*
• Gelsemium, for shaking and weak legs and knees, and overall apprehension. *(See page 195.)*
• Chamomilla, for a child who throws a tantrum about seeing the dentist. *(See page 204.)*

FLOWER ESSENCES
• Mimulus, for fear of known things. Make a personal remedy, and take a few drops every time you think of the dentist. Take hourly before going for treatment. *(See page 235.)*
• Rescue Remedy or Emergency Essence will help to reduce feelings of fear and panic. Take hourly before treatment, and also during treatment. *(See page 244.)*

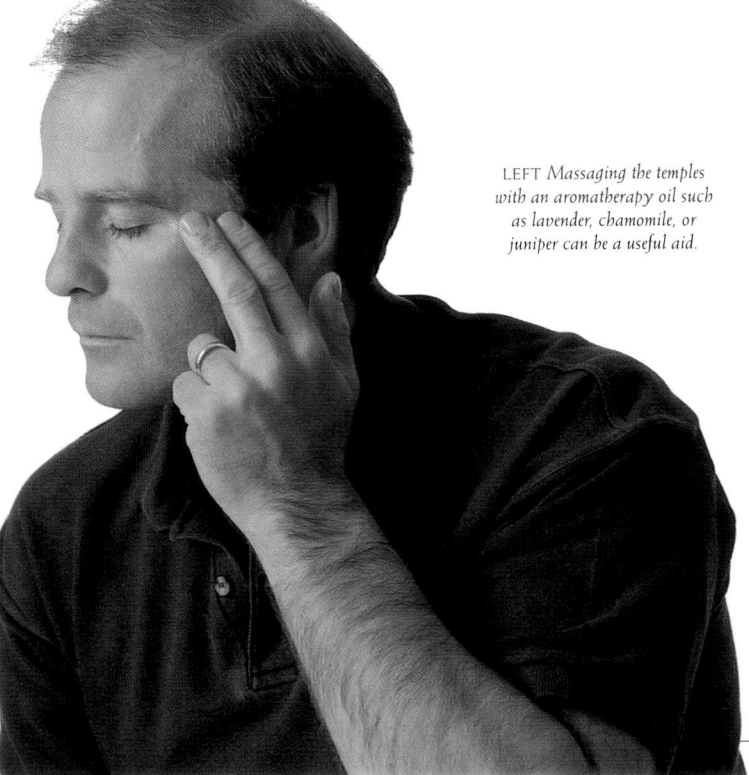

LEFT *Massaging the temples with an aromatherapy oil such as lavender, chamomile, or juniper can be a useful aid.*

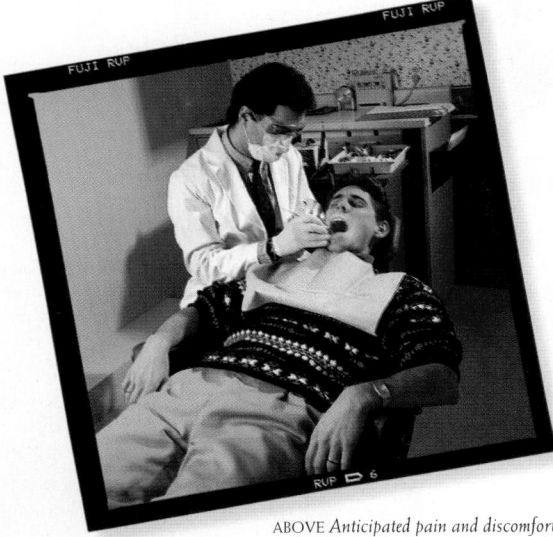

ABOVE *Anticipated pain and discomfort can lead to dental phobia. Taking remedies to overcome feelings of fear, tension, and apprehension can help.*

MOUTH AND THROAT PROBLEMS

Sore Throat

A sore throat (or pharyngitis) is an inflammation of the pharynx – the area of the throat between the back of the nose and the beginning of the trachea and vocal cords. It is usually caused by infection, which can be viral or bacterial in origin. A sore throat is a feature of illnesses such as tonsillitis and may also signal the onset of glandular fever, flu, or scarlet fever. If scarlet fever is not treated with antibiotics it may lead to rheumatic flu or kidney failure. Inflammation of the throat can also be caused by heavy smoking or drinking, abuse of gargles or mouthwashes, general vitamin deficiency, or food allergy; it can also be a symptom of blood disorders such as anemia. A sore throat will usually resolve itself in a few days, but infection, accompanied by high fever and malaise, may take up to three weeks. Streptococcal sore throat, or strep throat, is an inflammation of the throat and tonsils caused by bacteria and is the most common type of strep infection. Onset is usually sudden and is accompanied by pain, redness, and swelling in throat tissues, pus on the tonsils, fever, headache, and malaise. If left untreated, strep throat can lead to rheumatic fever.

SYMPTOMS

• *hoarseness and thirst* • *pain, causing difficulty in swallowing* • *possibly a burning sensation* • *slight fever* • *enlarged and tender lymph nodes in the neck* • *possibly earache*

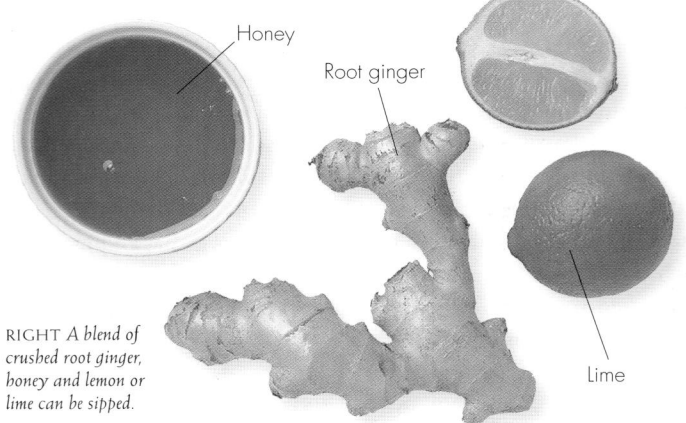

RIGHT *A blend of crushed root ginger, honey and lemon or lime can be sipped.*

Honey

Root ginger

Lime

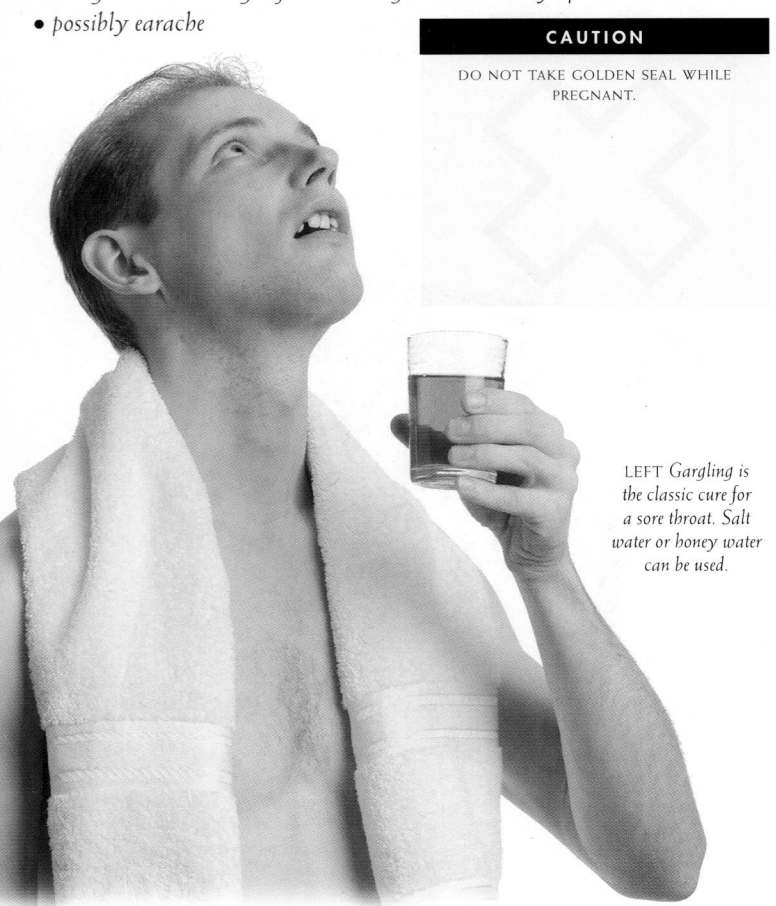

CAUTION

DO NOT TAKE GOLDEN SEAL WHILE PREGNANT.

LEFT *Gargling is the classic cure for a sore throat. Salt water or honey water can be used.*

TREATMENT

AYURVEDA
• Dasamoola rasayna, an oral syrup, will treat a sore throat.
• Crush a piece of root ginger to extract the juice, and add to a tablespoon of honey and 3 tablespoons of lime. Sip 4 times a day.
(See page 47.)

CHINESE HERBALISM
• Yin Qiao Jie du Pian pills, for a sore throat accompanied by flu symptoms, swollen lymph nodes, and headaches.
• Sang Ju Gan Mao Pian or Sang Ju Yin Pian, for a sore throat with symptoms of cold.
• Liu Wei di Huang Wan, for Kidney Yin-Deficient sore throat. Also for chronic dry sore throat, with hot palms and soles, and night sweats.
• Honeysuckle tea may be useful. *(See page 65.)*

TRADITIONAL HOME AND FOLK REMEDIES
• Gargle with salt water to ease symptoms and reduce inflammation. *(See page 103.)*
• Apply an apple cider vinegar compress to the throat to ease symptoms. *(See page 102.)*
• Gargle with honey water, which acts to encourage healing and deal with infection. *(See page 101.)*

• White cabbage juice is anti-inflammatory and will draw out infection. *(See page 85.)*
• A hot honey and lemon drink will reduce symptoms and encourage healing. *(See pages 87 and 101.)*

HERBALISM
• Eat fresh garlic whenever possible, to absorb its antibacterial and antiviral properties. *(See page 113.)*
• A gargle of red sage will help to soothe a sore throat. *(See page 129.)*
• Golden seal powder, added to a cup of hot water, can be infused and drunk as required.
• Tincture of calendula can be added to a cup of boiled water for a mouthwash to encourage healing and treat infection. *(See page 117.)*
• Burdock or comfrey teas will ease the pain. *(See pages 115 and 132.)*

AROMATHERAPY
• A steam inhalation of benzoin, lavender, or thyme will ease the discomfort and help to treat the infection. *(See pages 146–71.)*
• Massage a little lavender oil, blended in a light carrier oil, into the neck. *(See page 161.)*

• Dab the throat with diluted tea tree oil on a cotton bud – it is analgesic and fights infection, which will help to ease symptoms and treat the cause. *(See page 162.)*

HOMEOPATHY
• Belladonna, for sore throat accompanied by a red face and fever. *(See page 183.)*
• Gelsemium, when swallowing is painful, with weakness, exhaustion, pain in the neck and ears. *(See page 195.)*
• Apis, when the pain is worse on the right side of the body, and improves after cold drinks. *(See page 180.)*
• Lachesis, when pain is worse on the left side, there is a feeling of constriction, and pain is worse when swallowing saliva but better when swallowing food. *(See page 216.)*
• Aconite, for a sore throat that comes on suddenly, with a burning throat and swollen tonsils. *(See page 178.)*

VITAMINS AND MINERALS
• Increase vitamin C intake. *(See page 256.)*
• Suck a zinc lozenge. *(See page 265.)*

Tonsillitis

Tonsillitis is an inflammation of the tonsils located at the back of the throat. It is generally due to either viral or bacterial infection (often by the streptococcal bacteria), and causes swelling and redness of the tonsils, possibly with white or yellow spots of pus. The adenoids may also become inflamed and infected. Tonsillitis can occur at any time but is particularly common during childhood. In rare cases complications such as quinsy (an abscess behind the tonsil), kidney inflammation, or rheumatic fever may develop.

SYMPTOMS

• *swelling and tenderness of the lymph nodes in the neck* • *sore throat with pain on swallowing* • *headache, earache, and general weakness and malaise* • *fever* • *bad breath* • *constipation*

DATA FILE

• Tonsillitis is more common in children than in adults.

• Tonsillitis usually develops suddenly as a result of a streptococcal infection but may also be caused by a viral infection.

• In chronic tonsillitis the tonsils tend to flare up in episodes of acute infection, causing scarring that makes them difficult to treat in subsequent attacks.

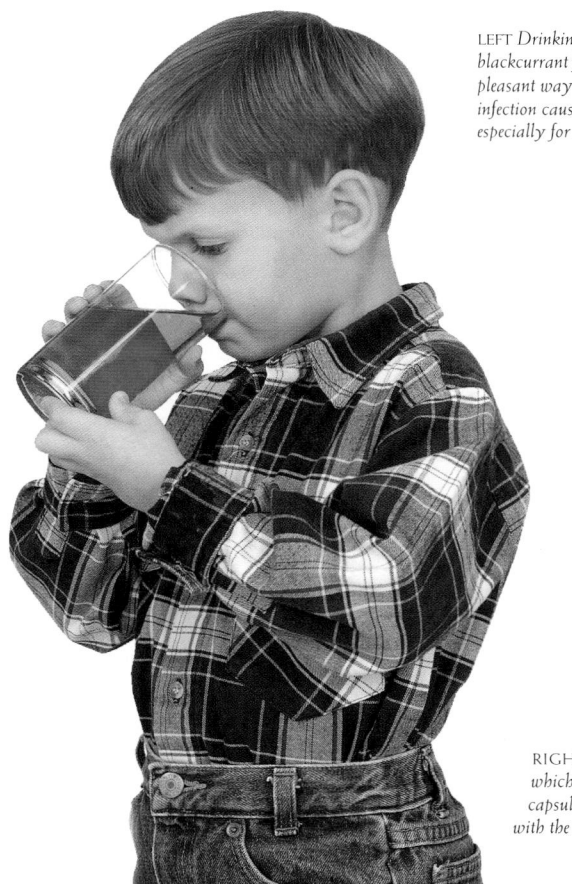

LEFT *Drinking hot blackcurrant juice is a pleasant way to treat the infection causing tonsillitis, especially for children.*

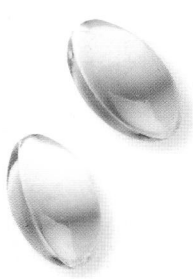

RIGHT *Cod liver oil, which can be taken in capsule form, can help with the healing process.*

TREATMENT

AYURVEDA
• Apply a cloth with mustard oil to the forehead to ease the pain and reduce fever. *(See page 30.)*
• Root ginger can be chewed, and mixed with honey and lemon to make a soothing drink. *(See page 47.)*

CHINESE HERBALISM
• Treatment would be aimed at Fire, Poison, Wind, and Heat. Avoid spicy food and drink honeysuckle tea. *(See page 65.)*

TRADITIONAL HOME AND FOLK REMEDIES
• Blackcurrant tea or juice (hot) will treat infection and relieve the sore throat.
• Drink plenty of hot honey and lemon or honey and apple cider vinegar to fight infection and boost immunity. *(See pages 87, 101, and 102.)*

HERBALISM
• A red sage gargle will address infection and reduce symptoms. *(See page 129.)*
• Herbs to boost the immune system include echinacea, garlic, myrrh, sage, and wild indigo. *(See pages 113, 129, and 130.)*
• Cleavers, marigold, and poke root will help the lymphatic system. *(See page 117.)*
• Herbs to reduce fever by inducing sweating are chamomile, elderflowers, yarrow, and limeflowers. *(See pages 112, 119, 130, and 134.)*

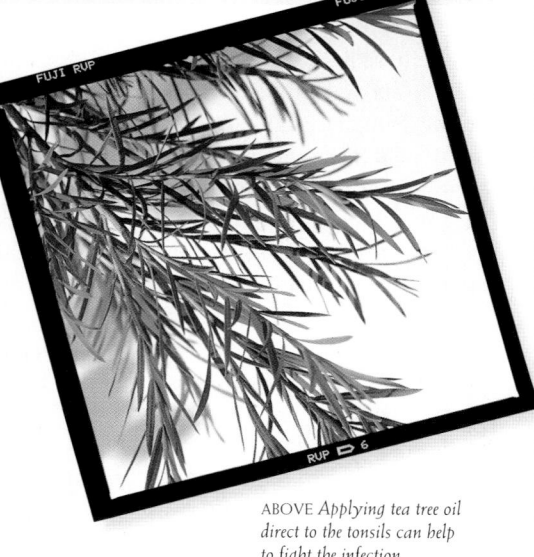

ABOVE *Applying tea tree oil direct to the tonsils can help to fight the infection.*

• Agrimony, elderflowers, plantain, and raspberry leaves tone the mucous membranes, and clear the catarrh and inflammation. *(See pages 112, 126, 128, and 130.)*
• Herbs to soothe painful tonsils include comfrey, marshmallow, and mullein. *(See pages 114, 132, and 137.)*

AROMATHERAPY
• Thyme oil is a powerful antiseptic and has a local anesthetic effect to reduce the discomfort. Use in a vaporizer, and add to a light carrier oil and massage into the neck. *(See page 170.)*
• Lavender and benzoin can be added to a cup of cooled, boiled water and gargled. *(See pages 161 and 170.)*
• Tea tree oil, applied neat to the tonsils on the end of a cotton bud, fights infection and discomfort. *(See page 162.)*

HOMEOPATHY
Chronic tonsillitis must be treated constitutionally, but for acute conditions try:

• Belladonna, for a sore, tender throat, with shooting pains and a stiff neck. *(See page 183.)*
• Hep. sulf., for a feeling that there is a fishbone caught in the throat, and when pain is alleviated by warm drinks, the breath is foul, and there is yellow pus. *(See page 198.)*
• Lycopodium, for a throat sore on the right side, and where the tongue is dry and puffy but not coated, the throat is better after cold drinks, and worse between 4 and 8 A.M. or P.M. *(See page 203.)*
• Mercurius, when the throat is dark red, swollen, and sore, and worse on the right side, and when the breath smells and there are hot sweats. *(See page 205.)*
• Phytolacca, for a rough, constricted, hot throat, with red, swollen tonsils and pain extending to the ears. The throat is worse on the right side and with heat.

VITAMINS AND MINERALS
• Cod liver oil tablets, along with vitamin C and garlic, will speed up the healing process. *(See page 256.)*

Laryngitis

Laryngitis is an inflammation of the voice box (the larynx) in which the larynx and vocal cords become swollen and sore, distorting the vocal apparatus. Acute laryngitis is usually a complication of a sore throat, cold, or other upper respiratory tract infection, and should last for only a few days. It can also be an allergic reaction to inhaled pollen. Chronic laryngitis is more persistent and may be caused by long-term irritation from smoking, overuse of the voice, or excessive coughing. It can be an occupational hazard for singers and teachers.

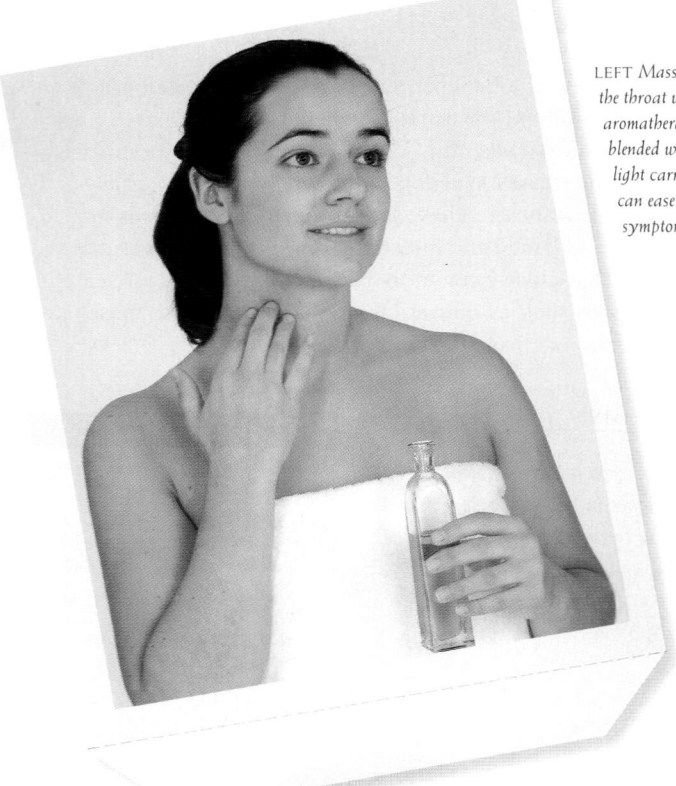

LEFT *Massaging the throat with aromatherapy oils blended with a light carrier oil can ease the symptoms.*

SYMPTOMS

- *the throat is inflamed and mucus-coated in acute laryngitis*
- *the larynx is dry and inflamed in chronic laryngitis* • *hoarseness*
- *difficulty in raising the voice above a whisper*
- *dry, irritating cough*

LEFT *Plenty of vitamin C is required in the diet to combat infection. Drinking freshly pressed orange juice can help.*

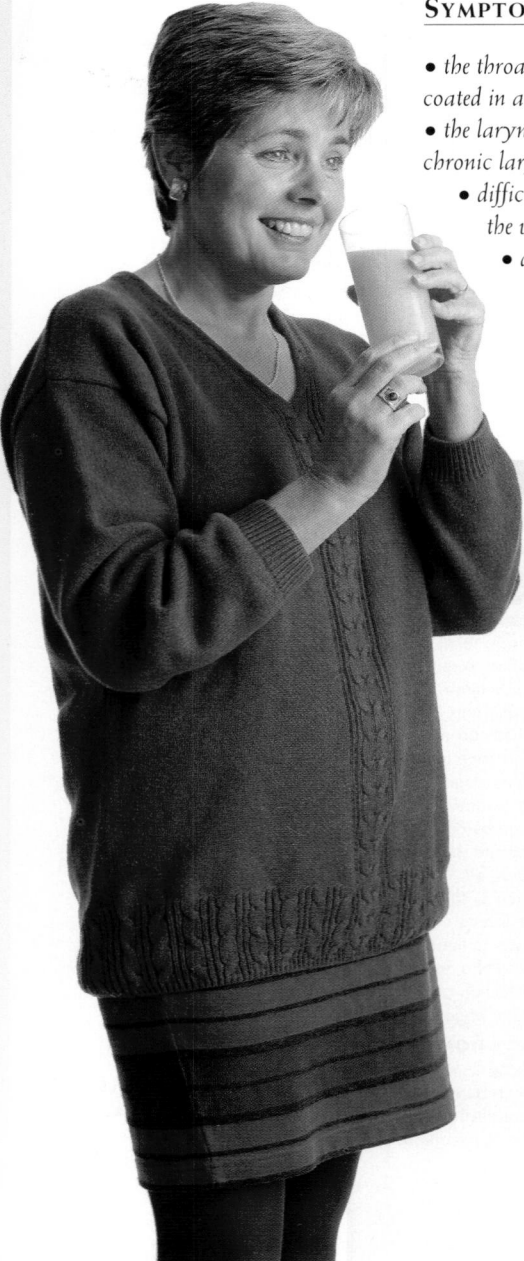

TREATMENT

AYURVEDA
• Hollyhock is useful for throat inflammation.

CHINESE HERBALISM
• Treatment would address poisoned Heat in the lungs, and the following herbs may be appropriate: peppermint, honeysuckle flowers, mulberry, lily, and licorice. *(See pages 64 and 65.)*

TRADITIONAL HOME AND FOLK REMEDIES
• Drink a glass of honey and lemon or honey and apple cider vinegar in hot water as required to reduce any inflammation and infection, and encourage healing. *(See pages 87, 101, and 102.)*

RIGHT *A glass of warm lemon and honey is a tried and tested home treatment.*

HERBALISM
• Drink an infusion of red sage, or gargle, to reduce inflammation. *(See page 129.)*
• Echinacea both treats and prevents laryngitis – drink infusion 3 times daily. *(See page 120.)*

AROMATHERAPY
• Gargle with a drop of geranium, pepper, rosemary, or tea tree oil in a glass of boiled water, as required, to prevent and treat inflammation and infection. *(See pages 146–71.)*
• Massage the throat area with a drop of lavender or tea tree oil in a light carrier oil.

(See pages 161 and 162.)
• Try a steam inhalation of sandalwood or thyme to ease inflammation and reduce infection. *(See pages 169 and 170.)*

HOMEOPATHY
Treatment would be constitutional, but some of the following remedies may help:
• Aconite, when symptoms come on suddenly, and there is restlessness and anxiety. *(See page 178.)*
• Spongia, for a dry, barking cough – particularly useful for croup. *(See page 213.)*
• Lachesis, for chronic laryngitis, particularly if you talk a

great deal. *(See page 216.)*
• Hep. sulf., when symptoms are worse in the morning and after exposure to cold; symptoms are accompanied by a loose cough and a choking feeling. *(See page 198.)*
• Apis, where the problem has been caused or exacerbated by allergy, and there is redness and swelling. *(See page 180.)*
• Ignatia, when the condition sets in after a trauma of some sort. *(See page 200.)*
• Baryta carb., when you lose your voice often, without any obvious cause. *(See page 185.)*

VITAMINS AND MINERALS
• Eat a diet rich in vitamin C to increase resistance to infection. *(See page 256.)*
• Avoid alcohol.

Oral Thrush

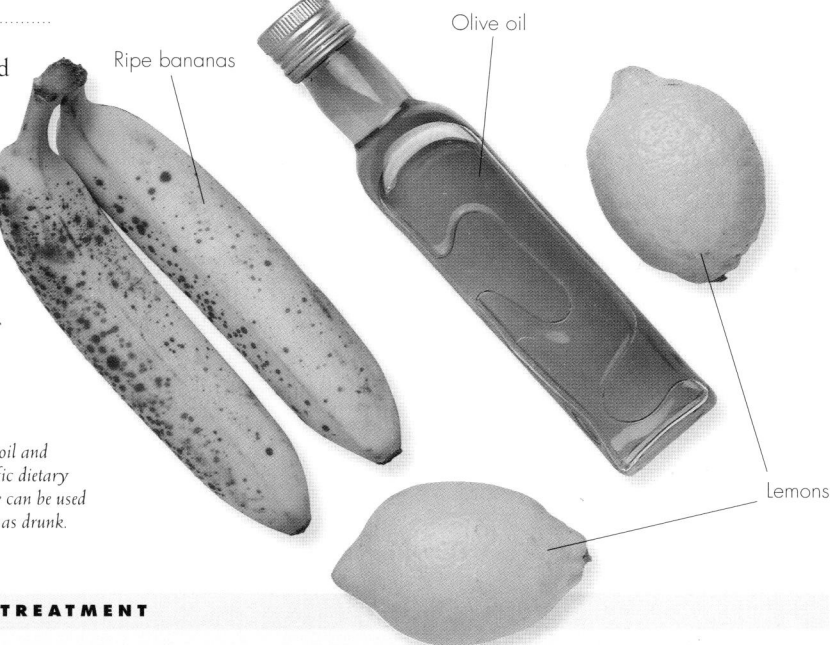

Ripe bananas

Olive oil

Lemons

Oral thrush is a fungal infection which appears as raised creamy spots on the lining of the mouth, lips, and throat. The Candida albicans fungus occurs naturally in the mouth and other moist, warm areas of the body, but if excessive growth is allowed to take place infection can result. This may occur if the bacteria that usually keep it in check are themselves under attack by antibiotics, or if the immune system is compromised for any other reason. Oral thrush is most common in the young and elderly, and in people who wear dentures. Women also appear to be more susceptible than men.

SYMPTOMS

- *pain, soreness, and irritation in the affected area*
- *raised creamy spots in the mouth*

RIGHT Olive oil and bananas are specific dietary aids, and lemon juice can be used externally as well as drunk.

TREATMENT

CHINESE HERBALISM
- Gentian and Oriental wormwood may be prescribed to treat fungal infections of the mouth.

TRADITIONAL HOME AND FOLK REMEDIES
- Eat fresh live yogurt, and dab on to the affected patches, as required. *(See page 93.)*
- Olive oil prevents yeast becoming fungus in the body, and should be drunk or used in cooking, as often as possible. *(See page 95.)*
- Rub raw garlic on to the affected areas, and incorporate plenty of raw garlic into your diet. *(See page 82.)*

- Lemon will help to soothe discomfort and encourage healing. Drink a cup of hot lemon and honey in water 3 times daily. *(See page 87.)*

HERBALISM
- Aloe vera mouthwash has an antifungal effect. *(See page 114.)*
- Barberry prevents the growth of fungus, and stimulates the immune system. Take 3 times daily.
- Caprylic acid is a good antifungal agent. Take 3 capsules with each meal.
- Chew fresh juniper berries to reduce inflammation and attack the Candida fungus.

AROMATHERAPY
- Add a few drops of myrrh, tea tree, or lavender oil to a cup of boiled water and rinse the mouth several times daily to destroy fungal infection. *(See pages 146–71.)*

HOMEOPATHY
Constitutional treatment to boost immunity will be offered, but the following remedies may also be useful:
- Capsicum, when patches are hot and sore and worse after cold drinks.
- Borax, at first symptoms.
- Arsenicum, for thrush associated with mouth ulcers and which occurs when you are run down. *(See page 182.)*

- Mercurius, when your tongue is hot and trembling, and you have more saliva than usual. *(See page 205.)*

VITAMINS AND MINERALS
- Take acidophilus tablets, and eat plenty of ripe bananas to encourage the growth of healthy bacteria in the body, which will reduce the severity of attacks and act to prevent them. *(See page 271.)*

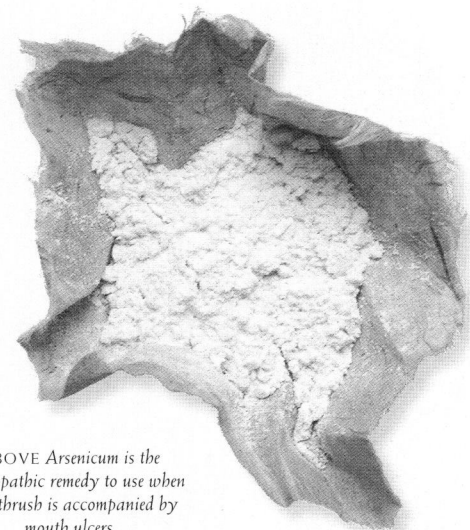

ABOVE Arsenicum is the homeopathic remedy to use when oral thrush is accompanied by mouth ulcers.

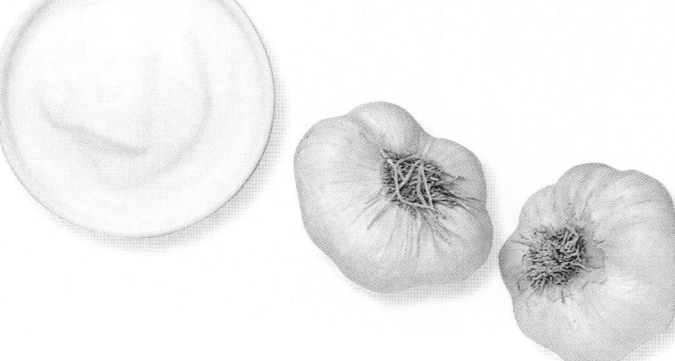

RIGHT Yogurt and garlic are both beneficial. They can be applied to the sore area and added to the diet.

Mouth Ulcers

Mouth ulcers are white, gray, or yellow open sores with an outer ring of red inflammation, and occur when the mucous membrane or skin surface becomes pitted, resulting from an erosion or disintegration of the tissues. They appear on the inside of the lips, cheeks, or floor of the mouth, and may occur as a result of aggressive tooth brushing, ill-fitting dentures, accidentally biting the side of the mouth, or eating very hot food. They can also be triggered by stress or being run down, and can be a feature of Crohn's disease, ulcerative colitis, and celiac disease, or food allergy. Women may be particularly prone to mouth ulcers around menstruation. In children, contact with the herpes simplex virus that causes cold sores may manifest itself as mouth ulcers. Mouth ulcers are common, affecting one in five U.S. adults.

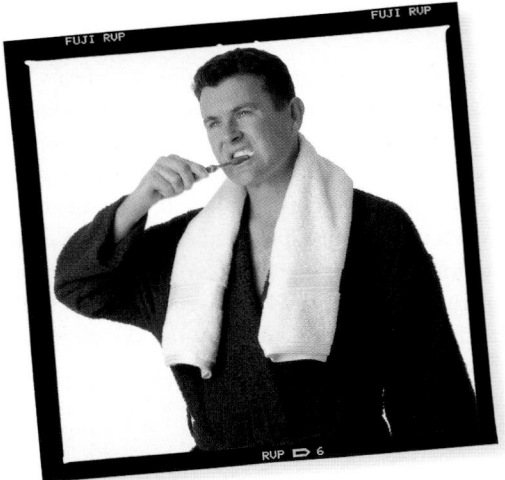

ABOVE *Mouth ulcers can occur as a result of brushing the teeth too vigorously.*

SYMPTOMS

• *pain and stinging in affected area, particularly when eating acidic or spicy foods* • *dry mouth*

TREATMENT

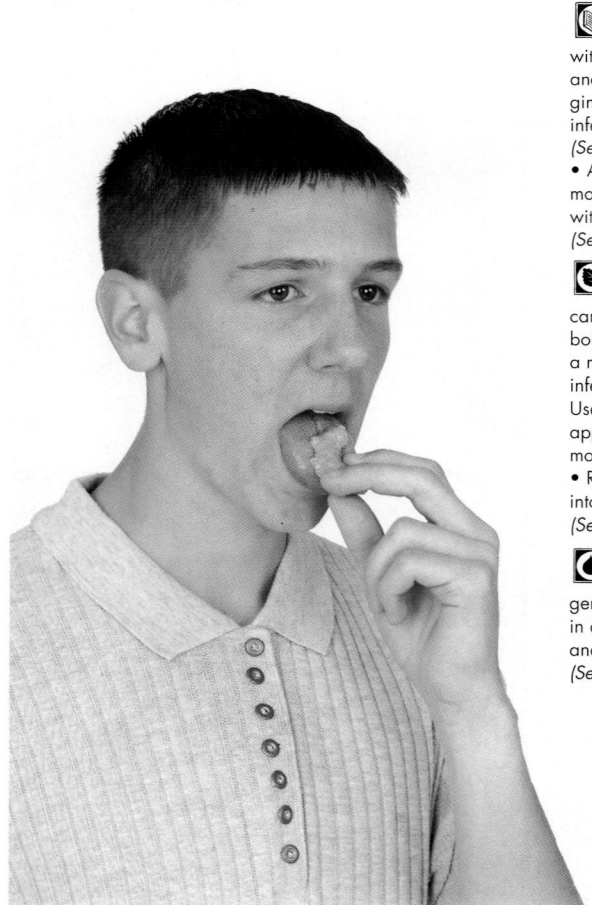

LEFT *Rubbing the tongue with a piece of fresh ginger root is good for some infections of the mouth.*

AYURVEDA
• Rub the tongue with a piece of ginger, and chew fresh root ginger to treat fungal infections of the mouth. (See page 47.)
• Aloe vera is useful for mouth ulcers associated with the herpes virus. (See page 27.)

HERBALISM
• Tincture of myrrh can be added to a cup of boiled water and used as a mouth rinse to destroy infection or infestation. Use the tincture neat and apply to sores in the mouth with a cotton bud.
• Rub a little aloe vera gel into the affected area. (See page 114.)

AROMATHERAPY
• Mix a drop of geranium and lavender oil in a cup of boiled water and gargle as required. (See pages 161 and 165.)

HOMEOPATHY
• Arsenicum, when ulcers are on the edges of the tongue, with burning pains. (See page 182.)
• Mercurius, for ulcers that erupt on the palate or tongue, and which are yellow and spongy. (See page 205.)
• Kali bich., for ulcers that feel thick and firm, and sting. (See page 200.)

VITAMINS AND MINERALS
• Take supplements of vitamin A, E, and B2. (See pages 252, 253, and 257.)
• Vitamin E oil can be applied directly to the ulcers. (See page 257.)

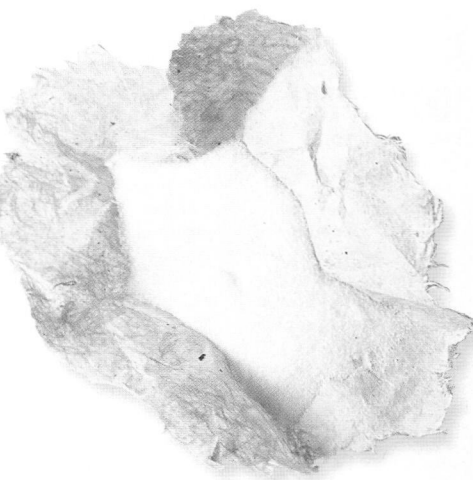

ABOVE *Use the homeopathic remedy Kali bich. when ulcers feel thick and firm, and sting.*

Bad Breath

Bad breath (or halitosis) is often caused by accumulated food debris as a result of poor dental hygiene, smoking, and alcohol consumption. It may be accompanied by dribbling during sleep and a yellowish, thickly coated tongue. Bad breath can also be a symptom of many disorders including gingivitis, tonsillitis, sinusitis, oral thrush, diabetes, acute bronchitis, liver failure, cancer of the mouth, throat, larynx, lungs, or esophagus, chronic gastritis, underproduction of saliva, and constipation.

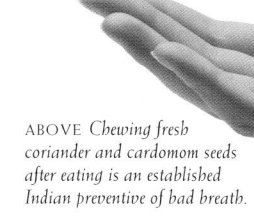

ABOVE *Chewing fresh coriander and cardomom seeds after eating is an established Indian preventive of bad breath.*

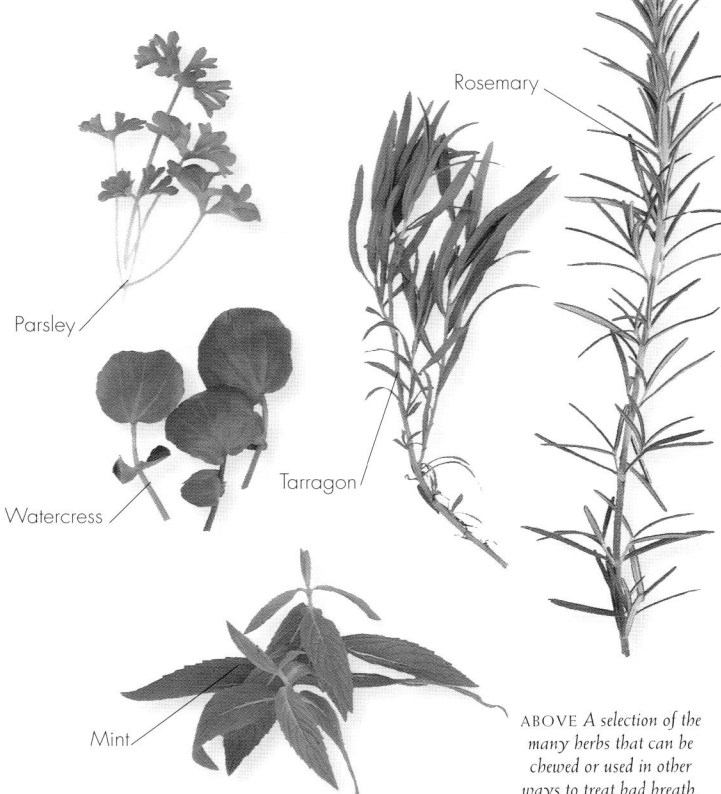

Rosemary

Parsley

Tarragon

Watercress

Mint

ABOVE *A selection of the many herbs that can be chewed or used in other ways to treat bad breath.*

TREATMENT

AYURVEDA
• Chew fresh coriander or cardamom seeds after meals – they will act as a digestive and discourage bad breath. *(See pages 35, 38.)*

CHINESE HERBALISM
• Treatment would be aimed at stomach damp heat, using golden thread, peppermint tea, giant hyssop, and radish seeds. *(See page 54 and 61.)*

TRADITIONAL HOME AND FOLK REMEDIES
• Drink a combination of fresh carrot, celery, watercress, and cucumber juice with some paprika. *(See pages 83, 86, 89, and 94.)*

HERBALISM
• Chew fresh rosemary leaves, or make a mouthwash with a pinch of cloves, cinnamon, anise seed, and rosemary. Steep in a cup of sherry for a week, and then strain. Use daily as required. *(See page 127.)*
• Chew fresh watercress, which is rich in chlorophyll and vitamin C.
• Chew walnut bark and rub it on the gums, then gargle with lemon water.
• Chew fresh parsley, thyme, mint, or tarragon. *(See page 135.)*

AROMATHERAPY
• Add a drop of myrrh essential oil to a cup of cool, boiled water, and rinse the mouth daily. *(See page 155.)*
• Thyme or fennel oil will be equally effective. *(See pages 159 and 170.)*

HOMEOPATHY
• Nux vomica, for breath that smells sour, particularly after meals or drinking alcohol. *(See page 214.)*

• Petroselinium, for breath that smells of onions.
• Nitric acid for bad breath with loose teeth and mouth ulcers.
• Pulsatilla for bad breath after eating fatty foods, and which is accompanied by a dry mouth and no thirst. *(See page 209.)*
• Mercurius, for breath that smells, with copious saliva and a yellow, furry tongue. *(See page 205.)*

VITAMINS AND MINERALS
• Store your toothbrush in grapefruit seed extract to destroy bacteria and other germs which may be encouraging bad breath.

Cold Sores

Cold sores are fluid-filled blisters which crust over after bursting. They usually appear on the mouth and around the lips, sometimes in clusters. They are caused by viral infection (herpes simplex). Most of us are exposed to the herpes simplex virus by the age of five, and can carry an immunity to it. In children who do not successfully fight off the virus, cold sores are manifested as painful mouth ulcers, which appear when the sufferer is run down, or when the immune system is depressed or overstressed. Once you succumb to the virus, you may carry it for the rest of your life, and attacks may be triggered by extremes of weather, or by being run down. In some women, cold sores are worse, or appear more often, during menstruation. There is some evidence that cold sores may be linked to atherosclerosis. Cold sores are highly contagious. *(See under Skin and Hair, page 308.)*

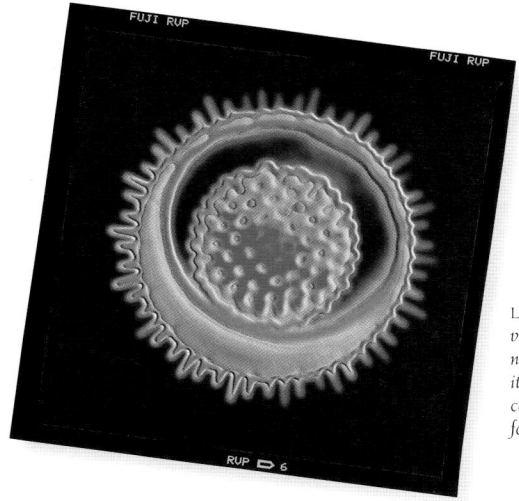

LEFT *The herpes simplex virus. If immunity is not acquired to this virus, it may manifest itself as cold sores periodically for life.*

341

LUNG AND RESPIRATORY DISORDERS

Tuberculosis

More commonly known as TB, tuberculosis is an infectious disease caused by three species of bacteria. The infecting bacteria enter the body through the digestive tract (often in unpasteurized milk from infected cows), or may be spread by person-to-person droplet infection. The lungs are usually the first organs to be affected, but the lymph nodes, the skin, and bones are all possible targets. The disease is most common in areas where poor housing, diet, and sanitation are predisposing factors, or where the immune system is compromised (as in HIV/AIDS). Once established, TB can cause complications such as tuberculosis pleurisy and tuberculosis meningitis. In its latent phase, the disease causes a lesion at the infected site which leaves a characteristic scar but no associated symptoms. If the lesion does not heal, then progressive pulmonary tuberculosis (consumption) develops, causing symptoms in its active phase.

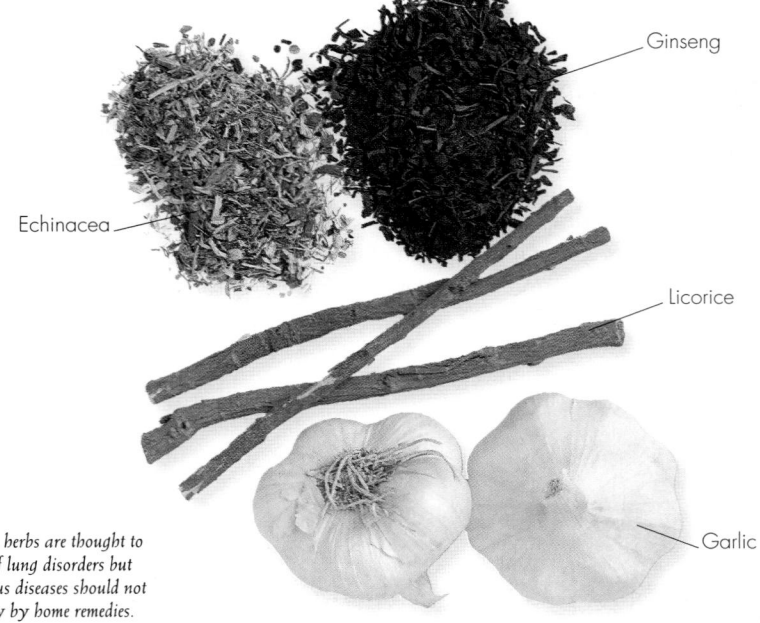

Echinacea

Ginseng

Licorice

Garlic clo

ABOVE *Several herbs are thought to help in cases of lung disorders but potentially serious diseases should not be treated solely by home remedies.*

SYMPTOMS

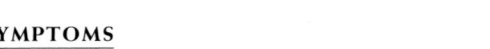

- *loss of appetite* • *fever* • *persistent cough with blood-stained mucus*
- *night sweats* • *fatigue*
- *marked weight loss*

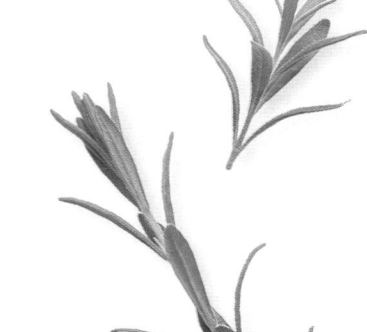

ABOVE *Lavender oil is one of the antibacterial oils that can help to prevent infections.*

CAUTION

IF TB IS SUSPECTED, SEE YOUR PHYSICIAN IMMEDIATELY.

TREATMENT

AYURVEDA
- Stramonium will help with bronchial spasm and congestion.

HERBALISM
Herbs to boost the immune system would be most appropriate:
- Licorice helps recovery, stimulating formation and efficiency of white blood cells and antibodies.
- Garlic helps to prevent many infections, including those which have become immune to antibiotics. *(See page 113.)*
- Echinacea is widely used for chronic and acute infections, cleansing the blood and lymphatic

system, stimulating the production of white blood cells and antibodies. *(See page 120.)*
- Ginseng can boost immunity, as well as stimulating white blood cell production and aiding recovery after illness. *(See page 126.)*

AROMATHERAPY
- Anti-infectious oils which can be used in a vaporizer include: garlic, tea tree, and lavender. *(See pages 146–71.)*
- Use antibacterial oils to prevent further infection, such as juniper, rosemary, bergamot, or eucalyptus. *(See pages 146–71.)*

HOMEOPATHY
The following remedies may help alongside conventional treatment, or alone under the guidance of an experienced homeopath:
- Baccillinum, for fever and weight loss.
- Arsenicum, for exhaustion, chilliness, and a thirst for small sips of water. *(See page 182.)*
- Calcarea, for weakness, fever, cold hands and feet. *(See page 186.)*

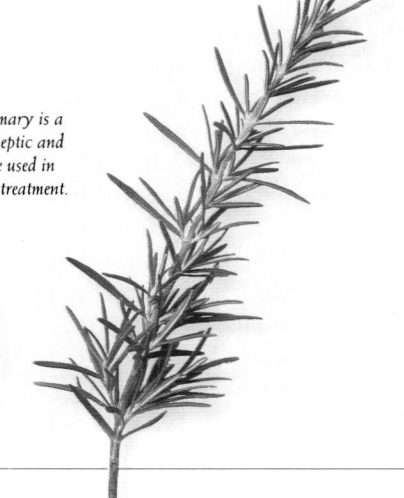

RIGHT *Rosemary is a powerful antiseptic and the oil can be used in aromatherapy treatment.*

DATA FILE

- The bacilli can remain dormant for years before becoming active.

- The disease is not spread through a single exposure to infected droplets, but by extended contact with someone who is infected.

- In the mid-1980s there was a resurgence of tuberculosis in the U.S., first noticed among prison populations and in AIDS patients.

- The further spread of TB may in part be related to crowded urban living conditions.

- Since the mid-1980s, a drug-resistant strain has spread, in part because some patients do not follow the long-term treatment regime once they feel better.

- TB may also be acquired by drinking unpasteurized animal milk.

- A vaccine known as BCG (Bacille Calmette-Guerin), prepared from a living but weakened strain of bacilli, confers some protection against tuberculosis.

- Most at risk in the U.S. are Mexican, African, South American, and Asian immigrants, American men between the ages of 25 and 44, drug and alcohol users, anyone with a weakened immune system, and residents in institutions.

- Experts say that up to 90 percent of the U.S. population have encountered the bacteria, but most are able to fight off the infection.

- The U.S. Lung Association estimates that approximately 14 in 100,000 are affected by TB.

- One tubercule bacillus can replicate itself billions of times in one month.

Pneumonia

Pneumonia is an infection of the lung caused by bacteria or viruses entering the lungs via the upper respiratory tract, leading to inflammation of the lung tissue. There are two main types of the disease: bronchopneumonia, which is usually confined to areas of tissue surrounding the bronchi, and lobar pneumonia, which affects a whole lobe (or more) of the lung. Pneumonia begins with irritation of lung tissue. The walls of air sacs (alveoli) swell or are destroyed, and plasma, red blood cells, and white blood cells from lung capillaries fill the alveolar spaces. The portion of the lung involved becomes relatively solid and basically is rendered temporarily nonfunctional.

SYMPTOMS

• *rapid, shallow breathing* • *chest pain* • *sore throat and headache* • *cough with mucus and possibly blood* • *fever, sweating, and attacks of shivering*

CAUTION

SEEK URGENT MEDICAL ATTENTION IF PNEUMONIA IS SUSPECTED – IT CAN BE FATAL AMONG THE ELDERLY OR VERY YOUNG, OR PEOPLE ALREADY ILL FROM OTHER CAUSES, SUCH AS A STROKE OR HIV/AIDS.

DATA FILE

• Viruses are believed to cause about half of all types of pneumonia.

• The most common form of bacterial pneumonia is caused by Pneumococcus. Staphylococcus, Bacteroides, or Klebsiella.

• Primary atypical pneumonia is a special type of pneumonia that occurs frequently in children and young adults, caused by the micro-organism Mycoplasma pneumoniae.

• Pneumocystis carinii causes pneumonia in those with depressed immune systems and is commonly associated with AIDS.

• Children under one, and people over 60, diabetics, smokers, and alcoholics are most at risk of infection.

• There are over 2 million cases in the U.S. each year.

• Between 40,000–70,000 people die of pneumonia in the U.S. every year.

• Positive diagnosis can only be made with X-ray.

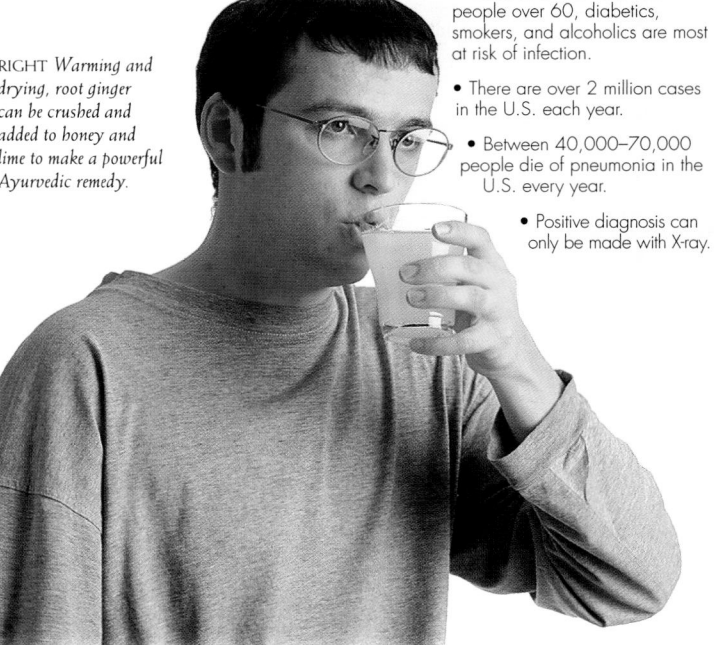

RIGHT *Warming and drying, root ginger can be crushed and added to honey and lime to make a powerful Ayurvedic remedy.*

TREATMENT

AYURVEDA
• Heat mustard oil and apply as a compress to the head to reduce fever. *(See page 30.)*
• Crush root ginger, add to a little honey and lime, and drink as required. *(See page 47.)*

CHINESE HERBALISM
• The problem is believed to be Mucus and Heat in the Lungs, and can be treated with peach kernel, skullcap, and fritillary bulb. *(See pages 63, 72, and 74.)*

HERBALISM
• Try an infusion of coltsfoot, which soothes coughs and helps to fight infections, particularly respiratory infections.
• Raw garlic and onions will help to expel phlegm and fight infection. *(See page 113.)*
• Drink an infusion of boneset to clear congestion and relieve aches and pains.
• Fenugreek with lemon and honey will help to bring down fever and deal with any infection.
• Ginseng is a great all-round restorer and will help to bring down body temperature and fight infection. *(See page 126.)*

AROMATHERAPY
• A steam inhalation of eucalyptus and tea tree will aid breathing, open the lungs, and help fight infection. *(See pages 159 and 162.)*
• A massage of niaouli or cajeput can be used to fight infection and ease symptoms, but this should not be used when there is fever. *(See pages 162 and 163.)*

HOMEOPATHY
Constitutional treatment is necessary after and during the illness, but the following remedies may help in a case of mild pneumonia:
• Aconite, for sudden onset with anxiety and fever. *(See page 178.)*
• Bryonia, for sharp chest pains which are made worse by moving about. *(See page 185.)*
• Sanguinaria, for pneumonia after flu, with right lung affected and accompanied by rust-colored phlegm.
• Phosphorus, for rust-colored phlegm, weakness, trembling, and a thirst for cold drinks. *(See page 208.)*

VITAMINS AND MINERALS
• Include plenty of fluids and foods rich in vitamin C and zinc, which will encourage the immune system. *(See pages 256 and 265.)*

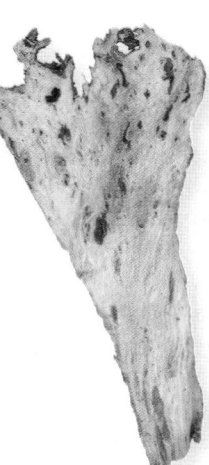

ABOVE *Skullcap, one of the "Three Yellows" of Chinese herbalism used to clear severe infections with signs of Heat.*

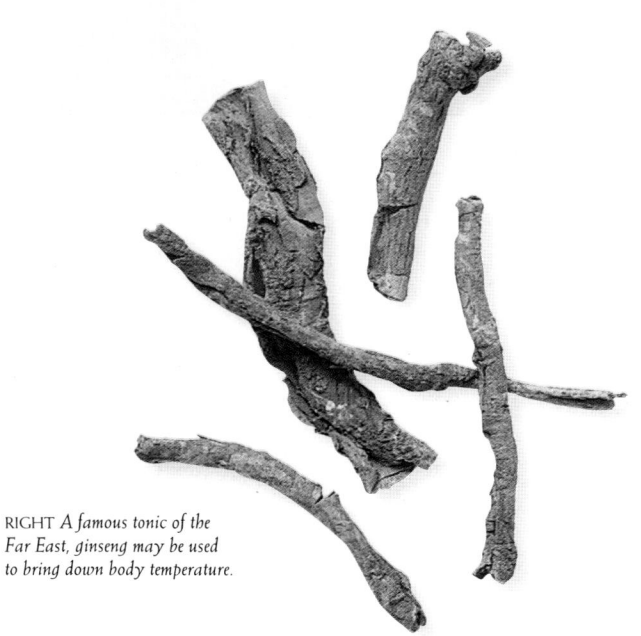

RIGHT *A famous tonic of the Far East, ginseng may be used to bring down body temperature.*

Asthma

Asthma is a condition in which the muscles of the bronchi (the air tubes of the lung) contract in spasm, obstructing the flow of air and making breathing out, in particular, very difficult. Asthma is becoming increasingly common, especially among children, and may be triggered by a number of factors, including allergens (such as house dust or pets), pollution, infection, emotional trauma, or physical exertion. Asthma is divided into two categories: intrinsic, for which there is no identifiable cause for attacks, and extrinsic, which is caused by something, usually inhaled, that triggers an attack.

In many asthma patients, inflammation of the lining of the airways leads to increased sensitivity to a variety of environmental triggers that can cause narrowing of the airways, resulting in obstruction of airflow and breathing difficulty. In some patients, the mucous glands in the airways produce excessive thick mucus, further obstructing airflow.

An asthma attack may be brief or last for several days. Typically, an attack begins within minutes after exposure to a triggering agent. Some patients have only occasional or "seasonal" symptoms, while others have daily symptoms.

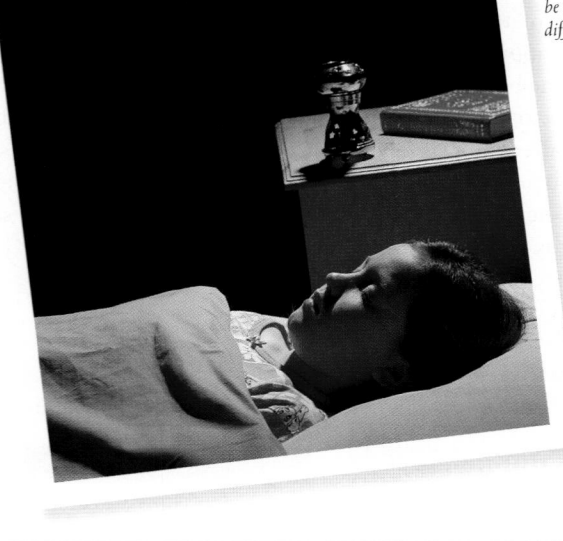

LEFT *Antispasmodic aromatherapy oils can be inhaled from a diffuser.*

SYMPTOMS

• *difficulty in breathing* • *an increase in pulse rate* • *wheezing, especially on breathing out* • *a persistent dry cough* • *a sensation of tightness around the chest*

DATA FILE

• The prevalence of asthma is only about 1 or 2 percent worldwide, but in the U.S. asthma affects about 6 percent of children.

• In the U.S. asthma affects 1 in 20 adults, affecting over 7 million adults and 3 million children, or roughly 4 percent of the population.

• Children under 16 and adults over 65 are most commonly affected.

• The incidence of hospitalization for children suffering from asthma and asthma-related illness has increased by 500 percent over the last 30 years.

• The incidence of asthma in the U.K. population has increased 30 times over the last 30 years.

• Asthma is on the increase in the Western world, and although orthodox medicine can control all the worst symptoms, there is no sign of a cure being found.

• Drinking caffeine is said to open the airways and reduce symptoms by one-third in asthma sufferers.

CAUTION

A PROLONGED ATTACK OF SEVERE ASTHMA THAT DOES NOT RESPOND TO SIMPLE REMEDIES REQUIRES IMMEDIATE MEDICAL ATTENTION.

IF A COUGH LASTS FOR MORE THAN 10 DAYS, OR IS ACCOMPANIED BY FEVER, DIFFICULT BREATHING, BLUE LIPS, DROWSINESS, OR DIFFICULTY IN SPEAKING, CONTACT YOUR PHYSICIAN.

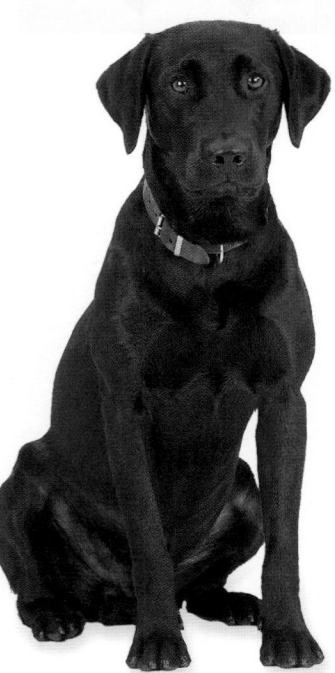

ABOVE *Asthma sufferers may find attacks are brought on by proximity to the family pet.*

TREATMENT

AYURVEDA
• Common ginger and stramonium may be used to treat asthma. *(See page 47.)*

CHINESE HERBALISM
• The cause of the illness is considered to be Phlegm produced by weakness of the Spleen and Kidneys. Almond and ephedra may be prescribed to open the Lungs.

HERBALISM
• Any of the herbs suggested for stress *(see page 284)* will help you to relax, which should decrease the incidence of attacks.
• Elecampane can be infused to treat asthma. Drink daily if you are prone to attacks.
• During a mild attack, grindelia, hyssop, wild cherry bark, and motherwort will help. *(See page 124.)*
• Turmeric has a broncho-dilatory effect, and it can be sipped sprinkled in a cup of warm water.

AROMATHERAPY
• A steam inhalation of chamomile, eucalyptus, or lavender essential oils can be taken during an attack and immediately afterwards to ease panic and to help open the airways. *(See pages 146–71.)*
• Pine oil in the bath or a vaporizer will reduce the incidence of attacks. *(See page 166.)*
• Bergamot, clary sage, neroli, chamomile, and rose are antispasmodic, as well as being relaxant, and they will be particularly useful for attacks brought on by stress. *(See pages 146–71.)*

HOMEOPATHY
Chronic asthma must be treated constitutionally, but the following remedies can be used for mild attacks, while waiting for medical attention:
• Ipecac., for wheezy children who cough until they vomit up a little mucus. *(See page 189.)*

• Arsenicum, for waking between midnight and 2 A.M., accompanied by difficult breathing. *(See page 182.)*
• Bryonia, for asthma at the end of a cold, with a hard, dry cough. *(See page 185.)*
• Nat. sulf., for asthma in damp weather, with a loose cough and yellowish mucus. *(See page 207.)*
• Lachesis, for asthma that starts in spring or autumn, or at the menopause. *(See page 216.)*

FLOWER ESSENCES
• Take Rescue Remedy when you feel symptoms coming on. This will ease symptoms and prevent a full-blown attack. *(See page 244.)*

VITAMINS AND MINERALS
• Increase your intake of vitamin B6, which is said to reduce the frequency and severity of attacks. *(See page 254.)*

Coughs

Coughs are necessary to expel foreign bodies and mucus from the trachea and airways of the lungs. Coughing is a symptom rather than an illness, and can indicate sinusitis, croup, bronchitis, pneumonia, flu, viruses, the early stages of measles, asthma, whooping cough, or an excess of catarrh from the nose or sinuses, due to irritation or infection.

A dry cough may be caused by mucus from infections or colds, chemicals in the atmosphere, a foreign object or nervousness which constricts the throat. A loose, wetter cough is caused by inflammation of the bronchial tubes produced by an infection or allergy. A constant nighttime cough, or one which recurs with each cold and is hard to get rid of, may indicate asthma.

DATA FILE

Various terms describe the type of cough:

- An acute cough starts suddenly, and is usually resolved within a day or two.

- A chronic cough persists, sometimes for many weeks.

- A productive cough brings up lots of catarrh or mucus.

- A nonproductive cough brings up very little or no mucus, and usually sounds harsh and hard.

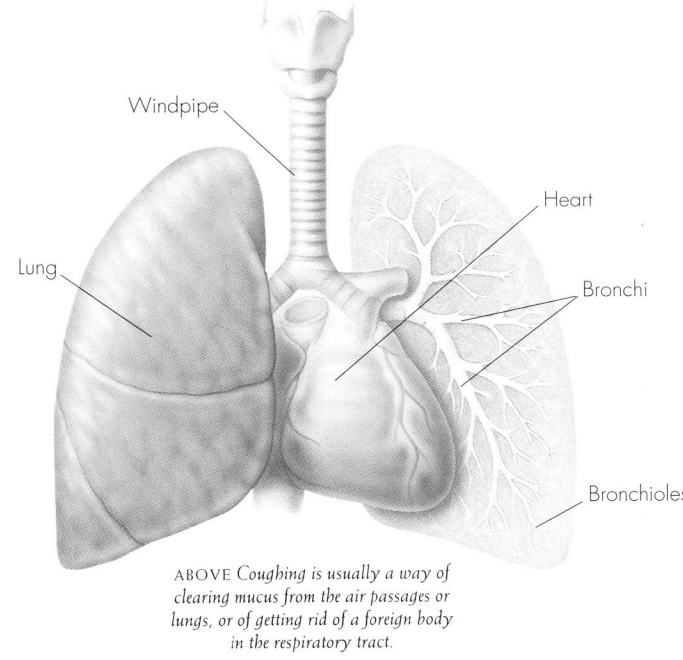

ABOVE *Coughing is usually a way of clearing mucus from the air passages or lungs, or of getting rid of a foreign body in the respiratory tract.*

TREATMENT

AYURVEDA
- Brown 4 tablespoons of coriander seeds in a frying pan, then boil with 4 cups of water, with 4 slices of root ginger. Reduce to 2 cups of liquid, strain, and drink. *(See page 35.)*
- Other herbs to consider are sunflower, henbane, and stramonium.

TRADITIONAL HOME AND FOLK REMEDIES
- A tincture of garlic (place several garlic cloves in brandy and leave for 2 or 3 weeks, then strain) or garlic syrup (tincture, or fresh garlic mixed with a little honey) will help the body to fight infection. It also works to cleanse the blood. *(See page 82.)*
- Ginseng in hot herbal tea warms the body and eases symptoms.
- Honey and lemon will ease coughs and encourage healing. *(See pages 87 and 101.)*
- Mustard powder, mixed with a little water, can be made into a poultice and applied to the chest area. *(See page 98.)*
- Apply a warm roasted onion poultice to the chest, or drink a warm onion broth to cleanse and reduce congestion. *(See page 82.)*

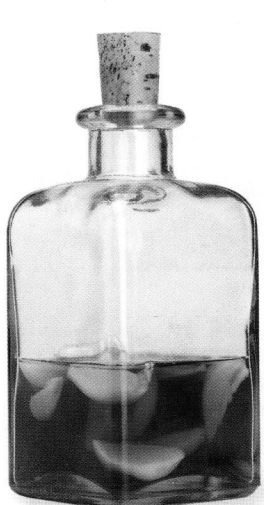

LEFT *Tincture of garlic is made by steeping garlic cloves in a jar of brandy.*

HERBALISM
- Peppermint tea can be drunk to soothe. *(See page 125.)*
- Add lightly macerated licorice root sticks to your herbal drink to ease. *(See page 122.)*
- Aniseed, marshmallow, and wild cherry bark are useful for unproductive, irritating coughs. *(See page 114.)*
- Use golden seal, plantain, and thyme if infection is present. *(See pages 126 and 135.)*

AROMATHERAPY
- Inhale the steam from a few drops of eucalyptus oil in boiling water, as it is expectorant and decongestant. *(See page 159.)*
- Pine oil, in a vaporizer, will ease coughing and act to restore the lungs. *(See page 166.)*
- Massage frankincense or sandalwood into the chest and back. *(See pages 147 and 169.)*
- Essential oil of myrrh reduces mucus and phlegm. *(See page 155.)*

HOMEOPATHY
- Pulsatilla, for a loose, wet, rattling cough, which is worse in the morning and when in bed at night. *(See page 209.)*
- Ant. tart. is especially useful for elderly people who suffer from persistent rattling cough, and are full of loose mucus but cannot seem to bring it up. *(See page 179.)*
- Rumex, for a very tickly cough, when cold air irritates the nose and throat.
- Bryonia, for a dry cough where the chest feels sore from coughing. *(See page 185.)*
- Phosphorous, for a tickling cough in delicate people with weak chests. *(See page 208.)*
- Drosera, for a violent tickly cough with retching and pain in the ribs. *(See page 193.)*
- Chamomilla, for a dry, irritating cough with wheezing, and which is worse at night and makes you feel irritable. *(See page 204.)*

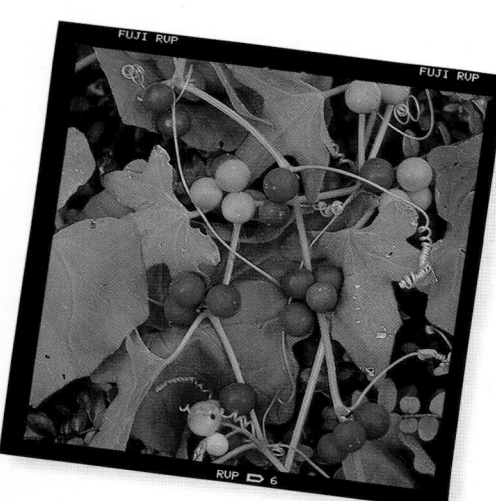

ABOVE *Bryony, the source of the homeopathic remedy Bryonia, useful for a dry cough with a sore chest.*

CAUTION

IF A COUGH LASTS FOR MORE THAN 10 DAYS, OR IS ACCOMPANIED BY FEVER, DIFFICULT BREATHING, BLUE LIPS, DROWSINESS OR DIFFICULTY SPEAKING, CONTACT YOUR PHYSICIAN.

Flu

More properly known as influenza, flu is a viral disease of the upper respiratory tract, spread by the contaminated droplets (via coughing and sneezing) of other sufferers. The three main types of flu are caused by three different viruses – A, B, and C. Type C, once caught, confers immunity. Types A and B, however, are constantly mutating so that our bodies cannot build up resistance against them. Incubation of the virus is generally one or two days, during which time it is highly infectious, and therefore notoriously impossible to contain.

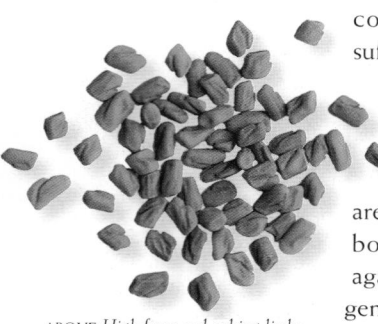

ABOVE *High fever and aching limbs can be relieved by taking fenugreek, mixed with lemon and honey.*

DATA FILE

• When new strains of influenza virus arise, they spread rapidly around the world, infecting millions of people and causing many deaths.

• Flu victims 50 years old or older, children, and immune-deficient people are at risk of developing pneumonia and other secondary infections.

• Over the age of 65, pneumonia and flu are the fifth leading cause of death.

• The disease is produced by any one of three types of Orthomyxovirus virus (A, B, and C), of which there are many strains.

• Vaccines have been developed that have been found to be 70–90 percent effective for at least six months against either A or B types, and a genetically engineered live-virus vaccine is under development.

• Vaccination is considered especially important for older people, patients with cardiac or respiratory diseases, and pregnant women.

• The incidence of infection is highest among school-age children, partly because of their lack of previous exposure to various strains.

• Approximately every ten years, influenza pandemics have been caused by new strains of type-A virus.

• Epidemics, or regional outbreaks, have appeared every 2 to 3 years for influenza A, and every 4 to 5 years for influenza B.

SYMPTOMS

• *high fever, possibly accompanied by shivering* • *sore throat, and possibly a dry, unproductive cough* • *runny nose and sneezing* • *breathlessness and general weakness* • *headache, stiff and aching joints, and muscular pain* • *nausea and loss of appetite* • *possibly insomnia and depression*

TREATMENT

AYURVEDA
• Heat mustard oil and apply as a compress to the head to reduce fever. *(See page 30.)*
• Crush root ginger, add to a little honey and lime, and drink as required. *(See page 47.)*
• Bitter orange, sunflower, and coriander may be useful in treating flu. *(See pages 35, 40.)*

TRADITIONAL HOME AND FOLK REMEDIES
• Some warmed apple juice (preferably fresh) can ease the fever. *(See page 94.)*
• Barley water is a traditional remedy for high fever – particularly one caused by infection and inflammation. *(See page 92.)*
• Ginseng powder can be added to herbal teas to restore.
• Drink hot lemon and honey in a cup of warm water to ease inflammation and fever. *(See pages 87 and 101.)*
• Gargle with lemon juice to kill germs and help to stop the spread of the virus. *(See page 87.)*

HERBALISM
• Drink an infusion of boneset to relieve aches and pains and clear congestion.

• Fenugreek with lemon and honey will help to bring down fever and soothe aching limbs.
• Ginseng is a great all-round restorer and will help to bring down body temperature to normal. *(See page 126.)*
• Use wormwood, sage, and licorice to prevent flu. *(See pages 122 and 129.)*

AROMATHERAPY
• Gargle with tea tree oil to prevent the spread of infection. *(See page 162.)*
• Use a eucalyptus or peppermint inhalation to unblock sinuses and the chest. *(See pages 159 and 164.)*
• Massage tea tree and geranium oil into the chest and head to reduce symptoms and fight infection. *(See pages 162 and 165.)*
• Oils which act to bring down fever include bergamot, chamomile, melissa, and tea tree. *(See pages 146–71.)*

HOMEOPATHY
• Gelsemium, for occasions when muscular weakness, aching, and heaviness predominate. *(See page 195.)*
• Rhus tox., for flu that starts after getting wet, where there is a lot of aching in joints rather than muscles.

Accompanied by restlessness and inability to get comfortable. *(See page 210.)*
• Bryonia, for a bad headache and dry cough, with a desire to lie quite still. *(See page 185.)*
• Eupatorium perfoliatum, for intense aching in the back and limbs, together with shivery chills.
• Arsenicum, when you feel debilitated, often with loss of fluids, and with accompanying watery diarrhea and sometimes vomiting. *(See page 182.)*
• Baptisia, for gastric flu, when you feel very "wiped out," and your body feels bruised, or scattered around the bed; also with sudden bouts of diarrhea or vomiting. *(See page 184.)*

VITAMINS AND MINERALS
• Eat plenty of foods rich in vitamin C, bioflavonoids and zinc, which will encourage healing, help to fight infection, and boost the action of the immune system. *(See pages 256, 272, and 265.)*
• Royal jelly acts as a tonic and an antiviral agent. *(See page 276.)*

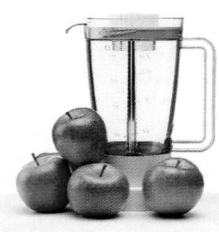

ABOVE *Freshly made apple juice is a good home remedy, providing vitamin C to help to combat infection. Using a juice extractor enables this to be made quickly and easily.*

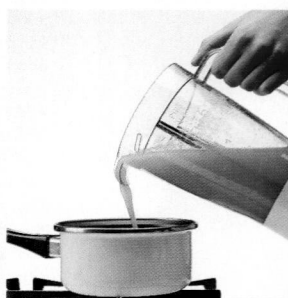

ABOVE *The apple juice can be poured into a pan and gently warmed, but it must not be boiled or overheated or the vitamin content will be severely reduced.*

LEFT *Flu is characterized by a high fever with a runny nose and sneezing.*

Emphysema

Emphysema is a progressive disease in which the tiny air sacs in the lungs (alveoli) break down, reducing the area available for gas exchange. This means that insufficient oxygen reaches the vital organs, and too much carbon dioxide enters the bloodstream. Emphysema is particularly common among heavy smokers and sufferers of asthma and chronic bronchitis. Industrial pollutants may also be a cause, as well as hereditary factors.

The exact cause of pulmonary emphysema is unknown. Cigarette smoking is closely associated with the disease, and in some cases a genetic link is suspected, in that a significant number of people with emphysema lack a gene that controls the liver's production of a protein called alpha-1 antitrypsin, or AAT. Emphysema rarely occurs before the age of 40, and women appear to be less prone, although with the increase in the numbers of women smoking this may change.

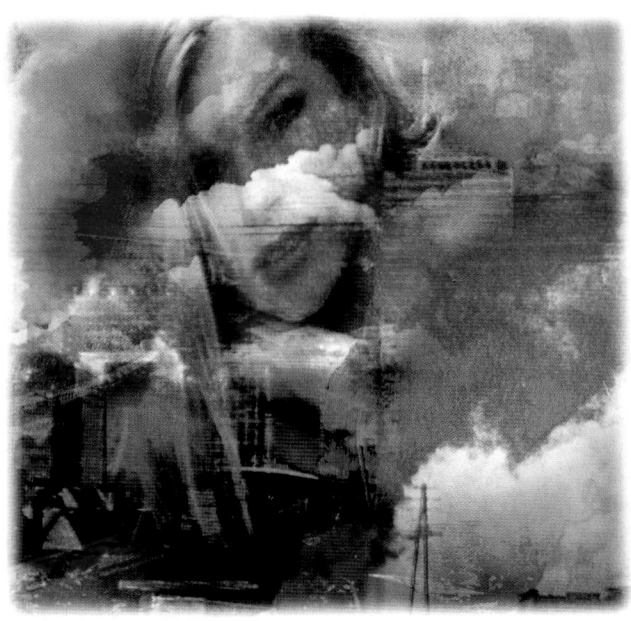

ABOVE *The exact causes of this disease are not known, but smoking and breathing polluted air are two major contributors.*

SYMPTOMS

- *breathlessness, especially on exertion* • *a cough producing sputum*
- *the chest may become barrel-shaped as the disease progresses*
- *a blue tinge to the skin (cyanosis)* • *respiratory failure may eventually occur*

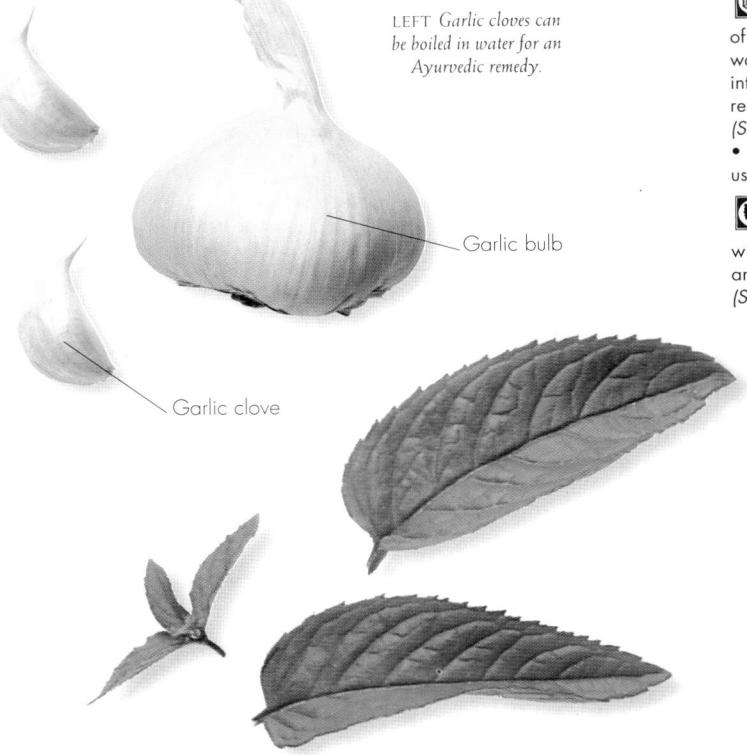

LEFT *Garlic cloves can be boiled in water for an Ayurvedic remedy.*

Garlic bulb

Garlic clove

TREATMENT

AYURVEDA
- Boil 2 or 3 cloves of garlic in 2 cups of water until tender. Crush into the water and drink to relieve chest pain. *(See page 26.)*
- Stramonium may be useful.

HERBALISM
- Peppermint tea will soothe inflammation and help to open lungs. *(See page 125.)*

- Slippery elm bark soothes the chest and lungs, and can be added to any herbal tea. *(See page 136.)*

AROMATHERAPY
- Massage oils of cedarwood, peppermint, or eucalyptus into the chest daily, to open lungs and reduce coughing. *(See pages 146–71.)*
- Make an inhalation of eucalyptus, and use as required to expel phlegm. *(See page 159.)*

HOMEOPATHY
- Emphysema cannot be cured, but the symptoms can be alleviated and the condition arrested by constitutional treatment.
- See coughs *(page 345)*, bronchitis *(page 349)*, and asthma *(page 344)* for remedies that fit specific symptoms.

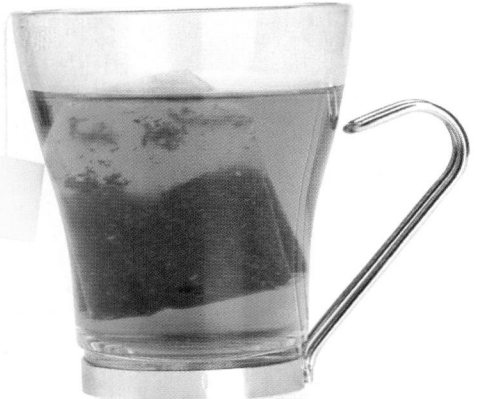

LEFT and RIGHT *Peppermint leaves can be used to make a soothing tea.*

347

Pleurisy

Pleurisy (or pleuritis) is an infection, viral or bacterial in origin, caused by an inflammation of the pleura – the sac-like membrane surrounding the lungs. The two layers of the inflamed pleura rub together to cause the characteristic creaking noise in the chest that makes diagnosis so easy. A surplus of pleural fluid may also be produced by the inflammation, causing a pleural effusion which can be detected on physical examination. In a very few cases, pleurisy may be an indication of more serious diseases such as lung cancer or pulmonary embolism, while chronic pleurisy may be a symptom of tuberculosis. Before the advent of antibiotics, pleurisy was a life-threatening condition and one of the most common causes of death, particularly in children. Today, the condition is usually easily diagnosed and treated in the early stages.

SYMPTOMS

• *stabbing pain, usually at a particular point in inhalation or on coughing*

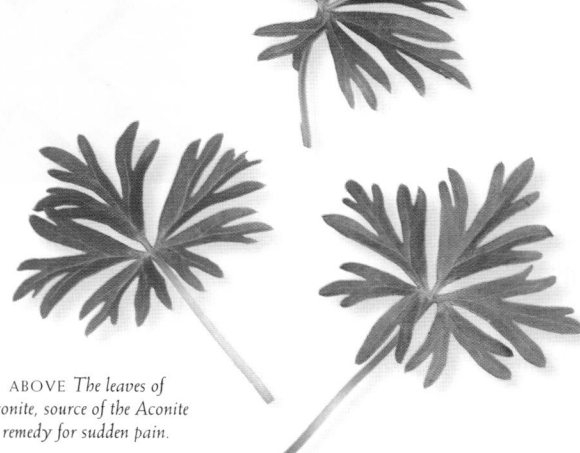

CAUTION

IF YOU DO NOT FEEL BETTER AFTER A DAY (TAKING DOSES EVERY HOUR), SEE YOUR PHYSICIAN.

ABOVE *The leaves of aconite, source of the Aconite remedy for sudden pain.*

TREATMENT

TRADITIONAL HOME AND FOLK REMEDIES
• Apple cider vinegar compresses will reduce inflammation and encourage healing. *(See page 102.)*

HERBALISM
• Comfrey root or leaf tea compresses can be applied to the chest to ease inflammation. *(See page 132.)*
• Wrap a bruised wet plantain leaf across the chest to soothe symptoms. *(See page 126.)*
• Combine a handful of sage leaves and corn silk to strengthen the kidneys and expel water from the system. *(See page 129.)*

AROMATHERAPY
• The following anti-inflammatory oils can be used in gentle massage of the chest and back, or in the bath or an inhaler to encourage healing: bergamot, calendula, chamomile, myrrh. *(See pages 146–71.)*
• Lavender can be sniffed during an attack to calm you and help fight infection. *(See page 161.)*

HOMEOPATHY
During an acute attack, the following remedies may be useful:
• Aconite, for a sudden sharp pain, usually after exposure to cold wind. *(See page 178.)*

• Cantharis, for breathlessness and burning pains with mild fever and a dry cough. *(See page 188.)*
• Belladonna, for sudden pain and a hot flushed face accompanied by thirst. *(See page 183.)*
• Hep. sulf., for slower recovery, with fluid on the lungs. *(See page 198.)*
• Bryonia, for pain that is made worse by movement, and which is accompanied by thirst and general irritability. *(See page 185.)*
• Sulfur, for sharp, cutting pains that are made worse by movement. *(See page 215.)*

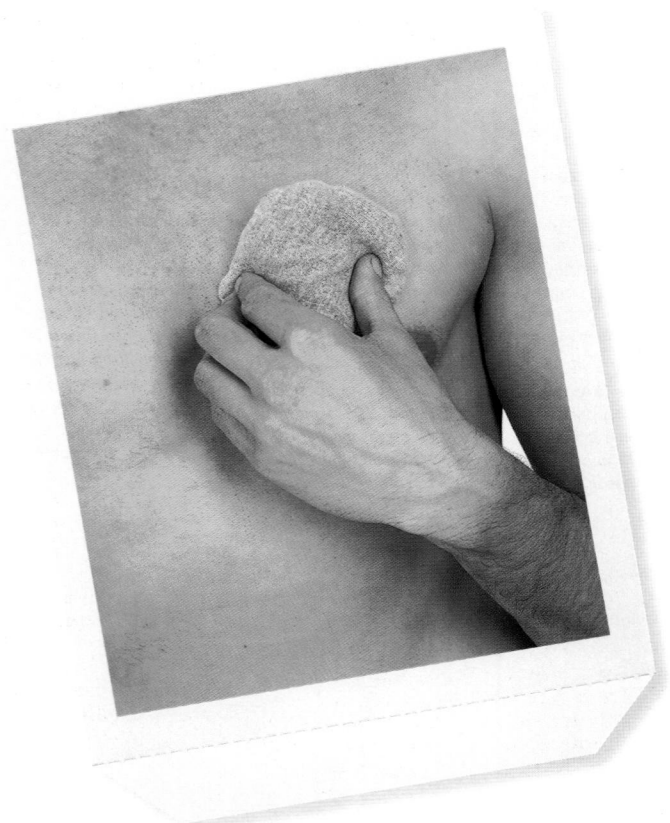

ABOVE *An inflammation of the pleura causes a sharp, stabbing pain in the chest. Apply a leaf tea compress to relieve symptoms.*

RIGHT *An excellent herbal remedy for pleurisy may be made from corn silk and sage.*

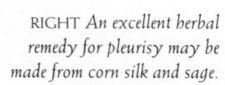

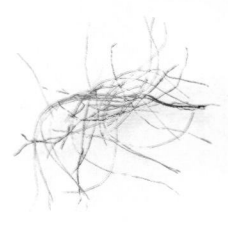

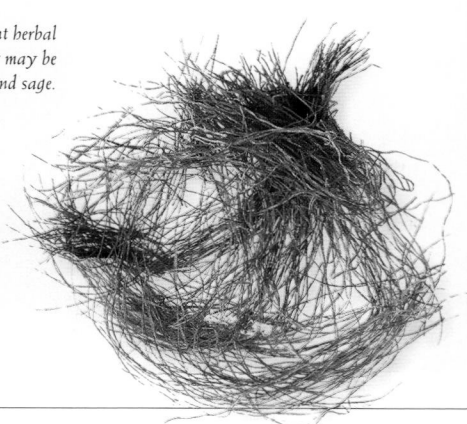

Bronchitis

Bronchitis is an inflammation of the lining of the bronchi (the air tubes of the lungs). Acute bronchitis, in which mucus infected with bacteria is expelled from the lungs, often follows a viral illness such as a cold or flu. Smoking and a damp, dusty, or foggy atmosphere can lead to chronic bronchitis resulting from long-term irritation of the air passages.

ABOVE *Mustard powder can be used to make a warming poultice for the chest.*

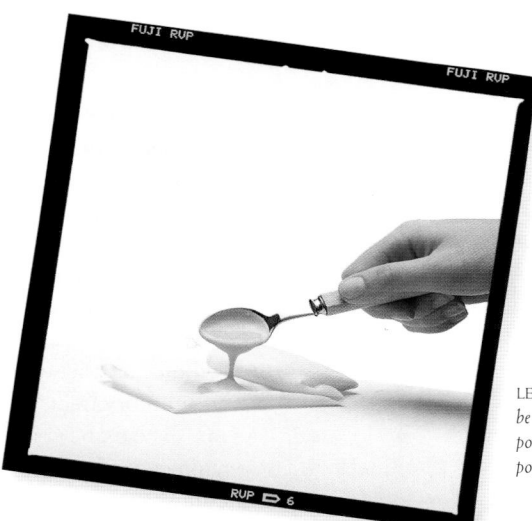

LEFT *Chest congestion may be relieved by applying a poultice of mustard seed powder and water.*

SYMPTOMS

• *a cough, dry at first but with gradually increasing sputum* • *possibly chest pain* • *fever* • *shortness of breath and wheezing* • *in cases of chronic bronchitis symptoms may begin in winter, but then persist throughout the year*

DATA FILE

• Smokers are 50 times more susceptible to bronchitis.

• Male sufferers outnumber female sufferers by ten to one.

• Ayurvedic breathing exercises and yoga generally assist breathing and shortness of breath.

• Acute bronchitis is usually caused by infection by one of the many viruses that cause the common cold or influenza, and is frequently associated with measles.

• Acute chemical bronchitis may be caused by the inhalation of irritating fumes, such as smoke, chlorine, ammonia, and ozone.

• Chronic bronchitis results from prolonged irritation of the bronchial membrane, causing coughing and the excessive secretion of mucus for extended periods. By far the most common cause of chronic bronchitis is cigarette smoking, but air pollution, industrial fumes, and dust are also recognized lung irritants.

CAUTION

IF YOUR TEMPERATURE RISES ABOVE 39 DEGREES, OR IF YOU COUGH BLOOD, CALL YOUR PHYSICIAN.

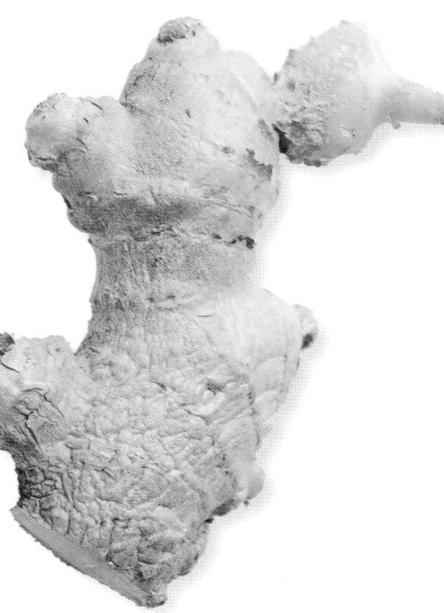

RIGHT *Ginger root is a warming treatment, and in Ayurveda it is mixed with honey and lime juice to make a curative drink.*

TREATMENT

AYURVEDA
• Heat mustard oil and apply as a compress to the head to reduce fever. *(See page 30.)*
• Crush root ginger, add to a little honey and lime, and drink as required. *(See page 47.)*
• Hollyhock may be appropriate, as well as bitter orange and stramonium.

CHINESE HERBALISM
• The source is believed to be external Wind, Cold, or Heat in cases of acute bronchitis, and internal Deficient Spleen or Lung, or internal Mucus for chronic bronchitis.
• Acute conditions will respond to fritillary bulb, plantain seed, and balloon flower root. *(See pages 63 and 69.)*
• Chronic conditions would respond to honeysuckle flowers, mulberry leaves, gardenia fruit. *(See page 65.)*

TRADITIONAL HOME AND FOLK REMEDIES
• Honey and lemon work to fight infection and ease coughs. *(See pages 87 and 101.)*
• Combine mustard seed powder and water to make a poultice to decongest the chest. *(See page 98.)*

• Onions will soothe inflamed membranes and induce perspiration. *(See page 82.)*

HERBALISM
• Anise diluted in a small amount of water soothes a hacking cough.
• Wild cherry bark extract added to any herbal drink relieves coughing.
• Coltsfoot can be added to licorice and honey to alleviate coughs.
• Rub garlic oil into the chest to fight infection and encourage healing. *(See page 113.)*
• Drink ginseng in hot water, as it will help to eliminate infection and ease coughing fits. *(See page 126.)*
• Peppermint tea will soothe the cough and help to bring out the infection. *(See page 125.)*

AROMATHERAPY
• Oils to help clear the congestion include eucalyptus and thyme, which can be inhaled as required. *(See pages 159 and 170.)*
• Ginger oil can be diluted and rubbed into the chest for chronic bronchitis, to dispel mucus. *(See page 171.)*
• Juniper, myrrh, and rosemary will help to prevent mucus, and act to detoxify the body. *(See pages 146–71.)*

HOMEOPATHY
The following remedies can be offered for acute bronchitis; chronic bronchitis must be treated constitutionally:
• Pulsatilla, for symptoms that are worse in stuffy rooms, and for a cough which is dry at night and loose in the morning. *(See page 209.)*
• Ipecac., for nausea, vomiting, and suffocation feelings. *(See page 189.)*
• Bryonia, for a dry, stabbing cough accompanied by a headache and great thirst. *(See page 185.)*
• Phosphorus, for a tight, tickly cough, when you are pale, anxious, and thirsty for cold water. *(See page 208.)*
• Aconite, for sudden onset bronchitis, with a dry cough and chills. *(See page 178.)*

VITAMINS AND MINERALS
• Increase your intake of vitamins B, C, and A, and zinc. *(See pages 252–5, 256 and 265.)*

Tracheitis

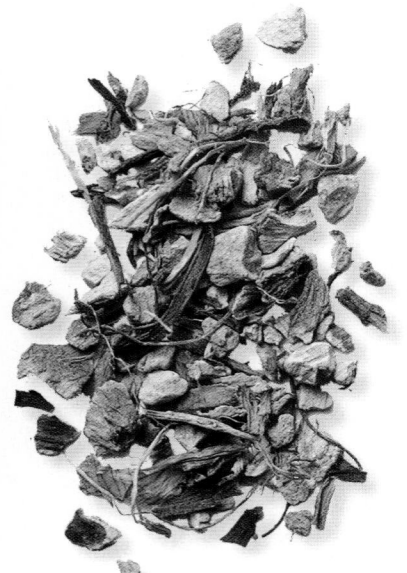

ABOVE *Rumex is the homeopathic treatment for certain types of sore throat.*

Tracheitis is an acute inflammation of the lining of the trachea (windpipe). It is usually viral in origin but can sometimes be bacterial. It is often associated with an infection elsewhere in the upper respiratory tract, such as bronchitis or influenza. Tracheitis is the most common cause of painful attacks of croup in young children. In cases where the bronchi of the lungs become infected (laryngotracheobronchitis), the walls of the airway swell, which can lead to asphyxia in small children.

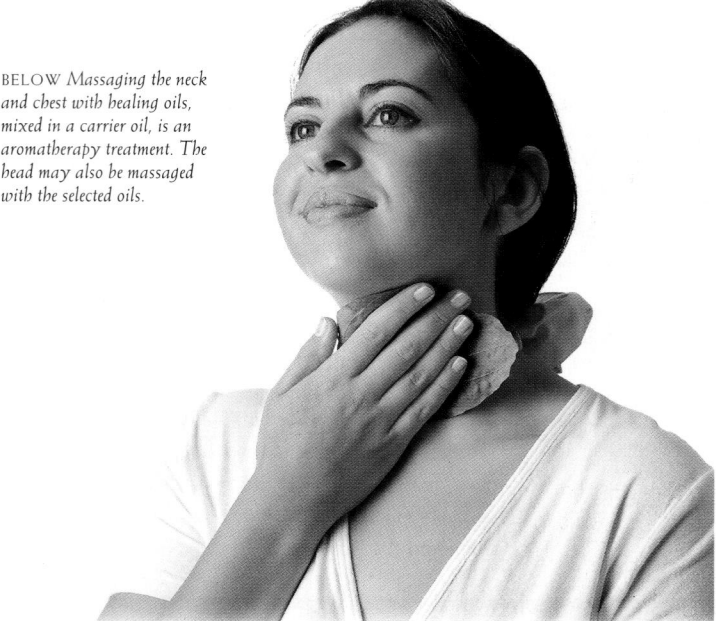

BELOW *Massaging the neck and chest with healing oils, mixed in a carrier oil, is an aromatherapy treatment. The head may also be massaged with the selected oils.*

TREATMENT

AYURVEDA
• Hollyhock may be useful for throat irritation.

HERBALISM
• Comfrey root or leaf tea compresses on the throat and neck will help ease inflammation. *(See page 132.)*
• Wrap a bruised, wet plantain leaf across the throat to soothe symptoms. *(See page 126.)*

AROMATHERAPY
• Anti-inflammatory oils can be used in gentle massage of the chest, neck, and head, or in the bath or an inhaler to encourage healing. Try bergamot, calendula, chamomile, and myrrh. *(See pages 146–71.)*

HOMEOPATHY
• Rumex, for a raw feeling in the throat, a tickly cough, and where the throat is sore to the touch.
• Stannum, when there is sweet yellow phlegm and pain after coughing.
• Bryonia, when pain is made worse by talking, smoke, and warm rooms. *(See page 185.)*
• Phosphorus, for a hacking cough, thirst for cold drinks, and a raw feeling. *(See page 208.)*
• Kali bich., for sticky phlegm that is difficult to expel. *(See page 200.)*

VITAMINS AND MINERALS
• Take extra vitamin C and zinc to boost the immune system. *(See pages 256 and 265.)*

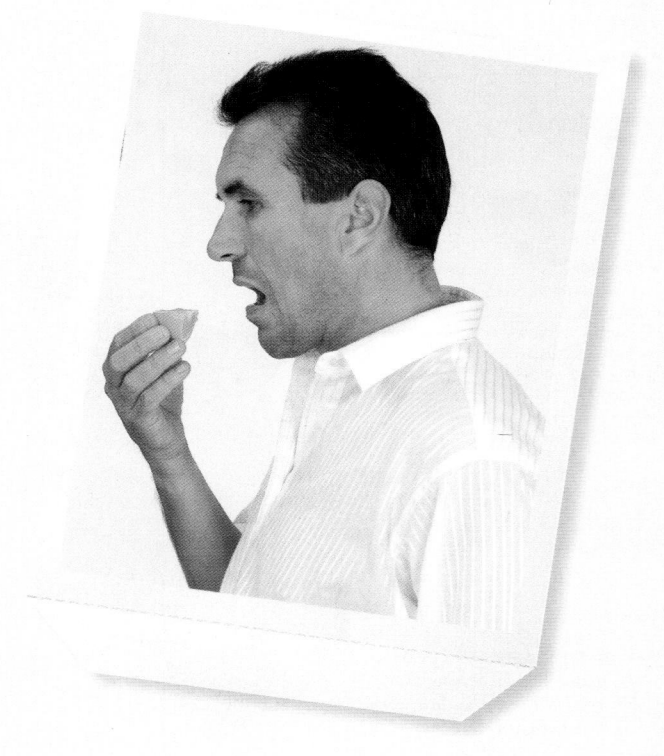

RIGHT *Boosting the immune system by taking extra vitamin C in the form of oranges will help fight infections, such as tracheitis, and prevent further occurrences.*

Hyperventilation

Hyperventilation is the term used to describe the act of breathing more quickly and deeply than normal, and which causes excessive loss of carbon dioxide from the blood. This can lead to alkalosis (an increase in blood alkalinity). It can occur at high altitudes, as a result of heavy exercise, during panic attacks, or as a response to poisoning (as in an aspirin overdose). Hyperventilation associated with uncontrolled diabetes or with kidney failure represents the body's efforts to eliminate excess carbon dioxide in dealing with acidosis. Chronic hyperventilation is association with a combination of fatigue and over-arousal (lack of sleep, plus stress, for instance); it may also stem from organic problems in the brain, or in the lungs themselves. Acute attacks are usually a reaction to emotional or physical trauma.

SYMPTOMS

• *a feeling of not getting enough air* • *the muscles of the forearms and calves may go into spasm, causing involuntary bending and extension of the wrists and ankles*

TREATMENT

AYURVEDA
• An Ayurvedic medical practitioner would balance the tridoshas, and use panchakarma for balancing the vátha. *(See page 22.)*

CHINESE HERBALISM
• A Chinese herbalist might suggest ginseng, Chinese angelica, and white peony root with thorowax root for relaxation. Treatment would be designed to strengthen the Spleen and enliven Liver. *(See pages 56 and 67.)*

TRADITIONAL HOME AND FOLK REMEDIES
• Oats contain thiamine and pantothenic acid, which act as gentle nerve tonics. *(See page 84.)*

HERBALISM
• Herbal remedies would be used to calm the nervous system and to relax you. Skullcap and valerian are useful herbs, blended together for best effect. Drink this as a tea three times daily while suffering symptoms. *(See pages 131 and 136.)*
• Lady's slipper and limeflowers may also work to ease factors which may be causing the condition. *(See page 134.)*

AROMATHERAPY
• A relaxing blend of essential oils of lavender, geranium, and bergamot in sweet almond oil or peach kernel oil may be used in the bath at times of great stress and anxiety. *(See pages 146–71.)*

HOMEOPATHY
• Take Aconite every 5 minutes for up to six doses in an acute attack. *(See page 178.)*
• Constitutional treatment will be necessary for chronic conditions.

FLOWER ESSENCES
• Rescue Remedy or Emergency Essence will help to calm you in an attack. *(See page 244.)*
• Elm, for an attack linked to anxiety accompanying a feeling of being unable to cope. *(See page 241.)*
• Aspen, for an attack caused by anxiety for no apparent reason. *(See page 236.)*

VITAMINS AND MINERALS
• Increase your intake of B vitamins, which work on the nervous system. *(See pages 252–5.)*
• Avoid caffeine in any form.

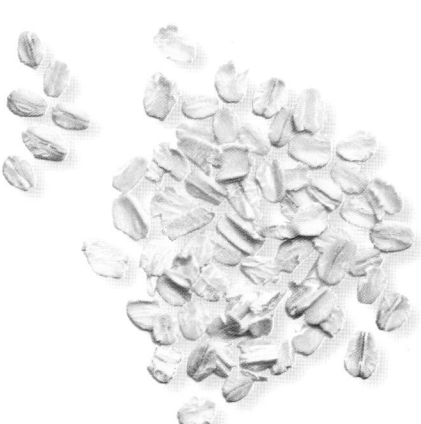

ABOVE *Oats contain a gentle nerve tonic and eating them regularly can be of great help for people who suffer panic attacks.*

RIGHT *Physical trauma, even being overactive and overaggressive in sport, can lead to hyperventilation.*

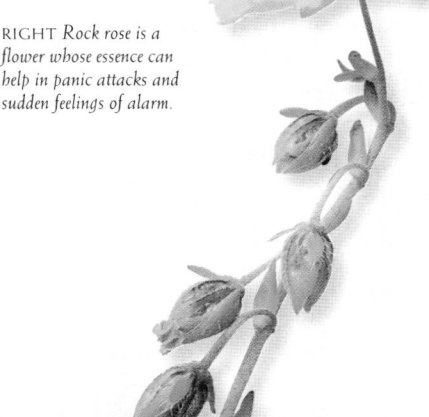
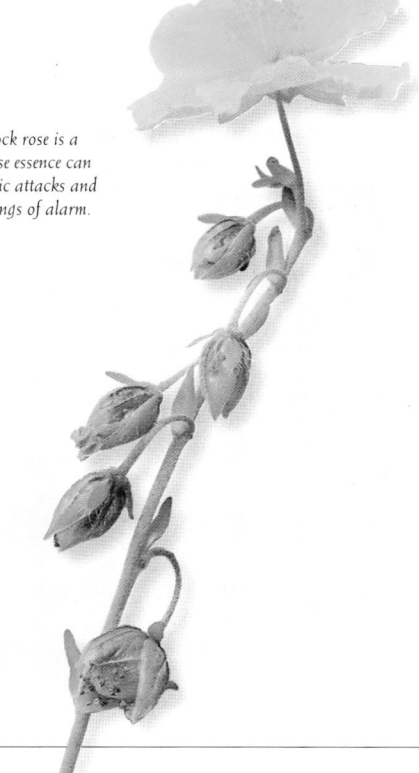

RIGHT *Rock rose is a flower whose essence can help in panic attacks and sudden feelings of alarm.*

Hiccups

A hiccup is a common irritation of the diaphragmatic nerves which causes involuntary inhalation of air. A lowering of the diaphragm and the sudden closure of the vocal cords result in the characteristic hiccup sound. Hiccups may be brought on by indigestion and drinking carbonated drinks, and can also occur during pregnancy and as a result of alcoholism. Most attacks last only a few minutes, usually with a brief interval in between attacks. Frequent, prolonged attacks of hiccups, which are extremely rare, may lead to severe exhaustion.

CAUTION

WHILE HICCUPS ARE USUALLY QUITE INNOCUOUS, THEY MAY BE A FEATURE OF MORE SERIOUS DISORDERS SUCH AS PLEURISY, HIATUS HERNIA, AND PNEUMONIA.

SYMPTOMS

- *prolonged episodes of hiccups may be accompanied by chest pain*
- *if persistent, hiccups can eventually be extremely exhausting*

TREATMENT

CHINESE HERBALISM
- The cause is thought to be Heat, Cold, or Food Stagnation. Berilla stems, rhubarb, and ginger will be used to treat hiccups. *(See page 73.)*

TRADITIONAL HOME AND FOLK REMEDIES
- Squirt some lemon juice to the back of your throat, or suck a piece of fresh lemon. *(See page 87.)*
- Give babies a sip of water with honey. *(See page 101.)*

HOMEOPATHY
Take one of the following remedies every 15 minutes for up to 6 doses:
- Nux vomica, for hiccups after eating, and accompanied by belching. *(See page 214.)*
- Arsenicum, for hiccups which are worse after cold drinks and accompanied by a chilly feeling. *(See page 182.)*
- Ignatia, when hiccups come on after emotional upset, eating, drinking, or smoking. *(See page 200.)*
- Mag. phos., for a sore chest and retching. *(See page 204.)*
- Cicuta, for violent, noisy hiccups.

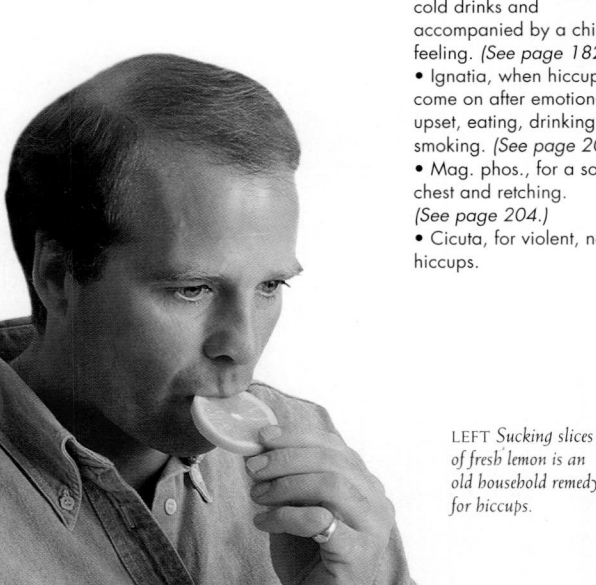

LEFT *Sucking slices of fresh lemon is an old household remedy for hiccups.*

Common Cold

The common cold is an infection of the upper respiratory tract which may be caused by any one of up to 200 strains of virus. These are spread either by inhaling droplets coughed or sneezed by others, or, more probably, by direct hand-to-hand contact with sufferers. When infection occurs, the walls of the respiratory tract swell and produce excess mucus, giving rise to the typical cold symptoms of stuffy or runny nose, throat discomfort, malaise, and occasional coughing. Colds can produce fevers of up to 39°C (102°F) in infants and children, but such fevers in adults indicate that the infection is probably influenza. The incubation period is from 1–3 days, after which symptoms occur, and most colds run their course in 3–10 days. Infants and elderly people are susceptible to complications such as sinusitis, ear inflammations, and pneumonia.

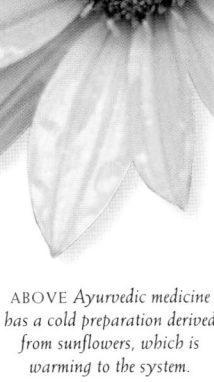

ABOVE *Ayurvedic medicine has a cold preparation derived from sunflowers, which is warming to the system.*

In conventional medicine, colds are treated with rest and fluids, in addition to antihistamines, decongestants, and cough medicines, as needed. Aspirin is recommended only when symptoms are severe, because it increases viral shedding and makes the sufferer more contagious. Vaccines are of little use in prevention because so many kinds of viruses are involved. Research suggests that interferon (a protein produced by animal cells when they are invaded by viruses, which is released into the bloodstream or intercellular fluid to induce healthy cells to manufacture an enzyme that counters the infection) could prevent the spread of colds and may prove useful to people at high risk of complications.

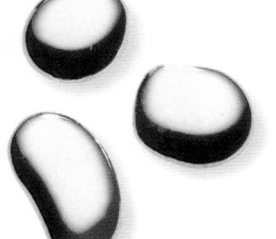

SYMPTOMS

- *sneezing and runny nose* • *mild fever*
- *headache* • *coughing and a burning or sore throat* • *catarrh*

LEFT *Mercury or quicksilver is the source of a homeopathic remedy used when the cold starts with a sore throat and affects the glands.*

TREATMENT

AYURVEDA
• Brown 4 tablespoons of coriander seeds in a frying pan, then boil with 4 cups of water, with 4 slices of root ginger. Reduce to 2 cups of liquid, strain, and drink. *(See page 35.)*
• Sunflower may be useful. *(See page 40.)*

CHINESE HERBALISM
• Plantain seed, peppermint, mulberry, honeysuckle, and skullcap may be prescribed to address weakness of the Lung, Cold, and Wind. *(See pages 65 and 74.)*

TRADITIONAL HOME AND FOLK REMEDIES
• Barley water with lemon and honey will encourage healing and shorten the duration of a cold. *(See page 92.)*
• Cinnamon is an excellent warming herb, and can be added to food and drinks, or as an oil to a vaporizer, to treat and prevent colds and flu.
• Fresh garlic, eaten daily, will discourage the onset of a cold. Garlic will also work to reduce fever. *(See page 82.)*
• Honey, eaten fresh or added to herbal teas, will encourage healing and prevent secondary infections occurring. *(See page 101.)*
• Steep lemons in hot water, and a little honey; drink regularly in the cold season, or during a cold, to restore yourself and prevent infection. This will also treat coughs. *(See pages 87 and 101.)*
• A mustard poultice on the chest or mustard added to a foot bath will act as a decongestant. *(See page 98.)*

HERBALISM
• Ginger promotes perspiration and helps soothe the throat. *(See page 139.)*
• The herb echinacea will encourage immune response, and acts as a natural antibiotic. *(See page 120.)*
• Peppermint helps to reduce the symptoms of a cold. *(See page 125.)*
• Ginseng powder, added to any warming herbal tea, will boost the immune system and help the body to fight the infection. *(See page 126.)*

AROMATHERAPY
• Tea tree and lemon oils help to fight infection. Massage, in a light carrier oil, into the chest and head, or place in the bath or a burner. *(See pages 146–71.)*
• Lavender oil in the bath will help you sleep, to aid recovery – particularly good if there is a cough. *(See page 161.)*
• Eucalyptus oil can kill bacteria and soothe inflamed mucous membranes. *(See page 159.)*

HOMEOPATHY
• Aconite, in the first stage of a cold. *(See page 178.)*
• Belladonna, for colds with a high temperature and great thirst. *(See page 183.)*
• Mercurius, for colds that begin with a sore throat, with swollen glands. *(See page 205.)*
• Gelsemium, for flu-like symptoms, weakness, and achiness. *(See page 195.)*
• Allium, for streaming nose and eyes where the discharge makes the nose red raw. *(See page 178.)*
• Pulsatilla, for runny nose with thick, yellow or green mucus. *(See page 209.)*
• Nat. mur., for colds with a crop of cold sores; sneezing and watery eyes. *(See page 206.)*
• Dulcamara, when the nose is stuffed up with catarrh in rainy or windy weather. *(See page 213.)*
• Bryonia, if you feel like a bear with a sore head. *(See page 185.)*

VITAMINS AND MINERALS
• Citrus fruit is rich in vitamin C, which will help the body to fight infection. *(See page 256.)*
• Zinc is known to reduce the duration of a cold; suck a zinc lozenge at the first signs. *(See page 265.)*
• Royal jelly acts as a tonic and an antiviral agent. *(See page 276.)*

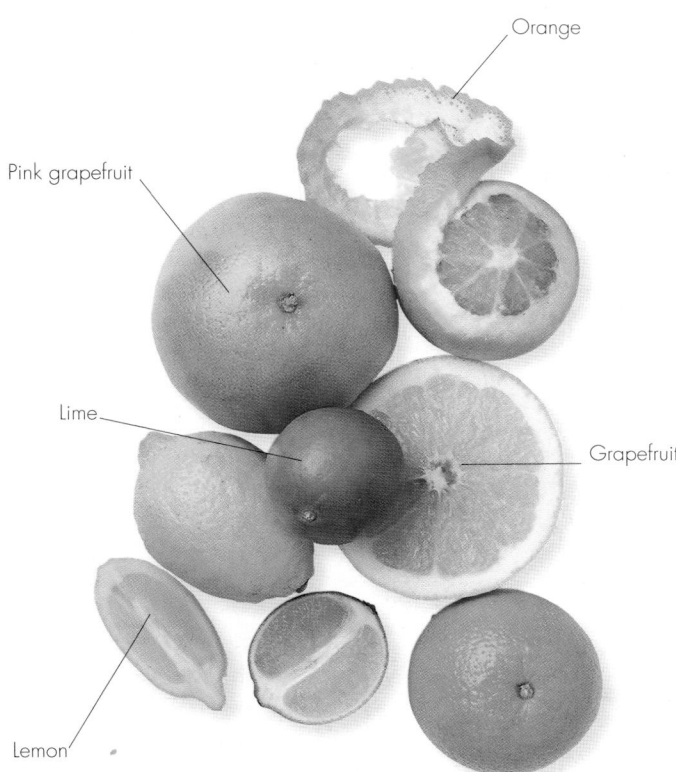

ABOVE Citrus fruits are the favorite natural remedy for a cold. They are the perfect source of vitamin C, which helps the body to fight infection.

Orange

Pink grapefruit

Lime

Grapefruit

Lemon

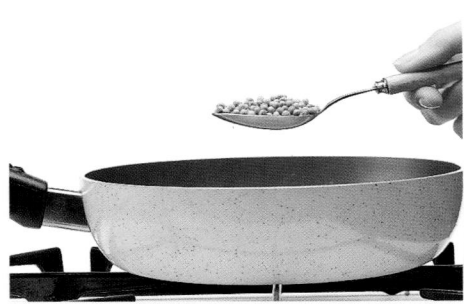

Both ginger and coriander are useful in treating colds. To make a decoction, brown 4 tablespoons of coriander seeds.

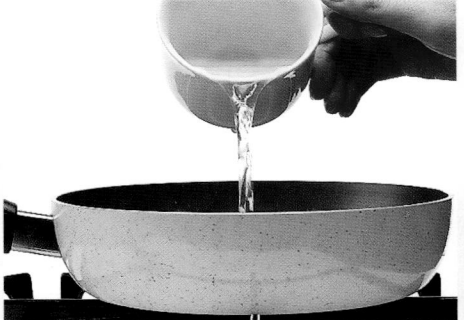

Once the seeds are browned, add 4 cups of water and bring to the boil.

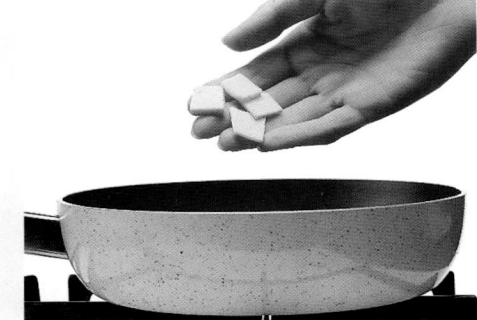

Add 4 slices of root ginger and reduce the liquid to 2 cups and strain. Drink to reduce a fever.

HEART, BLOOD, AND CIRCULATORY DISORDERS

High Blood Pressure

Blood pressure is the force with which the blood presses against the arterial walls as it circulates. In a person with high blood pressure, or hypertension, this force is greater than normal and causes the arterial walls to narrow and thicken, putting extra strain on the heart. Blood pressure fluctuates even in healthy individuals. It tends to increase with physical activity, excitement, fear, or emotional stress, but such elevations are usually transient. Most physicians will not make the diagnosis of hypertension unless the pressure is high on at least three separate occasions. Obesity, alcohol and sugar intake, and hereditary and ethnic factors all contribute, as will diabetes, kidney disease, and pregnancy. It is usually only when the secondary complications – damage to the arteries, brain, eyes, or elsewhere in the body – have developed that symptoms occur, by which time the condition is serious.

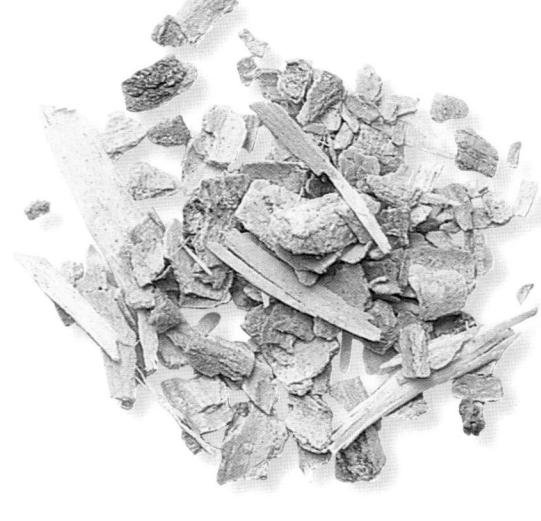

LEFT *Cramp bark is a useful herbal remedy for high blood pressure as it helps the arteries to dilate.*

DATA FILE

• In the U.S. at least 50 million people have hypertension.

• Hypertension is usually described as being a systolic pressure greater than 139, or a diastolic pressure greater than 89, or both. The World Health Organization defines it as being consistently above 160mm. Hg. systolic, and 95mm. Hg. diastolic.

• In the U.K. high blood pressure is extremely common, affecting 10–20 percent of the adult population.

• High blood pressure is more frequent and more severe in African Americans than in the white U.S. population, and in both races in the south-eastern United States than in the rest of the nation.

• It is uncommon but not unheard of in children and adolescents.

• In young adulthood and early middle age, high blood pressure occurs more frequently in men than in women; thereafter the reverse is true.

• Hypertension occurs worldwide and is most prevalent in Japan and northern China.

• In societies that consume little or no salt the incidence of hypertension is extremely low.

SYMPTOMS

• *mild hypertension has no symptoms*
• *severe hypertension: headaches – shortness of breath – visual disturbances – giddiness*

LEFT *Garlic is one of the most healing plants known to humankind. It has been shown to lower blood pressure, so if you suffer from hypertension eat plenty of raw garlic.*

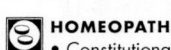

TREATMENT

AYURVEDA
• The Ayurvedic products Dashamoola and Sarpaganda are used for treating high blood pressure.

CHINESE HERBALISM
• Internal Wind is believed to be the cause, and treatment will calm Liver Yang and Blood Wind. The herbs used might include chrysanthemum flowers, peony root, astragalus. *(See page 67.)*

TRADITIONAL HOME AND FOLK REMEDIES
• Eat plenty of fresh raw garlic, which acts as a tonic to the circulatory system and maintains its health. *(See page 82.)*

HERBALISM
• Hawthorn berries, infused, are a good heart tonic. *(See page 119.)*
• Cramp bark can be used to encourage the arteries to dilate. *(See page 138.)*
• Limeflowers and yarrow are also useful in the treatment of high blood pressure. *(See pages 112 and 134.)*

AROMATHERAPY
• Lavender will soothe and relax. *(See page 161.)*
• Regular massage with oils of lavender, marjoram, and ylang ylang can have a beneficial effect. *(See pages 146–71.)*

HOMEOPATHY
• Constitutional treatment is appropriate.

VITAMINS AND MINERALS
• Increase your intake of dietary fiber, and of potassium, calcium, and magnesium, which have a balancing effect on the circulation and encourage the action of the heart. *(See pages 258 and 262.)*

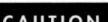

CAUTION

ROUTINE BLOOD PRESSURE CHECKS SHOULD BE UNDERTAKEN BY EVERYONE AS A MATTER OF COURSE. SUSTAINED HIGH BLOOD PRESSURE CAN CAUSE SEVERE DAMAGE TO THE HEART, KIDNEYS, AND EYES, AND SHOULD NOT BE IGNORED. DO NOT TAKE HERBAL REMEDIES WHILE TAKING CONVENTIONAL MEDICATION WITHOUT CONSULTING YOUR PHYSICIAN.

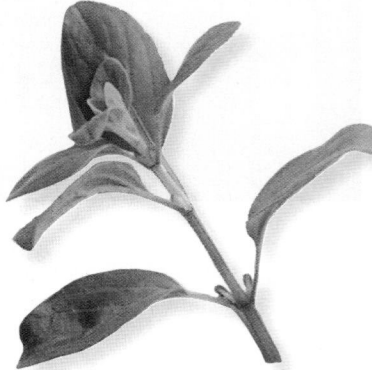

ABOVE *A relaxing massage with aromatherapy essential oils, such as marjoram, may be of benefit in cases of hypertension.*

Low Blood Pressure

L ow blood pressure, or hypotension, is an abrupt fall in blood pressure due possibly to the heart's failure to maintain it or to severe loss of fluid from the circulation. It is perhaps most commonly noticed on standing up suddenly from a sitting or prone position, but can also result from severe hemorrhage, burns, gastroenteritis, or dehydration.

SYMPTOMS

• *fainting (due to the blood volume circulating being insufficient to supply the brain and lungs); older people in particular and those taking drugs against hypertension may experience fainting episodes, accompanied by paleness, a weak pulse, and dilated pupils*

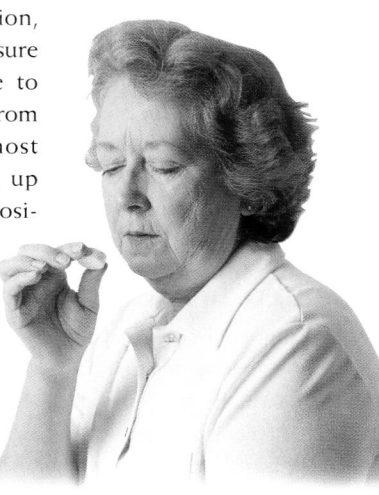

ABOVE *Many homeopathic treatments, such as Ignatia or Aconite, are excellent remedies for hypotension.*

DATA FILE

Blood pressure is conventionally written as two numbers, systolic pressure over diastolic pressure. Systolic pressure is the maximum blood pressure that occurs during the contraction of the heart; diastolic pressure is the lowest pressure measured during the interbeat period. The medically acceptable upper limit for blood pressure in an adult has been lowered in recent years and is now considered to be 140/90mm. Hg.

TREATMENT

CHINESE HERBALISM
• Treatment would be aimed at Deficient qi in the Blood and Heart. Ginseng and Chinese angelica might be used. *(See pages 56 and 67.)*

HERBALISM
• Broom is useful for treating low blood pressure, as it tones the arteries.
• Ginger, hawthorn tops, and rosemary will also be useful as they are stimulating and work to encourage circulation. *(See pages 119, 127, and 139.)*

AROMATHERAPY
• Regular massage with oils of black pepper, lemon, sage, or rosemary, which stimulate and warm, will be useful. *(See pages 146–71.)*

HOMEOPATHY
Treatment would be constitutional, but the following remedies may help if you feel a tendency to faint:
• Veratrum, for fainting caused by anger.
• Coffea, for fainting brought on by excitement. *(See page 192.)*
• Ignatia, for fainting caused by an emotional shock or trauma. *(See page 200.)*
• Aconite, for fainting caused by fright, and characterized by tension and pale, clammy skin. *(See page 178.)*
• Cocculus, when caused by lack of sleep.
• Gelsemium, when you feel weak and shaky. *(See page 195.)*

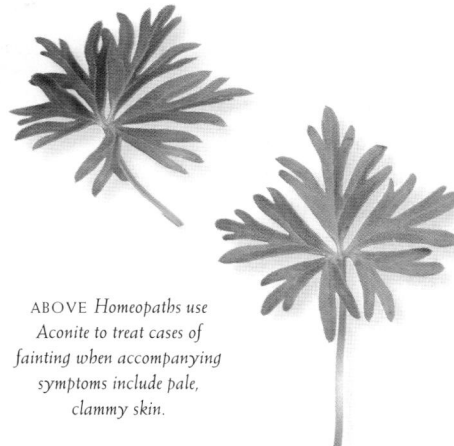

ABOVE *Homeopaths use Aconite to treat cases of fainting when accompanying symptoms include pale, clammy skin.*

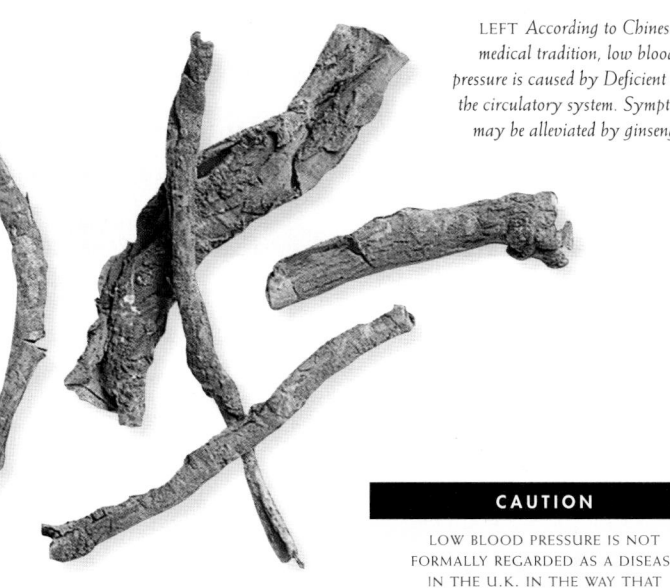

LEFT *According to Chinese medical tradition, low blood pressure is caused by Deficient qi in the circulatory system. Symptoms may be alleviated by ginseng.*

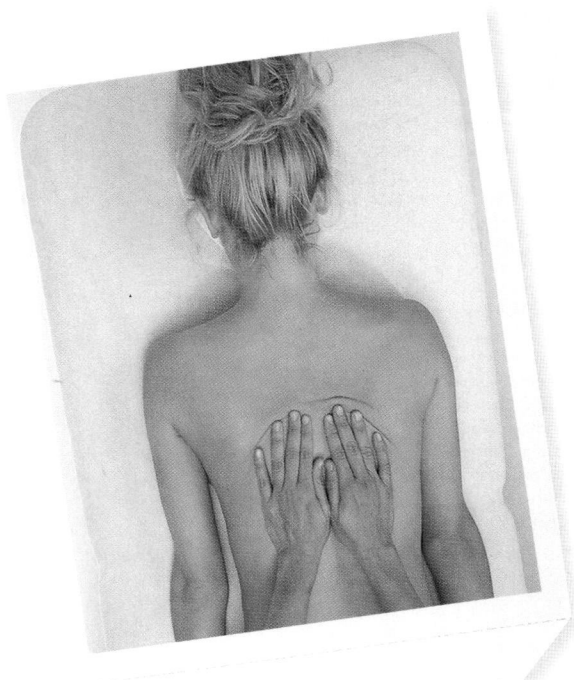

LEFT *Regular massage with stimulating essential oils such as black pepper, lemon or sage, may help regulate blood pressure.*

CAUTION

LOW BLOOD PRESSURE IS NOT FORMALLY REGARDED AS A DISEASE IN THE U.K. IN THE WAY THAT HYPERTENSION, OR HIGH BLOOD PRESSURE, IS. GENUINE HYPOTENSION CAN, HOWEVER, BE FATAL, AND MUST BE GIVEN URGENT MEDICAL ATTENTION.

Leukemia

Leukemia is the name given to a group of serious diseases in which certain white blood cells reproduce arbitrarily, replacing and interfering with the blood's normal components. Untreated, this disorder will lead to a fatal shortage of red blood cells, bleeding, or infection. Leukemia can be classified into two main groups – acute and chronic. Acute leukemia is rapid in onset, affecting children in particular, while chronic leukemia is slower in onset, with a much greater life expectancy for sufferers.

DATA FILE

• Acute and chronic leukemias, together with the other types of tumors of the blood, bone cells (myelomas), and lymph tissue (lymphomas), cause about 10 percent of all cancer deaths and about 50 percent of all cancer deaths in children and adults less than 30 years old.

• Lymphoblastic leukemia is more common in children, with 50 cases per 1 million of the population occuring between the ages of two and four.

• In the U.K. there are 10 cases per million of the population up to the age of 75, then 50 cases per million thereafter.

• When untreated, acute leukemia is fatal in one to two years and often fatal within about six months of onset.

SYMPTOMS

• *acute leukemias are most common in children and are characterized by: general aching and tiredness – susceptibility to infection – bleeding gums – sore throat – swelling of glands in the neck, groin, and armpits – appetite and weight loss – severe anemia* • *chronic leukemias are characterized by: slow onset of fatigue – gradual enlargement of the spleen until it is so big as to cause a dragging sensation and pain in the upper left abdomen – gradual weight loss – nosebleeds – painful and prolonged erections in men – fever and night sweats*

TREATMENT

AROMATHERAPY
• Essential oils can be very supportive, but massage must not be used if you are suffering from leukemia. Add a few drops of niaouli or bergamot to the bath, or place in a vaporizer. *(See pages 153 and 163.)*

HOMEOPATHY
• Chronic and acute leukemia are given constitutional treatment, to help the body to cope with the effects of conventional medication.

FLOWER ESSENCES
• Remedies are very useful in helping with accompanying negative feelings.
• Mimulus, for fear and concern. *(See page 235.)*

• Rescue Remedy or Emergency Essence, for trauma and shock. *See page 244.)*
• Agrimony, for hiding true feelings of distress behind a cheerful face. *(See page 225.)*
• Elm, for times when the pressures of responsibility seem overwhelming. *(See page 241.)*

CAUTION

A PRECISE MEDICAL DIAGNOSIS OF THE TYPE OF WHITE BLOOD CELL INVOLVED MUST BE MADE IN ORDER TO TREAT THE DISEASE EFFECTIVELY SINCE DIFFERENT CELLS CALL FOR DIFFERENT TREATMENTS.

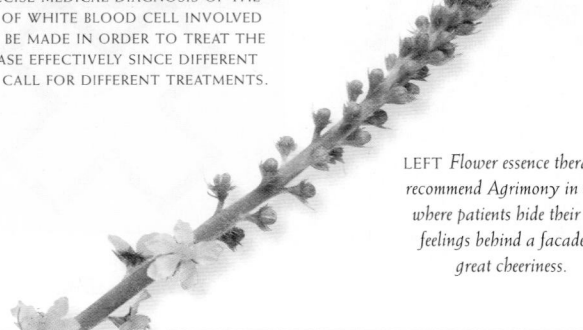

LEFT *Flower essence therapists recommend Agrimony in cases where patients hide their true feelings behind a facade of great cheeriness.*

Enlarged Spleen

The spleen is located on the left side of the body below the ribs and is responsible for removing dead blood cells from the blood. It varies in size and weight according to the amount of blood it contains in storage and its immune functions. In adult humans the spleen functions both as an immunologically active organ and as a filter for white and red blood cells. All of the blood in the human body passes through the spleen approximately every 90 minutes. Slight enlargement of the spleen is normal during and after digestion, and the size of the spleen in adults usually ranges from 3 ½–8oz. (100–250g.). Abnormal enlargement, or splenomegaly, may occur in the course of a number of diseases, including: malaria, typhoid, hemolytic anemia, leukemia, Hodgkin's disease, glandular fever, septicemia, and syphilis. An enlarged spleen becomes firmer and can easily be felt on physical examination.

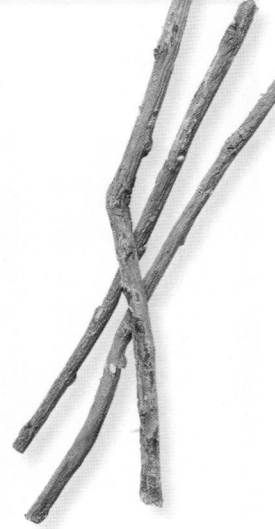

ABOVE *Oak, the source of Quercus. It is used homeopathically to treat an enlarged spleen.*

CAUTION

AN ENLARGED SPLEEN IS FAR MORE LIKELY TO RUPTURE THAN A NORMAL, HEALTHY SPLEEN. IN THE EVENT OF A RUPTURE, THE MAIN DANGER IS FROM SEVERE HEMORRHAGE, WHICH CAN BE FATAL IF IT IS NOT TREATED IMMEDIATELY.

SYMPTOMS

• *symptoms will vary according to the cause of enlargement, but the general area of the spleen will be very tender*

TREATMENT

HERBALISM
Any of the herbs that help the immune action will be useful, including the following:
• Licorice can enhance recovery, stimulating white blood cell and antibody formation and efficiency. *(See page 122.)*
• Garlic helps to prevent infections of all kinds, including those which have become resistant to a dose of antibiotics. *(See page 113.)*
• Echinacea is widely used to treat chronic and acute infections, cleansing the blood and lymphatic system, and stimulating production of white blood cells and antibodies. *(See page 120.)*

• Ginseng can boost immunity and encourage the body to deal efficiently with stress, as well as stimulating white blood cell production and aiding recovery after illness. *(See page 126.)*

HOMEOPATHY
Treatment would be constitutional, but the following may help, depending on the cause:
• Quercus, for an enlarged spleen associated with cirrhosis of the liver, and swollen ankles.
• Nat. mur., for a swollen spleen with constipation, salt cravings, and oversensitive reactions. *(See page 206.)*

ABOVE *Licorice, which stimulates the formation of white blood cells, will help the immune system to recover from an enlarged spleen.*

Anemia

Anemia is a deficiency of hemoglobin – the chemical that carries oxygen – in the red cells of the blood. The most common cause of anemia is iron deficiency resulting from excessive blood loss (through trauma, surgery, childbirth, or heavy menstrual bleeding), poor diet, or failure to absorb iron from food. Other causes of anemia include: excessive destruction of red blood cells (hemolytic anemia); vitamin B12 deficiency (pernicious anemia); and the inherited disorders of sickle cell anemia and thalassemia.

DATA FILE

• Of all sufferers, 20 percent are women, and 50 percent are children.

• The most common type of anemia is iron deficiency anemia, most often resulting from chronic blood loss; also from lack of iron in the diet, impaired absorption of iron from the intestine, or an increased need for iron, as occurs during pregnancy.

• Iron is an essential component of the hemoglobin, which carries oxygen to the tissues in chemical combination with its iron atoms.

• Pernicious anemia is a chronic inherited disease of middle-aged and older people in which the stomach fails to produce a factor needed for the absorption of vitamin B12, which is essential for mature red blood cells.

• Aplastic anemia is the result of the failure of bone marrow cells to manufacture mature red cells. It is usually caused by toxic chemicals (for example, benzene) or by radiation.

SYMPTOMS

• *weakness and fatigue*
• *breathlessness on minimal exertion*
• *pale skin and lips* • *headaches, dizziness, and possibly fainting in severe cases* • *in pernicious anemia there may be: nosebleeds – a sore tongue – "pins and needles" in the hands and feet*

TREATMENT

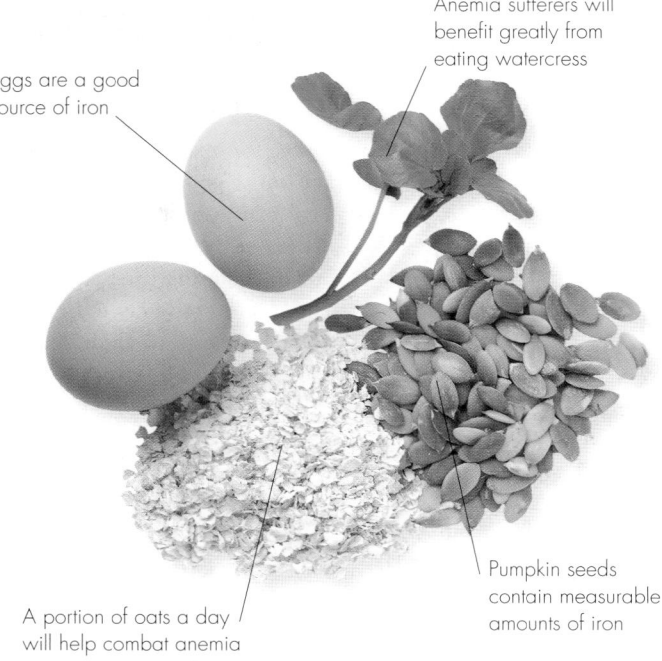

Eggs are a good source of iron

Anemia sufferers will benefit greatly from eating watercress

Pumpkin seeds contain measurable amounts of iron

A portion of oats a day will help combat anemia

ABOVE *Eating foods rich in iron will help the hemoglobin levels in your blood to rise.*

CAUTION

IRON DEFICIENCY IN POST-MENOPAUSAL WOMEN AND IN MEN SHOULD ALWAYS BE INVESTIGATED.

RIGHT *If you are suffering from anemia try drinking carrot juice, a traditional remedy for iron deficiency.*

AYURVEDA
• There are a number of Ayurvedic products available, including Kalyanaka ghritha (oral ghee), Kishor (oral pills) and Avipathi choorna (oral powder), which would complement a treatment program.

CHINESE HERBALISM
• The cause would be attributed to a Spleen not transforming qi, and Gui Pi Wan (return spleen tablets) would be useful.

TRADITIONAL HOME AND FOLK REMEDIES
• Nettle tea is rich in iron; drink daily.
  • Beet and carrot juice may be drunk to treat the condition. *(See page 89.)*

HERBALISM
• Chinese angelica root may be helpful. Take as tincture, decoction, or tea. *(See page 115.)*
• Alfalfa, dandelion root, nettles, watercress, and yellow dock are rich in iron. *(See pages 128, 134, and 137.)*

AROMATHERAPY
• Lavender essential oil is helpful where the anemia is associated with palpitations and dizzy spells. *(See page 161.)*
• Massage with Roman chamomile essential oil. *(See page 150.)*

HOMEOPATHY
• Ferr. phos. helps assimilation of iron from food. *(See page 194.)*
• Nat. mur., for anemia with constipation, headache, and a tendency to cold sores. *(See page 206.)*

• Calc. phos., for anemia during a growth spurt, and irritability. *(See page 186.)*
• Picric acid, for anemia with mental overload.

VITAMINS AND MINERALS
• Iron-rich foods include oats, egg yolks, pumpkin seeds, and watercress. *(See page 260.)*
• Calcium, copper, vitamin C, and B vitamins must be present for the body to assimilate iron; ensure you have a sufficient intake in your diet. *(See pages 252–5, 256, 258, and 259.)*
• Vegetarians should take extra vitamin B12. *(See page 255.)*
• Avoid drinking tea at mealtimes as this makes iron absorption less efficient.

Angina

Angina (known medically as *angina pectoris*) is chest pain caused by a narrowing of the arteries, with the result that the blood supply to the heart muscle is not enough to meet its demands for oxygen and nutrients. The pain most commonly occurs after physical exertion, a heavy meal, cold weather, or various other circumstances requiring the heart to work harder. Groups likely to be susceptible to angina include smokers, diabetics, and the overweight.

ABOVE *Hawthorn is a good herbal tonic for angina and may be taken with most orthodox drugs (except dioxin).*

SYMPTOMS

• *severe pain in the chest, often spreading up to the neck and down the left arm* • *a feeling of tightness in the chest* • *there may also be pain between the shoulder blades*

TREATMENT

CHINESE HERBALISM
• Treatment would be aimed at stagnant qi in the Blood and Heart. Herbs used may include safflower, cinnamon twigs, red sage root, peony root, and macrosten onion bulb. *(See pages 58, 59, and 67.)*

HERBALISM
• Hawthorn berries, made into an infusion, are a good tonic for the heart. *(See page 119.)*
• Motherwort is useful for the treatment of angina. Sip a motherwort decoction 3 times daily. *(See page 124.)*

• Balm and limeflowers are tonics for the heart and the circulatory system, and regular infusions will help ensure their healthy functioning. *(See page 134.)*

HOMEOPATHY
Treatment would be constitutional, but the following remedies may help in mild attacks:
• Cactus, for a constricted chest and consequent trouble breathing.
• Lilium, for a bursting feeling in the heart, with palpitations and some pain in the right arm.
• Naja, for an irregular pulse, accompanied by anxiety and fearfulness.

• Glonoinum, for a fluttering heart, a sensation of blood rushing, difficulty breathing, and faintness, which are made worse by heat. *(See page 196.)*

VITAMINS AND MINERALS
• Increase your intake of dietary fiber and oily fish (such as sardines, herring, salmon, and mackerel).
• Raw garlic aids the functioning of the circulatory system, and helps treat the condition.

DATA FILE

• Cardiovascular diseases such as angina have been a major health problem in the U.S. for years and comprise the leading cause of death.

• Nearly 1 million people die each year of cardiovascular disease.

• The death rate from cardiovascular diseases has declined since the mid-1970s, due to modification of risk factors for disease, and improvements in diagnosis and treatment.

• At first, angina may only be evident during periods of exercise or emotional stress, resolving when the activity ceases. Later, it may occur even at rest.

• An estimated 50 million Americans have cardiovascular disease and are unaware of it.

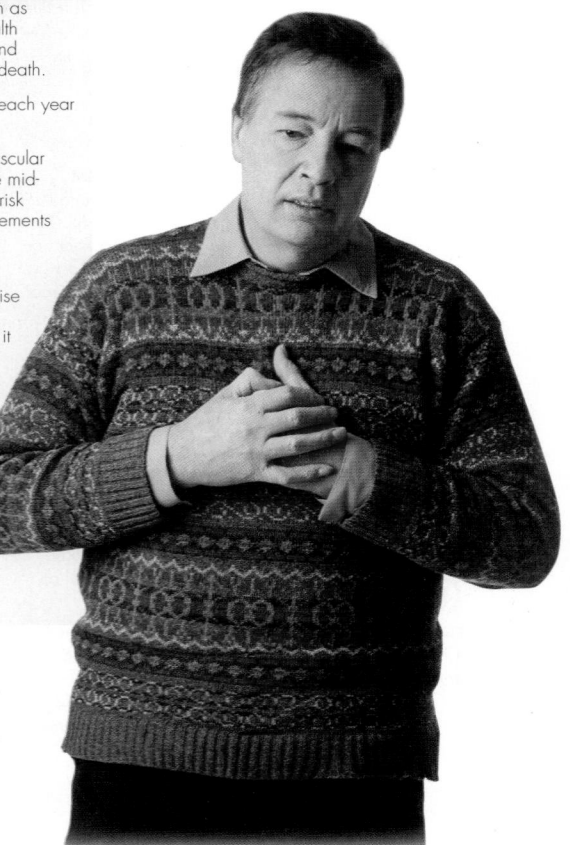

RIGHT *Angina is characterized by severe chest pain that often spreads to the neck and the left arm. The chest will also be constricted.*

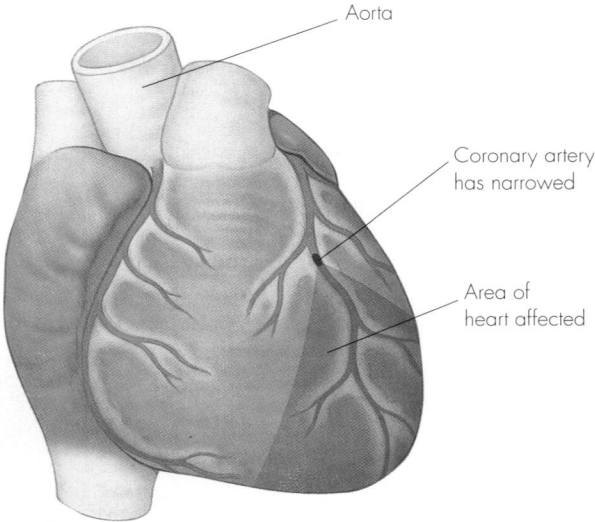

Aorta

Coronary artery has narrowed

Area of heart affected

ABOVE *Angina occurs when the muscular wall of the heart becomes short of oxygen.*

CAUTION

PROLONGED OR MORE SEVERE CASES OF ANGINA CAN BE A PRECURSOR TO A HEART ATTACK AND SHOULD RECEIVE URGENT MEDICAL ATTENTION.

Palpitations

The average heart beats about 72 times a minute and pumps about 3,600 gallons (13,640l.) of blood a day. During exercise, the pumping action automatically increases three- or fourfold, in response to the tissues' demand for increased oxygen. Palpitation refers to a fast or irregular heartbeat. Palpitations are quite common and usually harmless, often brought on by physical exertion or fright. Frequent or prolonged palpitations, however, may be an indication of heart disease, particularly if accompanied by dizziness, fainting, or chest pain. The sensation of a "missed" beat is due to a premature ectopic beat followed by a compensatory gap before the next beat. This can be induced by excitement, anxiety, or stimulants such as caffeine and nicotine.

SYMPTOMS

- *pounding in the chest following exercise*
- *uncomfortable awareness of a rapid heart rate when anxious*

TREATMENT

CHINESE HERBALISM
- Treatment would be aimed at addressing a Heart Blood deficiency, and may include the use of asparagus root and wild jujube seed. *(See page 75.)*

HERBALISM
- Motherwort, drunk as an infusion, may help if palpitations are linked to anxiety or stress. *(See page 124.)*
- Broom, limeflowers, mistletoe, and valerian are useful herbs for treating palpitations. *(See pages 134 and 136.)*

AROMATHERAPY
- If your palpitations are linked to emotional causes, calming oils such as ylang ylang, marjoram, lavender, and mandarin will help. Place a few drops in the bath, or use in regular massage. Carry a bottle with you, and sniff in times of distress. *(See pages 146–71.)*
- Peppermint, aniseed, lavender, melissa, rosemary, and neroli essential oils can be used separately or combined in a good massage oil to treat palpitations. *(See pages 146–71.)*

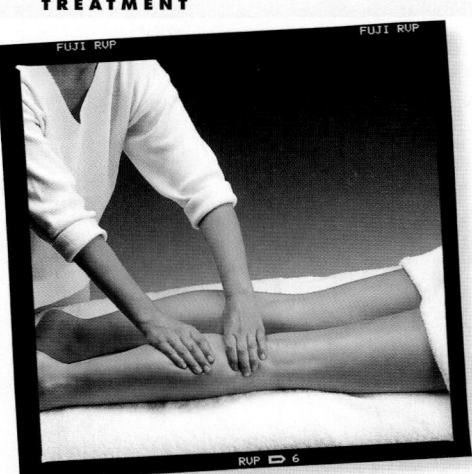

ABOVE *Soothing essential oils, such as ylang ylang or mandarin, may be used in aromatherapy massage to calm palpitations.*

HOMEOPATHY
- Nux vomica, when palpitations are brought on by overindulgence. *(See page 214.)*
- Nat. mur., for strong palpitations and chest constriction, made worse by heat. *(See page 206.)*
- Cactus, for violent palpitations which are worse before menstruation, with dizziness, shortness of breath, and flatulence.

- Pulsatilla, when palpitations are brought on by heat or rich fatty foods. *(See page 209.)*
- Lachesis, for fainting, a constricted feeling, and anxiety. *(See page 216.)*

FLOWER ESSENCES
- Rescue Remedy or Emergency Essence will help to calm panic and anxiety associated with the onset of palpitations. *(See page 244.)*

Gangrene

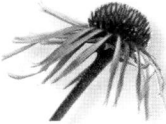

ABOVE *The* Echinacea *species is used to make a homeopathic remedy for persistent, festering, septic wounds.*

Gangrene is the decay and eventual death of tissue as a result of inadequate blood supply. This may be caused by injury, burns, frostbite, or by disorders such as atherosclerosis, embolism, thrombosis, and diabetes. Excessive smoking can also lead to gangrene.

SYMPTOMS

- *if the affected area is not infected, it will typically be dry, and brown or black in color* • *if bacteria have entered the affected tissue, festering occurs, leading to "wet" gangrene* • *infection of the affected area by one of the clostridia family of gas-producing soil bacteria leads to "gas" gangrene. This is characterized by swelling of the tissues, particularly the muscles, which spreads rapidly to healthy tissues, discoloration, and severe illness* • *antibiotics can sometimes prevent gangrene from spreading*

CAUTION

TREATMENT IS URGENT, AND YOU SHOULD BE SEEN BY YOUR PHYSICIAN.

TREATMENT

HOMEOPATHY
The following symptoms can be used on an emergency basis, for up to 10 doses:
- Echinacea, when the wound turns septic and also smells foul.
- Euphorbia, for wet gangrene in a chronic ulcer.
- Lachesis, for pain which is worse after sleeping, and when the affected area is blue or purple. *(See page 216.)*
- Arsenicum, when the skin is ulcerated, cold makes the pain worse, and you feel restless. *(See page 182.)*

VITAMINS AND MINERALS
- Vitamin E taken orally and applied to the wound or gangrenous area will promote healing. *(See page 257.)*

BELOW *Vitamin E will promote healing. It can be taken by mouth or applied externally.*

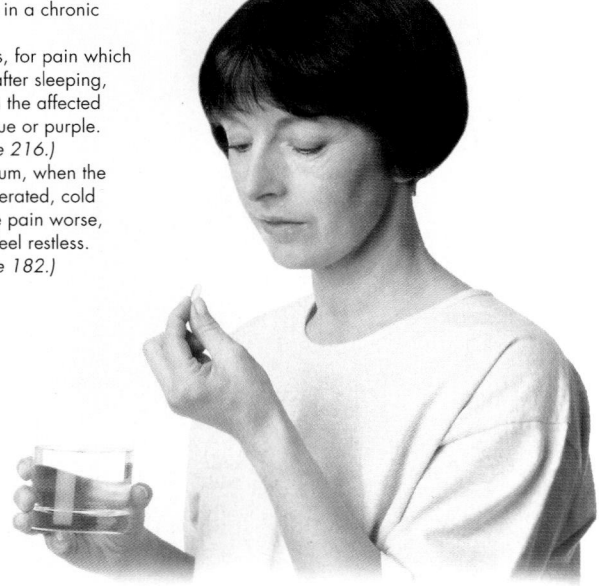

Atherosclerosis

Atherosclerosis is a degenerative disease of the arteries in which a fatty patch (atheroma) consisting mainly of cholesterol builds up on the wall of an artery. This eventually hardens and partially blocks the artery, causing the formation of a blood clot behind it. It is a progressive condition, generally worsening with age, and is most dangerous when the arteries supplying blood to the heart and brain are affected. Contributing factors to the development of atherosclerosis include smoking, high blood pressure, high blood cholesterol, heredity, and diabetes.

DATA FILE

Atherosclerosis can lead to:

• heart attack and angina, where the coronary arteries (supplying the heart) are affected

• stroke, where the carotid arteries (supplying the brain) are affected

• severe pain in the legs on walking when the femoral arteries (supplying the legs) are affected

• severe anemia

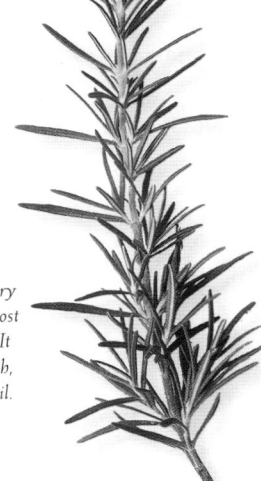

RIGHT *Rosemary can be used to boost the circulation. It can be taken fresh, dried, or as an oil.*

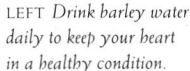

LEFT *Drink barley water daily to keep your heart in a healthy condition.*

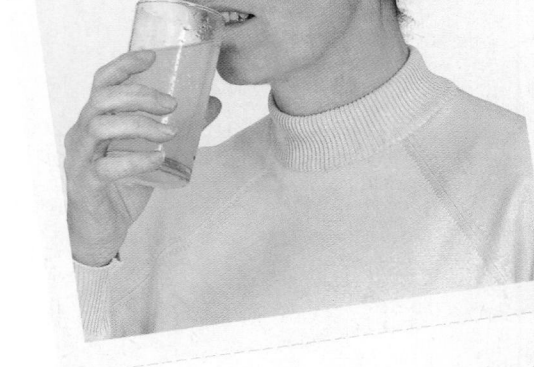

TREATMENT

TRADITIONAL HOME AND FOLK REMEDIES
• Increase your intake of olive oil, which breaks down cholesterol and fatty deposits in the blood. *(See page 95.)*
• Drink barley water daily to ensure that your heart is healthy. *(See page 92.)*
• Garlic, onions, and yogurt all have a beneficial effect on the heart. *(See pages 82 and 93.)*

HERBALISM
• Lavender oil helps to regulate the heart and may prevent heart attack. Use the herb in the bath, or the oil in a vaporizer or gentle massage.
• Rosemary – fresh, dried, or as an oil – can be used to stimulate the circulatory system. *(See page 127.)*
• Hawthorn berries and tops, and limeflowers are both useful herbs for arterial diseases. *(See pages 119 and 134.)*

AROMATHERAPY
• Regular massage with juniper and lemon can help to break down fatty deposits in the body. *(See pages 154 and 160.)*

HOMEOPATHY
• Baryta carb., if you suffer from high blood pressure and palpitations. *(See page 185.)*
• Phosphorus, for treating fainting spells, salt cravings, and nervousness. *(See page 208.)*
• Glonoinum, for tight congested headache and pounding arteries. *(See page 196.)*

• Vanadium, for fainting, dizziness, liver problems, feeling that the heart is being compressed.

VITAMINS AND MINERALS
• Increase your intake of dietary fiber, and reduce your intake of salt and sugar.
• Increase your intake of foods with bioflavonoids, to improve artery health. *(See page 272.)*

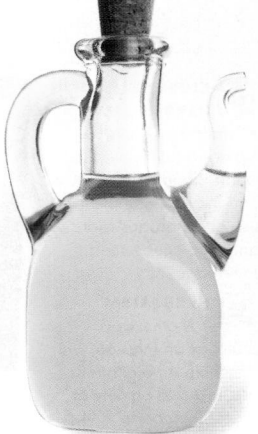

RIGHT *Scientific studies have proved that consumption of olive oil lowers cholesterol levels in the blood.*

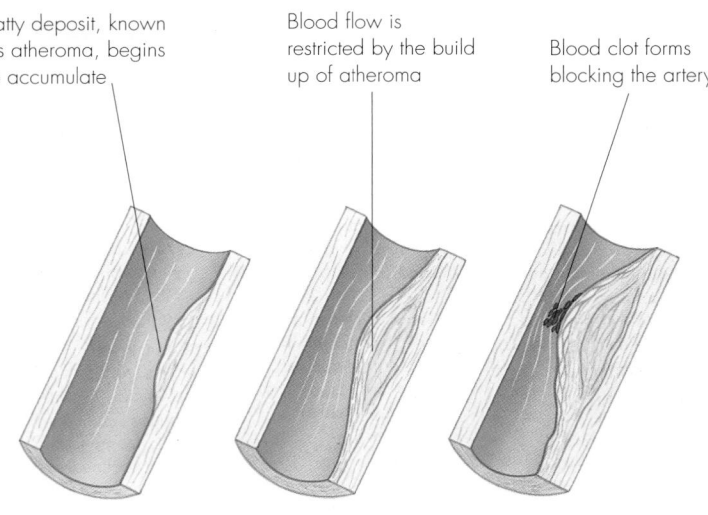

Fatty deposit, known as atheroma, begins to accumulate

Blood flow is restricted by the build up of atheroma

Blood clot forms blocking the artery

ABOVE *Atherosclerosis occurs when fatty deposits build up in the wall of an artery, restricting blood flow, and leading to the formation of a blood clot.*

Aneurysm

An aneurysm is a swelling or bulge in the wall of an artery that can vary in shape, size, and cause. A potentially fatal complication is rupture of the vessel, resulting in massive hemorrhage. It may occur in the main artery, the aorta, as a result of weakness in the muscular wall, possibly through atherosclerosis, syphilis, or a congenital defect. It can eventually rupture, causing fatal internal bleeding. It can also develop in the left ventricle of the heart (ventricular aneurysm) following a heart attack, and can lead to heart failure or an embolism. Aneurysms can also occur in the blood vessels of the brain. These are often congenital.

SYMPTOMS

• *severe headaches* • *painful spine from the pressure of the swelling in the aorta, which can also cause: — a cough — voice loss — and difficulty in swallowing* • *in a dissecting aneurysm the wall of the affected artery splits, forcing blood between the layers*

BELOW *Oily fish, such as mackerel, contain fatty acids that are believed to be a valuable protection against cardiovascular disease.*

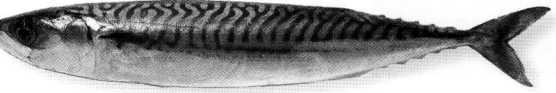

DATA FILE

There are many different types of aneurysms:

• Arterial aneurysms may be due to atherosclerosis, trauma, infectious injury, or a congenital defect. They occur most often in elderly people.

• Aortic aneurysms usually occur in the abdominal portion of the aorta, generally below the arteries leading to the kidney.

• A relatively common type of aneurysm – giant aneurysms – cause a hemorrhage in the brain.

• Defects in eye arteries may result in multiple aneurysms of the retina.

• Dissecting aneurysms, also called aortic dissection, begin suddenly as a tear in the inner vessel lining followed by entry of blood.

• A ventricular aneurysm may occur following a heart attack. Scar tissue forms over the dead heart cells and creates a patch over the weakened area, which may then bulge when the heart contracts.

TREATMENT

AROMATHERAPY
• Oils like chamomile and cypress will bring about the contraction of the capillaries. Use in the bath or in a vaporizer. *(See page 150.)*

HOMEOPATHY
• For a burst aneurysm, ring for emergency help and take aconite every 5 minutes until help arrives. *(See page 178.)* Constitutional treatment is appropriate for a developing aneurysm, but the following treatments will help until you receive treatment:

• Baryta carb., for raised blood pressure, palpitations, possible atherosclerosis, and pallor. *(See page 185.)*
• Lycopodium, for aneurysm of the aorta, where symptoms worsen between 4 and 8P.M. *(See page 203.)*
• Kali iod., for bone pain, which is worse at night and when in warmth.

VITAMINS AND MINERALS
• Eat plenty of garlic and brewer's yeast, which will encourage the healthy functioning of the circulatory system. *(See page 272.)*

• Increase your intake of oily fish.
• Vitamins C and E will encourage the healthy functioning of the circulatory system. *(See pages 256 and 257.)*

Varicose Veins

Varicose veins are swollen and twisted veins, most commonly found in the legs but also in the rectum (where they are known as hemorrhoids), the scrotum, and the esophagus. The swelling is caused by a weakness in the valves of the veins, which leads to increased pressure on the vein walls. This can be the result of deep vein thrombosis, obesity, pregnancy, prolonged sitting or standing, constipation, prolapse, or it may be hereditary.

ABOVE *Raw beetroot is said to help varicose veins and should be eaten daily for its value as a powerful tonic.*

SYMPTOMS

• *extremely sore, swollen, and tender veins* • *swelling of the legs* • *bruising and discoloration* • *burning sensation* • *aching calves* • *irritated and flaky skin* • *ulcers* • *in severe cases, a vein may rupture and bleed*

TREATMENT

CHINESE HERBALISM
• The source of the problem is bad circulation, stagnant qi, and stagnant Blood, and the following herbs would be used: angelica, cinnamon twigs, and astragalus; honey might be used externally. *(See pages 56, 57, and 59.)*

TRADITIONAL HOME AND FOLK REMEDIES
• Raw beetroot should be eaten daily, for its healing and strengthening action.
• A mustard poultice, may help to encourage circulation in the area. *(See page 98.)*

HERBALISM
• Calendula oil, or marigold tea as a compress can be applied. *(See page 117.)*

• Herbs to repair and tone the veins include hawthorn berries, horse chestnut, prickly ash and yarrow – all of which can be infused and drunk. *(See pages 112 and 119.)*

AROMATHERAPY
• Rosemary oil, blended with a light carrier oil, can be massaged into the legs. *(See page 68.)*
• Essential oils of juniper and lavender can be diluted and massaged into the surrounding area, or used in the bath. *(See pages 160 and 161.)*

HOMEOPATHY
• Hamamelis, for bruised, sore veins, and piles. *(See page 197.)*
• Carb. veg., for mottled and marbled skin. *(See page 188.)*

• Pulsatilla, especially during pregnancy, and if warmth makes symptoms worse. *(See page 209.)*
• Ferr. phos., for pale legs that redden easily, but are better on walking. *(See page 194.)*

VITAMINS AND MINERALS
• Increase your intake of vitamins E and C, and bioflavonoids, which improve blood vessel health. *(See pages 257, 256 and 272.)*
• Increase your intake of dietary fiber, which will prevent constipation.
• Rutin helps to keep the vein walls in good shape.

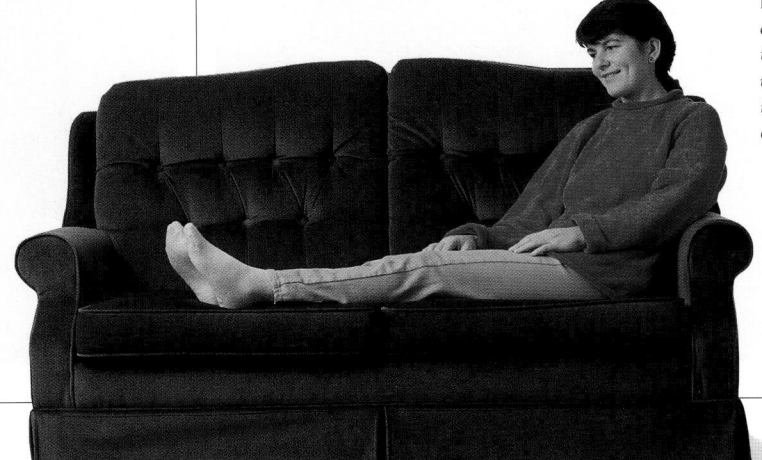

LEFT *Poor circulation, often the cause of varicose veins, may be improved by elevating the legs.*

Raynaud's Disease

Raynaud's disease is a disorder in which the arteries of the fingers and (less often) the toes go into spasm on exposure to cold. Raynaud's disease is more common in women than men, and its onset usually occurs in young adulthood. It affects mainly young women, has no known cause, and is rarely serious. Raynaud's phenomenon, however, caused by disease or occupational hazard, is more problematic: inflammation of the arteries of the fingers and toes occurs, some-times leading to the formation of a blood clot.

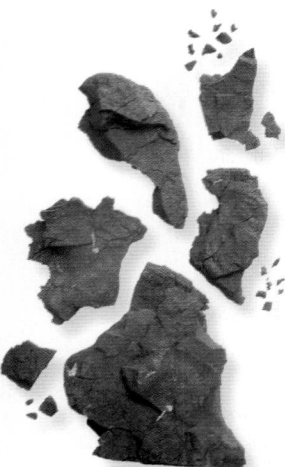

ABOVE *The homeopathic remedy Carbo vegitabilis is used to treat conditions where the symptom picture is characterized by icy mottled skin.*

SYMPTOMS

• *tingling sensation, burning, and numbness in fingers or toes* • *affected areas turn white, then blue, then red* • *painful ulcers or even tissue death (gangrene) can occur in cases where the disease persists for years*

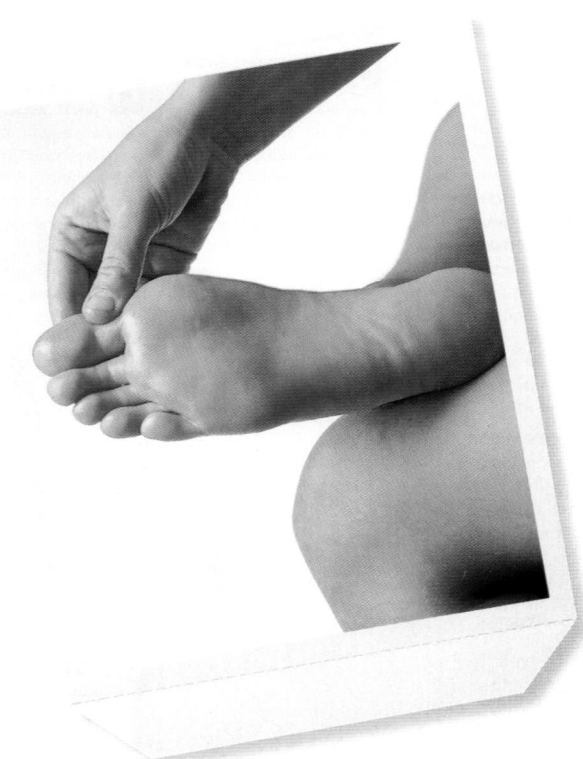

ABOVE *In Ayurvedic medicine, hands and feet are massaged with warm mustard and sesame oils to stimulate the circulation.*

TREATMENT

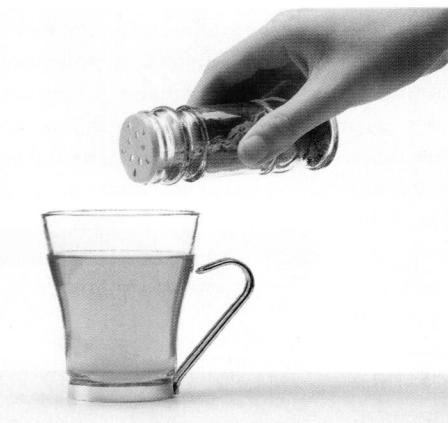

ABOVE *Herbalists add cayenne pepper to herbal tea to treat conditions when there is poor circulation.*

AYURVEDA
• Massage hands and feet with a mixture of warm mustard and sesame seed oils. *(See page 30.)*

CHINESE HERBALISM
• Cinnamon twigs and Chinese angelica may be useful. *(See pages 56 and 59.)*

HERBALISM
• Cayenne pepper can be added to any herbal tea to stimulate the circulation and warm the body. *(See page 118.)*

• Fresh ginger can be chewed, and the juices swallowed, to improve circulation and act as a tonic to the heart. *(See page 139.)*

AROMATHERAPY
• Rubefacient oils such as black pepper, lemon, and rosemary can be massaged into the affected area to increase circulation and warmth. *(See pages 146–71.)*

HOMEOPATHY
Constitutional treatment is advised, but the following may help:
• Carb. veg., for icy, mottled-looking skin. *(See page 188.)*
• Lachesis, for blue or purple skin, worse after sleep. *(See page 216.)*
• Pulsatilla, for symptoms that are made worse by heat or hanging the limb. *(See page 209.)*
• Arsenicum, for swelling, burning and itching made worse by exposure to cold. *(See page 182.)*
• Cactus, for icy cold, swollen hands and feet.
• Secale, for burning sensation in fingers or toes.

VITAMINS AND MINERALS
• Increase your intake of iron, and ensure that you take plenty of foods rich in vitamin C alongside, which helps the absorption of iron. *(See pages 260 and 256.)*

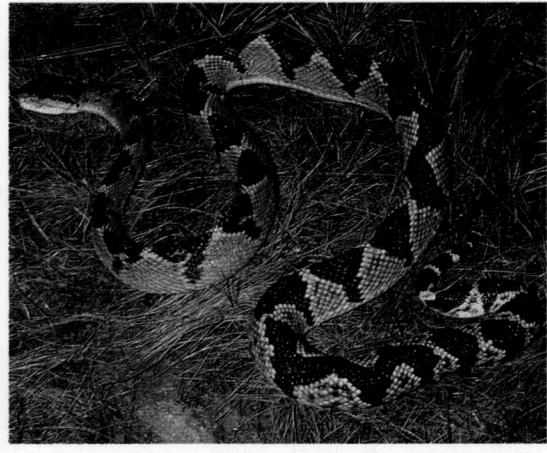

ABOVE *Lachesis is prepared from the bushmaster snake. It is used to treat complaints where there is mottled, purplish skin.*

Bruising

Bruising (or ecchymosis) results from the release of blood from the capillaries into the tissues under the skin. The characteristic bluish-black mark on the skin lightens in color and eventually fades as the blood is absorbed by the tissues and carried away. Bruising usually occurs as a result of an injury, but can occasionally be spontaneous and an indication of an allergic reaction, or more serious diseases such as leukemia and hemophilia.

SYMPTOMS

- *pain on pressure*
- *in severe cases, pain on attempting to move the affected area*

CAUTION

A CASE OF BRUISING WITHOUT ANY OBVIOUS CAUSE REQUIRES MEDICAL INVESTIGATION AS IT MAY BE AN OUTWARD SYMPTOM OF A MORE SERIOUS CONDITION.

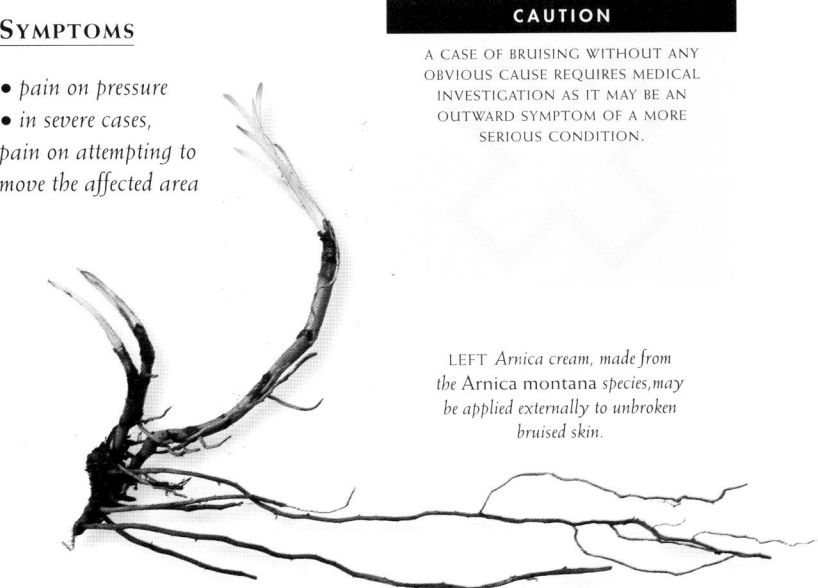

LEFT *Arnica cream, made from the* Arnica montana *species, may be applied externally to unbroken bruised skin.*

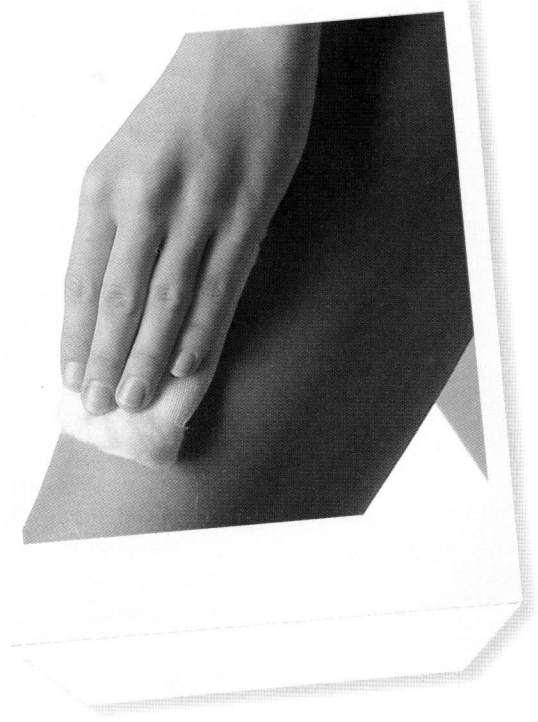

ABOVE *Apply a cold vinegar compress to relieve bruises and swelling.*

TREATMENT

✋ TRADITIONAL HOME AND FOLK REMEDIES

- Macerated and heated cabbage leaves can be applied to the affected area. *(See page 87.)*
- A mustard poultice or black pepper oil draws the blood away from the bruise. *(See pages 97 and 98.)*
- A vinegar compress can be used for all bruises or swelling. Avoid the eye area. *(See page 102.)*
- Witch hazel tincture can be used to relieve swellings and bruises. Apply to a cool compress. *(See page 91.)*
- Use roasted onions in a poultice to help heal bruising. *(See page 82.)*

🌿 HERBALISM

- Bathe the area in witch hazel, which disperses the blood and encourages healing. *(See page 123.)*

⊙ HOMEOPATHY

- Arnica, where there is bruising due to trauma or injury. *(See page 182.)*
- Hamamelis, for bruising with broken skin, or due to poor circulation. *(See page 197.)*
- Ruta. grav., for bruising that feels as if it is in the bone. *(See page 210.)*
- Hypericum, when bruising involves nerve endings, such as fingers and toes. *(See page 199.)*

- Homeopathic remedy and tincture of Calendula will ease symptoms. *(See page 187.)*

✳ FLOWER ESSENCES

- Rescue Remedy can be applied to the bruised area, to encourage healing and prevent the negative effects of trauma. *(See page 244.)*
- Crushed agrimony roots and leaves can be used as a compress for bruises or taken internally. *(See page 225.)*
- Comfrey is exceptional for healing, and can be applied as a compress or poultice on the bruise.

- Daisy is also known as bruisewort; bruise the leaves and flowers and add them to wheat germ oil.
- Crushed yarrow can be placed on fresh cuts or bruises.

💊 VITAMINS AND MINERALS

- Increase your intake of vitamin C and bioflavonoids, to help the health of the capillaries. *(See pages 256 and 272.)*
- Zinc strengthens the integrity of the capillaries. *(See page 265.)*

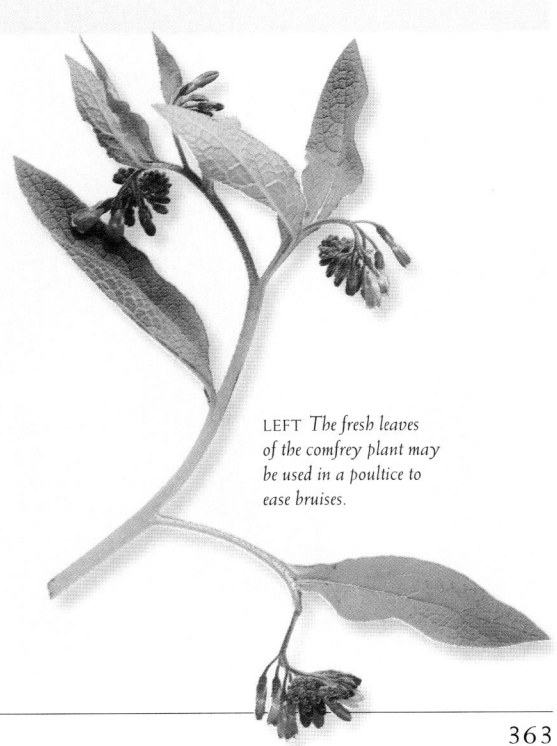

LEFT *The fresh leaves of the comfrey plant may be used in a poultice to ease bruises.*

DISORDERS OF THE DIGESTIVE SYSTEM

Nausea and Vomiting

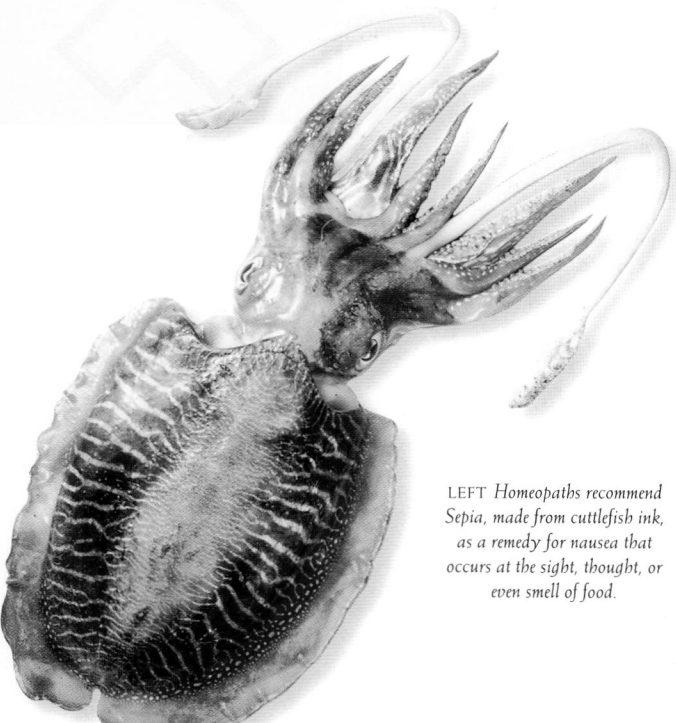

ABOVE *Nausea may be relieved by chewing a piece of crystallized ginger.*

Nausea (a feeling of sickness) and vomiting are symptoms of various disorders, which include gastroenteritis, inner ear infection, migraine, excessive food or alcohol intake, hiatus hernia, pancreatitis, indigestion, food poisoning, gallstones, or liver disease. They may also be caused by hormonal changes in pregnancy and menstruation, travel, or by certain smells and sights. Nausea may be accompanied by a feeling of faintness and dizziness. Vomiting is usually preceded by nausea, and may be accompanied by sweating, excessive salivation, and a slowing of the heart rate. A constant feeling of nausea with no vomiting, but with a headache and abdominal pain, is most likely to be stress- or anxiety-related.

LEFT *Homeopaths recommend Sepia, made from cuttlefish ink, as a remedy for nausea that occurs at the sight, thought, or even smell of food.*

TREATMENT

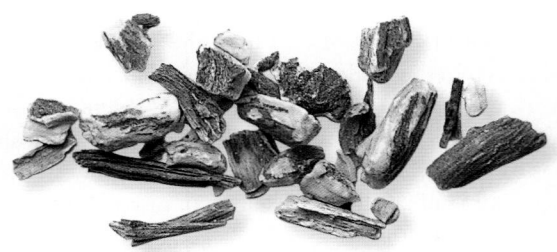

ABOVE *Dandelion root is a liver stimulant and tonic. Drink dandelion coffee when nausea may be a result of liver problems.*

CHINESE HERBALISM
• Treatment would be aimed at ascending Stomach qi, and useful herbs may include root ginger, Ren Dan, Shen Chu Cha, Xiang Sha Yang Wei Pian, or Bu Zhong Yi Qi Wan.
• Er Chen Wan pills, a classical formula to dissolve Phlegm, resolve Spleen Damp and harmonize the center (digestive organs), as well as symptoms brought on by food retention in the Stomach.

HERBALISM
• Drinking ginger tea or chewing a piece of crystallized ginger warms the stomach and allays cold nausea. This can be used for relief of sickness in pregnancy or during travel. *(See page 139.)*
• Persistent nausea may indicate liver trouble: seek advice. Take decoction or coffee made of dandelion root. *(See page 134.)*

HOMEOPATHY
• Sepia, when you feel nauseous at the thought or smell of food, but feel better for eating. *(See page 212.)*
• Nux vomica, when nausea is made better by vomiting, and may be caused by overindulgence. *(See page 214.)*
• Lactic acid, when there is profuse salivation and a history of anemia.
• Tabacum, for nausea and vomiting relieved by uncovering the abdomen.
• Arsenicum, when nausea and vomiting are accompanied by diarrhea, and symptoms are worse between midnight and 2 A.M. *(See page 182.)*
• Phosphorus, for cravings for cold water, which is then vomited, with blood in the vomit and burning pains in the stomach. *(See page 208.)*

• Pulsatilla, for vomiting after rich, fatty food, with some tearfulness. *(See page 209.)*
• Arnica, when vomiting follows a head injury. *(See page 182.)*
• Aconite, when vomiting and severe pain last for more than one hour, and are not relieved by vomiting. *(See page 178.)*

FLOWER ESSENCES
• Rescue Remedy or Emergency Essence will be useful for prolonged or distressing vomiting; it will help to reduce panic and calm the mind and body. *(See page 244.)*

VITAMINS AND MINERALS
• Take vitamin B6 for morning sickness (consult your doctor first) and for travel sickness. It is appropriate for children if given in half-doses. *(See page 254.)*

BELOW *Star of Bethlehem, as one of the five ingredients of Bach's Rescue Remedy, is used to treat cases of prolonged or distressed nausea.*

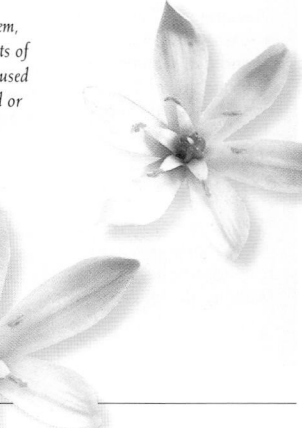

Jaundice

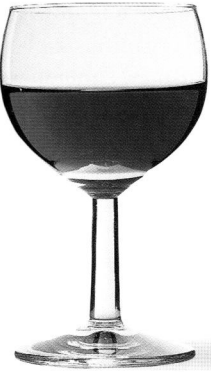

ABOVE *Avoid drinking alcohol if you have jaundice.*

Jaundice refers to a yellowing of the whites of the eyes and of the skin caused by bilirubin – a natural coloring substance. Under normal circumstances, bilirubin is released by red blood cells and passed to the intestine in bile, via the liver. If the liver is diseased, however, or if there is bile duct blockage, it accumulates in the blood, causing the characteristic yellow staining of tissue.

Newborn infants frequently develop mild jaundice, which lasts several days until a normal excess of red blood cells is destroyed. This condition is not normally considered to be serious. But erythroblastosis fetalis, a serious form of jaundice in infants, generally is due to a Rh factor incompatibility. Adolescents and young adults who have a viral inflammation of the liver often develop jaundice; jaundice in middle-aged adults is commonly due to gallstones. In older adults jaundice may signal cancer of the liver or the bile ducts. It is often the first symptom of liver damage in heavy drinkers.

SYMPTOMS

- *yellowing of the skin and the whites of the eyes*
- *darkened urine* • *pale-colored stools*

CAUTION

JAUNDICE IS NOT A DISEASE IN ITSELF, BUT IS AN INDICATION OF AN UNDERLYING DISORDER SUCH AS HEPATITIS, GALLSTONES, HEMOLYTIC ANEMIA, CIRRHOSIS OF THE LIVER, PANCREATITIS, OR PANCREATIC CANCER. THE CAUSE OF JAUNDICE SHOULD ALWAYS BE INVESTIGATED IMMEDIATELY.

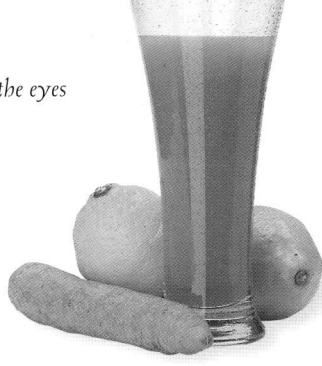

ABOVE *A daily drink of carrot and lemon juice will help relieve jaundice.*

TREATMENT

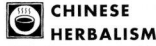 **CHINESE HERBALISM**
- Treatment would be aimed at Dampness in the Gall Bladder and Liver, and useful herbs may include gardenia fruit, oriental wormwood, and the bark of the cork tree. *(See page 68.)*

HERBALISM
- Any of the following herbs can be used to tonify the liver: golden seal, verbena, barberry, blue flag, dandelion, and wild yam. *(See pages 120 and 133.)*

AROMATHERAPY
- Oils that strengthen the liver include chamomile, cypress, lemon, peppermint, rosemary, and thyme. Use one or a blend of these oils in massage, or in a vaporizer in your room. *(See pages 146–71.)*

HOMEOPATHY
- Constitutional treatment would accord with the cause of the jaundice.
- Crotalus is appropriate for jaundice caused by hemolytic anemia.

VITAMINS AND MINERALS
- Drink fresh carrot and lemon juice daily.
- Avoid alcohol and caffeine.
- Eat plenty of fresh fruit and vegetables, as well as whole grains and cereals.

Hiatus Hernia

A hiatus hernia occurs when part of the stomach slides up through the esophageal opening in the diaphragm into the chest. As a result of this the stomach's contents regurgitate into the esophagus, which may cause damage and inflammation (esophagitis). The underlying cause of hiatus hernia is unknown, but this common condition tends to occur more often in obese people (and especially in women in later middle age), and in those who smoke. In some cases it is present at birth.

SYMPTOMS

- *severe heartburn (a burning pain behind the breastbone) that worsens on bending, straining, and lying down* • *if esophagitis occurs there may be associated symptoms of acid in the mouth, difficulty in swallowing, and ulceration*

RIGHT *A hiatus hernia is characterized by severe heartburn that becomes more painful if you bend forward or lie down.*

TREATMENT

CHINESE HERBALISM
- Treatment would be individual, but there are a number of herbs which will restore the balance. *(See pages 48–75.)*

HOMEOPATHY
- Constitutional treatment would be suggested, but the remedies for indigestion will be appropriate. *(See page 368.)*
- Calc. fluor., a tissue salt, will help elasticity.

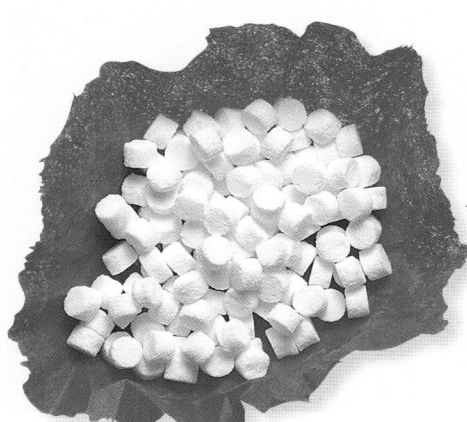

LEFT *The homeopathic remedy Calc. fluor. will help maintain tissue elasticity and so may be a useful treatment for a hiatus hernia.*

Appendicitis

The appendix is 1–8in. (2–20cm.) long, about as thick as a pencil, and hollow. It consists mostly of lymphoid tissue, like the tonsils and adenoids, and is easily invaded by micro-organisms. One out of every 15 people develops appendicitis, the inflammation of an infected appendix. This is a medical emergency that usually requires the surgical removal of the appendix. For many years the appendix was regarded as a vestigial organ with no function in the human body, but it is now thought to be one of the sites where immune responses are initiated. Appendicitis is particularly common in adolescents and young adults.

SYMPTOMS

• *pain and tenderness beginning in the center of the abdomen, then moving to the right and down towards the groin*
• *possibly nausea and vomiting*
• *fever*

CAUTION

PERFORATION OF THE APPENDIX CAN LEAD TO PERITONITIS – A SERIOUS, POTENTIALLY FATAL INFLAMMATION OF THE MEMBRANE LINING THE ABDOMINAL CAVITY.

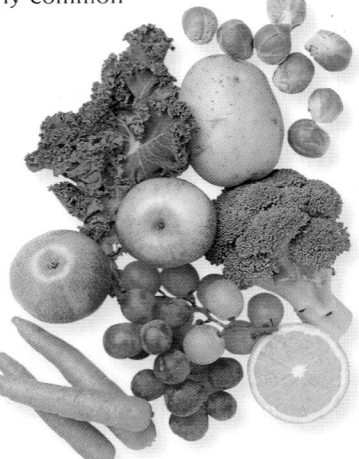

ABOVE *To avoid constipation make sure you eat plenty of fresh fruit and vegetables.*

TREATMENT

HERBALISM
• Treatment is aimed at preventing the condition in people who have a "grumbling" appendix, with inflammation and recurring abdominal pain. The following herbs will help to resolve inflammation and irritation: agrimony, chamomile, echinacea, licorice, and wild yam. These can be combined or taken separately, up to 3 times a day.
(See pages 112–139)

HOMEOPATHY
Urgent medical treatment will be required, but the following remedies can be offered, every 15 minutes, while waiting for help:
• Lachesis, for cutting, tearing pains, a distended abdomen and irritability. *(See page 216.)*
• Bryonia, for intense pain over the appendix area. *(See page 185.)*
• Belladonna, for pain that is made worse by movement, accompanied by a red, flushed face. *(See page 183.)*
After an operation, the following remedies help:
• Arnica, to prevent bruising and encourage healing. *(See page 182.)*
• Phosphorus, to relieve nausea caused by the effects of the anesthetic. *(See page 208.)*

FLOWER ESSENCES
• Rescue Remedy or Emergency Essence can be given while waiting for help, to calm and reduce anxiety. *(See page 244.)*

VITAMINS AND MINERALS
• Eat plenty of fresh fruits and vegetables, and avoid getting constipated.
• Never use laxative preparations, which will aggravate the condition.

Gastroenteritis

Gastroenteritis is an acute inflammation of the stomach and intestine, causing violent upset. It may be due to bowel organisms such as salmonella or other bacterial toxins or viruses that may contaminate food or water; food intolerance; or excessive alcohol intake. The symptoms and their severity will vary according to the cause. It can also be a side-effect of certain drugs. Gastroenteritis is most serious in the elderly and in babies because of the danger of dehydration through vomiting and diarrhea.

SYMPTOMS

• *fever* • *abdominal pain* • *nausea and vomiting*
• *diarrhea* • *in severe cases there may be shock and collapse*

TREATMENT

TRADITIONAL HOME AND FOLK REMEDIES
• Very ripe bananas will ease nausea, act as a gentle constipant, and help to restore the healthy bacteria in the intestines.
• Live yogurt, taken by the teaspoon throughout the day, can help to restore bacteria to the stomach and digestive tracts. *(See page 93.)*
• Honey is a natural antibiotic and anti-inflammatory. Mix a few teaspoonfuls in a cup of warm water and sip. Freeze into ice cubes if you find hot drinks difficult to manage. *(See page 101.)*

HERBALISM
• Make an infusion of comfrey root and meadowsweet to treat the infection and relieve the associated symptoms. *(See pages 121 and 132.)*
• Arrowroot or slippery elm tea can be sipped during the worst symptoms to soothe the digestive tract, and afterwards to help restore bowel health. *(See page 136.)*

AROMATHERAPY
• Massage chamomile and geranium essential oils into the abdomen to bring relief from pain and discomfort. *(See pages 150 and 165.)*

HOMEOPATHY
The following remedies can be taken hourly, as required:
• Arsenicum, for burning abdominal pains, accompanied by great thirst. *(See page 182.)*
• Pulsatilla, for symptoms which are worse at night, and tearfulness. *(See page 209.)*
• Baptisia, if a salmonella infection is suspected – stools dark, bloody, and smelly, nearly liquid. *(See page 184.)*
• Mercurius for diarrhea, where there is blood and mucus in the stools. *(See page 205.)*
• Phosphorus, for a burning sensation when stools are passed, with vomiting and cravings for cold water, which is then vomited. *(See page 208.)*
• Sulfur for burning diarrhea which is at its worst around 5a.m., with a red, itchy anus. *(See page 215.)*

VITAMINS AND MINERALS
• Take acidophilus to restore the healthy flora in the intestines, which will help to fight infection. *(See page 271.)*

LEFT *Live yogurt contains Lactobacillus bulgaris, which can help restore equilibrium in the gut.*

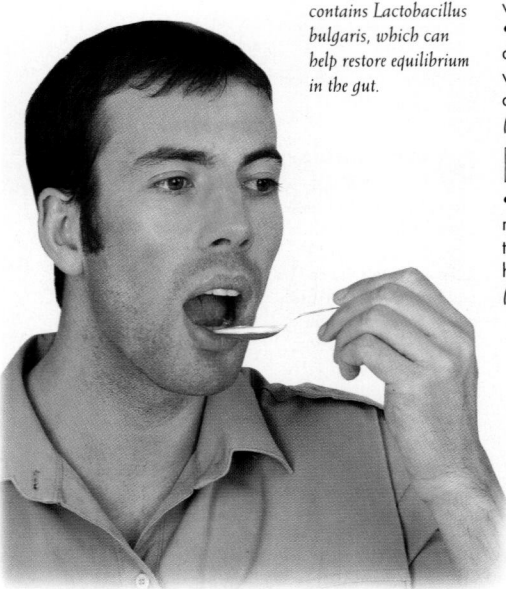

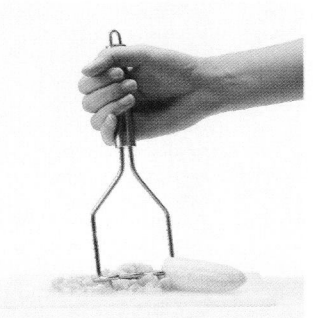

ABOVE *Bananas are easily digestible and will ease the discomfort of diarrhea. They are best eaten ripe and may be mashed to ease digestion.*

Stomach Ulcers

Peptic ulcers occur most commonly in the duodenum, near the junction with the stomach, and in the stomach wall. They usually occur singly as round or oval wounds. The erosions are usually shallow, but can penetrate the entire wall, leading to hemorrhage and possibly death. When gastric juices (consisting of hydrochloric acid, mucus, and a digestive enzyme called pepsin) act upon the walls of the digestive tract, a peptic ulcer results. Peptic ulcers tend to become chronic.

The peptic ulcer develops when there is imbalance between the normal "aggressive" factors, the acid-peptic secretions, and the normal "resistance" factors, such as mucus and rapid cellular replacement. Physical and mental stress are thought to be triggers, as are hereditary factors, smoking, excessive alcohol intake, and non-steroidal anti-inflammatory drugs (NSAIDs). Gastric (stomach) ulcers affect both men and women, usually over the age of 40, while duodenal ulcers are more common in men. Ulcers in the lower esophagus are relatively rare and are usually associated with hiatus hernia (see page 365) and esophagitis. Peptic ulcers affect approximately 10 percent of the U.S. population. Duodenal ulcers are two to three times more common than gastric ulcers, and people with blood group O are more likely to get them.

SYMPTOMS

• *gastric ulcers: a gnawing, burning pain, which is worse during or after eating, nausea, and vomiting* • *duodenal ulcers: intermittent upper abdominal pain characteristically relieved by eating; pain usually begins around mid-morning and sufferers are often woken up by it at night* • *peptic ulcers: may bleed, causing blood in vomit and dark, blackish stools; occasionally a peptic ulcer perforates, causing severe pain and shock*

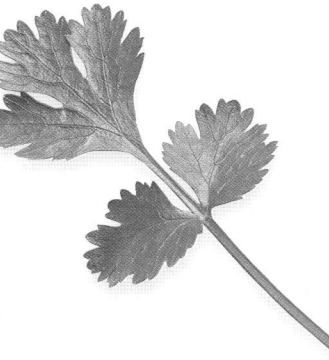

ABOVE *Coriander is given in Ayurvedic medicine for peptic ulcers.*

BELOW *A decoction of licorice can be given three or four time daily to relieve symptoms.*

TREATMENT

AYURVEDA
• Suitable herbs which might be suggested include bitter orange, coriander, and kalanchoe. *(See page 35.)*

CHINESE HERBALISM
• Treatment would be aimed at unblocking stagnant Stomach qi, excess Heat, and a weak Spleen. Suitable herbs may include dandelion, ginseng, and corydalis tuber. *(See page 67.)*

HERBALISM
• Licorice has a soothing effect on the stomach and the mucous membranes, and a decoction can be drunk three or four times each day to ease symptoms. *(See page 122.)*

• A decoction of marshmallow root is healing. *(See page 114.)*
• Comfrey or slippery elm may also be of help. *(See pages 119 and 136.)*

AROMATHERAPY
• Oils of chamomile, frankincense, geranium, and marjoram can be diluted and massaged into the abdomen. *(See pages 146–71.)*

HOMEOPATHY
Treatment would be constitutional, but the following remedies may be appropriate:
• Nux vomica, for pain which is worse after eating. *(See page 214.)*
• Anacardium, when pain is relieved by eating. *(See page 179.)*

• Kali bich., for pain in a small, distinct position in the stomach area. *(See page 200.)*
• Phosphorus, for burning pains and vomiting which are better for cold drinks. *(See page 208.)*
• Bryonia, for a feeling of a stone in the stomach and sensitivity to touch. *(See page 185.)*

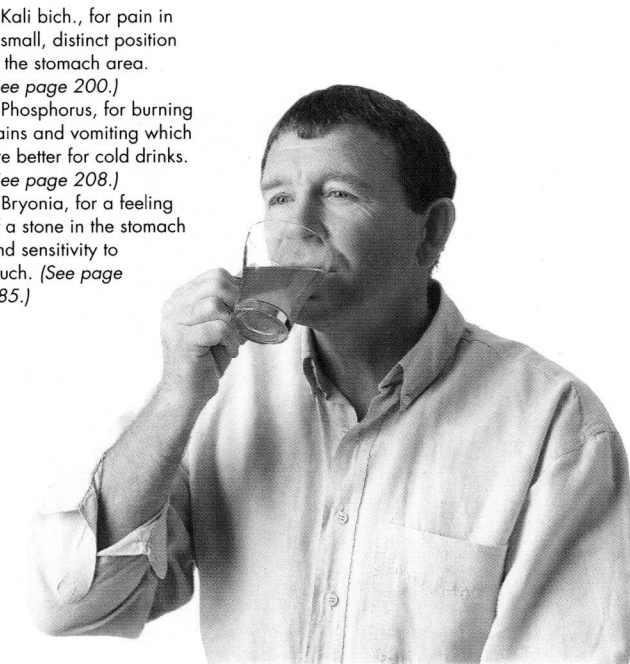

Indigestion

Indigestion (or dyspepsia) is a general term which usually refers to abdominal discomfort, nausea, heartburn (burning sensation or pain behind the breastbone), hiccups, and flatulence. Indigestion refers to discomfort in the upper abdomen – gastric distress – often brought on by eating too much, by eating too quickly, or by eating very rich, spicy, or fatty foods. Nervous indigestion is a common effect of stress. Indigestion is also commonly caused by excessive smoking, excessive alcohol or caffeine consumption, pregnancy, or anxiety. It can also be a feature of several diseases, including esophagitis (inflammation of the lining of the esophagus), gastroenteritis (see page 366), peptic ulcer (see page 367), and gallstones (see page 369).

SYMPTOMS

• *abdominal discomfort* • *nausea* • *heartburn (burning sensation or pain behind the breastbone)* • *hiccups* • *flatulence*

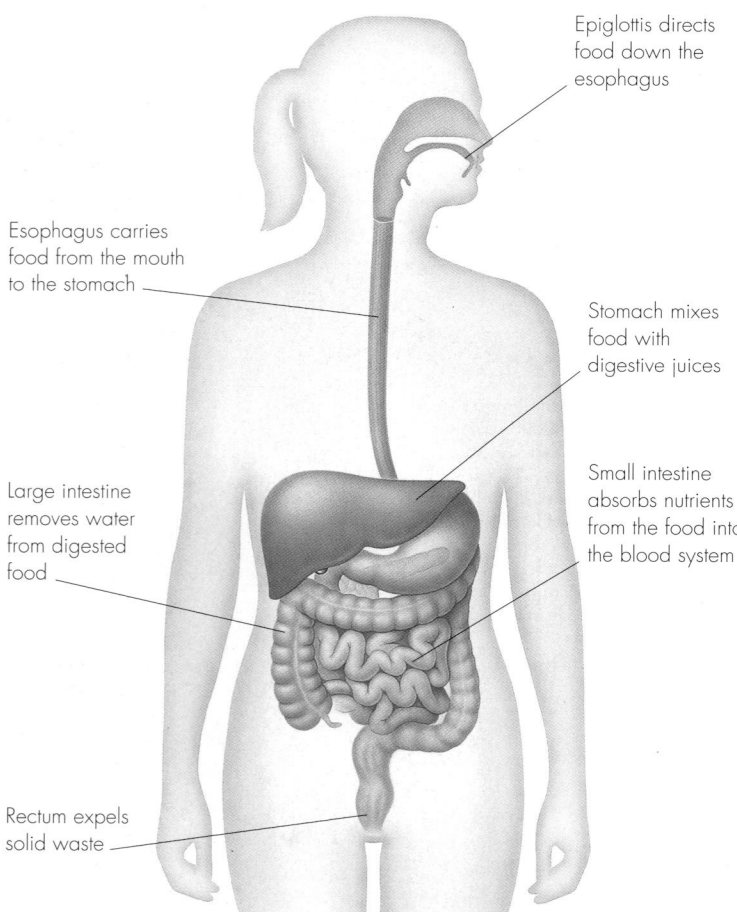

Epiglottis directs food down the esophagus

Esophagus carries food from the mouth to the stomach

Stomach mixes food with digestive juices

Small intestine absorbs nutrients from the food into the blood system

Large intestine removes water from digested food

Rectum expels solid waste

ABOVE *There are many natural remedies that can be used for digestive complaints, including homeopathic and herbal remedies.*

AYURVEDA
• Crush fresh root ginger to extract the juice. Mix with the juice of a lime and a lemon, add a pinch of salt, and drink. *(See page 47.)*

CHINESE HERBALISM
• Treatment would address a weakness of the Spleen and Stomach. Rice and wheat sprouts would be used.

HERBALISM
• Try an infusion of peppermint or fennel tea after meals or when feeling full and windy. *(See pages 121 and 125.)*
• Improve the general tone of the digestive tract with bitter aperient herbs such as dandelion, gentian, and wormwood, taken 20 minutes before food. *(See page 133.)*
• A cold stomach can be warmed by eating 3 cardamom pods, or a pinch of ginger or cayenne. *(See pages 118 and 139.)*
• Fresh dill, added to boiling water and steeped, will reduce flatulence and gas pains.

TRADITIONAL HOME AND FOLK REMEDIES
• Eat a slice of fresh pineapple after meals to ease symptoms.
• Clove tea and cinnamon tea are both digestive and will soothe away the symptoms. *(See page 90.)*
• Fennel, eaten raw or cooked, or the bruised seeds infused and drunk, acts as a digestive.
• Peppermint leaves can be infused and drunk to relieve indigestion, and to soothe any gas pains. Peppermint oil can be rubbed into the abdomen for instant relief.
• Drink a little warmed vinegar and honey in a cup of hot water to ease digestive complaints. *(See pages 101 and 102.)*

HOMEOPATHY
Chronic indigestion should be treated constitutionally, but the following remedies may be useful during an attack:
• Carb. veg., after rich foods, with gas and belching. *(See page 188.)*
• Nux vomica, after spicy food, and overindulgence in cigarettes and alcohol. *(See page 214.)*
• Arsenicum, when there is burning pain, particularly between midnight and 2 A.M. *(See page 182.)*
• Pulsatilla, for an attack brought on by rich food, and accompanied by a bad taste in the mouth, nausea, and weepiness. *(See page 209.)*
• China, for windy stomach, and a bloated and sluggish feeling, and where stools have the appearance of chopped egg. *(See page 190.)*

• Lycopodium, for a bloated stomach with heartburn, and a full feeling even when hungry, especially where food causes instant discomfort. *(See page 203.)*
• Graphites, for burning pains which are relieved by food or milk, but followed by ingestion. *(See page 196.)*
• Bryonia, for a heaviness in the stomach, which is worse after food, with heartburn, nausea, and faintness; and which is made worse by movement but improved by lying down. *(See page 185.)*

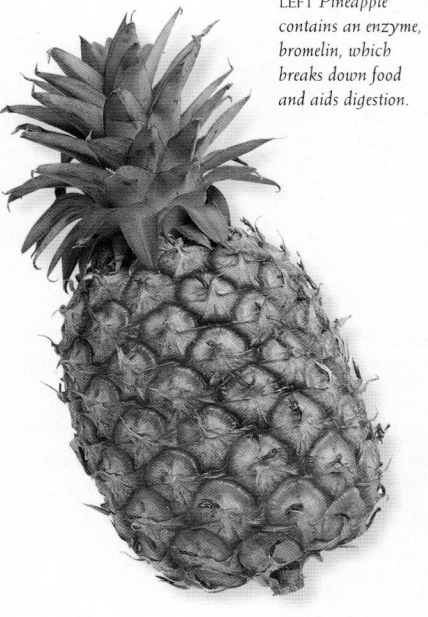

LEFT *Pineapple contains an enzyme, bromelin, which breaks down food and aids digestion.*

Travel Sickness

Travel or motion sickness is a sensitivity to the constant passive movement of the body while in a car, boat, airplane, train, or bus. Some people may even experience it in lifts. Why only some people experience travel sickness is unclear. The syndrome appears to arise from sensory mismatch, when the information coming to the brain from various sensory inputs does not add up, as when the eyes report a steady horizon, but the balancing (vestibular) system reports a rocking motion. Travel sickness appears to be more common in women, and children under the age of two. Elderly people do not seem to be so troubled by the problem. Severe travel sickness can cause a complete lack of coordination.

SYMPTOMS

• progressive nausea • vomiting • pallor, faintness, and dizziness • abdominal discomfort • headache • sweaty palms and face • increased salivation

TREATMENT

AYURVEDA
• Ginger, chewed fresh, may help symptoms. *(See page 47.)*
• Oral syrup of Vilwadi lehya will be useful.

CHINESE HERBALISM
• Sipping a warm drink with grated root ginger may be helpful.

HERBALISM
• Chew fresh angelica leaves, and hang them in the car while traveling. *(See page 115.)*

• Chew fresh or crystallized ginger to ease nausea. *(See page 139.)*
• Fennel or chamomile tea will ease the symptoms. *(See pages 119 and 121.)*
• Fresh peppermint leaves can be chewed, or drink an infusion to soothe and settle the stomach. *(See page 125.)*

HOMEOPATHY
Take the following remedies hourly when symptoms begin:
• Nux vomica, for a feeling of chilliness, which is improved by vomiting. *(See page 214.)*

• Arnica, when you are overtired and irritable. *(See page 182.)*
• Cocculus, for nausea with a metallic taste in the mouth.
• Sepia, when nausea is made worse by the smell of food and improved by eating. *(See page 212.)*
• Tabacum, for nausea with giddiness, and pale, cold sweat, with a band around the head.

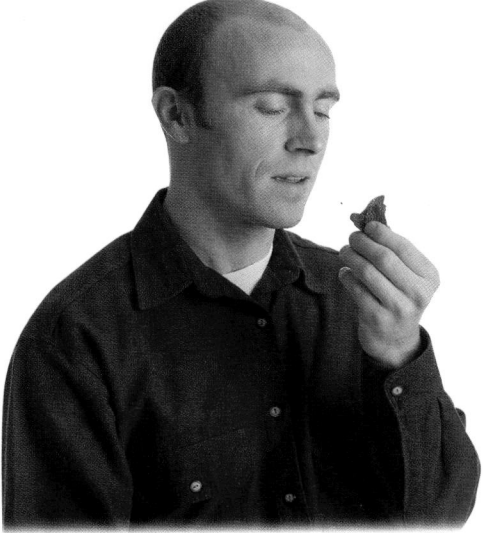

RIGHT *Chewing a piece of ginger may relieve travel sickness.*

Gallstones

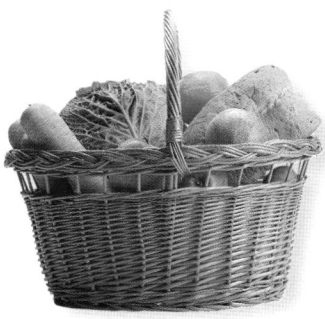

ABOVE *To minimize the risk of gallstones, increase your intake of dietary fiber.*

Gallstones are hard stone-like masses occurring in the gall bladder or in the bile duct. They are usually about the size of a pebble, and most are composed of cholesterol, calcium, or both. Abnormal composition of bile (too much cholesterol, for example), blockage of bile outflow, infection, or hereditary factors may all cause gallstones. Risk factors include obesity, advancing age, a high-fat diet, and food intolerance. Far more women than men are affected by gallstones. Gallstones occur in about 10 percent of the U.S. population, particularly in women. There may be from one to ten or more stones, ranging in size, about 1–25mm. across. Gallstones are rare in childhood, but become progressively more common with age. Autopsies show that 20 percent of all women have gallstones when they die. The use of oral contraceptives may cause gallstones to form earlier than they would have otherwise.

SYMPTOMS

• acute upper abdominal pain • possibly high fever • inflammation of the gall bladder (cholecystitis) • there may be some jaundice if the stones cause bile duct obstruction • severe pain if a stone passes from the bile duct into the duodenum (biliary colic)

TREATMENT

AYURVEDA
• Kalanchoe can be used to treat gallstones.

CHINESE HERBALISM
• Herbs such as lysimachia, pyrrosia leaf, and rhubarb may break up and dissolve small stones. *(See page 73.)*

HERBALISM
• The following herbs will dissolve the gallstones, but it will take several months. Blend infusions of balmony, dandelion leaves, stone root, and fringetree bark. Take 2 or 3 times a day. *(See page 133.)*

AROMATHERAPY
• Massage lavender and rosemary oils over the gall bladder area to relieve the pain. *(See page 161.)*

HOMEOPATHY
Treatment would always be constitutional, but the following remedies may help until you are able to seek advice:
• Berberis, for relief of normal symptoms.
• China, if berberis is not effective. *(See page 190.)*

VITAMINS AND MINERALS
• Reduce your intake of all fats, except olive oil, which has been proved to break up gallstones.
• Increase your intake of dietary fiber, and ensure that you drink plenty of water.

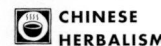

LEFT *Increasing your intake of water is crucial to prevent gallstones.*

Hepatitis

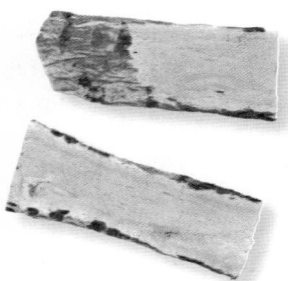

ABOVE *Astragalus is used by Chinese herbalists to strengthen the liver and treat deficient qi.*

Hepatitis is a disorder involving inflammation of the liver. Hepatitis A, once called infectious hepatitis, is the most common cause of acute hepatitis and is usually transmitted by food and water contaminated by human waste. Hepatitis B is spread mainly by blood or blood products, but can be transmitted from mother to fetus, and by intimate contact, including sexual intercourse. It often causes an initial episode of liver disease and occasionally leads to chronic hepatitis. Hepatitis C is the most common form of viral hepatitis. Type C is transmitted in blood and blood products (which are now screened for the virus), and it may be present in the body for many years before it damages the liver. Hepatitis C is a leading cause of chronic hepatitis and is considered a serious public health threat.

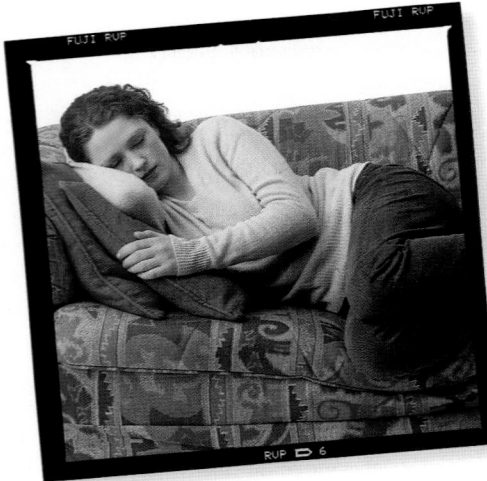

LEFT *Hepatitis leaves the sufferer feeling extremely weak and tired.*

SYMPTOMS

• *loss of appetite* • *dark urine* • *fatigue* • *sometimes fever* • *the liver may become enlarged* • *jaundice may occur, giving the skin a yellow tinge* • *hepatitis may be acute or chronic: the acute form can subside after about two months or, rarely, can result in liver failure*

DATA FILE

• Hepatitis C accounts for 10–40 percent of all hepatitis, and 90–95 percent get the disease from blood transfusions.

• Another strain of hepatitis C is uncommon in Europe and the U.S., but common in Mexico, Africa, and Asia, and usually contracted from contaminated water.

• According to recent research, 25 percent of people in the U.S. who receive blood transfusions will develop hepatitis.

• Of those contracting chronic hepatitis, most are women under the age of 45.

• Chronic hepatitis leads to cirrhosis and liver damage.

• Acute hepatitis may arise secondary to various infections that involve the liver.

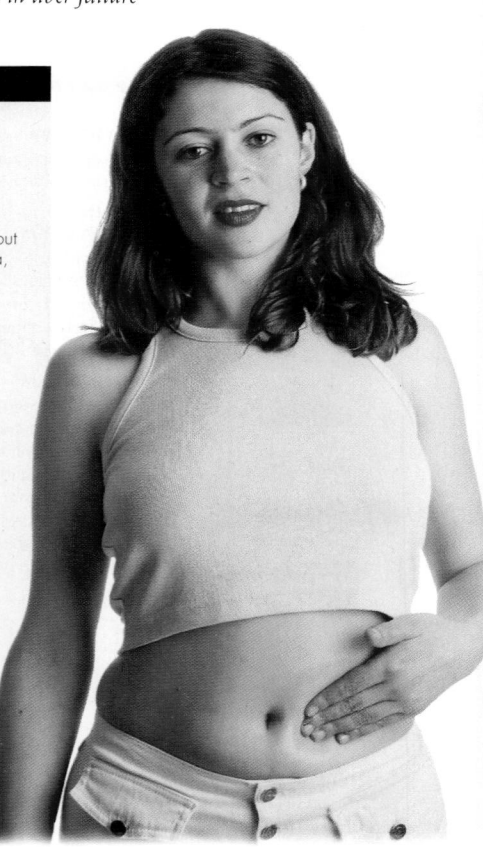

LEFT *Certain essential oils rubbed on the abdomen, act as tonics to the liver.*

TREATMENT

CHINESE HERBALISM
• Hepatitis A would require treatment for excess liver and gall bladder Damp Heat. Suitable herbal remedies include gardenia fruit and oriental wormwood.
• Hepatitis B would require treatment for deficient qi and a weakened liver. Suitable herbs include peony root, mulberry, ginseng, licorice, and astragalus. *(See pages 57, 64, 67, and 116.)*

HERBALISM
• Liver tonics may be taken daily to encourage healing and rejuvenation. Any of the following herbs can be used: golden seal, verbena, barberry, blue flag, dandelion, and wild yam. *(See pages 120 and 123.)*

TRADITIONAL HOME AND FOLK REMEDIES
• Drink barley or rice water as an overall tonic. *(See pages 92 and 96.)*

AROMATHERAPY
• Oils which act as tonics to the liver include juniper, grapefruit, chamomile, and cypress. Massage them, in a little carrier oil, into the abdominal area, or add a few drops to your bath. *(See pages 146–71.)*

HOMEOPATHY
Chronic hepatitis, which is rare, will be treated constitutionally. Cases of acute hepatitis may respond to the following:
• Bryonia, for symptoms that come on after exposure to cold, with sharp pain in the liver area. *(See page 185.)*

• Mercurius, for a yellow tongue and bad breath, with jaundice and sensitivity to cold and heat. *(See page 205.)*
• Hydrastis, for swollen, tender liver, and catarrh.
• Lachesis, when the liver feels tender and swollen, and the abdomen is distended and painful. *(See page 216.)*

VITAMINS AND MINERALS
• Plenty of fluids are necessary to cleanse the system.
• Extra vitamin C will help overcome the infection. *(See page 256.)*

Cirrhosis of the Liver

The liver is the second-largest organ in the human body, after the skin. It is a spongy, reddish brown gland that lies just below the diaphragm in the abdominal cavity, and it serves to metabolize carbohydrates and store them as glycogen; metabolize lipids (fats, including cholesterol and certain vitamins) and proteins; manufacture a digestive fluid, bile; filter impurities and toxic material from the blood; produce blood-clotting factors; and destroy old, worn-out red blood cells.

ABOVE *Taking a bath containing a few drops of the recommended essential oils, such as chamomile, relieves pain associated with liver damage.*

The liver is able to regenerate itself after being injured or diseased; but if a disease progresses beyond the tissue's capacity to regenerate new cells, the body's entire metabolism is severely affected. Severely impaired livers are sometimes replaced, and in the early 1990s the one-year survival rate was 76 percent.

Cirrhosis of the liver is the replacement of normal tissue by nonfunctioning fibrous tissue, causing scarring (or fibrosis). Cirrhosis occurs as the last stage in a range of liver disorders which have been so damaging as to cause a breakdown in the liver's regeneration process. Normal liver function is prevented and any remaining healthy liver cells are cut off from the blood supply they need. Cirrhosis may be caused by hepatitis B, poisoning, and long-term alcohol abuse.

SYMPTOMS

• *appetite and weight loss* • *continuous indigestion* • *nausea and vomiting with general malaise* • *loss of muscle power* • *itching of the skin* • *bad breath* • *bleeding varicose veins (caused by the blood's attempt to use an alternative route from the liver back to the heart)* • *vomiting blood*

TREATMENT

HERBALISM
• Good liver tonics include barberry, dandelion root, golden seal, vervain, wild yam, and yellow dock. Make an infusion of one or more and sip 2 or 3 times daily. *(See pages 120, 128, 134, and 138.)*

AROMATHERAPY
• Oils which work as a tonic to the liver and improve its function include chamomile, cypress, grapefruit, juniper, lemon, and orange. Mix a few drops in a warm carrier oil and massage into the abdomen, or add a few drops to your bath. *(See pages 146–71.)*

HOMEOPATHY
Constitutional treatment with an experienced homeopath will be necessary, but the following remedies will help until you have arranged treatment:
• Arsenicum, when there is fluid retention, and the patient feels chilly, restless, and worse between midnight and 2 A.M. *(See page 182.)*
• Phosphorus, when there is jaundice, a craving for cold water (which makes symptoms worse), and a tendency to bleed easily. *(See page 208.)*
• China, when the liver is swollen and painful, and you feel chilly and full of wind. *(See page 190.)*

Pancreatitis

A long, thin organ, the pancreas has both digestive and endocrine functions, and for this reason contains two completely different types of cells. It measures about 5–6in. (12–15 cm.) in length and is situated within the curve of the duodenum.

Pancreatitis is an inflammation of the pancreas which can be either acute or chronic. Acute pancreatitis may be caused by interference (often from gallstones) with the outflow of digestive juices from the pancreas, as a result of which the pancreas begins to digest itself. Heavy drinking is another cause, and is almost always responsible for cases of chronic pancreatitis. Chronic pancreatitis is more common in men than in women and is most commonly due to heavy drinking. The dominant feature of chronic pancreatitis is upper abdominal and back pain. Diagnosis of pancreatitis can be difficult since it closely resembles peptic ulcer and acute appendicitis. Pancreatic cancer is the fourth leading cause of cancer death in the U.S.

SYMPTOMS

• *acute pancreatitis: severe central abdominal pain, spreading to the back and shoulder, then the whole abdomen — nausea, vomiting, and shock* • *chronic pancreatitis: constant pain, often in the back — weight loss* • *if bile duct obstruction occurs there will be jaundice*

RIGHT *An infusion of yellow dock is recommended for an inflamed pancreas.*

TREATMENT

HERBALISM
• Soothing herbs include licorice and yellow dock, drunk as an infusion in an attack. *(See pages 122 and 128.)*
• Treatment would be individual, according to the cause of the illness.

HOMEOPATHY
• For acute pancreatitis, ring for emergency medical attention, and give Aconite, every 10 minutes, until help arrives. *(See page 178.)*
• For chronic pancreatitis, constitutional treatment is necessary, but the following remedies may help in an attack:
• Phosphorus, when there is jaundice and a craving for cold drinks that are then vomited up. *(See page 208.)*
• Iris, for watery stools, a burning sensation in the bowels, and cutting pains in the abdomen.
• Mercurius, for stabbing pains in the abdomen, a chilly feeling, jaundice, and offensive sweat. *(See page 205.)*
• Arsenicum, for burning pains which are worse between midnight and 2 A.M., feeling chilled and restless. *(See page 182.)*

Crohn's Disease

For sufferers of Crohn's disease, segments of the bowel become inflamed, ulcerated, and greatly thickened, while the sections in between remain normal. Any part of the bowel may be affected, but usually it is the last part of the small intestine, the terminal ileum, that is involved. It is a chronic disease whose cause is unknown, although there may be a genetic factor. Complications of Crohn's disease include arthritis, red swellings on the skin, mouth ulcers, eye inflammation, gallstones, urinary infections, and kidney stones. Crohn's most often affects young adults and people over sixty.

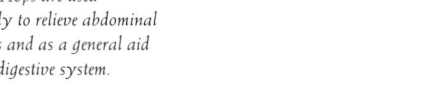

White rice

White sliced bread

Sugar

White flour

ABOVE *Diet may be a contributory factor to Crohn's disease. Avoid sugar and other refined carbohydrates and seek advice from a professional nutritionist as you may be allergic to some foods.*

SYMPTOMS

- *spasms of lower abdominal pain • diarrhea • appetite and weight loss*
- *anemia • rectal bleeding in older sufferers*

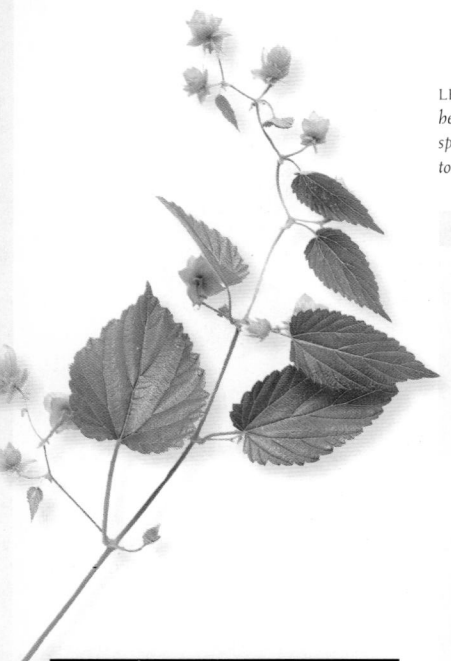

LEFT *Hops are used herbally to relieve abdominal spasms and as a general aid to the digestive system.*

DATA FILE

- Commonly occurs between the ages of 20 and 40.

- Four times more common in Caucasians and Jews than any other ethnic group.

- Crohn's may be hereditary, affecting multiple family members.

- Crohn's mainly affects the small intestine, but can occur anywhere along the digestive tract.

- Bowel obstruction and various other complications which arise may require surgical intervention.

- The cause of the potentially fatal disorder remains unknown.

TREATMENT

AYURVEDA
- Henbane can be used for bowel spasms and colic. It has sedative and antispasmodic actions.
- Coriander can help with diarrhea and the pain of Crohn's disease. It is an anti-inflammatory. *(See page 35.)*
- Hollyhock is often used to treat bowel irritation.

HERBALISM
- An infusion of peppermint can help protect the gut lining from irritation, and help to soothe the griping of the condition. The bitters stimulate and cleanse the bowels, and have an antiseptic and antibacterial action. *(See page 125.)*
- Hops have an antispasmodic action which reduces tension in the body, relieving colic and spasm in the gut. The bitters in hops also enhance the action of the digestive system.

AROMATHERAPY
- Lavender oil will help you to relax and to reduce the effects of stress. Add it to your bath water, or use in an overall body massage for best effect. *(See page 161.)*
- Roman chamomile oil, rubbed into the abdomen, may help to soothe pain. *(See page 150.)*

HOMEOPATHY
Treatment would be constitutional, but some of the following remedies may be appropriate:
- Colocynthis, for diarrhea accompanied by griping pains, and also copious, thin, frothy stools. *(See page 191.)*
- Pulsatilla, for symptoms made worse by onions, rich food, and cold drinks, with diarrhea worse at night. *(See page 209.)*

VITAMINS AND MINERALS
- You may need to take extra vitamin A, B, and D, and zinc supplement daily. *(See pages 252–5 and 256.)*
- You may be allergic to some foods, such as dairy produce or wheat – see a nutritional therapist for advice.
- Avoid sugar and other refined carbohydrates.

RIGHT *Some herbs, such as peppermint, have a soothing effect on the digestive system and may be drunk as a tea.*

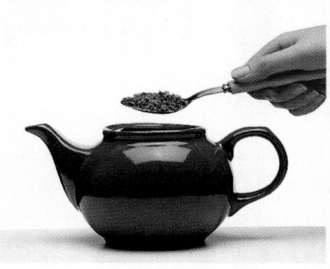

Place chopped peppermint leaves in a pot and pour boiling water over the herb. Cover with a lid.

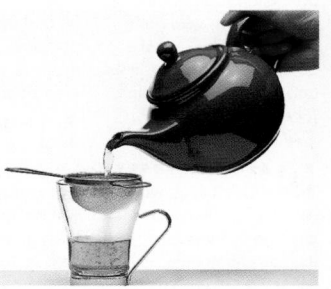

Allow the peppermint to infuse for approximately 4 minutes before pouring.

Constipation

Constipation refers to unduly infrequent or irregular bowel movements, with difficulty, discomfort, and sometimes pain on passing dry, hard feces. It is usually harmless but may be an indication of an underlying disorder, especially in adults over the age of 40. Constipation may result from: insufficient fiber in the diet, immobility, hemorrhoids *(see page 377)*, an anal fissure *(see page 376)*, iron tablets, hypothyroidism *(see pages 404–405)*, or hormonal changes, such as those in pregnancy. Dietary causes include inadequate fluid intake; a lack of vitamin B1, B5, B6, potassium, magnesium, and zinc; too much animal protein, too many dairy products; too much vinegar, pepper, salt, spices, and aluminum. If the diet is not at fault, the cause may be eating meals too fast, not taking enough exercise, tension, anxiety, depression, taking antibiotics, abusing laxatives, or abuse of certain over-the-counter drugs, such as cough mixtures.

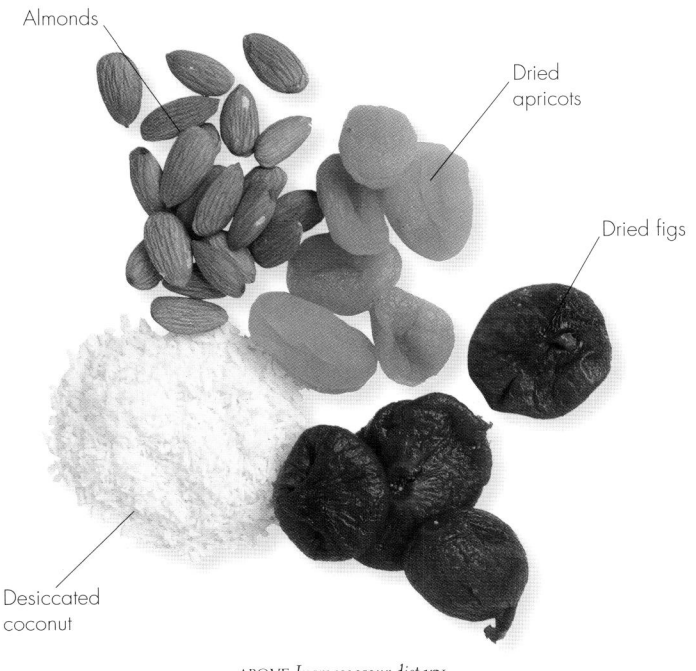

Almonds

Dried apricots

Dried figs

Desiccated coconut

ABOVE *Increase your dietary fiber intake by choosing foods that contain a high fiber content.*

SYMPTOMS

- *pain during bowel movements*
- *weight loss* • *sufferers may experience headaches, furred tongue, loss of appetite, nausea, fatigue and depression, all arising largely from anxiety about constipation*

ABOVE *Senna leaves act as a stimulating laxative and will help with constipation.*

TREATMENT

CHINESE HERBALISM

Constipation is believed to be caused either by Heat, stagnation of qi, Deficiency (of qi, yang, Blood, or yin), or interior Cold. Some suitable pills include:
- Ma Ren Wan, for Heat (dry stools, thirst, dark urine).
- Run Chang Wan, for chronic constipation of any kind, especially in old age or after childbirth.
- Mu Xiang Shun Qi Wan, for qi stagnation.

HERBALISM

- Laxative herbs, which can be drunk as herbal infusions up to 3 times daily, include licorice, marshmallow root, rhubarb root, buckthorn, and senna leaves. *(See pages 114, 122, and 127.)*

AROMATHERAPY

- Massage a few drops of marjoram, rosemary, or fennel oil, diluted in grapeseed oil, into the abdomen, to relieve constipation. *(See pages 146–71.)*

HOMEOPATHY

Constipation is regarded as a constitutional problem, but the following remedies can help with occasional symptoms:
- Lycopodium, when there is flatulence but no need to open bowels for long periods of time; then stools are hard, and passed with pain. *(See page 203.)*
- Nux vomica, for constipation that alternates with diarrhea. *(See page 214.)*

- Sepia, when the belly feels full. *(See page 212.)*
- Opium, when there is no desire to pass stool. *(See page 207.)*
- Silicea, when there is a burning sensation after a bowel movement. *(See page 211.)*
- Causticum, for a stitch-like pain accompanying a bowel movement. *(See page 189.)*
- Bryonia, for large, hard, dry stools, with congestion in the abdomen causing distension, and a burning feeling in the rectum. *(See page 185.)*
- Alumina, when there is no desire to open bowels until the rectum is full; the stool may be covered in mucus.

VITAMINS AND MINERALS

- Increase your intake of dietary fiber, which will help to bulk out stools.
- Acidophilus will encourage the health of the intestines and make bowel movements more normal. *(See page 271.)*
- Chronic constipation may respond to an increased intake of B-complex vitamins, particularly if it follows a course of antibiotics. Vitamin B1 is most effective. *(See page 252.)*

BELOW *Rhubarb root contains a natural laxative. Drink an infusion 3 times a day to relieve constipation.*

Diarrhea

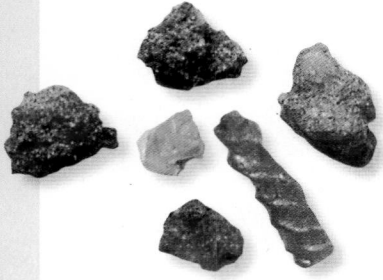

ABOVE *Myrrh is an old herbal remedy for diarrhea. Add a few drops of myrrh tincture to water to relieve symptoms.*

Diarrhea occurs when normal reabsorption of water from the stools has not taken place, so that stools are characteristically loose and runny. The two basic mechanisms involved in diarrhea, which may operate independently or together, are excessive accumulation of fluid in the intestinal tract and excessive propulsive action in the intestines. Excessive fluid in the intestines can result from conditions that decrease the absorption of water from the colon, or from conditions that cause water to be secreted into the intestines, as in cholera and other infections. The body secretes excess water in order to "flush" disease and toxins. Excessive propulsive action may be caused by nervous and chemical factors or by partial obstruction of the intestine.

Diarrhea is a feature of many conditions, including dysentery, food poisoning, cholera, typhoid, gastroenteritis, and parasitic infestation. It can also be brought on by stress or anxiety, and in babies it may be caused by lactose intolerance. Chronic diarrhea may be caused by Crohn's disease (see page 372), ulcerative colitis, or cancer of the colon.

CAUTION

CONSULT A PHYSICIAN REGARDING EPISODES OF DIARRHEA LASTING MORE THAN 48 HOURS, PARTICULARLY IF THERE IS FEVER AND/OR VOMITING.

SYMPTOMS

- *Depending on the cause, associated symptoms may include:*
- *abdominal cramps* • *vomiting*
- *wind*

RIGHT *Make sure that you drink enough fluids as you are at risk of dehydration with diarrhea. Restrict your food intake to soups as they are easily digestible.*

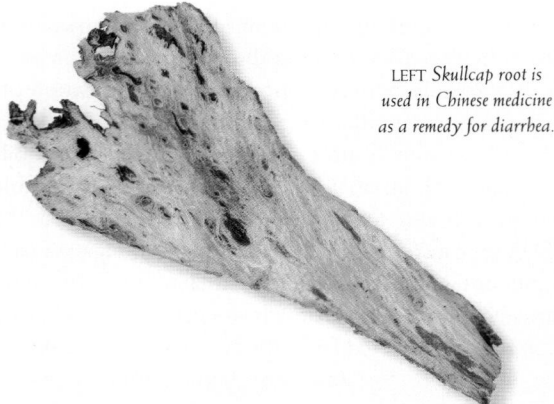

LEFT *Skullcap root is used in Chinese medicine as a remedy for diarrhea.*

AYURVEDA
• Cassia pods, henbane, and coriander can be used to treat diarrhea.
(See pages 32 and 35.)

CHINESE HERBALISM
• The full condition is caused by Cold Damp or Damp Heat; the empty condition is due to a Spleen, Stomach, or Kidney yang deficiency. *(See page 48.)*
• Skullcap root may be suitable for acute diarrhea, as well as golden thread, kapok flowers, and dandelion root. *(See pages 61 and 74.)*
• For chronic diarrhea, a treatment of psoralea fruit, codonopsis root, and astragalus may be given. *(See pages 57 and 60.)*
• Huo Xiang Zheng Qi Wan/Agastache upright qi powder, for gastric flu. *(See page 54.)*
• Mu Xiang Shun Qi Wan and Shen Ling Bai Zhu Wan, 2 pills taken together for alternating diarrhea and constipation (Liver qi stagnation with Spleen qi deficiency). The latter can be taken for chronic loose stools with poor appetite, tiredness, etc. *(See page 57.)*

• Liu Jun Zi Pian, or Six Gentlemen Tablet, for loose stools, diarrhea, indigestion resulting from Spleen qi deficiency.
• Xiang Sha Liu Jun Zi Wan, for loose stools, diarrhea, and indigestion, accompanied by nausea.

TRADITIONAL HOME AND FOLK REMEDIES
• Carrot juice or soup is very helpful, especially for infants. *(See page 89.)*

HERBALISM
• For acute diarrhea take a gentle laxative such as dock to clear away the cause of the irritant.
• A few drops of myrrh tincture in water will clear many infections.
• For chronic and nervous diarrhea use chamomile or marigold mixed with a soothing, astringent herb such as raspberry leaf. *(See pages 117, 119, and 128.)*

HOMEOPATHY
Chronic diarrhea should be treated constitutionally, but acute attacks may be treated with one of the following remedies:
• Aconite, for diarrhea that comes on suddenly, where the patient has a distended abdomen. *(See page 178.)*
• Pulsatilla, for diarrhea which is worse at night and made worse by rich foods. *(See page 209.)*

• Colocynthis, for diarrhea accompanied by griping pains, with yellowish, thin, and copious stools. *(See page 191.)*
• Arg. nit., for diarrhea caused by anxiety, characterized by episodes of belching and cravings for sweet and salty food. *(See page 181.)*
• China, for stools accompanied by wind, and made worse by fruit. *(See page 190.)*
• Phosphoric acid, when stools contain undigested food and you feel better after passing them.

VITAMINS AND MINERALS
• Increase your intake of potassium, which is easily lost in diarrhea and vomiting. *(See page 262.)*
• Increase your intake of vitamins B1 and B3, which will address the digestive system. *(See pages 252 and 253.)*
• Drink plenty of water, to flush the system.
• Take a multivitamin and mineral supplement with food when you are able to eat properly again, to replace lost nutrients. *(See page 248.)*
• Take plenty of fresh acidophilus for at least a month after an attack, to ensure the health of the bowels. *(See page 271.)*

Irritable Bowel Syndrome (IBS)

Irritable bowel syndrome (or spastic colon) is a very common disorder with recurrent abdominal pain, intermittent diarrhea alternating with constipation. This may be caused by a disturbance in the muscle movement in the large intestine, triggered by anxiety, stress, or food intolerance. IBS affects far more women than men.

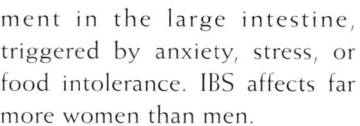

DATA FILE

- 10–20 percent of the population suffers or has suffered from IBS.

- Up to 50 percent of all health cases dealt with by gastroenterologists are caused by IBS.

- The vast majority of sufferers are women, and the young to middle-aged are particularly vulnerable.

SYMPTOMS

- *cramp-like abdominal pain, usually after eating, relieved by going to the toilet* • *swelling of the abdomen* • *excessive wind and abdominal rumblings* • *headache and back pain* • *general malaise* • *a sensation of fullness halfway through a meal* • *undue awareness of bowel action* • *anxiety*

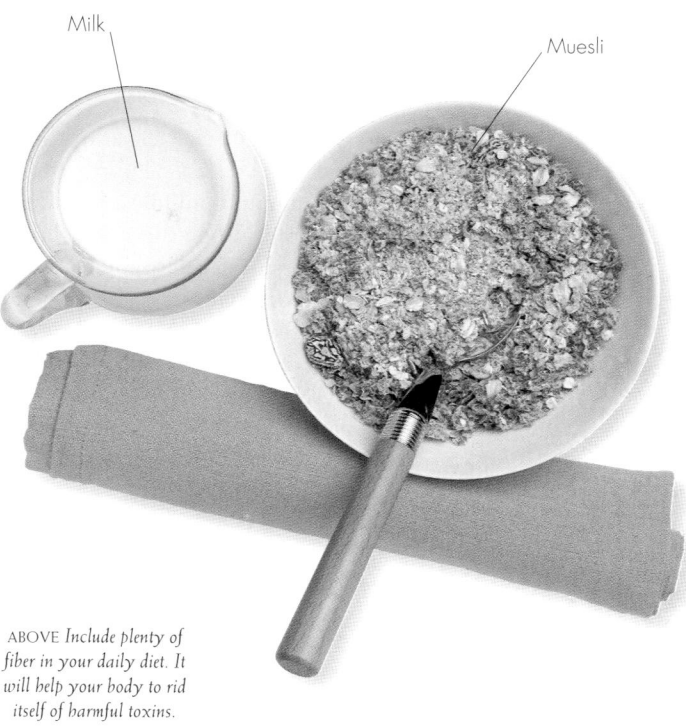

Milk

Muesli

ABOVE *Include plenty of fiber in your daily diet. It will help your body to rid itself of harmful toxins.*

TREATMENT

AYURVEDA
- Coriander and hollyhock are suitable herbs to treat IBS. *(See page 35.)*

CHINESE HERBALISM
- Treatment would address weakness of the Kidneys and Spleen, excess Damp in the intestines, and stagnation of Liver qi. Some suitable herbs might include rhubarb, dandelion, magnolia, and angelica. *(See pages 65 and 73.)*

HERBALISM
- Slippery elm has a soothing action along the length of the gut. *(See page 136.)*
- Try calming herbal teas such as chamomile, peppermint, and balm, all of which have an antispasmodic action. *(See pages 119 and 125.)*
- Chew fresh ginger to help relieve spasms. *(See page 139.)*

AROMATHERAPY
- Massage the abdomen with lavender or chamomile oils, which have antispasmodic qualities. *(See pages 161 and 150.)*
- Detoxifying oils include juniper, garlic, fennel, and rose; add to your bath water or use in massage. *(See pages 146–71.)*

HOMEOPATHY
Treatment must be constitutional, but the following remedies may provide some relief:
- Arg. nit., when there is flatulence, constipation alternating with diarrhea, and mucus in the stools. *(See page 181.)*
- Cantharis, for burning pain in the abdomen, great thirst, nausea, and accompanying cystitis. *(See page 188.)*
- Colocynthis, for griping pains brought on by anger. *(See page 191.)*
- Colchicum, for water stools, and tearing pains and nausea made worse when food is smelt.

FLOWER ESSENCES
- Consider whether or not your condition is stress-related *(see Stress, page 284)* and choose a remedy that fits your emotional symptoms. *(See page 219.)*
- Rescue Remedy is useful during attacks, to calm. *(See page 244.)*
- Mimulus will help if you are frightened by the thought of eating or of experiencing another attack. *(See page 235.)*

VITAMINS AND MINERALS
- Vitamin A is necessary to keep the intestinal tract healthy. *(See page 252.)*
- Take acidophilus to encourage the growth of healthy bacteria. *(See page 271.)*
- A deficiency of zinc and vitamin B6 is indicated in many cases; ensure that your intake is adequate. *(See pages 265 and 254.)*
- Dietary fiber helps to detoxify.

LEFT *Stress and anxiety may act as triggers for irritable bowel syndrome. Take Bach's Rescue Remedy during attacks to calm you.*

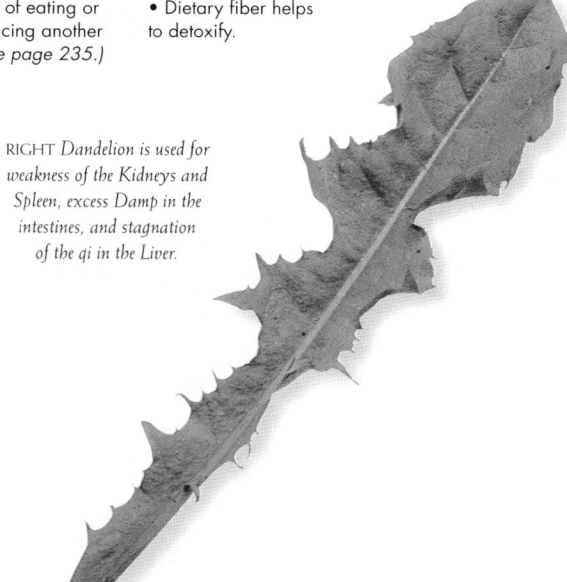

RIGHT *Dandelion is used for weakness of the Kidneys and Spleen, excess Damp in the intestines, and stagnation of the qi in the Liver.*

Anal Fissure

An anal fissure is a tear in the lower anal canal, close to the anal sphincter, and is often associated with internal hemorrhoids. The condition is fairly rare, but is most common in middle age, although it affects some children. When the stool is passed, the split is irritated, causing the sphincter muscles to go into painful spasm. Constipation is the root cause in most cases. Usually it heals quickly without complications but occasionally it may be chronic, spreading to the sphincter muscle and ending in infection. In some cases an anal fissure may be linked with other gut diseases.

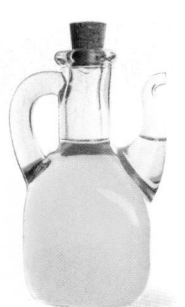

ABOVE *Relieve pain by dabbing olive oil onto the affected areas.*

SYMPTOMS

- *pain during bowel movements* • *minor bleeding*
- *irritation and discomfort*

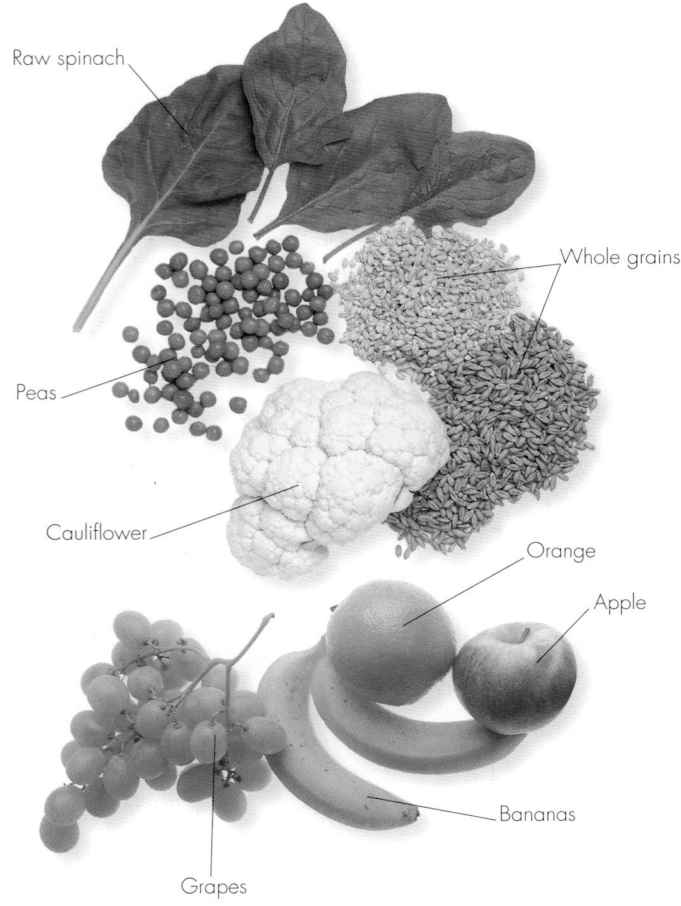

Raw spinach

Whole grains

Peas

Cauliflower

Orange

Apple

Grapes

Bananas

ABOVE *Eating fiber-rich foods will prevent constipation which is the major cause of anal fissures.*

TREATMENT

AYURVEDA
• The following preparations may be helpful if the fissure is caused by constipation: Abhayarishta (an oral tonic), Gin (oral pills), or Sukumara ghritha (oral ghee).

TRADITIONAL HOME AND FOLK REMEDIES
• Dab a little olive oil on to the fissure to encourage healing and relieve pain. *(See page 95.)*
• Fresh lemon juice, applied to the fissure, will prevent infection and dull the pain. *(See page 87.)*

HERBALISM
• Dandelion coffee is a mild laxative, and can be drunk, as required, on a daily basis. *(See page 134.)*
• Take a drink made of a cup of psyllium or flax seeds in a cup of water before bedtime to moisten stools and encourage regular bowel movements.
• Butternut, cascara, licorice, and yellow dock, decocted and mixed with a little honey, can help to stimulate bile, which will help produce normal bowel movements. *(See pages 122 and 128.)*
• Slippery elm and cinnamon will lubricate. *(See page 136.)*
• Comfrey root can help to heal the sore and inflamed tissues. *(See page 132.)*

AROMATHERAPY
• Apply a few drops of neat lavender or tea tree oil to the fissure to encourage healing and prevent infection. It may sting. *(See pages 161 and 162.)*

HOMEOPATHY
• Constitutional treatment would be appropriate, particularly if you are prone to fissures, but the following remedies, taken four times daily, may help:
• Nitric acid, for sharp pains during the passing of stools, also afterwards; constipation, irritability.
• Ratanhia, for relieving a burning sensation in the rectum which worsens after a bowel movement (loose or constipated).

• Aesculus, for sore, burning pain in the fissure, and an aching lower back, with stools large and hard.

VITAMINS AND MINERALS
• Acidophilus encourages the health of the bowels, and so should be taken daily as required. *(See page 271.)*
• Eat plenty of foods that are high in dietary fibers, including whole grains, fresh, raw vegetables and fruits, and dried fruits.

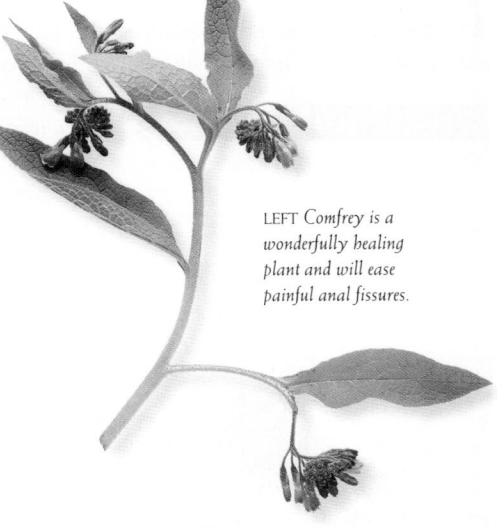

LEFT *Comfrey is a wonderfully healing plant and will ease painful anal fissures.*

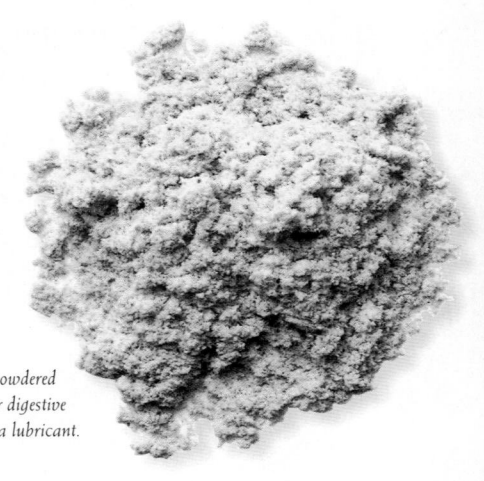

RIGHT *Use powdered slippery elm for digestive disorders and as a lubricant.*

Piles (Hemorrhoids)

Piles are swollen (or varicose) veins in the lining of the anus. The varicosity may be just above the anal canal, causing "internal" hemorrhoids, or at the lower end of the canal, causing "external" hemorrhoids. The latter may even protrude outside the anus ("prolapsed" hemorrhoids). Piles are caused by increased pressure on the veins of the anus, most commonly as a result of chronic constipation with straining, pregnancy, and childbirth. There may, however, be a congenital predisposition. Piles affect 50–75 percent of the U.S. population, and become more common with age.

ABOVE *As its common name suggests, pilewort is a good treatment for piles.*

SYMPTOMS

• *pain and bleeding during bowel movements* • *soreness and itching around the anus* • *possibly a mucus discharge from prolapsed hemorrhoids*

TREATMENT

AYURVEDA
• There are several Ayurvedic preparations available from health food stores, including Abhayarishta, which is an oral tonic, and Dadimadi ghritha (oral ghee).

TRADITIONAL HOME AND FOLK REMEDIES
• Red potato can be cut into a slim cigar shape and inserted into the anus to relieve symptoms. *(See page 98.)*
• Sit on a cold bowl of water, or use a cold bidet, several times daily to reduce inflammation and swelling. *(See page 103.)*

HERBALISM
• Make a small witch hazel compress, and keep it on the affected area for as long as possible to reduce inflammation and encourage healing. *(See page 123.)*
• Pilewort ointment is useful, and should be applied 2 or 3 times daily.
• Bayberry and yellow dock are both astringent herbs, and can be added to cocoa butter, which can then be shaped into a suppository and placed in the anus. *(See page 128.)*
• Internally, a course of dandelion root, horse chestnut, stone root, or yarrow can be helpful. *(See pages 112 and 134.)*
• Externally, horse chestnut can be applied.
• Clear congestion in the area with a good diet and teas of bitter herbs such as dock or dandelion root. *(See page 134.)*

AROMATHERAPY
• Apply a local compress of astringent essential oils of cypress, frankincense, lavender, or myrrh. *(See pages 146–71.)*
• Add a little rosemary oil to a warm bath to improve the circulation. *(See page 168.)*

HOMEOPATHY
• Ratanhia, for pain that feels like splinters on the anus when passing a stool.
• Hamamelis, for a bruised, sore, and congested feeling.
• Sulfur, for hot, burning, and itching piles. *(See page 215.)*
• Sepia, for the sensation of having a ball in the rectum, along with a tendency to prolapse. *(See page 212.)*

Wind

Wind (or flatulence) refers to the expulsion from the body of an excessive amount of air or gas, via the anus (breaking wind) or the mouth (belching or burping). Gas discharged via the anus is called flatus and comprises a number of gases, including hydrogen sulfide, which is responsible for the characteristic unpleasant smell. Wind can be caused by excessive swallowing of air (aerophagy), which may be a response to stress, or a consequence of eating too quickly. It is also a feature of disorders such as indigestion and irritable bowel syndrome. Certain foods such as pulses and beans produce more flatus than others. Gas is formed in the large intestine as a result of the action of bacteria on carbohydrates and amino acids in digested food; the gas consists of hydrogen, carbon dioxide, and methane. Gas formed in the intestine is passed only through the anus.

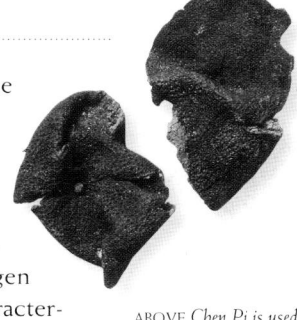

ABOVE *Chen Pi is used to treat Wind as it invigorates stagnant qi.*

CAUTION

EXCESSIVE FLATULENCE ACCOMPANIED BY WEIGHT LOSS, SEVERE ABDOMINAL PAIN, OR BLEEDING DURING BOWEL MOVEMENTS REQUIRES MEDICAL ATTENTION.

SYMPTOMS

• *besides its characteristic sounds, flatulence can also often cause abdominal discomfort*

TREATMENT

AYURVEDA
• Ayurvedic preparations available include Digesic, which is an oral tablet, as well as Gasex and Ramabana.
• Henbane may also be useful.

CHINESE HERBALISM
• Treatment would be aimed at stagnant Stomach energy, and suitable herbs include magnolia bark, and orange or lemon peel.

TRADITIONAL HOME AND FOLK REMEDIES
• Charcoal is excellent for reducing gas in the stomach and intestines.
• Celery seeds can reduce flatulence. *(See page 83.)*

HERBALISM
• Fresh dill, added to boiling water and steeped, will reduce flatulence and gas pains.
• Try making an infusion of sweet flag, drinking half a cup before meals.

HOMEOPATHY
The following remedies can be taken in every 30 minutes, for up to 6 doses:

• Lycopodium, when gas feels stuck, is painful, and is made worse by onions, garlic, and fried foods. *(See page 203.)*
• Arsenicum, for a burning discomfort. *(See page 182.)*
• Arg. nit., for the feeling that the stomach is full of gas. *(See page 181.)*

BELOW *If you suffer from gas in the intestine, try taking charcoal or celery seeds.*

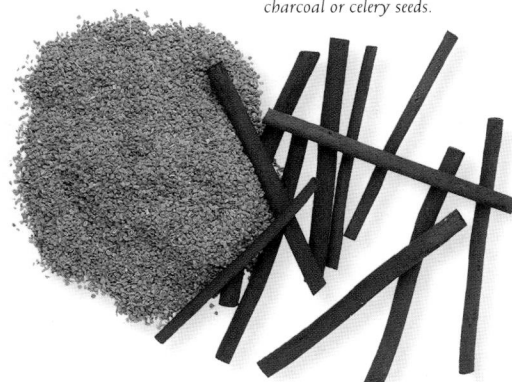

DISORDERS OF THE URINARY SYSTEM

Kidney Stones

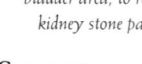

ABOVE *Add a few drops of juniper essential oil to your bath, or massage into the bladder area, to relieve kidney stone pain.*

Kidney stones (calculi) may occur anywhere in the kidneys or ureters and are the result of the crystallization of various substances in the urine, often when the body is dehydrated, causing the urine to be more concentrated. Dehydration alone, however, will not cause the formation of stones, and there is usually some other factor involved, such as kidney disease, infection, a bodily disturbance, or certain drugs. Most stones are combinations of calcium, magnesium, phosphorus, and oxalate. Collections of small kidney stones are known as "gravel," while much larger ones are called "staghorn" calculi.

SYMPTOMS

• *if a stone is lodged in the ureter it may cause agonizing pain – ureteric colic – through muscle contractions – the pain may spread to the lower abdomen and the groin* • *often there is blood in the urine* • *if stones cause blockage of the urinary tract, this can cause serious damage to kidney function*

DATA FILE

• The most common types of stones contain various combinations of calcium, magnesium, phosphorus, or oxalate. Up to 80 percent of stones are formed mainly of calcium.

• Kidney stones affect approximately 1 in 1,000 Americans – an estimated 10 percent of U.S. men and 3 percent of U.S. women.

• Most common in the south-eastern U.S., known as the "stone belt."

• Less common types are due to inherited disorders characterized by excretion of abnormal amounts of cystine or xanthine.

• Recurrence of most stones can be prevented by therapy based on analysis of the stones, the urine, and the blood.

• Kidney stones range in size from less than ⅔in. (5mm.) to over 1in. (2.5cm.) in diameter.

• They tend to run in families, and four out of every five patients with kidney stones are male, usually between the ages of 20 and 30.

• Differences in dietary and fluid intake may put certain people at higher risk for kidney stones.

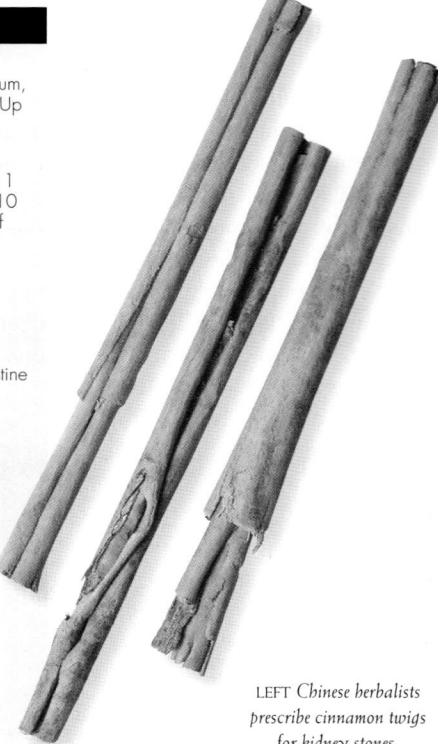

LEFT *Chinese herbalists prescribe cinnamon twigs for kidney stones.*

TREATMENT

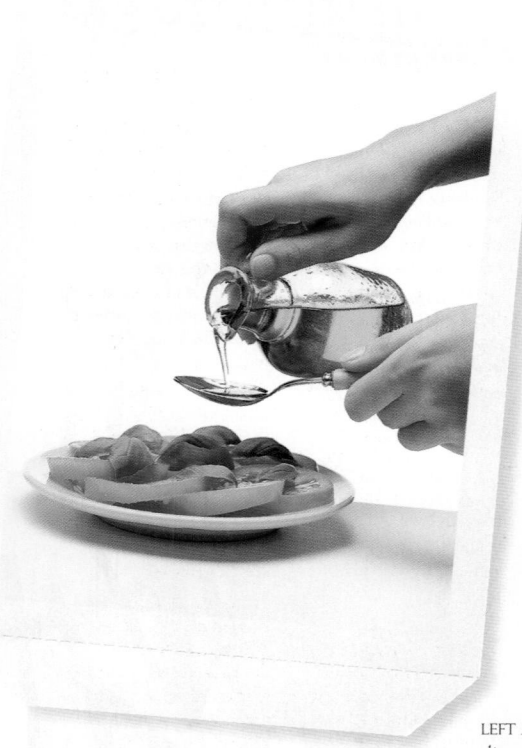

LEFT *Include at least 2 tablespoons of olive oil in your daily diet. If you can afford it, choose extra virgin olive oil.*

CHINESE HERBALISM
• Herbs which may help with correcting Kidney deficiency include ginseng, water plantain, poria, cinnamon twigs, and ephedra. *(See pages 59, 67, and 71.)*

TRADITIONAL HOME AND FOLK REMEDIES
• Include 2 tablespoons of extra virgin olive oil in your diet each day. *(See page 95.)*
• Fresh lemon juice, drunk in a little hot water every morning, will help to flush the kidneys and break down kidney stones. *(See page 87.)*

HERBALISM
• Herbs that can be used to dissolve the stones include celery seed, gravel root, parsley, and stone root. Sip a

decoction 3 times daily.
• During an acute attack, try infusions of corn silk, coughgrass, or yarrow. *(See page 112.)*

AROMATHERAPY
• Oils used to treat kidney stones include fennel, geranium, juniper, and lemon. These can be added to a light carrier oil and massaged into the bladder area, or used in the bath. *(See pages 146–71.)*

HOMEOPATHY
Treatment would be constitutional, but the following remedies may be useful for up to 10 doses:
• Tabacum, for pains shooting to the urethra, causing nausea and cold sweat.
• Nux vomica, for right-sided pain, causing nausea and vomiting, or

an urgent need to empty the bowels, accompanied by weak urine flow and irritability. *(See page 214.)*
• Berberis, for stitching pain in the lower ribs and hips when urinating, which worsens if moving about.
• Lycopodium, for pain in the right side which stops at the bladder, and which is worse between 4 and 8P.M. *(See page 203.)*

VITAMINS AND MINERALS
• Drink plenty of water (about 6pt. [3l.] a day) to flush the kidneys.
• Avoid long-term use of vitamin C, calcium, or vitamin D supplements. *(See pages 256 and 258.)*
• Extra magnesium and vitamin B6 will help. *(See pages 262 and 254.)*

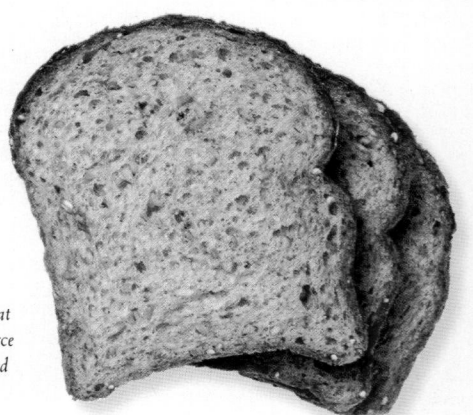

RIGHT *Whole wheat bread is a good source of magnesium needed for a healthy diet.*

Bladder Stones

Most bladder stones (calculi) are made up of crystals of calcium oxalate or uric acid. They are caused by the precipitation from solution of substances present in the urine. The stones may cause obstruction to urinary output, resulting in infection, although often they remain unrecognized. They occur with greater frequency in developing countries, and may be a result of a diet low or deficient in phosphate and protein. Bladder stones mainly affect men. Gout sufferers may experience bladder stones, and any disease which causes a high level of calcium in the blood and urine, such as hyperparathyroidism, may contribute to the formation of stones.

SYMPTOMS

• *difficulty in passing urine*
• *stress incontinence* • *if infection develops there may also be: — burning pain on passing urine — small amounts of urine, cloudy in appearance and with an unpleasant smell — fever — a dull ache in the lower abdomen*

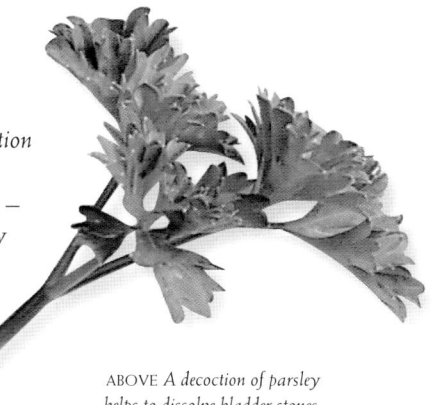

ABOVE *A decoction of parsley helps to dissolve bladder stones. Sip three times daily.*

TREATMENT

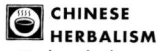 **CHINESE HERBALISM**
• Herbs which may help include ginseng, water plantain, poria, cinnamon twigs, and ephedra. *(See pages 59, 67, and 71.)*

TRADITIONAL HOME AND FOLK REMEDIES
• Fresh lemon juice, drunk in a little hot water every morning, will help to flush the bladder and break down bladder stones. *(See page 87.)*
• Barley or rice water will help to encourage the flow of urine and act as a tonic to the urinary system. *(See pages 92 and 96.)*

HERBALISM
• Herbs that can be used to dissolve the stones include celery seed, gravel root, parsley, and stone root. Sip a decoction 3 times daily.

• During an acute attack, try infusions of corn silk, couchgrass, or yarrow. *(See page 112.)*

AROMATHERAPY
• A number of essential oils work on the urinary tract, including tea tree, sandalwood, juniper, and eucalyptus. They should be applied in repeated hot compresses over the bladder area. *(See pages 146–71.)*

HOMEOPATHY
Treatment would be constitutional, but the following remedies may be useful for up to 10 doses:
• Lycopodium, for red sediment in the urine and a frequent urge to urinate, particularly at night. *(See page 203.)*
• Sarsaparilla, for slimy, sandy urine, with severe pain around the urethra when the flow stops.

• Uva ursi, when stones stop the flow of urine, which contains blood and mucus.

VITAMINS AND MINERALS
• Drink plenty of water (about 6pt. [3l.] a day) to flush the bladder.
• Extra vitamin C acts as a natural diuretic and will help to flush the urinary system. *(See page 256.)*

Cystitis

Cystitis is inflammation of the urinary bladder and/or urethra (the tube through which urine passes from the bladder out of the body). Inflammation usually occurs as a result of infection, bruising, or irritation. In the case of infection the bacteria involved are most often Escherichia coli, which will have traveled from the anus, via the urethra, to the bladder. Irritation and bruising can be caused by barrier contraceptives and sexual intercourse. Other causes of cystitis include chemical irritants (soap, bubble bath, bath oils), poor hygiene, insufficient drinking, food irritants, fruit juices, pregnancy, and the menopause. Cystitis is far more common in women than in men.

SYMPTOMS

• *burning pain on passing water* • *frequent and urgent need to pass water, although little if any is passed* • *dragging pain in lower abdomen and lower back* • *nausea and possibly vomiting* • *possibly unpleasant smelling urine, which may contain blood*

TREATMENT

AYURVEDA
• Hollyhock is a diuretic, and can treat cystitis.
• Boil 4 tablespoons of coriander seeds in 4 cups of water until the liquid is reduced to 2 cups. Strain and drink with a little honey. *(See page 35.)*

BELOW *Cranberry juice is an excellent remedy for cystitis. Drink as much as possible to flush the urinary system.*

 CHINESE HERBALISM
• Plantain seeds would be used to address Damp Heat.

TRADITIONAL HOME AND FOLK REMEDIES
• Eat live yogurt; use as a douche to ease symptoms and prevent recurrence. *(See page 93.)*
• Cranberry juice discourages bacteria from sticking to the walls of the bladder. *(See page 99.)*
• Garlic tincture added to food or warm drinks eases cystitis. *(See page 82.)*
• Drink barley water and lemon juice daily. *(See page 92.)*

HERBALISM
• Herbs used to treat cystitis include urinary antiseptics and diuretics. Drink infusions of buchu, corn silk, couchgrass, uva ursi, and yarrow. *(See pages 112 and 116.)*

AROMATHERAPY
• Add antiseptic bergamot, lavender, and sandalwood to the bath. *(See pages 146–71.)*

HOMEOPATHY
Chronic cystitis should be treated constitutionally, but take the following in an attack:
• Cantharis, for burning urine. *(See page 188.)*
• Staphisagria, for cystitis after intercourse.
• Mercurius, for violent pain with blood in the urine. *(See page 205.)*
• Apis, for stinging pain that is better for cold water. *(See page 180.)*
• Sarsaparilla, for burning after urinating.

VITAMINS AND MINERALS
• Drink plenty of water to flush the urinary system.
• Take 1g. of vitamin C daily, which acts as a natural diuretic and boosts the immune system. *(See page 256.)*

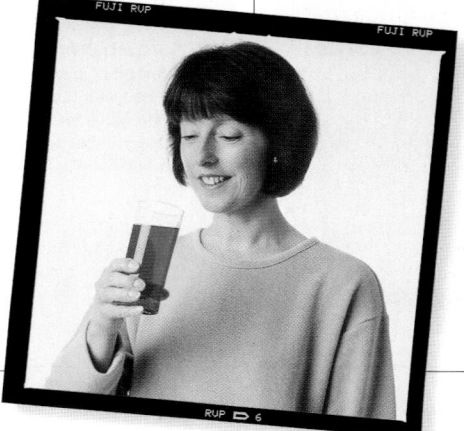

Urethritis

Urethritis is an inflammation of the urethra (the tube through which urine passes out of the body). In women it is usually caused by a bladder infection, while in men it may be a symptom of other diseases, including gonorrhea and Reiter's syndrome. It may also result from damage to the urethra, from a catheter for example. Nonspecific urethritis (NSU) is a milder form thought to be caused in most cases by chlamydia, although the cause may not be established. NSU may be caused by a large number of different types of micro-organisms, including bacteria and yeasts. Other possible causes include exposure to irritant chemicals, such as antiseptics and some spermicidal preparations. Urethritis may be followed by scarring and the formation of a urethral stricture (narrowing of a section of the urethra), which can make the passing of urine difficult.

CAUTION

ALL SUSPECTED CASES SHOULD BE INVESTIGATED BY A PHYSICIAN, IN CASE THE CAUSE IS CHLAMYDIA OR A SIMILAR INFECTION.

SYMPTOMS

• *burning sensation and sometimes severe pain on passing urine* • *blood in urine and possibly a pus-filled yellow discharge* • *in NSU the symptoms are milder and the discharge in men is usually clear* • *in women there may be no symptoms, with occasionally increased discharge*

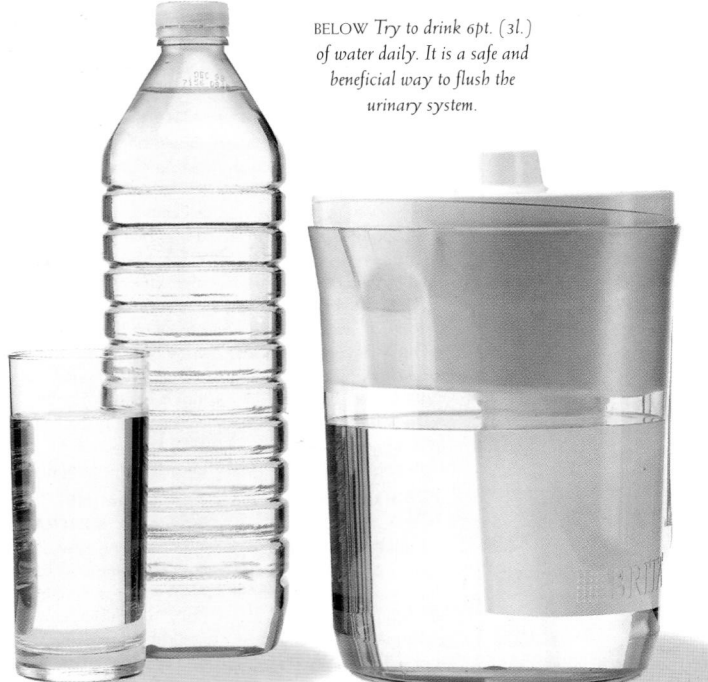

BELOW *Try to drink 6pt. (3l.) of water daily. It is a safe and beneficial way to flush the urinary system.*

TREATMENT

AYURVEDA
• Hollyhock is diuretic, and can be used to treat urethritis.
• Boil 4 tablespoons of coriander seeds in 4 cups or water until the liquid is reduced to 2 cups. Strain and drink with a little honey. *(See page 35.)*

TRADITIONAL HOME AND FOLK REMEDIES
• Eat live yogurt, and use as a douche to ease the symptoms of infection and inflammation, and prevent recurrence of the urethritis. *(See page 93.)*
• Cranberry juice, drunk daily, discourages bacteria from sticking to the urinary tract. It treats and prevents urethritis. *(See page 99.)*
• Garlic tincture, added to food or warm drinks, will ease inflammation and fight infection. *(See page 82.)*
• Drink barley water, several cups a day, with some lemon juice. *(See pages 87 and 92.)*

HERBALISM
• Herbs used to treat urethritis include urinary antiseptics and diuretics. You may drink infusions of any of the following herbs, alone or in combination: buchu, corn silk, coughgrass, uva ursi, and yarrow. *(See pages 112 and 116.)*
• Buchu will help to clear infection. Take as a tea, three times daily.

AROMATHERAPY
• Bergamot, lavender, and sandalwood are soothing and antiseptic. Add them to the bath water every evening. *(See pages 146–71.)*

HOMEOPATHY
For NSU, antibiotics should be taken, as prescribed, but the following may be helpful if it is not NSU:

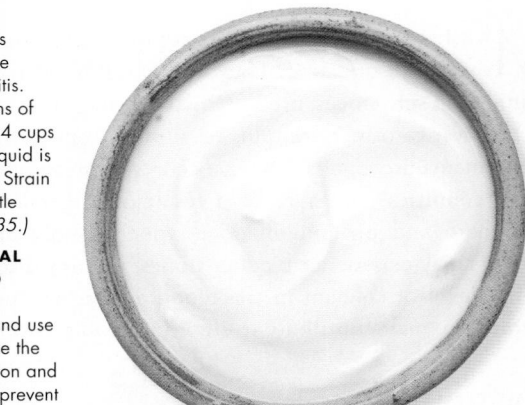

ABOVE *Antibiotics destroy good as well as bad bacteria in the intestinal tract. Eat plain live yogurt after taking antibiotics to restore the good bacteria.*

• Cantharis, when the urine burns and is violently painful. *(See page 188.)*
• Staphisagria, for cystitis after intercourse.
• Mercurius, for violent pain with blood in the urine. *(See page 205.)*
• Apis, for stinging pain that is better for cold water. *(See page 180.)*
• Sarsaparilla, for burning pain which comes on after urinating.

VITAMINS AND MINERALS
• Drink plenty of water (6pt. [3l.] daily) to flush the urinary system.
• Take 1g. of vitamin C daily, which acts as a natural diuretic and boosts the immune system. *(See page 256.)*
• Vitamin C builds healthy mucous membranes. *(See page 256.)*
• Take acidophilus after a course of antibiotics. *(See page 271.)*

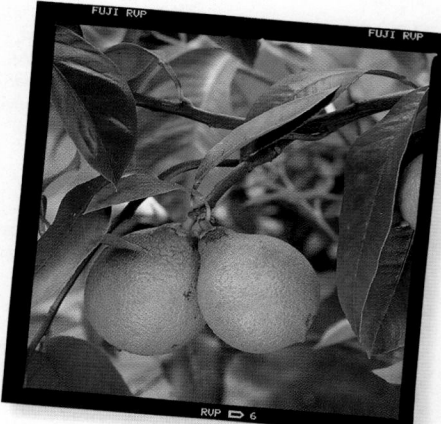

ABOVE *Vitamin C, contained in citrus fruits, will boost your immune system as well as building healthy mucous membranes.*

Incontinence

Incontinence is the inability to retain feces in the rectum, or an uncontrollable involuntary passing of urine. Incontinence, or involuntary urination, is extremely common. The most common form is stress incontinence, in which a small quantity of urine is "leaked" when there is increased pressure in the abdomen, as in laughing, sneezing, or coughing. Stress incontinence is often experienced after childbirth, as a result of injury or strain to the pelvic floor muscles, whose function it is to support the bladder and keep the urethra closed. Other causes include senile dementia, prostate enlargement, damage to nerve control as a result of stroke, multiple sclerosis, or local cancer, and bladder stones.

Fecal incontinence (lack of normal control over passing feces) may occur in diarrhea, or if the controlling muscles have been damaged by disease or childbirth. Another cause is fecal impaction, which is often caused by long-standing constipation. *(See Constipation on page 373 and Diarrhea on page 374 for treatment of fecal incontinence.)*

ABOVE *Use a decoction or tincture of horsetail for incontinence of urine. It has toning properties that help strengthen the bladder.*

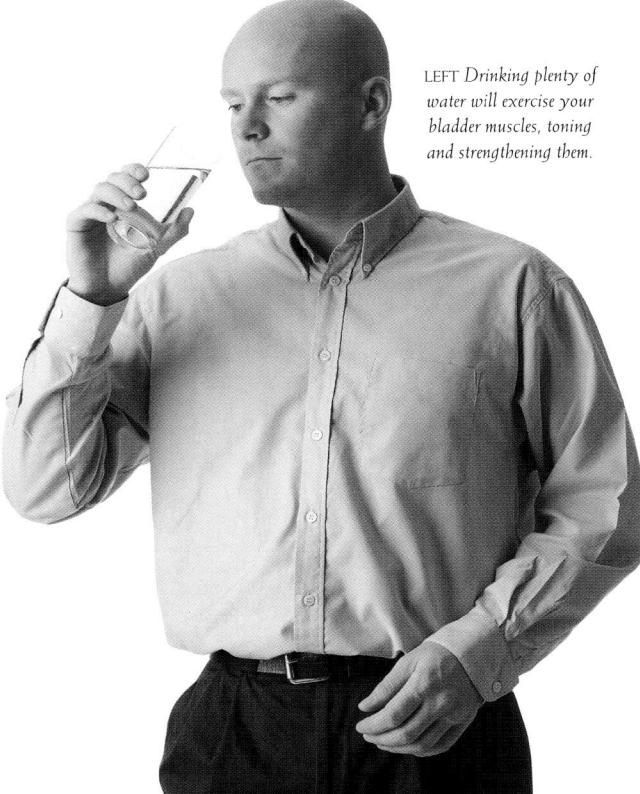

LEFT *Drinking plenty of water will exercise your bladder muscles, toning and strengthening them.*

TREATMENT

CHINESE HERBALISM
• Treatment would address Kidney Yang Deficiency with internal Cold, and the best herb to use is golden lock, taken as a tea. *(See page 61.)*
• If the condition accompanies prolapse, treatment will be given for Deficient qi, using central qi pills. This will help with the control of fecal and urinary incontinence.

HERBALISM
• The seeds of the ginkgo biloba plant act as a tonic to the kidneys and bladder, and have been used for incontinence and excessive urination. *(See page 122.)*
• Horsetail has toning and astringent properties, which make it useful both for incontinence and frequent urination. *(See page 120.)*

HOMEOPATHY
Treatment would be based on the cause of the incontinence, but some of the following might be useful:
• Causticum, for incontinence made worse by coughing or laughing. *(See page 189.)*
• Ferr. phos., for an inability to control the bladder, with pain and a frequent urge to urinate. *(See page 194.)*
• Nux vomica, for irritability and involuntary dribbles of urine. *(See page 214.)*
• Pulsatilla for stress incontinence which is made worse by sitting down. *(See page 209.)*
• Sepia, for incontinence related to weak pelvic floor muscles, accompanied by the feeling that the abdomen is falling out of the vagina. *(See page 212.)*

FLOWER ESSENCES
A number of the remedies will help with negative emotions and distress. Some to try are:

• Walnut, if incontinence is the result of change, such as pregnancy, a new baby, or menopause. *(See page 232.)*
• Sweet Chestnut, if you suffer from despair. *(See page 227.)*
• Agrimony, if you hide behind a cheerful face. *(See page 225.)*
• Crab Apple if you feel unclean. *(See page 234.)*

VITAMINS AND MINERALS
• Increase your intake of dietary fiber, which will prevent constipation and straining, a common cause of incontinence.
• Drink plenty of water to ensure regular use of the bladder muscles.

SWEET CHESTNUT

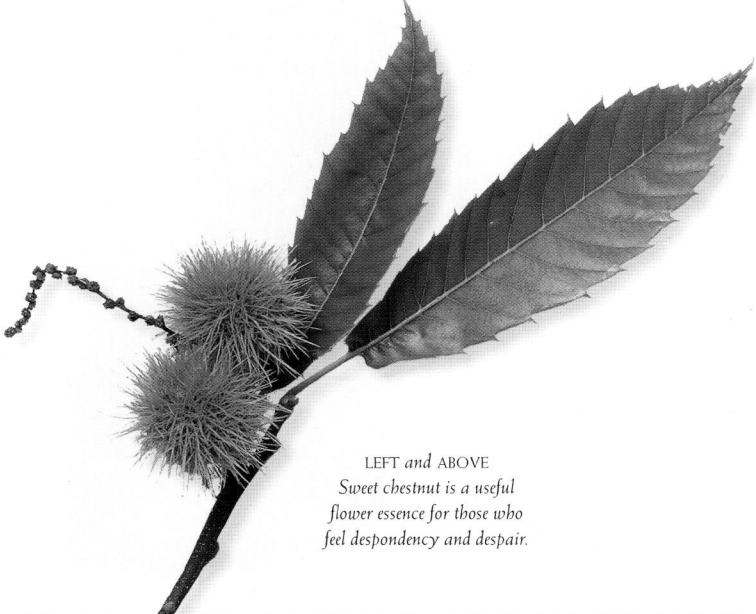

LEFT *and* ABOVE *Sweet chestnut is a useful flower essence for those who feel despondency and despair.*

Breast Problems

The female breast consists mainly of a round mass of glandular tissue comprising about 15–20 lobes, each having a duct leading to an opening on the nipple; the duct system and glandular tissue develop fully with pregnancy. The amount of fat sheathing the glandular tissue determines the size of the breast. Connective tissues, or stroma, form the foundation or framework of the breast. The layer of ligaments directly beneath the breast sends strands into the breast itself, providing the firm consistency of the organ. The deep layer of connective tissue sends strands in the opposite direction into the covering of the chest muscles.

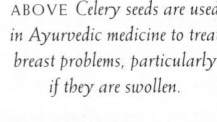

ABOVE *Celery seeds are used in Ayurvedic medicine to treat breast problems, particularly if they are swollen.*

DATA FILE

Breast cancer is an important medical problem, with women of age 35 or older at increasing risk of developing some form of the disease. Physicians urge that women conduct monthly self-examinations of their breasts to detect potentially cancerous lumps, because the disease is more easily curable when found at an early stage. Another screening method is the X-ray process called mammography. Medical groups agree that women of 50 and older should have a yearly mammograph test. Some groups also advise an initial test for women between 35 and 40, and a test every one or two years for women between 40 and 50.

Some typical breast problems are:

• Tenderness, associated with pregnancy and PMS.

• Abscesses, which start as a bacterial infection in the breast tissue, producing swelling, redness, pain, and possibly fever. They usually occur in women who are breast-feeding. *(See also Breast-feeding Problems, page 383.)*

• Cysts, non-cancerous fluid-filled capsules in the ducts of the breast, appearing in groups or singly, occur mainly between the ages of 30 and 50, and in many women they cause one or more breasts to become lumpy and tender in the week or so before a menstrual period starts.

• Duct ectasia, blockage and inflammation of the milk ducts, is one of the most common causes of breast pain, particularly in women aged 40 to 50. It produces hot, red areas on the breast, a lump, and sometimes a watery discharge.

• Duct papillomas are benign, wart-like tumors in the ducts which, if not removed, may turn malignant. Their cause is uncertain, but may be hormonal.

• Fat necrosis, when fatty material released from the fat cells as a result of a blow to the breast forms into a hard lump of scar tissue, causing dimpling on the skin.

• Fibroadenoma, a benign breast tumor which is usually round, firm, and rubbery, causing no pain, can be moved around beneath the skin using the fingertips. These lumps are very common and most women will have one at some stage.

CAUTION

PREGNANT WOMEN SHOULD NOT TAKE CELERY SEED WITHOUT A PHYSICIAN'S APPROVAL.

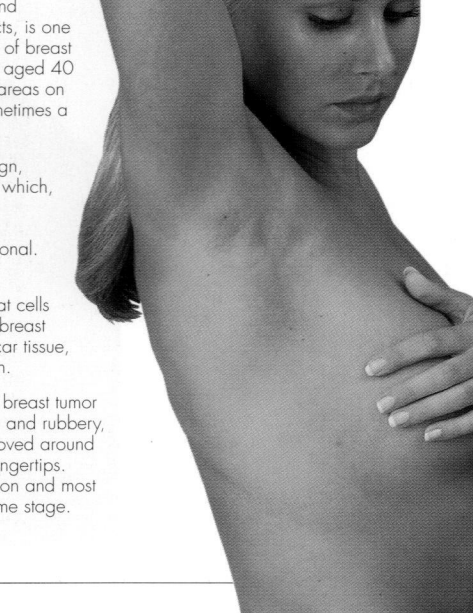

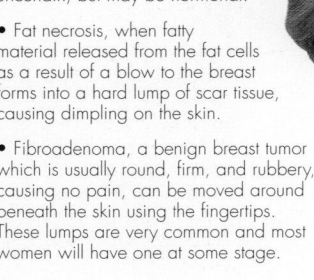

LEFT *Regular self-examinations of your breasts will reveal any abnormalities.*

TREATMENT

AYURVEDA
• Barberry can be applied externally for its antibiotic and antifungal action. It also shrinks tumors (benign and cancerous), when it is taken internally. *(See page 29.)*
• Calamus oil will stimulate lymphatic drainage, and can be used for treating most breast problems. *(See page 24.)*
• Celery seed is diuretic, and can be useful when breast problems are related to swellings. *(See page 29.)*

CHINESE HERBALISM
• A poultice made from powdered dried rhubarb root can be applied to the breast to ease pain and swelling. *(See page 73.)*
• Madder root and dandelion may also be useful.

TRADITIONAL HOME AND FOLK REMEDIES
• Apply a bruised white cabbage leaf to the breast when there is infection, to heal and draw out the pus. *(See page 85.)*

• Apply continuous compresses of strong peach tea to the affected area for infection.
• Bruised parsley leaf poultices can be used for hard and lumpy breasts.

HERBALISM
• The herbs that are most useful for preventing and treating breast problems are those that encourage the action of the lymphatic system: cleavers, golden seal, marigold, marshmallow, nettles, and yellow dock. *(See pages 114, 117, 128, and 137.)*
• Consider taking the herb agnus castus for breast problems related to hormones (particularly premenstrually, and during the menopause). *(See page 139.)*

AROMATHERAPY
• Geranium oil can be used in the bath for relief of tenderness and edema, or massage it, blended into a little carrier oil, into the affected area. *(See page 165.)*
• Juniper, rosemary, lavender, and fennel oils will help to regulate hormone imbalance and relieve the symptoms of breast diseases. *(See pages 146–71.)*

HOMEOPATHY
For pain associated with PMS, try:
• Carb. an., for breast enlargement with shooting pains.
• Conium, for swelling, pain, and tenderness.
• Nat. mur., when the breasts are retaining water. *(See page 206.)*
• Calcarea, for heavy, pendulous breasts. *(See page 186.)*
Cysts should be dealt with constitutionally, but the following remedies may be useful in the short term:
• Pulsatilla, for sudden, inexplicable pains. *(See page 209.)*
• Conium, when the affected area is hard and painful.

• Phytolacca, for breasts that are more tender premenstrually, and when you are stressed.
For an abscess, try:
• Bryonia, for the early stages, with hardened breasts and pain. *(See page 185.)*
• Belladonna, for the early stages when there are red streaks. *(See page 183.)*
• Hep. sulf., for localized pain with irritability. *(See page 198.)*
• Silicea, for cracked, oozing nipples and feelings of exhaustion. *(See page 211.)*
For lumps, the following may be useful:
• Graphites, for hard, swollen, thickened breasts with blistered and sore nipples. *(See page 196.)*
• Belladonna, when the breasts are red, throbbing, and heavy. *(See page 183.)*
• Mercurius, for when the breasts are painful and full of milk at the time of menstruation. *(See page 205.)*

VITAMINS AND MINERALS
• Cut down on salty food to prevent water retention.
• Supplements of evening primrose oil and vitamin B6 may be useful. *(See pages 270 and 254.)*
• Cut down on caffeine, which can encourage the formation of cysts and lumps in the breast.
• Breast pain and lumps may be alleviated by increasing your daily intake of vitamin A. *(See page 252.)*
• Women with low levels of selenium may have a greater risk of suffering fibrocystic breast disease. *(See page 264.)*
• Apply vitamin E cream to heal cracked nipples. *(See page 257.)*

Breast-feeding Problems

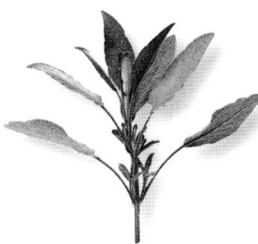

ABOVE *If you need to stop producing milk quickly try red sage as a safe alternative to drugs.*

After the birth of a child a mother's breast begins to produce milk, a natural process designed to provide complete nourishment for a baby for several months after its birth. Before milk is produced the mother's breast produces colostrum, a deep-yellow liquid containing high levels of protein and antibodies. A newborn baby who feeds on colostrum in the first few days of life is better able to resist the bacteria and viruses that cause illness. The mother's milk, which begins to flow a few days after childbirth when the mother's hormones change, is a blue-white color with a very thin consistency. If the mother is well nourished the milk provides the baby with the proper balance of nutrition. The fat contained in human milk, compared with cow's milk, is more digestible for infants and allows for greater absorption of fat-soluble vitamins into the bloodstream from the baby's intestine. Calcium and other important nutrients in human milk are also better utilized by infants. Antigens in cow's milk can cause allergic reactions in a newborn child, whereas such reactions to human milk are rare. Human milk also promotes growth, largely due to the presence of certain hormones and growth factors.

Breast-fed babies have a very low risk of developing meningitis or severe blood infections, and have a 500–600 percent lower risk of getting childhood lymphoma. Breast-fed babies also suffer 50 percent fewer middle ear infections.

DATA FILE

Typical breast-feeding problems are:

• Aching breasts, usually caused by engorgement either through increased blood pressure or overproduction of milk. Symptoms include fever, with hard, lumpy, and painful breasts.

• Blocked duct, a small red lump on the breast or a white lump on the nipple caused by rushed feeds, or by not emptying the breast properly.

• Cracked nipples, possibly caused by poor feeding position or by using damp breast pads.

• Mastitis, inflammation of the breast, usually caused either by a blocked duct or by infection. Symptoms include fever, redness and pain in the affected breast.

• Slow let-down reflex, that is to say a delay in the breast's milk-releasing response.

• Sore nipples, tenderness caused by prolonged suckling.

• Vaginal dryness caused by the suppression of estrogen production during lactation.

BELOW *A drink of dill tea can help prevent wind or colic in a baby, making it easier for the baby to suckle.*

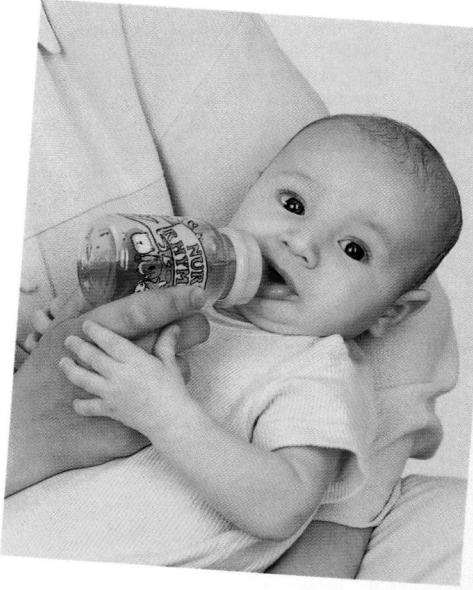

TREATMENT

AYURVEDA
• Cumin can increase milk production. *(See page 36.)*
• Fenugreek seeds will increase milk production. *(See page 45.)*

CHINESE HERBALISM
• Dandelion, peony bark, Chinese gentian, and madder root can be used for relieving mastitis. *(See page 67.)*

TRADITIONAL HOME AND FOLK REMEDIES
• Bruise parsley leaves, and apply them to hardened or knotty breasts during breast-feeding.
• Feed your baby a little diluted dill tea to prevent wind, which may be causing his or her breast-feeding problems.

HERBALISM
• Calendula cream will soothe and encourage the healing of sore and cracked nipples, and is safe for the baby to swallow. *(See page 117.)*
• Caraway, aniseed, dill, and fennel promote the flow of best milk, and can be taken in the form of teas or infusions. *(See page121.)*
• Compresses of marshmallow and slippery elm can often help with engorgement. *(See pages 114 and 136.)*
• Red sage will dry up breast milk almost instantly, if necessary. *(See page 129.)*
• Dilute tinctures of St. John's wort and marigold in boiled water and dab on to cracked nipples after each feed. *(See pages 117 and 124.)*
• Take echinacea for any infection. *(See page 120.)*

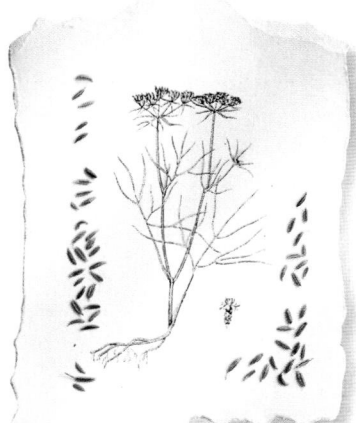

ABOVE *Ayurvedic practitioners give cumin to promote the flow of breast milk.*

AROMATHERAPY
• Lavender oil, in the bath or in a vaporizer, can encourage the let-down reflex. Better still, try massaging your baby with 1 drop in a little light carrier oil before a feed, to relax you both. *(See page 161.)*
• Caraway and verbena oils can be massaged into the breasts to stimulate the production of milk. *(See pages 146–71.)*
• Calendula and chamomile oils are anti-inflammatory, and can be applied to the breasts to ease inflammation and pain. Wash off before feeding. *(See pages 148–150.)*
• Peppermint oil, in cold compresses, can reduce the flow of milk when there is engorgement. *(See page 164.)*

HOMEOPATHY
• Chamomilla, Pulsatilla, Sulfur, and Graphites for sore and cracked nipples. *(See pages 204, 209, 215, and 196.)*
• Pulsatilla and Calcarea, for hard, engorged breasts. *(See page 209.)*
• Agnus will help with loss of breast milk.
• Calcarea, for poor-quality milk, when the mother is prone to chills. *(See page 186.)*

• Aconite, for sudden, excessive milk production, or, equally, sudden loss of milk caused by shock. *(See page 178.)*
• Bryonia, for hard and swollen breasts. *(See page 185.)*
• China, for exhaustion from breast-feeding. *(See page 190.)*
• Ignatia, for loss of milk due to grief or trauma. *(See page 200.)*

FLOWER ESSENCES
• Apply Rescue Remedy or Emergency Essence cream to the nipples when they are sore or cracked, to soothe and encourage healing. *(See page 244.)*
• Take either essence internally for distress caused by pain. *(See page 244.)*
• Olive is useful for overwhelming fatigue. *(See page 235.)*
• Walnut is useful for helping with change – in this case, the birth of your baby. *(See page 232.)*

VITAMINS AND MINERALS
• Breast-feeding mothers need plenty of protein, vitamins, and iron. *(See page 260.)*
• Drink plenty of fluids while breast-feeding.
• Apply vitamin E oil to sore and cracked nipples to help them heal. *(See page 257.)*

Menstrual Problems

The most common menstrual problems are dysmenorrhea (painful menstruation), menorrhagia (heavy menstrual bleeding), and amenorrhea (no menstrual bleeding). In primary dysmenorrhea there is either an increased level of or increased sensitivity to prostaglandin, the hormone-like substance that produces uterine contractions. Secondary dysmenorrhea (unusual menstrual cramps) begins at least three years after menstruation begins and may be caused by endometriosis, fibroids, a pelvic infection, stress, or a thyroid disorder. The symptoms for both include sharp pain or a dull ache in the lower abdomen and lower back, headaches, sweating, diarrhea. In severe cases there may be vomiting and fainting. Menorrhagia is best described as bleeding that is so heavy that it interferes with normal life. It may be caused by fibroids, polyps, pelvic infection, endometriosis, hypothyroidism, blood-clotting disorders, stress, or use of an IUD or injectable contraceptive. Primary amenorrhea refers to menstruation not starting by the age of 18. This is usually due to low body weight or heredity. Secondary amenorrhea occurs when menstruation stops for more than six months due to pregnancy, weight loss, starting oral contraceptives, severe shock, stress, anemia, thyroid disorder, or a fibroid.

ABOVE *Take bioflavonoids to regulate your menstrual cycle. They will also balance your hormone levels.*

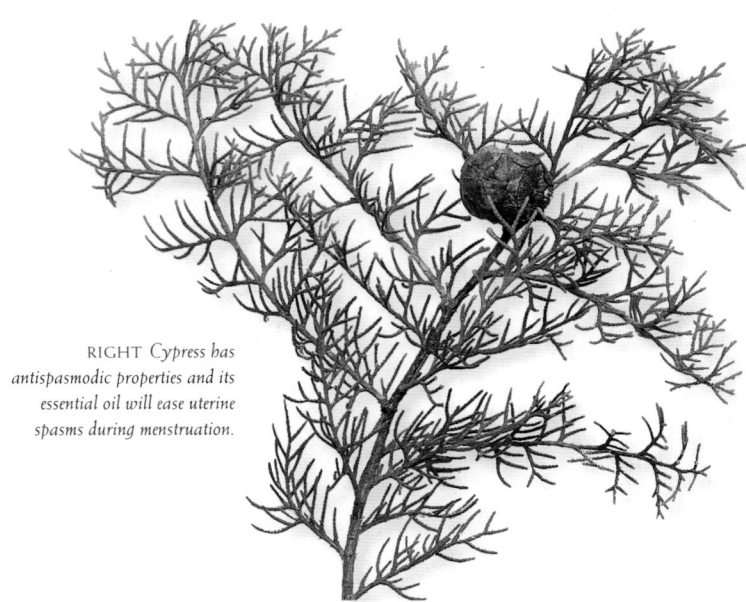

RIGHT *Cypress has antispasmodic properties and its essential oil will ease uterine spasms during menstruation.*

AYURVEDA
• Aloe vera can induce menstruation. *(See page 27.)*
• Basil can be used to promote menstruation. *(See page 42.)*
• Caraway relaxes uterine tissue and is beneficial for menstrual cramps. *(See page 30.)*
• Cardamom will help digestive problems associated with menstruation. *(See page 38.)*
• Cedar stimulates the menstrual cycle, and celery seeds can treat irregular menstruation. *(See page 32.)*

CHINESE HERBALISM
• Excessive flow is considered to be caused by Heat in the Blood; scanty flow, late menstruation, and painful menstruation are due to Cold in the Blood.
• Warming herbs, such as ginger, ginseng, and cinnamon, may be used. *(See pages 59 and 67.)*
• Cornelian Asiatic cherry can be used in the treatment of heavy menstrual bleeding. *(See page 60.)*

TRADITIONAL HOME AND FOLK REMEDIES
• Dried carrot powder taken daily may help to regulate the menstrual cycle. *(See page 89.)*
• Cayenne pepper regulates bleeding. Add a few grains to any herbal tea.
• Cinnamon bark will help to control menstrual flow.
• Diluted lemon juice cleanses the system and helps to control bleeding. *(See page 87.)*
• Beets help to regulate menstrual problems.
• Strawberry leaves, taken over a long period, can help to regulate menstrual flow and ease pain.

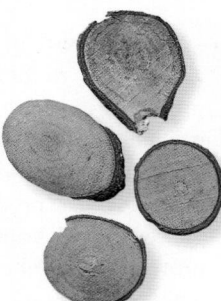

ABOVE *The Chinese use warming herbs, such as cinnamon, for menstrual problems.*

HERBALISM
• Cramp bark is helpful for menstrual cramps. *(See page 138.)*
• Lady's mantle is an astringent and is useful for heavy menstrual bleeding. Take 3 times daily, as required. *(See page 113.)*
• Yarrow will help to regulate menstruation. *(See page 112.)*
• Raspberry leaves can help to control an excessive flow of blood. *(See page 128.)*
• Thyme tea, drunk each morning and evening, can control excessive flow. *(See page 135.)*
• Angelica root can help to promote menstruation which is delayed. *(See page 115.)*
• Catnip tea, drunk each evening and morning during menstruation, will help to ease pain.
• Peppermint tea will ease any bloating and pain during menstruation. *(See page 125.)*

AROMATHERAPY
• Antispasmodic oils, such as clary sage, cypress, and lavender, will help to ease cramps. *(See pages 146–71.)*
• Clary sage and fennel oils, massaged into the lower back, can help to regulate hormone balance, and, through that, the menstrual cycle. *(See pages 146–71.)*

• Heavy menstrual bleeding can be treated with geranium, rose, or cypress essential oils. Add to the bath water or use in a local massage. *(See pages 146–71.)*

HOMEOPATHY
• China, for spasmodic bleeding with dark clots and cramps. *(See page 190.)*
• Belladonna, for pain, bright red blood, and nagging headache. *(See page 183.)*
• Ipecac., for heavy bleeding and bright red blood with nausea. *(See page 189.)*
• Sepia, for a bearing-down type pain. *(See page 212.)*
• Aconite, for menstruation that stops after an emotional shock. *(See page 178.)*
• Ignatia, for menstruation that stops after grief, trauma, or loss. *(See page 200.)*
• Colocynthis, for cramping pain which is improved by pressure. *(See page 191.)*
• Sabina, for pain and dark red blood with clots.
• Chamomilla, for pains that resemble labor pains. *(See page 204.)*

VITAMINS AND MINERALS
• Vitamin B6, taken twice daily, can help prevent menstrual cramps. *(See page 254.)*
• Iron and zinc will help in cases of heavy menstrual bleeding. *(See pages 260 and 265.)*
• Take vitamin A and B6 for heavy bleeding. *(See pages 252 and 254.)*
• Bioflavonoids can help to balance hormone levels and regulate the menstrual cycle. *(See page 272.)*
• Deficiencies of zinc and vitamin B6 can result from absence of menstruation. *(See pages 265 and 254.)*

Premenstrual Syndrome (PMS)

Premenstrual syndrome is the term used to describe a huge range of symptoms, at least some of which are experienced by most women (especially those over 30) every month between ovulation and menstruation. The symptoms may be physical, emotional, or behavioral in character and are thought to be caused either by hormonal imbalance (possibly due to recent childbirth or a gynecological disorder) or by marginal (sub-clinical) nutritional deficiencies which can affect the fine hormone balance in the body. Interestingly, women who regularly consume caffeine are more likely to suffer from severe PMS, and there is sometimes a connection with a thyroid condition.

SYMPTOMS

- *physical: breast enlargement and tenderness – bloated abdomen – headaches/migraines – pelvic discomfort – fluid retention and weight gain – constipation or diarrhea – greasy hair and skin – tiredness* • *emotional: irritability and confusion – anxiety – disturbed sleep – depression and, in severe cases, suicidal thoughts* • *behavioral: clumsiness and lack of coordination – poor concentration – violent or aggressive outbursts*

LEFT *Eating fresh apples, celery, and grapes will help to prevent bloating in the week before your menstrual period is due.*

RIGHT *The Mediterranean shrub* agnus castus *is a useful remedy for the emotional and physical symptoms of premenstrual syndrome (PMS).*

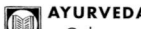 **AYURVEDA**
- Calamus root stimulates the adrenals, which will help PMS associated with stress. *(See page 24.)*
- Caraway is useful for digestive problems associated with PMS, and is a natural diuretic. *(See page 30.)*
- Myrrh is used for treating many conditions relating to menstruation. *(See page 34.)*
- Angelica is specific for PMS. *(See page 28.)*

CHINESE HERBALISM
- PMS is believed to be caused by an imbalance of Spleen, Kidneys, and Liver, and can be treated with angelica, peony, hoelen, and skullcap. *(See pages 56, 67, 71, and 74.)*

TRADITIONAL HOME AND FOLK REMEDIES
- Swelling can be prevented by eating plenty of fresh, crunchy apples in the week prior to menstruation. *(See page 94.)*
- Celery is also a good diuretic, and acts on the kidneys to encourage their action. *(See page 83.)*
- Eat fresh grapes to prevent bloating.
- Barley water, which is rich in B vitamins, can be drunk freely throughout your menstrual cycle to ease symptoms. *(See page 92.)*
- To ease irritability and other emotional symptoms, eat plenty of oats. *(See page 84.)*

HERBALISM
- Try an infusion (herbs steeped in boiling water) of agnus castus or false unicorn, which have a balancing effect on the hormones. *(See page 139.)*

- Herbs which help to reduce some of the symptoms of stress and anxiety include oats, vervain, and passiflora. *(See pages 117 and 138.)*
- Water retention can be eased with couchgrass or dandelion teas, drunk two or three times each day during the premenstrual phase. *(See page 133.)*
- Rosemary, oats, cinnamon, and lemon balm will help to lift the spirits. *(See pages 117 and 127.)*
- Skullcap, wood betony, and vervain are good for addressing tension, anxiety, and depression. *(See pages 131 and 138.)*
- Cornsilk and burdock are useful for symptoms associated with bloating. *(See page 115.)*
- Cleavers and poke root will help with monthly breast tenderness.
- Take valerian for extreme tension. *(See page 136.)*
- Chamomile, cinnamon, and peppermint will help with nausea and vomiting. *(See pages 119 and 125.)*
- Yellow dock and wormwood will balance the blood sugar levels. *(See page 128.)*

AROMATHERAPY
- Try essential oils of geranium and rosemary in your bath to relieve symptoms, including water retention and irritability. *(See pages 165 and 168.)*
- Clary sage and rose may help with depression. *(See pages 169 and 168.)*
- A light massage (whole body, or over the abdominal area) with lavender oil or clary sage will balance hormones and ease symptoms. *(See pages 161 and 169.)*

HOMEOPATHY
Treatment will be constitutional, but useful remedies include:

- Lachesis, for symptoms which are worse first thing in the morning; also good for painful breasts. *(See page 216.)*
- Nux vomica., for irritability and chilliness, constipation, frequent urination, and various food cravings. *(See page 214.)*
- Sepia, for irritability, weepiness, emotional flatness, feeling turned off by sex, and cravings for sweet or salty foods. *(See page 212.)*
- Kali carb., for tension, exhaustion, feeling overweight, and where the symptoms become worse around 3A.M.
- Pulsatilla, for suddenly bursting into tears, nausea, depression, irregular menstruation, and painful breasts. *(See page 209.)*
- Lycopodium, for bad temper, depression, and a craving for sweet things. *(See page 203.)*
- Sulfur, when the main symptom is a craving for sweets. *(See page 215.)*

FLOWER ESSENCES
- Mustard, for depression. *(See page 239.)*
- Scleranthus, for mood swings. *(See page 239.)*
- Olive, for fatigue. *(See page 235.)*
- Crab Apple, for feeling repulsive and unliked. *(See page 234.)*

VITAMINS AND MINERALS
- Evening primrose oil, with the following supplements: vitamins C, E, and B6, magnesium, zinc, iron, and chromium. These should be taken continuously for one month, and subsequently during the fortnight preceding menstruation. *(See pages 270, 256, 257, 254, 265, 260, and 259.)*

Infertility

The term infertility, or failure to reproduce, is generally applied when failure to conceive follows regular, unprotected sex over an 18-month period. Infertility indicates a fault in the reproductive system and is very often treatable.

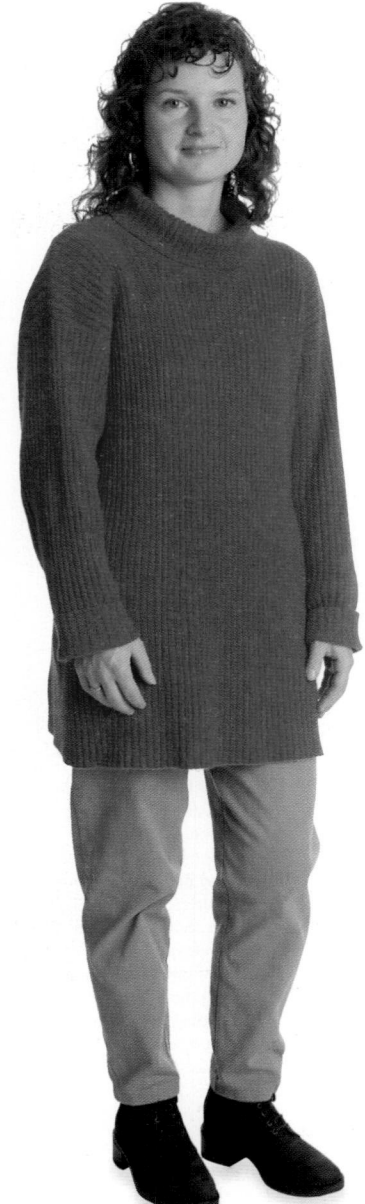

ABOVE *White Chestnut is an excellent flower essence to take if the problems of infertility are causing you great anxiety.*

TREATMENT

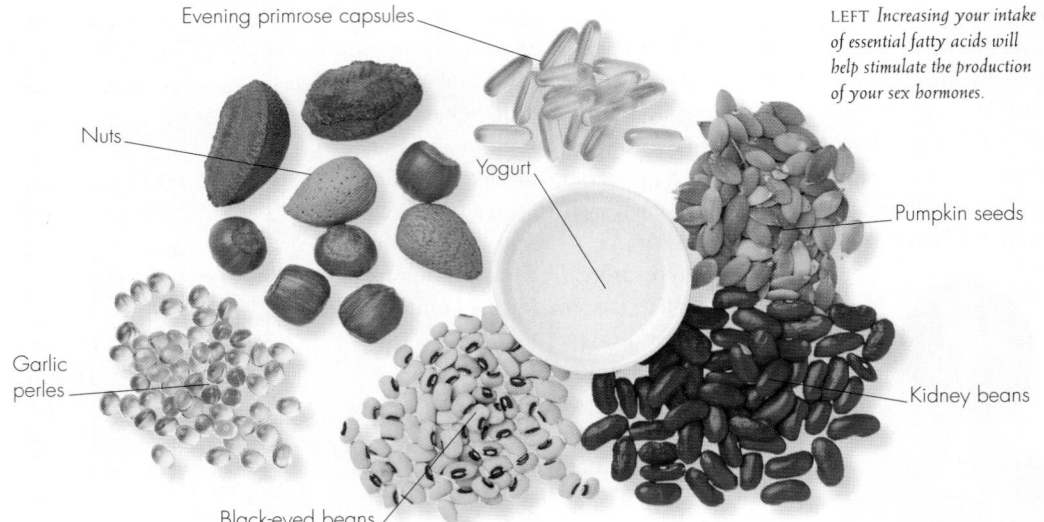

Evening primrose capsules

Nuts

Yogurt

Garlic perles

Black-eyed beans

Pumpkin seeds

Kidney beans

LEFT *Increasing your intake of essential fatty acids will help stimulate the production of your sex hormones.*

AYURVEDA
• Cloves can tone the uterus, and garlic has a rejuvenating effect on the reproductive system. *(See page 38.)*
• Saffron is aphrodisiac, and can help when infertility is associated with sexual problems. *(See page 36.)*

CHINESE HERBALISM
• Infertility is believed to be caused by Damp Heat and imbalance of yin and yang. Golden lock tea may be useful, but treatment is always individually prescribed, so see a practitioner.

TRADITIONAL HOME AND FOLK REMEDIES
• Oats are calming, and can help with the effects of stress, as well as toning the body. Eat as often as possible. *(See page 84.)*

HERBALISM
• Agnus castus is an excellent hormone regulator and will help if your menstruation is irregular, or you are not ovulating for hormonal reasons. It may also be useful if you are prone to early miscarriage. *(See page 139.)*

• False unicorn root helps to regulate the ovaries and strengthen the endometrium.
• Balm, passiflora, and skullcap will help to reduce the effects of stress, which may be causing the condition. *(See page 131.)*

AROMATHERAPY
• Rose oil is said to increase sperm count and quality, as well as acting as a mild aphrodisiac. Add a few drops to your partner's bath, or perhaps engage in a little gentle massage, with 2 or 3 drops of rose essential oil in a mild carrier oil such as sweet almond oil. *(See page 168.)*
• A few drops of geranium and melissa can be used neat in the bath, or diluted in a gentle carrier oil and massaged over the abdomen on a regular basis. *(See pages 165 and 163.)*
• Tea tree and lavender oils are anti-infective and anti-inflammatory, and can be useful in abdominal massage, for treating any pelvic infection or inflammation which may be preventing the woman conceiving. *(See pages 161 and 162.)*

• If infertility is causing the patient great anxiety, one of the relaxing oils, such as lavender, marjoram, or chamomile, can be used in the bath, or try it in a vaporizer. *(See pages 150, 161, and 165.)*
• When repeated attempts to get pregnant have failed and you need a little encouragement to continue with love-making, ylang ylang is a lovely, relaxing oil that acts as an aphrodisiac. Use as a massage oil or in the bath. *(See page 148.)*

HOMEOPATHY
Treatment would be constitutional, but the following remedies may be helpful:
• Conium, when breasts are tender, with areas of hard swelling, and sexual desire is suppressed.
• Saline, for previous miscarriages before 12 weeks.
• Sepia for irregular menstruation, and a feeling of chilliness, weeping, and irritability. *(See page 212.)*

FLOWER ESSENCES
• White Chestnut may be useful if you are extremely upset or tormented by the problem. *(See page 224.)*

• For despondency, try Gorse. *(See page 240.)*

VITAMINS AND MINERALS
• Cutting out alcohol, smoking, and drugs may be suggested for the period before conception.
• Eating plenty of whole foods rich in vitamins and minerals will not only ensure that sperm and egg are healthy, but that the woman's body is a welcoming home for the growing embryo. Good nutrition increases the chances of conception and gives the baby every chance of being healthy.
• Vitamin E and B6 may be supplemented, as low intake is often linked to a low sperm count. Vitamin E may regulate the production of cervical mucus in women. *(See pages 257 and 254.)*
• Increase intake of EFAs (essential fatty acids): in oily fish, fish liver oils, seeds, nuts, pulses, beans, evening primrose oil, unrefined vegetable oils), to stimulate sex hormone production.
• Zinc deficiency has been linked to infertility. *(See page 265.)*

Miscarriage

Spontaneous abortion, or miscarriage, occurs when the embryo fails to develop, when there is complete or incomplete expulsion of the embryo or fetus, and placenta, or when the fetus dies prior to 20 weeks. If fetal death occurs at 20 weeks or more after the last period, it is termed a late fetal death or a stillbirth.

Up to three-fourths of conceptions abort spontaneously. Most occur before the woman's pregnancy can be confirmed, prior to six weeks after her last period. These constitute about one-fifth of confirmed pregnancies and about one-tenth of all pregnancy hospitalizations in the United States.

In many cases the womb sheds an embryo because it is not developing normally. Often, however, there is no explanation for miscarriage at all, although the following may be at greater risk: women over 40, pregnancies resulting from fertility treatment, twin or multiple pregnancies, and pregnancies where the placenta is faulty.

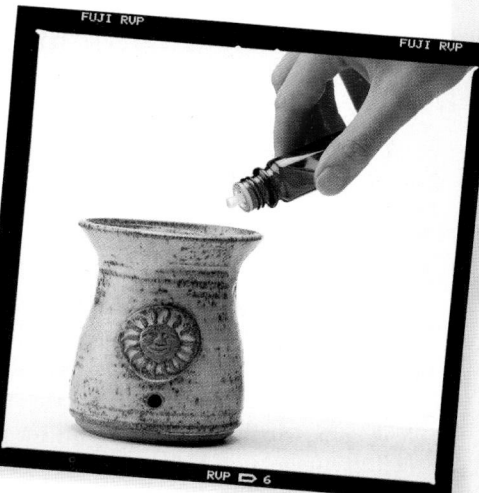

ABOVE *The therapeutic vapors of essential oils such as lavender can help you through the grieving period that follows the loss of a baby.*

SYMPTOMS

• *of a threatened miscarriage: — bleeding, clots or a dark discharge from the vagina — mucus in the vaginal blood — abdominal pain, possibly cramp-like pain similar to menstrual cramps — back pain* • *of inevitable miscarriage: — opening of the cervix and continuous bleeding (inevitable abortion) — emptying of the uterus, after which the cervix closes and bleeding stops (complete abortion) — partial emptying of the uterus, after which the cervix remains open and bleeding continues (incomplete abortion)*

TREATMENT

AYURVEDA
• Herbs to tone the uterus and improve circulation may be useful, but treatment must be undertaken by a registered practitioner. *(See page 20.)*

CHINESE HERBALISM
• Dodder seeds are used to prevent miscarriages. *(See page 62.)*

HERBALISM
• Herbs for threatened miscarriage include false unicorn root decoction, which should be sipped every few minutes.

• Cramp bark can help to relax the uterus and prevent miscarriage. *(See page 138.)*
• Black haw can be used to avert miscarriage and ensure relaxation.
• Tonic herbs to prevent miscarriage include red raspberry leaves mixed with a little vervain. *(See pages 128 and 138.)*
• Following miscarriage, you can use raspberry leaves to aid the healing of the uterus, and antiseptic herbs such as thyme or echinacea to help prevent infection. *(See pages 120, 128, and 135.)*
• Rosemary and wild oats will help to support the nervous system following

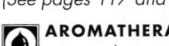

LEFT *Raspberry is an excellent healing remedy for the uterus after a miscarriage.*

the trauma of miscarriage. *(See pages 117 and 127.)*

AROMATHERAPY
• Lavender is relaxing, and can be used daily in the bath to calm – particularly if you are concerned about miscarriage. Use only in a vaporizer if you have a history of miscarriage. It will be useful following a miscarriage to help your body get back to normal. *(See page 161.)*
• Rose has an affinity with the reproductive system, and can be used in a vaporizer (not applied) to help prevent miscarriage. *(See page 168.)*

HOMEOPATHY
• Arnica, where there is risk of miscarriage following an accident or injury. *(See page 182.)*
• Take Hypericum, following amniocentesis,

to prevent miscarriage. *(See page 199.)*
• Ipecac., for threatened miscarriage, when the blood is bright red with abdominal cramps. *(See page 189.)*
• Sabina, if the blood is dark and clotting, usually at the end of the first trimester.

FLOWER ESSENCES
• Rock Rose, for helplessness and terror. *(See page 231.)*
• Mimulus, for gnawing fear of miscarriage. *(See page 235.)*
• Star of Bethlehem, for shock. *(See page 235.)*
• Gentian, for despondency following a very early miscarriage. *(See page 230.)*
• Walnut, to help you adjust to the new situation. *(See page 232.)*

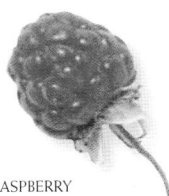

RASPBERRY

Pregnancy Problems

Women may experience problems during pregnancy, often as a result of hormonal changes. Some of the most common problems women experience are:

• ANEMIA *(see page 357)*

• BACKACHE, due either to postural changes made to accommodate the extra weight, or to the position in which the baby is lying

• BLEEDING GUMS, caused by hormonal changes which lead to a thickening and softening of the gums

• CONSTIPATION, when normal bowel action is slowed down by an increase of progesterone

• CRAMPS, which occur mainly in the feet, calves, and thighs due to inefficient circulation (as a result of increased progesterone), and possibly calcium deficiency

• FAINTING, caused by a shortage of blood to the brain due to lowered blood pressure and an increased demand for blood to the womb

• FLATULENCE, since digesting food is moved more slowly, which allows wind to build up

• FLUID RETENTION, when an upset in the balance of salt and potassium in the cells causes swelling in the hands, legs, and feet

• HEARTBURN, a burning sensation in the upper chest, and possibly a sour taste in the mouth, which are caused by acidic juices rising back up the esophagus

• INSOMNIA, caused by general inevitable bodily discomfort towards the end of pregnancy

• MORNING SICKNESS, nausea and/or vomiting usually in the first three months of pregnancy, but not necessarily confined to the morning

• PELVIC PAIN, pain in the groin or inside of the thighs when walking, caused by pressure on the pelvic nerves

• PILES *(see page 377)*

• STRETCH MARKS, fine red lines (which eventually turn silver) appearing on the breasts, abdomen, and thighs, and caused by stretching of the skin

• VARICOSE VEINS

• TIREDNESS, characterized by a desire to sleep a lot in the first three months

• INCREASED VAGINAL DISCHARGE, probably thickish and white

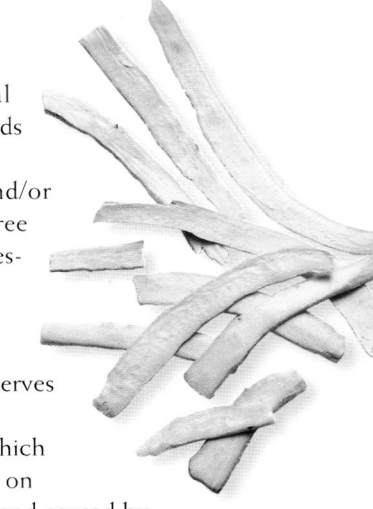

ABOVE *Bai Shao or white peony is considered one of the best women's tonics in Chinese medicine.*

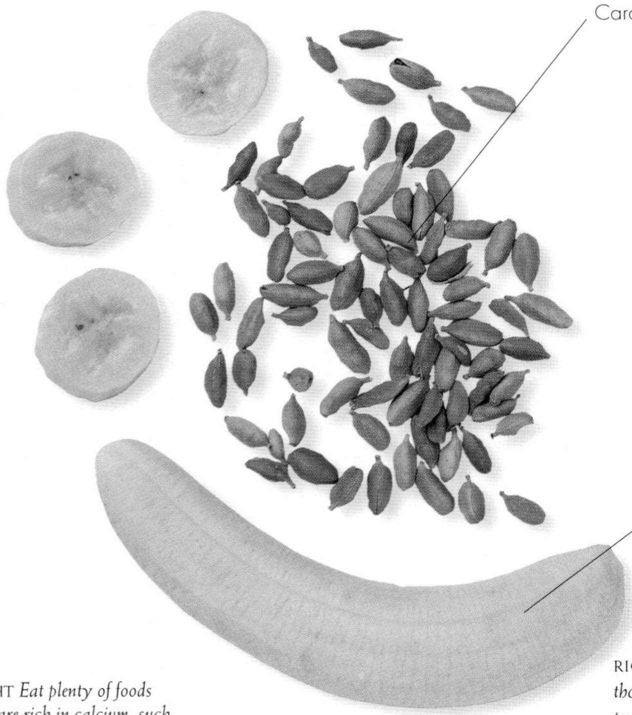

Cardamom seeds

Banana

RIGHT *Eat plenty of foods that are rich in calcium, such as bananas and cardamom, to prevent cramps.*

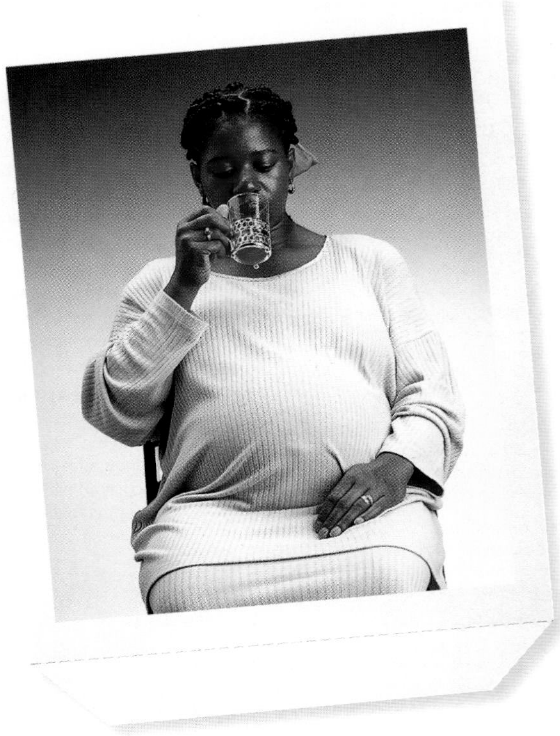

RIGHT *To get you to sleep during those last uncomfortable months of pregnancy, drink a glass of honey and apple cider vinegar in warm water before you retire.*

TREATMENT

AYURVEDA
• Aloe vera can be applied externally to prevent stretch marks. *(See page 27.)*
• Ginger, for recurrent nausea in pregnancy. *(See page 47.)*
• Eating caraway seeds deals with constipation and digestive problems. *(See page 30.)*
• Cardamom suppresses vomiting when eaten with a banana. *(See page 38.)*
• Cayenne, used externally, can ease muscle pain. *(See page 31.)*
• Clove tones muscles and expectant mothers are recommended to eat them in the last month of pregnancy to strengthen the uterus. *(See page 38.)*
• Licorice, for constipation, and digestive problems. *(See page 39.)*
• Long pepper, for muscle soreness, digestive problems, and constipation. *(See page 43.)*
• Mustard can help with muscle and joint pain, and acts as a laxative. *(See page 30.)*

CHINESE HERBALISM
• Teasel root, ginseng, and acanthopanax root, for persistent back pain. *(See page 54.)*
• Peony root and astragalus, for high blood pressure. *(See pages 57 and 67.)*
• Ginseng, licorice, and tangerine peel, for an acid stomach. *(See pages 59, 64, and 67.)*
• Gui Pi Wan, for anemia.
• Astragalus, for overwhelming exhaustion. *(See page 57.)*
• Wild jujube and fleece-flower stem, for insomnia. *(See pages 71 and 75.)*
• Dittany bark, for itching.
• Ginger, for morning sickness.
• Water plantain, poria, cinnamon twigs, and ephedra, for edema. *(See pages 59 and 71.)*
• Gentian and oriental wormwood, for thrush.

TRADITIONAL HOME AND FOLK REMEDIES
• Eating yogurt will cool the pain of heartburn. *(See page 93.)*
• Use a witch hazel compress on varicose veins – either in the legs or the vulva. *(See page 91.)*
• For relief of varicose veins in the legs or vulva, apply neat lemon juice. *(See page 87.)*
• Garlic helps the circulation, and can prevent cramping, varicose veins, and piles.*(See page 82.)*
• Apply a witch hazel compress to piles to reduce inflammation and encourage healing. *(See page 91.)*
• Drink a glass of honey and apple cider vinegar in warm water before bed to help you sleep peacefully. *(See pages 101 and 102.)*
• Celery juice can help you sleep when taken before bedtime. *(See page 83.)*
• Chamomile, fennel, and thyme have antifungal properties, and can be used as a compress and pressed against the vagina to ease and treat thrush.

HERBALISM
• Dandelion tea is a mild diuretic, and so will help with edema. *(See page 133.)*
• Chamomile or peppermint tea will ease heartburn. *(See pages 119 and 125.)*
• Dandelion leaves, nettles, chives, sorrel, and coriander leaves are rich in iron, which will prevent anemia. *(See pages 133 and 137.)*
• Chamomile, fennel, burdock, and ginger are gentle laxatives, safe for preventing constipation. *(See pages 115, 119, 121, and 139.)*
• Lavender, vervain, and lemon balm will soothe the nerves and relax muscles. *(See page 138.)*
• Nettles, meadowsweet, and celery seeds are rich in calcium, which can help to prevent cramping. *(See pages 121 and 137.)*

• Lemon balm and chamomile tea can help prevent nausea, as can ginger and fennel. Take as infusions as required. *(See pages 119, 121, and 139.)*
• Slippery elm helps to soothe the digestive tract, and can help morning sickness and weak digestion. *(See page 136.)*
• Hops can be used for treating severe vomiting.
• False unicorn root and agnus castus can balance the hormones, which will prevent many symptoms. *(See page 139.)*
• Calendula, marjoram, and comfrey are astringent and can be applied to the legs or vulva as required. *(See pages 117 and 132.)*
• Peppermint and cleavers can be drunk as an infusion to improve circulation and treat varicose veins. *(See page 125.)*
• Chamomile, catnip, and vervain can help with insomnia, when taken before bedtime or during the night. *(See pages 119 and 138.)*
• Chamomile, dandelion root, nettle, and licorice can be taken three times daily for piles. *(See pages 119, 122, 134, and 137.)*
• Calendula flowers can be infused, added to coconut oil, and rubbed into the skin to prevent stretch marks. *(See page 117.)*

AROMATHERAPY
• Lavender oil can be rubbed into the temples for headaches, and into the back for muscle pains. *(See page 161.)*
• Geranium, fennel, marjoram, and ylang ylang can be added to the bath to prevent constipation. *(See pages 146–71.)*
• Roman chamomile and marjoram are excellent in a full-body massage to ease the muscular pains of pregnancy. *(See pages 150 and 165.)*
• Thyme, cypress, lavender, and lemon oils can be added to the bath water to strengthen the veins and increase circulation. *(See pages 146–71.)*

• Essential oil of geranium can be added to the bath for piles. *(See page 165.)*
• A gentle massage with lavender, chamomile, or lemon balm can relax and help you sleep. *(See page146–71.)*
• Add a few drops of tea tree or cinnamon oil to a cup of cool water and apply to the vaginal area on a clean cloth to treat thrush. *(See pages 162 and 150.)*
• A light massage of lavender and neroli, in a carrier oil, can prevent stretch marks. *(See pages 162 and 152.)*
• Massage lavender, geranium, or ginger oils into the lower back to ease pain and reduce tension. *(See pages 146–71.)*

HOMEOPATHY
• Nat. mur., for help with water retention. *(See page 206.)*
• For anemia *(see page 357)*, try Kali carb., when the back feels weak and tired, and there are unpleasant dragging pains.
• Belladonna, when there is a hard tense feeling in the lower abdomen. *(See page 183.)*
• Nux vomica., for nausea that is worse in the morning, and when the vomit contains mucus. *(See page 214.)*
• Ipecac., for nonstop nausea and vomiting. *(See page 189.)*
• Pulsatilla, for nausea which comes on in the evening. *(See page 209.)*
• Ferr. phos., for nausea a few hours after eating. *(See page 194.)*
• Nat. mur., for nausea with an aversion to bread and fat, with a craving for salt and great thirst. *(See page 206.)*
• Capsicum, for heartburn with a burning sensation behind the breastbone.
• Phosphorus, for heartburn with a craving for cold drinks that are then vomited. *(See page 208.)*

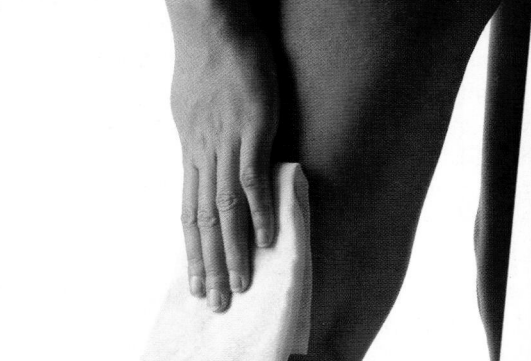

ABOVE *A witch hazel compress will help relieve painful varicose veins.*

• Sulfur, for heartburn that is worse around 11 A.M. *(See page 215.)*

FLOWER ESSENCES
• Olive is useful for dealing with general exhaustion. *(See page 235.)*
• Crab Apple may help with relief of nausea. *(See page 234.)*
• Rescue Remedy or Emergency Essence may be useful for vomiting. *(See page 244.)*

VITAMINS AND MINERALS
• Ensure you get plenty of iron, to prevent and treat anemia. Take vitamin C together with iron, in order to aid iron absorption. *(See pages 256 and 260.)*
• Folic acid is necessary during pregnancy for the healthy development of the fetus. *(See page 255.)*
• Dietary fiber will help to prevent constipation.

• Eat plenty of foods rich in calcium to prevent cramp. *(See page 258.)*
• Supplements of vitamin B6, zinc, and magnesium may help with nausea. *(See pages 254, 265, and 262.)*
• Vitamins C and E, and bioflavonoids, zinc, and brewer's yeast will help to heal damaged blood vessels which are the cause of varicose veins. *(See pages 256, 257, 265, and 272.)*
• Take acidophilus for thrush. *(See page 271.)*
• Ensure you have plenty of vitamins E, C, zinc, silica, and pantothenic acid, which can help to prevent stretch marks. *(See pages 257, 256, 263, 264, and 254.)*
• Vitamin E oil can be applied neat to areas that are likely to become stretched, including the perineum. *(See page 257.)*

Labor Pains

Labor pains are caused by womb contractions. In the first stage of labor the contractions slowly dilate the cervix until it is wide enough to allow the baby's head to pass through. During the second stage, more powerful and more frequent contractions push the baby into the lower part of the birth canal and into the world. In the third stage, continued contractions help to expel the placenta. The pain itself varies at different stages. At first it may be no more than a dull discomfort eased by moving around. Later it may be likened to severe menstrual cramps which reach a peak then die out as the contraction ends. Pain may be felt in the lower abdomen, lower back, and the legs. The pain experienced appears to be different between women, and is related to their "pain threshold." Most women describe severe, in many cases almost unbearable, pain.

LEFT *Add a few drops of relaxing lavender essential oil to a bathing pool to relieve labor pains.*

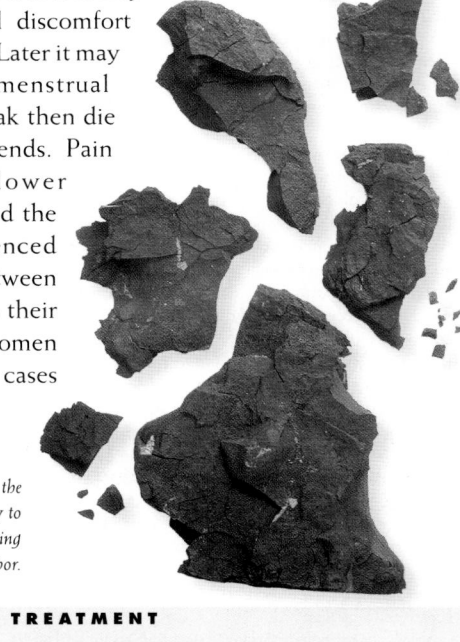

RIGHT *Carb. veg. is the homeopathic remedy to try for exhaustion during the first stage of labor.*

TREATMENT

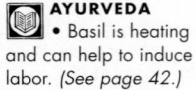

AYURVEDA
• Basil is heating and can help to induce labor. *(See page 42.)*

CHINESE HERBALISM
• Chinese angelica and peony root, for abdominal pains experienced during and after childbirth. *(See pages 56 and 67.)*
• Jing Jie may be useful as a painkiller, and will help to prevent hemorrhaging.

HERBALISM
• Blue cohosh can be taken throughout labor to tone the uterus and help keep contractions strong.

• Raspberry leaf, black cohosh, and motherwort can help during the second stage of labor. *(See page 128.)*
• Angelica root and raspberry leaf can help with the delivery of the placenta. *(See pages 115 and 128.)*
• Chamomile tea can be sipped to soothe and calm. *(See page 119.)*
• Ginger may be used to speed up a slow labor. *(See page 139.)*

AROMATHERAPY
• Clary sage, jasmine, and rose can be massaged into the lower back to relax the mother between contractions. *(See pages 146–71.)*

• Melissa oils can help to relieve the pain of childbirth, and should be used throughout the labor. *(See page 163.)*
• Rub lavender oil into the lower back, or add it to the water of a birthing pool to ease pain. *(See page 161.)*

HOMEOPATHY
• Coffea, for violent, unbearable pain when the mother cries out and is understandably nervous between contractions. *(See page 192.)*
• Belladonna, for violent contractions, with delirium and staring eyes. *(See page 183.)*
• Nux vomica., when the pains are accompanied by a need to pass water or a stool, and the mother is irritable. *(See page 214.)*

• Secale can speed a slow labor, when the uterus seems unable to contract any longer.
• Carb. veg. is useful when the mother becomes exhausted during labor. *(See page 188.)*
• Caulophyllum for weak, irregular contractions.
• Gelsemium, if the mother is anxious and trembles, and contractions are not productive. *(See page 195.)*

FLOWER ESSENCES
• Rescue Remedy can be sipped for anxiety and tension. *(See page 244.)*
• Olive, for overwhelming fatigue. *(See page 235.)*
• For overstraining, use Vervain. *(See page 241.)*
• Sweet Chestnut is good for utter despair, and for the feeling that the baby will never be born. *(See page 227.)*
• Impatiens, when things do not seem to be happening fast enough. *(See page 233.)*

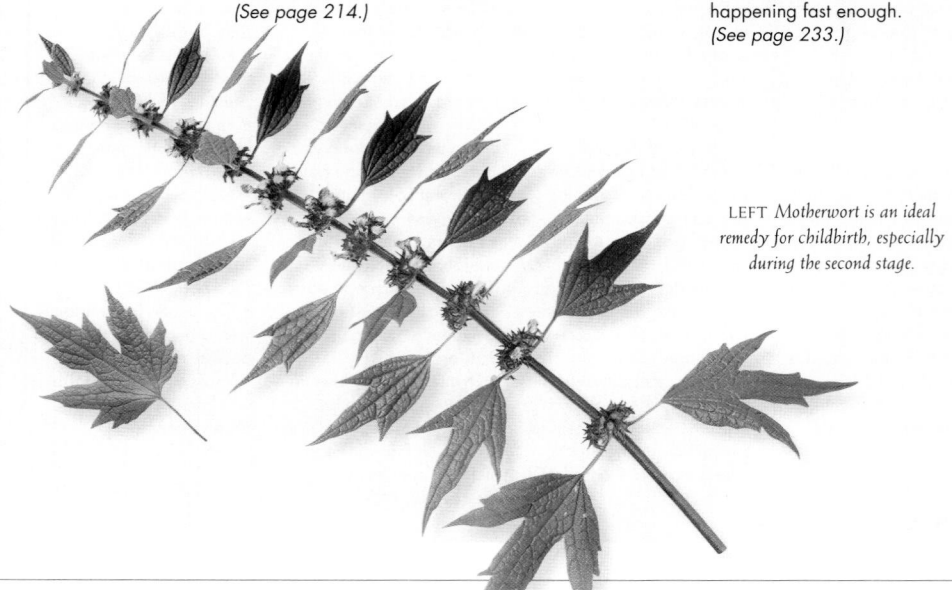

LEFT *Motherwort is an ideal remedy for childbirth, especially during the second stage.*

Post-delivery Problems

Almost all women suffer from problems of some kind following the trauma of childbirth, whether physical or emotional. These may include:

• ABDOMINAL SORENESS, usually resulting from a Cesarean section, from which it can take up to 12 weeks to recover

• ANEMIA caused by blood loss during delivery (see page 357)

• BACKACHE, which may very well relate to back strain during the birth process

• BREAST-FEEDING PROBLEMS (see page 383)

• EXHAUSTION as a result of the birth, coupled with sheer lack of sleep due to the needs of a crying baby

• HAIR LOSS caused by normal hormonal changes after the birth

• HEADACHE, which may be severe and last up to 48 hours after the delivery, for those who have an epidural injection

• PILES (see page 377)

• POSTNATAL DEPRESSION (see page 392)

• PROLAPSE (see page 394)

• SORENESS in the genital area, caused by stitches from a tear or episiotomy, which may last for some days

ABOVE *In Ayurveda, saffron is traditionally prescribed for postnatal problems.*

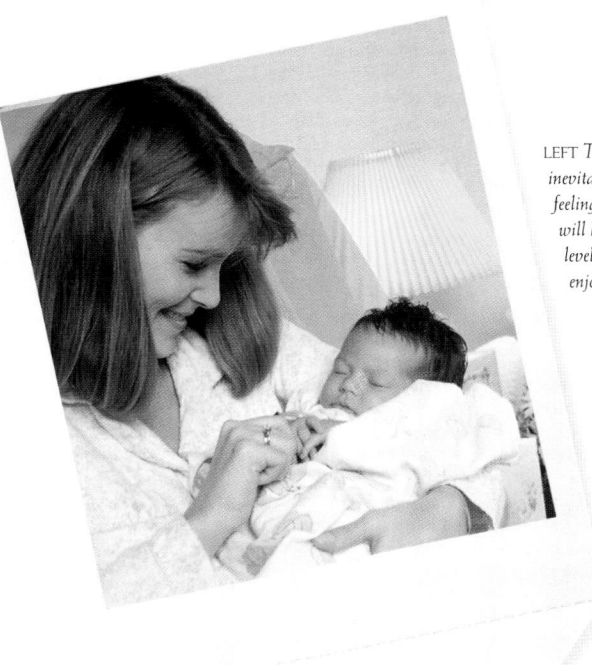

LEFT *The birth of a baby inevitably leaves you feeling exhausted. Ginseng will boost your energy levels and help you to enjoy motherhood.*

TREATMENT

AYURVEDA
• Aloe vera will encourage healing, and soothe spasm and inflammation. *(See page 27.)*
• Vetovert is excellent for exhaustion and depression. *(See page 46.)*
• Turmeric can be used for bruising. *(See page 37.)*
• Saffron is a good overall herb for postnatal problems. *(See page 36.)*

CHINESE HERBALISM
• San Qi will relive swelling, stop hemorrhaging, and disperse bruising. *(See page 68.)*
• Tian Ma (castrodia rhizome) will help relieve headaches which come on after childbirth. *(See page 62.)*
• Ginseng will help to restore, boost energy levels, prevent infection, and encourage healing. *(See page 67.)*

HERBALISM
• Good pain-relieving herbs include pulsatilla, black cohosh, lavender, and wild yam. *(See page 120.)*
• St. John's wort and calendula will help healing. *(See page 124.)*
• An infusion of calendula can be used to assist in healing the perineum. *(See page 117.)*
• Witch hazel can be applied to the perineum to encourage healing and soothe pain. *(See page 123.)*
• A comfrey compress can be applied to the perineum to speed healing. *(See page 132.)*
• Golden seal will help with bleeding, as will beth root and false unicorn root.
• Golden seal and myrrh are excellent for dispelling uterine infections.

• Cramp bark will help with uterine infections, pain, and cramping. *(See page 138.)*
• Black haw is useful for any afterpains suffered.
• Beth root and horsetail can be added to the bath for incontinence and weak pelvic floor muscles. *(See page 120.)*
• Nettles, chickweed, and coriander will act as tonics for fatigue. *(See page 137.)*

AROMATHERAPY
• Geranium, rose, and clary sage act as uterine tonics and help the pelvic tissues to regain their elasticity after the birth. *(See pages 146–71.)*
• Lavender is useful for relief of afterpains. *(See page 161.)*
• Chamomile, massaged into the abdomen, helps relieve pain and cramps. *(See page 150.)*
• Jasmine has a tonic action on the womb. *(See page 161.)*
• Apply lavender and chamomile, diluted in a little apricot kernel oil, to the affected area for sore stitches. *(See pages 161 and 150.)*

HOMEOPATHY
• Coffea, for sharp afterpains and exhaustion. *(See page 192.)*
• Nux vomica., for afterpains associated with an urgent need to pass water. *(See page 214.)*
• Pulsatilla, for pains if part of the placenta is retained. *(See page 209.)*

RIGHT *Dab witch hazel on the perineum to encourage healing and relieve pain.*

• China, for exhaustion following loss of blood. *(See page 190.)*
• Carb. veg., for exhaustion with sweating. *(See page 188.)*
• Sepia, for exhaustion with bearing-down pains. *(See page 212.)*
• Belladonna, for troublesome incontinence. *(See page 183.)*
• Pulsatilla, for piles. *(See page 209.)*
• Ferr. phos., for bleeding (the blood is bright red, clots easily), accompanied by a burning face. *(See page 194.)*
• Secale, for a post-partum hemorrhage.
• Pulsatilla, for continuing labor pains and dark red blood. *(See page 209.)*
• Arnica, to encourage healing and prevent bruising. *(See page 182.)*
• Hypericum or Arnica tincture, diluted in water, to cleanse the perineum and any stitches. *(See pages 199 and 182.)*
• Ledum, where stitching has been necessary. *(See page 202.)*

VITAMINS AND MINERALS
• Ensure that you are getting plenty of iron, which can help with fatigue. *(See page 260.)*
• Vitamin B and chromium stabilize energy levels. *(See pages 252–5 and 259.)*
• Vitamin E will encourage healing, and can be applied to stitches. *(See page 257.)*

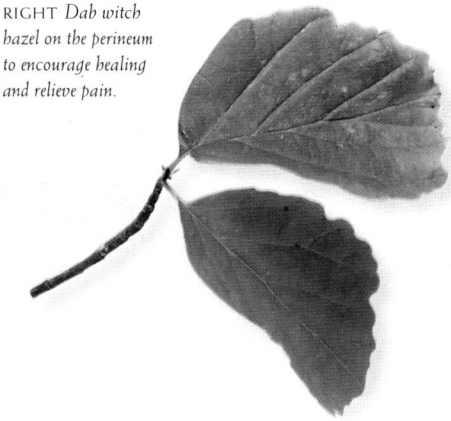

Postnatal Illness (PNI)

The term postnatal illness covers the varying degrees of anxiety, fearfulness, and depression experienced by women after the birth of a baby. Its cause is thought to be the massive drop in pregnancy hormones, aggravated by general exhaustion and discomfort in the days following delivery. Mild "baby blues" usually begin three to four days after delivery, and last only a few days. Some women experience symptoms for several weeks. Many women suffer from baby blues, but in a few women the symptoms, initially a natural response to a new situation, last for much longer than a few weeks and seriously undermine their ability to cope. Postnatal depression (PND) generally starts within weeks of the birth and may last for a year or more. In extreme cases there may be postnatal psychosis, characterized by virtual breakdown. Postnatal depression is most common in women with other stresses – marriage or relationship problems, anxiety about coping with a new baby, financial problems – as well as hormonal imbalances, blood sugar problems, and previous episodes of postnatal depression.

ABOVE *Known as the women's ginseng in China, angelica is a good tonic for PNI.*

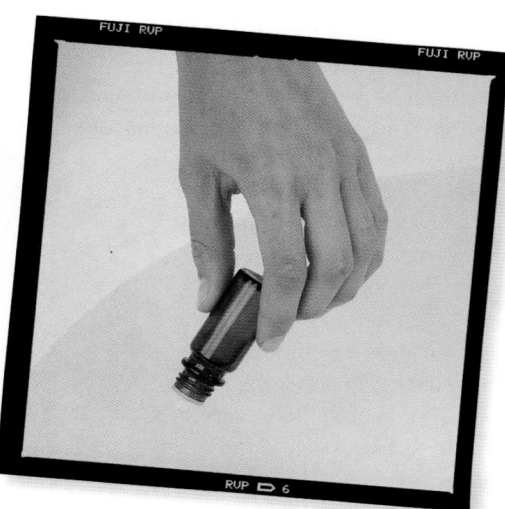

RIGHT *If you are suffering from PND relax in a warm bath with a few drops of ylang ylang or neroli oils.*

SYMPTOMS

• baby blues: irritability – tearfulness and vulnerability – mild depression and anxiety – fears about responsibility • postnatal depression: constant feeling of sadness – feeling unable to cope – feelings of guilt and inadequacy – loss of sex drive – excessive worrying • postnatal psychosis: hyperactive, manic and euphoric – depressive, with panic attacks and insomnia – almost schizophrenic behavior – hallucinations

RIGHT *Flower essence therapists recommend Olive for the sheer exhaustion that follows the birth of a baby.*

TREATMENT

AYURVEDA
• Camphor clears the mind and helps the nervous system. *(See page 33.)*
• Cumin may be useful. *(See page 36.)*
• Licorice strengthens the nerves. *(See page 39.)*
• Individual treatment will be necessary to lift the spirits and to address any hormonal problems. *(See page 22.)*

CHINESE HERBALISM
• Angelica, peony root, licorice, and thorowax root may be useful. *(See pages 56, 64, and 67.)*
• Ginseng will help to restore and to strengthen the whole person. *(See page 67.)*
• Chinese senega can reduce insomnia and bouts of depression. *(See page 70.)*
• Dodder seed may help to restore hormone imbalances to normal. *(See page 62.)*

HERBALISM
• Agnus castus can help to restore the hormone balance in the body. *(See page 139.)*
• St. John's wort and oats are nervine, and will help to reduce stress symptoms and anxiety. *(See page 124.)*

• Rosemary or lemon balm teas or tinctures will help the nervous system and lift depression. *(See page 127.)*
• False unicorn root balances the hormones and can be added to any herbal preparation.

AROMATHERAPY
• Clary sage has a balancing effect on hormones, and so can help to treat and prevent post-natal illness. *(See page 169.)*
• Jasmine and bergamot are overall tonics and relaxants, and can be used daily, either in the bath or in massage, to ease symptoms. *(See pages 161 and 153.)*
• Ylang ylang and neroli are specific to PND, and can be used in a long, enjoyable, warm bath in order to ease symptoms. *(See pages 148 and 152.)*

HOMEOPATHY
Treatment would be constitutional, but the following remedies may help:
• Pulsatilla, for curtailing episodes of weepiness. *(See page 209.)*
• Nat. mur., for coping with feelings of irritation, guilt, and withdrawal. *(See page 206.)*

• Sepia, for allaying exhaustion, lack of interest, and irritability. *(See page 212.)*

FLOWER ESSENCES
• Rescue remedy or Emergency Essence will help after the trauma of the birth. *(See page 244.)*
• Gorse is good for feelings of hopelessness. *(See page 240.)*
• Mustard, when you feel as if you are under a dark cloud for no apparent reason. *(See page 239.)*
• Olive will help to address exhaustion. *(See page 235)*
• Walnut will help you to deal with change. *(See page 232.)*
• Sweet Chestnut is for fits of utter despair. *(See page 227.)*

VITAMINS AND MINERALS
• Some experts believe that nutritional deficiencies are at the root of the problem; ensure you eat plenty of foods rich in vitamins C and B, calcium, iron, magnesium, and also potassium. *(See pages 256, 252–5, 258, 260, and 262.)*
• Tyrosine and tryptophan, amino acids, can help to ease post-natal depression. *(See page 269.)*

Menopause Symptoms

Menopause is the cessation of menstruation and a woman's reproductive capacity. It usually occurs around the age of 50, but may happen prematurely, or artificially after removal of the ovaries. Most symptoms that occur during menopause result directly from the estrogen deficiency produced by the failing ovaries. Interestingly, Japanese women suffer far fewer symptoms of the menopause because they eat more plant estrogens like tofu, soya, and miso.

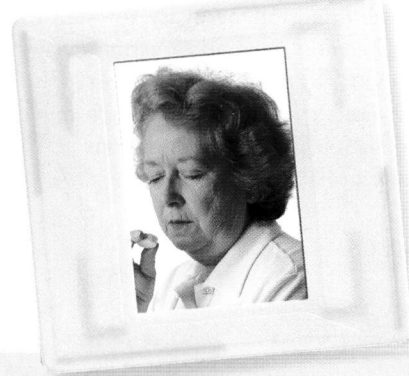

LEFT *Menopausal symptoms, including hot flushes and depression, may be relieved with homeopathic remedies.*

SYMPTOMS

- *back pain* - *dry, thinning hair and dry skin* - *very heavy periods (flooding)* - *very light periods* - *hot flushes, mostly affecting the face and neck, and varying in frequency and duration* - *incontinence, one of the most common menopausal symptoms; through wear and tear, childbearing, and lack of estrogen* - *osteoporosis* - *psychological problems such as irritability, anxiety, insomnia, and poor memory* - *increased hair growth on the face, stomach, or chest, due either to an increase in the male hormone, androgen, or the drop in estrogen production* - *vaginal looseness, a feeling of slackness, or of something protruding into the vaginal passage — possibly a prolapsed uterus, or a section of the urethra, bladder or rectum dropping downward as a result of lost muscle tone* - *about 20–25 percent of menopausal women experience pain during intercourse, called dyspareunia. Mostly, this is due to thinning of the vaginal wall and a lack of lubrication, both caused by estrogen deficiency*

TREATMENT

AYURVEDA
- Calamus root can be good for memory problems and mental stress. *(See page 24.)*
- Celery seeds and cedar are balancing, and may help with menstrual problems. *(See page 29.)*
- Cinnamon is especially powerful during menopause, and is particularly useful for low libido and edema. *(See page 34.)*
- Coriander is cooling, and acts as a diuretic and diaphoretic. It is also thought to be aphrodisiac. *(See page 35.)*
- Aloe vera cools and cleanses the liver when taken internally, helping with any "hot" symptoms of menopause, including flushes, sweats, and swelling. *(See page 27.)*

CHINESE HERBALISM
- Shan Zhu Yu can be used for flooding, with ginseng for heavy sweating and hot flushes. *(See pages 60 and 67.)*
- Chinese senega may be useful for irritability, insomnia, and depression. *(See page 70.)*
- Angelica, peony root, and thorowax root are the ideal herbs to treat the symptoms of menopause, which is believed to be a weakness of the Kidneys, deficient Blood, and an imbalance between Kidney and Liver. *(See pages 56 and 67.)*

HERBALISM
- Valerian will help with anxiety and tension, and combined with skullcap relaxes the nervous system. *(See pages 131 and 136.)*
- Ginseng will help with anxiety and irritability, and increases mental alertness. It will also boost vitality and prevent feelings of fatigue. *(See page 126.)*
- Herbal laxatives include butternut, blue flag, and senna.
- Shepherd's purse, lady's mantle, yarrow, golden seal, beth root, and periwinkle help with heavy bleeding. *(See pages 112 and 113.)*
- Dandelion cleanses the liver and helps the body to detoxify, which can reduce the risk of breast growths and other cell changes. *(See page 133.)*
- Milk thistle can be used to treat lumpy and painful breasts. *(See page 131.)*
- Agnus castus can be used for breast tenderness and any problems of the menopause, as it works to normalize the levels of female hormones. *(See page 139.)*

- Black cohosh can restore female hormonal balance and help to prevent night sweats and hot flushes. Other herbs to consider are licorice, alfalfa, and Dong Quai. *(See page 122.)*
- American ginseng can increase libido, as can agnus castus and black cohosh. *(See pages 126 and 139.)*
- Ginkgo biloba can help with memory and concentration problems. *(See page 122.)*
- Cramp bark is antispasmodic and will help with painful menstruation. *(See page 138.)*
- Burdock root helps with dry and scaly skin, and licorice or chamomile, applied directly to the skin, will soothe and soften. *(See pages 115, 119, and 122.)*
- Valerian can help improve the quality of sleep and treat insomnia. *(See page 136.)*
- Passiflora will help you to sleep.
- Motherwort can restore thickness and elasticity to the walls of the vagina, and dong quai can help with dryness. *(See page 124.)*
- Dandelion is a natural diuretic and will help with any swelling associated with water retention. *(See page 133.)*

AROMATHERAPY
- Clary sage will lift your mood and help to deal with fluctuating hormones. *(See page 169.)*
- Chamomile, diluted in a little carrier oil, is adaptogenic, and will balance hormone levels causing night sweats, hot flushes, and other symptoms. *(See page 150.)*
- Essential oils of damian, and geranium or ylang ylang are aphrodisiacs for low libido. *(See pages 146–71.)*
- Fennel can be massaged into the abdomen for water retention and symptoms of hormonal imbalance. *(See page 159.)*

HOMEOPATHY
- Sepia is enormously useful, and can treat hot flushes, headaches, irritability, and heavy menstrual bleeding. *(See page 212.)*
- Conium, for loss of libido.
- Graphites, for weight gain, hot flushes, and scanty menstrual bleeding. *(See page 196.)*
- Lachesis, for flooding, irritability, memory loss and concentration problems, hot flushes, and headaches. *(See page 216.)*
- Pulsatilla, for depression, weepiness and changeable moods. *(See page 209.)*

- Sanguinara, for tender breasts and flooding.

FLOWER ESSENCES
- Mustard, for depression with no identifiable cause. *(See page 239.)*
- Olive, for fatigue. *(See page 235.)*
- Mimulus, for fear of aging and death. *(See page 235.)*
- Walnut, for life changes. *(See page 232.)*

VITAMINS AND MINERALS
- Take magnesium and vitamin B-complex for anxiety and irritability. *(See pages 262 and 252–5.)*
- Vitamin E, linseed oil, acidophilus, and vitamin B-complex will help with tender and lumpy breasts. *(See pages 257, 271, 252–5.)*
- For constipation, try extra vitamin C. *(See page 256.)*
- Co-enzyme Q10 will help lack of energy and fatigue; check that you are not anemic.
- Quercetin can help with migraine and headaches

associated with menopause, as can vitamin C and E. *(See pages 256 and 257.)*
- Vitamin C can help regulate heavy bleeding (flooding) when combined with bioflavonoids. *(See page 256.)*
- Vitamin A, zinc, iron, and vitamin B-complex can also help with heavy menstrual bleeding. *(See pages 252, 265, 260, and 252–5.)*
- Selenium may help to reduce hot flushes and night sweats, as will vitamin C, which is a more effective preventive than HRT. *(See pages 264 and 256.)*
- Zinc, vitamin C, vitamin E, and magnesium will help with painful menstruation. *(See pages 256, 265, 257, and 262.)*
- Linseed oil, evening primrose, vitamin B-complex and zinc can be taken for skin problems. *(See pages 270, 252–5, and 265.)*
- Magnesium is helpful for insomnia and sleep problems. *(See page 262.)*
- A vitamin E capsule can be placed inside the vagina for vaginal dryness. *(See page 257.)*

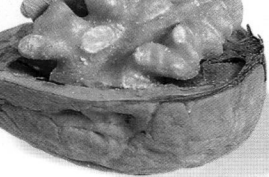

LEFT *Walnut is an excellent flower essence to take during important life transitions.*

Prolapse

Prolapse occurs when the uterus and/or vagina slip downward due to a weakening or stretching of the structures that would normally keep them in place. It occurs when ligaments and muscles which hold the uterus and vagina in place become weak or slack with age, or as a result of childbirth, allowing the uterus to bulge into the vagina and press on the bladder or rectum. If prolapse is complete a large part of the vagina or uterus may actually protrude through the vaginal opening, causing soreness or ulceration, and encouraging infection. The risk of a prolapse may be heightened by a chronic cough, chronic constipation, or obesity. Neither prolapse is serious at first, but may become so if neglected. Surgery to tighten pelvic floor muscles may be necessary if exercises do not improve the muscle tone. A ring pessary, fitted behind the pubic bone, may be necessary in an elderly woman. Sixty-five percent of all women who prolapse do so before the age of 55. Women who have had several children, or a difficult labor, seem to be more prone to prolapse.

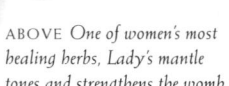

ABOVE *One of women's most healing herbs, Lady's mantle tones and strengthens the womb.*

SYMPTOMS

• a sensation of something dropping down • dragging feeling in lower abdomen • backache • fatigue • in addition to the above, prolapse of the vagina may involve: frequent urge to pass water — stress incontinence — possibly urine infections

TREATMENT

CHINESE HERBALISM
• Treatment would be aimed at Deficient qi, and Central qi pills would be useful. *(See page 49.)*

HERBALISM
• Motherwort, lady's mantle, and life root can help to restore the tone of the uterus and vagina. *(See pages 113 and 124.)*
• Use astringent herbs such as horsetail, shepherd's purse, false unicorn, and bayberry. These can be taken as teas, tisanes, decoctions, pills, etc. They can also be used as a poultice and applied to the abdomen. Barberry stimulates the uterus to contract: do not use in pregnancy. *(See page 119.)*

• For a prolapse after the menopause, try sage, calendula, ginseng, and wild yam: all estrogenic. *(See pages 117, 120, 126, and 129.)*
• Chickweed ointment or douche can soothe and heal soreness of the vagina or cervix.
• Pessaries with glycerin and golden seal can be helpful.

AROMATHERAPY
• Massage the lower abdomen and back with diluted oils of rosemary and lemon to improve the circulation and tighten tissues. *(See pages 168 and 154.)*

HOMEOPATHY
• Sepia, for a pressing feeling that something is coming out. *(See page 212.)*
• Aloe, for long-standing prolapse with a feeling of fullness and sometimes morning diarrhea.

VITAMINS AND MINERALS
• Uterus glandular tissues give support to your uterus.
• Vitamin E increases the elasticity of the tissues, and helps them respond to stress more effectively. *(See page 257.)*

Ovarian Cysts

A cyst is an abnormal sac or cavity that contains liquid or semi-solid material enclosed by a membrane. Ovarian cysts most commonly occur in women between the ages of 35 and 55. Usually they are benign, but they can sometimes cause problems because of their size. Ovarian cysts may be caused by slight ovulation disorders, or by swelling of the lining of the ovary through fluid collection. The most common ovarian cyst is a follicular cyst that contains watery fluid. Pseudomucinous cysts contain a thick mucous fluid and can lead to complications if they rupture or become infected.

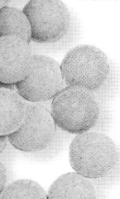

ABOVE *If you suffer from ovarian cysts, try taking vitamin E supplements.*

SYMPTOMS

• pain, once the cyst has grown large enough to cause problems • abdominal discomfort • possibly an increase in the size of the abdomen • breathlessness • may lead to varicose veins (see page 361) or piles (see page 377) • repeated or multiple cysts may affect fertility (see page 398)

TREATMENT

CHINESE HERBALISM
• Dodder seeds can balance the reproductive system. *(See page 62.)*
• San qi, for general relief of pain. *(See page 68.)*
• Tree peony may be useful. *(See page 67.)*

HERBALISM
• False unicorn root or blue cohosh can help to restore the function of the reproductive system.
• Kelp can be added to ensure normal thyroid function. *(See page 122.)*
• Take dandelion root to help the liver metabolize estrogen. *(See page 134.)*
• Agnus castus acts to restore estrogen levels. *(See page 139.)*

AROMATHERAPY
• Basil, marjoram, and lavender can be massaged into the abdomen to ease pain and restore balance. *(See pages 146–71.)*
• Clary sage will help to balance hormones. *(See page 169.)*

HOMEOPATHY
Treatment should be constitutional, but the following remedies may be useful.
• Colocynthis, is for small round cysts which cause boring pain which is improved by pressure. *(See page 191.)*
• Apis, for stinging pains, particularly in the right ovary. *(See page 180.)*
• Lachesis, for local pain which is worse in the morning, and occurs mainly in the left ovary. *(See page 216.)*
• Ledum, for driving pain through the ovary and womb. *(See page 202.)*

FLOWER ESSENCES
• Take Rescue Remedy or Emergency Essence to restore a sense of calm during pain and discomfort. *(See page 244.)*

VITAMINS AND MINERALS
• Increase your intake of iodine, since thyroid problems may be at the root of the cysts. *(See page 261.)*
• Vitamin E is helpful for preventing and treating cysts. *(See page 257.)*
• The B-complex vitamins will help to re-establish hormone balance and the metabolism of estrogen by the liver. *(See pages 252–5.)*

BELOW *Kelp stimulates the thyroid gland and may be taken to ensure normal function.*

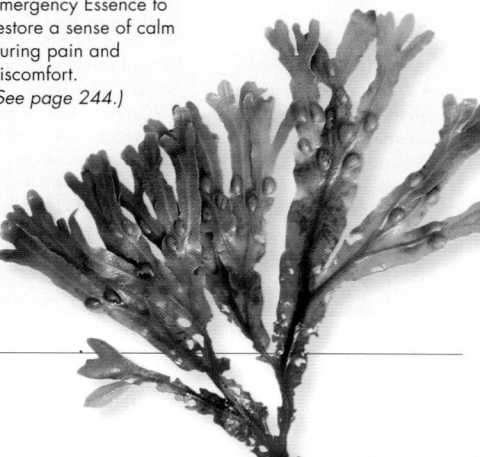

Pelvic Inflammatory Disease (PID)

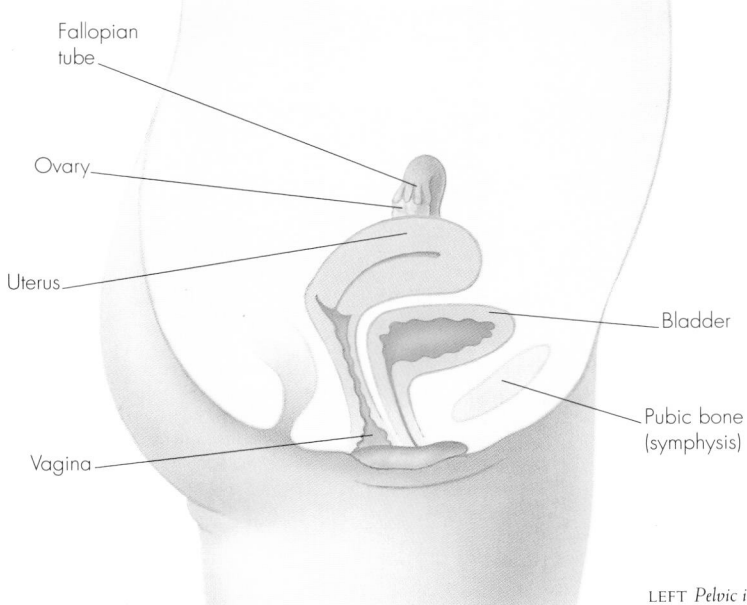

ABOVE *Use myrrh in conjunction with unicorn root. Its anti-inflammatory properties will relieve PID.*

Pelvic inflammatory disease (PID) is an umbrella term for infections and inflammations that have penetrated the reproductive system, i.e. the ovaries (ovaritis), Fallopian tubes (salpingitis), and the uterus (endometritis). Left untreated, these infections can develop and recur for years. Possible causes of PID are gonorrhoea and chlamydia cystitis (*see page 379*), various viruses, or the natural flora of the vagina. Triggers include anything that allows a lurking infection to travel, such as childbirth, abortion, surgery on the reproductive system or in the pelvic area, or an IUD (intrauterine device, which prevents pregnancy).

SYMPTOMS

• *acute: fever with shaking – painful intercourse – unusual vaginal discharge – vaginal bleeding after sex or in mid-menstrual cycle – severe lower abdominal pain – back pain*
• *chronic: weight loss – backache and lower abdominal pain – nausea – diarrhea – tiredness – pain on urination – reduced fertility (caused by scarring which blocks the Fallopian tubes)*

TREATMENT

AYURVEDA
• Aloe vera relieves inflammation, soothes muscle spasms, and purifies the blood. *(See page 27)*
• Angelica has antibacterial properties and can help with pain. *(See page 28.)*
• Gotu kola may be useful if the infection is linked to STDs. *(See page 33.)*

CHINESE HERBALISM
• Peony root can be used for abdominal pain. *(See page 67.)*
• Cinnamon treats pain and other symptoms. *(See page 59.)*
• Pseudoginseng root (San Qi) may be useful. *(See page 68.)*

TRADITIONAL HOME AND FOLK REMEDIES
• Peel a clove of garlic, wrap it in gauze, and tie a piece of string to one end. Place in the vagina and change daily. *(See page 82.)*

HERBALISM
• Fresh garlic, taken as often as possible throughout the day, can act to fight infection and boost the immune system. *(See page 113.)*
• Echinacea will help to boost immunity as well as addressing the infection. *(See page 120.)*
• Thyme and parsley will help to fight infection. *(See page 135.)*
• Blue cohosh has an affinity with the reproductive system. Take daily.
• False unicorn root and myrrh combine well.

AROMATHERAPY
• Add lavender, rosemary, or geranium oils to the bath water to relax and help to fight infection. *(See pages 146–71.)*

HOMEOPATHY
Treatment should be constitutional, but the following may help:
• Mercurius, for chills and sweat that is unpleasant, and where the condition is improved by rest. *(See page 205.)*
• Apis, for stinging, burning pains, mainly on the right side. *(See page 180.)*
• Aconite, for sudden onset, with mild fever and anxiety. *(See page 178.)*
• Belladonna, for sudden onset, with red face and burning. *(See page 183.)*
• Colocynthis, is for cramping pains relieved by pressure. *(See page 191.)*

VITAMINS AND MINERALS
• Include vitamin C, E, and zinc in your diet to boost the immune system. *(See pages 256, 257 and 265.)*
• Acidophilus encourages the growth of healthy bacteria, and is especially useful if you have taken a course of antibiotics. *(See page 271.)*

Fallopian tube
Ovary
Uterus
Vagina
Bladder
Pubic bone (symphysis)

LEFT *Pelvic inflammatory disease refers to any infections of the reproductive system.*

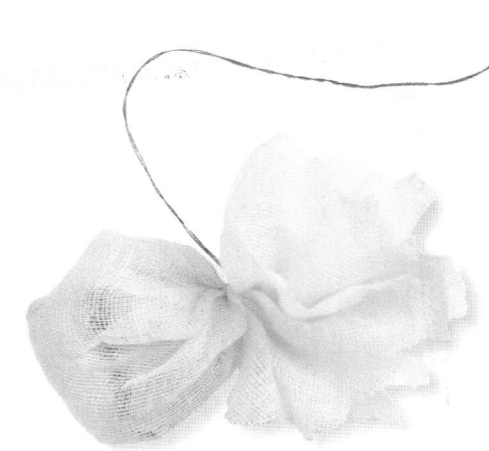

ABOVE *Place a piece of garlic wrapped in gauze inside the vagina. Its antibiotic and antiseptic actions may help to fight PID.*

Thrush

Thrush is caused by the yeast organism *Candida albicans*, which lives naturally in the vagina and also the mouth, bowel, and, to some extent, the skin. It only begins to cause problems when there is an overgrowth of it. Antibiotics, immuno-suppressive drugs, a compromised immune system, periods of hormonal change and stress can all encourage Candida growth, and thrush as a result. Other aggravating factors include a high sugar intake, tight clothing, poor personal hygiene, and scented bath oils. Women seem to suffer more frequently from thrush, or candidiasis, than men.

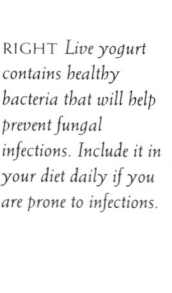

RIGHT *Live yogurt contains healthy bacteria that will help prevent fungal infections. Include it in your diet daily if you are prone to infections.*

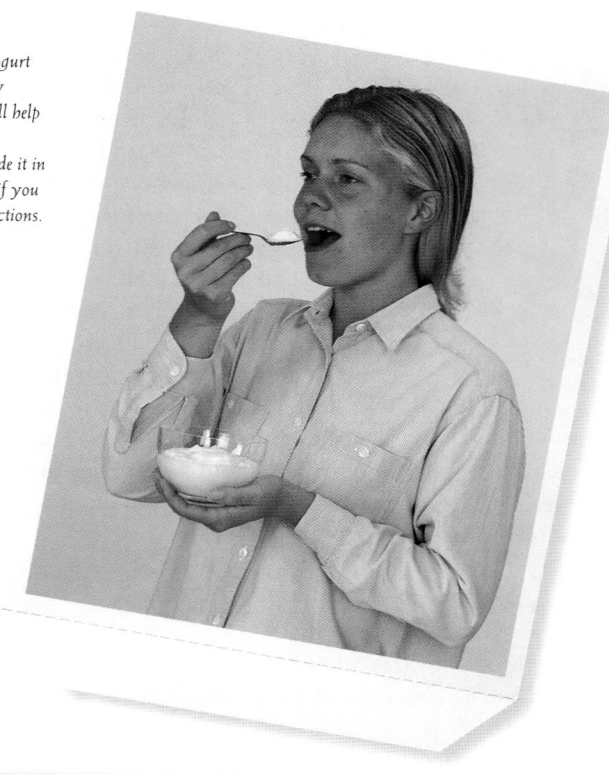

SYMPTOMS

- *an itchy, white vaginal discharge*
- *sore, red, dry, itchy vulva*
- *stinging pain on urination*
- *soreness and discomfort during intercourse* • *possibly a red rash extending down the thighs, or around to the anus*

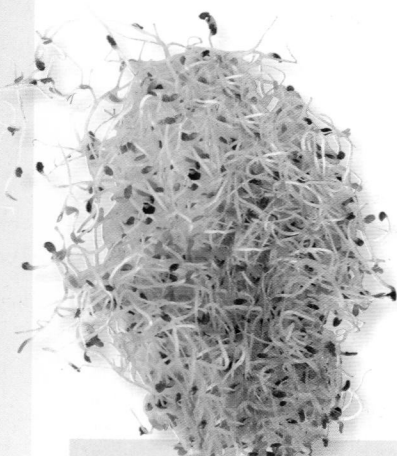

LEFT *Alfalfa has antifungal properties and is used in Ayurveda to treat thrush.*

TREATMENT

AYURVEDA
- Garlic is a useful anti-infective agent, and works against fungi. (See page 26.)
- The following herbs may be used in internal and external preparations, for their antifungal properties: barberry, alfalfa, basil, cinnamon, coriander, myrrh, and elecampane. (See pages 29, 34, 35, 40, 41, and 42.)
- Treatment would be individual, to balance the system.

CHINESE HERBALISM
- Treatment would address excess Damp and Damp Heat. Suitable herbs might include gentian and oriental wormwood.
- Dang Gui or ginger will be used when you feel generally depleted. (See page 56.)

TRADITIONAL HOME AND FOLK REMEDIES
- A live yogurt douche will encourage the growth of healthy bacteria (flora) which will prevent fungal infection. Use regularly if you are prone to thrush. Apply to patches of oral thrush, and include live yogurt in your daily diet. (See page 93.)

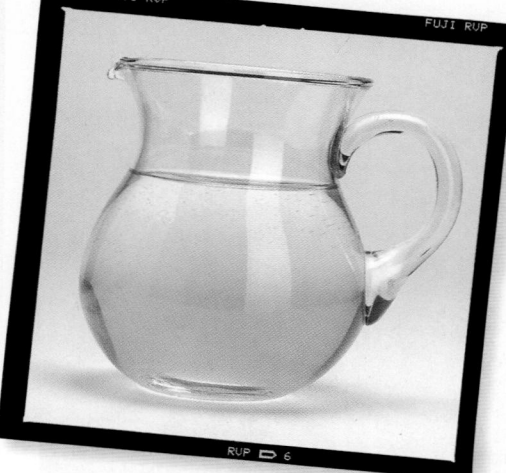

ABOVE *Use a douche of cider vinegar and warm water to treat vaginal thrush.*

- Apple cider vinegar, added to a pint of warm water, can be used as a douche. (See page 102.)
- Sit in a bowl of water to which a little vinegar or lemon juice has been added, to correct pH imbalance and maintain an acid environment. (See page 102.)

HERBALISM
- Drink an infusion of echinacea or marigold to encourage healing, boost the immune system, and clear infection. (See pages 117 and 120.)
- A douche of marigold or lavender flowers will ease symptoms. (See page 117.)
- Take echinacea 3 times daily for chronic cases of thrush, and every 2 hours in acute attacks, to boost the immune system. (See page 120.)
- Useful antifungal herbs include calendula, cinnamon, and rosemary. (See pages 117 and 127.)

- Chamomile cream and chickweed ointment can be applied externally to soothe itching and irritation. (See page 117.)
- Soak a tampon in water with a few drops of golden seal tincture and insert; remove after one hour.

AROMATHERAPY
- A tiny drop of tea tree oil, added to 2pt. (1.2l) of warm, already boiled water, can be used as a douche. (See page 162.)
- Massage with lavender or tea tree oil can boost the immune system and prevent further infections. (See pages 162 and 161.)

HOMEOPATHY
- Pulsatilla, for cloudy or watery discharge which causes smarting and soreness. (See page 209.)

- Lachesis, for burning discharge, with weariness, bloating, and symptoms that are worse around menstruation. (See page 216.)
- Graphites, for a sore vagina with small ulcers appearing on the labia. (See page 196.)
- Calcarea, if there is vaginal itching, a yellow or milky discharge, and increased itchiness around the time of menstruation. (See page 186.)
- Aluminia, for frequent, straw-colored discharge which causes itching and stiffens underwear.

VITAMINS AND MINERALS
- Take acidophilus tablets to restore the healthy bacteria in the body, which will fight the infection. (See page 271.)

Painful Intercourse

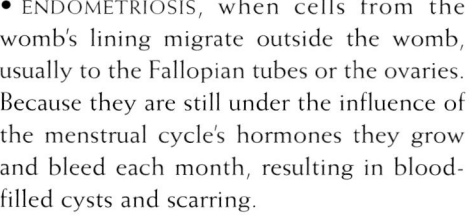

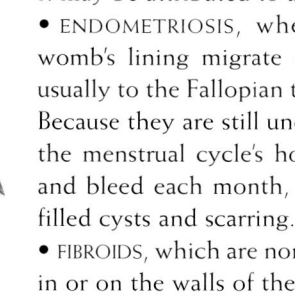

Many women experience pain or discomfort during sexual intercourse (called dyspareunia) at different points in their lives, and it may be attributed to a number of causes:

- ENDOMETRIOSIS, when cells from the womb's lining migrate outside the womb, usually to the Fallopian tubes or the ovaries. Because they are still under the influence of the menstrual cycle's hormones they grow and bleed each month, resulting in blood-filled cysts and scarring.
- FIBROIDS, which are noncancerous growths in or on the walls of the uterus.
- PELVIC INFLAMMATORY DISEASE (PID), an umbrella term for infections and inflammations that have penetrated deep into the reproductive system.
- SEXUALLY TRANSMITTED DISEASES (STDs).
- THRUSH (see page 439).
- CHILDBIRTH. The labor and delivery process can cause soreness and discomfort for some weeks, particularly if the woman has had an episiotomy.
- Menopause (see page 393).

ABOVE *Marjoram is a warm, relaxing, and sedative herb. Use the essential oil in a massage or burn in a vaporizer.*

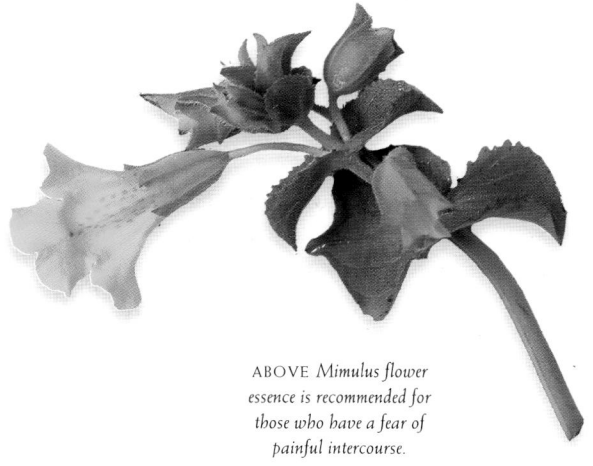

ABOVE *Mimulus flower essence is recommended for those who have a fear of painful intercourse.*

TREATMENT

(See treatment for Thrush on page 396, Menopause on page 393, Pregnancy Problems on page 388, and PID on page 395.)

AROMATHERAPY
- Lavender and marjoram are relaxing, and can help you to get over the emotional trauma of painful sex. Try a full-body massage with your partner before intercourse. (See pages 161 and 165.)

HOMEOPATHY
Treatment would be constitutional, and would depend on the cause of the pain.
- Calcarea iod., for treating small fibroids with a yellow discharge. (See page 186.)
- Aurum mur., for a swollen uterus and painful contractions of the vagina associated with fibroids.
- Aconite, for sharp pain that comes on suddenly.

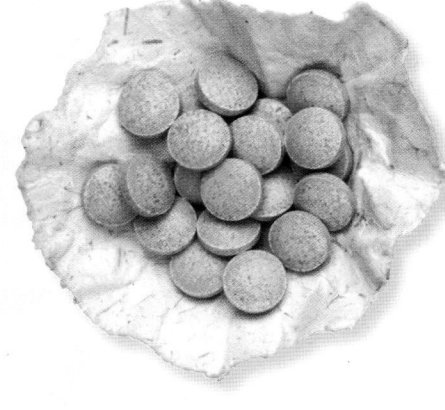

ABOVE *Supplement your diet with vitamins A and E to promote a healthy reproductive system.*

- Sepia or Belladonna, when the problem is associated with prolapse. (See pages 212 and 183.)

FLOWER ESSENCES
- Mimulus, for fear of pain during sex. (See page 235.)
- Rescue Remedy or Emergency Essence, taken before making love, to calm and reduce feelings of panic and anxiety. (See page 244.)

VITAMINS AND MINERALS
- Take plenty of vitamin A and E, which will help restore the health of the reproductive system. (See pages 252 and 257.)
- Acidophilus will help to maintain the balance of healthy flora in the body. (See page 271.)
- Vitamin E capsules can be placed in the vagina to ease pain and dryness. (See page 257.)

RIGHT *Give your partner a soothing massage prior to sexual intercourse if she fears pain. This will help her to relax and reduce negative emotions.*

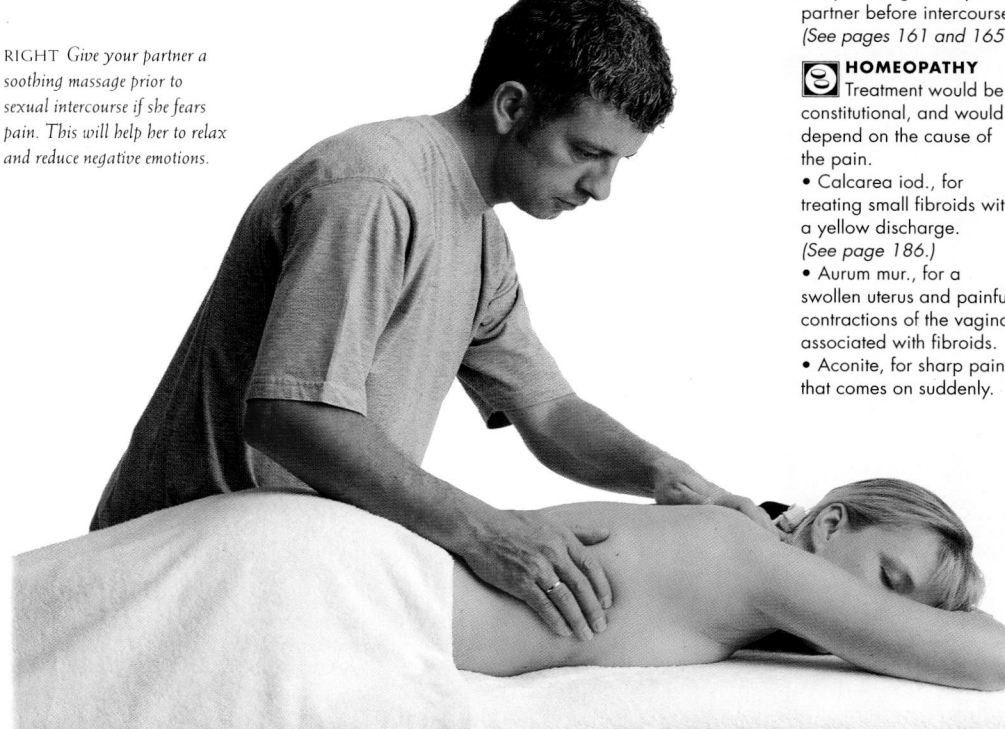

DISORDERS OF THE REPRODUCTIVE SYSTEM: MALE

Infertility

The term infertility is generally applied when failure to conceive follows an 18-month period of regular, unprotected sexual intercourse. It is usually a sign that something in the body is not working properly. The most common cause of infertility in men is a low sperm count (possibly due to environmental pollution). Poor sperm quality, inadequate mobility of sperm, no sperm at all, or an abnormality in the penis may also be responsible. In some cases the problem may be hormonal. Risk factors include smoking, excessive alcohol consumption, raised temperature around the testes (caused by tight trousers, or by varicose veins on the scrotum), certain prescription drugs, stress, or infection with mumps. A diet lacking in vitamins and minerals can also cause a man to be less fertile. One research study discovered that organic farmers had twice the sperm count of other men!

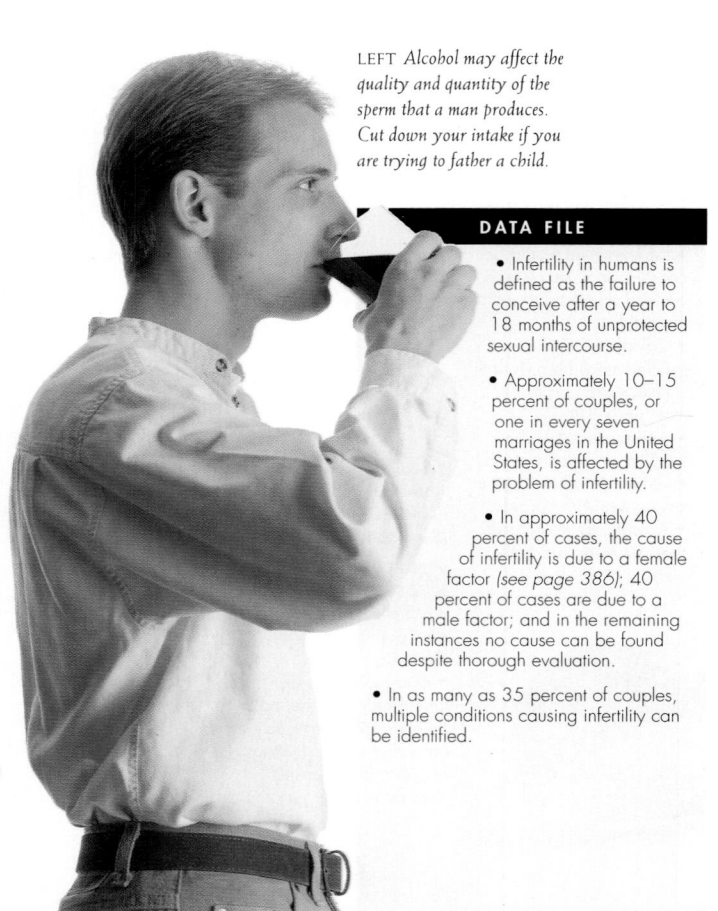

ABOVE *Low sperm counts, abnormal, or immobile sperm all contribute to male infertility.*

LEFT *Alcohol may affect the quality and quantity of the sperm that a man produces. Cut down your intake if you are trying to father a child.*

DATA FILE

• Infertility in humans is defined as the failure to conceive after a year to 18 months of unprotected sexual intercourse.

• Approximately 10–15 percent of couples, or one in every seven marriages in the United States, is affected by the problem of infertility.

• In approximately 40 percent of cases, the cause of infertility is due to a female factor (see page 386); 40 percent of cases are due to a male factor; and in the remaining instances no cause can be found despite thorough evaluation.

• In as many as 35 percent of couples, multiple conditions causing infertility can be identified.

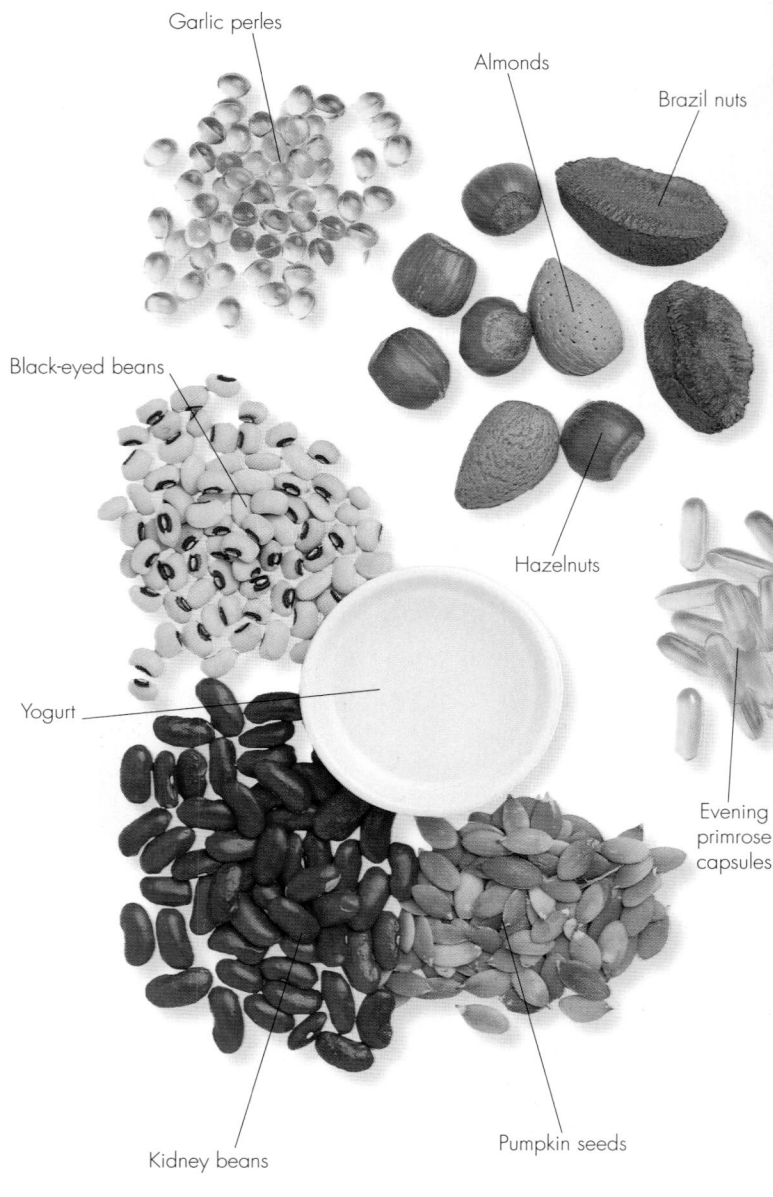

Garlic perles

Almonds

Brazil nuts

Black-eyed beans

Hazelnuts

Yogurt

Evening primrose capsules

Kidney beans

Pumpkin seeds

ABOVE *Foods that contain essential fatty acids, such as these, are believed to stimulate the production of sex hormones.*

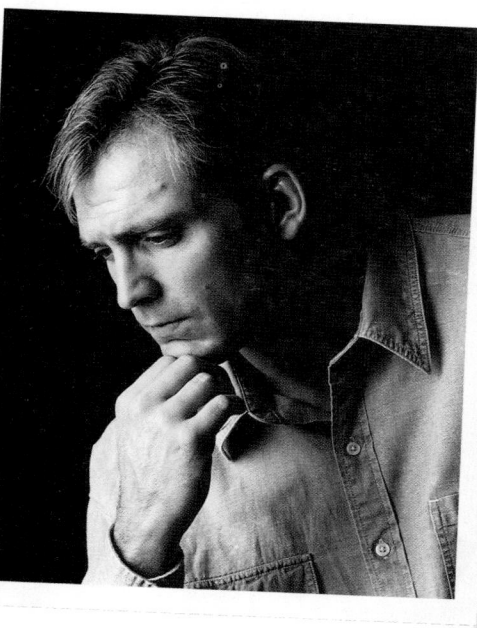

ABOVE *White Chestnut flower essence is useful to calm persistent worrying thoughts.*

AYURVEDA
• Saffron is used for the treatment of infertility. *(See page 36.)*
• Sandalwood can help with impotence and acts as an aphrodisiac. *(See page 44.)*
• Clove, ginger, cardamom, cinnamon, vetiver, and coriander are aphrodisiac, which may help. *(See pages 34, 35, 38, 46, and 47.)*

CHINESE HERBALISM
• Infertility is believed to be caused by Damp Heat, and an imbalance of yin and yang; treatment will be according to the nature of your infertility. The following combinations may be useful: Yi Zhi Ren, He Shou Wu, Gou Qi Zi, Du Zhong, and Wu Wei Zi, for problems associated with sperm. *(See pages 63, 66, 70, and 74.)*

TREATMENT

HERBALISM
• Remedies such as damiana and saw palmetto have hormonal effects, stimulating the male reproductive system while also acting as useful nerve restoratives. *(See pages 131 and 135.)*

AROMATHERAPY
• Rose oil is said to increase sperm count and quality, as well as acting as a mild aphrodisiac. Add a few drops to your partner's bath, or perhaps engage in a little gentle massage, with 2 or 3 drops of rose essential oil in a mild carrier oil such as sweet almond oil. *(See page 168.)*
• If infertility is causing anxiety, any of the relaxing essential oils, such as lavender, marjoram, or chamomile, can be vaporized or used in a bath. *(See pages 146–71.)*
• When repeated attempts to get pregnant have failed and you need a little encouragement to continue with love-making, ylang ylang is a lovely, relaxing oil that will act as an aphrodisiac. *(See page 148.)*

HOMEOPATHY
• Treatment would be constitutional, but the following remedies may be helpful:
• Conium, for inability to sustain an erection.
• Lycopodium, for an increased desire for sex, but where intercourse is spoiled by anticipation of failure. *(See page 203.)*
• Sepia, for a dragging sensation in the genitals, and no desire for sex. *(See page 212.)*

FLOWER ESSENCES
• Willow can be taken for resentment, bitterness, and self-pity about the problem. *(See page 239.)*

• White Chestnut, for worrying thoughts. *(See page 224.)*
• Pine, for guilty feelings. *(See page 236.)*
• Olive, for exhaustion and overwhelming fatigue. *(See page 235.)*

VITAMINS AND MINERALS
• There is a possibility that a zinc deficiency might cause problems with male fertility. Studies in the U.S. have shown that zinc is essential for sperm formation, and men who have zinc deficiencies may produce zero or reduced sperm counts. Zinc is also linked to a man's sex drive. *(See page 265.)*

• Cutting out alcohol, smoking, and drugs may be suggested for both couples for the period before conception.
• Vitamins E and B6 may be supplemented, as a deficiency is often linked to a low sperm count. *(See pages 257 and 254.)*
• An increased intake of EFAs (essential fatty acids, found in oily fish, fish liver oils, seeds, nuts, pulses, beans, evening primrose oil, and unrefined vegetable oils) stimulates sex hormone production.

BELOW *Rose essential oil has aphrodisiac qualities, well as relaxing the mind.*

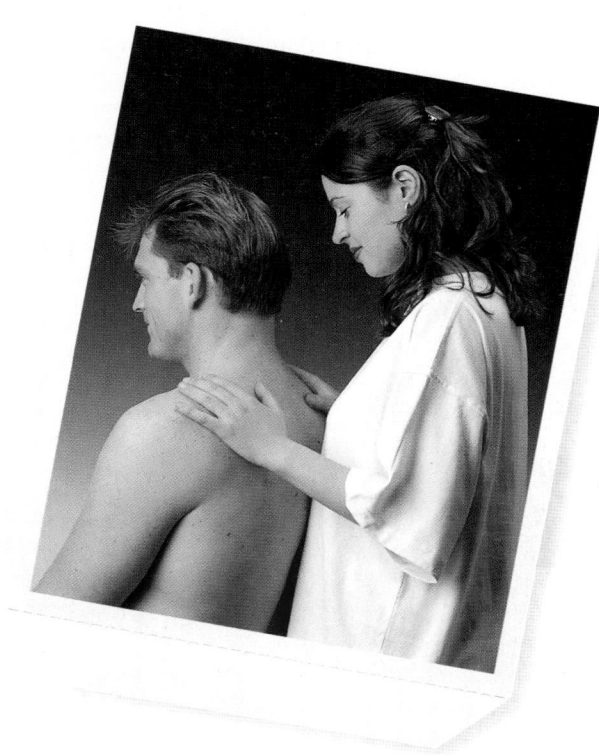

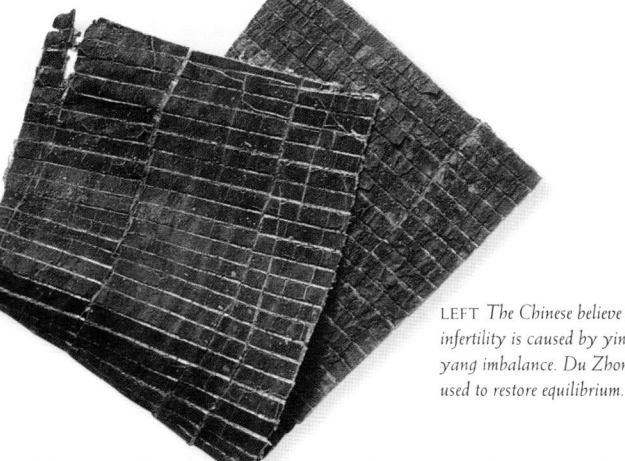

LEFT *The Chinese believe that infertility is caused by yin/yang imbalance. Du Zhong is used to restore equilibrium.*

Prostate Problems

The prostate is a small sex gland which surrounds the urethra (urine tube) under the bladder. Its function is to produce the fluid which transports and nourishes sperm as it is ejaculated. Common prostate problems include:

• BENIGN PROSTATIC HYPERPLASIA (BPH), a slow, noncancerous enlargement of the prostate, progressively constricts the urethra, causing obstruction in the flow of urine. Incomplete emptying of the bladder as a result causes a frequent urge to urinate at night as well as during the day.

• PROSTATITIS, inflammation of the prostate gland, is common in younger men and may be chronic or acute. Symptoms include a frequent urge to urinate, burning pain, and difficulty in urinating, lower back pain, painful ejaculation, and inflamed testes.

• PROSTATE CANCER, the second most common form of cancer in men. The prostate is enlarged, as in BPH, but is felt to be hard on examination. As well as an urge to urinate more frequently, there may be blood in the urine and pain on urinating. If the cancer is advanced there may also be bone pain and weight loss.

• CANCER of the prostate occurs in 1 of 8 American men. Prostate cancer is more common after the age of 55; approximately 80 percent of all cases occur in men over 65; by the age of 80, 80 percent of all men have the cancer to some degree. Cancer of the prostate also becomes increasingly common in men over the age of 60; its development is stimulated by male hormones and retarded – to a variable extent – by female hormones. A male baby has a 13 percent chance of contracting prostate cancer, and a 3 percent chance of dying from it. For early detection of prostate cancer, the ACS (American Cancer Society) recommends that men over age 40 should have an annual digital rectal examination. After age 50, men should have an annual prostate-specific antigen blood test.

• BENIGN PROSTATIC HYPERTROPHY occurs in half of all men over the age of 50, and in three-quarters over the age of 70 – a total of about 10 million men.

Watercress has powerful antibiotic properties and will help fight urinary infections

LEFT *Certain foods, such as those shown here, may be of particular benefit to the prostate gland.*

Sesame seeds are believed to enhance sexual vigor

Pumpkin seeds act as a male sexual tonic and protect the prostate

TREATMENT

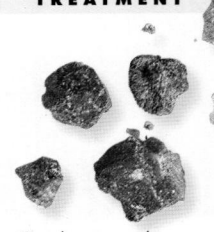

LEFT *Benzoin has diuretic properties and can be used in the bath or for a massage to relieve the prostate.*

AYURVEDA
• Gotu kola is cooling, rejuvenating, and diuretic. *(See page 33.)*
• Cedar and celery seed are natural diuretics and will encourage urination. *(See pages 29 and 32.)*
• Cinnamon is diuretic and analgesic, which will help ease the discomfort. *(See page 34.)*
• Coriander is diuretic and aphrodisiac, which will help address the low libido that is associated with this condition. *(See page 35.)*

CHINESE HERBALISM
• Prostate problems are believed to be caused by excess dampness and stagnant qi. The herbs cinnamon bark, cork tree bark, and water plantain will be useful treatments. *(See pages 59 and 68.)*
• Panax ginseng is recommended for an enlarged prostate. *(See page 67.)*

TRADITIONAL HOME AND FOLK REMEDIES
• Watercress leaves are tonic and should be eaten as often as possible to help alleviate the problem. *(See page 94.)*
• Sesame seeds have a beneficial effect in maintaining and enhancing sexual vigor.
• Pumpkin seeds are a male sexual tonic, and are used in the treatment of prostate problems.

HERBALISM
• Saw palmetto is able to reduce inflammation of the prostate. *(See page 131.)*

• Couchgrass and horsetail can be given to help encourage urination, and can be drunk freely throughout the day as a natural diuretic.

AROMATHERAPY
• Clary sage and geranium, which have estrogen-like oils, can be used in whole-body massage or in the bath to treat the condition. *(See pages 165 and 169.)*
• Bergamot, chamomile, and myrrh are anti-inflammatory, and will ease symptoms, particularly of prostatitis. *(See pages 146–71.)*
• Benzoin, sandalwood, frankincense, and cedarwood are all diuretic, and can be used both in the bath and for a full-body massage. *(See pages146–71.)*

HOMEOPATHY
Constitutional treatment would be required, but in the meantime the following remedies can be taken 4 times daily for 3 to 4 weeks:
• Arg. nit., for impotence because erection is lost on penetration, and for pain on intercourse and low libido. *(See page 181.)*
• Sabal, for difficult or painful urination, and spasms of pain. Also for enlarged prostate, and if intercourse is painful.

• Pulsatilla, for thick yellow discharge from the penis and an urgent desire to urinate. *(See page 209.)*
• Thuja, for burning at the neck of the bladder and a frequent need to urinate. *(See page 216.)*
• Baryta carb., for a frequent urge to urinate, a slow stream of urine, and premature ejaculation. *(See page 185.)*
• Iodum, for loss of potency, with shrunken testicles and hard prostate gland.

VITAMINS AND MINERALS
• Lecithin, calcium, and magnesium may help treat prostate disorders. *(See pages 271, 258, and 262.)*
• An increased intake of zinc can help to prevent and treat prostatitis. *(See page 265.)*
• Evening primrose has been successfully used for prostate problems. *(See page 270.)*
• Cold-pressed linseed oil can help if the condition is mild but recurrent.
• Flower pollen is widely used to treat problems of the prostate gland. *(See page 271.)*

Erection Problems

Failure to achieve an erection that is firm enough, or sustained for long enough, to allow normal sexual intercourse is generally known as impotence. Its cause may be physical (organic), psychological, or a combination of both. Organic impotence may be due to an imperfect blood supply to the penis, an age-related loss of male sex hormones, diabetes, medicinal drugs, or various neurological conditions. Psychological factors such as lack of desire, depression, or fear of failure may be responsible for impotence, and alcohol, while enhancing sexual desire, can actually impede performance.

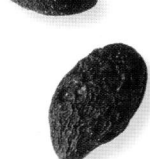

ABOVE *Saw palmetto is a strengthening tonic and will help the male reproductive system.*

DATA FILE

• Approximately 30 million men in the U.S. suffer from impotence.

• It is now believed that up to 85 percent of cases have a physical cause.

• The Association for Male Sexual Dysfunction recognizes over 200 drugs that may cause it, including alcohol, antihistamines, antidepressants, narcotics, diuretics, sedatives, nicotine.

• Primary impotence is the case in which the male has never maintained an erection of long enough duration to engage in sexual intercourse.

• Secondary impotence is when a previously potent male loses the ability to maintain an erection during intercourse.

• Fear of failure and performance anxiety are frequently underlying negative psychological sources of impotence.

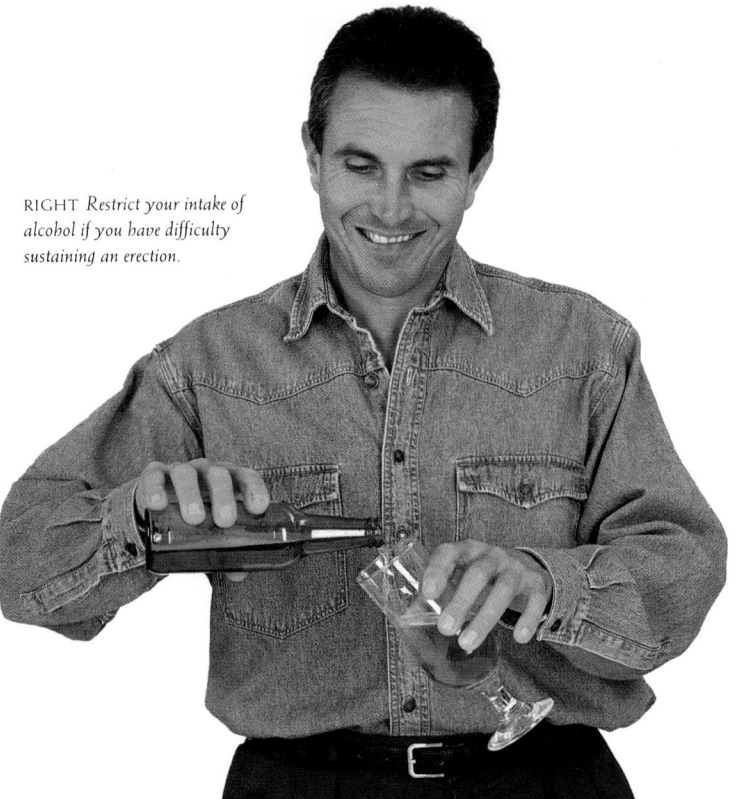

RIGHT *Restrict your intake of alcohol if you have difficulty sustaining an erection.*

TREATMENT

AYURVEDA
• Sandalwood is good for impotence, and accompanying anxiety and nervousness. *(See page 44.)*
• Cinnamon tones the muscles and is noted for treating impotence. *(See page 34.)*
• Ginger is warming and can help improve matters. *(See page 47.)*
• Saffron is used for impotence and anxiety. *(See page 36.)*
• Clove, ginger, cardamom, cinnamon, vetiver, and coriander are aphrodisiac, which may help. *(See pages 34, 35, 38, 46, and 47.)*

CHINESE HERBALISM
• Ginseng can improve vitality and help to reduce feelings of anxiety. *(See page 67.)*
• Impotence is believed to be caused by weakness of the Kidneys and Liver, with Liver qi stagnation, and cibot root may be useful.
• Chinese angelica, white peony root, and thorowax will help feelings of anxiety. *(See pages 56 and 67.)*

TRADITIONAL HOME AND FOLK REMEDIES
• Watercress leaves are tonic and should be eaten as often as possible to help alleviate the problem. *(See page 94.)*
• Sesame seeds have a beneficial effect in maintaining and enhancing sexual vigor.

• Pumpkin seeds are a male sexual tonic.
• Avocado pear is excellent if you suffer from sexual problems. *(See page 96.)*

HERBALISM
• Peppermint leaves stimulate and warm the body, and will help to reduce feelings of anxiety. *(See page 125.)*
• Anise is a powerful tonic: drink small amounts to treat impotence.
• Remedies like damiana and saw palmetto have dual hormonal effects, stimulating and toning the male reproductive system, and restoring nerves. *(See pages 131 and 135.)*

AROMATHERAPY
• Essential oils of clary sage, sandalwood, and ylang ylang are natural aphrodisiacs and will help you to relax. Try a full-body massage, or a few drops in the bath. *(See page 146–71.)*

HOMEOPATHY
• Lycopodium, when you feel surges of desire, but anticipate failure. *(See page 203.)*
• Agnus, for an erection that is not firm enough for successful penetration.
• Conium, for an erection which does not last.
• Caladium, for erections which occur during sleep, but disappear on waking, and a lack of erection even when sexually excited. *(See page 91.)*

FLOWER ESSENCES
• Larch, for lack of sexual confidence and feelings of inadequacy. *(See page 233.)*
• Gentian, for a sense of failure. *(See page 230.)*
• Sweet Chestnut, for despair and hopelessness. *(See page 227.)*
• Crab Apple, for feeling unclean on any level. *(See page 234.)*

VITAMINS AND MINERALS
• Avoid alcohol, drugs, and caffeine, which constrict the blood vessels and inhibit the blood flow needed to achieve an erection.
• Molybdenum can prevent impotence and sexual difficulties. *(See page 263.)*
• Zinc is required for the healthy functioning of the reproductive organs, and should be included in a varied, healthy diet. *(See page 265.)*
• L-tryptophan may help to prevent feelings of anxiety from causing sexual difficulties. *(See page 269.)*

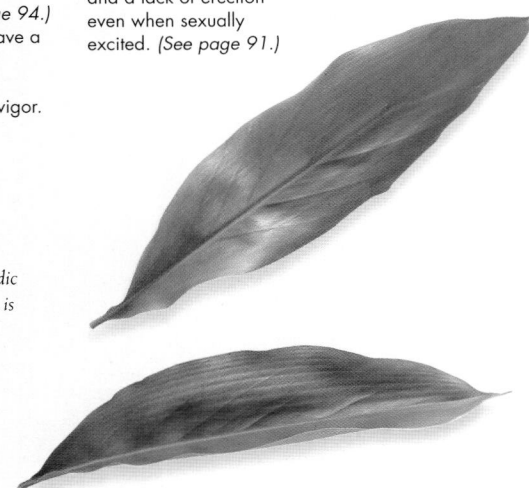

RIGHT *In Ayurvedic medicine cardamom is recommended as an aphrodisiac.*

Ejaculation Problems

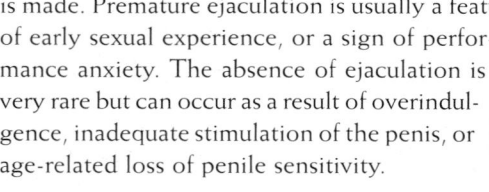

For men, orgasm is usually accompanied by ejaculation. A single ejaculate contains about 300 million sperm in a fluid medium called semen. Ejaculation is a two-phased process. In the emission phase seminal fluid accumulates in the bulb of the prostate. In the expulsion phase the neck of the urinary bladder closes to ensure that no urine will mix with the semen, and the muscles at the base of the penis and of the penile urethra contract to force the semen out of the urethral opening. Some men experience a "retrograde," or dry, ejaculation as a result of genetics, illness, medication, surgery, or damage to the valves of the urethra that control the flow of semen.

In most cases ejaculation problems are psycho-sexual in origin, and not due to any physical abnormality, so that a man may experience sexual failure with one partner, but function quite normally with another. There are two main problems: premature ejaculation and absence of ejaculation. Premature ejaculation is very common indeed and refers to the occurrence of the male orgasm at the time of penetration, or very soon after. In extreme cases it may even take place before physical contact is made. Premature ejaculation is usually a feature of early sexual experience, or a sign of performance anxiety. The absence of ejaculation is very rare but can occur as a result of overindulgence, inadequate stimulation of the penis, or age-related loss of penile sensitivity.

ABOVE Ginseng works as an aphrodisiac and is recommended for men who have sexual problems due to anxiety.

RIGHT Most ejaculation problems have a psychological origin. Eat oats, which have relaxing and therapeutic qualities.

TREATMENT

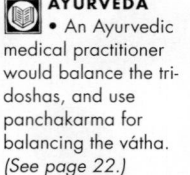 **AYURVEDA**
• An Ayurvedic medical practitioner would balance the tridoshas, and use panchakarma for balancing the vátha. *(See page 22.)*
• Sandalwood may help to relieve anxiety, and has an anesthetic effect on the area which can reduce premature ejaculation. *(See page 44.)*
• Saffron may be helpful. *(See page 36.)*

CHINESE HERBALISM
• Treatment may address weakness of the Kidneys and Liver, and deal with Liver qi stagnation. Cibot root may work well.
• Problems causing or associated with anxiety may be treated with ginseng, Chinese angelica, white peony root, and thorowax root. *(See pages 56 and 67.)*

TRADITIONAL HOME AND FOLK REMEDIES
• Oats contain thiamine and pantothenic acid, which act as gentle tonics for the nerves and will relax and calm you. Take regularly. *(See page 84.)*

HERBALISM
• Herbal remedies would be used to calm the nervous system and to relax. *(See page 104.)*
• Skullcap and valerian are useful herbs, and should be blended together for best effect. Drink this as a tea three times daily to calm. *(See pages 131 and 136.)*
• Lady's slipper and lime blossom may also work to ease anxiety and tension associated with the condition.

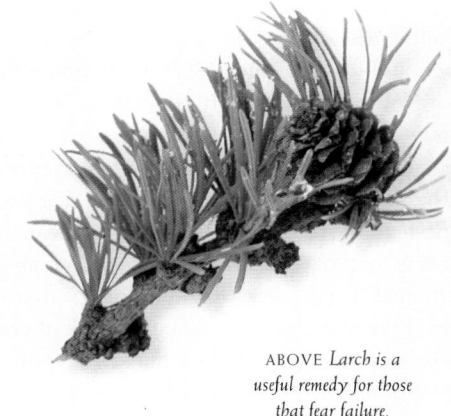

ABOVE Larch is a useful remedy for those that fear failure.

• Remedies like damiana and saw palmetto have hormonal effects, stimulating and toning the male reproductive system and restoring nerves. *(See pages 131 and 135.)*

AROMATHERAPY
• A relaxing blend of essential oils of lavender, geranium, and bergamot in sweet almond oil or peach kernel oil may be used in the bath at times of great stress and anxiety. *(See pages 146–71.)*

HOMEOPATHY
Constitutional treatment will be necessary, but the following remedies may be of some use:
• Lycopodium, for an increased sexual desire; lack of self-confidence and expectation of failure with premature ejaculation. *(See page 203.)*
• Nux vomica., for impatience, craving excitement, short temper, and use of stimulating drugs. *(See page 214.)*
• Graphites, for loss of sex drive, premature or non-existent ejaculation. *(See page 196.)*
• Nitric acid, for irritability, self-criticism, and extreme sensitivity.

• Ignatia, for problems caused by grief or disappointment. *(See page 200.)*
• Mercurius, when thrush or urethritis causes the problem. *(See page 205.)* *(See also Prostate Problems, page 400).*

FLOWER ESSENCES
• Try Elm for anxiety accompanying a feeling of being unable to cope. *(See page 241.)*
• Larch may help with lack of self-confidence. *(See page 233.)*
• Gentian may be useful for a sense of failure. *(See page 230.)*
• Rescue Remedy or Emergency Essence, taken before intercourse, can help to calm and relax you. *(See page 244.)*

VITAMINS AND MINERALS
• Increase your intake of B vitamins, which work on the nervous system, and avoid caffeine or other stimulants in any form. *(See pages 252–5.)*

Priapism

Priapism is the name given to prolonged and painful erection in the absence of sexual interest. It is caused by failure of the blood to return from the penis to the circulation after a period of sexual activity. This may be because of a disturbance in the nervous system's control of blood flow, due to a disease of the spinal cord or brain. It may also be caused by clotting due to leukemia or sickle-cell anemia, inflammation of the prostate, bladder stones, or urethritis.

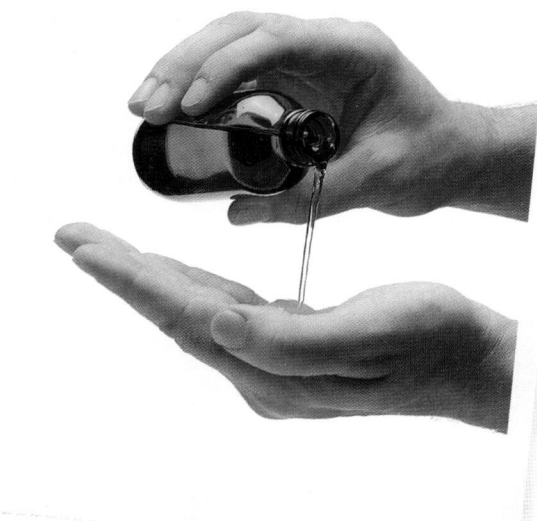

CAUTION

LONG-SUSTAINED ERECTION CAN BE DANGEROUS AS THERE IS A RISK OF THROMBOSIS, WHICH MAY CAUSE PERMANENT LOSS OF ERECTILE FUNCTION.

LEFT *Bergamot oil is recommended for priapism as it is anti-inflammatory. Massage the area or use the oil in a bath.*

Dang Gui reduces pain and stimulates the circulation

Gui Zhi regulates the movement of bodily fluids

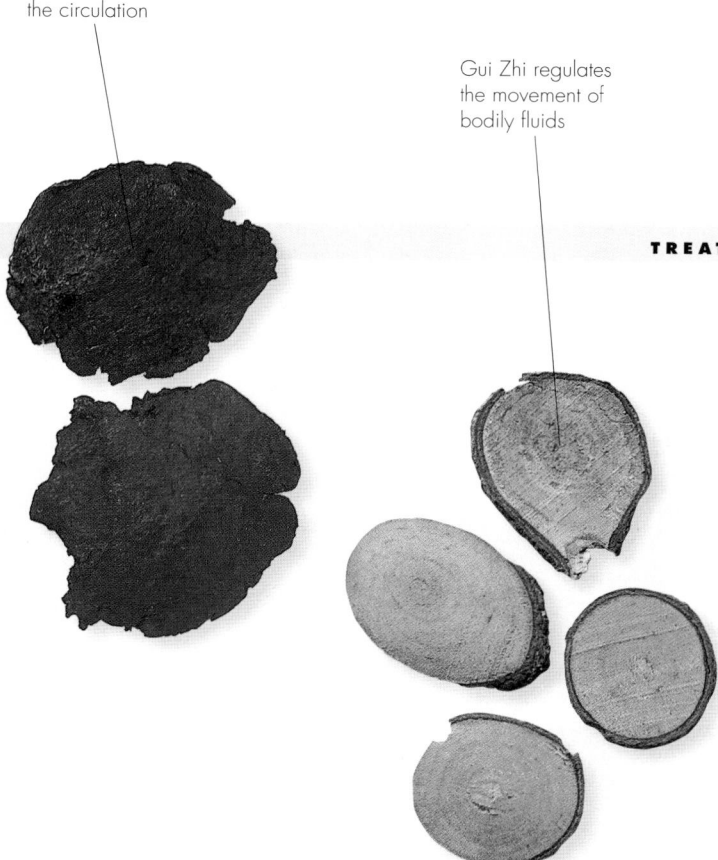

ABOVE *Chinese medicines that are used to treat priapism include Gui Zhi and Dang Gui.*

TREATMENT

AYURVEDA
• Angelica can improve circulation. *(See page 28.)*
• Black pepper increases blood circulation and feeds the nervous system. *(See page 44.)*
• Calamus oil massage will improve circulation in the area. *(See page 24.)*
• Cayenne pepper is analgesic and warming. *(See page 31.)*

CHINESE HERBALISM
• Gui Zhi may be useful when the yang qi has failed to move fluids through channels. *(See page 59.)*
• Dang Gui will reduce pain and invigorates blood circulation. *(See page 56.)*

HERBALISM
Herbs which encourage circulation include:
• Broom, which tones the arteries.
• Ginger, hawthorn tops, and rosemary, which are stimulating and work to encourage circulation. *(See pages 119, 127, and 139.)*
• Lavender and vervain, which are calming, and can be sipped during an attack to ease symptoms. *(See page 138.)*
See also the sections on *Prostate problems, page 400; Urethritis, page 380; and Bladder Stones; page 379.*

AROMATHERAPY
• Local massage with rosemary or peppermint is stimulating and will help normalize the blood flow in the area. *(See pages 164 and 168.)*
• Massage the area with diluted juniper, marjoram, myrrh, or tea tree, which will act as a tonic. *(See pages 146–71.)*

• Bergamot is anti-inflammatory, and may be used in local massage or in the bath to ease inflammatory conditions causing priapism. *(See page 153.)*

HOMEOPATHY
Treatment would be constitutional, but during an attack the following remedies may help:
• Carb. veg., for sluggish circulation, and possibly piles and varicose veins. *(See page 188.)*
• Kali brom., for the treatment of impotence.
• Cantharis, for a painful erection. *(See page 188.)*

VITAMINS AND MINERALS
• Vitamin E is suggested. *(See page 257.)*
• Vitamin C, which affects the health of the circulatory system, may be useful. *(See page 256.)*

DISORDERS OF THE ENDOCRINE SYSTEM

Thyroid Problems

The thyroid gland, found in the neck, is responsible for controlling the general level of activity of the body. An overactive gland (hyperthyroidism) causes a racing heart, increased digestion, and enormous physical energy. Untreated, this condition can lead to heart failure and extreme weight loss, among other things. An underactive gland (hypothyroidism) leads to apathy, overwhelming fatigue, heart problems, menstrual problems, and weight gain. Thyroid problems are very common and, fortunately, they can be diagnosed long before they become serious, and various remedies can then be applied. Occasionally thyroid disease forms part of a wider disease process, including diabetes and rheumatoid arthritis. Other causes of thyroid disease include iodine deficiency, which may exist from birth and features in mental retardation, enlargement of the thyroid gland (goiter), inflammation, and, rarely, cancer.

TREATMENT

AYURVEDA
• An Ayurvedic medical practitioner may suggest panchakarma Method for detoxification. *(See page 22.)*

CHINESE HERBALISM
• Hyperthyroidism is believed to be caused by Heat in the Liver, and marine plants and seaweed are prescribed.

HERBALISM
• Bugleweed is excellent, and should be drunk 3 times daily for hyperthyroidism.
• Bladderwrack helps to regulate the function of the thyroid gland. Take 3 times daily, in any form. *(See page 122.)*

AROMATHERAPY
• Geranium oil balances hormone production, and will help to ensure that the thyroid gland is working effectively. Use the oil in the bath, or in an overall massage for best effect. *(See page 165.)*

HOMEOPATHY
Treatment will be constitutional and aimed at controlling acute symptoms. Long-term control of the condition should be undertaken by a physician. However, specific remedies which may help control symptoms are:
Hyperthyroidism:
• Iodum, when the sufferer feels hot, cannot stop activity, is obsessive, and probably dark-haired and brown-eyed.

• Nat. mur., for symptoms accompanied by constipation, palpitations and earthy-colored complexion. *(See page 206.)*
• Belladonna, when symptoms include a flushed face and staring eyes. *(See page 183.)*
• Lycopus, when the heart is pounding and racing.
Hypothyroidism:
• Arsenicum can be taken for up to five days, twice daily, while constitutional treatment is being sought. *(See page 182.)*

VITAMINS AND MINERALS
• Nutritional deficiencies (for example, zinc, Vitamin A, selenium, and iron) and a toxic overload are thought to be the main factors involved in the onset of hypothyroidism. Ensure that you eat a good healthy diet, with plenty of fresh organic vegetables, seafood, and onions.
• Garlic and onions are both particularly valuable if the patient's thyroid gland is underactive.

• Supplement your diet with natural thyroid hormones created from iodine, and the amino acid tyrosine for hypothyroidism. *(See pages 261 and 269.)*
• Garlic is a rich source of iodine, which can help regulate thyroid function. *(See page 261.)*

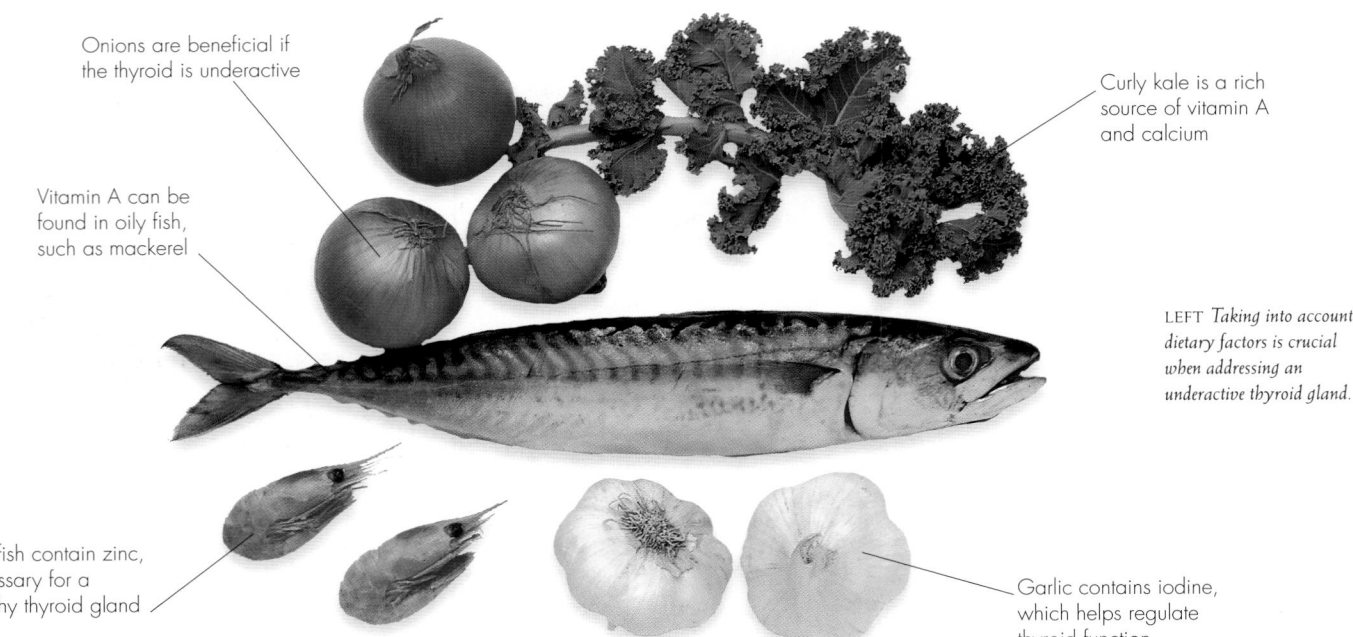

Onions are beneficial if the thyroid is underactive

Vitamin A can be found in oily fish, such as mackerel

Curly kale is a rich source of vitamin A and calcium

LEFT *Taking into account dietary factors is crucial when addressing an underactive thyroid gland.*

Shellfish contain zinc, necessary for a healthy thyroid gland

Garlic contains iodine, which helps regulate thyroid function

Disorders of the thyroid include:

• Iodine deficiency. Iodine is an essential element in the thyroid hormone. Deficiency of iodine is rare, but can cause cretinism – physical and mental retardation featuring poor feeding, constipation, a characteristic cry, and a large tongue.

• Hypothyroidism, underaction of the thyroid. Features slowing of physical and mental processes, sensitivity to cold, obesity, no sweating, loss of hair, a puffy face, coronary artery disease. Untreated, hypothyroidism may lead to coma.

• Hyperthyroidism, overaction of the thyroid. Features weight loss, increased appetite, palpitations, anxiety, irritability, dislike of heat, sweating, and infrequent menstruation. Untreated it may lead to heart failure.

• In the U.K. researchers discovered that one in ten people suffering from Parkinson's disease also suffered from hyperthyroidism.

• Over 5 million people in the U.S. suffer from thyroid problems; 90 percent of them are women.

• Goiter. Various conditions can cause goiter, an enlargement of the thyroid gland

• If goiter is caused by a low dietary intake of iodine, it is termed endemic (colloid) goiter.

• Overproduction of hormones in the thyroid gland, which may follow emotional or physical stress, results in toxic diffuse goiter (Grave's disease) or toxic nodular goiter (Plummer's disease), both of which are characterized by nervousness, sweating, weight loss, and hyperactivity.

• Cancer. Thyroid cancer is quite rare and is usually found as a single firm lump in the neck. It may spread to the lymph nodes in the neck and can involve the vocal cords, causing hoarseness or loss of the voice.

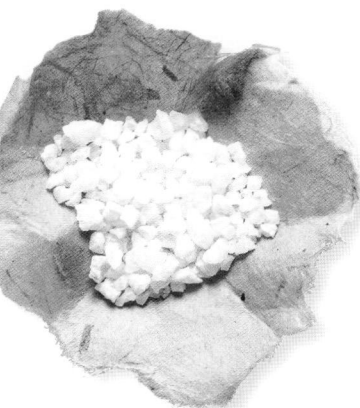

ABOVE *Nat. mur., made from rock salt, is a possible homeopathic remedy for thyroid problems.*

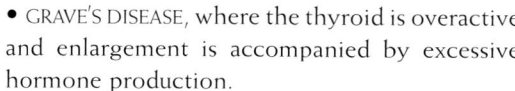

ABOVE *Clary sage oils helps to balance hormones, which may stimulate an underactive thyroid.*

Goiter

Goiter is an enlargement of the thyroid gland, visible as a swelling on the neck, and is fairly common. In order for the thyroid to produce hormones it requires iodine in the diet for their synthesis. If there is insufficient iodine in the diet the gland increases its activity and swells, resulting in a goiter. The nontoxic enlargement of the thyroid due to insufficient iodine is common and easily remedied by eating more fish and iodized salt, thereby increasing iodine intake. Conditions of which goiter is a feature are:

• GRAVE'S DISEASE, where the thyroid is overactive and enlargement is accompanied by excessive hormone production.

• HASHIMOTO'S THYROIDITIS, where the thyroid is underactive due to antibodies to thyroid hormone. Causes an ache in the neck and difficulty in swallowing.

• SUB-ACUTE THYROIDITIS, probably a viral infection which causes inflammation and pain.

• DYSHORMONOGENESIS, a genetic enzyme deficiency which interferes with normal hormone synthesis.

• TUMORS of the thyroid gland, which may be benign or malignant.

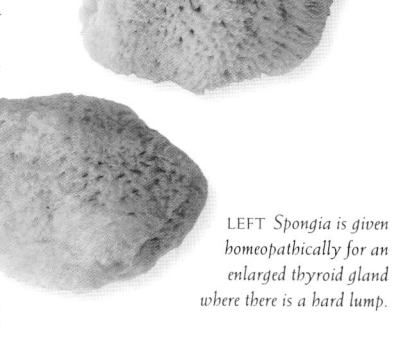

LEFT *Spongia is given homeopathically for an enlarged thyroid gland where there is a hard lump.*

SYMPTOMS

• *swelling at the front of the neck, which may vary from a small lump to a very large mass* • *difficulty in swallowing or breathing in severe cases* • *hyperthyroidism (overactive thyroid): weight loss – increased appetite – warm, dry skin – tremor – insomnia – bulging eyes –*
• *hypothyroidism (underactive thyroid): tiredness – muscle weakness – weight gain – flaky skin – hair loss – deepening voice*

TREATMENT

HERBALISM
• Bladderwrack, brown seaweed, can help goiter caused by an underactive thyroid. *(See page 122.)*
• Bugleweed is used to treat an overactive thyroid.

AROMATHERAPY
• Clary sage has a balancing effect on hormones, and since it is now believed that an underactive thyroid may be linked to an excess of female hormones, this may be a useful oil. *(See page 169.)*

HOMEOPATHY
The following remedies, taken twice daily for up to 2 weeks, should improve the condition:

• Iodum, for someone who is always in a hurry and feeling hot.
• Spongia, for a long-standing condition, where there is a hard lump. *(See page 213.)*
• Calcarea, for a pale, chilly, overweight person. *(See page 186.)*
• Fluoric acid, for elderly sufferers who are young-thinking, vigorous, and with varicose veins.

VITAMINS AND MINERALS
• Increase your intake of salt, fish, seafish, and kelp to ensure adequate iodine. *(See page 261.)*

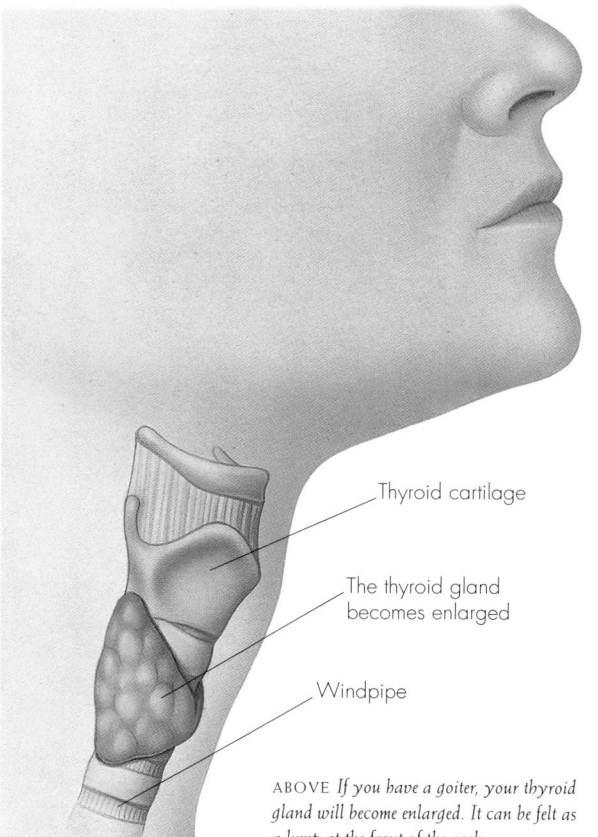

Thyroid cartilage

The thyroid gland becomes enlarged

Windpipe

ABOVE *If you have a goiter, your thyroid gland will become enlarged. It can be felt as a lump at the front of the neck.*

Diabetes

The most common form of diabetes is diabetes mellitus. It is caused by a lack of, or insufficient, insulin (the hormone produced by the pancreas), as a result of which the body is unable to process glucose. This causes a high level of glucose in the blood, and low absorption of the vital energy-producing glucose by the tissues. In Type I (insulin-dependency) diabetes the sufferer produces little or no insulin and requires lifelong monitoring. Blood sugar levels can swing wildly between hypoglycemia (featuring strange feelings, abnormal behavior, and a risk of coma) and hyperglycemia (causing overproduction of ketones, and coma). Type I usually first appears in those who are under the age of 35, particularly adolescents, and develops rapidly. Type II, maturity-onset diabetes, is thought to be caused by the body's cells' lack of response to insulin. It usually affects people aged 40 and over, and there is an association with obesity and pregnancy. The onset of Type II is gradual and may go unnoticed for some time.

ABOVE Scientific studies have shown that onions reduce blood sugar levels for longer periods than insulin, but more slowly.

SYMPTOMS

- *excessive thirst* • *excessive urination* • *weight loss* • *fatigue, weakness, and apathy* • *hunger* • *bad breath* • *complications include: nerve damage (causing damage to the eye muscles and double vision as a result) – damage to blood vessels affecting the eyes (sometimes causing blindness), kidneys, circulation in the legs – organic impotence – arterial disease and gangrene*

RIGHT Try to ensure that you include garlic in your diet. If you do not like the taste, take garlic oil supplements.

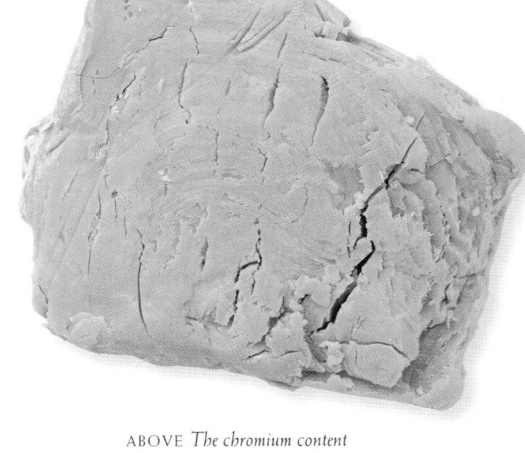

ABOVE The chromium content of brewer's yeast may help blood sugar levels to remain constant.

TREATMENT

AYURVEDA
- An Ayurvedic practitioner would recommend oral preparations from herbs that act upon the levels of glucose in the blood. There have been good results from treatment, with some cases being resolved within as little as 2 months. *(See page 22.)*
- For non-insulin-dependent diabetes, boil and cut one karella into small pieces and eat with the seeds every morning and evening.

CHINESE HERBALISM
- Lilyturf root, grassy privet, lotus seed, and Chinese yam are suggested.
- Treatment aimed at nourishing the Spleen, Kidneys, and Stomach would use Chinese yam, lotus seed, and mulberry.

HERBALISM
- Onions and garlic lower blood sugar levels. Ensure that you have plenty in your diet; take garlic oil supplements if not. *(See page 113.)*
- Fenugreek seed works to control blood sugar levels. Drink daily.

- Alfalfa is recommended for diabetics, and it should be taken daily.

HOMEOPATHY
Constitutional treatment will be balancing and can be taken alongside conventional medication. In some cases the condition has been completely cured through homeopathy, but it must be undertaken by a registered practitioner.

VITAMINS AND MINERALS
- Brewer's yeast contains chromium, which helps to normalize blood sugar levels and metabolism. Take 2–3 tablespoons daily. *(See page 272.)*

RIGHT Fenugreek seeds regulate blood sugar levels. Drink a decoction daily.

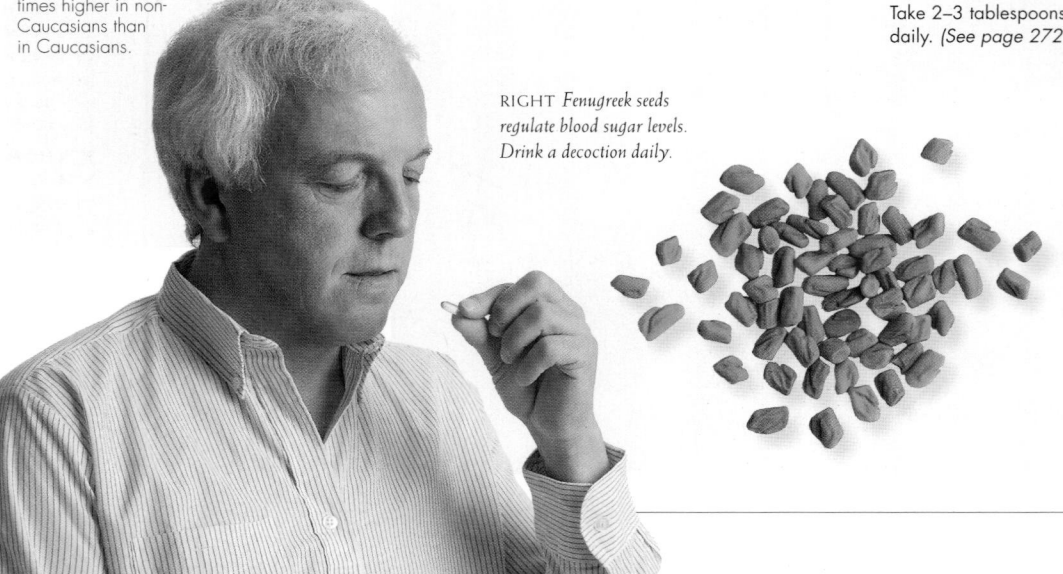

Addison's Disease

Addison's disease is a disorder of the adrenal glands which leads to insufficient output of cortisol and aldosterone – the steroid hormones which help the body to react to stress and control water balance, respectively. The disease is caused by an inflammation followed by atrophy of the outer layer (cortex) of the adrenal gland. This in turn is caused by abnormal action of the immune system in which it behaves towards the gland tissue as though it were foreign. Addison's is therefore known as an auto-immune disease. Addison's disease is usually due to damage by an auto-immune reaction, tuberculosis, or fungal infections. Addison's disease is rare, and generally has a slow onset and chronic course, with symptoms developing gradually over months or years. Acute episodes, called Addisonian crises, can be brought on by infection, injury, or other stresses, and they occur because the adrenal glands cannot increase their production of steroid hormones which normally help the body to deal with stress. The condition was invariably fatal before hormone treatment became available in the 1950s.

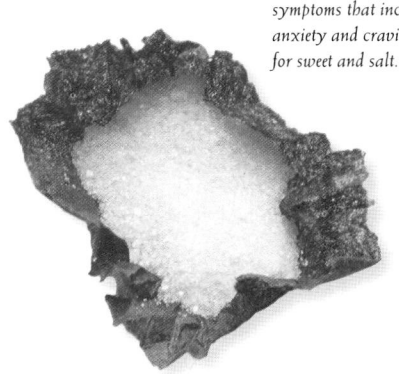

BELOW *Argentum nitricum is the homeopathic remedy for symptoms that include anxiety and cravings for sweet and salt.*

SYMPTOMS

• *weakness* • *fatigue* • *low blood pressure* • *excessive urination*
• *dehydration* • *skin discoloration, as the pituitary gland attempts to compensate for insufficient adrenal output by overproducing another hormone which stimulates the pigment cells*

TREATMENT

HERBALISM
• Treatment to stimulate the endocrine system; herbs to boost the immune system may also be appropriate. Treatment would be individual.

AROMATHERAPY
• Oils which strengthen the adrenal system include: rosemary, ginger, and lemongrass. *(See pages 146–71.)*

HOMEOPATHY
Treatment would be constitutional; however, the following treatments may help. If you don't feel any better after a week or so, see your doctor.
• Silicea, when your feet are sweaty and smelly, cold weather makes the symptoms worse, and you feel really exhausted. *(See page 211.)*

• Nat. mur., for when you have constipation, dry lips, a craving for salt, and symptoms which are made worse by sun. *(See page 206.)*
• Arg. nit., for apprehension, salt and sweet cravings, and tremors. *(See page 181.)*

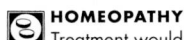

LEFT *Lemongrass essential oil is used by aromatherapists to strengthen the adrenal system.*

Hypoglycemia

Hypoglycemia is a condition in which there is an abnormally low level of glucose in the blood. It is extremely dangerous because the brain is dependent on a constant supply of glucose. The most common cause of hypoglycemia is a relative insulin overdose by diabetics (i.e. the actual amount of insulin taken may be correct, but the intake of carbohydrate or the amount of exertion may have used up the supply too quickly). Excessive exercise and insufficient carbohydrate may, in fact, lead to hypoglycemia in non-diabetics.

SYMPTOMS

• *headache and faintness* • *rapid pulse and palpitations* • *profuse sweating* • *mental confusion and loss of memory* • *irrational and disorderly behavior* • *slurred speech* • *numbness, temporary paralysis* • *fits and, eventually, potentially fatal coma*

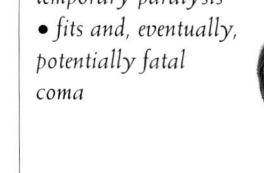

RIGHT *Eating onions will help to regulate blood sugar levels.*

DATA FILE

• The condition occurs in association with a number of diseases, most notably insulin overdose in diabetics.

• Repeated severe attacks can cause permanent brain damage.

• There are two main types of hypoglycemia: organic and functional.

• Any endocrine malfunction in the pancreas and adrenal glands, as well as the pituitary, thyroid, or sex glands, may result in organic hypoglycemia. Alcoholism, which impairs the liver's ability to produce glucose, can also lead to organic hypoglycemia, as can other disorders of the liver and tumors of the liver or pancreas.

• Functional hypoglycemia is a temporary condition of markedly lowered blood sugar, most commonly occurring 2–3 hours after a meal high in carbohydrates.

• 50 percent of sufferers over the age of 50 have a thyroid problem.

TREATMENT

AYURVEDA
• Plants which act on blood sugar levels will be prescribed, as well as detoxification treatment to ensure that the system is working efficiently. *(See page 22.)*

TRADITIONAL HOME AND FOLK REMEDIES
• Onions and garlic will help to regulate blood sugar levels. Eat raw or cooked, as often as possible. *(See page 82.)*

CHINESE HERBALISM
• Chinese yam and lotus seed will help to normalize blood sugar levels.

HOMEOPATHY
• Homeopathic treatment would be constitutional, but well worth it, because in many cases the condition can be cured completely.

FLOWER ESSENCES
• Take Rescue Remedy if you feel an attack coming on. It will calm you and help to reduce the severity. *(See page 244.)*

VITAMINS AND MINERALS
• Take extra Vitamin C and B-complex tablets, chromium (to regulate blood sugar levels), magnesium, potassium, zinc, and manganese. *(See pages 256, 252–5, 259, 262, 265, and 263.)*

Obesity

Obesity is the excessive storage of energy in the form of fat, and applies to a bodyweight that is more than 20 percent over the recommended maximum for a person's height. The main cause of obesity is excessive calorie intake, but other factors include a low basal metabolic rate, genetic factors, emotional problems, metabolic disorders such as thyroid problems, taking steroids or insulin. Obesity can aggravate or trigger other conditions such as heart attack, gallstones, arthritis, hiatus hernia, varicose veins, kidney disorders, and fertility problems. In particular, the chances of suffering from high blood pressure, stroke, and maturity-onset diabetes are greatly increased by obesity. Obese women are more likely to be at risk from cancer of the ovaries, womb, and breast; obese men are at risk from cancer of the colon, rectum and prostate. The strain on the joints of the back, knees, and hips from extra weight can also cause problems.

ABOVE *Increase your intake of pungent foods, such as peppers, to encourage the body to eliminate waste more easily.*

THE BODY MASS INDEX

• The Body Mass Index (BMI) is reached by dividing your weight in kilograms by your height in meters squared. So, if you weigh 80kg. and are 2m. tall, your BMI is 80 divided by 2x2 – 80 divided by 4 – which is 20. The graphic below shows how the index works.

• If you have a BMI of 27 or more, you double the risk of high blood pressure, heart disease, and gallstones, and are 14 times more likely to contract diabetes.

• If it is over 30, you have 4 times the risk of heart disease, high blood pressure, and gallstones, and are 30–50 times more likely to contract diabetes. You are also 4 times more likely to get degenerative arthritis.

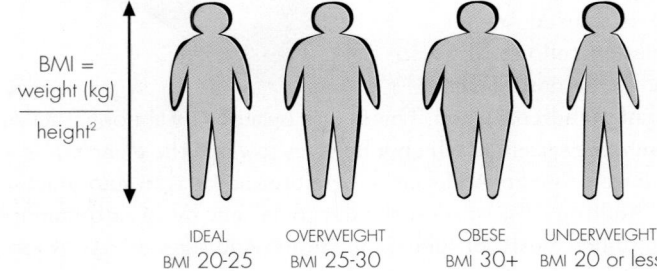

$$BMI = \frac{weight\ (kg)}{height^2}$$

| IDEAL | OVERWEIGHT | OBESE | UNDERWEIGHT |
| BMI 20-25 | BMI 25-30 | BMI 30+ | BMI 20 or less |

ABOVE *People are judged to be obese if they weigh more than 20 percent above their ideal bodyweight.*

DATA FILE

• Affects approximately 20–30 percent of the U.S. population.

• Fat should account for up to 25 percent of body weight in a healthy woman, and 17 percent in a healthy man.

• Individuals who weigh more than 20 percent above their supposed "ideal bodyweight" according to the standard height and weight tables of the Metropolitan Life Insurance Company may be judged as obese.

• At least one-third of Americans are 20 percent or more overweight.

• 25–50 percent of adult Americans are currently on a diet; $30 billion is spent on diet aids annually.

• One in every four U.S. teenagers carries enough weight to put them at risk of later health problems.

• Obesity may be classified according to the age of onset, family history, degree of obesity, and adipose tissue cell size and distribution.

• Obesity significantly increases the risk of premature death, heart attack, diabetes mellitus, hypertension, atherosclerosis, gall bladder disease, osteoarthritis, and certain cancers.

• Obese individuals with an apple shape (fat in the upper body or abdomen) are at greater risk of medical diseases than those with a pear shape (fat confined to the lower body or hips).

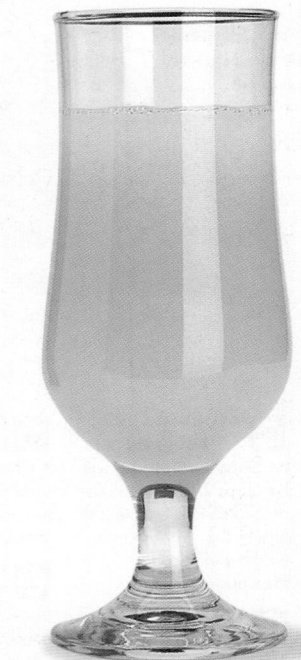

ABOVE *A daily glass of grapefruit juice will suppress the appetite and help break down fats.*

TREATMENT

AYURVEDA
• Treatment would be aimed at addressing an addiction to food, accompanied by marma puncture and a diet modified to your dosha type. *(See page 22.)*
• A complete detoxification will encourage weight loss naturally.

CHINESE HERBALISM
• Increase your intake of foods that are bitter, pungent, astringent, and hot, which will encourage your body to eliminate waste more efficiently.
• Cut down on salty, sweet, and sour foods.

TRADITIONAL HOME AND FOLK REMEDIES
• Drink a glass of freshly squeezed grapefruit juice every morning to cleanse, help break down fats, and suppress appetite. *(See page 88.)*

HERBALISM
• Bladderwrack may help to encourage the metabolism. *(See page 122.)*
• Nettles are good diuretics and generally help the metabolism. Try drinking nettle tea before meals. *(See page 137.)*

HOMEOPATHY
Constitutional treatment is most appropriate, but some of the following remedies might be useful:
• Graphites, if you suffer from constipation and skin problems, and feel cold. *(See page 196.)*
• Kali carb., if you are clogged with catarrh, have backache, and feel cold.
• Ferr. phos., if you are oversensitive and flush easily. *(See page 194.)*
• Capsicum, if you are lazy, have a red face, and suffer from burning sensations in the digestive tract.

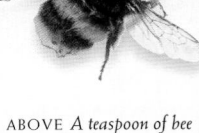

ABOVE *A teaspoon of bee pollen will stimulate the body's metabolism.*

• Calcarea, if you suffer from indigestion, and crave hot food and eggs. *(See page 186.)*

VITAMINS AND MINERALS
• Bee pollen stimulates the metabolism and helps to curb appetite. Take up to 1 teaspoon daily. *(See page 271.)*
• Brewer's yeast will help to reduce various cravings for food and drink. *(See page 272.)*
• Chromium supplements will help to ensure that your blood sugar levels are stable, and regulate appetite. *(See page 259.)*
• Phenylalanine, taken on an empty stomach before bed, encourages weight loss. *(See page 268.)*

Gout

Gout is an acute disease of the joints. It is caused by the deposition of chalky crystals around the joints, tendons, and other body tissues when there is an abnormally high level of uric acid in the body. Severe inflammation and tissue damage result, and possibly structural damage to the kidneys and stone formation. Gout affects more than 1 million Americans, mostly men between the ages of 40 and 50. Primary gout appears to involve a hereditary factor.

SYMPTOMS

The first sign of gout is usually excruciating pain and inflammation of the innermost joint of the big toe (or, less frequently, the ankle, knee joint, hand, wrist, or elbow). An attack can last for days or weeks and then subsides, but usually there are recurrences, until eventually gout is a constant presence.

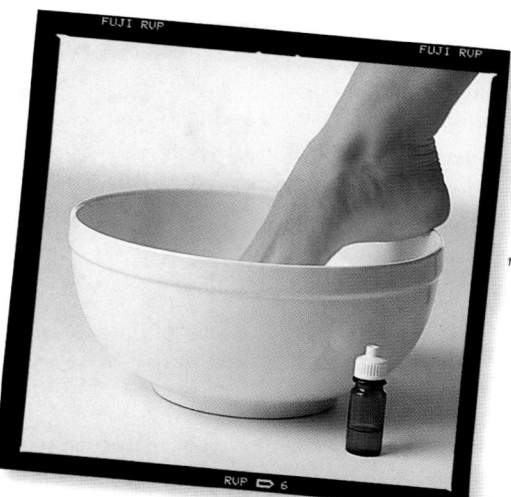

LEFT *Add a few drops of a recommended essential oil such as pine to a foot bath. This will increase the circulation and relieve the painful symptoms associated with gout.*

TREATMENT

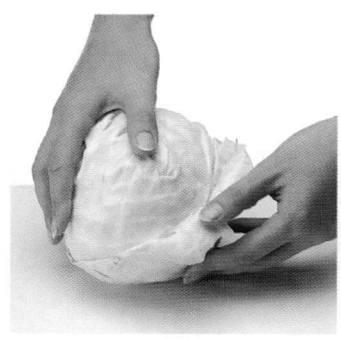

To make a soothing compress, take a few cabbage leaves.

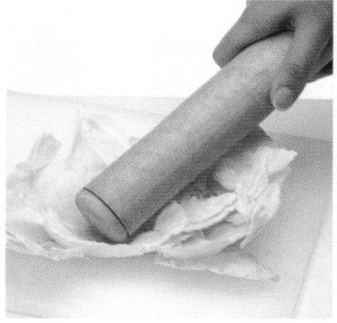

Crush the leaves with a rolling pin. Apply in a compress to the inflamed area.

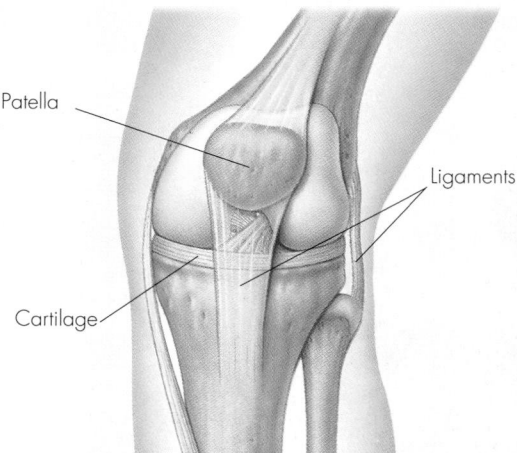

ABOVE *The symptoms of gout include acute pain in the affected joints as a result of uric acid deposits.*

Patella

Ligaments

Cartilage

CHINESE HERBALISM
• Painful joints are said to be caused by Wind Cold, and some of the most useful herbs to relieve Cold and Damp include cinnamon, aconite root, angelica root, and wild ginger.
(See pages 56 and 59.)

TRADITIONAL HOME AND FOLK REMEDIES
• Raw apple and cucumber juice will help to reduce the severity and incidence of attacks.
(See pages 89 and 94.)

HERBALISM
• Drink plenty of water and cleansing infusions such as celery seed tea.
• Bring down the acute inflammation with a compress made of crushed cabbage leaf.
• Nettle tea is helpful in preventing attacks.
(See page 137.)

AROMATHERAPY
• Rub a few drops of lavender and frankincense, mixed in a little grapeseed oil, into the affected joints.
(See pages 146–71.)
• Pine, rosemary, or juniper oils, which increase circulation, can be added to the bath or added to a foot-bath to ease the condition. Rub them neat into the affected joints.
(See pages 146–71.)

HOMEOPATHY
Homeopathic treatment would be constitutional, but in an attack one of the following remedies may be appropriate:
• Pulsatilla, for fleeting pains. *(See page 209.)*
• Lycopodium, for symptoms that are worse between 4–8P.M.
(See page 203.)
• Urtica, for joints that feel hot and itchy.
(See page 217.)

• Arnica, for painful joints which feel bruised.
(See page 182.)
• Ledum, for joints that are cold and swollen, and are improved by moving about. *(See page 202.)*

VITAMINS AND MINERALS
• A good diet is the key. Eat plenty of fresh, green vegetables and avoid high-protein foods such as red meat and seafood.
• Eat food containing plenty of vitamin C (or take supplements of 1g. daily). *(See page 256.)*
• Avoid alcohol, which increases uric acid.
• Charcoal tablets may help to reduce the levels of uric acid in the body.
(See page 273.)

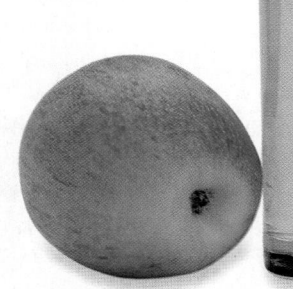
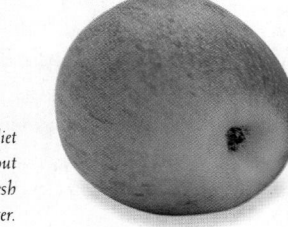
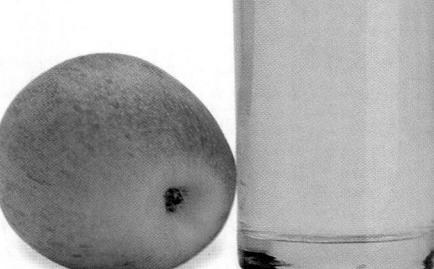

RIGHT *A change of diet will help symptoms of gout to subside. Include fresh fruit and plenty of water.*

DISORDERS OF THE IMMUNE SYSTEM

HIV and AIDS

HIV is the human immunodeficiency virus, which makes the immune system unable to fight off infections. HIV is believed to be responsible for AIDS (acquired immune deficiency syndrome). Once acquired, HIV remains in the body for life, although there may be no symptoms for years. HIV may be contracted from transfusion of contaminated blood; from infected blood passing through the skin barrier via a deep graze, needle puncture, or a wound; in the womb or at birth; by breast-feeding; or through unsafe sex. When the immune system reaches a particular stage of deterioration due to HIV, certain bacteria which are usually kept in check by healthy immune functioning are able to thrive (opportunistic infections). AIDS is diagnosed when one or more of these infections is present, but AIDS is not a disease in itself. Previously an AIDS diagnosis suggested that death would follow quickly, but improvement in drugs treatments may change the implications of an AIDS diagnosis.

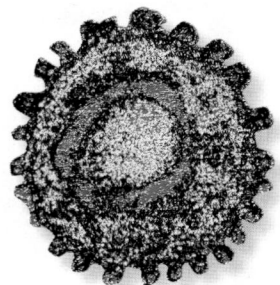

ABOVE *The HIV virus, which weakens the human immune system, leaving it open to infection.*

DATA FILE

• Since the first AIDS cases were reported in 1981, through mid-1995, more than 476,000 AIDS cases and more than 295,000 deaths have been reported in the U.S.

• Nearly 1 million Americans were infected with HIV through the mid-1990s but do not yet have clinical symptoms.

• AIDS cases have also been reported in almost every country in the world, with an estimated cumulative 19 million adults and children infected worldwide since the late 1970s.

• Many of those infected with HIV may not even be aware that they carry and can spread the virus.

• 90 percent of HIV-positive children under the age of 13 acquired HIV from their infected mothers; around one child in twelve born to infected women is HIV-positive. All babies born to infected mothers will test positive for HIV at birth, because the test is for antibodies to HIV and the baby has the mother's antibodies in its blood. Babies who test positive after 18 months (when the baby has developed its own antibodies) are actually infected with the virus.

• The period between initial infection and production of antibodies is three to six months.

• Estimates indicate that somewhere between 26–46 percent of the infected individuals will go on to develop AIDS within a little more than seven years following infection with HIV.

• Once AIDS is diagnosed, the clinical course generally follows a rapid decline; most people with AIDS die within three years. However, recent scientific advances in triple-drug therapy may extend life expectancy.

SYMPTOMS

• *flu-like symptoms when HIV first enters the system (seroconversion)*
• *once the virus has begun to work on the immune system there will be: night sweats and fevers – exhaustion – weight loss – diarrhea – thrush and herpes – mouth ulcers and bleeding gums* • *conditions associated with AIDS itself include: neurological problems – fits and confusion – yellow skin and swollen painful joints – Kaposi's sarcoma, a rare form of skin cancer characterized by raised purple blotches – eye infections, particularly cytomegalovirus (CMV), which can lead to blindness – gut infections – pneumocystis carinii pneumonia (PCP)*

TREATMENT

CHINESE HERBALISM
• Tonic herbs, such as astragalus, ganoderma, and ginseng will help your overall constitution. *(See page 57 and 67.)*
• Salvia, millettia, and peony will improve the Blood and help promote good circulation. *(See page 67.)*
• Chinese angelica can restore energy and stimulate white blood cells and antibody formation. *(See page 56.)*

HERBALISM
Treatment will always be tailored to the individual, but there are a number of herbs which can be used to boost immunity, including:
• Licorice, to enhance recovery, stimulating the formation and efficiency of white blood cells and antibodies. It is also useful in preventing stress. *(See page 122.)*
• Garlic, to prevent infections of all kinds, including those which have now become immune to antibiotics. *(See page 113.)*
• Echinacea, widely prescribed for treatment of chronic and acute infections – it cleanses the blood and lymphatic system, stimulating production of white blood cells and antibodies. *(See page 120.)*

• Ginseng, to boost immunity and encourage the body to deal efficiently with stress, as well as stimulating white blood cell production, and aiding recovery after illness. *(See page 126.)*

AROMATHERAPY
• Antiviral oils include tea tree, niaouli, eucalyptus, and thyme, and they can be used in any form – lymphatic massage is particularly recommended for its ability to stimulate the immune system. *(See pages 146–71.)*
• Lavender, tea tree, and bergamot stimulate production of white blood cells, and are active against one or more bacteria and viruses. *(See pages 146–71.)*
• Tea tree in particular has antiviral, antibacterial, and fungicidal properties, with a stimulating action on the immune system. *(See page 162.)*
• Mood-enhancing and uplifting oils, such as bergamot, lavender, geranium, rose, sandalwood, and ylang ylang, may be useful. *(See pages 146–71.)*

HOMEOPATHY
• Homeopathic remedies are designed to encourage the immune system to fight for itself, increasing the number of white blood cells in the body, and allowing you to reach a state of mental and emotional balance, which makes your body more responsive. Constitutional treatment is often aimed at the present ailment, as well as tendencies and symptoms which have not yet become proper ailments. Your homeopath will suggest improved nutrition, fresh air, exercise, and rest, which can restore the ability of the immune system to cope. Homeopathic remedies will be prescribed in conjunction with this advice.

VITAMINS AND MINERALS
• Include a variety of vegetables each day, with wholegrain cereals like brown rice and whole wheat bread, fruit, pulses (beans and lentils), and a few nuts and seeds for their oils.
• A daily multivitamin and multimineral preparation – especially one containing high amounts of the antioxidant nutrients – acts to boost immune activity. *(See page 251.)*
• Vitamin C stimulates immunity and is antiviral. *(See page 256.)*
• Acidophilus will encourage the healthy bacteria in your gut, which will help to fight off infections and infestations. *(See page 271.)*
• Zinc stimulates the immune system, and acts as an antiviral agent. *(See page 265.)*

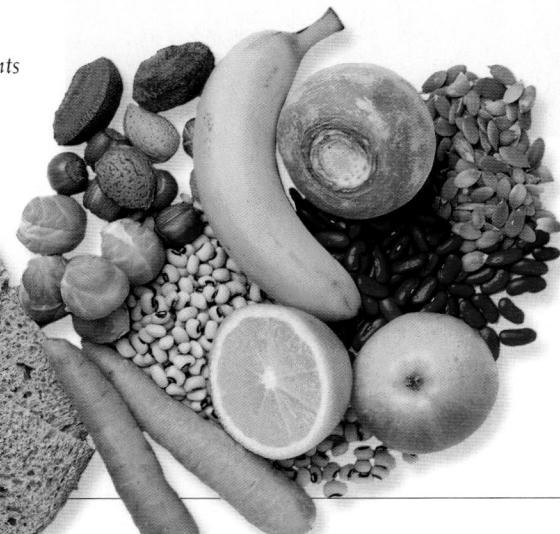

LEFT *Certain foods such as fresh vegetables, wholegrains, nuts, and seeds will boost the immune system. Include as many of them as possible in your diet.*

Glandular Fever

Glandular fever, or infectious mononucleosis as it is also known, is caused by the Epstein-Barr virus (a herpes virus). The virus multiplies in the white blood cells, eventually harming the immune system's efficiency. Glandular fever is usually transmitted via saliva, hence its nickname of the "kissing disease." While symptoms may last for only six weeks, recovery is slow and fatigue and low energy levels may linger for months. The disease occurs most commonly in adults 15–30 years old, but one attack confers immunity.

SYMPTOMS

• *flu-like symptoms, including fever, sore throat, headache* • *fatigue and lethargy* • *swollen lymph glands in the neck, armpits, and groin* • *a rash of small, slightly raised red spots* • *chest pain, with breathing difficulty and a cough* • *enlarged spleen and possibly damaged liver, causing jaundice*

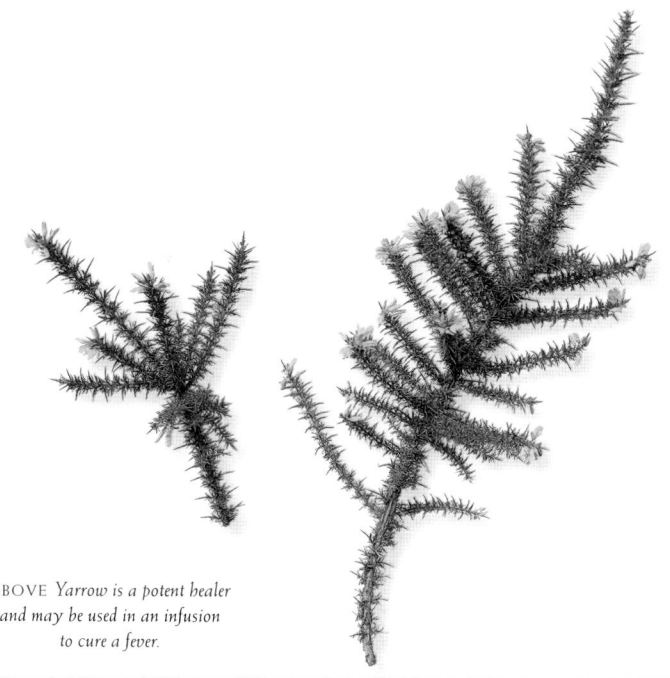

ABOVE *Yarrow is a potent healer and may be used in an infusion to cure a fever.*

BELOW *For an easy home remedy for glandular fever, try applying apple cider vinegar to the neck glands.*

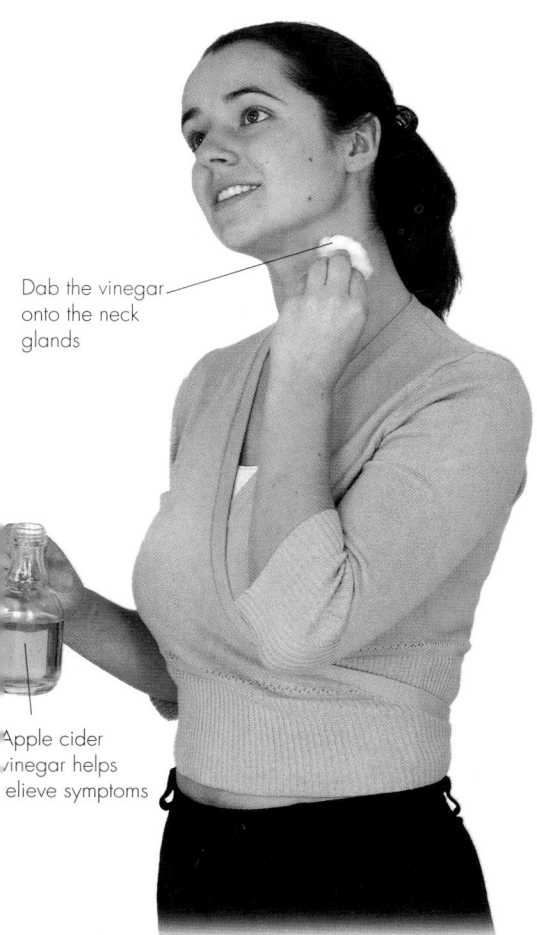

Dab the vinegar onto the neck glands

Apple cider vinegar helps relieve symptoms

TREATMENT

CHINESE HERBALISM
• Tonic herbs such as astragalus, ganoderma, and ginseng will help your overall constitution. *(See pages 57 and 67.)*
• Salvia, millettia, and peony will improve the Blood, and give the circulation a boost. *(See page 67.)*
• Chinese angelica can restore energy and stimulate white blood cells and antibody formation. *(See page 56.)*

TRADITIONAL HOME AND FOLK REMEDIES
• Apply apple cider vinegar to the neck glands daily. Drink it in a cup of warm water to encourage healing. *(See page 102.)*
• Ginseng acts to balance the glands. Chew the fresh or dried root, or add the powder to hot herbal teas. It will prevent fatigue and stimulate you.

HERBALISM
• Herbs to promote healing include cleavers, echinacea, and nettles, all of which stimulate immune activity as well as fighting infection. *(See pages 120 and 137.)*
• Balm, oats, and skullcap, if depression accompanies the fever. *(See pages 117 and 131.)*
• Infusions of yarrow and elderflower will help to control fever and also induce sweating. *(See pages 112 and 130.)*

AROMATHERAPY
• Essential oils can be used in the bath, or in massage, which also has therapeutic benefits. Oils to consider are eucalyptus, lavender, rosemary, and tea tree, which will encourage immune activity and fight the virus. *(See pages 146–71.)*

HOMEOPATHY
Constitutional treatment is recommended, but the following remedies may be useful, taken up to six times daily, for two days.
• Belladonna, for sudden high fever, with a reddish face and agitation. *(See page 183.)*
• Mercurius, for tender glands and smelly sweat. *(See page 205.)*
• Calcarea, for chilliness, sweating, a sour taste in the mouth, and fatigue. *(See page 186.)*
• Cistus, for a chilly feeling, with painful neck and glands, exacerbated by cold air and mental exertion.
• Baryta carb., for swollen glands. This is particularly useful for children. *(See page 185.)*

FLOWER ESSENCES
• Flower essences are often used by practitioners to help you cope with the physical and emotional effects of glandular fever.
• Olive will help if you feel exhausted on all levels. *(See page 235.)*
• Mustard controls feelings of depression that have no identifiable cause. *(See page 239.)*
• Gorse will help with feelings of hopelessness. *(See page 240.)*

VITAMINS AND MINERALS
• Take extra vitamin C, B-complex, and zinc. *(See pages 256, 252–5, and 265.)*
• Evening primrose oil will help to encourage healing. *(See page 270.)*
• Royal jelly will help fight feelings of fatigue and depression, and stimulate the immune system. *(See page 276.)*
• Eat plenty of foods containing antioxidants. *(See page 251.)*

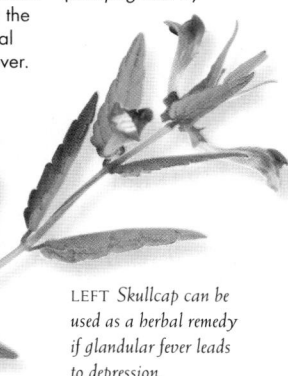

LEFT *Skullcap can be used as a herbal remedy if glandular fever leads to depression.*

Allergies

An allergy is the immune system's abnormal response to contact with a specific substance. The system overreacts when faced with foreign substances or organisms – allergens – and deals with them as if they were harmful, as it would with invading bacteria, for example. The result is an allergic reaction, also known as a histamine reaction (histamine being the substance produced in response to attack). Common allergens include certain foods, grass pollens, spores, fabrics, drugs, household chemicals, and stress. Some of the most common allergic responses are urticaria (see page 303),

BELOW *Dermatitis is a common allergy. It is characterized by red, itchy patches on the skin.*

dermatitis (see page 300), asthma (see page 344) and hay fever/rhinitis (see page 330). An estimated 35 million people in the United States suffer from various allergies, some of which are mistaken for the common cold.

SYMPTOMS

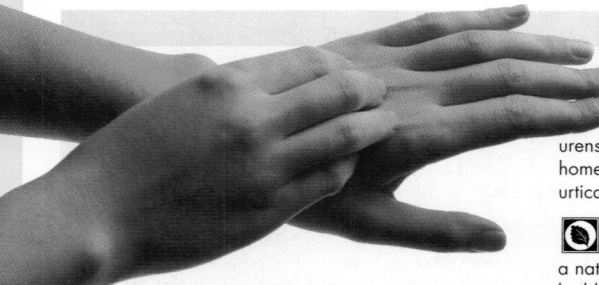

RED
CLOVER

• *sneezing and runny nose* • *wheezing* • *excess catarrh*
• *urticaria* • *anaphylactic shock (sometimes fatal), causing breathing difficulty, edema, constriction of air tubes, and heart failure*

TREATMENT

AYURVEDA
• Cleansing and detoxification will be followed by a varied diet of organic foods.
• Herbal preparations to boost immunity may be appropriate, including Chebulic myrobalan (Harithaki), which helps in cases of eczema; bitter orange for asthma and other respiratory allergies; and stramonium. *(See page 22.)*

CHINESE HERBALISM
• Bi Yan Pian/Nose inflammation pills, for Wind Cold or Wind Heat to the face, indicated by sneezing, itchy eyes, facial congestion and sinus pain, acute and chronic rhinitis, and nasal

allergies. Herbal prescriptions will be offered. *(See page 52.)*
• Yu Ping Feng San/Jade screen helps prevent hay fever and guards against allergies.
• Cang Er Zi Tang/xanthium powder, for allergic rhinitis, with thick yellow catarrh or blocked nose.

TRADITIONAL HOME AND FOLK REMEDIES
• Eat the local honey if you suffer from hay fever. *(See page 101.)*
• Honey and apple cider can be drunk in a glass of warm water to restore and prevent allergies. *(See pages 101 and 102.)*
• Drink nettle tea to increase resistance.

• Apply nettle tea to skin, or use Urtica urens cream or homeopathic remedy for urticaria.

HERBALISM
• Echinacea acts as a natural antibiotic while building the immune system. Take three times daily, as an infusion, or a few drops of tincture in a glass of warm water, during attacks or when you are run down. *(See page 120.)*
• Other useful herbs include chamomile, elderflower, red clover, yarrow. *(See pages 112, 119, and 130.)*
• Add a small amount of ginseng powder to herbal drinks to overcome the tendency to allergic attacks, such as hay fever. *(See page 126.)*
• Eat the local honey in a cup of warm water with 2 tablespoons of apple cider vinegar to reduce the reaction to allergens. This is particularly useful during the hay fever season.
• Herbs to boost immunity include garlic, angelica, borage, wild yam. *(See pages 113, 115, and 120.)*
• Strengthen the weakened area with tonic teas, 2 cups taken over a period of time: the sinuses

with elderflower tea; the stomach with chamomile, linden, and a warming digestive like cardamom; the skin with chamomile washes and rosemary in the bath. *(See pages 119, 127, and 134.)*

AROMATHERAPY
• Place a few drops of Roman chamomile in a vaporizer or on a light bulb to treat an allergic reaction, including asthma. *(See page 150.)*
• Melissa, in the bath or a vaporizer, soothes and reduces a reaction's severity. *(See page 163.)*
• Lavender essential oil, in a light carrier oil, can be massaged into the chest or other affected area to reduce spasm and generally boost immunity. *(See page 161.)*

HOMEOPATHY
Homeopathic treatment has proved to be very successful in the treatment of allergies. Remedies will be prescribed according to your individual case, so it is best to see a registered practitioner to ensure that prescription is exact.
• Urtica, for urticaria. *(See page 217.)*
• Pulsatilla or Arg. nit., for relief of conjunctivitis. *(See page 209.)*
• Apis, for bee stings. *(See page 180.)*

Anaphylactic shock is a medical emergency, and you must summon emergency medical care immediately. The following remedies can be given until help arrives:
• Aconite, when the patient is frightened and restless. *(See page 178.)*
• Veratrum, when the skin is cold and mottled, and the victim is in a cold sweat.
• Arnica, for shock brought on by injury. *(See page 182.)*

FLOWER ESSENCES
• If suffering a sudden allergic reaction, take Rescue Remedy or Emergency Essence. *(See page 244.)*

VITAMINS AND MINERALS
• Take steps to boost immunity, by increasing intake of magnesium (seafood, beans, and nuts), B vitamins (yeast extract, meat, or yeast), zinc (eggs, nuts, and seeds), vitamin A (fish and yellow and green vegetables), iron (liver, sesame seeds, and dried fruit) and vitamin C (fresh fruit and vegetables). *(See pages 262, 252–5, 265, 252, 260, and 256.)*
• A diet high in protein will help to build up immunity, while roughage from fruit, vegetables,

nuts, seeds, and pulses will keep the digestive tract working and encourage the growth of beneficial bacteria in the gut (called flora), which helps the body to resist infection.
• Acidophilus, taken daily, will also work to encourage bowel health. *(See page 271.)*
• Evening primrose oil and blackcurrant seed oil are rich sources of essential fatty acids, which can prevent allergies in susceptible people. *(See page 270.)*
• Pollen supplements are useful for preventing allergies, in particular hay fever. *(See page 271.)*

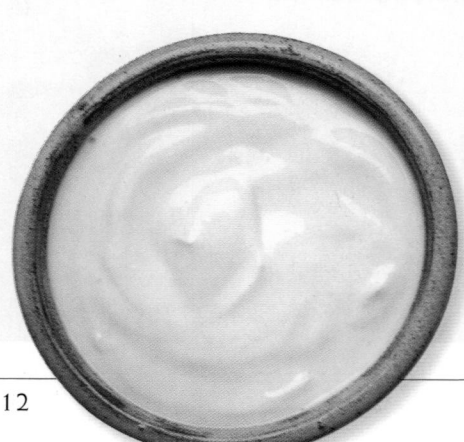

LEFT *Live natural yogurt will encourage the growth of beneficial bacteria in the gut.*

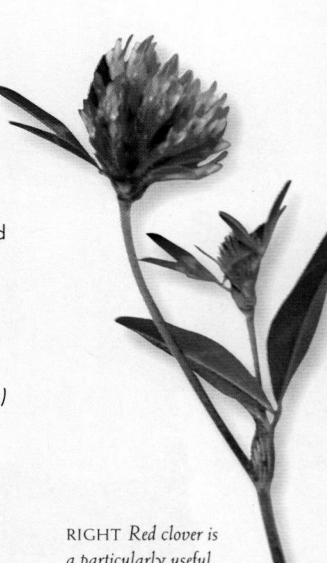

RIGHT *Red clover is a particularly useful remedy for skin allergies.*

Hodgkin's Disease

Hodgkin's disease (or Hodgkin's lymphoma) is a cancer that attacks the lymphatic tissue and the lymph nodes in particular. As the tissue becomes more and more damaged, relatively minor infections may become life-threatening. Late in the disease's development the bone marrow may also be affected. The cause of Hodgkin's is unknown, although it is thought that cancer-causing viruses are involved. In the United States, about 30 people out of every million have this ailment; it is more common in males between the ages of 20 and 40, although both sexes can suffer from the condition. Untreated, Hodgkin's disease is invariably fatal. (*See also Cancer, page 457*)

SYMPTOMS

• painless enlargement of lymph nodes, which acquire a rubbery feel • liver and spleen enlargement • anemia and fever • appetite and weight loss • night sweats • possible secondary effects caused by pressure on other structures from enlarged nodes: – neurological damage – obstruction to veins – difficulty in swallowing and breathing – jaundice

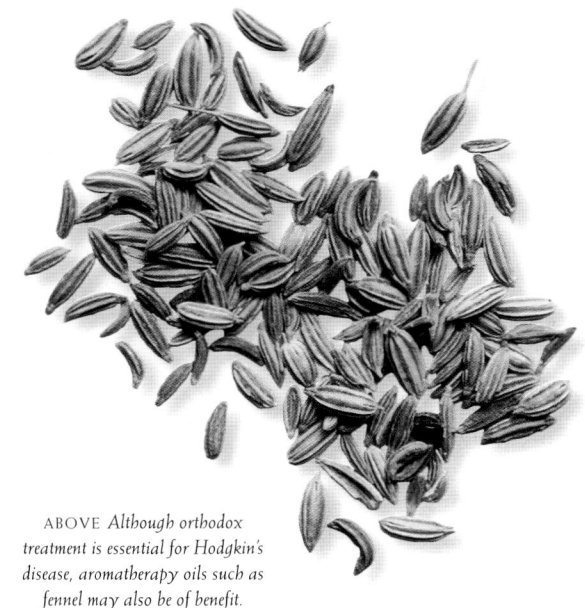

ABOVE *Although orthodox treatment is essential for Hodgkin's disease, aromatherapy oils such as fennel may also be of benefit.*

TREATMENT

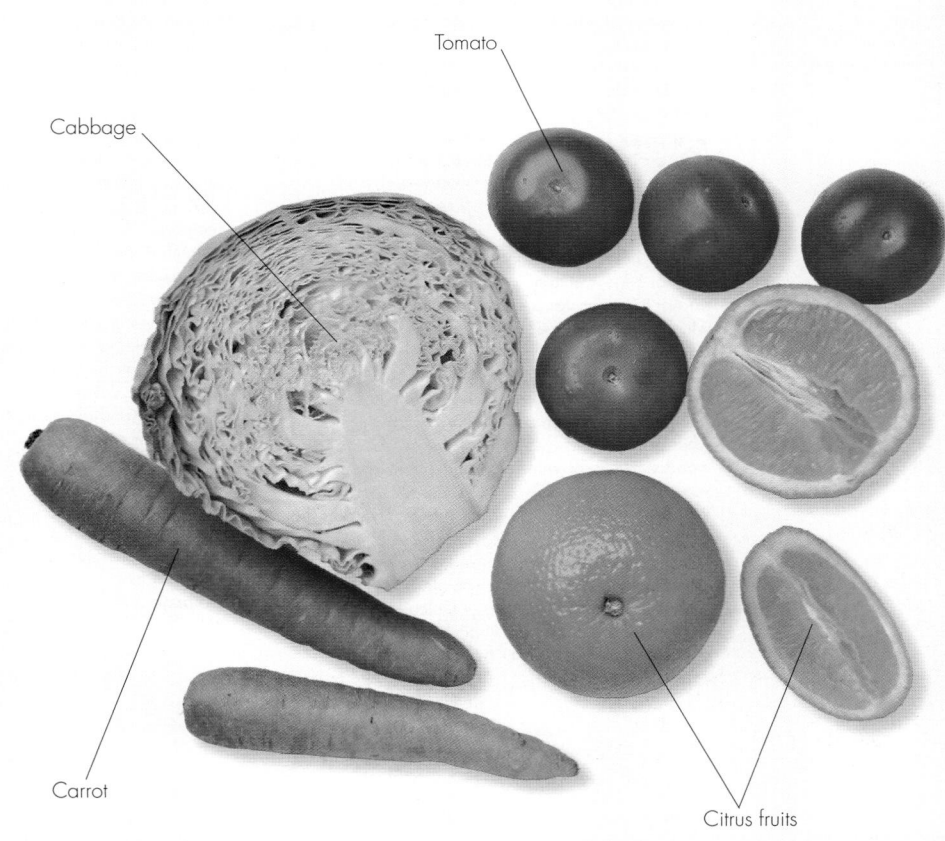

Tomato

Cabbage

Carrot

Citrus fruits

AROMATHERAPY
• Extra treatments to try are fennel, garlic, juniper, and rose, which can be used in the bath or in a vaporizer to detoxify the body.
(See pages 146–71.)
• Tea tree and lavender essential oils strengthen the body's defenses.
(See pages 161 and 162.)
• Oils which strengthen the action of the adrenals include geranium and rosemary, along with peppermint and thyme.
(See pages 146–71.)

VITAMINS AND MINERALS
• Eat as much fresh fruit and vegetables as you can, paying particular attention to those containing antioxidants.
(See page 251.)

• Reduce your intake of animal fats and avoid processed foods.
• A deficiency of vitamin C has been found in conjunction with certain tumors. Ensure you get plenty in your diet.
(See page 256.)
• Vitamin A can protect against cancer in smokers to some degree.
(See page 252.)
• Digestive enzymes may be offered to halt activities of trophoblastic cancer cells.
• Vitamin E is said to prevent a number of cancers. Ensure that you get plenty in your diet or take supplements.
(See page 257.)

LEFT *Eat foods that contain antioxidants to strengthen your immune system.*

DISORDERS OF THE MUSCULOSKELETAL SYSTEM

Osteoporosis

In osteoporosis (meaning porous bones) the bones lose their density, becoming fragile and brittle. This is caused by alterations, with age, of the amounts of the various growth and sex hormones which control chemical changes in the bones, leading to progressive calcium and protein loss. Osteoporosis affects far more women than men, and may be triggered or accelerated by a sedentary lifestyle, loss of activity, a low-calcium diet, smoking, heavy alcohol consumption, hereditary factors, or prolonged lack of estrogen. An overactive thyroid gland, chronic liver disease, and prolonged use of corticosteroids all predispose a person to osteoporosis.

SYMPTOMS

• *loss of height from shrinkage of the spinal bones* • *sudden breakage of a bone in the spine, with severe pain and disfigurement* • *reduced ribcage movement, causing shortness of breath and pain* • *wrist, forearm, neck, or hip fractures resulting from minor stumbles or falls*

DATA FILE

• Bone mass reaches a peak in women between the ages of 30 and 45; between the ages of 55 and 70, a woman will have lost 30–40 percent of her bone mass.

• Most common in white women after menopause.

• Affects more women than heart disease, stroke, diabetes, breast cancer, and arthritis.

• 50 percent of women between the ages of 45 and 75 suffer from some osteoporosis; 30 percent of these suffer from serious bone deterioration.

• Costs approximately $3.8 billion in treatment in the U.S. each year.

• Aggravated by a variety of factors, including smoking, excessive alcohol consumption, and a sedentary lifestyle.

• A dowager's hump is an abnormal curvature of the spine in the upper back. Typically affecting older women, the curvature is a result of collapse of the spinal column, caused by osteoporosis.

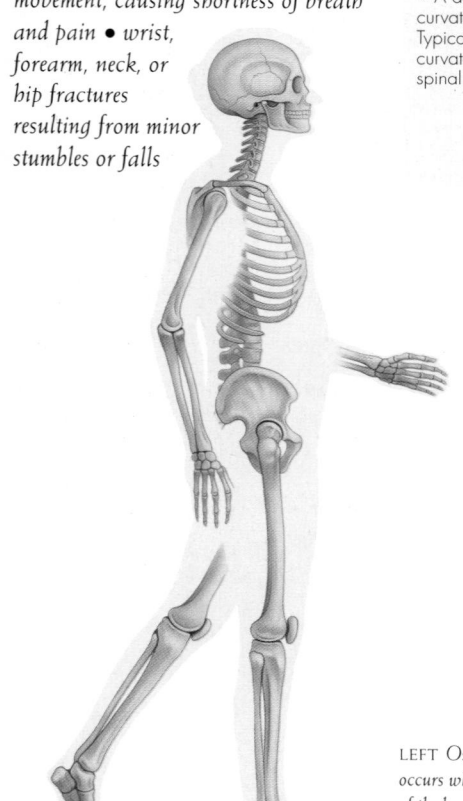

LEFT *Osteoporosis occurs when the density of the bones is reduced, causing them to become thin and weak.*

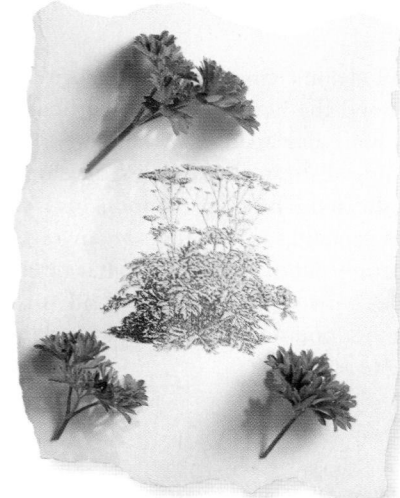

LEFT *Drink an infusion of parsley as a herbal remedy for osteoporosis. Its high calcium content will be of benefit.*

TREATMENT

CHINESE HERBALISM
• The condition is believed to be caused by Kidney Deficiency, and can be treated with cibot rhizome, drynaria tuber, and eucommia bark. *(See page 63.)*
• Cinnamon twigs will help to reduce pain. *(See page 59.)*

HERBALISM
• Drink a cup of comfrey leaf and bay leaf tea three times a day. *(See page 132.)*
• Many herbs, such as hops or sage, contain estrogen-like substances which can protect the bones against loss. *(See page 129.)*
• If you are in pain, use analgesic herbs such as white willow, meadowsweet, or wild yam. *(See pages 120, 121, and 129.)*
• Herbs that contain calcium include nettles, parsley, dandelion leaves, kelp, and horsetail, which can be drunk as often as possible. *(See pages 120, 122, 133, and 137.)*

• Take estrogenic herbs, which discourage the loss of calcium from the bones, including calendula, ginseng, false unicorn root, sage, hops, blue cohosh, wild yam, and licorice. *(See pages 120, 122, 126, and 129.)*
• Herbs which encourage the digestion and absorption of minerals from food include yellow dock root, rosemary, wormwood, and yarrow. *(See pages 112, 127, and 128.)*

HOMEOPATHY
Constitutional treatment will be necessary, but the following remedies may be useful to deal with bone pain:
• Ruta grav., for pain at the nape of the neck and in the lumbar region. *(See page 210.)*
• Aurum, for pains that are worse at night, mainly in the skull, nose, or palate. *(See page 184.)*
• Calcarea phos., for limbs that feel achy, numb, and chilly. *(See page 186.)*
• Fluoric ac., for stabbing pain.

VITAMINS AND MINERALS
• Recent evidence suggests that an increased intake of magnesium may help prevent the worst effects of osteoporosis. Magnesium sources include soybeans, nuts, and brewer's yeast. *(See page 262.)*
• Calcium can also be very helpful. Recommended doses are between 1,000mg. and 1,500mg. a day. *(See page 258.)*
• Vitamin D helps the body absorb calcium. *(See page 256.)*
• Increase your intake of foods containing boron, which reduces the body's excretion of calcium and magnesium, and increases the production of estrogen. *(See page 258.)*
• Fluoride may be useful for preventing and treating the condition because it stimulates new bone formation. *(See page 260.)*

Rheumatism

Rheumatism is a very general term applied to aches, pains, and stiffness in bones and muscles, occurring as a result of viral infection, food allergy, emotional stress, or an underlying joint disease. The following may all come under the umbrella term rheumatism:

- FIBROSITIS (see page 423)
- HYPERTHYROIDISM (see page 405)
- MYOSITIS, in which inflammation of muscles causes pain and weakness. It may develop from a bacterial or viral infection
- POLYMYALGIA RHEUMATICA, featuring pain and stiffness in the shoulders, neck, back, and arms, possibly due to a blood disorder
- VITAMIN D DEFICIENCY, which causes bone pain and muscle weakness

LEFT *The symptoms of rheumatism may be relieved by chewing horseradish leaves.*

DATA FILE

- Palindromic rheumatism is a disease that causes frequent and irregular attacks of joint pain, especially in the fingers, but leaves no permanent damage to the joints.

- Psychogenic rheumatism is common in women between the ages of 40 and 70, although men also contract this disease. Symptoms include complaints of pain in various parts of the musculoskeletal system that cannot be substantiated medically.

- One of the commonest forms of rheumatism is rheumatoid arthritis, affecting 1–3 percent of the population. Rheumatoid arthritis usually occurs between ages 35 and 40, but can occur at any age. It characteristically follows a course of spontaneous remissions and exacerbations, and in about 10–20 percent of patients remission is permanent.

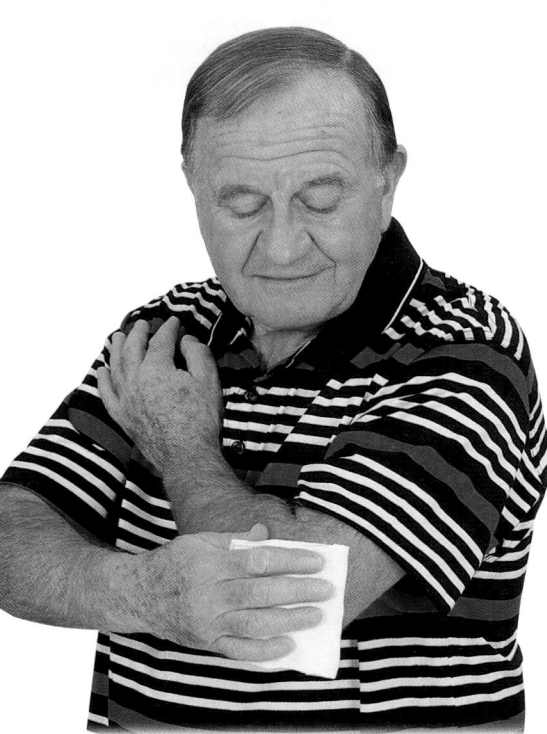

ABOVE *A poultice made from slippery elm may be applied to the part of the body affected by rheumatism.*

TREATMENT

AYURVEDA
- Ginger, coriander, and aloe vera (when there are hot pains) can be used to treat rheumatism. (See pages 27, 35, and 47.)
- Angelica is a good tonic and is warming for stiffness and discomfort. (See page 28.)
- Barberry, taken as a tea or applied as a compress, can be used to treat rheumatic ailments. (See page 29.)
- Basil relieves arthritis and rheumatism. (See page 42.)
- Rub calamus oil into the affected joints to improve circulation and drainage. (See page 24.)
- Camphor is indicated for arthritis, rheumatism, and many other musculoskeletal problems. (See page 33.)

CHINESE HERBALISM
- The condition is thought to be caused by qi stagnation, excess Wind, Damp, and Heat. Chinese herbalists use achyranthus root and cork tree bark. (See page 68.)

TRADITIONAL HOME AND FOLK REMEDIES
- Chew a tiny quantity of horseradish leaves, which is said to prevent attacks. (See page 84.)

HERBALISM
- Useful herbs, which may be taken internally or applied as a compress to the affected part of the body, include bogbean, feverfew, meadowsweet, and white willow. (See pages 121, 129, and 133.)
- Use a little cayenne pepper oil to warm the area and reduce pain and stiffness. (See page 118.)
- A poultice of slippery elm may be of benefit. (See page 136.)
- An infusion of celery seed may help reduce the level of acid in the blood, which is a contributory factor in rheumatism.

AROMATHERAPY
- Bergamot and myrrh reduce inflammation. Use in the bath, or massage the local area. (See pages 135 and 153.)
- There are many oils which can reduce swelling and inflammation and encourage the healing process. Try massage with pine, lemon, or juniper, in a suitable carrier oil. (See pages 146–71.)
- Massage with oil of black pepper or eucalyptus can stimulate the circulation and relieve stiffness. (See pages 159 and 167.)
- Lavender oil calms pain and helps to relieve stiffness. (See page 161.)

HOMEOPATHY
- Aconite, for sharp pains which tend to come on suddenly. (See page 178.)
- Bryonia, for pains that are worse in dry cold weather and on movement. (See page 185)
- Pulsatilla, for pains that move from joint to joint, and muscle to muscle. (See page 209.)
- Rhus tox., for stiffness that is worse in the morning or after rest. (See page 210.)
- Mercurius, for pain that is worse at night and for heat. (See page 205.)
- Calcarea hypophos., for sharp pains in the wrists and hands.
- Causticum, for pains in the jaw and neck, with spasm. (See page 189.)

FLOWER ESSENCES
- Rub a little Rescue Remedy, or the cream, into the affected area. (See page 244.)

VITAMINS AND MINERALS
- Many cases of rheumatism respond to a dietary change, and it is suggested that the following foods are eaten as often as possible to reduce muscular and joint inflammation: cabbage, celery, turnip, lemon, dandelion, and oily fish.
- Drink plenty of water, which will flush the system and act as a detoxicant.
- Eliminate members of the "nightshade" family of plants from your diet, as these can cause joint problems. These include potatoes, peppers, eggplant (aubergine), and paprika.
- Evening primrose oil is a rich source of gamma-linolenic acid, which is necessary for the production of prostaglandins, which may have an anti-inflammatory effect. (See page 270.)

Fractures

A fracture is a break or crack in a bone. It may occur as a result of excessive force through injury (particularly in sport), an accident such as a car crash, or disease. A simple fracture is one where the soft tissue overlying the broken bone is still intact; a compound fracture is one where the skin is damaged so that the fractured bone is exposed and therefore vulnerable to infection. Fractures caused by disease (such as osteoporosis, or a tumor or cyst) are known as pathological fractures. In such cases there is a weakening of bones that predisposes them to break more easily. An estimated 200,000 hip fractures occur in people over the age of 65 each year. The tendency to fracture increases with age.

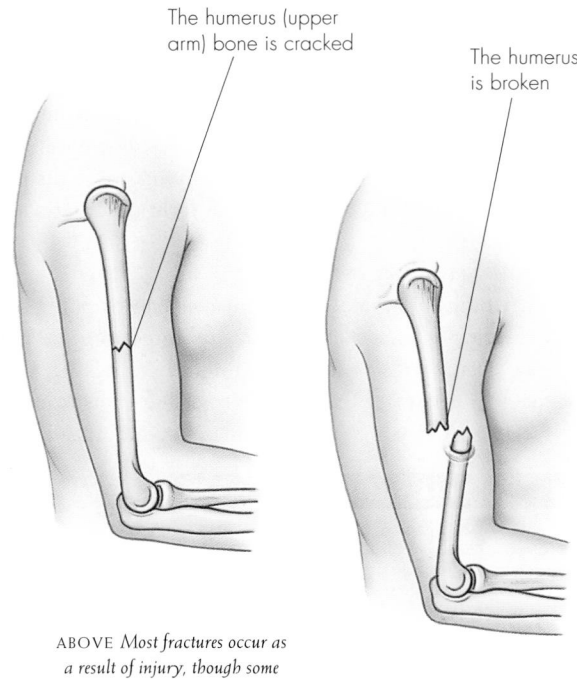

The humerus (upper arm) bone is cracked

The humerus is broken

ABOVE *Most fractures occur as a result of injury, though some are caused by disease.*

SYMPTOMS

• *swelling, pain, and tenderness* • *inability to move the affected part* • *possibly a protruding bone, deformity, and discoloration*

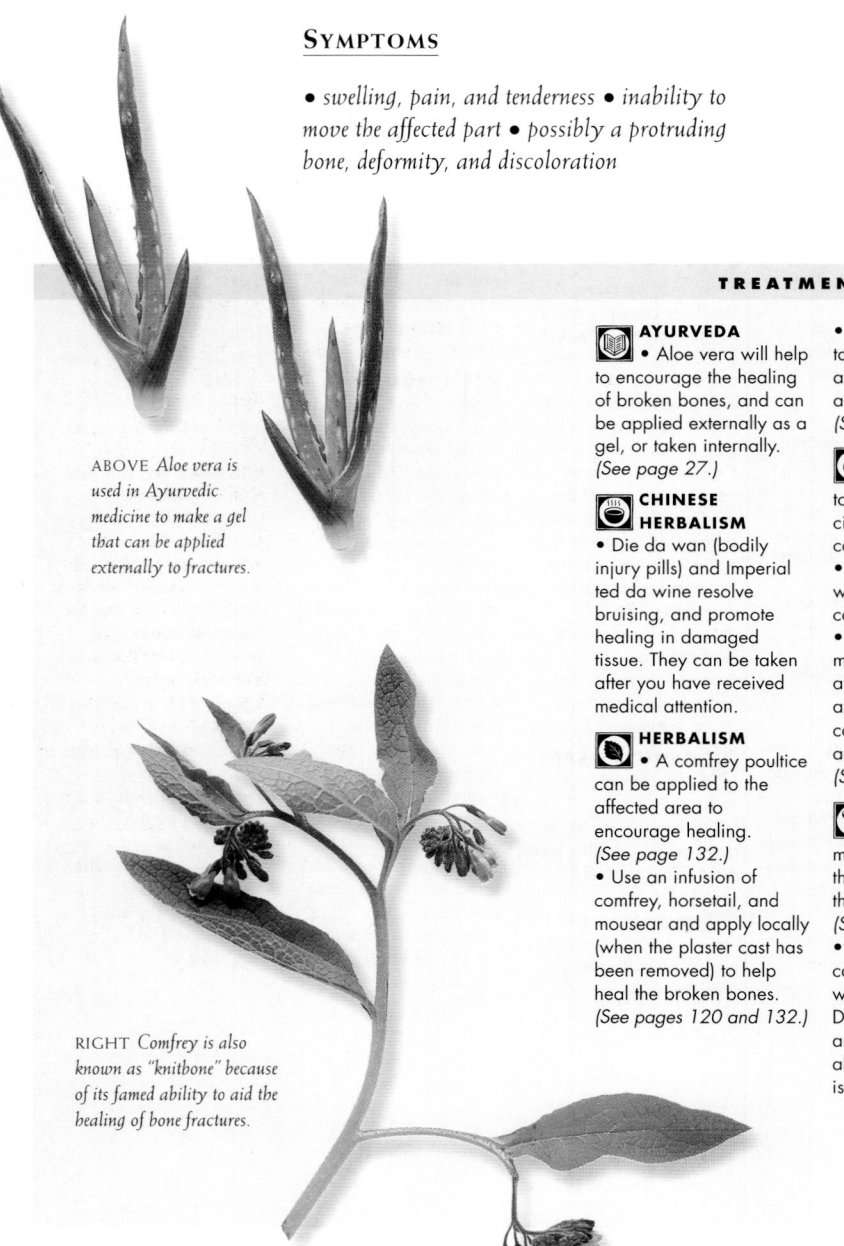

ABOVE *Aloe vera is used in Ayurvedic medicine to make a gel that can be applied externally to fractures.*

RIGHT *Comfrey is also known as "knitbone" because of its famed ability to aid the healing of bone fractures.*

TREATMENT

AYURVEDA
• Aloe vera will help to encourage the healing of broken bones, and can be applied externally as a gel, or taken internally. *(See page 27.)*

CHINESE HERBALISM
• Die da wan (bodily injury pills) and Imperial ted da wine resolve bruising, and promote healing in damaged tissue. They can be taken after you have received medical attention.

HERBALISM
• A comfrey poultice can be applied to the affected area to encourage healing. *(See page 132.)*
• Use an infusion of comfrey, horsetail, and mousear and apply locally (when the plaster cast has been removed) to help heal the broken bones. *(See pages 120 and 132.)*

• Comfrey root can be taken internally (in small amounts) to set the bone and encourage healing. *(See page 132.)*

AROMATHERAPY
• Elemi oil can help to encourage the circulation after a plaster cast has been removed.
• Lavender in a vaporizer will help to relax and calm. *(See page 161.)*
• Thyme, rosemary, and marjoram can be diluted and massaged into the area, or applied as a compress, to soothe pain and promote healing. *(See pages 146–71.)*

HOMEOPATHY
• Arnica, every 10 minutes after the injury, then every 8 or 10 hours thereafter, as necessary. *(See page 182.)*
• Symphytum (bone knit) can be used for up to 3 weeks to promote healing. Do not take this unless you are sure the bone is aligned, for the healing is profound.

FLOWER ESSENCES
• Rescue Remedy or Emergency Essence can be given at the time of the injury, and taken as required to calm and to treat any shock. *(See page 244.)*

VITAMINS AND MINERALS
• Increase your calcium, magnesium, and phosphorus intake. *(See pages 258, 262, and 263.)*
• Increase your intake of vitamin A. Foods such as carrots are a good source. *(See page 252.)*

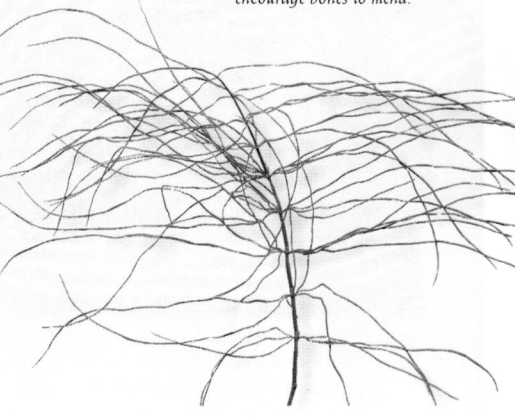

BELOW *An infusion of comfrey, horsetail (shown here), and mouse ear may be applied externally to the fracture to encourage bones to mend.*

Sprains and Strains

A sprain is the result of an overstretching or tearing of the ligaments which bind the joints together, caused by a sudden pull. Severe sprains may lead to dislocation of the affected joint (particularly common in the case of the shoulder), and repeated injury of this nature can cause a loss of the ligaments' elasticity. The most commonly strained or sprained joint is the ankle, which is usually sprained as a result of going over on the outside of the foot so that the complete weight of the body is placed on the ankle. The back, fingers, knees, and wrists are also commonly sprained.

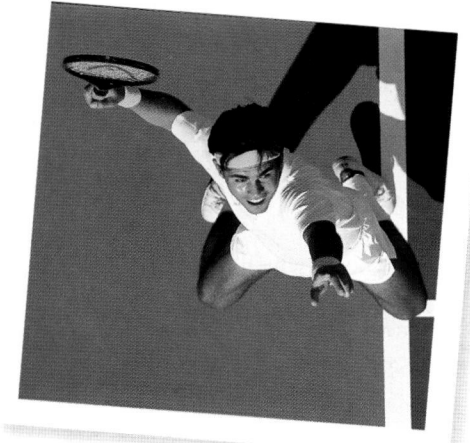

LEFT *Sprains and strains often occur during sports activities. Make sure you warm up muscles properly beforehand to minimize the chance of injury.*

SYMPTOMS

• *swelling in the affected area* • *pain in the affected joint, sometimes severe*

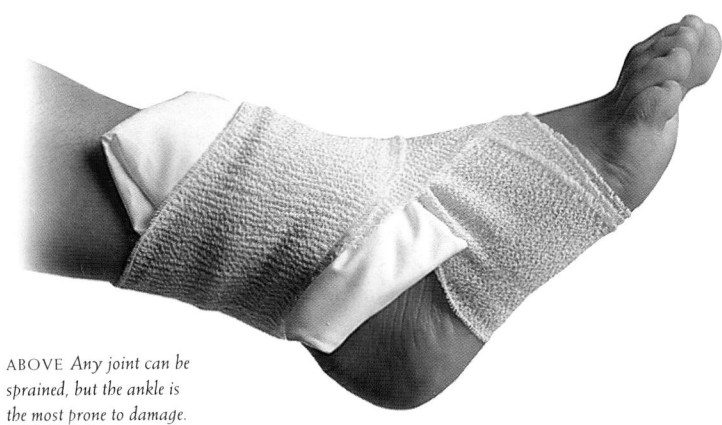

ABOVE *Any joint can be sprained, but the ankle is the most prone to damage.*

CAUTION

IF YOU SUSPECT A FRACTURE, SEE YOUR PHYSICIAN IMMEDIATELY.

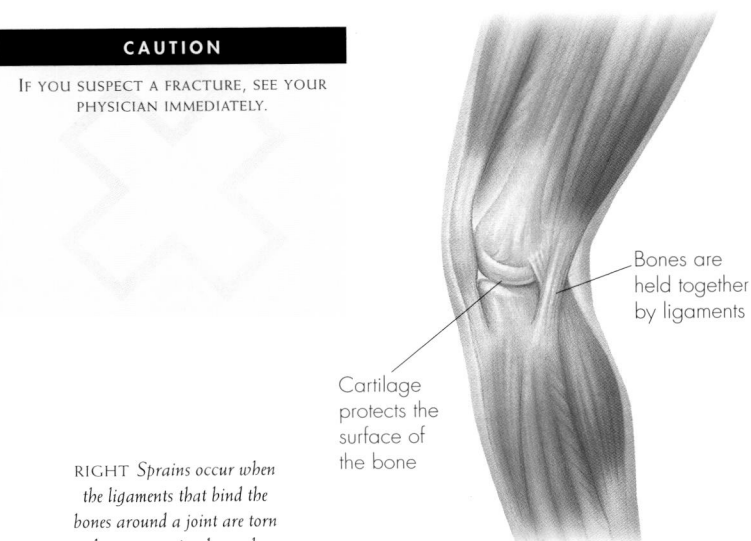

Bones are held together by ligaments

Cartilage protects the surface of the bone

RIGHT *Sprains occur when the ligaments that bind the bones around a joint are torn due to excessive demands made on the joint.*

TREATMENT

CHINESE HERBALISM
• San Qi is useful after injury, for swelling and pain. *(See page 68.)*
• Die Da Wan will help with injuries to the soft tissues, inflammation, and bruising.

TRADITIONAL HOME AND FOLK REMEDIES
• Cider vinegar can be used as a compress in order to relieve pain and swelling. *(See page 102.)*
• Apply a poultice of raw onions to the sprain. *(See page 82.)*
• Raise the affected limb and apply a cold compress as soon as possible. Strains should be bandaged with an elastic bandage to provide support, but take care not to bind too tightly and cut off circulation. Keep the limb elevated until the swelling goes down and some normal movement is possible.

HERBALISM
• Burdock can be taken internally in the form of a tea, or applied as a poultice to the affected area. *(See page 115.)*
• Ginger can be added to bath water or a foot bath, or applied as a compress to encourage healing. *(See page 139.)*
• Chamomile can be taken internally to calm and reduce pain. *(See page 119.)*

AROMATHERAPY
• Use a little lavender oil in a foot bath, or on a cold compress applied to the area. Avoid massaging the area, which will increase inflammation. *(See page 161.)*
• A compress with essential oils of sweet marjoram and rosemary can be used to heal and to reduce inflammation. *(See pages 165 and 168.)*

HOMEOPATHY
• Arnica should be taken internally until the injury has healed. *(See page 182.)*
• Ruta grav. can be taken the day after the injury occurs. *(See page 210.)*
• A cold compress with Arnica tincture should be applied hourly for the first 8 hours to reduce swelling. *(See page 182.)*

FLOWER ESSENCES
• Rescue Remedy can be taken internally to reduce shock and to calm. A few drops on a cold compress, applied to the injury, can help to reduce pain. When the swelling has gone down, a little Rescue Remedy cream can be massaged into the joint area. *(See page 244.)*

VITAMINS AND MINERALS
• The following nutrients help to encourage healing in the body: vitamin C, beta carotene, zinc, selenium, and vitamin E. *(See pages 256, 265, 264, and 257.)*

Neck Problems

Constant movement of the neck, along with its position and the number of structures within it, makes it particularly vulnerable to problems, which include:

• CERVICAL OSTEOARTHRITIS – the cartilage of the vertebrae of the neck wear away, most commonly in middle age, causing pain, stiffness, and sometimes tenderness to touch.

• CERVICAL RIB – this is an abnormal floating rib or pair of ribs attached to the lowest vertebra of the neck, which can cause compression of various nerves and arteries.

• CERVICAL SPONDYLOSIS – neurological damage is caused in the neck region as a result of compression of the spinal cord or nerve roots by an outgrowth of bone. Sufferers develop a walking disorder (spastic gait) and weakness in the arm muscles. Cervical spondylosis can begin from the age of 25 onward.

• LOCKED NECK – overstrain of ligaments or muscle spasms caused by an awkward or sudden movement, often occurring during sleep.

• NECK RIGIDITY – stiffness and pain on movement caused by neck muscle spasms. A classic symptom of meningitis.

• NECK SWELLING – swelling of any of the structures in the neck may be caused by tumors, allergy, bleeding, or inflammation. It can be extremely dangerous, seriously interfering with breathing. It may also affect swallowing.

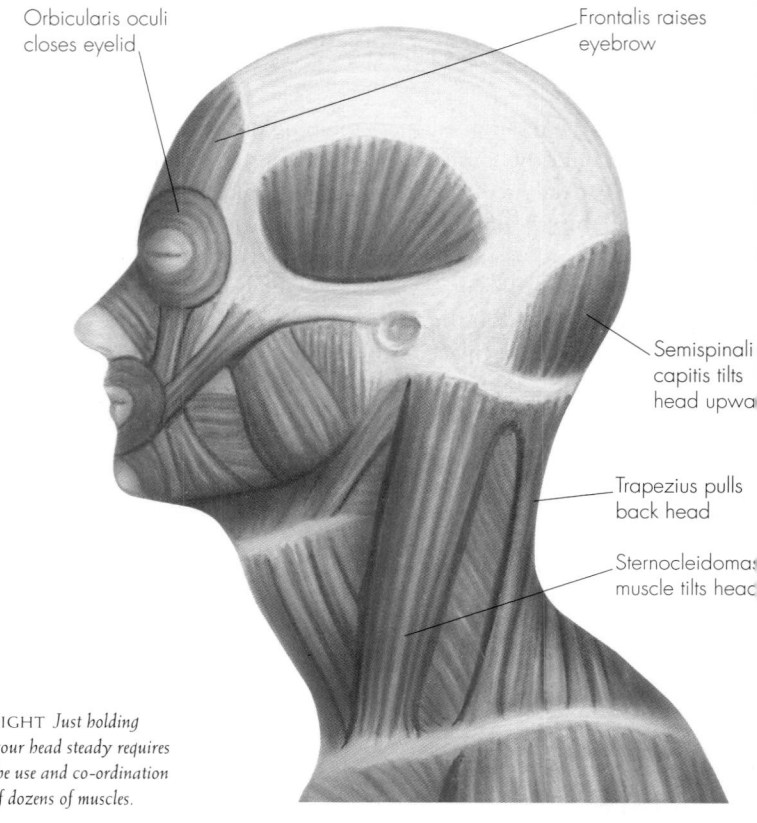

Orbicularis oculi closes eyelid

Frontalis raises eyebrow

Semispinali capitis tilts head upwa

Trapezius pulls back head

Sternocleidomas muscle tilts heac

RIGHT *Just holding your head steady requires the use and co-ordination of dozens of muscles.*

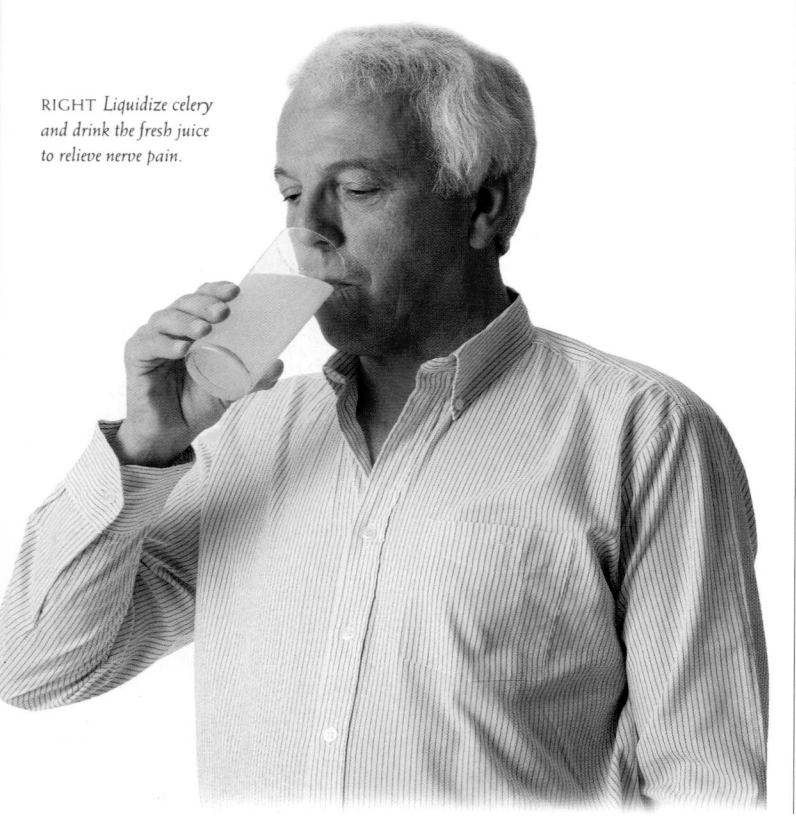

RIGHT *Liquidize celery and drink the fresh juice to relieve nerve pain.*

• TORTICOLLIS (WRY NECK) – an abnormality in the head's position caused by permanent twisting of the neck, due possibly to muscle damage sustained at birth, a whiplash injury, a visual problem, or shortening of the skin of the neck through scarring.

• WHIPLASH INJURY – a sudden force (such as a car collision) causes a violent bending of the neck in one direction, followed by reflex muscle contraction which throws the neck in the opposite direction. The ligaments connecting the vertebrae are stretched or torn, causing prolonged pain and disability.

BELOW *Barberry has anti-inflammatory properties and is used internally for pain in the Ayurvedic tradition.*

CAUTION

A STIFF NECK ACCOMPANIED BY HEADACHE, NAUSEA, VOMITING, AND ABNORMAL SLEEPINESS MAY INDICATE MENINGITIS, AND IMMEDIATE MEDICAL ATTENTION IS REQUIRED.

TREATMENT

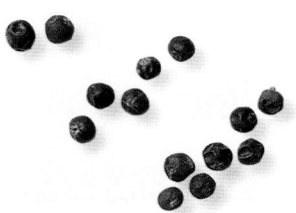

ABOVE *Use crushed juniper berries externally to relieve pain.*

AYURVEDA
• Barberry can be taken internally for pain. *(See page 29.)*
• Mustard oil relieves muscular pains and stiffness. *(See page 30.)*
• Turmeric and St. John's wort are also excellent for relieving stiffness, pain, and inflammation. *(See pages 37 and 40.)*

CHINESE HERBALISM
• The cause of stiffness and "freezing" may be caused by weak yang qi, external Cold and Damp. Useful treatments include cinnamon twigs and turmeric. *(See page 59.)*

TRADITIONAL HOME AND FOLK REMEDIES
• Drink celery juice to ease nerve pain. *(See page 83.)*
• Apply fresh horseradish to the affected area (do not leave on for long, or it will numb and burn). *(See page 84.)*
• Apply bruised juniper berries to muscular swellings for effective relief.
• Local heat will help to relax tense muscles.

HERBALISM
• St. John's wort has sedative, painkilling properties. It can be drunk as an infusion or applied to the affected area in an oil. *(See page 124.)*
• Valerian can reduce tension and help you to sleep. *(See page 136.)*
• The following herbs reduce inflammation and relieve pain: Jamaican dogwood, St. John's wort, vervain, and white willow. *(See pages 124, 129, and 138.)*

AROMATHERAPY
• A drop of juniper, mustard, or pepper oils, diluted in some carrier oil, can be massaged into the affected area. Wrap warmly afterwards. *(See pages 146–71.)*
• Wintergreen oil is good for muscular pains: massage into the affected area.
• Rosemary is stimulating and analgesic, and can be massaged into the area to relieve pain and stiffness. *(See page 168.)*

• Take hot baths with lavender, juniper, pine, or nutmeg to warm, reduce pain, and encourage the healing process. *(See pages 146–71.)*

HOMEOPATHY
• Cimicifuga, for a stiff neck, with the chin fixed in a raised position. *(See page 190)*
• Causticum, for dull pain at the nape of the neck, together with stiffness between the shoulders. *(See page 189.)*
• Bryonia, for pain made worse by the slightest touch. *(See page 185.)*
• Dulcamara, for pain at the top of the nape of the neck, as if from lying in an awkward position. *(See page 213.)*

• Lacnanthes, for pain down the right side of the neck, and in the upper arm and elbow.

FLOWER ESSENCES
• Rub Rescue Remedy cream into the affected area. *(See page 244.)*
• Star of Bethlehem can be taken internally after an injury to reduce the effects of shock and trauma. *(See page 235.)*
• Olive, if you feel exhausted and drained of spirit. *(See page 235.)*

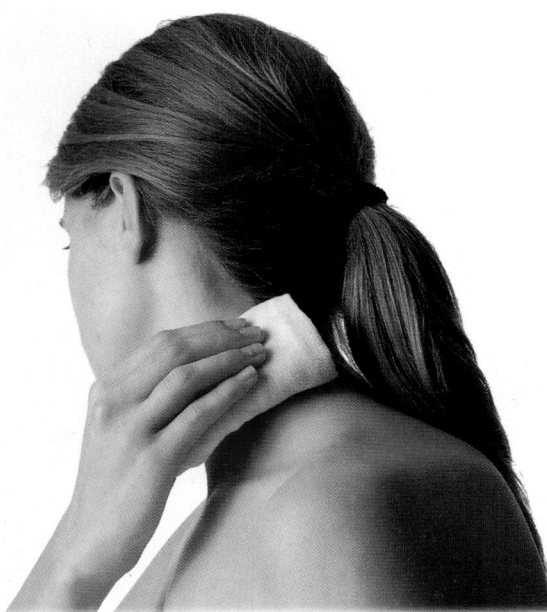

ABOVE *Essential oils, such as juniper or rosemary, can be added to a carrier oil and massaged into the painful area.*

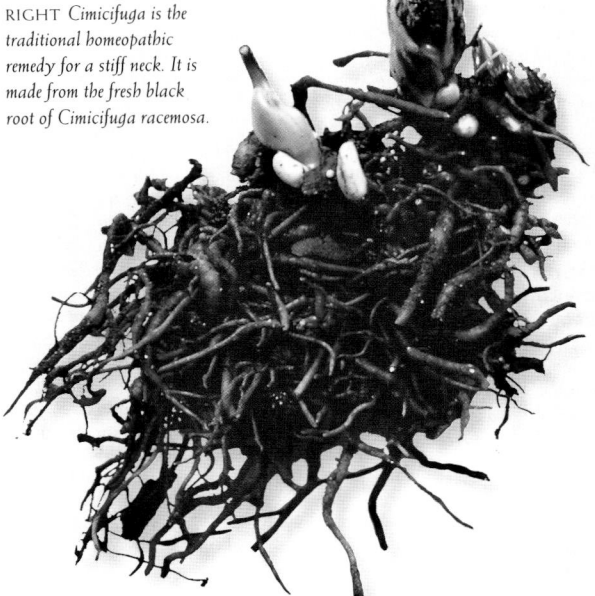

RIGHT *Cimicifuga is the traditional homeopathic remedy for a stiff neck. It is made from the fresh black root of Cimicifuga racemosa.*

RIGHT *Healing herbs, such as vervain or valerian, may be made into a compress and applied to the affected area of the neck.*

Back Problems

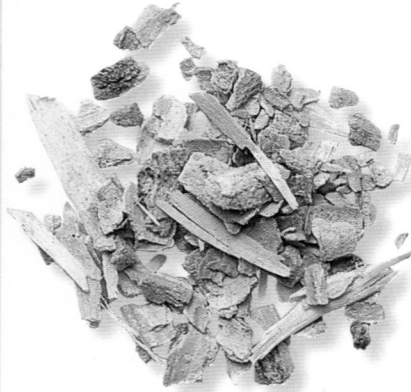

ABOVE *Cramp bark relaxes muscular spasms. It can be made into a cream, decoction, tincture, or capsules.*

Aches or pains in the back are due to mechanical disorders, which may cause or arise from damage to ligaments, muscles, vertebral joints, or disks. These may occur as a result of poor posture, lack of exercise, obesity, unaccustomed lifting or maneuvers, pregnancy, stress, or depression. A slipped disk is one of the most common causes of back pain, and this in turn may cause sciatica. Types of back pain vary according to the underlying cause.

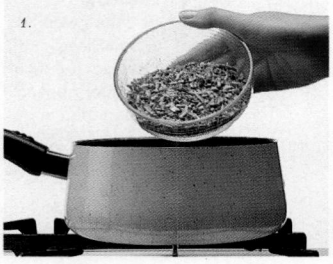

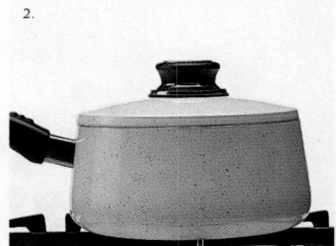

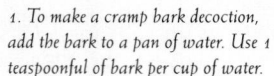

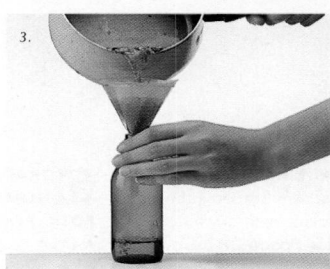

1. To make a cramp bark decoction, add the bark to a pan of water. Use 1 teaspoonful of bark per cup of water.

2. Cover the pan, bring the mixture to the boil, and simmer for about 10 to 15 minutes.

3. Pour the decoction through a strainer and store it in a dark glass bottle if you are not using it immediately.

DATA FILE

• A slipped disk does not, in fact, slip, but it herniates when the outer layer of the disk degenerates and the soft interior material extrudes into the spinal column, causing pain and sciatica.

• Most back pain is caused by a muscle strain. Injuries are the second most common cause of pain.

• Nearly 80 percent of all adults suffer from back pain at some time.

• The U.S. National Center for Health Statistics reports that back pain is the sixth most common reason for visits to the emergency room, and accounts for 13 million visits to general physicians' offices each year.

• In the U.K., the Back Pain Association estimates that every year over 3 million Britons consult a family physician because of back trouble.

• In the U.S., around 60 million working days are lost each year through back pain, and that figure is rising. Those days cost the economy around $5.2 billion (£3 billion) each year.

SYMPTOMS

• *muscle spasms* • *lower back pain, ranging from mild to excruciating* • *stiffness* • *referred pain or pins and needles in other areas*

AYURVEDA
• Aloe vera can be taken for inflammation, and applied externally for pain and inflammation. *(See page 27.)*
• Massage the painful area with mustard oil to reduce pain and aching. *(See page 30.)*
• Use cayenne externally for muscle soreness and stiffness. *(See page 31.)*

CHINESE HERBALISM
• Teasel root, ginseng, and acanthopanax can be used to relieve pain. *(See pages 54 and 67.)*
• Jing Jie can be used to stop swelling and to kill pain.
• Pseudoginseng root can be used to relieve swellings and for general relief of pain. *(See page 68.)*

TRADITIONAL HOME AND FOLK REMEDIES
• It may be helpful to chew a small quantity of horseradish leaves every day to ease pain. *(See page 84.)*
• A mustard poultice, applied to the area, will ease pain and reduce any congestion in the area. *(See page 98.)*

HERBALISM
• Massage cramp bark cream into the back. Or take cramp bark decoction, tincture, or capsules. *(See page 138.)*
• Rub macerated comfrey or St. John's wort into the back to relieve pain. *(See page 124.)*
• The following herbs reduce inflammation and relieve pain: Jamaican dogwood, St. John's wort, vervain, and white willow. *(See pages 124, 129, and 138.)*

AROMATHERAPY
• Relaxing in a warm bath to which lavender oil has been added can be very soothing. *(See page 161.)*
• Pain due to fatigue or tension can be treated with a massage of ginger, juniper, marjoram, or rosemary; the same oils can be added to the bath. *(See page 146–71.)*
• Massage with ginger or black pepper can be used when there is acute pain. *(See pages 167 and 171.)*
• Marjoram can help to treat the muscular problem in the longer term, as well as reducing pain. *(See page 165.)*

• Bergamot and myrrh are anti-inflammatory, useful for massage or in the bath. *(See pages 153 and 155.)*

HOMEOPATHY
Treatment would be constitutional, but the following remedies may be useful:
• Calc. fluor., for backache that is worse when starting to move but eases if you continue to move.
• Arnica, for bruising and pain resulting from an injury. *(See page 182.)*
• Ruta grav. helps relieve pain at the nape of the neck and in the lumbar region. *(See page 210.)*
• Aconite, for sharp pain made worse by exposure to cold or dry weather. *(See page 178.)*
• Rhus tox., when the lower back feels stiff and bruised, especially after resting and in damp weather. *(See page 210.)*
• Sulfur, for violent sharp pain on stooping. *(See page 215.)*
• Bryonia, for pain that comes on in cold dry weather and is made worse by movement. *(See page 185.)*

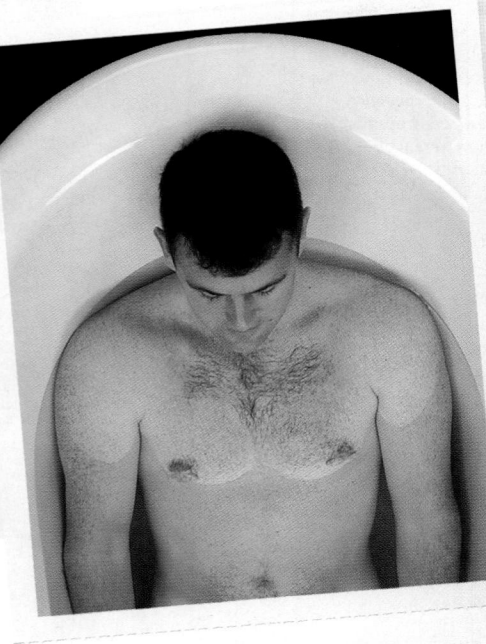

RIGHT *A relaxing bath with lavender oil can be extremely beneficial. It is one of the key oils for muscular pain.*

Lumbago

Lumbago is the term used to describe any persistent or recurrent lower back pain. It is muscular in origin and usually concerns the large group of muscles surrounding the spine. Lumbago may vary in severity from a dull ache to severe pain; often it is experienced as a sudden excruciating pain on bending, on standing up from sitting, on twisting round, or on lifting heavy objects. It is generally brought on or exacerbated by cold, damp weather conditions, muscle strain, poor posture, obesity, and pregnancy. Lumbago is one of the most commonly reported complaints and it generally becomes more frequent with age.

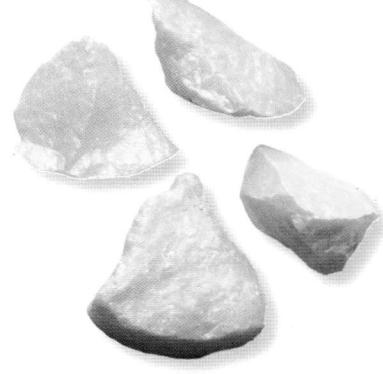

ABOVE *Sulfur is used to treat lower back pain that occurs from prolonged standing, stooping, or sitting.*

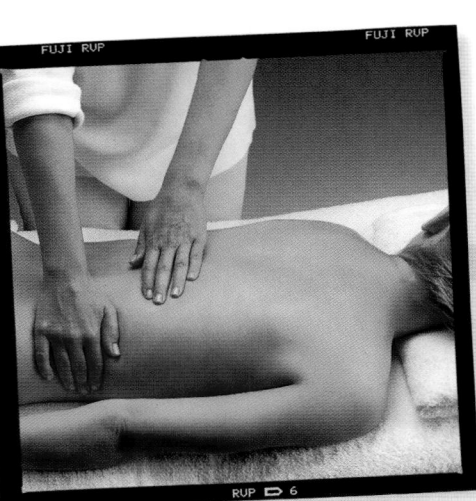
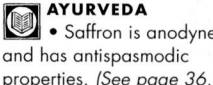

LEFT *Relieve lumbago by rubbing a little oil made from comfrey or St. John's wort onto the affected area.*

ABOVE *Lumbago pain is centred in the small of the back and may be quite severe.*

TREATMENT

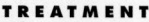

AYURVEDA
• Saffron is anodyne and has antispasmodic properties. *(See page 36.)*

CHINESE HERBALISM
• Apart from physical injury, the cause may be excess internal Cold. Treatment would include tincture of achyranthes root and acanthopanax bark.

HERBALISM
• Rub a little oil made from comfrey or St. John's wort into the affected area, to relieve the pain. *(See pages 124 and 132.)*
• The following herbs reduce inflammation and relieve pain: Jamaican dogwood, St. John's wort, vervain, and white willow. *(See pages 124, 129, and 138.)*

AROMATHERAPY
• Add a little mustard, rosemary, and thyme oils to the bath to relieve pain. Hot baths are most effective. *(See pages 146–71.)*
• Juniper, oregano, pine, and rosemary poultices ease inflammation and pain. *(See pages 146–71.)*

HOMEOPATHY
• Aconite can be taken when the pain comes on suddenly and is made worse by cold dry weather. *(See page 178.)*
• Arnica, for pain that comes on after injury. *(See page 182.)*
• Rhus tox., for a painful lower back that feels bruised and stiff, and that improves with movement. *(See page 210.)*

• Sulfur, for violent sharp pain on stooping. *(See page 215.)*
• Bryonia, for pain that comes on in cold dry weather and is made worse by movement. *(See page 185.)*
• Ant. tart., for continuous pain with nausea and vomiting. *(See page 179.)*
• Dulcamara, for pain which is aggravated by stooping and exertion. *(See page 213.)*

FLOWER ESSENCES
• Agrimony is useful for those who make light of the pain and do not let it show in front of others. *(See page 225.)*
• Hornbeam, for weariness at the prospect of doing daily tasks that cause pain. *(See page 227.)*

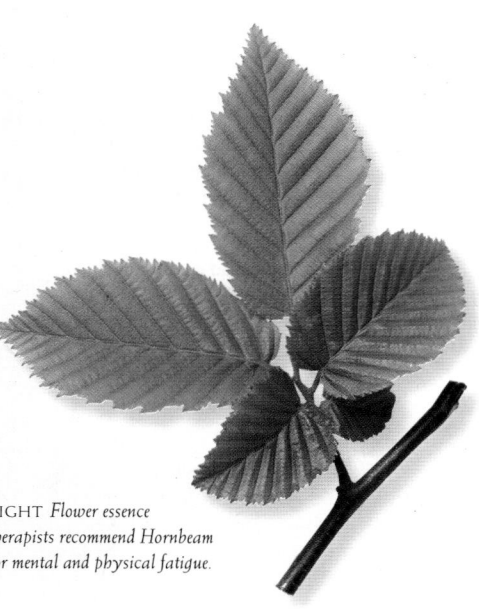

RIGHT *Flower essence therapists recommend Hornbeam for mental and physical fatigue.*

Sciatica

Sciatica is the name given to the aching or pain along the route of the sciatic nerve. This is the largest nerve in the body, running from the spinal cord, through the buttock and the back of each leg. Sciatica is usually caused by pressure on the roots of the sciatic nerve, most commonly from a prolapsed disk (*see page 420*), but other possible causes include pregnancy and childbirth, heavy lifting, stress, or a tumor. The type of pain varies from mild to more severe and "shooting" in nature. There may also be associated symptoms. Sciatica and other back pains may be eased by lying on the floor for 15 minutes. Prop the head up on a small pile of paperback books and keep the knees bent. Repeat daily.

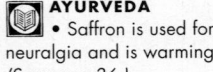

ABOVE *Gou Teng is recommended by Chinese herbalists as a remedy for sciatica.*

CAUTION

SEE YOUR PHYSICIAN IF YOU HAVE PROLONGED SCIATICA.

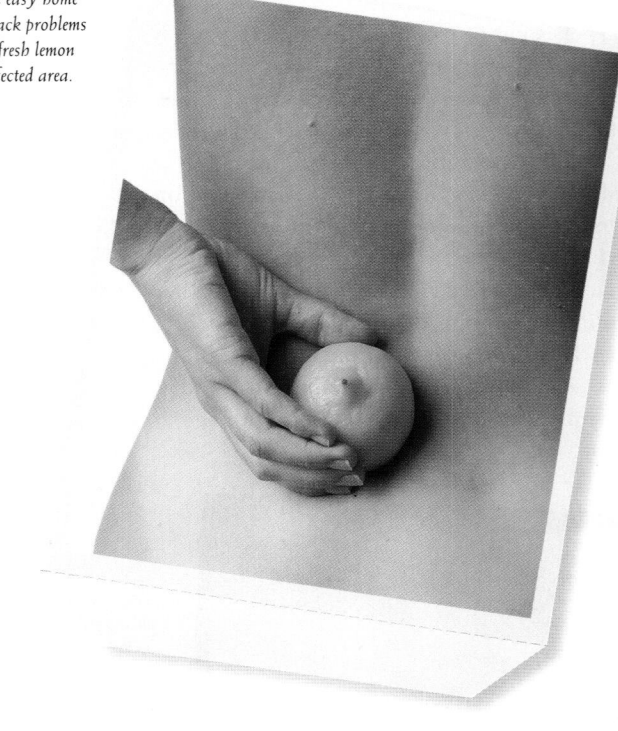

RIGHT *An easy home remedy for back problems is to rub a fresh lemon over the affected area.*

SYMPTOMS

• *a burning sensation and muscle weakness* • *numbness or pins and needles in the leg, foot, or toes* • *muscle spasms in buttock or leg* • *diminished reflexes in knees and ankles*

TREATMENT

AYURVEDA
• Saffron is used for neuralgia and is warming. (*See page 36.*)
• Mustard oil can be rubbed into the affected area to warm it. (*See page 30.*)

CHINESE HERBALISM
• Sciatica is believed to be caused by Heat stagnation in the Liver. Gou Teng may be useful, and San Qi can help with the general relief of pain. A practitioner will select herbs specific to your symptoms and the cause of the condition. (*See page 68.*)

TRADITIONAL HOME AND FOLK REMEDIES
• Take a warm bath to which nettles have been added to help relieve the pain.
• Celery juice or tea can alleviate some forms of sciatica. (*See page 83.*)
• Rub fresh lemon over the affected area – it works! (*See page 87.*)

HERBALISM
• Apply bruised juniper berries to the affected area for pain relief

• Coltsfoot leaf or tincture can be used in a soothing compress (hot) and applied on the affected area.
• Elderberry wine is a traditional remedy for sciatica. (*See page 130.*)
• For pain relief, try cajeput cream or ointment rubbed on the affected area.

AROMATHERAPY
• Lavender oil is antispasmodic and anti-inflammatory. Use in the bath or in local massage. (*See page 161.*)

• Chamomile compresses or massage will reduce the irritation and lessen the pain. (*See page 150.*)
• Mix a few drops of juniper, mustard, or pepper essential oil in a little carrier oil and rub into the affected area. Cover with warm clothing. (*See pages 146–71.*)
• Oregano and thyme can be added to the bath to relieve the symptoms. (*See page 170.*)

HOMEOPATHY
• Colocynthis, is for shooting pains down the right leg to the foot, causing numbness. (*See page 191.*)
• Rhus tox., for tearing pain which is better for heat and movement. (*See page 210.*)

• Arsenicum, for sciatic pain in an elderly person. (*See page 182.*)
• Lycopodium, for pain in the right leg, and which is worse between 4 and 8P.M. (*See page 203.*)
• Carbon sulf., for pain in the left leg, which is worse for heat and cold.
• Gelsemium, for burning pains which are worse at night. (*See page 195.*)

LEFT *To relieve sciatica, lie on the floor with your knees bent and your head on a small pile of books. Spend 15 minutes a day in this position.*

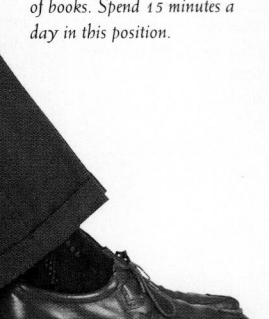

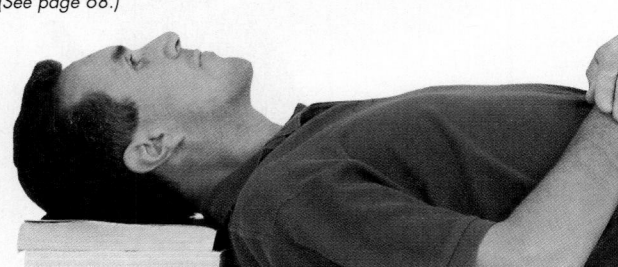

Fibrositis

Fibrositis (or fibromyalgia) is a chronic stress- or occupation-induced condition in which a series of muscular spasms causes intermittent aches and pain, usually in the back and trunk. It seems to be triggered by cold weather conditions or emotional upset. Fibrositis is most common in middle-aged and elderly people, and may occur more often in anxious people, and in those who spend time sitting in a cramped position. Tender areas (there are nine specific spots) are felt on the affected muscles. Pain and stiffness may be felt in the neck, shoulders, chest, buttocks, knees, and back. In some cases the attacks are accompanied by exhaustion and disturbed sleep. Fibrositis is not considered to be a medical term, and some doctors refuse to recognize the condition because investigation usually fails to reveal any detectable reason for the symptoms.

ABOVE *Basil is known as tulsi in Ayurvedic medicine and is used for pain relief.*

SYMPTOMS

• *aches and pain in muscles or tendons* • *tenderness in particular spots on the affected muscles* • *possibly stiffness*

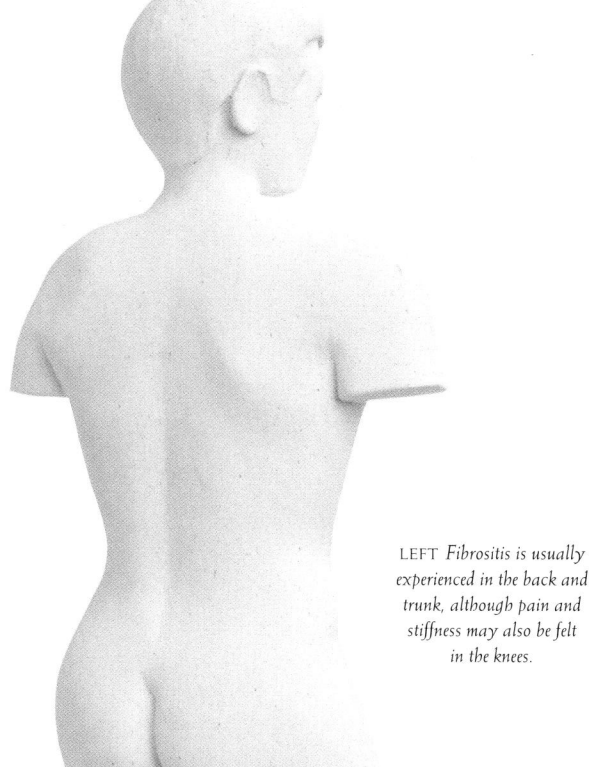

LEFT *Fibrositis is usually experienced in the back and trunk, although pain and stiffness may also be felt in the knees.*

TREATMENT

AYURVEDA
• Barberry, taken as a tea or applied as a compress, treats fibrositis. *(See page 29.)*
• Basil can provide pain relief. *(See page 42.)*
• Rub calamus oil into the affected joints to improve circulation and drainage. *(See page 24.)*
• Camphor can be rubbed into the affected area to warm and encourage healing. *(See page 33.)*

CHINESE HERBALISM
• Gan Caeo is good for spasm in the legs. *(See page 64.)*
• Bai Shao helps spasm in the feet and hands. *(See page 67.)*
• Ginseng will be useful as an overall tonic. *(See page 67.)*

TRADITIONAL HOME AND FOLK REMEDIES
• Apply compresses of apple cider vinegar to the affected area; use several cups of vinegar in bath water. *(See page 102.)*
• Make a honey and vinegar drink, with 1 tablespoon of each in a cup of hot water, and drink. *(See pages 101 and 102.)*

HERBALISM
• A decoction of cramp bark taken 4 or 5 times a day should bring relief. Cramp bark can also be taken as a tincture or in capsule form. The ointment is useful for massaging into the affected area. *(See page 138.)*

• Make a fresh peppermint poultice and apply to the area of spasm. *(See page 125.)*

AROMATHERAPY
• Essential oil of lavender relieves pain and reduces inflammation. Use in the bath or in a gentle massage of the affected area. *(See page 161.)*
• Chamomile, lavender, and rosemary are anti-inflammatory and pain-relieving, and are good for local massage or using in compresses. *(See page 146–71.)*
• Black pepper, eucalyptus, marjoram, and benzoin will improve the circulation in the area and reduce stiffness. *(See page 146–71.)*

HOMEOPATHY
• Aconite, for pain that starts suddenly and worsens with movement. *(See page 178.)*
• Arnica, for muscles that feel bruised and are made worse by movement. *(See page 182.)*
• Bryonia, for fibrositis in the back, neck, and limbs, which worsens with movement. *(See page 185.)*
• Chamomilla, for pain, stiffness, and bad temper. *(See page 204.)*
• Ledum, for a cold feeling in the muscles, with pain and stiffness alleviated by cold.

(See page 202.)
• Nux vomica., for pain and stiffness which are worse in damp weather and improved by pressure. *(See page 214.)*
• Rhus tox., for muscles stiff from overuse, which are better for movement. *(See page 210.)*
• Causticum, for tearing pains in the muscles, with stiffness, and which are made worse by cold. *(See page 189.)*

FLOWER ESSENCES
• Rub a little Rescue Remedy cream into the affected area to encourage healing and provide pain relief. *(See page 244.)*
• Take Rescue Remedy or Emergency Essence during an attack to calm and restore. *(See page 244.)*

VITAMINS AND MINERALS
• Royal jelly may help to relieve symptoms. *(See page 276.)*
• Take extra calcium, magnesium, and vitamin C to encourage the health of the muscles and joints. *(See pages 258, 262, and 256.)*

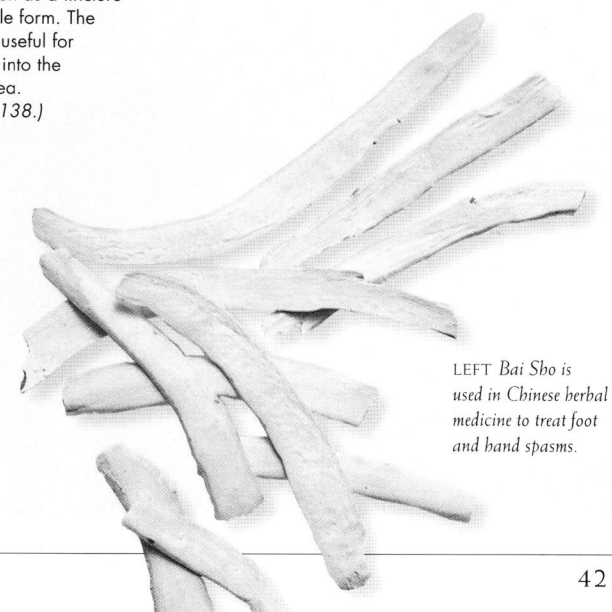

LEFT *Bai Sho is used in Chinese herbal medicine to treat foot and hand spasms.*

Arthritis

Arthritis is an inflammation of the tissues of one or more joints, usually with pain, swelling, and redness. The two most common forms of arthritis are osteoarthritis and rheumatoid arthritis. Other disease processes and infections which cause arthritis include gout, psoriasis, tuberculosis, rubella, and gonorrhea.

Osteoarthritis is a degenerative disorder in which the cartilage between the joints wears away. The body attempts to repair this damage by producing bony outgrowths at the margins of affected joints, but these, in fact, cause pain and stiffness. It is usually age-related and affects the hips, knees, spine, and shoulders in particular. Obesity is an aggravating factor.

Rheumatoid arthritis is a chronic, progressive disorder. It most commonly arises between the ages of 30 and 40, affecting women more often than men. Its exact causes are not clear, but it is thought that there may be immunological (perhaps triggered by infection) and genetic factors at work. The synovial membrane lining the joint becomes inflamed, spreading over and eroding the cartilage, causing the characteristic pain and stiffness. Anemia, joint infections and pericarditis are all complications of rheumatoid arthritis.

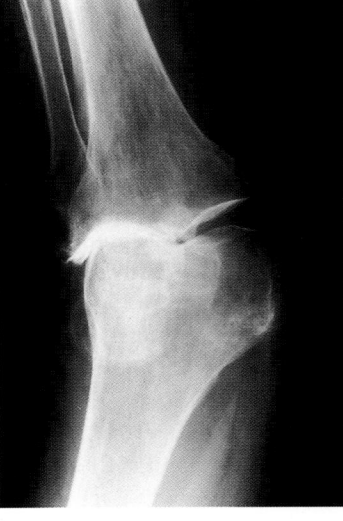

ABOVE *Arthritis is characterized by painful, swollen, and inflamed joints. As the disease progresses, the joints often become deformed.*

SYMPTOMS

• *osteoarthritis: intermittent pain in affected joints, gradually becoming more frequent — progressive movement limitation — audible creaking in affected joints — swelling and redness* • *rheumatoid arthritis: morning stiffness, taking up to an hour for the joints to loosen — weakness and inflammation of the ligaments, tendons, and muscles — eventually there may be deformity of joints (typically the fingers/hands), causing pain and debility — eye inflammation — bursitis — general feelings of being unwell include lethargy, appetite and weight loss, muscle pain*

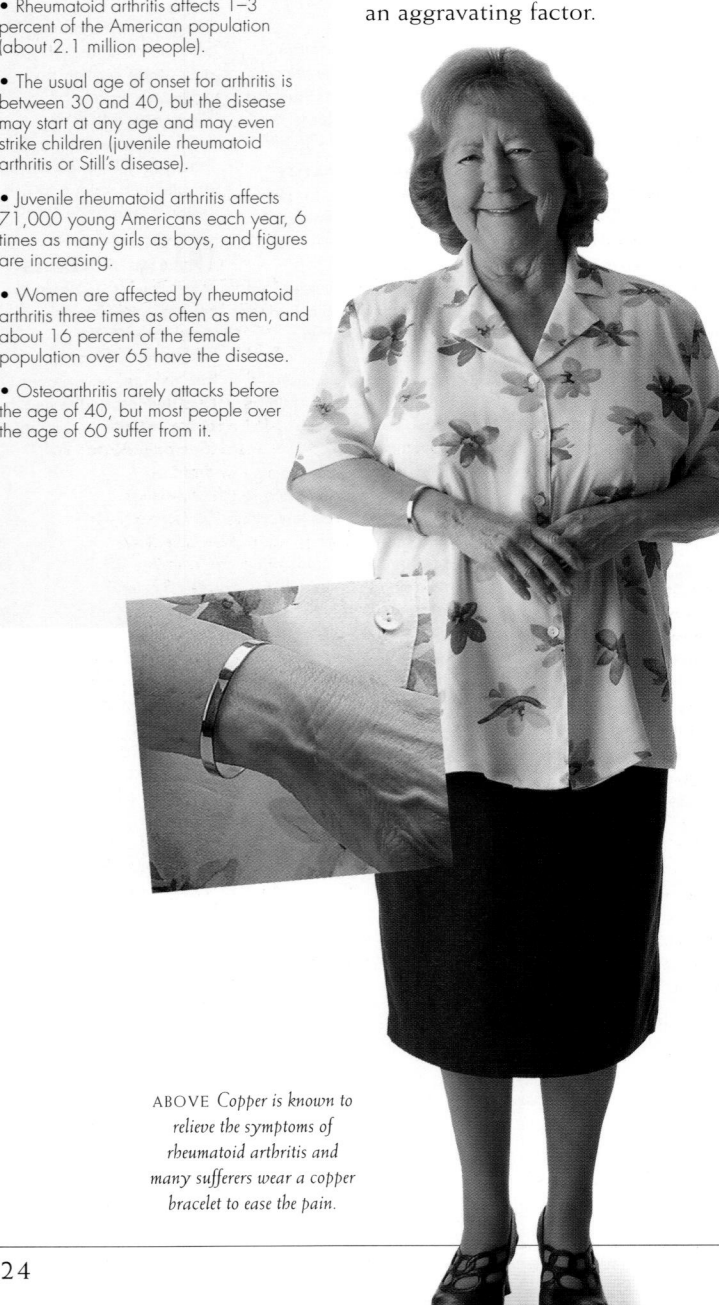

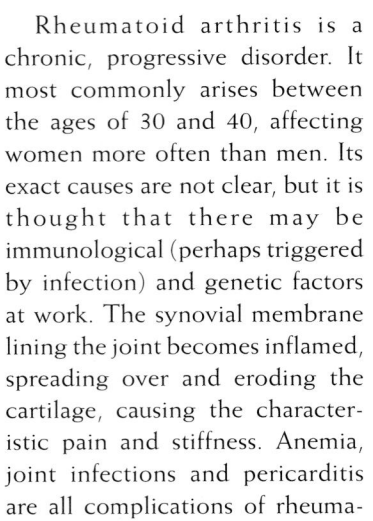

ABOVE *Copper is known to relieve the symptoms of rheumatoid arthritis and many sufferers wear a copper bracelet to ease the pain.*

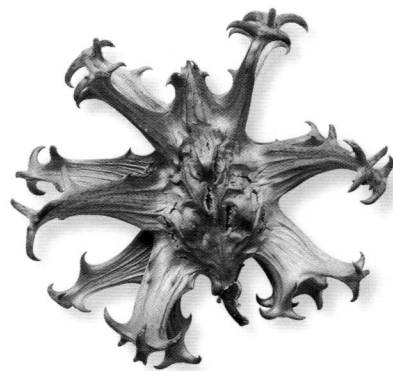

ABOVE *A tincture made from the Devil's claw tuber is used to treat all kinds of arthritis.*

TREATMENT

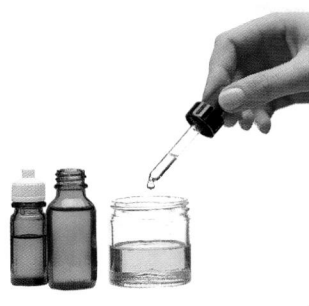

Make a liniment with comfrey tincture and black pepper oil. Pour some olive oil into a small jar.

Add a few drops each of comfrey tincture and black pepper oil. Leave the liniment to mature.

AYURVEDA
• Ginger, coriander, and aloe vera can be used to treat arthritis. *(See pages 27, 35, and 47.)*
• Angelica is a good tonic and is warming. *(See page 28.)*
• Barberry, taken as a tea or applied as a compress, can be used to treat arthritis. *(See page 29.)*
• Basil can provide relief from the pain of arthritis and rheumatism. *(See page 42.)*
• Rub calamus oil into the affected joints to improve circulation and drainage. *(See page 24.)*
• Camphor is indicated for the treatment of arthritis and rheumatism, and many other musculoskeletal problems. *(See page 33.)*

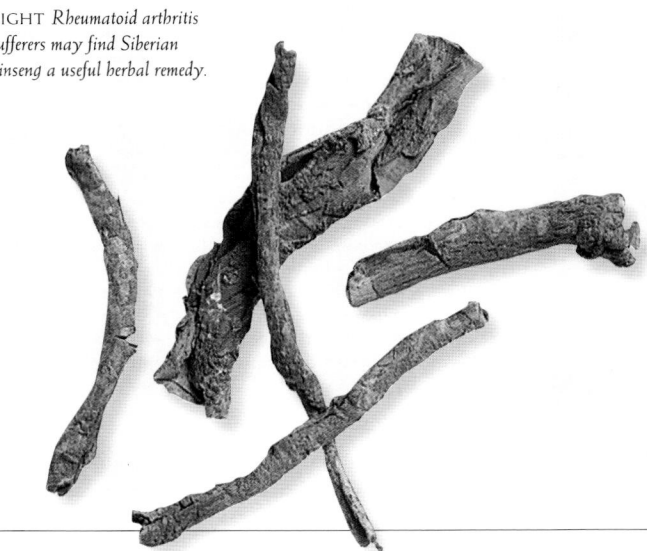

RIGHT *Rheumatoid arthritis sufferers may find Siberian ginseng a useful herbal remedy.*

CHINESE HERBALISM
• The source of the problem is considered to be Wind Damp. Painful joints are caused by Wind Cold. Arthritis with hot, swollen, but not painful, joints is considered to be caused by Wind Heat.
• Treatment would include cinnamon twigs to release qi; aconite root, angelica root, and wild ginger to relieve Cold and Damp. *(See pages 56 and 59.)*
• Gentian and cork bark tree can be used for Wind Heat. *(See page 68.)*
• Pupleuri root, licorice, and Chinese skullcap are recommended for their powerful anti-inflammatory effects. *(See pages 64 and 74.)*

TRADITIONAL HOME AND FOLK REMEDIES
• Eating nettles or drinking nettle tea is an old remedy for arthritis. The "stings" in stinging nettles contain histamine, which is anti-inflammatory.
• Vinegar and honey is another old remedy. *(See pages 101 and 102.)*
• Apple cider baths or ginger root baths can help to reduce symptoms and encourage healing. *(See page 102.)*

• Apples are good detoxifiers. Eat them daily to improve symptoms and cure the condition. *(See page 94.)*

HERBALISM
• Apply a poultice of slippery elm and cayenne to the affected joints. *(See pages 118 and 136.)*
• Herbs that work to heal arthritis include feverfew, meadowsweet, celery seed, and white willow. They can be taken internally, or used externally, as required. *(See pages 121, 129, and 133.)*
• Bladderwrack capsules, tablets, or powder used regularly may prevent the progress of the disease. *(See page 122.)*
• For aching joints, try a liniment made with tincture of comfrey and a few drops of black pepper essential oil. *(See page 132.)*
• Dandelion root and horsetail tea or tincture is recommended for degenerative arthritis. *(See pages 120 and 134.)*
• For inflamed hand joints, take a decoction or tincture of devil's claw. *(See page 123.)*
• Siberian ginseng is beneficial for rheumatoid arthritis. *(See page 126.)*

AROMATHERAPY
• Use juniper oil in the bath or in a massage oil blend. It is stimulating and anti-rheumatic. *(See page 160.)*
• Massage petitgrain into the limbs for osteoarthritis. *(See page 152.)*
• Lemon and cypress oils are detoxifying, and can be used in the bath and in massage to help the body eliminate poisons. *(See pages 154 and 156.)*
• Chamomile, lavender, and rosemary are anti-inflammatory and

• Osteoarthritis is thought to be a weakness in the Kidneys, and Blood stagnation. Use cinnamon twigs, tinospora stem, angelica, and ledebouriella root. *(See pages 56 and 59.)*

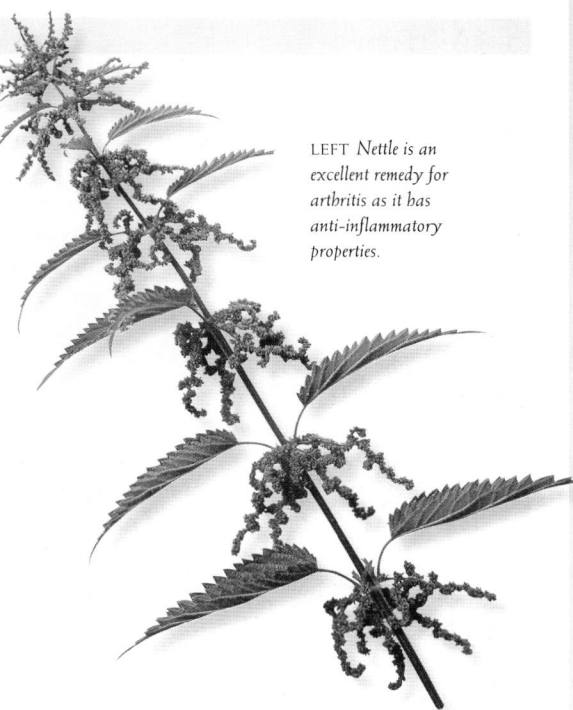

LEFT *Nettle is an excellent remedy for arthritis as it has anti-inflammatory properties.*

pain-relieving; use in local massage or compresses. *(See pages 146–71.)*
• Black pepper, eucalyptus, marjoram, and benzoin will improve the circulation in the area and reduce stiffness. *(See pages 146–71.)*

HOMEOPATHY
• Bryonia is useful for arthritis where stitching pains occur in swollen pale or red joints. *(See page 185.)*
• Colchicum, when it is worse in warm weather, with inflamed joints, irritability, and sensitivity to touch.
• Rhododendron, when it is worse in stormy weather.
• Rhus tox., when the arthritis symptoms include pain and stiffness, and are made worse after rest and in cold damp weather, as well as improving with movement. *(See page 210.)*

• Pulsatilla, when pain moves from one joint to another. *(See page 209.)*
• Apis, for hot, stinging pain. *(See page 180.)*

VITAMINS AND MINERALS
• There is some evidence to show that the antioxidants – Vitamins A, C, and E, plus selenium – may have beneficial effects on arthritis. *(See pages 252, 256 and 257.)*
• Magnesium is required to form the synovial fluid which surrounds the joints, and an adequate intake will ensure health. *(See page 262.)*
• Cod liver oil and evening primrose oil capsules are reported to help rheumatoid arthritis. *(See pages 269 and 270.)*
• Copper may help relieve the symptoms of rheumatoid arthritis, and many sufferers use copper bracelets as a result. *(See page 259.)*

Cramp

Cramp is a painful muscular spasm which occurs most frequently in the feet and legs, but can also affect the abdomen, arms, and hands (writer's cramp). Excess salt loss through sweating is the most common cause, and pregnancy, prolonged sitting or standing, strenuous or unaccustomed exercise, or lying in an unusual position may all be triggers. The muscle contraction is usually short-lived, lasting minutes only, but in some cases it may be prolonged, and repeated. Many old people suffer from night cramps. Some research indicates that a vitamin E deficiency may be partly to blame, and there may also be an imbalance of magnesium and calcium in the body.

ABOVE *One traditional remedy for cramp that works well is to take lemon with a pinch of salt. If taken before bed, it will help to prevent night cramps.*

CAUTION

SEEK MEDICAL ADVICE IF CRAMP IN THE CHEST OCCURS DURING OR AFTER EXERCISE, AS THIS MAY BE ANGINA.

SYMPTOMS

• *twitching, followed by severe pain and a sensation of contortion in the affected muscle*

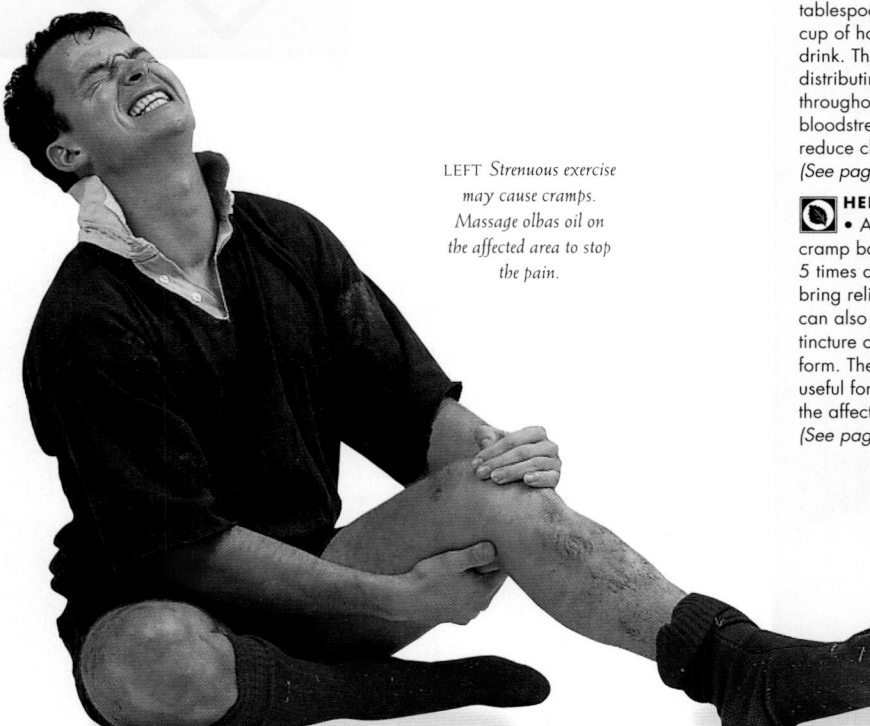

LEFT *Strenuous exercise may cause cramps. Massage olbas oil on the affected area to stop the pain.*

TREATMENT

AYURVEDA
• Yarrow is antispasmodic and can help to prevent and treat cramp. *(See page 24.)*
• Aloe vera, taken internally and applied externally, can soothe muscular spasm. *(See page 27.)*
• Basil, caraway, celery seed, garlic, and myrrh all help. *(See pages 26, 29, 30, 34, and 42.)*

CHINESE HERBALISM
• Gan Caeo is good for spasm and cramps in the abdomen and legs. *(See page 64.)*
• Bai Shao helps cramps in the feet and hands. *(See page 67.)*

TRADITIONAL HOME AND FOLK REMEDIES
• Apply compresses of apple cider vinegar to the affected area, and use several cups of vinegar in the bath. *(See page 102.)*
• A pinch of salt and a sip of lemon juice before bed may prevent night cramps. *(See page 87.)*
• Make a honey and vinegar drink, with 1 tablespoon of each in a cup of hot water, and drink. This works by distributing calcium throughout the bloodstream, which can reduce chronic cramp. *(See pages 101 and 102.)*

HERBALISM
• A decoction of cramp bark taken four or 5 times a day should bring relief. Cramp bark can also be taken as a tincture or in capsule form. The ointment is useful for massaging into the affected area. *(See page 138.)*

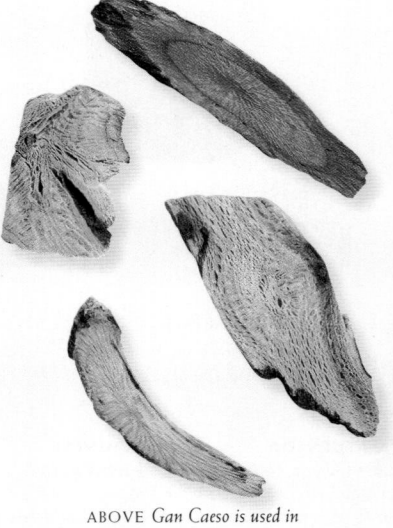

ABOVE *Gan Caeso is used in Chinese medicine to stop spasms and relieve pain.*

• Make a fresh peppermint poultice and apply directly to the area affected by the spasm. *(See page 125.)*
• Olbas oil is effective for sports-induced muscle cramps and spasm.

AROMATHERAPY
• Lavender is antispasmodic and can be usefully employed for cramp as a massage oil. *(See page 161.)*
• Rub the affected area with geranium essential oil. *(See page 165.)*
• Use melissa and chamomile oils for abdominal cramps, diluted in a light carrier oil. *(See pages 150 and 163.)*

HOMEOPATHY
• Take Mag. phos. (6c) every five minutes when cramp occurs. It is especially useful for writer's cramp and cramp that occurs after excessive exercise. *(See page 204.)*
• For menstrual cramp, take Mag. phos. every 30 minutes. *(See page 204.)*
• Cuprum metallicum, for the spasm and subsequent pain. *(See page 192.)*

• Arnica, for cramps caused by muscle fatigue following prolonged exercise. *(See page 182.)*

FLOWER ESSENCES
• Rub a little Rescue Remedy cream into the affected area to encourage healing and provide pain relief. *(See page 244.)*
• Take Rescue Remedy or Emergency Essence during an attack to calm and restore. *(See page 244.)*

VITAMINS AND MINERALS
• Increase your intake of calcium if you are susceptible to cramp. *(See page 258.)*
• Vitamin D is essential for the absorption of calcium. *(See page 256.)*
• Vitamin E supplements have been proved to help prevent night cramps. *(See page 257.)*
• Increase your intake of salt and magnesium. *(See page 262.)*
• Calcium tablets taken with vitamin C are said to prevent night cramps. *(See page 258.)*

Restless Legs

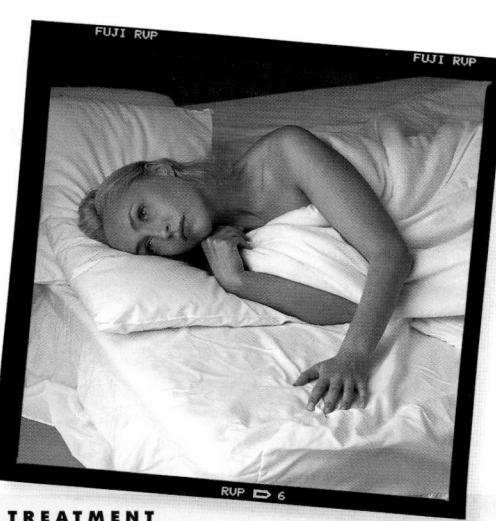

RIGHT *If you have trouble sleeping, try using sedative oils such as chamomile or ylang ylang. They may be inhaled safely from a vaporizer as you sleep.*

Restless legs is the term used to describe a condition associated with insomnia in which the legs ache and are constantly moved about in order to achieve comfort. It is thought to be due either to problems in the nervous system, or to hereditary factors. It is more common in older people and smokers, and it may be triggered by cold, damp weather conditions or overexertion of muscles. There is also an association with diabetes, vitamin B and iron deficiency, excess caffeine intake, and withdrawal from drugs.

ABOVE *Add a few drops of ylang ylang essential oil to a vaporizer in your bedroom to help you sleep.*

SYMPTOMS

• *tickling sensation under the skin* • *burning or prickling sensation* • *aching, twitching, and jerking* • *restlessness relieved by movement*

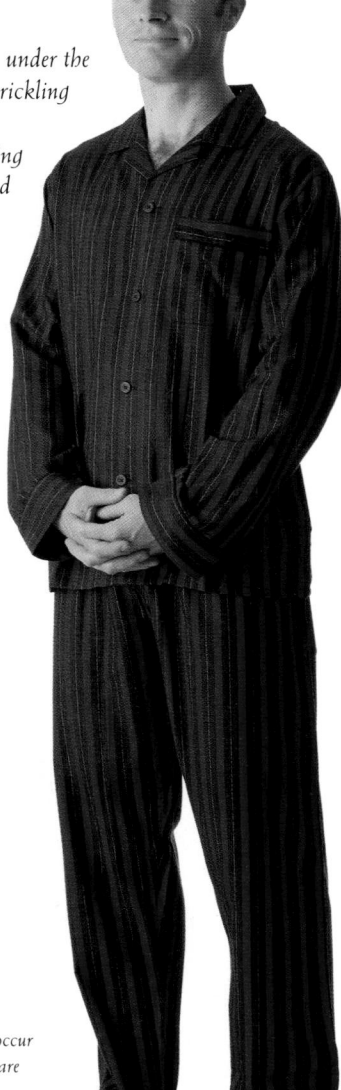

RIGHT *Restless legs occur at nighttime as you are trying to sleep.*

TREATMENT

AYURVEDA
• Warming herbs such as mustard (seeds and oil) and turmeric may be recommended. *(See pages 30 and 37.)*
• Black pepper stimulates circulation and the nervous system. *(See page 44)*
• Camphor stimulates the nervous system and body tissues. *(See page 33.)*
• Cumin is useful for nervous conditions and is generally warming. *(See page 36.)*

CHINESE HERBALISM
• Restlessness is thought to be caused by yin or Blood Deficiency, and possible treatments are lotus seed sprouts and felskrone root tea.

HERBALISM
• A chamomile infusion or compress can help dispel the condition. *(See page 119.)*
• Valerian root works on the nervous system and can help to calm. *(See page 136.)*
• Bruised cloves can be added to any tea to relieve nervous conditions.

AROMATHERAPY
• Benzoin, bergamot, and frankincense have a calming action on the nervous system and can be used in the bath, in a vaporizer, or in local massage to ease. *(See pages 146–71.)*
• If you have trouble sleeping, try using a few drops of chamomile, lavender, marjoram, and ylang ylang, which are hypnotic. *(See pages 146–71.)*

HOMEOPATHY
• Arsenicum, for general restlessness and feelings of chilliness. *(See page 182.)*
• Sepia, for twitching which is worse during the day, and better for taking exercise. *(See page 212.)*
• Belladonna, for legs that jerk into spasm, and for feeling hot, with cold extremities. *(See page 183.)*
• Ignatia, when the problem comes on after grief or a broken love affair. *(See page 200.)*

FLOWER ESSENCES
• Rescue Remedy cream can be rubbed into the muscles of the legs, as required, to calm. *(See page 244.)*

VITAMINS AND MINERALS
• Vitamin E will help to control the condition. *(See page 257.)*
• Iron or vitamin B deficiency may be at the root of the condition, so ensure that you include plenty in your diet. *(See pages 260 and 252–5.)*
• Cut consumption of stimulants, such as caffeine, alcohol, and tobacco.
• Keep the affected muscles warm, and take plenty of hot baths.
• Zinc, for trembling, twitching feet, and restless legs, even while sleeping.

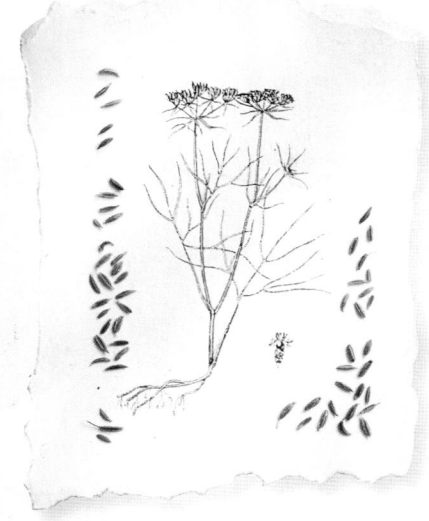

ABOVE *Problems of the nervous system are treated with cumin in Ayurvedic medicine.*

Bursitis

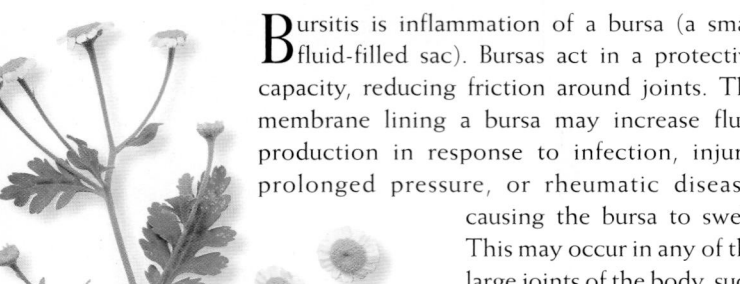

Bursitis is inflammation of a bursa (a small fluid-filled sac). Bursas act in a protective capacity, reducing friction around joints. The membrane lining a bursa may increase fluid production in response to infection, injury, prolonged pressure, or rheumatic disease, causing the bursa to swell. This may occur in any of the large joints of the body, such as the ankle or shoulder, and is commonly associated with bunions at the joint between the big toe and the foot. The build-up of calcium deposits on tendons associated with a joint is a frequent precipitating cause. The calcium deposits trigger an inflammatory reaction that can spread to a nearby bursa and even rupture it. Constant kneeling is a trigger for bursitis, causing a condition known as "housemaid's knee."

ABOVE *A compress of feverfew will relieve painful and hot joints.*

SYMPTOMS

- *restricted movement in the affected joint, caused by swelling*
- *pain and tenderness in the affected area*

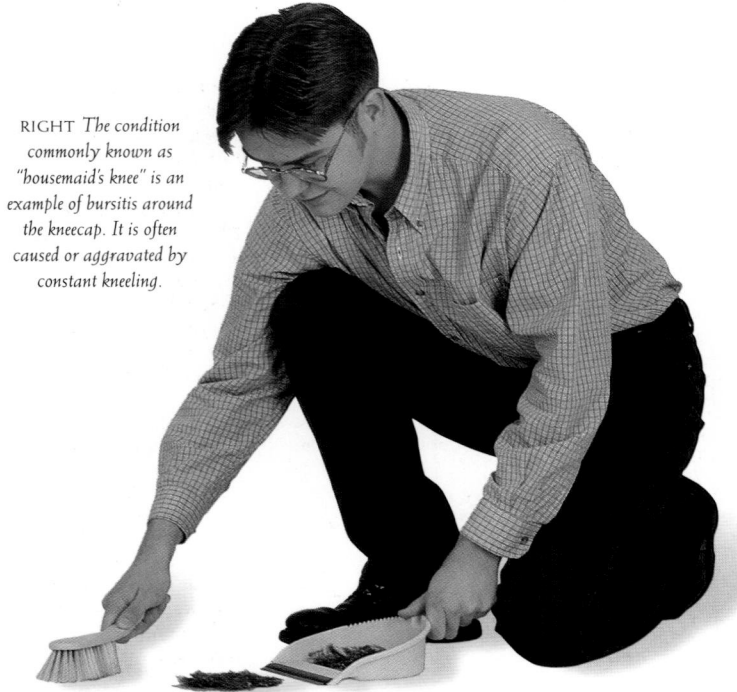

RIGHT *The condition commonly known as "housemaid's knee" is an example of bursitis around the kneecap. It is often caused or aggravated by constant kneeling.*

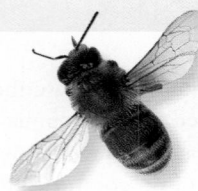

ABOVE *The honey bee, the source of the Apis homeopathic remedy.*

AYURVEDA
- Ginger, coriander, and aloe vera can be used to treat bursitis. *(See pages 27, 35, and 47.)*
- Angelica is a good tonic and is warming. *(See page 28.)*
- Barberry, taken as a tea or applied as a compress, can be used to treat pain and inflammation. *(See page 29.)*
- Rub calamus oil into the affected joints to improve circulation and drainage. *(See page 24.)*

CHINESE HERBALISM
- Pupleuri root, licorice and Chinese skullcap are recommended for their powerful anti-inflammatory effects. *(See pages 64 and 74.)*
- Cinnamon twigs, tinospora stem, angelica, and ledebouriella root may also be helpful. *(See pages 56 and 59.)*

TRADITIONAL HOME AND FOLK REMEDIES
- Eating nettles, or drinking nettle tea, is a traditional remedy for pain and inflammation. The "stings" in stinging nettles contain histamine, which is anti-inflammatory.
- Apple cider foot baths or ginger root baths can help to reduce symptoms and encourage healing. *(See page 102.)*
- Hot or cold compresses on the area will help to disperse swelling. *(See page 80.)*

HERBALISM
- Apply a poultice of slippery elm and cayenne to the affected joints. *(See pages 118 and 136.)*
- Herbs that work to heal bursitis include feverfew, meadowsweet, celery seed, and white willow. They can be taken internally, or used externally, as required. *(See pages 121, 129, and 133.)*
- For relief of aches and pains, try a liniment made with tincture of comfrey and a few drops of black pepper essential oil. *(See page 132.)*
- For improving inflamed joints, take a decoction or tincture of devil's claw. *(See page 123.)*
- Siberian ginseng is a beneficial herb. *(See page 126.)*

AROMATHERAPY
- Use juniper oil in the bath or as part of a massage oil blend. It has stimulating and anti-rheumatic qualities. *(See page 160.)*
- Chamomile, lavender, and rosemary are anti-inflammatory and relieve pain. Use on a compress or for local massage. *(See page 146–71.)*
- Black pepper, eucalyptus, marjoram, and benzoin will improve the circulation in the area and reduce stiffness. *(See pages 146–71.)*

HOMEOPATHY
- Belladonna, for pain which is made worse by the slightest movement, with red hot joints that are swollen and throbbing. *(See page 183.)*
- Kali iod., for pains that are worse at night.
- Rhus tox., for tearing pains with stiff, swollen joints, and which are made worse by heat and cold. *(See page 210.)*
- Pulsatilla, for dragging pain and tightness over the bursa, with chilliness. *(See page 209.)*
- Apis, for burning, stinging pain made worse by heat. *(See page 180.)*
- Sticta, for shooting pains.
- Bryonia, for pain made worse by movement or heat. *(See page 185.)*

FLOWER ESSENCES
- Rub a little Rescue Remedy cream into the affected area to encourage healing and provide pain relief. *(See page 244.)*
- Take Rescue Remedy or Emergency Essence during an attack to calm and restore. *(See page 244.)*

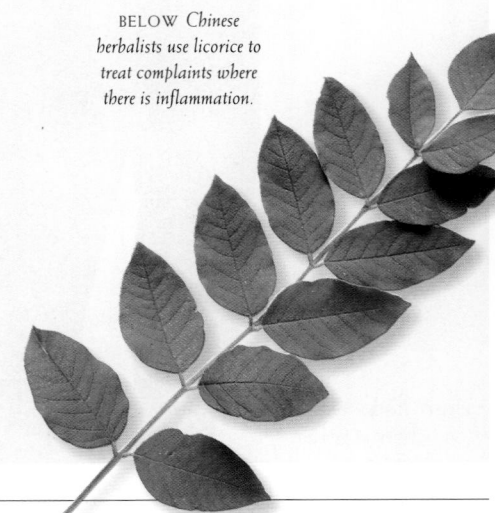

BELOW *Chinese herbalists use licorice to treat complaints where there is inflammation.*

Tendinitis

Tendinitis is an inflammation and thickening of the tendons, usually caused by an injury or overuse of the muscles. There is some association with bursitis (*see page 428*), and indeed the diagnosis is often difficult to make. Bursitis is characterized by a dull pain, whereas the pain of tendinitis is sharp.

SYMPTOMS

• *sharp pain and limited movement in the affected area* • *swelling* • *pins and needles and numbness*

LEFT *Turmeric has anti-inflammatory properties and may be used to treat tendinitis.*

TREATMENT

AYURVEDA
• Turmeric is anti-inflammatory, can be used externally, as an infused oil, or taken internally, 3 times daily, between meals. *(See page 37.)*

TRADITIONAL HOME AND FOLK REMEDIES
• Apply a vinegar compress to reduce areas of inflammation. *(See page 102.)*
• Wrap a bruised wet plantain leaf around the affected area to reduce swelling and stiffness, and to encourage healing.

HERBALISM
• Apply a poultice of slippery elm and cayenne to the affected joints. *(See pages 118 and 136.)*

• Herbs that work to heal arthritis include feverfew, meadowsweet, celery seed, and white willow. They can be taken internally or used externally, as required. *(See pages 121, 129, and 133.)*
• For aching joints, try a liniment of tincture of comfrey and a few drops of black pepper essential oil. *(See page 132.)*
• For inflamed joints in the hand, take a devil's claw decoction or tincture. *(See page 123.)*

AROMATHERAPY
• Chamomile, lavender, and rosemary are anti-inflammatory and pain-relieving. Use in local massage or compresses. *(See pages 146–71.)*

• Black pepper, eucalyptus, marjoram, and benzoin improve the circulation in the area and reduce stiffness. Use as cold or warm compresses. *(See pages 146–71.)*

HOMEOPATHY
• Ruta grav., for tearing pains and lameness. *(See page 210.)*
• Rhus tox., for tearing pains made worse by rest, damp, and movement. *(See page 210.)*

VITAMINS AND MINERALS
• The following nutrients in the diet help encourage healing of the soft tissues: vitamin C, beta carotene, zinc, selenium, vitamin E. *(See pages 256, 264, and 257.)*
• Bromelain, a digestive enzyme, is an anti-inflammatory agent.

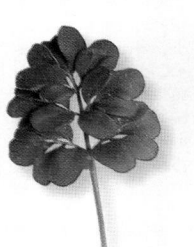
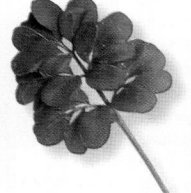
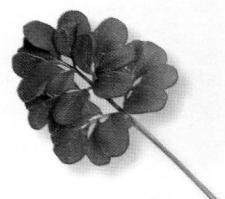

ABOVE *Ruta grav. is used homeopathically to treat bruised, aching, and inflamed tendons.*

Bunions

A bunion (or hallux valgus) is an inflammation of the soft tissue at the base of the big toe due either to ill-fitting shoes or an inherited weakness. Women are more prone to bunions than men, and there is also an association with flat feet. A bunion pushes the big toe outward at the base and in towards the other toes at the top. In some cases a bunion is so large it may distort the sufferer's shoe. Bunions are known as bursitis (*see page 428*).

Ensure that shoes fit properly and are designed to suit the foot, not the fashion. High-heeled shoes and shoes with narrow toes are especially bad for the feet. Go barefoot as often as is practical, walking on a variety of surfaces to exercise the small bones in the feet. Practice picking up small objects, such as marbles, with the toes.

SYMPTOMS

• *pain and discomfort in the affected foot* • *the bunion is aggravated by continuous and prolonged pressure*

TREATMENT

Make a warming mustard foot bath to reduce pain and inflammation. Crush some mustard seeds in a pestle and mortar and add to a bowl of warm water (as hot as is comfortable).

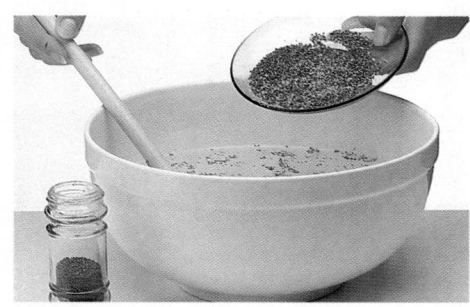

AYURVEDA
• Cedarwood can be used as a rub for sore joints and pain. *(See page 32.)*
• Camphor can be used externally to ease the pain caused by bunions. *(See page 33.)*
• St. John's wort can be taken internally and also used externally in the treatment of bunions. *(See page 40.)*
• Mustard, used in a footbath, will reduce pain and inflammation, and encourage healing. *(See page 30.)*

CHINESE HERBALISM
• Ginger is a useful anti-inflammatory agent.

• Other herbs to try, for external use, include: San Qi, for general relief of pain and swelling, and Jing Jie for inflammation, stiffness, and pain. *(See page 68.)*

HERBALISM
• Treatment to ease inflammation and swelling includes compresses of marshmallow, linseed, comfrey, and slippery elm. *(See pages 114, 132, and 136.)*
• Chamomile infusions, taken internally, will help. *(See page 119.)*

AROMATHERAPY
• For inflamed bunions, add a drop of melissa or chamomile essential oil to the massage oil and rub in

gently. *(See pages 150 and 163.)*
• Lavender or marjoram oil will relieve pain. *(See pages 161 and 165.)*

HOMEOPATHY
• Antimonium is the most effective remedy. *(See page 179.)*
• Apis, for burning, stinging pain made worse by heat. *(See page 180.)*
• Sticta, for shooting pains.
• Kali iod., for pain which is much worse at night.
• Ruta grav., when the bunion feels bruised and painful. *(See page 210.)*
• Rhus tox., when the skin is itchy, red, swollen, and burning and the joints are stiff, but pain decreases with moving about. *(See page 210.)*

COMMON CHILDHOOD AILMENTS

Sleep Problems

All babies and children need different amounts of sleep, and most of them experience some difficulty sleeping at some point. Common causes of sleep problems in babies are diaper rash, teething, colic, illness, being too hot or cold, or simply being wakeful. Older children may be worried about something at school, or a stressful event in the family home. Illness usually disrupts sleep patterns in some way. Some children experience night terrors, which may cause the child to waken suddenly, screaming.

BELOW *Babies will enjoy a gentle massage to help them drift off to sleep.*

CAUTION

IF YOU ARE CONCERNED ABOUT THE CAUSE OF YOUR CHILD'S SLEEP PROBLEMS, SEE YOUR PHYSICIAN.

BELOW *If your child is kept awake by worries about the next day, try White Chestnut flower essence.*

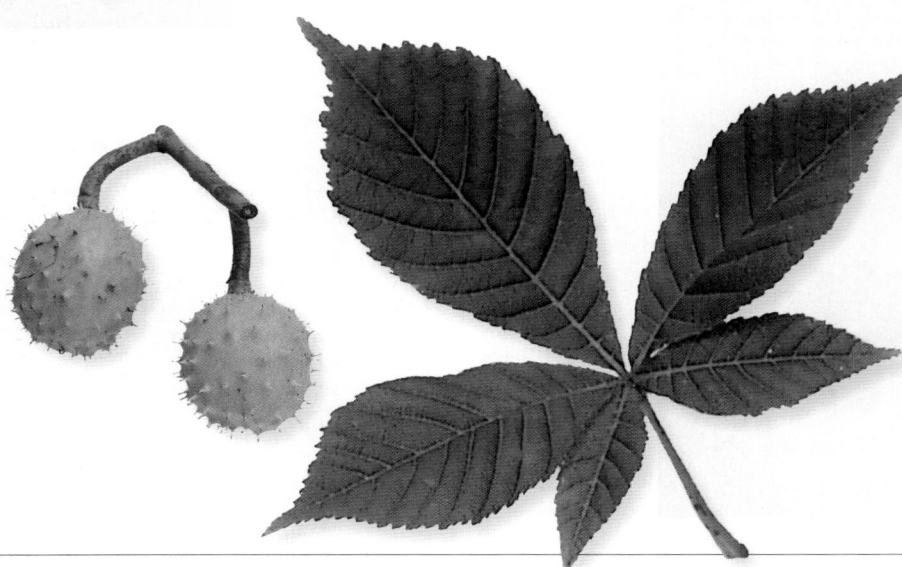

TRADITIONAL HOME AND FOLK REMEDIES
• A little brewer's yeast, mixed with honey and warm milk, makes a soothing bedtime drink for children from the age of four upwards. *(See page 101.)*

HERBALISM
• Vervain is a gentle sedative, and can help children fall asleep – particularly if they are fighting against it. *(See page 138.)*
• Limeflowers will be useful for calming nervous, sensitive children. *(See page 134.)*
• Motherwort can be useful for calming a frightened child or baby. *(See page 124.)*
• A crying baby may be soothed with an infusion of chamomile, offered an hour or so before bedtime or upon waking. *(See page 119.)*
• A strong infusion of chamomile, hops, lavender, or limeflower can be added to a warm bath to soothe and calm a baby or child. *(See pages 119 and 134.)*
• Tincture of catmint, added to a little honey, can be given to a distressed child as and when required.

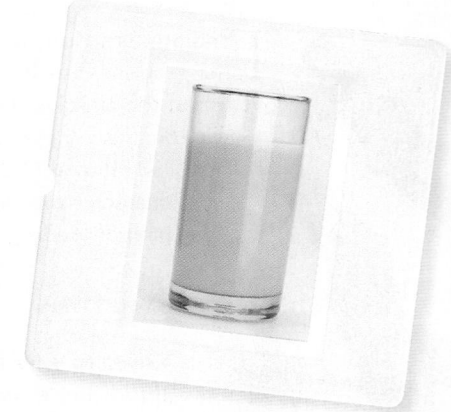

ABOVE *The traditional bedtime drink of warm milk gets extra power from the addition of yeast and honey.*

AROMATHERAPY
• A few drops of chamomile, geranium, rose, or lavender can be added to the bath water. *(See pages 141–71.)*
• Lavender oil, on a handkerchief tied near the cot or bed, will help your baby or child to sleep. *(See page 161.)*
• Lavender or chamomile can be used in a vaporizer in your child's room. *(See pages 150 and 161.)*
• A gentle massage before bedtime, with a little lavender or chamomile blended with a light carrier oil, may ease any tension or distress. *(See pages 150 and 161.)*

HOMEOPATHY
• Ant. tart. for night terrors. *(See pages 186 and 179.)*
• For constant crying use Colocynthis or Bryonia. *(See pages 191 and 185.)*
• Phosphorus, for thirst, and alternating anger and affection. *(See page 208.)*
• Pulsatilla, for a weepy and clingy child. *(See page 209.)*
• Chamomilla, if sleep is being disturbed by teething. *(See page 204.)*
• Nux vomica, for irritability, and after a busy, stressful day. *(See page 214.)*

FLOWER ESSENCES
• White Chestnut will be helpful for children with overactive minds. *(See page 224.)*
• A distressed child or baby can be given Rescue Remedy, which will calm him or her. *(See page 244.)*
• Rock Rose, for night terrors. *(See page 231.)*
• Aspen, for anxiety for no identifiable cause. *(See page 236.)*
• Walnut will be useful for change – a new baby, school, or house. *(See page 232.)*
• A few drops of Mimulus will soothe a child who is afraid of the dark. *(See page 235.)*

VITAMINS AND MINERALS
• Avoid cold-energy foods such as bananas and cucumbers, which can cause colic and digestive problems.
• A warm glass of goat's milk will encourage sleep without causing any digestive disturbance.
• Older children may suck a zinc lozenge before bedtime to help them to go to sleep. *(See page 265.)*

Hyperactivity

Hyperactivity is a behavioral disorder which appears to be becoming more common. A hyperactive child has an excessively high energy level, being restless, inattentive, and easily frustrated. There are often prolonged and regular tantrums, and fidgeting. Intelligence is common among hyperactive children, but there is such a short attention span that they often do not do well at school. Psychiatrists have labeled the problem attention-deficit hyperactivity disorder, or ADHD. (Some children display attention-deficit disorder, or ADD, without hyperactivity.) ADHD appears in children before the age of four, but its signs are often missed until the child attends school.

There is a widespread belief that food additives, such as preservatives, are at the root of the problem, but this has not been conclusively proved. Others believe that minor brain damage may be the cause of hyperactivity.

ABOVE *Sandalwood essential oil calms the nervous system and soothes a restless child.*

SYMPTOMS

• *restlessness* • *inattentiveness*
• *tantrums* • *fidgeting*

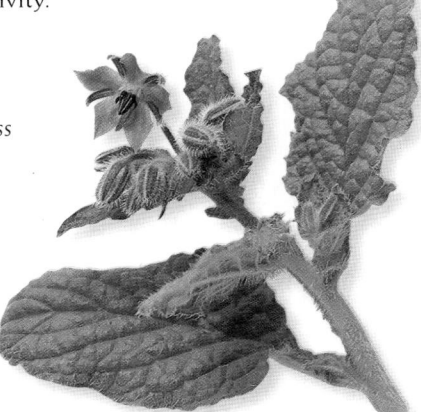

RIGHT *The adrenal gland is overworked by stress; borage helps redress the balance.*

ABOVE *Tantrums may be caused by food additives – try to eliminate them from your child's diet.*

TREATMENT

HERBALISM
• Black root and fringe tree may be useful herbs if poor digestion is causing hyperactivity.
• Herbs to support a stressed nervous system include vervain and skullcap. *(See pages 131 and 138.)*
• Oats act as a tonic to the nervous system. *(See page 117.)*
• Chamomile, limeflowers, and skullcap, for tense and anxious children. *(See pages 119, 131, and 134.)*
• Borage and licorice will work to address an overworked adrenal gland. *(See page 122.)*

AROMATHERAPY
• Massage may calm hyperactivity in children. If the child can be persuaded to lie quietly for a few minutes, both mother and child may benefit from the feeling of peace and calm created during the massage. Use a little lavender or Roman chamomile oil to calm. *(See pages 150 and 161.)*
• Neroli, rose, and sandalwood essential oils have a calming action on the nervous system. *(See pages 146–71.)*
• Add a few drops of Roman chamomile to the bath water to soothe and encourage sleep. *(See page 150.)*

HOMEOPATHY
• Constitutional treatment is recommended, but China may be appropriate if food allergies or digestive problems are at the root. *(See page 190.)*
• Chamomilla will calm an overexcited, demanding child. *(See page 204.)*

FLOWER ESSENCES
• Vervain, for an over-enthusiastic child. *(See page 241.)*
• Impatiens, for a child who is talkative, quick thinking, and impatient. *(See page 233.)*
• Cherry Plum, for loss of control. *(See page 236.)*

VITAMINS AND MINERALS
• Include plenty of vitamin B-complex, vitamin C, zinc, and essential fatty acids in the diet, which help behavioral problems. *(See pages 252–5, 256 and 265.)*
• It will probably be necessary to take a good multivitamin and mineral tablet each day.

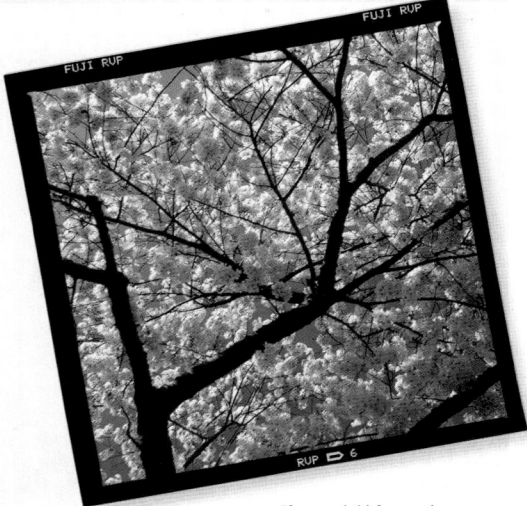

ABOVE *If your child frequently loses self-control, the flower essence Cherry Plum may help.*

Bedwetting

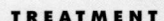

ABOVE *Sudden bedwetting, after a shock, may respond to Star of Bethlehem.*

Bedwetting is not considered to be a problem until your child is at least five years old. Many children, boys in particular, are slow in getting the message that they should get up to use the toilet at night, but that is no reflection on the state of their health – mental or otherwise. If a child sleeps heavily it may take longer for night dryness, but many children manage it by two or three years of age. Bedwetting in children who have already established a pattern of dry nights is usually caused by stress of some sort, like moving house, changing schools, or family fighting. Children who have never been dry at night may suffer from immature nerves and muscles controlling bladder function. Other medical causes include diabetes, urinary infection, a structural abnormality, nutritional deficiencies, and food allergies.

TREATMENT

HERBALISM
• Offer St. John's wort and horsetail teas throughout the day, sweetened with honey, to soothe an irritable bladder and encourage control of the bladder. *(See page 124.)*
• If the bedwetting stems from an emotional upset or disturbance, vervain and lemon balm relax and soothe. *(See page 138.)*

AROMATHERAPY
• Massage oil of chamomile into the lower back and tummy while settling your child down to sleep. *(See page 150.)*

HOMEOPATHY
• Equisetum, when the wetting occurs during dreams.
• Belladonna, when it occurs early in the night. *(See page 183.)*
• Kreosotum, when wetting occurs during dreams early in the night and during deep sleep.
• Causticum, for wetting in first sleep, and when the problem is worse in clear weather or when your child has a cough. *(See page 189.)*
• Plantago, when all else fails.

FLOWER ESSENCES
• Try Wild Rose if your child drifts through life. *(See page 238.)*
• Walnut will help if the bedwetting is brought on by change, such as a new house, school, or baby. *(See page 232.)*
• Chestnut Bud, if the child does not seem to learn from the experience. *(See page 224.)*
• Star of Bethlehem, if bedwetting is related to a trauma or shock. *(See page 235.)*
• Mimulus, when the problem is linked to fear. *(See page 235.)*

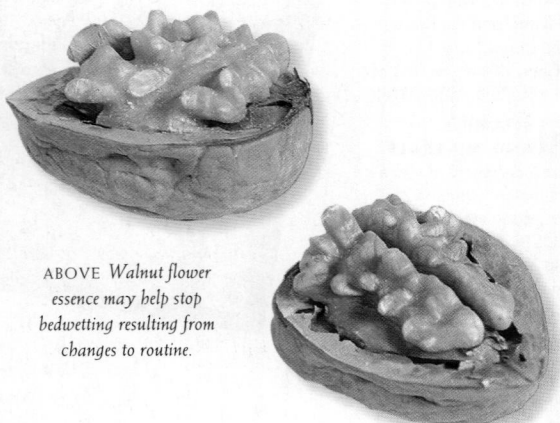

ABOVE *Walnut flower essence may help stop bedwetting resulting from changes to routine.*

Cradle Cap

Cradle cap (seborrheic eczema) is common during the first three months of life and is characterized by a thick encrusted layer of skin on the baby's scalp. Nearly 90 percent of all babies will suffer from cradle cap at some point during the first few months. There will be yellow scales, which form in patches, especially on the top of the head. In severe cases, cradle cap can last for up to three years. Like dandruff, cradle cap is a condition in which the seborrheic glands are overactive, and it is often associated with seborrheic dermatitis, a skin condition in which there are red, scaly areas on the forehead and eyebrows, among other places.

CAUTION

TRY NOT TO LOOSEN CRUSTS THAT HAVE NOT PULLED AWAY ON THEIR OWN – BLEEDING AND INFECTION MAY RESULT.

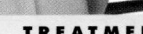

RIGHT *Calendula ointment is useful for many kinds of skin inflammation.*

TREATMENT

TRADITIONAL HOME AND FOLK REMEDIES
• Massage olive oil into the scalp each evening, and then gently shampoo away in the morning. *(See page 95.)*
• Mash an avocado, apply to the scalp, and then gently rinse. Rub the skin of the avocado across the head to moisten and heal. *(See page 96.)*
• Over-washing will make the condition much worse. Gently brush away loosened crusts with a soft brush.

HERBALISM
• Rinse the scalp after washing with an infusion of meadowsweet, which acts as an anti-inflammatory and will reduce any itching. *(See page 121.)*
• Burdock may also be used to rinse the scalp after washing your baby's hair. *(See page 115.)*
• Butternut can be taken internally (1 drop, 3 times daily, mixed in water) to encourage healing.

AROMATHERAPY
• Massage a few drops of lavender or lemon oil, mixed in a light carrier oil, into the scalp before bedtime. Rinse gently each morning. *(See pages 154 and 161.)*

HOMEOPATHY
• Massage the scalp with Calendula ointment. *(See page 187.)*
• Lycopodium, taken internally, is useful if the skin is dry but uninfected. *(See page 203.)*

FLOWER ESSENCES
• Rock Rose is useful if the itching causes distress. Rescue Remedy cream may be massaged into the scalp to reduce symptoms. *(See page 231.)*
• Add 2 drops of Rescue Remedy to the rinse water, and use after a shampoo. *(See page 244.)*

Impetigo

(See under Skin and Hair, page 311).

Sticky Eye

Sticky eye is a mild infection of the eyes which causes a yellowish discharge and crusting. It is most common in the first week of life, and is usually the result of a foreign object entering the eye during birth, or from the blood or amniotic fluid. This condition is not serious and usually rights itself without treatment. In an older child, sticky eyes are usually a sign of conjunctivitis, which is a condition in which the conjunctiva of the eye becomes infected *(see page 318)*. It may indicate a blocked tear duct.

ABOVE *Distilled witch hazel is an old standby. Dilute with water and apply to the eyelid.*

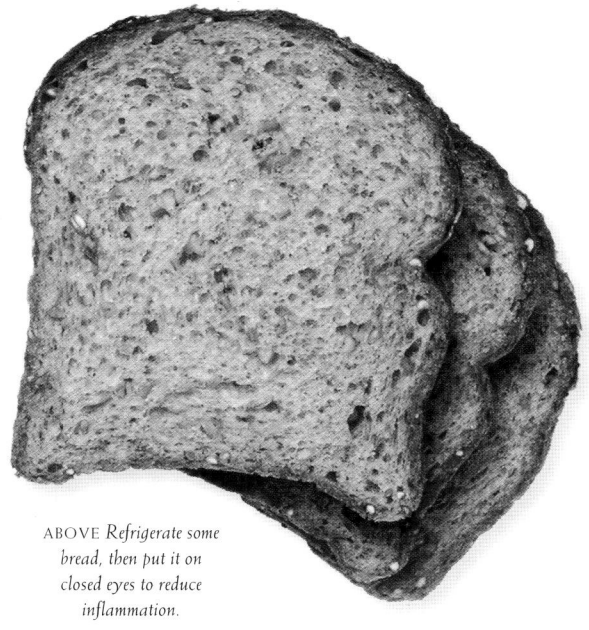

ABOVE *Refrigerate some bread, then put it on closed eyes to reduce inflammation.*

CAUTION

ALWAYS USE VERY WEAK HERBAL INFUSIONS FOR BABIES AND TODDLERS – ONE-FIFTH OF THE DOSE FOR ADULTS. CHILDREN SHOULD HAVE HALF DOSES BETWEEN THE AGES OF 6 AND 12.

TREATMENT

TRADITIONAL HOME AND FOLK REMEDIES
• Apply cold bread to closed eyes to reduce the inflammation and soothe itching. *(See page 101.)*
• Boil fennel seeds to make an eyewash for conjunctivitis and sore and inflamed eyes.
• Honey water can be used to cleanse the eye; it acts to destroy any infection, soothe, and encourage healing. *(See page 101.)*

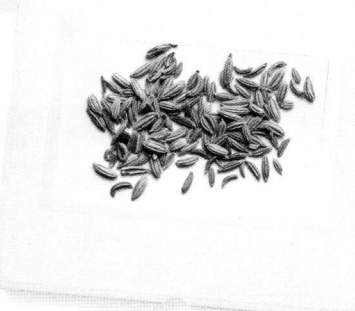

ABOVE *An eyewash made from fennel seeds reduces inflammation.*

HERBALISM
• Infusions of the following herbs can be taken internally to ease the condition: echinacea (which boosts the immune system and acts as a natural antibiotic), eyebright, and golden seal. *(See page 120.)*

• Infusions of chamomile, elderflower, eyebright, and golden seal can be applied externally. Some of these herbs can also be bought as a tincture and then used to make a soothing eyewash. *(See pages 119, 120 and 130.)*
• Soak a chamomile tea bag and hold to the eyelids to soothe. Use it to gently clean the eyes (a new bag for each eye). *(See page 119.)*
• Distilled rosewater or witch hazel can help. *(See page 123.)*

HOMEOPATHY
• Euphrasia, for burning, itching eyes. *(See page 194.)*
• 1 or 2 drops of Euphrasia tincture can also be used to bathe the eyes. *(See page 194.)*
• Pulsatilla can be used when there is mucus collecting in the corner of the eyes. *(See page 209.)*
• Hep. sulf. will be useful to draw out infection. *(See page 198.)*

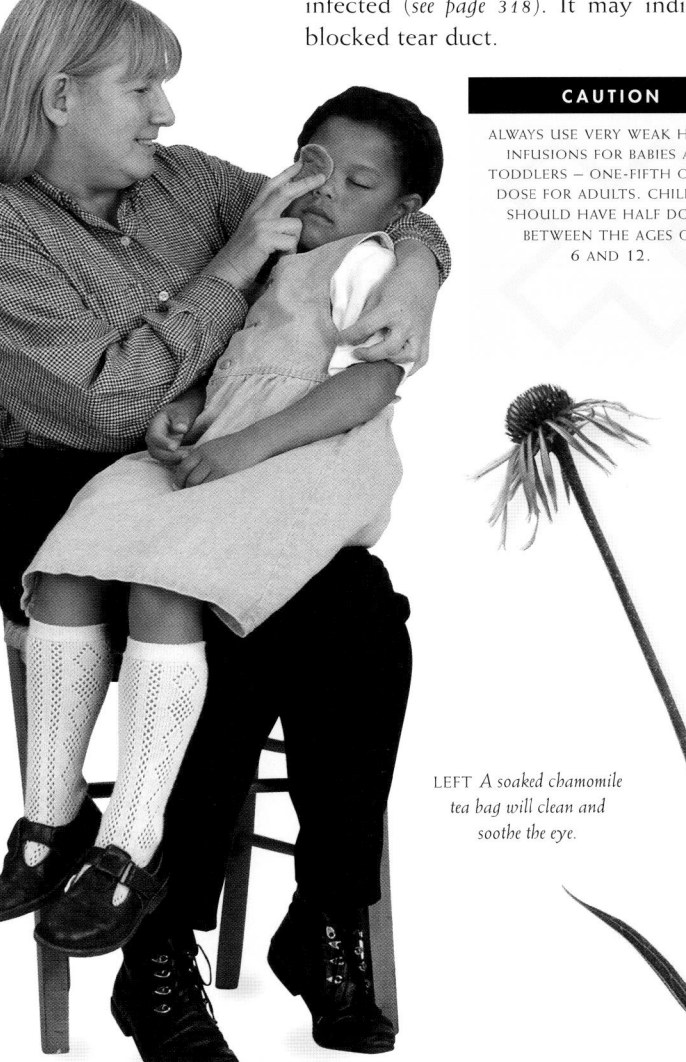

LEFT *A soaked chamomile tea bag will clean and soothe the eye.*

LEFT *Drinking echinacea infusion brings antibiotic benefits.*

Earache and Middle Ear Infections

Earache may be caused by inflammation of the lymph nodes in the neck, or by another illness like mumps. There may be an ear infection in the inner, middle, or outer parts of the ear. Occasionally a boil can crop up in the outer ear, which can be very painful. The most common ear infections in children are middle ear infections. These are usually caused by the transmission of infection from the nose or throat by the Eustachian tube. Because this tube is short and small in babies and young children, it is easily blocked, and infection does not have far to travel to the middle ear itself. Ear infections can cause a great deal of pain, and the pressure may burst the eardrum, causing a discharge. Earache is also occasionally a sign of dental problems.

SYMPTOMS

pain • possibly a discharge • possibly fever and a sore throat • malaise

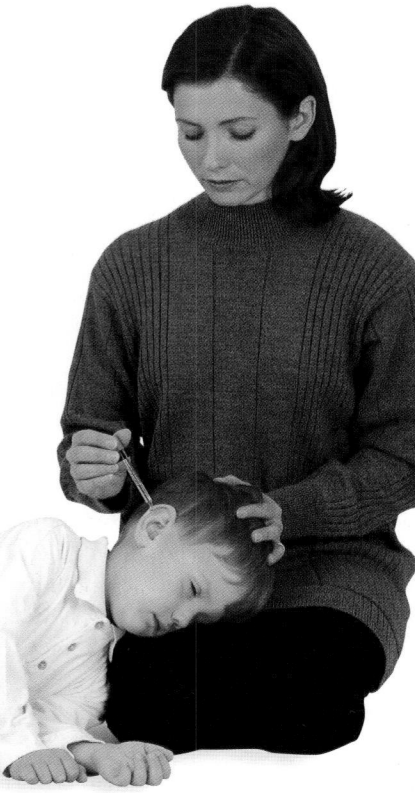

LEFT *Use a dropper to administer witch hazel and St. John's wort to relieve pain and inflammation.*

TREATMENT

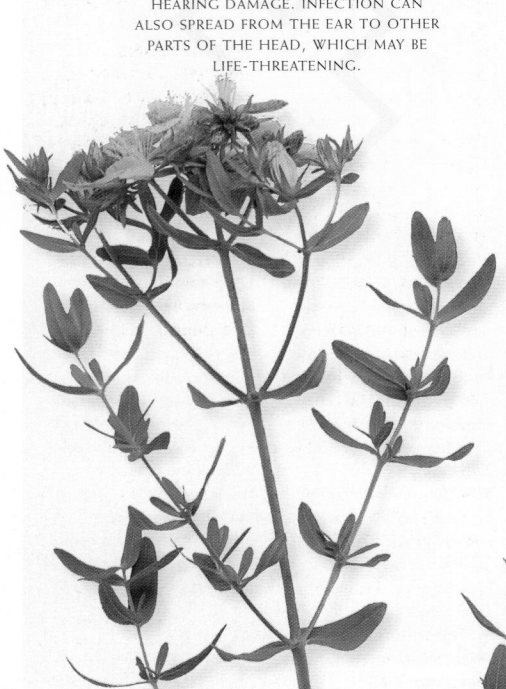

LEFT *A hot St. John's wort compress is anti-inflammatory and comforting.*

TRADITIONAL HOME AND FOLK REMEDIES
• Witch hazel can be added to a teaspoon of oil of St. John's wort and dropped into the ear. This will take away the pain and inflammation. *(See page 91.)*
• Crush fresh garlic and mix with a little honey to encourage the body to fight off the infection. *(See page 82.)*
• Drink honey and lemon, or a little cider vinegar in some warm water to help rid the body of catarrh and strengthen immunity. *(See pages 87, 101, and 102.)*
• Blackcurrant tea will help to boost the immune system and to reduce catarrh.

HERBALISM
• Passiflora will help if there is panic.
• Echinacea can be taken to boost the immune system and clear the pus. *(See page 120.)*
• Apply a hot compress or poultice to the neck and ears using mullein or St. John's wort, which are anti-inflammatory. *(See pages 124 and 137.)*
• Give chamomile tea to drink, to soothe pain and distress. *(See page 119.)*
• For an acute attack, use black root and hops to lower fever and reduce the inflammation present.
• A few drops of tincture of myrrh or golden seal can be added to a light oil, warmed, and dropped into the ear canal.
• Soak a cotton ball with a few drops of warmed garlic oil and press gently into the ear canal. *(See page 113.)*

AROMATHERAPY
• A few drops of neat lavender oil can be placed in the ear on a cotton ball, or gently eased in with a Q-tip. *(See page 161.)*
• Gently massage the neck and head around the ear with oil of mullein or lavender in a light carrier oil. *(See page 161.)*
• Tea tree or lavender oil can be used in a vaporizer for their antiseptic properties. *(See pages 161 and 162.)*
• Use a few drops of lavender oil on a handkerchief by the bed to help your child to stay calm and to sleep. *(See page 161.)*

HOMEOPATHY
• Hep. sulf. is useful for acute attacks, with an earache accompanying a sore throat; and where the child feels chilly. *(See page 198.)*
• Aconite can be used in the early stages, particularly when the symptoms set in suddenly. *(See page 178.)*

• Belladonna, when the affected ear is red and hot, and the child is feverish and perhaps delirious. *(See page 183.)*
• Chamomilla when the child is inconsolable and the pain is made worse if the child is in a draft. *(See page 204.)*

FLOWER ESSENCES
• Rub a little Rescue Remedy (stock or cream) into the painful parts just below the ears to stop the child panicking and reduce inflammation. *(See page 244.)*
• Rescue Remedy or Rock Rose will ease panic. *(See pages 244 and 231.)*
• Olive can be used during recuperation. *(See page 235.)*

VITAMINS AND MINERALS
• Make sure your child's diet is rich in foods containing vitamin C and zinc, which boost the immune system and help to treat infection. *(See pages 256 and 265.)*

Glue Ear

Glue ear is a chronic condition affecting a large number of children. It is characterized by a thick, often smelly, mucus which builds up in the middle ear, due to Eustachian tube obstruction. It impairs hearing, and causes the eardrum to perforate, allowing the mucus to be discharged. Glue ear is common in children who have frequent colds or other infections, which block the Eustachian tube (see *Middle Ear Infection on page 323 and Outer Ear Infection on page 324*). There is some indication that overuse of antibiotics may encourage the condition, and many children have excess or chronic catarrh (*see page 329*) which may be linked to food allergies or intolerance. Usually both ears are affected, and it is often accompanied by enlarged adenoids and frequently occurs with viral upper respiratory infections, such as the common cold. The first and often the only sign of glue ear is some degree of deafness.

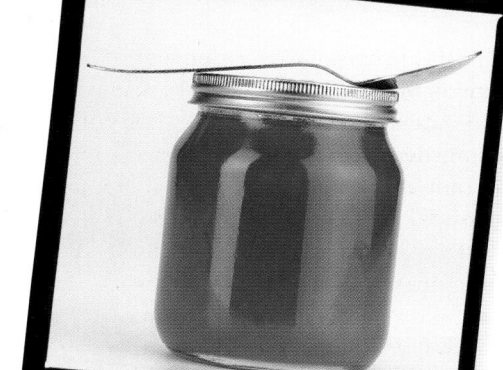
ABOVE *Eucalyptus is an antiseptic oil. Massage the ear and neck area.*

RIGHT *Make garlic-infused honey. It is an expectorant.*

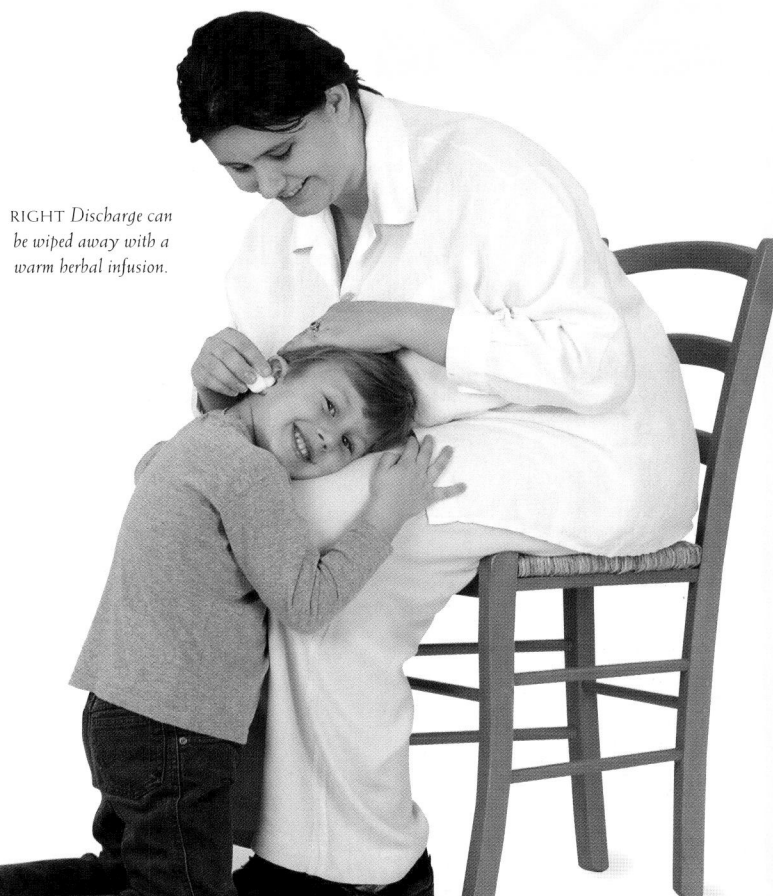
RIGHT *Discharge can be wiped away with a warm herbal infusion.*

TREATMENT

CHINESE HERBALISM
• Herbs to reduce inflammation and Mucus (Phlegm) would be Sheng di Huang or Chinese senega root/Polygala. (*See pages 70 and 72.*)

TRADITIONAL HOME AND FOLK REMEDIES
• Drink lemon and honey or cider vinegar to clear the mucus and to strengthen the immune system. (*See pages 87, 101, and 102.*)
• Garlic is excellent at shifting catarrh and cleansing the blood. Offer as garlic perles, or chop fresh garlic and serve with a teaspoon of honey. (*See page 82.*)
• Blackcurrant tea is excellent for catarrh and will encourage healing of the ear.

HERBALISM
• Chamomile and echinacea are antiseptic, and can be taken internally or added to a foot or hand bath to reduce subsequent infection and to relieve unpleasant symptoms. (*See pages 119 and 120.*)
• Clean away discharge with a warm infusion of antiseptic herbs, such as chamomile or golden seal. (*See page 119.*)
• Herbal remedies to boost the immune system include chamomile, echinacea, peppermint, and wild indigo. (*See pages 119, 120, and 125.*)
• Herbs to help clear the catarrh include elderflowers, euphrasia, golden rod, and hyssop. (*See page 130.*)
• Herbs which work to reduce catarrh include golden rod, ground ivy, and elderflower. (*See page 130.*)

AROMATHERAPY
• Dilute essential oils of lavender, chamomile, eucalyptus, or rosewood in a light carrier oil, warm, and massage around the ear and neck. (*See pages 146–71.*)
• Massage the ear area with a few drops of essential oil of lavender blended in a light carrier oil. (*See page 161.*)
• A steam inhalation of eucalyptus, chamomile, or lavender can help to reduce catarrh and ease accompanying symptoms. (*See pages 146–71.*)
• Apply a hot compress to the nose, ears, and throat made using diluted essential oils of lavender, rosewood, or chamomile. (*See pages 146–71.*)

RIGHT *Citrus fruits are high in vitamin C to help fight off infection.*

HOMEOPATHY
• Kali mur., when there are cracking sounds in the affected ear, accompanied by swollen glands in the neck.
• Lycopodium, when there is deafness and a roaring sound in the affected ear. (*See page 203.*)
• Pulsatilla, for a full feeling in the ear, and a feeling of weepiness. (*See page 209.*)
• Mercurius, when there is thick, smelly discharge. (*See page 205.*)

VITAMINS AND MINERALS
• Chronic infection can be caused by a build-up of catarrh (see page 329). Reduce consumption of dairy produce and any other possible allergens, including wheat.
• Take cod liver oil and vitamin C to boost the immune system. (*See page 269.*)

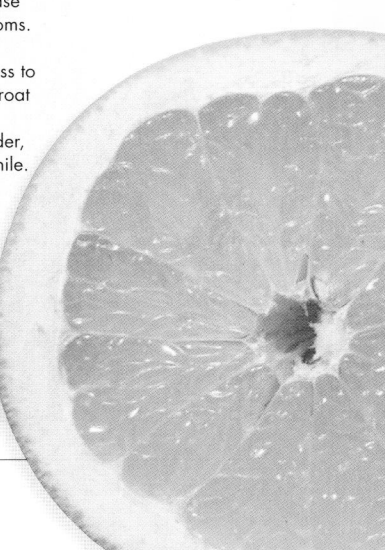

Colds

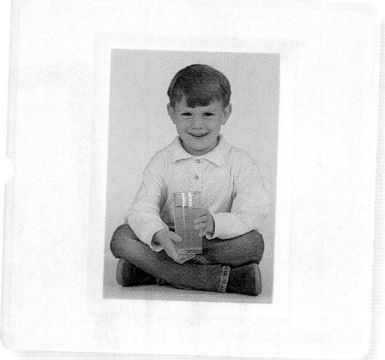

ABOVE *Hot lemon and honey is a tried and tested cold cure.*

Small children are more susceptible than adults to the viruses causing colds and flu because their immune systems are immature. Do not be surprised if your child seems to contract every cold he or she comes into contact with. Symptoms of a cold include a running nose, headache, and sometimes a cough. There may be a mild fever and a feeling of general malaise. Most colds run their course within 7–10 days. Some colds may be symptoms of allergy (particularly when the mucus remains clear) or common childhood illnesses and fevers, or part of a pattern of symptoms associated with asthma or cystic fibrosis. Recurrent colds (almost constantly suffering) may indicate a lowered immune capacity, which can be treated by complementary remedies. (*See Colds, page* 352.)

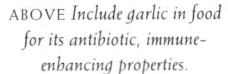

ABOVE *Include garlic in food for its antibiotic, immune-enhancing properties.*

SYMPTOMS

- *running nose* • *headache* • *sometimes a cough* • *possibly a mild fever and a feeling of general malaise*

LEFT *Steam inhalation improves congestion. Use a few drops of cinnamon oil.*

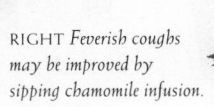

RIGHT *Feverish coughs may be improved by sipping chamomile infusion.*

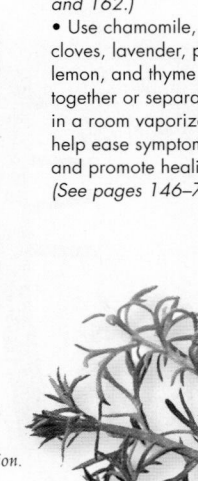

TREATMENT

TRADITIONAL HOME AND FOLK REMEDIES

- Blackcurrant tea is excellent for catarrh and infections.
- Eat plenty of fresh garlic and onions to reduce catarrh and cleanse the blood. Garlic is also antibiotic and boosts the immune system. *(See page 82.)*
- Hot lemon and honey will help to clear catarrh, prevent a secondary infection (such as tonsillitis or bronchitis), and soothe discomfort. *(See pages 87 and 101.)*

HERBALISM

- Blue flag or poke root, for swollen glands.
- Golden seal and elecampane, for chronic colds, to clear mucus from the lungs and nasal passages.
- Elderflowers, drunk as an infusion, will reduce catarrh and help to decongest. *(See page 130.)*
- Peppermint is another decongestant and will also work to reduce a fever. *(See page 125.)*
- Eucalyptus, rosemary, and thyme will help to clear congestion and work as antiseptics, which may help to prevent a secondary infection of the tonsils or bronchi (bronchitis). *(See pages 127 and 135.)*

- Chamomile will soothe an irritable child and help him or her to sleep. Chamomile also has antiseptic action, which will help to rid the body of infection, and it works to reduce fever and feverish symptoms. *(See page 119.)*
- Try adding a strong infusion of chamomile or yarrow to the bath. *(See pages 112 and 119.)*
- Mullein or comfrey can be drunk or used as a compress around the neck to soothe a sore throat. *(See pages 132 and 137.)*
- Herbs to strengthen the immune system, including echinacea, can be taken throughout a cold. *(See page 120.)*

AROMATHERAPY

- Place your child's head over a steaming bowl of water with a few drops of essential oil of cinnamon. Place a towel over her head to make a tent, and let her sit there for 4 or 5 minutes to ease congestion. *(See page 150.)*
- Massage a few drops of pine or eucalyptus, blended in a light carrier oil, into the chest area. *(See pages 159 and 166.)*
- Try a few drops of lavender or tea tree oil in a warm bath to encourage healing and open up the airways. *(See pages 161 and 162.)*
- Use chamomile, cloves, lavender, pine, lemon, and thyme together or separately in a room vaporizer to help ease symptoms and promote healing. *(See pages 146–71.)*

HOMEOPATHY

- Nat. mur., for dealing with watery colds. *(See page 206.)*
- Kali mur., for colds with catarrh.
- Ferr. phos., for hot colds. *(See page 194.)*
- Arsenicum, for watery colds, particularly if your child is prone to frequent colds. *(See page 182.)*
- Euphrasia, for colds affecting the eyes. *(See page 194.)*
- Pulsatilla is useful if your child is clingy and irritable, and when there is thick yellow discharge. *(See page 209.)*
- Bryonia, for an irritable child who is thirsty and wants to be left alone. *(See page 185.)*
- Mercurius, for a child with earache and swollen lymph nodes in the neck. *(See page 205.)*

FLOWER ESSENCES

- Rescue Remedy will soothe any distress. *(See page 244.)*
- Olive will help with fatigue. *(See page 235.)*
- Willow, if the child feels sorry for him or herself. *(See page 239.)*

VITAMINS AND MINERALS

- Eat plenty of foods with vitamin C and zinc, which will help discourage a cold and reduce its duration. *(See pages 256 and 265.)*

BELOW *Lavender oil, sprinkled on the pillow, promotes sleep.*

Coughs

Coughing expels foreign bodies and irritating mucus from the trachea and airways of the lungs. The membranes lining the whole respiratory tract are very sensitive and react to inhaled particles or infection by producing mucus, which is then coughed up. The color of the mucus or phlegm indicates the nature or the degree of irritation or infection. There are many types of coughs, some of which accompany a cold. Others are caused by chemicals, other infections, like ear and tonsil infections, excess catarrh, inflammation of the airways, and many other things. A chronic cough is one that lasts for more than 10 days, or one that recurs frequently.

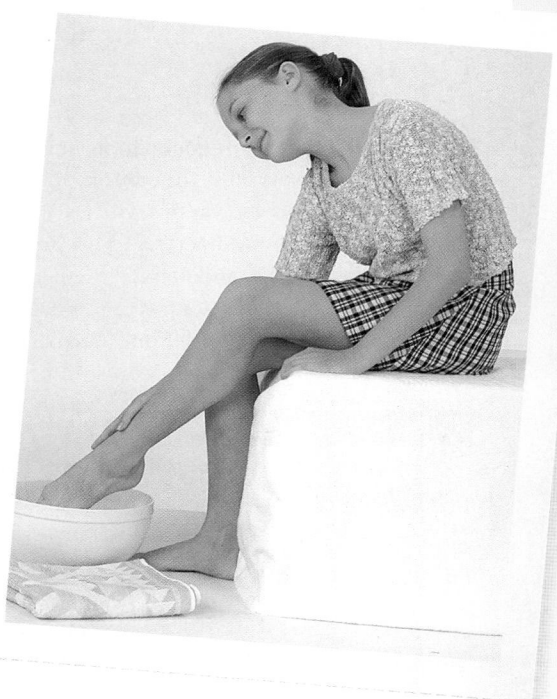

RIGHT *A thyme oil footbath helps shift stubborn catarrh.*

TREATMENT

TRADITIONAL HOME AND FOLK REMEDIES
• Fresh garlic should be eaten as often as possible to cleanse the blood, improve the immune response, and encourage healing. *(See page 82.)*
• Give your child lots of honey, which has antibacterial action and will also soothe a sore throat. *(See page 101.)*
• Blackcurrant tea will ease the pain of a sore throat and help to reduce catarrh.
• Ginger, added to meals, will help to get rid of any lingering catarrh.
• Pineapples are traditionally used for expelling excess catarrh.
• Lemon and honey will soothe a sore throat and ease a tickly cough. *(See pages 87 and 101.)*

HERBALISM
• Aniseed and fennel will warm the system and help to shift a cough. *(See page 121.)*

• Cayenne pepper can be added to food (a few grains) to stimulate the body's immune defenses and clear the wet secretions from the lungs. *(See page 118.)*
• Pasque flower and lobelia will clear fever and reduce inflammation.
• For fever, try infusions of chamomile, catmint, hyssop, and yarrow. *(See pages 112 and 119.)*
• Comfrey and coltsfoot help expel mucus from the lungs and airways. Mix 10 drops of each tincture with warmed honey. Serve by the teaspoonful. *(See page 132.)*
• Elecampane and thyme can be infused and used to treat a wet cough. *(See page 135.)*
• When the mucus is tough to shift, try strong infusions of ginger and fennel or thyme. *(See pages 121, 135, and 139.)*
• Elecampane root tea, sweetened with honey and ginger, will help to reduce inflammation and reduce mucus.

AROMATHERAPY
• Use lavender, myrrh, eucalyptus, or thyme in a vaporizer. *(See pages 146–71.)*
• A few drops of oil of thyme, pine, cinnamon, clove, or eucalyptus can be used in combination or on their own in a foot bath to ease congestion. *(See pages 146–71.)*
• Add a few drops of eucalyptus and sandalwood to a carrier oil or some petroleum jelly, and rub into the chest and upper back. *(See pages 159 and 169.)*
• Myrrh can be massaged into the body in the same way, to reduce mucus. Or put a few drops on a handkerchief and tie it to the bed. *(See page 155.)*
• Lavender oil on a handkerchief or pillow will encourage sleep and aid the healing process. *(See page 161.)*

HOMEOPATHY
• Belladonna can be taken when the cough is accompanied by a fever, and the child has bright red cheeks and neck. *(See page 183.)*
• Pulsatilla may be useful if there is a thick yellow discharge and your child is clingy and tearful. *(See page 209.)*
• Ant. tart., for a cough that causes the chest to rattle and makes breathing painful. *(See page 179.)*
• Bryonia, for a painful, dry cough which is made worse by movement. *(See page 185.)*
• Spongia is excellent for croup *(see page 438)* and for a loud, crowing cough. *(See page 213.)*
• Drosera, for a tickling cough which is worse when lying down. *(See page 193.)*
• Try aconite if the symptoms come on suddenly. *(See page 178.)*
• Chamomilla will soothe an inconsolable child, who is better for being held. *(See page 204.)*

FLOWER ESSENCES
• Use Rescue Remedy when your child experiences distress, or panics because breathing is difficult. Rescue Remedy may also help your child to sleep. A few drops can be taken internally or applied to pulse points. *(See page 244.)*
• Olive is good for a child who is overwhelmed by fatigue. *(See page 235.)*

VITAMINS AND MINERALS
• Plenty of fluids and bed rest will make it easier for your child to shift a cough. Offer fluids only for the first couple of days, and then just light meals. Avoid dairy produce altogether until the catarrh has shifted.

RIGHT *If your child is worn out by coughing, try Olive flower essence.*

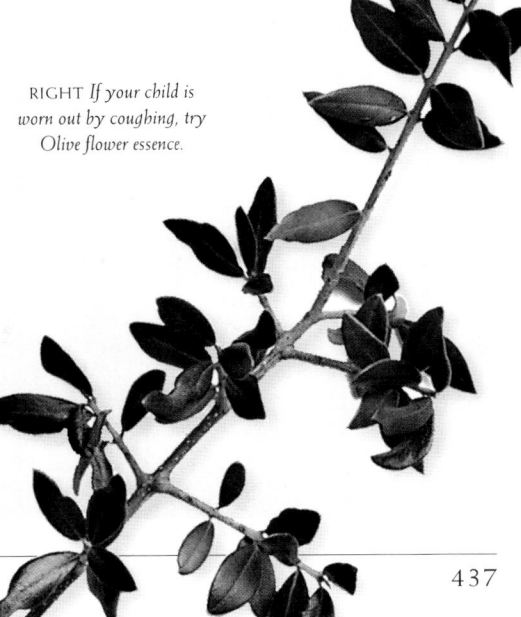

Croup

Croup is an acute inflammation and narrowing of the air passages, especially the larynx, in young children. The disorder is caused by various viruses, particularly the para-influenza virus, or by bacteria. The primary symptoms are coughing, hoarseness, and noisy, difficult breathing, which can sometimes be alleviated with steam inhalations. The characteristic cough of croup is a definite loud bark or whistle, caused by inflammation of the vocal cords. Infectious croup occurs mainly in the winter, when the larynx (voice box) or trachea (windpipe) become inflamed and swollen after what seems to be simply a cold. Other causes include allergy or the inhalation of a foreign body. Because the larynx swells and blocks the passage of air, breathing can be very difficult, which can panic a child.

CAUTION

IF YOUR CHILD TURNS BLUE, CALL A PHYSICIAN IMMEDIATELY.

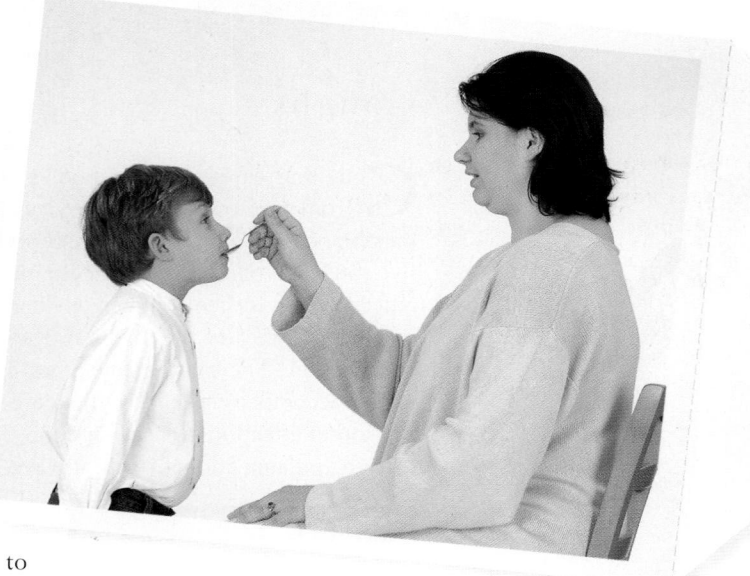

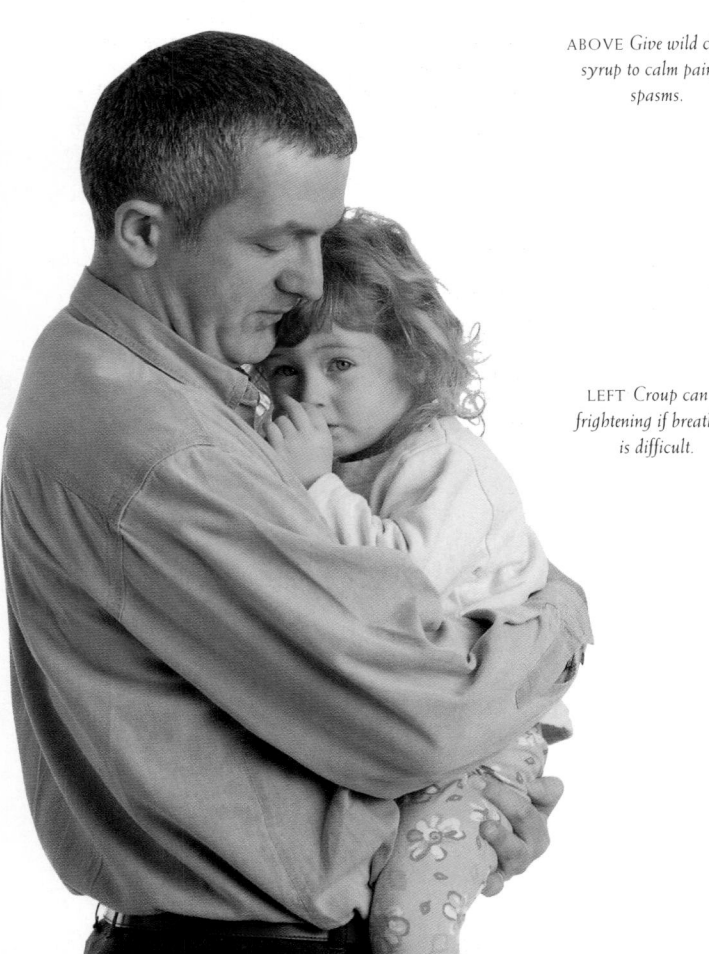

ABOVE *Give wild cherry syrup to calm painful spasms.*

LEFT *Croup can be frightening if breathing is difficult.*

TREATMENT

TRADITIONAL HOME AND FOLK REMEDIES

• Offer a hot honey and lemon drink to ease the symptoms. Honey has strong antibacterial properties and will be useful if the cause of the croup is bacterial infection. *(See pages 87 and 101.)*
• A little cider vinegar mixed with a mug of warm water can be sipped to ease symptoms. *(See page 102.)*
• Blackcurrant tea is helpful and restorative.
• Put your child in a bathroom with the door shut and the hot taps running, or fill a bowl with boiling water and gently place your child's head over it, covered by a towel. Steam will open the airways and reduce symptoms. Raise the upper end of the cot or bed so that breathing is easier. *(See page 103.)*

HERBALISM

• Lobelia and black cohosh will reduce spasm, soften the phlegm, and clear the lungs.
• Wild cherry syrup can reduce spasm and help deal with phlegm.
• Try infusing lavender flowers or chamomile in a bowl of hot water, then ask your child to lean over it, to help breathing. *(See page 119.)*

• Infuse some chamomile, catmint, or wild cherry, and give your child small sips before bedtime and during an attack. *(See page 119.)*
• Mix catmint, horehound, and wild cherry together with a little honey or licorice and give by the teaspoonful as necessary.
• A foot bath with some thyme or eucalyptus oil added should help. *(See page 135.)*

AROMATHERAPY

• Essential oils of eucalyptus, lavender, pine, chamomile, thyme and cinnamon can be added, together or individually, to a vaporizer or a foot-bath. *(See pages 146–71.)*
• A few drops of eucalyptus or lavender can be placed on a handkerchief by the child's cot or bed to ease breathing and encourage the child to relax. *(See pages 159 and 161.)*
• Rub a few drops of lavender oil mixed with petroleum jelly into your child's chest and upper back. *(See page 161.)*

HOMEOPATHY

• Spongia is the traditional treatment for croup, and can be taken every 20 minutes during an attack. *(See page 213.)*

• Aconite can be taken alongside Spongia. *(See page 178.)*
• Phosphorus may be useful when there is a thirst for cold drinks (which may be vomited up). *(See page 208.)*
• Drosera, for a deep hoarse-sounding cough, with gasping and retching. *(See page 193.)*

FLOWER ESSENCES

• Rescue Remedy will help to calm the child, which will make breathing easier. *(See page 244.)*
• Rock Rose will help if your child is frightened. *(See page 231.)*
• Olive can be taken following an attack, if the child is exhausted. *(See page 235.)*

Thrush

Thrush, or candidiasis, is a fungal, or yeast infection of the Candida albicans fungus, which is very common in those with immature immune systems, or those with immune systems that are compromised or very stressed. Thrush takes many forms, the most common of which are oral and that which develops in the diaper area.

The immune system can be impaired by poor diet, pollution, the overuse of drugs – which suppress it and upset the balance of the intestinal flora, causing Candida, or thrush, to flourish – injury, or surgery, among others. In babies, it usually occurs in conjunction with diaper rash. Oral thrush is characterized by sore, white, raised patches in the mouth. In the diaper area or skin folds it takes the form of an itchy red rash with a white top.

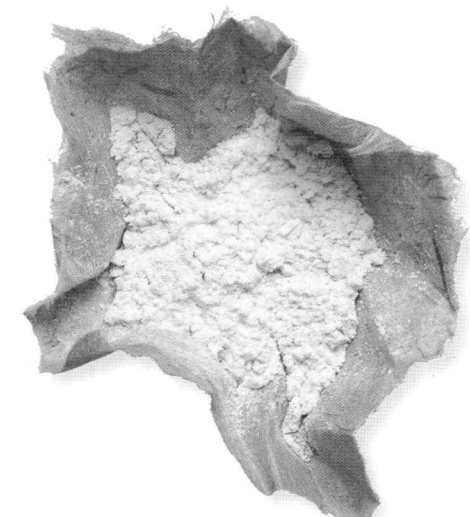

LEFT *Arsenicum is useful for sores on the mouth, especially if brought on by exhaustion.*

TREATMENT

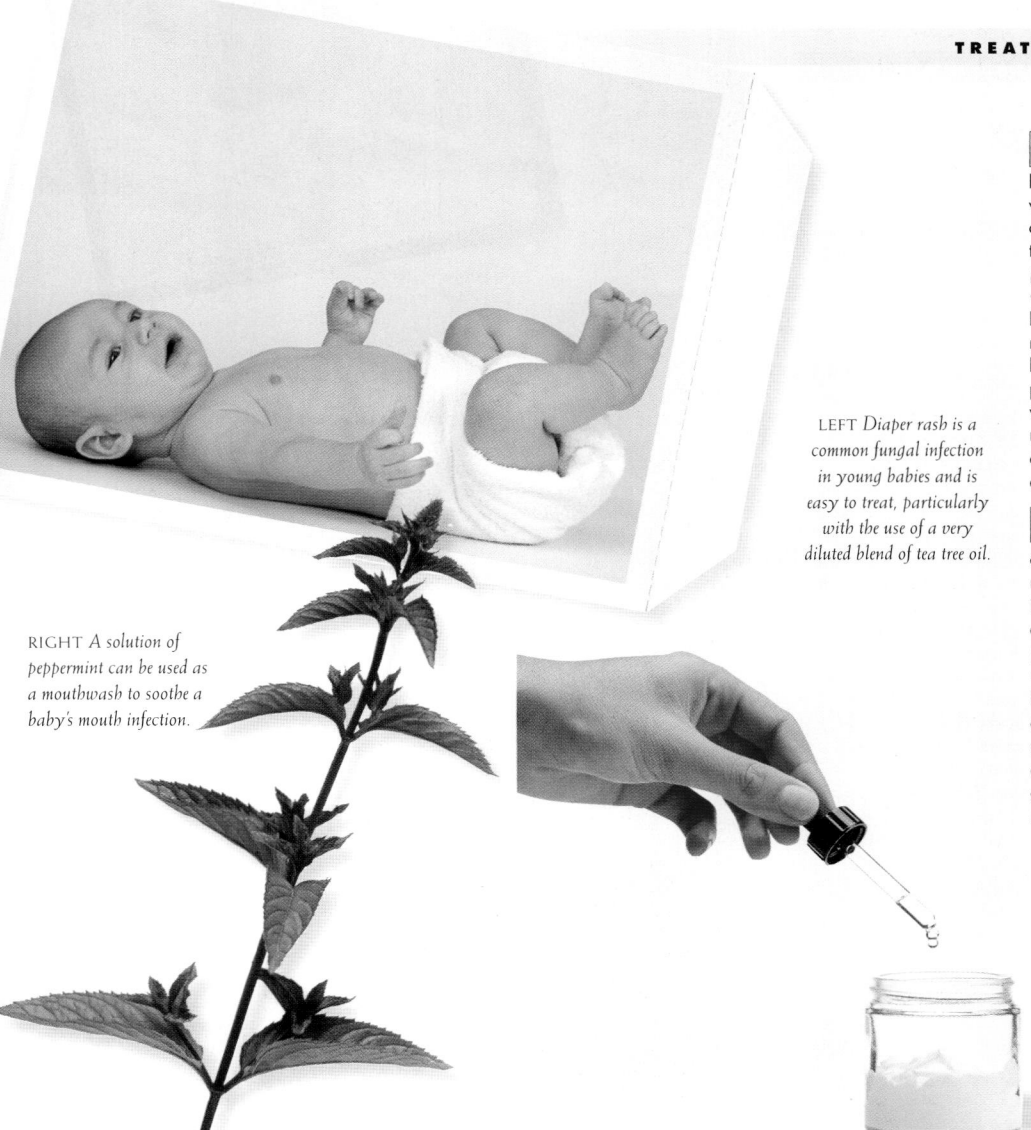

LEFT *Diaper rash is a common fungal infection in young babies and is easy to treat, particularly with the use of a very diluted blend of tea tree oil.*

RIGHT *A solution of peppermint can be used as a mouthwash to soothe a baby's mouth infection.*

LEFT *Rescue Remedy applied in a cream is a useful external application.*

HERBALISM
• Echinacea, to boost the immune system, will help to prevent chronic thrush and help the body to fight infection. *(See page 120.)*
• Oral thrush may be helped by preparing a mouthwash solution with lavender, lemon, or peppermint in spring water. Rinse the baby's mouth, or dab a few drops on the affected areas. *(See page 125.)*

AROMATHERAPY
• Use tea tree oil in a vaporizer in your child's room, to boost the immune system and act as an antifungal agent. *(See page 162.)*
• Extremely dilute lavender oil or tea tree oil can be dabbed on to patches in the mouth and on the bottom. Avoid the genitals. *(See pages 161 and 162.)*

HOMEOPATHY
Treatment will be constitutional, but the following remedies may be useful:
• Borax, at the first sign of an outbreak.
• Mercurius, when there is more saliva than usual and the tongue trembles. *(See page 205.)*
• Capsicum, for sore, hot patches.
• Arsenicum, for burning pains, mouth ulcers, and feeling worn out. *(See page 182.)*

FLOWER ESSENCES
• Apply a little Rescue Remedy cream to the affected area (externally) and a few drops of diluted stock remedy to sores in the mouth. *(See page 244.)*
• Olive can be useful if outbreaks are linked to exhaustion. *(See page 235.)*

Teething Problems

Your baby's first teeth will probably appear at about six months of age, and there may be problems with teeth coming through until the age of two or three. Most babies experience some discomfort, which can range from quite mild, which may make them clingy and fractious, to severe, accompanied by dribbling, loosened stools, and sleeping problems. A classic symptom is a red patch on one cheek.

ABOVE *A little honey, rubbed into the gums, lessens the discomfort of teething.*

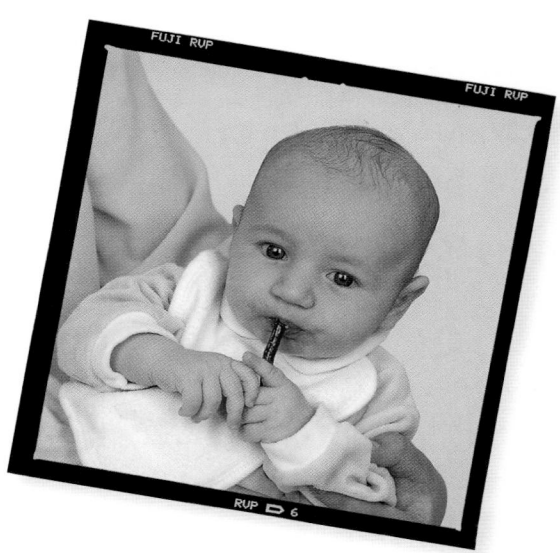

RIGHT *Try a piece of licorice root as a teether for your baby.*

TREATMENT

TRADITIONAL HOME AND FOLK REMEDIES
• Rub a little honey into the gums for relief. Make sure it is pasteurized. *(See page 101.)*
• Give your baby a cold licorice root to gnaw on. *(See page 91.)*
• Cold raw carrots are useful teethers, but watch your baby carefully to make sure he or she doesn't bite off a piece and choke on it. *(See page 89.)*

LEFT *Rock Rose is a component of Rescue Remedy which will soothe a child who seems inconsolable.*

HERBALISM
• Syrup made from the marshmallow root will soothe inflamed gums. Add a few teaspoons to your baby's normal meals. *(See page 114.)*
• Offer infusions of chamomile or fennel to calm and to soothe. *(See pages 119 and 121.)*

AROMATHERAPY
• Put a few drops of lavender oil on the bedclothes to help your baby to sleep. Essential oils of chamomile and lavender can be added to the bath water to calm a distressed baby. *(See pages 150 and 161.)*
• Rub the gums with a little chamomile oil mixed with a teaspoon of honey. Clove oil also acts as a local anesthetic, and a minute amount can be diluted and rubbed into the gums. *(See page 150.)*

HOMEOPATHY
• Chamomilla is the standard remedy for teething, and can be taken up to 6 times daily. *(See page 204.)*
• Calc. phos. may also be useful. *(See page 186.)*

BELOW *Make an infusion by pouring boiling water on lightly crushed fennel seeds. Leave for ten minutes.*

FLOWER ESSENCES
• Rub a little diluted Rescue Remedy directly into the gums, or apply to pulse points if your baby is crying inconsolably. A few drops at nighttime will keep your baby calm, enabling him or her to sleep. *(See page 244.)*
• Walnut will help the child through the transition. *(See page 232.)*

Colic

Colic is characterized by apparently unending frantic crying, usually at around the same time of day or night. The legs are drawn up to the abdomen, and the baby appears to be in severe pain. Excessive crying causes the baby to swallow air, which can exacerbate the problem and lead to abdominal bloating. The cause is unknown, but colic may be caused by contractions of the colon, an allergy to something in the formula (if bottle-fed) or the mother's diet (if breast-fed), or simply excessive air which is gulped in through repeated bouts of crying. The most common form of colic is three-month colic, typically coming on in the evening and lasting anything from a few minutes to several hours. Burping or laying the baby over the knee or shoulder usually has little effect.

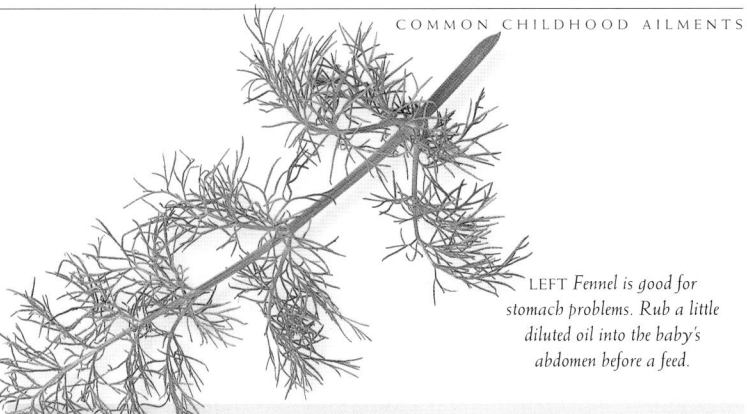

LEFT *Fennel is good for stomach problems. Rub a little diluted oil into the baby's abdomen before a feed.*

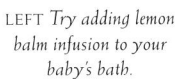

CAUTION

VOMITING OR DIARRHEA ARE NOT SYMPTOMS OF COLIC AND TREATMENT MUST BE SOUGHT IMMEDIATELY.

LEFT *Try adding lemon balm infusion to your baby's bath.*

TREATMENT

TRADITIONAL HOME AND FOLK REMEDIES
• Caraway water can be diluted and given to even a very young baby in a sterilized bottle. Offer a few sips just before a feed.

HERBALISM
• Because colic is exacerbated by tension, relaxing herbs are often suggested – used in the bath, or infused, cooled slightly and taken by bottle. Chamomile, lemon balm, and limeflowers are the most effective. *(See pages 119 and 134.)*
• A warm bath with an infusion of dill, fennel, marshmallow, or lemon balm will soothe a colicky baby. *(See pages 114 and 121.)*
• Catmint, infused and diluted, can be added to your baby's bath water to relax any abdominal spasm.

AROMATHERAPY
• Rub a little very dilute fennel oil into the abdomen before feeds to prevent colic. *(See page 159.)*
• A gentle massage of the abdominal area with one or a blend of essential oils of chamomile, dill, lavender, or rose will help to ease symptoms and calm a distressed baby. *(See pages 146–71.)*
• If your baby is wakened by discomfort, place a handkerchief with a few drops of lavender oil by the bed. *(See page 161.)*
• Try a few drops of lavender or chamomile oil in a warm bath, just before evening feeds. *(See pages 150 and 161.)*

HOMEOPATHY
• Chamomilla is useful for babies who seem better when they are held. *(See page 204.)*
• Pulsatilla is used for babies who are better in the fresh air and when they are rocked. *(See page 209.)*

• Cuprum met. is used when the tummy rumbles, and the child curls fingers and toes in discomfort. *(See page 192.)*

FLOWER ESSENCES
• Rock Rose is excellent for extreme fright. *(See page 231.)*
• Rescue Remedy can be used to calm and therefore help to reduce any spasm. *(See page 244.)*

VITAMINS AND MINERALS
• If you are breast-feeding, avoid dairy produce for a few days to see if this helps.
• Other foods which should be avoided are very spicy foods, citrus foods, gassy foods (beans, onions, cabbage, etc.), and sugar.

BELOW *Breastfeeding mothers should avoid dairy foods, which may cause colic in babies.*

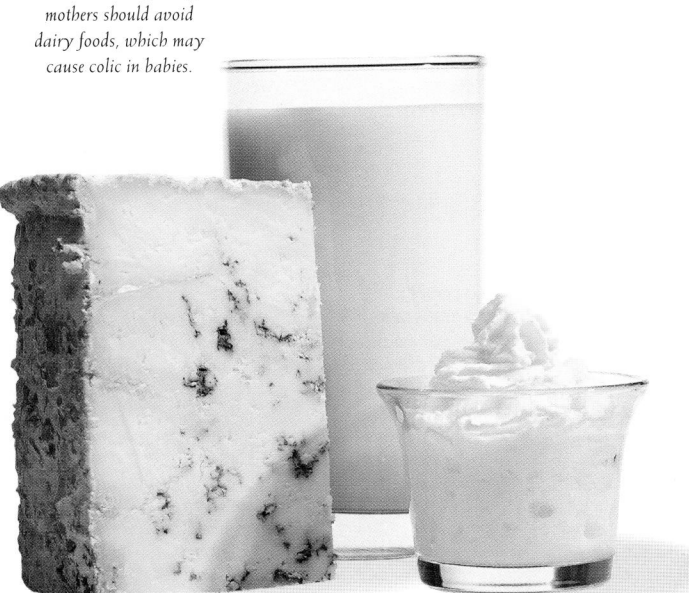

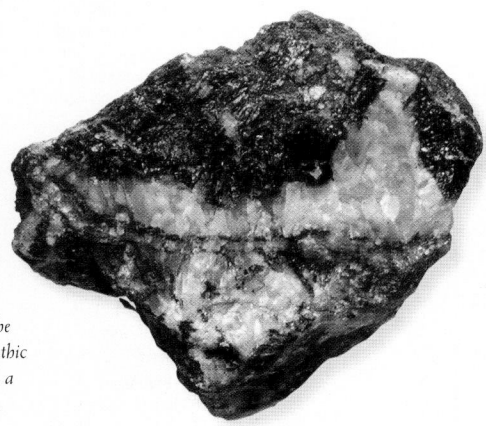

RIGHT *Copper is the source for the homeopathic remedy Cuprum met, a treatment for colic.*

Vomiting and Diarrhea

There are many causes of vomiting and diarrhea in children, including infections such as gastroenteritis, eating rich or fatty foods (or, indeed, overeating), emotional upsets, and food poisoning. These conditions are not usually serious, unless they recur. Gastroenteritis is usually present if there is fever of 38°C (100°F), vomiting, lack of enthusiasm for feeds, and torpor. Occasionally diarrhea is due to too early reintroduction of milk after an attack of gastroenteritis. Remember that babies and children can dehydrate quickly, and you must ensure that they drink plenty of liquids.

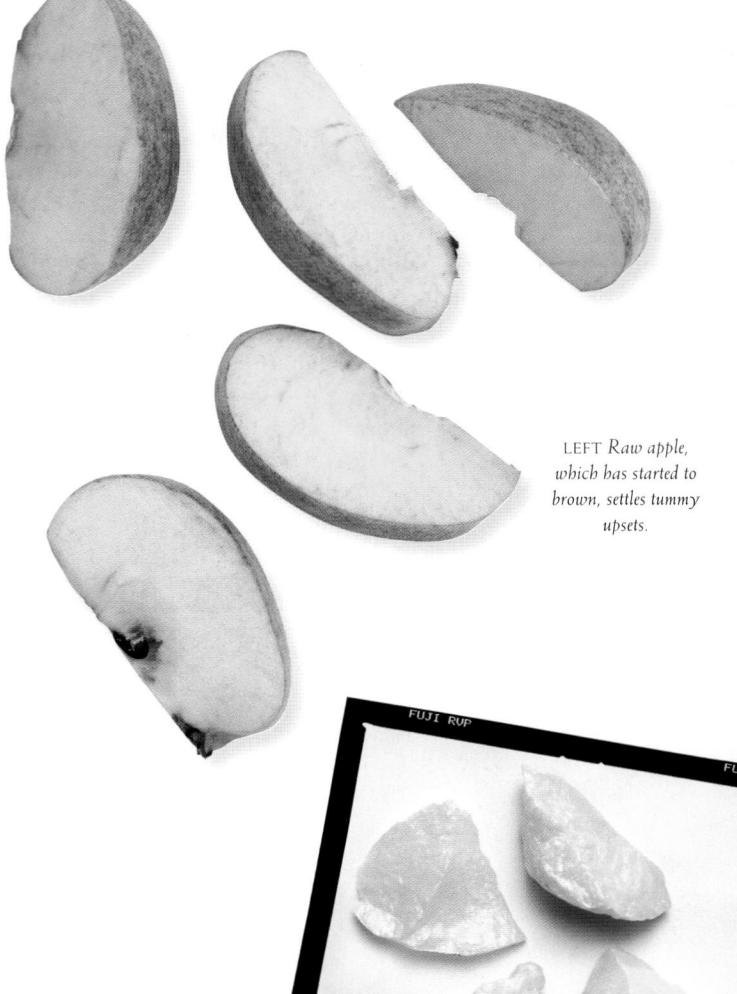

LEFT *Raw apple, which has started to brown, settles tummy upsets.*

CAUTION

BABIES AND CHILDREN CAN VERY EASILY BECOME DEHYDRATED BY VOMITING OR DIARRHEA, AND IT IS IMPORTANT THAT YOU SEEK MEDICAL TREATMENT URGENTLY. SEE YOUR PHYSICIAN IF THERE IS BLOOD IN THE VOMIT OR FECES.

LEFT *Very ripe bananas help restore beneficial intestinal bacteria.*

ABOVE *Sulfur, prepared as a homeopathic remedy, helps to drive toxins out of the body.*

TREATMENT

TRADITIONAL HOME AND FOLK REMEDIES
• Milk and honey are excellent for treating an attack of food poisoning. *(See page 101.)*
• Mustard is a natural emetic and can be taken internally, mixed with a few teaspoons of warm water. *(See page 98.)*
• Garlic is excellent to fight infection, boost immunities, and cleanse the blood. It is also a natural antibiotic, so is excellent in cases of bacterial infection. *(See page 82.)*
• Drink fresh lemon juice, warmed and mixed with a little honey, to cleanse the gut. *(See pages 87 and 101.)*
• Drink blackcurrant juice, as a gut astringent.

• Raw apple which has gone brown is useful for settling an upset stomach. Offer in small quantities. *(See page 94.)*

HERBALISM
• Chamomile or melissa tea will help to settle and calm an excited child. *(See page 119.)*
• Meadowsweet or marshmallow syrup can help with vomiting. *(See pages 114 and 121.)*
• Gentian and barberry can be added to water and sipped frequently.
• Chamomile and vervain can be taken internally to soothe a child whose illness is exacerbated or caused by emotional upset, or who is distressed by the vomiting. *(See pages 119 and 138.)*

• Try ginger, crushed or decocted, to ease nausea. *(See page 139.)*
• Chamomile, echinacea, peppermint, and thyme can be drunk as infusions or added to a foot-bath when infection causes the illness. *(See pages 119, 120, 125, and 135.)*

AROMATHERAPY
• Massage the tummy and chest with a few drops of lavender or chamomile essential oil in a light carrier oil. *(See pages 150 and 161.)*
• Use essential oil of thyme or tea tree in a vaporizer for their antiseptic properties. *(See pages 162 and 170.)*
• A few drops of lavender essential oil in the bath or by the bedside will calm. *(See page 161.)*

HOMEOPATHY
• Nux vomica may help if the child vomits after eating too much, or too quickly. *(See page 214.)*
• China, for diarrhea with wind, particularly when the child is very irritable. *(See page 190.)*
• Colocynthis, if diarrhea is copious, thin, and yellow, accompanied by episodic pain. *(See page 191.)*
• Arsenicum, when there is burning and the child is restless, anxious, and cold. *(See page 182.)*
• Veratrum alb., when there is vomiting and diarrhea with cold sweats.
• Pulsatilla, after a rich, fatty meal, when there is no thirst. *(See page 209.)*
• Sulfur, for red orifices, smelly burps, and cravings for sweets. *(See page 215.)*

FLOWER ESSENCES
• Rescue Remedy will relieve the distress caused by vomiting and diarrhea. *(See page 244.)*
• Olive flower essence is useful for recuperation. *(See page 235.)*
• If the vomiting is caused by emotional problems select a remedy that will help with those problems.

VITAMINS AND MINERALS
• Following an attack of vomiting or diarrhea, offer lots of live yogurt and very ripe bananas to restore the proper bacterial balance of the gut.
• An acidophilus tablet can be taken for the same purpose. These are available in vanilla flavor. *(See page 271.)*

Diaper Rash

Diaper rash is caused by contact with urine or feces, which cause the skin to produce less protective oil and therefore provide a less effective barrier to further irritation. It can also be caused by irritating chemicals in feces, not thoroughly rinsing soap or detergent out of diapers, and the chemicals contained in disposable diapers. The baby's buttocks, thighs, and genitals become sore, red, spotty, and weepy in areas touched by diapers. In boys, the foreskin may become inflamed, making urination painful. The rash may become secondarily infected with the Candida fungus if the baby has been given antibiotics or if breast milk has antibiotics in it, or if the mother has oral or genital thrush.

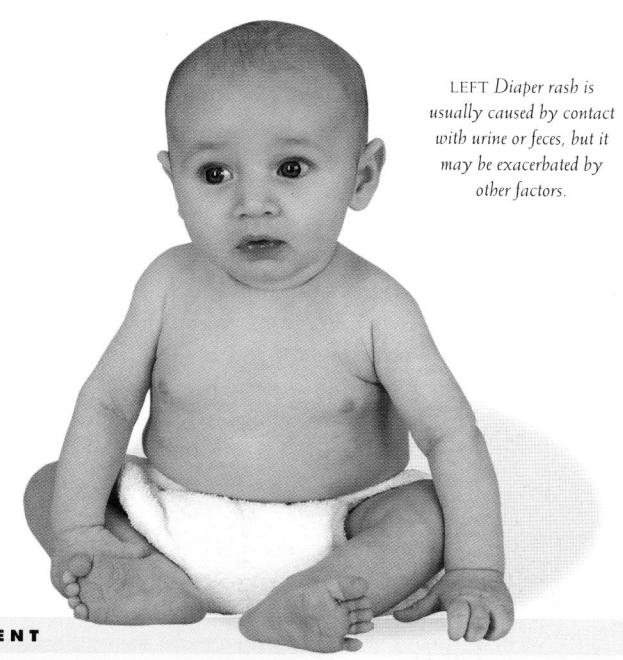

LEFT *Diaper rash is usually caused by contact with urine or feces, but it may be exacerbated by other factors.*

CAUTION

ANY DIAPER RASH WHICH DOES NOT HEAL WITHIN A WEEK OR SO SHOULD BE SEEN BY A PHYSICIAN.

TREATMENT

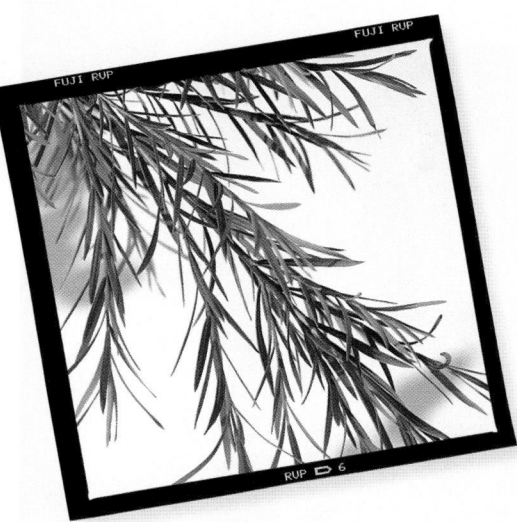

ABOVE *A natural disinfectant, tea tree oil can be added to rinsewater to get diapers extra clean.*

🖐 TRADITIONAL HOME AND FOLK REMEDIES

• Rub the skin of an avocado on the rash to encourage healing. *(See page 96.)*
• Wash the bottom with a little diluted cider vinegar and allow it to dry before putting on the diaper. *(See page 102.)*
• Live yogurt can be spread on the diaper area to soothe, and to prevent thrush from occurring in the folds of the skin. *(See page 93.)*

• Egg white can be painted on the sore bottom and allowed to dry before putting on a diaper. This will encourage the skin to heal and prevent further irritation.
• Avoid using soap or other detergents on the diaper area. Rinse carefully with clean water at each diaper change. Frequent diaper changes are suggested, and using a disposable diaper liner may help to reduce irritation. Allow your baby to go for as long as possible with a bare bottom, to allow it to dry and heal. Give plenty to drink.

🌿 HERBALISM

• Buchu will reduce the acidity of the urine.
• Marigold ointment can be rubbed on to the diaper area to soothe and to reduce inflammation. *(See page 117.)*
• Wash the diaper area with infusions of marigold, rosemary, or elderflower. *(See pages 117, 127, and 130.)*
• Powdered golden seal can be applied to a clean diaper area before putting on the new diaper.

• Give your baby lots of soothing drinks, such as diluted chamomile tea, to reduce the acidity of the urine. *(See page 119.)*

💧 AROMATHERAPY

• Add a few drops of tea tree to the rinse cycle of your machine when using cloth diapers to disinfect. Cloth diapers are much kinder to your baby's delicate skin. *(See page 162.)*
• A few drops of lavender or rose oil in a peach kernel carrier oil can be gently rubbed into the diaper area. Use this blend to protect against diaper rash as well. *(See pages 161 and 168.)*
• A drop of oregano or thyme oil, in a light carrier oil, can be used to discourage thrush. *(See page 170.)*

😊 HOMEOPATHY

• Calendula ointment can be applied to the diaper area. *(See page 187.)*
• Internally, you can try giving Rhus tox. for an itchy, blistered rash. *(See page 210.)*
• Sulfur may be appropriate if the skin is dry and scaled. *(See page 215.)*

• Merc. sol. can help to reduce the acidity of the urine. *(See page 205.)*
• Cantharis, when the urine is scalding and the skin is red and raw. *(See page 188.)*
• Rhus tox., when the rash appears as mounds or pimples. *(See page 210.)*

✸ FLOWER ESSENCES

• Rescue Remedy cream may be gently massaged into the affected area to reduce inflammation and ease pain or itching. A few drops of Rescue Remedy on pulse points will calm a distressed baby. *(See page 244.)*

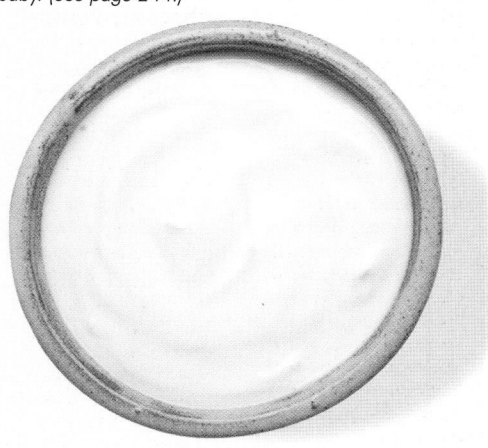

BELOW *Live yogurt cools the sore area and prevents the rash spreading.*

Worms

An infestation of worms in the digestive system is quite common, particularly in young children, who usually contract them at school. Worms can sometimes be seen around the anus, or in the feces, and they inflame the area of the bowel or rectum where they attach themselves. Several types of worms can exist as parasites in humans, ranging in size from microscopic to many meters in length. Most infestations are uncommon in the U.K. and the U.S., apart from threadworms. Threadworms, which are tiny, white threadlike worms which infest the rectum, are not dangerous, although they do tend to disturb sleep. They cause itching around the anus, and sometimes mild, colicky abdominal pain. Worms may be acquired by eating under-cooked, infected meat, by contact with soil or water contaminated by worm larvae, or by accidental ingestion of worm eggs (from the fingers or from food) from soil contaminated by infected feces.

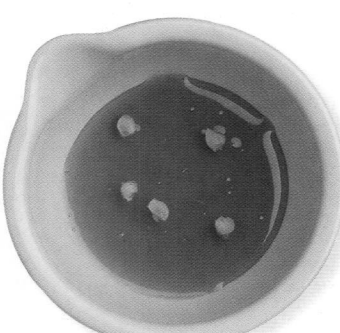

ABOVE *Grind lemon pips with honey for worm treatment.*

CAUTION

WHATEVER TREATMENT YOU GIVE, REPEAT IT AFTER TWO WEEKS TO EXPEL THE WORMS THAT WERE EMBRYOS AT THE FIRST TREATMENT.

TREATMENT

TRADITIONAL HOME AND FOLK REMEDIES
• Raw garlic, which is toxic to worms and parasites, can be eaten, or a small piece, wrapped in some gauze, can be inserted into the anus. (See page 82.)
• Give 5 lemon pips, ground and mixed with honey, daily for 5 days. (See pages 87 and 101.)

HERBALISM
• Cayenne pepper and senna can be combined; the former stuns the worms and the latter encourages them to be expelled. Mix in a little live yogurt, to avoid irritating the digestive tract. (See page 118.)
• Wormwood tea will stun worms.

AROMATHERAPY
• Rub a little black pepper oil, very diluted in grapeseed oil, into the abdominal area. (See page 167.)

HOMEOPATHY
• China may alter the balance of the body so that the child expels threadworms naturally. (See page 190.)
• Teucrium, for an itchy bottom and nose, which are worse in the evening and accompanied by restless sleep patterns.
• Santoninum, when all else fails.

FLOWER ESSENCES
• Rescue Remedy for distress caused by discomfort. (See page 244.)
• Crab Apple, if your child feels unclean or polluted. (See page 234.)

VITAMINS AND MINERALS
• Acidophilus tablets should be taken for several weeks to improve the health of the bowel. (See page 271.)

Whooping Cough (Pertussis)

CAUTION

THERE IS A RISK OF SECONDARY INFECTION, IN PARTICULAR PNEUMONIA AND BRONCHITIS. ALL CASES OF WHOOPING COUGH SHOULD BE SEEN BY A PHYSICIAN. IF THE COUGH IS ACCOMPANIED BY VOMITING, MAKE SURE THERE IS ADEQUATE INTAKE OF FLUID TO PREVENT DEHYDRATION. CALL YOUR PHYSICIAN IMMEDIATELY IF YOUR CHILD BECOMES BLUE AROUND THE LIPS.

Whooping cough is an acute, highly infectious, and quite serious illness which occurs mostly in children under the age of five. The incubation period of whooping cough is seven to ten days, and the condition can last for about six weeks – sometimes longer. Pertussis, as it is known, usually begins with a normal cold, which develops into a cough. The infection is bacterial and irritates the airways, causing them to become swollen and lined with thick, infected mucus. The coughing becomes severe, with long bouts that have a characteristic "whoop" sound to them. Vomiting often accompanies the coughing. Whooping cough is more dangerous in infants, who can suffer anxiety from being unable to breathe normally. Children should be kept away from others.

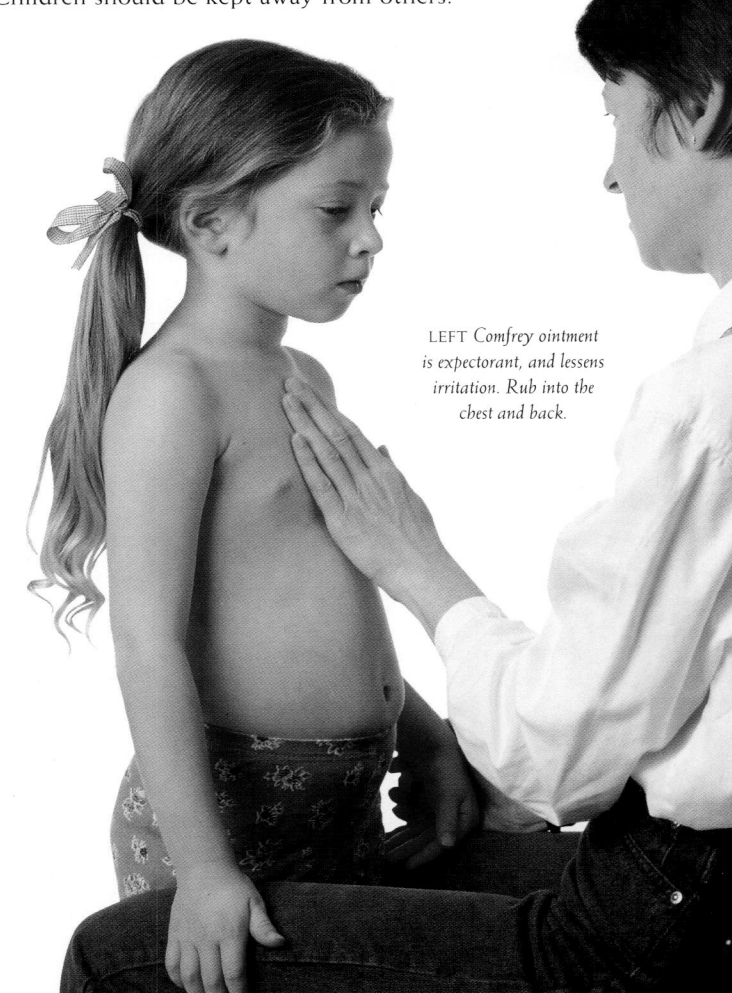

LEFT *Comfrey ointment is expectorant, and lessens irritation. Rub into the chest and back.*

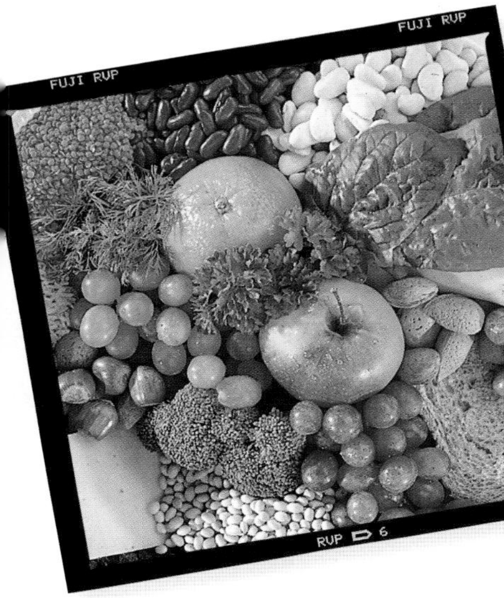

ABOVE *Make sure your child eats a good, balanced diet to cope with what can be a long illness.*

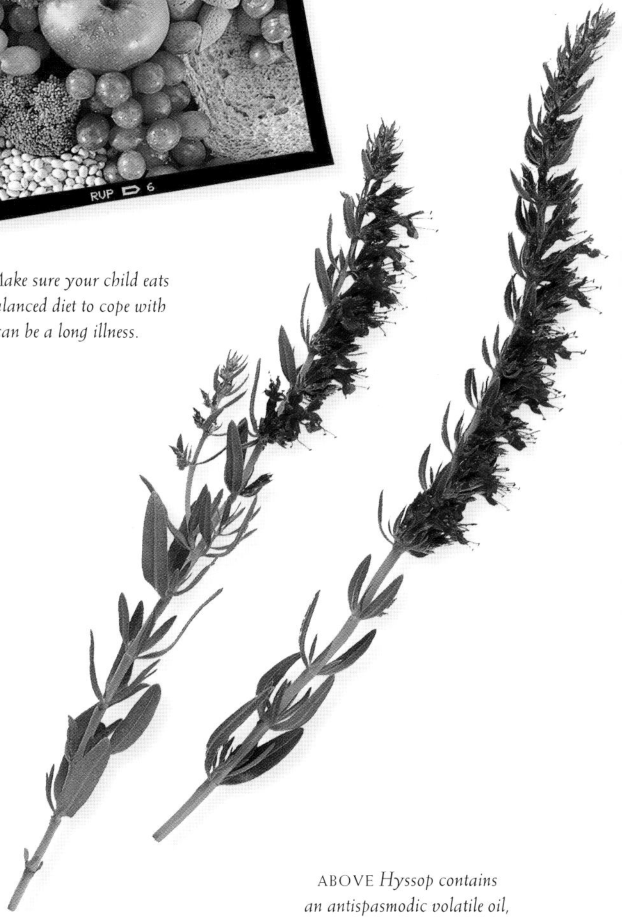

ABOVE *Hyssop contains an antispasmodic volatile oil, to ease a painful cough.*

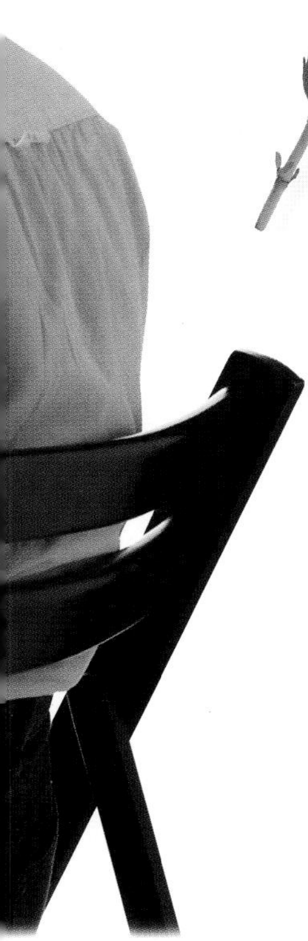

DATA FILE

• Whooping cough is caused by a bacteria, Bordetella pertussis.

• Because of mass vaccination of children, whooping cough is now relatively rare, affecting only a small proportion of the population.

• After an incubation period of about a week, symptoms at first resemble those of the common cold; after 7–10 days, coughing increases and takes on the distinctive attributes of whooping cough.

• The younger the patient, the greater the risk of serious illness; most deaths from whooping cough occur in the first six months of life.

TREATMENT

✋ TRADITIONAL HOME AND FOLK REMEDIES

• Honey and licorice can be mixed with a little hot water to make a drink to relieve the cough. *(See pages 91 and 101.)*
• A garlic poultice, placed on the chest and back area, is recommended to help expel the phlegm. Do not leave the poultice on for too long, because it can cause blistering. *(See page 82.)*

🌿 HERBALISM

• A combination of coltsfoot and elecampane can prevent the infection by strengthening the body and clearing phlegm.
• Sundew is very successful in treating a number of bacterial infections, and also works to relax the muscles of the breathing tubes. It should be made into an infusion and taken by the teaspoonful, as necessary.
• Hyssop and lobelia should be used to help allay the spasmodic cough.
• Coltsfoot can be used to loosen the cough and help to expel the mucus.
• The bark of the wild cherry has a profound effect on the cough reflex.
• Red clover will help to reduce any spasm of the bronchi.
• A few drops of tincture of thyme should be taken to loosen and expel the mucus. Thyme also works as an antiseptic. *(See page 135.)*
• Massage comfrey ointment into the chest and back to relax the lungs. *(See page 132.)*

• Lemon balm tea will soothe anxiety.
• Elecampane is commonly used for children's coughs, and can be purchased in easy-to-use syrup form.
• Offer a little black root if there is vomiting.
• After the bath, massage a little comfrey ointment into the chest and back to relax and expand the lungs. *(See page 132.)*

💧 AROMATHERAPY

• Mix a few drops of lavender and chamomile oils in a light carrier oil, and massage into the chest and back area to calm, and to relax tensed muscles. *(See pages 150 and 161.)*
• Tea tree, lavender, chamomile, and eucalyptus can be used in a vaporizer to help open up the lungs and reduce spasm. *(See pages 146–71.)*
• A few drops of oil of thyme, in the bath, will soothe and reduce the severity of the cough. *(See page 170.)*

🔵 HOMEOPATHY

• Pertussin may be given in one dose towards the end of the disease to prevent an "echo" effect.
• Aconite can be taken during an attack or at the beginning of the illness. *(See page 178.)*

• Ant. tart., when there is a rattling cough with gasping. *(See page 179.)*
• Sanguinaria, for a harsh, dry cough.
• Arnica, when there is bleeding, or the child is distressed before the coughing starts. *(See page 182.)*
• Drosera is useful when the cough is made worse by lying down and there are pains below the ribs. *(See page 193.)*
• Bryonia, when there is a dry, painful cough and vomiting. *(See page 185.)*

🌼 FLOWER ESSENCES

• Rescue Remedy is excellent for calming a child who has difficulty drawing breath, and who is frightened by the condition. A few drops on pulse points, or sipped in a glass of cool water, will help. *(See page 244.)*
• Cherry Plum will help if there is any serious spasmodic coughing. *(See page 236.)*
• Mimulus and olive are good during the later stages of the condition. *(See page 235.)*

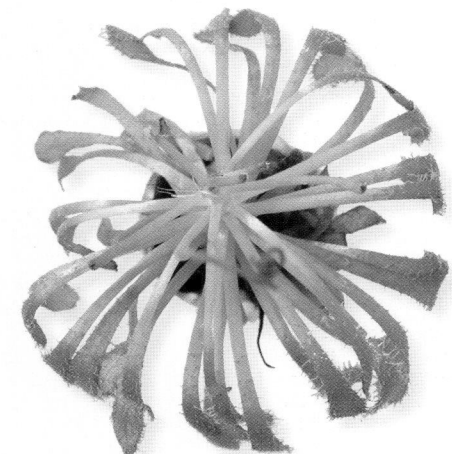

RIGHT *Drosera contains plumbagin, which fights streptococcus, pneumococcus, and staphylococcus bacteria.*

German Measles (Rubella)

Rubella, also called German measles, is a viral infection that begins with symptoms of a cold and loss of appetite, occasionally accompanied by a sore throat and swelling of the lymph nodes in the neck. The rash will appear about a day later and consists of tiny pink spots that may be so concentrated that the overall area appears red and inflamed. There may be mild fever. German measles is very infectious, with an incubation period of two or three weeks. The illness itself only lasts three to five days.

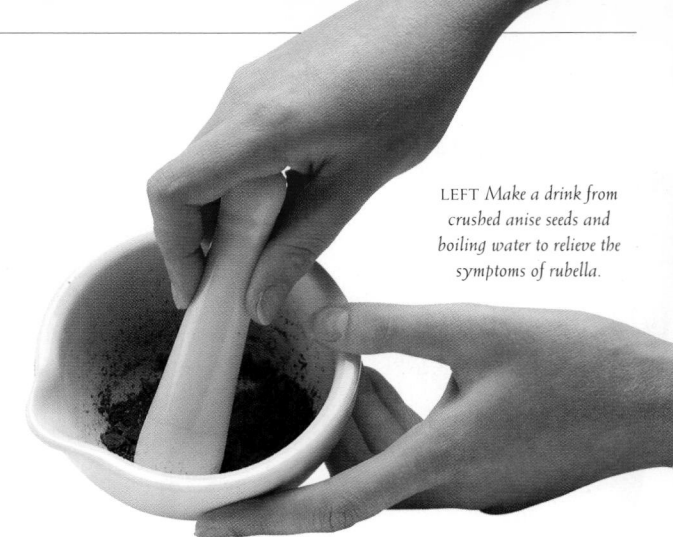

LEFT *Make a drink from crushed anise seeds and boiling water to relieve the symptoms of rubella.*

CAUTION

THE SYMPTOMS IN SMALL CHILDREN MAY BE MILD, BUT IF A PREGNANT WOMAN COMES INTO CONTACT WITH THE CONDITION THERE IS A SERIOUS RISK OF MISCARRIAGE AND BIRTH DEFECTS. SUFFERERS ARE INFECTIOUS FROM ONE WEEK BEFORE THE RASH APPEARS TO THREE WEEKS AFTERWARD.

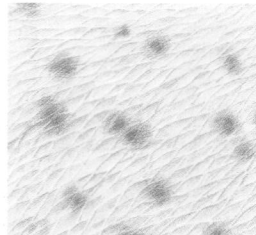

RIGHT *German measles produces a rash of pale pink, possibly itchy, spots that spread from the face.*

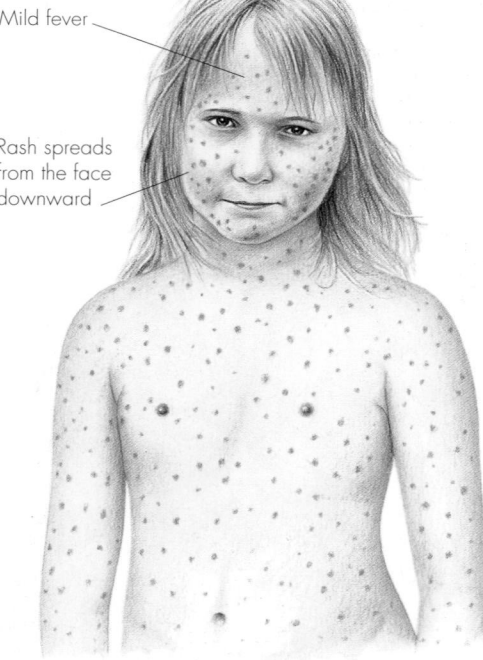

Mild fever

Rash spreads from the face downward

ABOVE *If rubella is not contracted in childhood, immunization is necessary for girls before puberty to protect their future offspring.*

TREATMENT

CHINESE HERBALISM
• Rubella is believed to be caused by external Wind and Heat. Use mulberry, honeysuckle, and chrysanthemum. *(See page 65.)*

TRADITIONAL HOME AND FOLK REMEDIES
Pound some anise seeds, allow them to steep in boiling water for about 30 minutes, and then offer the drink by the teaspoonful to relieve symptoms.
• Honey and lemon in a little hot water can be drunk to reduce discomfort of the cold-like symptoms. *(See pages 87 and 101.)*
• Frequent, cool baths will relieve any itchiness and bring down a fever. *(See page 103.)*

HERBALISM
• Borage stimulates the kidneys and can help when fever is present.
• Yarrow tea, cooled and drunk several times daily, will relieve symptoms. *(See page 112.)*
• An infusion of elderflower, combined with peppermint, will cool a fever and calm your child. *(See pages 125 and 130.)*
• Very high fever can be treated with an infusion of catmint, taken as required.

AROMATHERAPY
• A few drops of lavender oil on the bedclothes, or on a handkerchief near the bed, will help ease symptoms and calm the child. *(See page 161.)*
• If there is a build-up of phlegm, use a few drops of tea tree or eucalyptus essential oil in a vaporizer to assist easier breathing. *(See pages 159 and 162.)*

HOMEOPATHY
• Pulsatilla, when there is thick, yellow discharge and hot, red eyes. *(See page 209.)*
• Belladonna, for fever, a bright red rash, and a hot face. *(See page 183.)*
• Phytolacca, for painful ears and swollen glands which are improved by taking cool drinks.
• Aconite, if there is a high fever and not too much mucus present. *(See page 178.)*
• Merc. sol., where there is yellow discharge and a fever. *(See page 205.)*

FLOWER ESSENCES
• Rescue Remedy will ease distress and calm the child. *(See page 244.)*

VITAMINS AND MINERALS
• Eat a good amount of raw fruits and vegetables to cleanse the system.
• Increase the intake of foods containing vitamin C and zinc to aid the action of the immune system. *(See pages 256 and 265.)*
• Vitamin E oil can be applied to the spots to prevent scarring. Take vitamin E supplements for the same reason. *(See page 257.)*
• Acidophilus should be taken after any illness to encourage the production of healthy bacteria in the gut. *(See page 271.)*

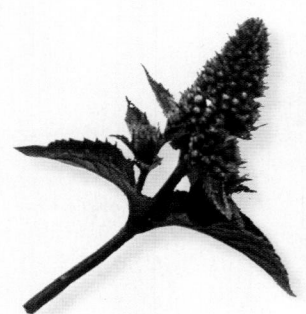

LEFT *Peppermint can be infused with elderflower to promote sweating and bring down a fever.*

DATA FILE

• German measles is highly contagious but mild.

• Symptoms usually disappear without complication in about a week.

• Many people may have had German measles without knowing it, because a skin rash is not always present.

• Natural infection apparently produces lifelong immunity.

• Pregnant women who become infected with rubella have a high risk of giving birth to a baby with serious defects, including blindness, cardiovascular disorders, deafness, or mental retardation.

Measles

Measles is a highly infectious disease caused by a virus which is normally inhaled. The incubation period is about 14 days, and just before the rash appears spots can be seen in the mouth. It begins like a cold, with runny nose or cough, then a fever, and occasionally conjunctivitis occurs. Fever tends to become high as the rash comes out. The rash is characterized by flat, brown-red spots, which usually begin behind the ears and on the face. The lymph nodes will become swollen and there will be little or no appetite; vomiting and diarrhea may occur in some cases. Measles spots are not itchy, but your child will feel profoundly unwell. Complications of measles are common, and they include pneumonia, middle ear infections, and bronchitis. Encephalitis may also occur.

DATA FILE

- Measles usually affects children, but the disease can occur at any age in susceptible people.

- The early symptoms – fever, malaise, sore muscles, headache, eye irritation, and sensitivity to light – occur about 11 days after infection.

- Nasal discharge, sneezing, and coughing develop rapidly.

- Measles reduces normal resistance, making a patient susceptible to more serious secondary bacterial infections.

- In rare cases, the virus enters the brain to cause a form of encephalitis.

- Measles was once common throughout the world, but in 1963 the measles vaccine was introduced, which greatly reduced the incidence.

- The 1980s saw a marked increase in measles cases in the U.S., which may have been due to the failure to vaccinate many infants at the age of 15 months.

- About 5 percent of vaccinated adults are not adequately protected by a single dose of vaccine.

- Infection confers lifelong immunity.

CAUTION

IF FEVER RECURS SEVERAL DAYS AFTER THE SPOTS HAVE BEGUN TO HEAL, SEE YOUR PHYSICIAN.

TREATMENT

CHINESE HERBALISM
- The source of the illness is believed to be excess Heat in the Blood and Stomach. Peppermint, safflower, and honeysuckle may be used to treat measles. *(See pages 58 and 65.)*

TRADITIONAL HOME AND FOLK REMEDIES
- Garlic will encourage the spots to "come out," which means that the body is expelling toxins. *(See page 82.)*
- Ginger can be used as a compress directly on the spots.
- Hot honey and lemon drinks are soothing and will encourage healing. *(See pages 87 and 101.)*

HERBALISM
- Garlic and echinacea can be taken to improve the action of the immune system. *(See pages 113 and 120.)*
- Catmint and yarrow teas can be sipped to bring down fever and ease discomfort. *(See page 112.)*
- Elderflower is also useful. *(See page 130.)*
- Add chamomile or marigold to the bath water to calm your child and soothe the symptoms. *(See page 117 and 119.)*
- A compress of ginger may be used to help encourage the toxins to be released from the body. *(See page 139.)*

AROMATHERAPY
- A few drops of Roman chamomile in the bath will ease symptoms and help encourage sleep. *(See page 150.)*
- Lavender oil can be dropped on the bedclothes or on a handkerchief by the bed to calm. It can also be applied neat to spots to encourage healing. *(See page 161.)*
- When there is a build-up of phlegm and other symptoms of a cold, a gentle chest massage with a few drops of tea tree oil in a light carrier oil base will help. *(See page 162.)*
- Use essential oil of eucalyptus, tea tree, or chamomile in a vaporizer. *(See pages 146–71.)*

HOMEOPATHY
- Aconite and Belladonna can be taken for a high fever. *(See pages 178 and 183.)*
- Pulsatilla, when there is diarrhea, yellow discharge, and a cough. *(See page 209.)*
- Bryonia, when there is a hard, painful cough, and a high temperature, accompanied by thirst. *(See page 185.)*
- Stramonium, when there is a high fever, a red face, and convulsions.
- Morbillinum can be taken for 3 days if your child has been in contact with a sufferer. This will help reduce the severity of the symptoms.

FLOWER ESSENCES
- Rescue Remedy eases distress and discomfort. *(See page 244.)*
- Cherry Plum, Hornbeam, and Chicory are suggested for all childhood illnesses. *(See pages 236, 227, and 228.)*

VITAMINS AND MINERALS
- Eat plenty of raw fruits and vegetables every day to cleanse the system.
- Increase the intake of foods containing vitamin C and zinc to aid the action of the immune system. *(See pages 256 and 265.)*
- Vitamin E oil can be applied to the spots to prevent scarring. Take vitamin E supplements for the same reason. *(See page 257.)*
- Acidophilus should be taken after any illness to encourage production of the healthy bacteria in the gut. *(See page 271.)*

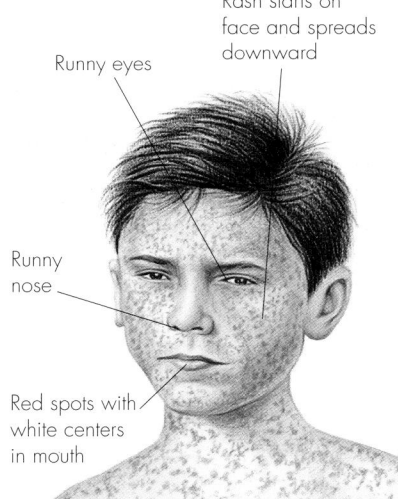

Rash starts on face and spreads downward

Runny eyes

Runny nose

Red spots with white centers in mouth

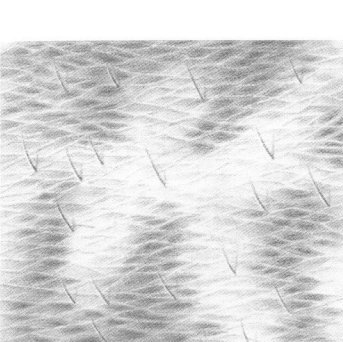

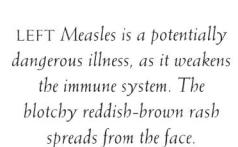

LEFT *Measles is a potentially dangerous illness, as it weakens the immune system. The blotchy reddish-brown rash spreads from the face.*

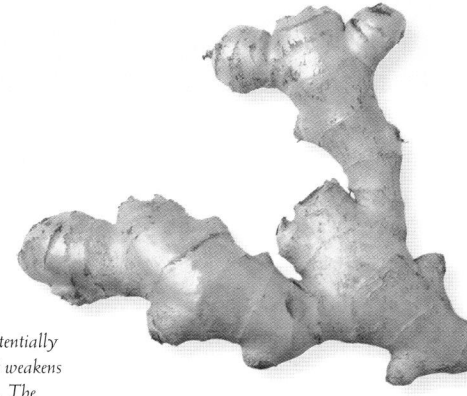

ABOVE *A ginger compress helps to relieve the rash of spots.*

Chicken pox

Chicken pox is an extremely contagious viral infection, which features headache, fever and general malaise, with spots starting usually on the trunk and spreading to most parts of the body, including the mouth, anus, vagina, and ears. They appear as pimples, which soon fill with fluid to become little blisters. Eventually the spots dry up and form a scab, which may cause scars. These spots are very itchy and it is important that the child does not scratch, for scarring and bacterial infection can result. The incubation period is 10 to 14 days, and sufferers are contagious from just before the spots appear.

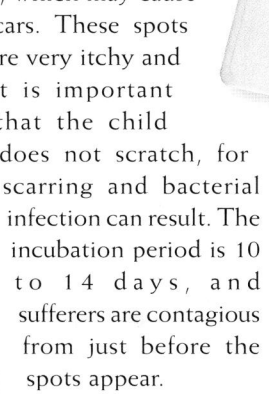

ABOVE *Make a witch hazel compress to help soothe the itchiness of the spots and to stop the child scratching.*

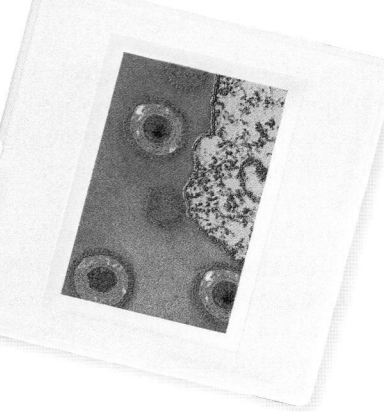

ABOVE *The chicken pox virus can cause shingles in adults.*

DATA FILE

• Chicken pox is usually contracted before the age of nine.

• The chicken pox virus, varicella zoster, usually lies dormant in the body. When immune activity is low, it can resurface as shingles.

• The rash develops into itching blisters that break in a few days and are covered by scabs, which leave no scars unless they become infected by bacteria from scratching.

• Chicken pox can be life-threatening to children with depressed immune systems.

• A mother with chicken pox may transmit the virus to her baby during the last days of her pregnancy.

• In 1995 a vaccine called Varivax was approved for use in children over the age of one. The vaccine is 70–90 percent effective in preventing chicken pox over the short term.

TREATMENT

CHINESE HERBALISM
• The illness is believed to be caused by Wind and Heat invasion. Safflower, cimicifuga, and honeysuckle may be used in the treatment. *(See pages 58 and 65.)*

TRADITIONAL HOME AND FOLK REMEDIES
• Add baking soda to the bath to ease itching. *(See page 100.)*

HERBALISM
• A witch hazel compress can be applied directly to the spots, or a little added to the bath, to ease discomfort.
• Tincture of comfrey or elderflower can be applied directly to the spots to encourage healing and to relieve the itching. *(See pages 130 and 132.)*
• Add burdock infusion to your child's bath. *(See page 115.)*
• Crushed peppermint leaves, applied to the spots, relieve symptoms. *(See page 125.)*

AROMATHERAPY
• A few drops of Roman chamomile can be used in the bath to soothe. *(See page 150.)*
• Essential oil of lavender can be dabbed directly on spots to ease the itching and encourage healing. Lavender also has an antibacterial action, which will help prevent a secondary infection. *(See page 161.)*

HOMEOPATHY
• Variolinum can be taken once before your child acquires the illness, during an epidemic of chicken pox, and symptoms should be less severe.
• Rhus tox. can be taken for a few days after contact with an infected child, and then again as soon as the first spots appear. *(See page 210.)*
• Aconite, in the early stages of the illness. *(See page 178.)*
• Belladonna, for fever. *(See page 183.)*

FLOWER ESSENCES
• If the child is unreasonably demanding of attention, Chicory may be helpful. *(See page 228.)*
• Impatiens can ease fractious behavior. *(See page 233.)*
• Crab Apple may be diluted and applied directly to the spots to encourage healing. *(See page 234.)*
• Olive will be useful for the convalescence period. *(See page 235.)*

Headache and fever

Spots first appear on the trunk, spreading to face and limbs

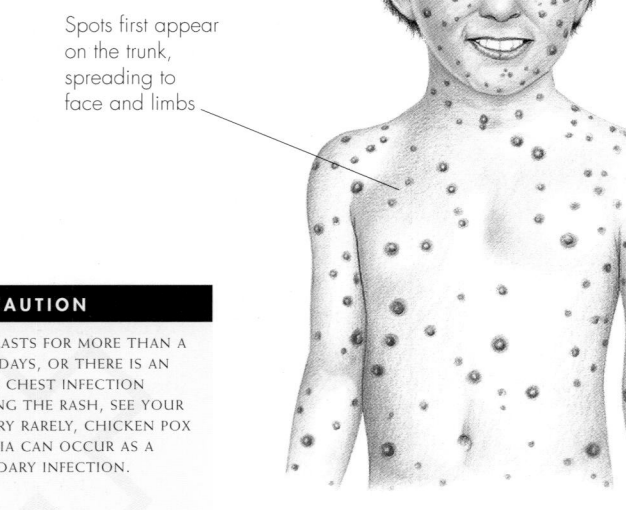

LEFT *Chicken pox rash is characterized by small, raised spots which develop into inflamed blisters. They become very itchy before drying to a scab.*

CAUTION

WHEN FEVER LASTS FOR MORE THAN A COUPLE OF DAYS, OR THERE IS AN OBVIOUS CHEST INFECTION ACCOMPANYING THE RASH, SEE YOUR PHYSICIAN. VERY RARELY, CHICKEN POX PNEUMONIA CAN OCCUR AS A SECONDARY INFECTION.

Mumps

Mumps is a viral infection which usually affects children, causing fever and swelling of the main salivary glands, the parotids. This swelling furnishes the sufferer with the characteristic "chipmunk" appearance. The condition rarely occurs in children under two or three years of age, and takes about two or three weeks to incubate. It is infectious from a day before the glands begin to swell until about a week after they have gone down. The virus is spread by coughing and sneezing.

SYMPTOMS

• *general malaise* • *fever* • *headache* • *pains around the neck*
• *swallowing will be painful*

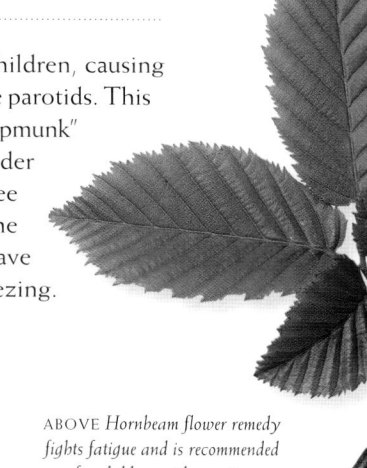

ABOVE *Hornbeam flower remedy fights fatigue and is recommended for children with mumps.*

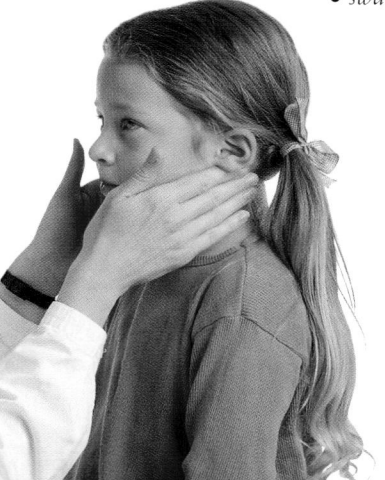

LEFT *A gentle neck massage with a chamomile oil blend will ease pain.*

DATA FILE

• Because mumps is a systemic infection, other parts of the body may also be affected, including salivary glands, the testicles, the ovaries, the pancreas, and the central nervous system.

• Mumps is communicable, though less so than measles, and occurs with great frequency in heavily populated areas.

• While the disease can occur at any age, it is children aged 5–15 who are primarily affected.

• Once a person has had mumps, this ensures permanent immunity.

• In adult males, inflammation and swelling may first occur in the testicles. Testicular inflammation, orchitis, occurs in about 20 percent of adult males who have mumps; it can be very painful and occasionally causes sterility.

• An infection involving the ovaries, oophoritis, occurs occasionally in women. Oophoritis causes high fever, chills, and lower back pain.

• A condition called aseptic meningitis sometimes occurs when the virus enters the central nervous system.

• Involvement of the pancreas occurs in less than 10 percent of cases.

TREATMENT

CHINESE HERBALISM
• The source of mumps is considered to be Wind and Damp Heat, and dandelion, honeysuckle, skullcap, and rhubarb may be suggested. *(See pages 65, 73, and 74.)*

TRADITIONAL HOME AND FOLK REMEDIES
• Chop fresh ginger and apply as a compress directly to the swollen glands to provide relief.
• Cayenne powder, mixed with vinegar, can be warmed and applied to the affected area. *(See pages 86 and 102.)*

HERBALISM
• Catmint, marigold, or chamomile infusions can be sipped to reduce fever, or added to a bath of cool water. *(See pages 117 and 119.)*
• Garlic, peppermint, and echinacea can be taken internally to boost immunity and encourage healing. *(See pages 113 and 120, and 125.)*
• Red clover and cleavers can help to reduce the inflammation and swelling. Drink both as a lukewarm infusion.
• A warm compress with poke root or marigold can be applied to the swelling. *(See page 117.)*

AROMATHERAPY
• Eucalyptus and thyme can be used for steam inhalations and in the bath (use sparingly). *(See pages 159 and 170.)*
• Massage the neck area with chamomile or lavender oil, diluted in a little grapeseed oil. Take care to do so gently. *(See pages 150 and 161.)*

HOMEOPATHY
• If your child has not had mumps, Phytolacca or Parotidium can be taken during an epidemic to reduce the severity of symptoms.
• Rhus tox., when the left glands are more severely affected than the right. *(See page 210.)*
• Belladonna, when there is high fever, shooting pains, and a bright red face and throat. *(See page 183.)*
• Merc. sol., when the patient sweats heavily and has a coated tongue. *(See page 205.)*

• Pulsatilla may help to prevent orchitis, and is useful if fever continues. *(See page 209.)*

FLOWER ESSENCES
• Rescue Remedy can be used to ease distress caused by discomfort. *(See page 244.)*
• Willow may be helpful if the child resents the fact that brothers and sisters are still well. *(See page 239.)*

VITAMINS AND MINERALS
• Eat a good selection of raw fruits and vegetables to cleanse the system.
• Increase the intake of foods containing vitamin C and zinc to aid the action of the immune system. *(See pages 256 and 265.)*
• Acidophilus should be taken after any illness to encourage production of the healthy bacteria in the gut. *(See page 271.)*

LEFT *Garlic oil capsules help revitalize a flagging immune system.*

COMMON AILMENTS IN THE ELDERLY

Depression

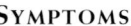

Many elderly people feel a sense of worthlessness as they age; they feel that they no longer matter to others, that their dependency is problematic, and that they have lost any sense of purpose or usefulness. Often this is exacerbated by the refusal of others to allow an elderly person to participate in daily chores, inadequate social intercourse, and lack of mental stimulation. A feeling of isolation develops, and withdrawal and depression are common responses to the dependency and loss of control that old age often brings. (*See also under Mind and Emotions, page 283.*)

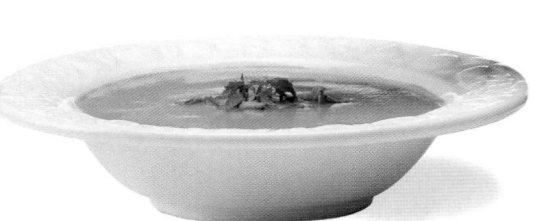

BELOW *Sage has stimulant qualities. Add fresh sage to food.*

SYMPTOMS

- *irritability or aggression*
- *bewilderment and disorientation*
- *fecal incontinence can be a feature of depression in the elderly*

LEFT *The value of human touch, received through massage, is of great reassurance in your twilight years.*

TREATMENT

AYURVEDA
- Detoxification treatment would be followed by specific oral medication to balance the three doshas. Treatment is always individual. *(See page 22.)*

CHINESE HERBALISM
- Depression is believed to be caused by stagnation of the Liver qi, and may be treated with angelica, peony root, licorice, and thorowax root. *(See pages 56, 64, and 67.)*

TRADITIONAL FOLK AND HOME REMEDIES
- Clove tea, or bruised cloves added to herbal teas such as chamomile or peppermint, are able to lift mild depression. *(See page 90.)*
- Drink sage tea, and add fresh sage to food, to fight depression.

HERBALISM
- The best antidepressant and nervine (with specific action for nerves) herbs include: balm, borage, limeflower, oats, rosemary, and vervain. These can be taken as herbal teas, added to the bath, or taken as tablets, or in tincture form (herbs suspended in alcohol). *(See pages 117, 127, 134, and 136.)*
- Ginseng is an antidepressant herb and will help with other problems accompanying old age, such as confusion, memory problems, and a weakening system. *(See page 126.)*

AROMATHERAPY
- Antidepressant oils include: bergamot, chamomile, clary sage, jasmine, geranium, lavender, melissa, neroli, orange, rose, sandalwood, and ylang ylang. These may be blended or used singly in massage (which will also be very therapeutic), or in the bath or a vaporizer. *(See pages 146–71.)*
- Basil, chamomile, juniper, marjoram, and tea tree will act as a general tonic, and can be used in any of the same ways. *(See pages 146–71.)*

HOMEOPATHY
Treatment should be constitutional, but some of the following remedies may help:
- Ignatia, for a depression which results from a trauma or a bereavement. *(See page 200.)*
- Arsenicum, for restlessness, chilliness, exhaustion, and obsessive tidiness. *(See page 182.)*
- Cadmium phos. for depression after illness, with exhaustion.
- Pulsatilla, for bursting into tears for no reason. *(See page 209.)*

FLOWER ESSENCES
- Cherry Plum, for "fear of the mind being overstrained, of doing dreaded things," and of doing violence to oneself or others. *(See page 236.)*
- Agrimony, for deeply held emotional tensions which are hidden from others. *(See page 225.)*
- Gorse, for feelings of great hopelessness. *(See page 240.)*
- Gentian, for relief of feelings of despondency or a mild depression. *(See page 230.)*
- Mustard, for blacker and deeper feelings that seem to have no identifiable cause. *(See page 239.)*
- Sweet Chestnut should be taken if the person is anguished and stretched beyond endurance. *(See page 227.)*

VITAMINS AND MINERALS
- Do not include an excessive amount of vitamin D, zinc, copper, or lead in the diet. *(See pages 256, 265, and 259.)*
- Ensure you have an adequate intake of vitamin C and the B vitamins, which help the health of the mind and nervous system. *(See pages 256 and 252–5.)*
- Calcium, potassium, and magnesium may also need to be supplemented. *(See pages 258 and 262.)*
- Take plenty of the antioxidant nutrients, which help to delay some of the effects of aging. *(See page 251.)*
- Some therapists may recommend using the amino acid tryptophan. *(See page 269.)*

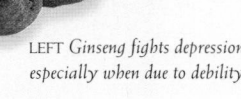

LEFT *Ginseng fights depression, especially when due to debility.*

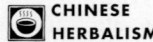

Confusion

One of the most common problems among elderly people is confusion. This may be a symptom of dementia (*see page 452*), hypothermia (very common among old people, who tend to economize on fuel and heating), or acute brain syndrome (caused by pneumonia, circulatory problems, or drug side-effects). Most often, however, it is a consequence of being cut off from the mainstream of life. Without visitors and possibly with no access to daily news, one day seems very much like another.

SYMPTOMS

• *self-neglect can be a natural consequence of confusion, with less attention paid to personal appearance and diet than previously* • *forgetfulness, sometimes with serious consequences* • *a lack of orientation, particularly in terms of time* • *bewilderment and agitation* • *depression and its associated symptoms (see page 450)* • *hallucinations (in acute brain syndrome)*

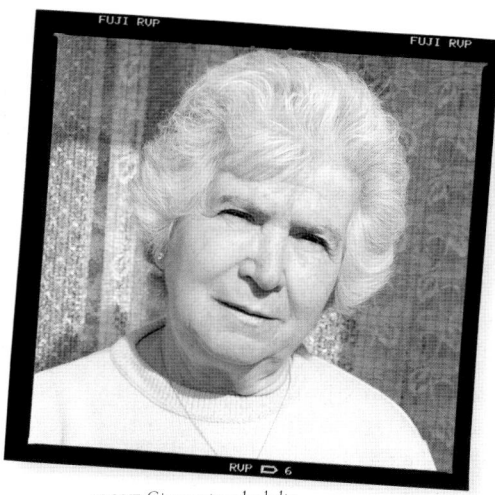

ABOVE *Ginseng powder helps improve powers of memory. Add it to herbal tea.*

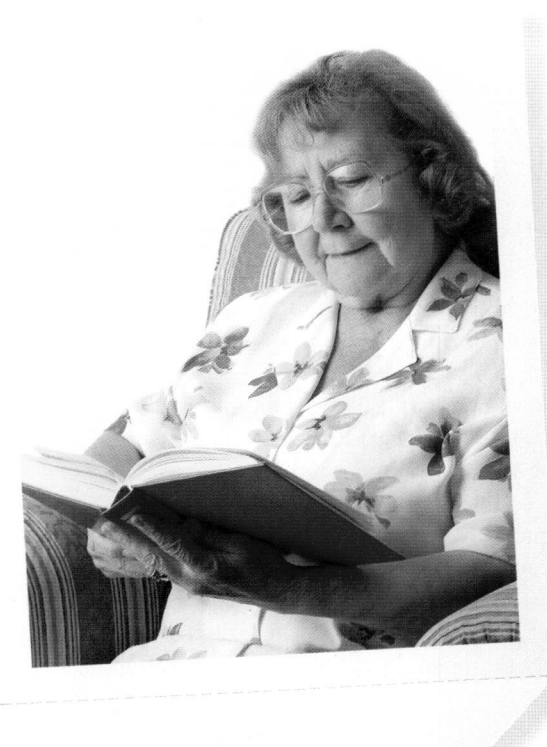

ABOVE *Keeping up interest in a subject or reading a novel will help to keep the mind sharp.*

TREATMENT

AYURVEDA
• Henbane may be suggested, as well as lemon or lime juice.

CHINESE HERBALISM
• Treatment might address deficient Kidney essence, and useful herbs include dodder seeds, mulberry, and black ginger seed. (See page 62.)

TRADITIONAL FOLK AND HOME REMEDIES
• Ginseng powder, added to herbal teas, will improve memory and help with symptoms of confusion and agitation.
• Gotu kola can revive memory and focus the mind. Add a small amount to your tea for a few days running, but discontinue use occasionally.

HERBALISM
• Rosemary is a tonic, particularly for the elderly, as it stimulates and nourishes the nervous system. It improves memory and concentration. Use fresh in food, or drink an infusion. (See page 127.)

• Orange blossom, particularly in the form of neroli oil, works on the nervous system and effectively counteracts nervous exhaustion, confusion, and depression.

AROMATHERAPY
• Geranium oil regulates the nervous system, and helps fight confusion, panic, and anxiety. (See page 165.)

HOMEOPATHY
• Acute confusion can be treated with Belladonna, particularly if accompanied by a red face and fever. Consult a physician if symptoms do not get any better after a day. (See page 183.) Chronic confusion can be treated with one of the following:
• Baryta carb., for confusion due to senile dementia. (See page 185.)
• Cannabis ind., for confusion, delusions.
• Alumina, for confusion, irritability, and obstinacy.

FLOWER ESSENCES
Flower essences have a tremendous effect on the mind and emotions. Some to try include:
• White Chestnut, a mind plagued by repetitive thoughts. (See page 224.)
• Wild Rose, if you drift through life resigned to accept any eventuality. (See page 238.)
• Gentian, for any feelings of despondency. (See page 230.)
• Scleranthus, if you suffer from indecision and cannot make up your mind. (See page 239.)

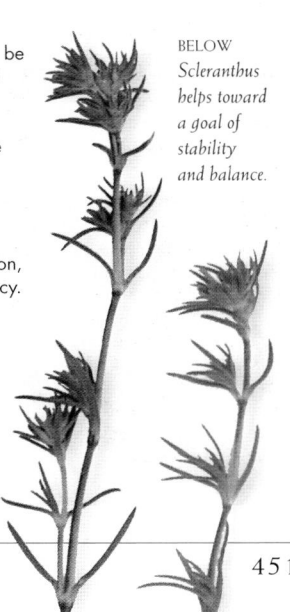

BELOW *Scleranthus helps toward a goal of stability and balance.*

Senile Dementia

Senile dementia is a form of chronic organic brain disease in which there is progressive loss of intellectual power due to shrinkage (atrophy) and deterioration of the brain in old age. The onset is subtle and is sometimes only identified retrospectively by slight personality changes. The risk of dementia increases with age, but not all older people will get dementia. Most dementias are irreversible, but people with dementia can function better with treatment of other medical or sensory problems, and optimal social and environmental support. Stimulation and activity can help people with dementia.

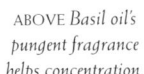

ABOVE *Basil oil's pungent fragrance helps concentration.*

SYMPTOMS

- *in the early stages: insomnia – restlessness – loss of interest in work or hobbies – forgetfulness, particularly of recent events – impaired judgment and reasoning*
- *later: progressive memory loss, until only events in the distant past may be remembered – mood swings to the point of character change – failure to follow even the most simple instructions – simplified vocabulary and repetitive conversation – delusions – apathy and indifference – sufferers fail to feed and warm themselves, which leads to total dependency – incontinence*

RIGHT *Rosemary is uplifting, and is a tonic for the nervous system.*

TREATMENT

CHINESE HERBALISM
- Dementia may be treated with herbs such as Chinese wolfberry or black ginger seed. *(See page 66.)*
- Treatment might be aimed at deficient kidney essence, and herbs to address this include mulberry and dodder seeds. *(See page 62.)*

AROMATHERAPY
- Basil and rosemary oils can be used in the bath, or in a massage, diluted in a little carrier oil, to clear the mind and stimulate mental activity. *(See pages 164 and 168.)*
- Chamomile, melissa, rosemary, marjoram, and lavender strengthen the nervous system, and can be used in any way. *(See pages 146–71.)*

- Tea tree acts as a general tonic, to help overall health and well-being. *(See page 162.)*

HOMEOPATHY
Treatment would be constitutional, but the following remedies may help:
- Phosphorus, for apprehension, cravings for salt, and accompanied by arteriosclerosis. *(See page 208.)*
- Baryta carb., for weakness, tiredness, when symptoms are worse in cold, and for degeneration of the blood vessels. *(See page 185.)*
- Ignatia, for symptoms stemming from a trauma or bereavement. *(See page 200.)*
- Lycopodium, for lack of self-confidence, use of the wrong words, particularly

in a person who was once sharp and ambitious. *(See page 203.)*
- Aurum iod., when there is partial paralysis.

FLOWER ESSENCES
- The flower essences work on the mind and emotions specifically, and there are a variety to choose from, according to your specific feelings. *(See page 219 for a full list.)*

VITAMINS AND MINERALS
- Ensure that your diet contains plenty of vitamins B and C, as well as zinc and magnesium. *(See pages 252–5, 256. 265, and 262.)*
- Taking lecithin, which contains phosphatidyl choline, improves memory when taken daily. *(See page 271.)*
- Take supplements which contain all 22 amino acids to improve brain function.

TREATMENT

AYURVEDA
- Add the juice of a lime or lemon to half a glass of soda water and sip in small doses.

CHINESE HERBALISM
- Fresh ginger, cinnamon twigs, and peppermint may be useful. *(See page 59.)*
- Mulberry will be used to nourish the blood.

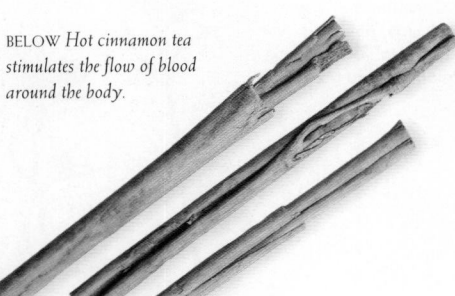

BELOW *Hot cinnamon tea stimulates the flow of blood around the body.*

HERBALISM
- Small sips of fresh ginger tea, made with root ginger, will help to ease the symptoms. *(See page 139.)*
- Teas of rock rose flowers or wild rose flowers, with a little honey, will be helpful.

HOMEOPATHY
Treatment will be constitutional, particularly if dizziness is a chronic problem, but some of the following may help:

- Causticum, when dizziness is worse in cold water and coughing causes urine to leak. *(See page 189.)*
- Silicea, for poor circulation, and when symptoms are worse when lying on the left side. *(See page 211.)*
- Arnica, when dizziness follows injury and occurs when standing suddenly. *(See page 182.)*
- Lycopodium, when it accompanies senile dementia, with an inability to concentrate, and when symptoms are worse between 4 and 8P.M. *(See page 203.)*

FLOWER ESSENCES
- If dizziness is associated with panic, stress, or anxiety, Rescue Remedy will be calming and restorative. Take as required. *(See page 244.)*

Dizziness

One of the most common features of aging is dizziness, often a cause of stumbles and falls. It may stem from age-related loss of orientation, side-effects of drugs, a failure in the balancing mechanism of the inner ear, or from neurological disturbances. (*See also page 299.*) It can also be a symptom of hypothermia, which is common among the elderly, partly because many tend to economize on fuel and heating, and partly because the brain's control of heat regulation is less efficient than that of younger people. Dizziness can be both frightening and debilitating, particularly for those elderly people who live alone.

CAUTION

CHRONIC, UNDIAGNOSED DIZZINESS SHOULD BE INVESTIGATED BY A PHYSICIAN.

SYMPTOMS

- *a spinning sensation* • *nausea and vomiting* • *headache*
- *pallor and sweating*

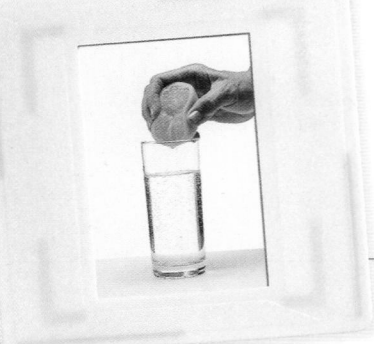

LEFT *Squeeze the juice of a lemon into soda water to sip.*

Falls and Accidents

Failing vision, unsteadiness, slower reflexes, dizziness, stiffness, and muscle weakness all contribute to the vulnerability of elderly people, making them more prone to falls and accidents. Often a stumble that would be little more than an inconvenience to a younger person is a serious hazard to the elderly, causing physical disability and, often, emotional complications. This may be partly explained by problems in the Data File alongside. (*See also First Aid, page 458.*)

DATA FILE

• Cataracts (*see page 317*).

• Osteoporosis (*see page 414*). Old people, and old women in particular, are susceptible to fractures even from minor accidents. The resulting immobility can trigger other problems, such as chest and urinary infections, and depression.

• Delicate skin. An older person's skin is more delicate and bruises or tears much more easily than previously.

• Slower healing processes. Muscular injuries are slow to heal among the elderly, causing long periods of disability and dependency. This in turn can lead to depression (*see page 450*).

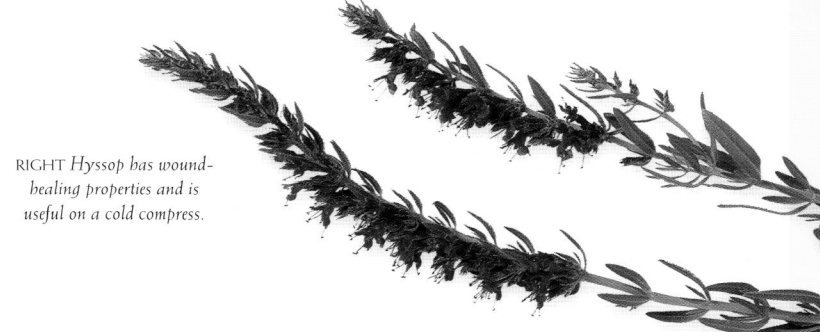

RIGHT *Hyssop has wound-healing properties and is useful on a cold compress.*

ABOVE *Finding hobbies which keep you active is one of the best ways of retaining mobility.*

TREATMENT

AYURVEDA
• Harithaki can help for conditions related to impaired vision, which can help to prevent accidents.

HERBALISM
• Use witch hazel on a cold compress for bruises. (*See page 123.*)
• Calendula cream will help healing of sprains, cuts, and bruises. (*See page 117.*)
• Compresses of herbs like hyssop, lavender, or fennel will reduce swelling and bruising. As it heals, essential oil of rosemary can be applied as a compress to encourage the circulation and, through that, the healing process. (*See page 121.*)
• Rosemary is a tonic, particularly for the elderly, as it stimulates and

nourishes the nervous system and will help keep you alert. (*See page 127.*)
• Orange blossom, particularly in the form of neroli oil, is an effective nervine tonic (for the nervous system), which can help prevent accidents that are caused by a lack of concentration, and general confusion.

AROMATHERAPY
• Oils that refresh and invigorate will help focus the mind, which prevents accidents. Use one or more of the following in the bath: rosemary, peppermint, geranium, eucalyptus. (*See page 146–71.*)
• Basil oil also clears the mind and stimulates mental activity. (*See page 164*)

• Bergamot, chamomile, lavender, marjoram, and rosemary will help to ease pain in the event of an accident. Do not apply to broken skin, but use in a vaporizer or in massage, avoiding the affected areas. (*See page 146–71.*)

HOMEOPATHY
• Arnica aids healing in someone who is constantly falling or having accidents. (*See page 182.*)
• Arnica followed by Symphytum, for fractures, to promote healing. (*See page 182.*)
• Aconite, for shock. (*See page 178.*)
• Veratrum, for shock, with cold pale skin and a cold sweat.
• Calendula will help heal deep and painful wounds. (*See page 187.*)

• Hypericum, for wounds that are characterized by shooting nerve pains. (*See page 199.*)

FLOWER ESSENCES
• Rescue Remedy or Emergency Essence can be used after an accident and in cases of shock. (*See page 244.*)

VITAMINS AND MINERALS
• Keeping physically and mentally active will help to prevent accidents. Ensure that you have a good intake of vitamin C and zinc, and B vitamins, which feed the nervous system. (*See pages 256, 265, and 252–5.*)
• Vitamin E will help healing. (*See page 257.*)

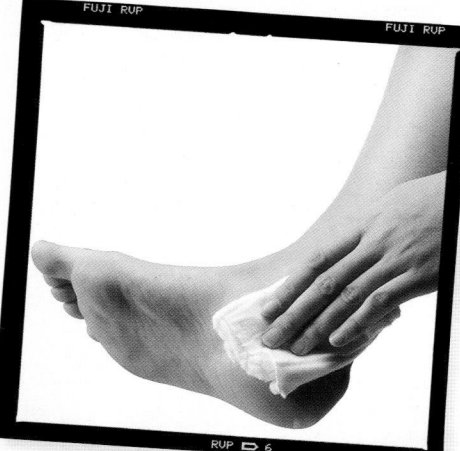

ABOVE *Distilled witch hazel, on a cold compress, treats a bruise.*

Trigeminal Neuralgia

Trigeminal neuralgia is a condition in which sudden nerve impulse discharges occur in the sensory nerve of the face on one side. These discharges cause severe pain and may be triggered by chewing, swallowing, or sometimes speaking. Usually there are repeated attacks over a period of some weeks, and the periods in between tend to become shorter. The cause of trigeminal neuralgia is unclear, but it is unusual under the age of 50. When the condition occurs in young people it may be associated with MS.

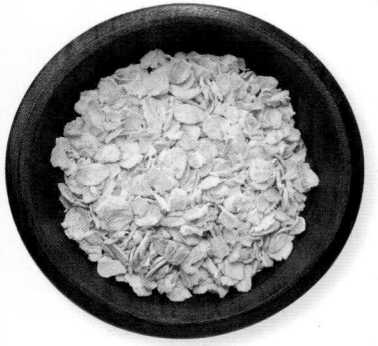

ABOVE *Cereals such as oats contain magnesium phosphate, itself the source of a homeopathic remedy.*

SYMPTOMS

- *excruciating pain lasting from a few seconds to one or two minutes*
- *a feeling of being on edge in constant anticipation of the next attack* • *a tic caused by the wincing of the facial muscles (hence trigeminal neuralgia is also known as tic douloureux)*

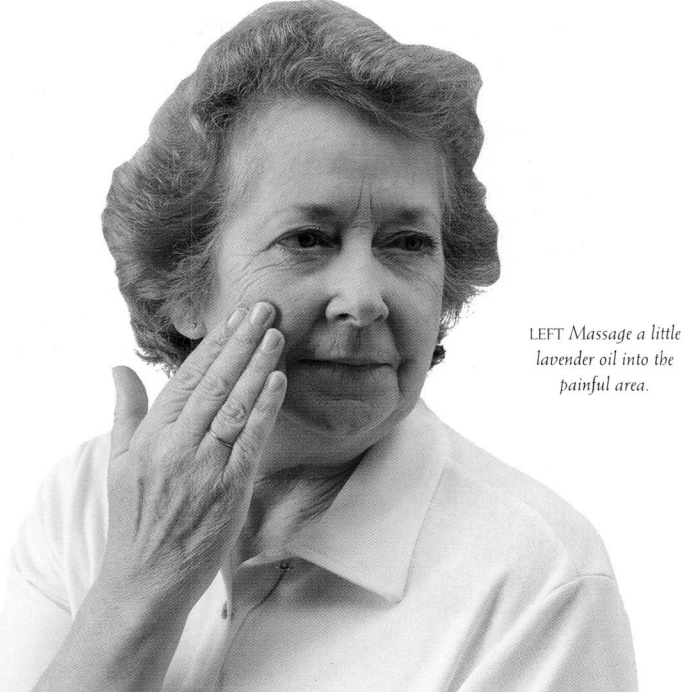

LEFT *Massage a little lavender oil into the painful area.*

TREATMENT

CHINESE HERBALISM
- Treatment would be aimed at addressing Wind, Damp, and Heat which have entered the meridians. Gentian and oriental wormwood may be useful.

LEFT *Brew up some celery seed tea by infusing 1-2 teaspoonsful of seeds in boiling water.*

TRADITIONAL HOME AND FOLK REMEDIES
- Celery juice or celery tea will help to ease the pain of neuralgia. *(See page 83.)*
- Rub lemons on the affected area for relief. *(See page 87.)*
- Rub peppermint oil into the affected area.
- Clove oil can be used where pain is experienced inside the mouth. *(See page 90.)*
- A compress of warm cider vinegar can bring relief. *(See page 102.)*

HERBALISM
- Ask a dentist to check your teeth, your bite, and jaw alignment.
- Drink rosemary and lavender infusions to relieve the pain. *(See page 127.)*
- Rub in cayenne-infused oil for neuralgia. *(See page 118.)*
- Warm chamomile compresses, applied to the affected area, will ease inflammation and pain. *(See page 119.)*

AROMATHERAPY
- Massage essential oil of eucalyptus, lavender, or chamomile into the affected area, or add the infused herbs to the bath. *(See pages 146–71.)*
- A compress of rosemary essential oil will invite the circulation to the area, which will encourage healing. *(See page 168.)*
- Blend 1 drop each of mustard and pepper oils in some grapeseed oil, and massage into the affected area. *(See pages 146–71.)*

HOMEOPATHY
Treatment should be constitutional, supervised by an experienced homeopath. Some of the following remedies may be helpful:
- Arsenicum, for an attack brought on by dry cold. You feel chilly, tired, restless, with burning pains. *(See page 182.)*
- Lachesis, for pain that is worse after sleep. *(See page 216.)*
- Mag phos., for pain that is relieved by heat and pressure. *(See page 204.)*
- Aconite, when symptoms come on suddenly, particularly after exposure to cold; the body feels congested and numb. *(See page 178.)*
- Colocynthis, for an attack brought on by cold or damp, and which is improved by heat. *(See page 191.)*

VITAMINS AND MINERALS
- Vitamins B1, B2, and biotin help nerve health. *(See pages 252, 253, and 257.)*
- Take extra vitamin E and chromium. *(See pages 257 and 259.)*

Incontinence

Incontinence, or involuntary urination, is extremely common among the elderly and usually has a physical cause. In men this may be prostate disease, and in women a prolapse of the bladder. Urinary infections or damage to the nervous system, such as acute or chronic brain disease, may also be responsible. Fecal incontinence is less common. It may be caused by constipation (if watery feces escape around the obstruction) or depression. Both types of incontinence are very distressing. (See also page 381.)

LEFT *Walnut flower essence helps with a change in life.*

BELOW *High fiber foods fight constipation, which may be the cause of incontinence.*

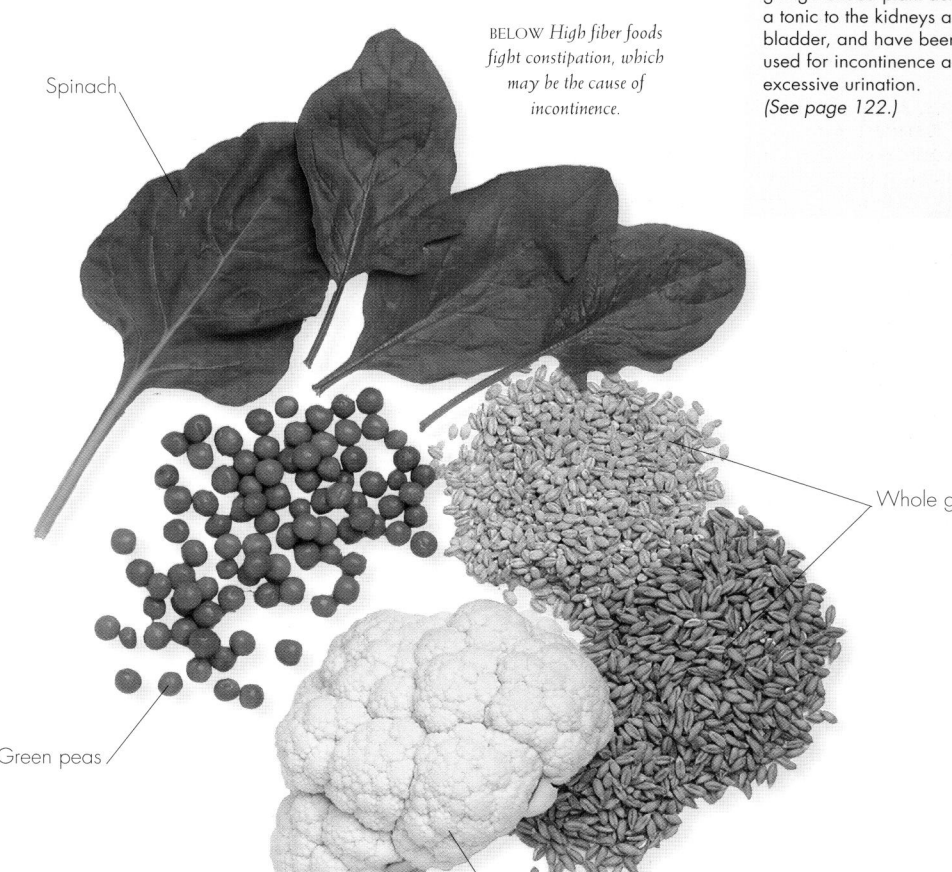

Spinach

Green peas

Cauliflower

Whole grains

TREATMENT

Fecal incontinence should be treated according to the cause (see constipation, senile dementia, depression, and gastroenteritis). Urinary incontinence can be treated in a variety of ways.

CHINESE HERBALISM
• Treatment would address Kidney Yang Deficiency with internal cold, and the best herb to use is golden lock, taken as a tea.
• If the condition accompanies prolapse, treatment will be given for deficient qi, using central qi pills. These will help with the control of fecal and urinary incontinence.

HERBALISM
• The seeds of the ginkgo biloba plant act as a tonic to the kidneys and bladder, and have been used for incontinence and excessive urination. *(See page 122.)*

• Horsetail has toning and astringent properties, making it useful for treating incontinence and frequent urination. *(See page 120.)*

HOMEOPATHY
Treatment would be based on the cause of the incontinence, but some of the following might be useful:
• Causticum, for incontinence made worse by coughing or laughing. *(See page 189.)*
• Ferr. phos., for an inability to control the bladder, with pain and a frequent urge to urinate. *(See page 194.)*
• Nux vomica, for irritability and involuntary dribbles of urine. *(See page 214.)*
• Pulsatilla, for stress incontinence which is made worse by sitting down. *(See page 209.)*
• Sepia, for incontinence related to weak pelvic floor muscles, with a feeling as if the abdomen is falling out of the vagina. *(See page 212.)*

FLOWER ESSENCES
A number of the remedies will help with negative emotions and distress. Some to try are:
• Sweet Chestnut, for feelings of despair. *(See page 227.)*
• Agrimony, if you hide behind a cheerful face. *(See page 225.)*
• Crab Apple, if you feel unclean. *(See page 234.)*

VITAMINS AND MINERALS
• Increase your intake of dietary fiber, which will prevent constipation and straining – a common cause of incontinence.
• Drink plenty of water to ensure regular use of the bladder muscles.

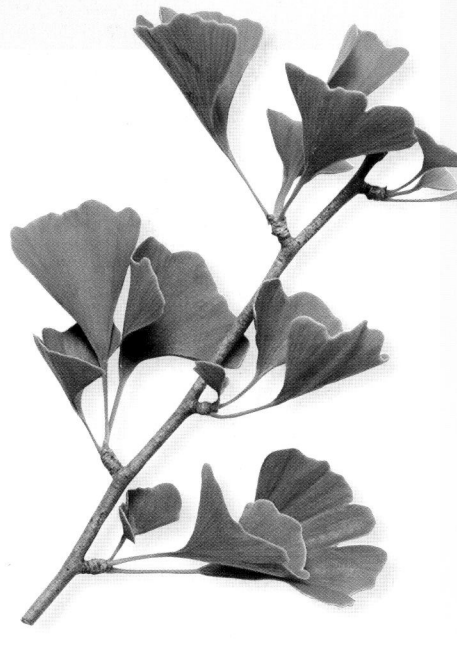

ABOVE *Gingko biloba seeds help to treat incontinence. The plant comes from China.*

CHRONIC ILLNESSES

Chronic Fatigue Syndrome (CFS)

Chronic fatigue syndrome (CFS) is also known as post-viral fatigue syndrome and myalgic encephalitis (ME), and its cause is the subject of controversy: it is thought by some to be caused by a viral infection (possibly herpes, polio, or Epstein-Barr), while others hold that it may be a psychological or neurological disorder, and others still that it is the result of damage to the immune system. There are recurrent acute attacks and rarely a full return to health in between. Symptoms may persist for years, aggravated by periods of stress or exertion.

SYMPTOMS

- *profound fatigue* • *fever* • *headache*
- *nausea and dizziness* • *muscle pain*
- *weight fluctuation* • *sleep disturbance*
- *depression* • *memory loss*

RIGHT *Olive flower essence is for those who cannot summon up interest in anything.*

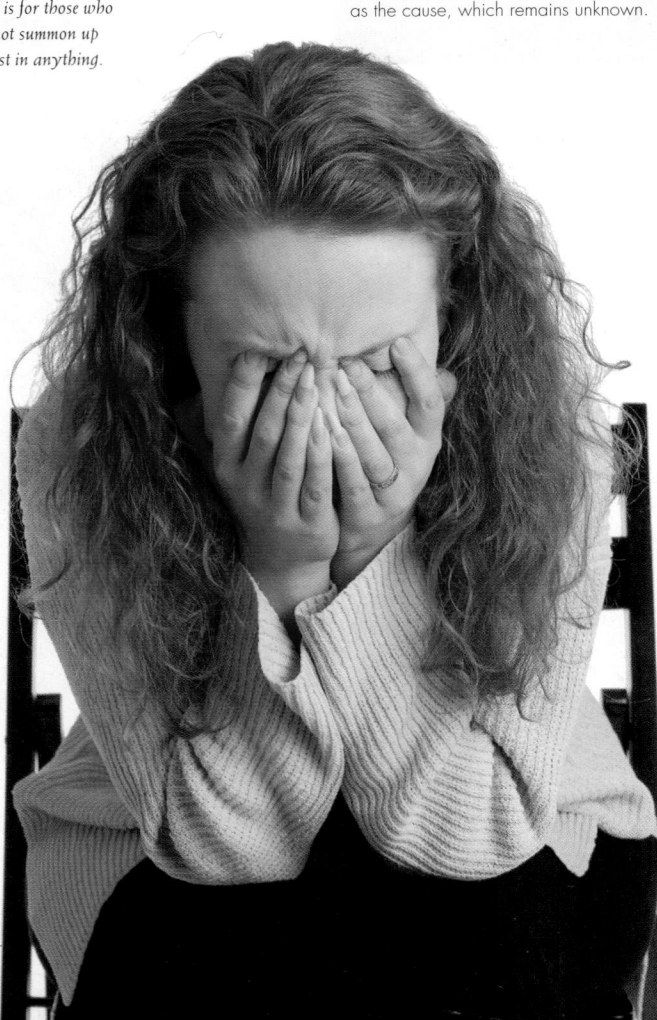

AYURVEDA
• Complete detoxification will help, along with oral preparations to strengthen the immune system and balance the doshas. Cluster fig and ginger may be useful to stimulate. *(See page 22.)*

CHINESE HERBALISM
• ME is believed to be caused by weakness of qi, Deficient Blood, and Damp Heat, and herbal treatment would be given accordingly, probably in conjunction with acupuncture. Chinese angelica can restore energy and stimulate white blood cells and antibody formation. *(See page 56.)*

HERBALISM
• Herbs that address the immune system, such as echinacea, will be most useful. *(See page 120.)*
• Ginseng and gingko biloba will encourage energy. *(See pages 122 and 126.)*
• Rosemary and sage wines act as an excellent tonic when you are run down and tired. *(See pages 127 and 129.)*
• Licorice can enhance recovery and stimulate the formation of white blood cells. *(See page 122.)*
• Astragalus can increase energy levels and resistance to disease. *(See page 116.)*

AROMATHERAPY
• Uplifting oils, such as bergamot, rose, and neroli, will help with flagging spirits. Use them in a massage or in the bath. *(See pages 146–71.)*
• Tea tree and niaouli will strengthen the immune system. Use these in a massage or in the bath. *(See pages 162 and 163.)*
• Rosemary is stimulating, and can be added to the bath, used in massage, or put in a vaporizer while you are working. *(See page 168.)*

HOMEOPATHY
• Homeopathic treatment would be constitutional, based on individual needs, but many promising studies have been done into its effects.
• China may be taken every 12 hours, for a few days, while waiting for constitutional treatment. *(See page 190.)*

BELOW *Add some deliciously fragrant rose oil to your bath: a treat for the senses.*

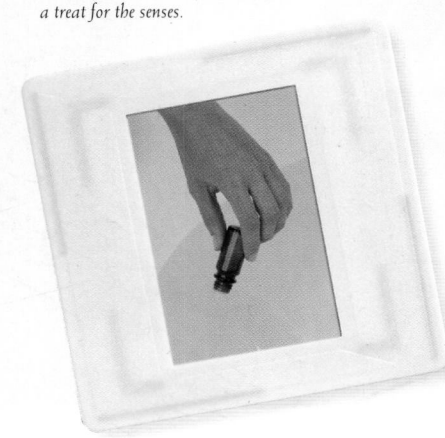

ABOVE *Astragalus root decoction fights chronic fatigue.*

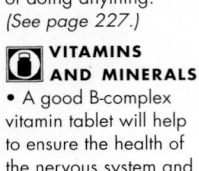

FLOWER ESSENCES
• Mustard, for depression, when you feel gloomy for no known reason. *(See page 239.)*
• Olive, when you are exhausted on all levels. *(See page 235.)*
• Rock Rose, for feelings of terror at the thought that you will never get better. *(See page 231.)*
• Crab Apple, if you feel unclean or impure on any level. *(See page 234.)*
• Hornbeam for exhaustion at the thought of doing anything. *(See page 227.)*

VITAMINS AND MINERALS
• A good B-complex vitamin tablet will help to ensure the health of the nervous system and give you more energy. *(See pages 252–5.)*
• Some sufferers have food allergies that may exacerbate or even cause the condition. Try an elimination diet to see if you are allergic to anything – in particular, dairy produce and wheat.
• Chronic yeast infection may be at the root of the condition. Taking an acidophilus supplement, or eating plenty of live yogurt will help fight the infection. *(See page 271.)*
• Evening primrose oil, taken over three months, has proved to be a useful treatment for ME. *(See page 270.)*

HIV/AIDS

(See under Immune System, page 410.)

Cancer

Cancer is a chronic disease that may occur anywhere in the body, beginning with a malignant tumor which may be either a carcinoma or a sarcoma. Carcinomas arise in the lining of the skin and internal organs. Sarcomas arise from solid tissues such as muscle, bone, lymph glands, blood vessels, and other connective tissues. Both are invasive – a cell becomes cancerous, divides, and forms an abnormal mass which grows until the healthy cells are outnumbered. The mass then spreads into adjacent tissues and structures, often destroying them. Secondary cancers occur if an invading cancer grows through the wall of a blood vessel so that the blood then carries cancerous cells to other parts of the body.

A tumor of low malignancy may take months or years to cause problems, whereas a high-malignancy tumor may have spread widely before the sufferer is aware of it.

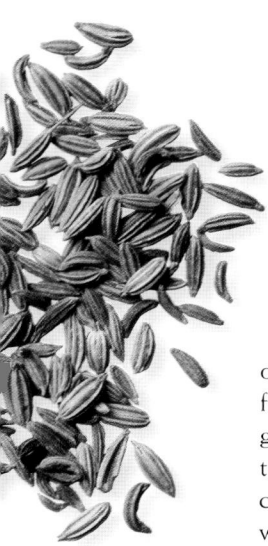

ABOVE *Use fennel essential oil for the nausea caused by chemotherapy.*

ABOVE *A healthy diet, high in antioxidants, helps the immune system.*

SYMPTOMS

- *It is impossible to enumerate all the symptoms of all cancers here, but awareness of signs that a change has occurred is important. They may have a harmless explanation, but include:*
- *unusual bleeding or discharge, especially from the vagina or rectum*
- *a lump or thickening in the breast or elsewhere*
- *a wound that does not heal* • *persistent change in bowel habits*
- *persistent hoarseness or coughing* • *persistent indigestion or difficulty in swallowing* • *change in the size or shape of a wart or mole*
- *persistent unexplained weight loss* • *nagging pain in the chest*

TREATMENT

CHINESE HERBALISM

- Treatment will be aimed at supporting the immune system and reducing the harmful effects of chemotherapy and radiotherapy.
- Ginseng protects the immune system and helps to restore vitality. *(See page 67.)*
- Dang Gui will protect the Liver. *(See page 56.)*
- Huang Qi will act as a tonic, support the nervous system, and invigorate the immune system, as will ginger and ginseng. *(See pages 57 and 67.)*
- Chinese angelica can restore energy, and stimulate white blood cells and antibody formation. *(See page 56.)*

HERBALISM

- Herbs that calm the nervous system will be useful. Try chamomile, valerian, and limeflowers. *(See pages 119, 134, and 136.)*
- Echinacea can be used to promote healing. *(See page 120.)*
- Sweet violet, cleavers, red clover, and burdock will help to boost the immune system. *(See page 115.)*

- St. John's wort is a mild antidepressant which acts as a restorative and helps treat depression. *(See page 124.)*
- There are several herbs which have been found to have anticancer properties, and which can be used in conjunction with conventional medical treatment. These include yellow dock, garlic, nettle, myrrh, cleavers, thyme, calendula, poke root, and plantain. *(See pages 113, 116, 117, 128, 135, and 137.)*

AROMATHERAPY

- An aromatherapy massage will restore the body's equilibrium.
- Geranium and rose, for lifting depression. *(See pages 165 and 168.)*
- Rosemary, bergamot, and sandalwood, for fatigue. *(See pages 146–71.)*
- Fennel, for nausea. *(See page 159.)*
- Do not massage the body immediately prior to or just after chemotherapy because it can encourage the spread of cancer cells throughout the body. In the early stages of cancer, use aromatherapy oils in the bath or in a vaporizer only. *(See page 144.)*

HOMEOPATHY

- Constitutional treatment will help you to cope with any treatment you are receiving, and there are specific remedies that will reduce the toxic effects of radiation and chemotherapy. There are some ongoing studies into homeopathic treatment of some cancers, but no evidence is available at the current time.

FLOWER ESSENCES

- Flower Essences are often used by practitioners to help you cope with the physical and emotional effects of cancer. *(See page 219 for a list of those that might be the most suitable.)*
- Mimulus is particularly good for feelings of fear. *(See page 235.)*
- Rock Rose is good if you feel helpless and experience terror or panic. *(See page 231.)*
- Olive will help if you feel exhausted on all levels. *(See page 235.)*

- Sweet chestnut will help if you feel there is no way out. *(See page 227.)*
- Gorse will help with feelings of hopelessness. *(See page 240.)*

VITAMINS AND MINERALS

- Eat as much fresh fruit and vegetables as you can, particularly those containing antioxidants. *(See page 251.)*
- Reduce animal fats and avoid processed foods.
- A deficiency of vitamin C has been found in conjunction with certain tumors. Ensure you get plenty in your diet. *(See page 256.)*
- Vitamin A can protect against cancer in smokers to some degree. *(See page 252.)*
- Digestive enzymes may be offered as a treatment to halt the activities of trophoblastic cancer cells.
- Vitamin E is said to prevent a number of cancers. Ensure that you get plenty in your diet or take supplements. *(See page 257.)*

DATA FILE

- In the 1990s nearly 6 million new cancer cases and more than 4 million deaths from cancer were being reported worldwide each year.
- The leading fatal cancer in the world today is lung cancer, which has risen rapidly because of the spread of cigarette smoking in developing countries.
- Stomach cancer, prevalent in Asia, is the second most fatal form of cancer in men, after lung cancer.
- Also on the increase is the leading killer of women, breast cancer, particularly in China and Japan.
- The fourth on the list is cancer of the colon or rectum, a disease that mainly strikes the elderly.
- In the U.S. in the early 1990s more than one-fifth of all deaths were caused by cancer; only cardiovascular diseases accounted for a higher percentage of deaths.
- In 1993 the American Cancer Society predicted that about 33 percent of Americans will eventually develop some form of cancer.
- Skin cancer is the most prevalent cancer in both men and women, followed by prostate cancer in men and breast cancer in women.
- Lung cancer, however, causes the most deaths in both men and women.
- Leukemia, cancer of the blood, is the most common type seen in children.
- An increasing incidence of cancer has been observed over the past few decades, due to improved cancer screening programs, the increasing age of the population, and also the large number of tobacco smokers.
- Researchers have estimated that if Americans stopped smoking, lung-cancer deaths could virtually be eliminated within 20 years.

FIRST AID

Bites and Stings

Insect bites and stings are common, and may cause discomfort, but unless you suffer from an allergic reaction, the best course of treatment is to soothe the pain and reduce swelling. The stinging insects inject a toxin through a stinger at the tail end of the abdomen. The reaction is usually local, but if the sting occurs in the mouth or throat, swelling can cut off the air supply and cause death by asphyxiation. Death can occur in individuals who are hypersensitive to bee venom. Animal bites should always be cleaned carefully and seen by a doctor. Dogs and other animals can transmit the infectious disease rabies through bites. Symptoms include fever and convulsions.

Bruises *See page* 363

Blisters

A blister occurs when a small area of the skin becomes raised and swollen by an accumulation of blood serum beneath it. If a blister is punctured the flesh beneath it becomes open to infection. It is therefore essential that it is kept clean and dry in order to heal effectively. Blisters can be caused by a number of things, including injuries – such as burns, scalds, or chafing (in new or ill-fitting shoes, for example) – insect bites, or infections. Some diseases will produce blisters, including chicken pox, herpes, eczema, and impetigo, and the disease can be transmitted by the virus particles inside the blisters.

AYURVEDA

- Aloe vera can be applied to the bite or sting to soothe; it also has anti-inflammatory and antiseptic properties. *(See page 27.)*
- Bitter orange is anti-inflammatory and bactericidal.
- Rub ghee on the affected area. *(See page 464.)*
- Place a slice of raw onion on the bite or sting for natural relief. *(See page 25.)*

- Aloe vera juice can be applied to the blister to encourage healing. *(See page 27.)*
- Barberry can be used for an infected blister. *(See page 29.)*
- Apply a basil oil poultice to the area. *(See page 42.)*
- Cedar is a natural insect repellent. Spray around the room in an atomizer half full of water. *(See page 32.)*

CHINESE HERBALISM

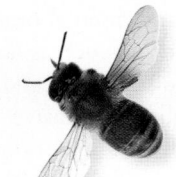

ABOVE *The homeopathic remedy Apis is made from bees and their venom.*

TRADITIONAL HOME AND FOLK REMEDIES

- The juice of a spring onion or a cucumber can be applied to stings to soothe and reduce inflammation. *(See page 82.)*
- The juice of daikon radish is useful for spider bites.
- Bathe stings in a bowl of water with several teaspoons of baking soda. *(See page 100.)*
- A slice of raw onion placed on an animal bite will discourage infection and draw out poison. *(See page 82.)*
- Apply garlic and onion to ant bites, and cucumber juice to ease the discomfort. *(See page 82.)*
- Make a compress from a pad of cotton wadding soaked in lemon juice or cider vinegar and apply to a wasp sting. *(See pages 87 and 102.)*
- Granulated sugar can be used to prevent a bite wound from scarring. Apply a poultice of sugar to the wound, after it has been cleaned, and bandage it with gauze.

- Boiled and mashed carrots can be applied to blisters to help to heal the area, and this is particularly good for infection. *(See page 89.)*
- Use roasted onions, applied as a poultice to blisters, particularly those which have become infected. *(See page 82.)*
- Peach pit tea is recommended to heal blisters. *(See page 103.)*
- Ice will also reduce inflammation and any itching or pain. *(See page 103.)*
- Bathe the blister with cold, salty water, which will discourage infection and help the blister to dry out. *(See page 103.)*
- You can also apply surgical spirit, and then petroleum jelly to areas which may be susceptible to blisters caused by chafing.
- Cover blisters in the daytime to prevent damage and infection. Remove bandages at night to allow them to dry out.

HERBALISM	AROMATHERAPY	HOMEOPATHY	FLOWER ESSENCES	CAUTION
• *Marigold petals are useful on a bee sting. (See page 117.)* • *Calendula cream will reduce swelling. (See page 117.)* • *The leaves of wormwood, sage, or rue can be macerated and applied to spider, scorpion, or jellyfish stings. (See page 129.)* • *Cover bites and stings with a wet, macerated plantain leaf. When it dries, replace with a wet leaf. (See page 126.)* • *Witch hazel is useful on mosquito bites. (See page 123.)*	• Use neat lavender oil on stings to reduce swelling and discomfort. *(See page 161.)* • 1 drop of tea tree oil can be rubbed into an insect bite or sting. *(See page 162.)* • A few drops of geranium oil, applied to water, can be used to clean a bite wound and encourage it to heal. *(See page 165.)* • Prevent insect bites by diluting essential oils of eucalyptus or citronella in half a mug of water, and then gently applying to exposed areas, avoiding the eyes and mouth. Use cider vinegar in the same way. *(See pages 158 and 159.)*	• *Ledum is useful for animal bites. (See page 202.)* • *Clean stings and animal bites with pure tincture of Hypericum. (See page 199.)* • *Aconite, for shock. (See page 178.)* • *Arnica, for bruising. (See page 182.)* • *Apis can be used for bee stings, after you have removed the sting with a pair of tweezers. (See page 180.)*	• Rescue Remedy or Emergency Essence, diluted in a few ounces of cool water, or the cream, can be applied to the sting or bite. Take orally for shock, pain, or distress, or apply to pulse points. *(See page 244.)*	

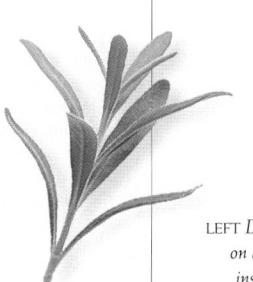

LEFT *Dab neat lavender oil on a sting. It has an insecticidal action.*

HERBALISM	AROMATHERAPY	HOMEOPATHY	FLOWER ESSENCES	CAUTION
• *Aloe vera can be applied to the blister to help it heal. (See page 114.)* • *Marigold (calendula) can be applied to a blister to promote healing. (See page 117.)* • *Witch hazel, applied neat to a blister, will quickly relieve pain and swelling, and encourage healing. (See page 123.)*	• Neat lavender oil can be applied to blisters. *(See page 161.)* • Benzoin, applied to areas which are susceptible to blisters, can prevent as well as heal them. *(See page 170.)* • Roman chamomile has antiseptic properties. Use a few drops in half a mug of water to cleanse punctured blisters and the area around them. *(See page 150.)*	• *Urtica urens ointment can be applied to blisters caused by infection or burns. (See page 217.)* • *Hypericum ointment will encourage the healing of blisters. (See page 199.)* • *Cantharis, for itching, burning blisters. (See page 188.)* • *Rhus tox., for red and itchy blisters, particularly those caused by the chickenpox virus. (See page 210.)* • *Punctured blisters can be cleansed with a few drops of tincture of calendula in clean water. (See page 187.)*	• Rescue Remedy or Emergency Essence can be diluted in water and applied directly to the blister. *(See page 244.)*	**CAUTION** TRY NOT TO BURST A BLISTER, WHICH WILL LEAVE THE SKIN OPEN TO INFECTION. THE TOP LAYERS OF THE SKIN ARE USUALLY AFFECTED BY BLISTERS. SEE YOUR PHYSICIAN IF BLISTERS BECOME VERY PAINFUL AND INFLAMED, OR IF BLISTERS APPEAR FOR NO REASON.

LEFT *Aloes produce a gel which is both soothing and healing.*

| | **AYURVEDA** | **CHINESE HERBALISM** | **TRADITIONAL FOLK AND HOME REMEDIES** |

Mild Shock

Injury or severe emotional trauma can lead to a potentially dangerous condition we call shock, in which the blood fails to circulate properly. In serious cases of shock, the brain and other organs can be deprived of oxygen. Causes of shock include extreme pain, severe vomiting or diarrhea, blood infection, or violent allergy.

Toothache *See page 333*

• Ginger and black pepper are *warming and will help to restore circulation in cases of mild shock.*

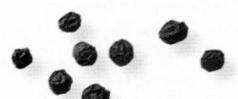

ABOVE Black peppercorns contain piperine, which helps to relieve pain.

Cuts and Abrasions

Minor cuts and abrasions should be cleaned with a mild antiseptic or cooled, previously boiled water to ensure that they do not become infected. More serious cuts, with damage to the skin and the structures below, should be seen by a physician.

Sprains *See page 417*
Travel Sickness *See page 369*
Nosebleed *See page 331*

• Aloe vera can be applied directly to cuts and grazes to encourage healing, reduce any inflammation, and prevent infection. *(See page 27.)*
• Yarrow improves blood clotting and may be useful for deeper wounds. *(See page 24.)*
• Myrrh can be used to clean the wound. *(See page 34.)*

• Lemon juice is an excellent styptic, and can be diluted and applied directly to a clean wound. *(See page 87.)*
• A compress made of peach pit tea can be used on infected wounds.
• Sugar is said to prevent scar tissue. Press a few teaspoons of granulated sugar into a clean wound and dress with gauze. Rinse the wound carefully and dress again. Repeat up to five times daily, but take care not to disturb the clotting action.
• Direct pressure should be applied to the bleeding area, and maintained until the flow of blood ceases.

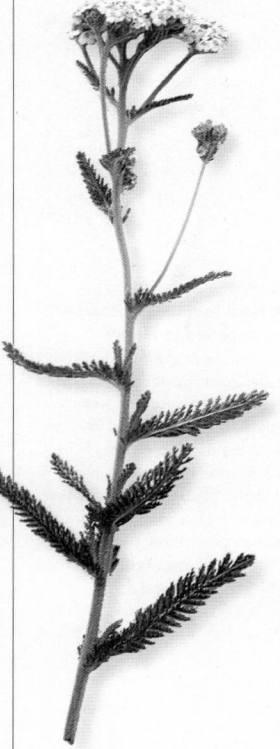

Burns and Scalds

A burn is an injury to the tissue of the body caused by heat, chemicals, electricity, or radiation. Serious burns must always be seen by a physician, as an emergency, but minor burns and scalds can be safely treated at home. Always cool a burn by letting cool water run over it until the pain has stopped. Try to avoid applying anything to the burn until it is cooled and you can see the extent of the damage. "Wet" burns should be dressed with a fabric, like gauze, which will "breathe." Change the dressing regularly.

Sunburn *See page 305*

• Aloe vera cools and prevents infection. *(See page 27.)*
• Onions may be used directly on the skin for instant relief. *(See page 25.)*
• St. John's wort can be used directly on the burn to cool and soothe. *(See page 40.)*

ABOVE Yarrow helps to stop bleeding. The whole plant is used.

• Crush blueberries and extract the juice. Keep in the refrigerator or freezer to use on burns or scalds in the case of an emergency.
• Honey can be applied directly to a burn to facilitate healing and to help prevent infection. *(See page 101.)*
• Raw potatoes can be placed on a burn to provide instant relief. *(See page 98.)*
• Immerse the area in cool (not freezing water) for at least 10 minutes. Then apply hypericum lotion (about 10 drops of mother tincture, in a cup of water).

HERBALISM	AROMATHERAPY	HOMEOPATHY	FLOWER ESSENCES	CAUTION
• Sip chamomile tea to calm. (See page 119.) • Add a little powdered ginseng to warm water with honey and lemon to restore. (See page 126.)	• Lavender, melissa, or peppermint can be dropped on a handkerchief and held under the nose until help arrives or the condition stabilizes. (See pages 146–71.)	• Aconite, for shock. Take every five minutes until it has subsided or help arrives. (See page 178.) • Arnica, for any bruising, injury, or trauma. (See page 182.) • Ignatia, for shock from an emotional upset or trauma. (See page 200.)	• Four drops of Rescue Remedy or Emergency Essence can be taken internally or applied to the temples and pulse points, to reduce the effects of shock and ease a feeling of panic. (See page 244.) • Rock Rose is suitable if you are experiencing terror or panic. (See page 231.) • Try Mimulus for fear. (See page 235.)	**CAUTION** ONLY MILD SHOCK SHOULD BE TREATED WITH NATURAL REMEDIES.
• Cayenne pepper is a very useful styptic, and a minute quantity can be applied directly to a clean wound to stop any bleeding. (See page 118.) • A few drops of marigold tincture in fresh, warm water can be used to clean the wound. This will help to prevent infection and encourage healing. (See page 117.) • Echinacea can be diluted and used directly on the wound to prevent infection. (See page 120.) • Comfrey ointment can be used on wounds which have become inflamed. (See page 132.) • Use a witch hazel compress on wounds and swellings. (See page 123.) • Tincture of myrrh is an excellent antiseptic. Apply a few drops to bandages before dressing a wound.	• Lavender oil, applied directly to the nostrils or massaged in a light carrier oil into the temples, will provide relief from any accompanying shock or pain. (See page 161.) • A few drops of tea tree oil, in clear, warm water, can be used to clean a wound and act as an antiseptic. (See page 162.) • Geranium oil can be dropped on to a dressing to encourage healing. (See page 165.)	• Ledum, for puncture wounds. This is particularly good if there is a risk of tetanus. (See page 202.) • Hypericum, for injuries that affect the nerve endings, such as the toes and fingers. (See page 199.) • Clean with calendula or hypericum tinctures. (See pages 187 and 199.) • Arnica should be used in the case of all injuries, to encourage healing and reduce the risk of bruising. (See page 182.)	• Rescue Remedy or Emergency Essence can be applied neat to a graze to encourage healing and reduce pain, or applied to the temples and pulse points to calm. Use diluted in water on cuts, as the brandy may sting. (See Shock, page 460.) (See page 244.)	**CAUTION** IF YOU ARE UNABLE TO STOP THE BLEEDING, SEEK EMERGENCY MEDICAL ATTENTION. DO NOT OFFER FOOD OR DRINK.

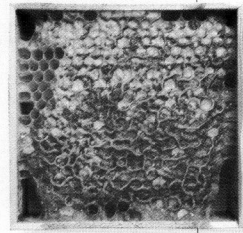

LEFT *Smear honey on burns, cuts or bruises, to help healing.*

HERBALISM	AROMATHERAPY	HOMEOPATHY	FLOWER ESSENCES	CAUTION
• Aloe can be applied directly to a burn in order to soothe and seal it from infection. It will also encourage healing. (See page 114.) • A few drops of echinacea tincture in a liter of water, poured over the burn, will help to prevent infection. (See page 120.) • Marigold tincture, applied sparingly to a dressing, is a useful healing agent. (See page 117.)	• Lavender oil is ideal for burns and can be applied neat (use sparingly). (See page 161.) • A few drops of geranium oil in a liter of cooled boiled water can be poured over a burn or scald to encourage healing. (See page 165.)	• Arnica can be taken to promote healing. (See page 182.) • Cantharis can help to relieve pain when taken immediately after the accident. (See page 188.) • Urtica can be used if the burn continues to be painful. (See page 217.) • Hypericum is useful for burns affecting the ends of fingers or toes, when there are sharp, stabbing pains. (See page 199.) • Aconite should be taken for shock. (See page 178.) • Urtica urens ointment may help to soothe a burn. (See page 217.) • Use hypericum ointment or calendula to prevent infection and encourage the burn to heal. (See page 199.)	• Rescue Remedy or Emergency Essence will help to calm. A little bit of diluted tincture can be applied directly to a minor burn. (See page 244.)	**CAUTION** DO NOT PUNCTURE BLISTERS CAUSED BY BURNS, WHICH CAN CAUSE INFECTION. BURNS CAUSED BY CORROSIVE SUBSTANCES MUST BE WASHED OVER AND OVER AGAIN.

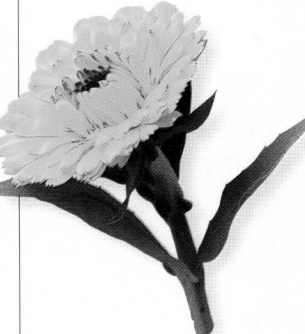

RIGHT *Calendula is antiseptic and promotes healing of any skin damage.*

	AYURVEDA	CHINESE HERBALISM	TRADITIONAL HOME AND FOLK REMEDIES

Sunstroke/Heatstroke

Sunstroke is a type of heat exhaustion, with symptoms that include headache, vomiting, fever, dizziness, and physical collapse. Heat exhaustion or sunstroke is usually caused by the excessive loss of water from the body that is the result of intensive heat. It is a mild form of shock. Sunstroke is also due to the body's inability to regulate internal heat. Heatstroke is a disorder that occurs when body-temperature regulating mechanisms are overwhelmed by excessive heat or fail in otherwise tolerable heat. Early nonspecific symptoms are faintness, dizziness, staggering, headache, dry skin, thirst, and nausea, which may be specifically related to heatstroke. In the latter stages of the condition, sweating ceases. Heatstroke is a medical emergency. The body temperature may be 40.5°C (105°F) or higher. Heatstroke differs from heat exhaustion, which lacks elevated body temperature and is characterized by persistent and heavy sweating.

AYURVEDA
• Add the juice of a lime or lemon to half a glass of soda water and sip in small doses.

CHINESE HERBALISM
• *Fresh ginger, cinnamon twigs, and peppermint may be useful.* *(See page 59.)*

TRADITIONAL HOME AND FOLK REMEDIES
• Sip a little fresh cucumber juice to cool. *(See page 89.)*

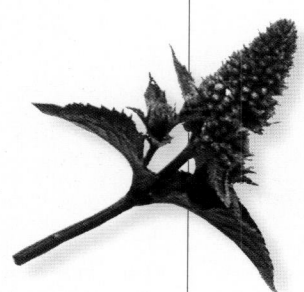

ABOVE *Peppermint soothes an upset stomach. Drink the tea as often as you like.*

Food Poisoning

Food poisoning is usually caused by eating food or drinking water that has been contaminated with bacteria, usually the salmonella strain. Symptoms of this kind of poisoning include diarrhea, fever, vomiting, and possibly pain in the abdomen. Gastroenteritis, an inflammation of the digestive system, can also result.

AYURVEDA
• Fresh lemon juice will help to cleanse, and fight infection.
• Strong spices like cayenne, curry, and turmeric have preventive properties against food poisoning.
• Combine 1 teaspoon of black pepper, 2 cloves of garlic, 1 tablespoon of cumin seeds, and a little salt in 4 cups of water. Boil until the liquid has reduced to 2 cups, and drink three times daily to cleanse and treat diarrhea.

CHINESE HERBALISM
• *Fresh ginger root will help to ease the nausea.*
• *Ping Wei Pian or Ren Dan may be useful.*

TRADITIONAL HOME AND FOLK REMEDIES
• Drink warm water with a little lemon juice to cleanse the system. *(See page 87.)*
• Add plenty of honey to a cup of warm water and sip for its antibacterial and immune-enhancing properties. *(See page 101.)*
• Chew ginger root to help ease the nausea.
• Cider vinegar, drunk with some warm water, will encourage vomiting to expel the poisons. *(See page 102.)*
• Drink plenty of cool fresh water, and avoid any food for at least twenty-four hours. *(See page 103.)*
• When the vomiting has ceased, ripe bananas can be eaten to help restore the bacterial balance in the gut. Live yogurt will have a similar effect. *(See page 93.)*

HERBALISM	AROMATHERAPY	HOMEOPATHY	FLOWER ESSENCES	CAUTION
• *Small sips of fresh ginger tea, made with root ginger, will help to ease the symptoms. (See page 139.)* • *Teas of rock rose flowers or wild rose flowers, with a little honey, will be helpful.*	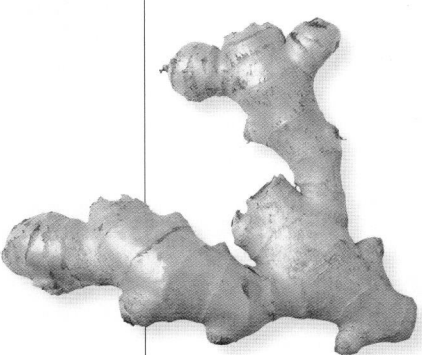 BELOW *Chinese herbalists use ginger to restore yang in the body.*	• *Take aconite initially, for symptoms of shock. (See page 178.) The following remedies will help in the aftermath:* • *Gelsemium, when there is accompanying trembling. (See page 195.)* • *Nux, when symptoms are made worse by flickering lights. (See page 214.)* • *Calcarea, when symptoms are worse on looking up. (See page 186.)* • *Borax, for symptoms made worse by downward motion.* • *Conium, when you feel worse lying down.*	• *Rescue Remedy or Emergency Essence should be offered as soon as possible to treat shock. (See page 244.)* • *Olive will help in the aftermath. (See page 235.)*	**CAUTION** FLUID MUST BE REPLACED AS SOON AS POSSIBLE, AND, IN SEVERE CASES, INTRAVENOUSLY. FIND A COOL PLACE AND SIT DOWN UNTIL ANY DIZZINESS SUBSIDES. IF YOU SUFFER FROM DIZZINESS THAT LASTS FOR MORE THAN AN HOUR OR FROM VOMITING, SEE YOUR PHYSICIAN.
• *Make a tea of comfrey root and meadowsweet to treat infection and relieve symptoms. (See pages 121 and 132.)* • *Arrowroot or slippery elm tea can be sipped during the worst symptoms to soothe the digestive tract, and afterwards to help restore bowel health. (See page 136.)* • *Golden seal and meadowsweet can also be drunk as tisanes. (See page 121.)* • *Licorice tea will help to flush out the toxins. (See page 122.)* • *Fresh garlic, or garlic capsules, should be taken to reduce infection. (See page 113.)* • *Chamomile, drunk as a tea, will help to ease digestion and reduce inflammation. (See page 119.)*	• Chamomile oil, sprayed in the air or rubbed into the temples, will help to calm and ease symptoms. (See page 150.) • Tea tree, garlic, eucalyptus, and juniper all work to kill bacteria, and can be added to a cool bath or placed on a burner to help fight infection. (See pages 146–71.) • Rub a little diluted lavender oil into the abdomen to reduce any spasm and to help encourage healing. (See page 161.) • Bergamot will help to reduce any fever. Place on a cold compress on the head. (See page 153.)	• *Aconite, for symptoms that come on swiftly, causing some distress and shock. (See page 178.)* • *Baptisia, for salmonella infections. (See page 184.)* • *Pulsatilla, when the symptoms are worse at night and the sufferer feels tearful. (See page 209.)* • *Phosphorus, when there is diarrhea with a burning sensation, vomiting, and a craving for cold drinks. (See page 208.)* • *Arsenicum is excellent for many cases, particularly when there are burning pains and diarrhea. (See page 182.)* • *Nux vomica will help when the pain improves upon passing stools and there is a feeling of chilliness. (See page 214.)*	• Take Rescue Remedy or Emergency Essence initially. *(See page 244.)* • Olive will be useful as symptoms improve, to ease overwhelming exhaustion. *(See page 235.)*	**CAUTION** ANY CASE OF FOOD POISONING WHICH LASTS LONGER THAN 48 HOURS SHOULD BE SEEN BY A PHYSICIAN. ALL CASES OF SALMONELLA SHOULD BE REPORTED TO THE MEDICAL AUTHORITIES.

THE HOME HEALING REMEDY CHEST

The best way to learn about natural medicines is to try them out on yourself, your family, and friends. Assemble a stock of home medicines. Keep them in a box or cupboard along with a thermometer, scissors, an eye bath, cotton balls, and a selection of bandages, plasters, and sterile dressings. Use them for first aid and to treat minor ailments. The more you use, them the easier it becomes.

The list below includes remedies that most people will find useful. Check through the rest of the book and add remedies that are more specific to your family's needs. What are the most common medical conditions that arise in your family? Make or assemble suitable remedies so that they are always available. Try to treat illnesses as soon as the first symptoms appear. Do not wait for a runny nose to turn into sinusitis or

bronchitis. Try to develop a general awareness of health. The aim of giving treatment at home should always be to prevent minor illnesses from turning into major ones – so avoiding visits to your practitioner.

Keep a notebook with the remedies to record your successes for future reference.

A short guide to indications and uses is given by each remedy below. Use this as a guide and consult the body of the book for more detailed information. The various remedies described can be used alone or in combination, but decide which is to be your main internal remedy for a specific situation, and use other suggestions as support. For example, use homeopathic Drosera for coughing attacks in children, and back this up with a drink of chamomile tea before bed, and eucalyptus essential oil in a vaporizer in the bedroom.

ABOVE *Remember to keep a record of treatments, to refer to.*

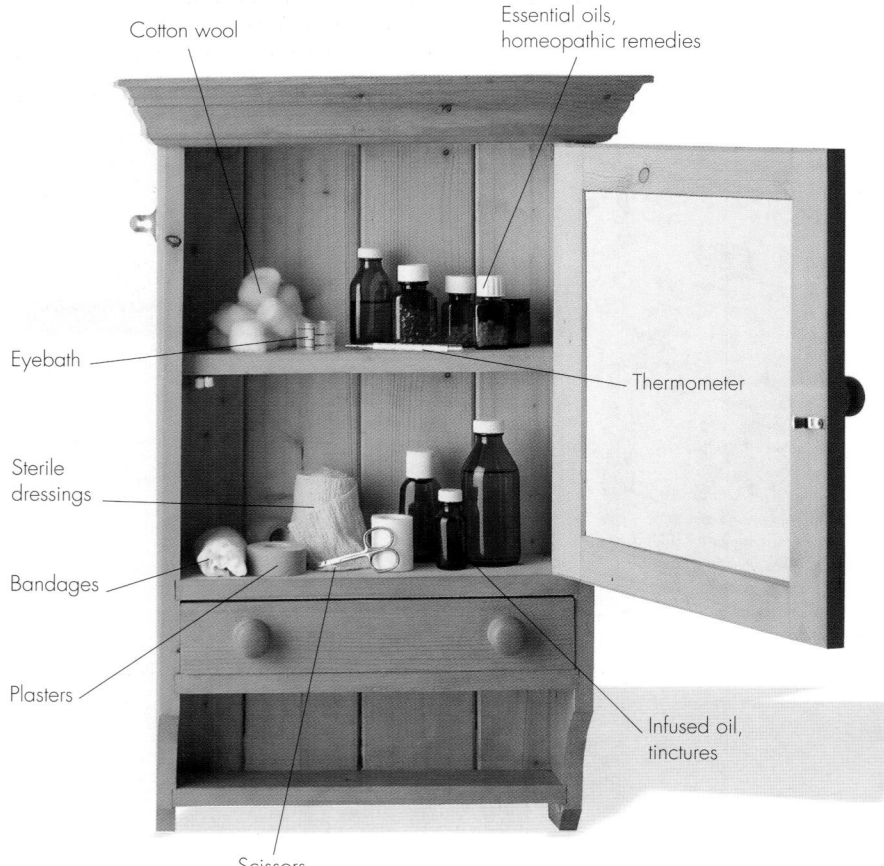

Cotton wool

Essential oils, homeopathic remedies

Eyebath

Thermometer

Sterile dressings

Bandages

Plasters

Scissors

Infused oil, tinctures

ABOVE *Be prepared! Keep a good stock of remedies and equipment at hand.*

Ayurveda

Coriander	USES	*Colds, flu, cystitis, sinus problems, and headaches.*
Mustard oil and seeds	USES	*Headaches, fever, rheumatism, sore feet, cold hands and feet.*
Curry leaves	USES	*Menstrual cramps.*
Garlic	USES	*Infections, chest pain, toothache.*
Ginger	USES	*Coughs and sore throats, indigestion, fungal infections.*
Black pepper	USES	*Diarrhea.*
Ghee	USES	*Bee and wasp stings, burning feet and hands.*
Karella	USES	*Tonic, calming.*
Lemon and lime juice	USES	*Dizziness.*
Aloe vera	ACTIONS	*Antiseptic, antibiotic, antiviral, anti-inflammatory and immune-enhancing.*
	USES	*Colds, colic, thrush, constipation, dermatitis, diabetes, water retention, ME, fungal infections, herpes, high blood pressure, inflammation, insomnia, indigestion, infections, menstrual cramps and irregularity, nausea, parasites, peptic ulcers, psoriasis, sprains, tinnitus.*

THE HOME HEALING REMEDY CHEST

Chinese Herbalism

Patent Chinese herbal remedies for minor ailments are recommended for short-term use only. If you do not see an improvement within a week, stop using them and see a practitioner.

	REMEDY	PROPERTIES
Burns	Jing Wan Hung ointment	*Stops pain, resolves inflammation, clears Heat, promotes healing. Excellent for all types of burns. Can also be helpful for bedsores.*
Colds and Flu	Yin Qiao Jie Du Pian (honeysuckle and forsythia febrifugal pills)	*Expels Wind Heat. Best for colds and flu where you feel hot, have a sore throat, sneezing, and thick catarrh. Best in the first few days of illness. Not for when you are feeling chilled and achy, with watery catarrh. Not so useful once a cold has settled on your chest.*
	Tong Xuan Li Fei Wan	*Expels Cold and Wind. Best for colds and flu where you feel chilled and achy, and there is sneezing, maybe with watery catarrh. Best in the first few days of a cold or flu. Not for when you are feeling hot or have a sore throat. Not so useful once the cold has gone on to your chest.*
Coughs and Bronchitis	Qing Qi Hua Tan Wan (clear breathing and transform phlegm pills)	*Clears Phlegm and Heat from the lungs, stops coughing. Take for chest congestion and tightness in the chest, a cough, and coughing up thick yellow phlegm. The symptoms may be acute or chronic and may be accompanied by fever. It should produce an improvement in a couple of days, if it does not, seek professional help. Stop taking if you become thirsty. Not suitable for a dry, unproductive cough.*
	Chuan Bei Pi Pa Lu (fritillaria and loquat extract, cough syrup)	*Clears Phlegm and Heat from the Lungs, stops coughing. Use for an acute and chronic cough which produces thick phlegm, maybe yellow mucus. Not so good for dry coughs.*
Digestive Disturbances	Huo Xiang Zheng Qi Wan (herba agastachis pills)	*Regulates digestive system qi, clears Cold and Damp. For acute attacks of nausea, vomiting, and diarrhea with abdominal pain, especially when there are chills. Useful for gastric flu and for vomiting caused by food poisoning. If there is no improvement within a day, seek professional advice.*
Muscular Injuries	Die Da Wan (bodily injury pills) and Imperial Ted Da Wine	*Moves Blood and qi, resolves bruising, promotes healing in damaged tissue. The remedy is taken internally for bruises and sprains. Also useful for fractures after you have received medical attention. Not to be taken during pregnancy or if there is copious bleeding.*
Menstrual Problems	Dang Gui Pian (angelica tea), Shi Chuan Da Bu Wan (ten flavor tea), Wu Ji Rai Feng Wan (white phoenix pills)	*Supplements qi and Blood. There may be many causes of menstrual problems. For persistent problems it is wise to consult a practitioner. Dang Gui Pian is good for pain, but is not for excessive bleeding. Do not use Shi Chuan Da Bu Wan if you feel too hot.*

RIGHT *Sprinkle cayenne pepper in herbal tea for relief of indigestion.*

LEFT *Patent Chinese medicines are classic formulas developed over centuries.*

Traditional Home and Folk Remedies

Barley water (with lemon)	USES	Digestive upsets, sore throats, cystitis.
Black pepper	USES	Congested head colds.
Cabbage leaves	USES	Mastitis, infections, hot swollen joints (crush and wrap around hot swollen joints).
Cinnamon sticks	USES	Colds, indigestion, circulatory problems.
Celery	USES	Neuralgia, headaches, muscle problems, spasm, kidney problems.
Cloves	USES	Neuralgia, indigestion, toothaches.
Carrot juice	USES	Stomach pains, children's diarrhea.
Garlic	USES	Internal and external infections and infestations.
Honey	USES	Weeping eczema, infected cuts, sore throats, flu, colds.
Mustard	USES	Colds, headaches, rheumatic pains, coughs.

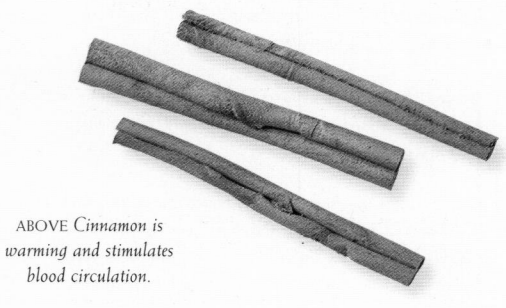

ABOVE *Cinnamon is warming and stimulates blood circulation.*

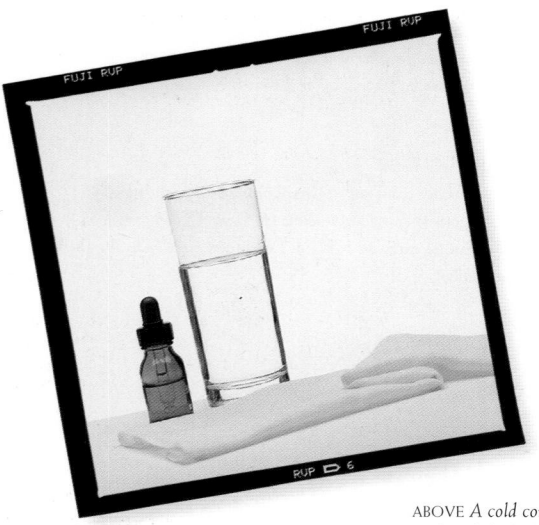

ABOVE *A cold compress, made with herbal tincture, has various uses.*

Aromatherapy

Keep essential oils in their original bottles. They last well but remember to screw the tops back on properly or they will slowly evaporate. If you buy them with the eyedropper attached, remember to keep them upright or the oil will eat away at the rubber top and leak. The home aromatherapist needs only a basic kit for minor ailments and first aid purposes. These ten oils are suitable for most people's needs.

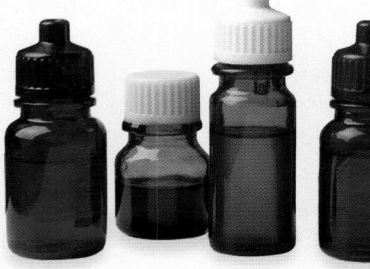

LEFT *Essential oils are usually diluted before skin application.*

Lavender	ACTIONS	Relaxing, antiseptic, generally therapeutic.
	USES	Dry skin, cuts, wounds, burns, bruises, insomnia, stress, indigestion, cystitis, headache.
Chamomile	ACTIONS	Calming, antiseptic, analgesic.
	USES	Pain, indigestion, acne, eczema, sensitive skin, diaper rash, hay fever, toothache.
Tea tree	ACTIONS	Antifungal, antiseptic.
	USES	Dandruff, mouthwash, cuts, insect bites, cystitis, thrush, colds, catarrh, infections.
Geranium	ACTIONS	Refreshing, relaxing, antidepressant, astringent.
	USES	PMS, menopause, apathy, anxiety, cuts, fungal infections, eczema, bruises.
Eucalyptus	ACTIONS	Antiseptic, decongestant, antiviral.
	USES	Colds, chest infections, aches and pains.
Rose	ACTIONS	Soothing, tonic, antiseptic, antidepressant.
	USES	Painful or irregular menstruation, menopause, insomnia, sensitive skin, sore throat, sinus congestion, depression.
Rosemary	ACTIONS	Stimulating, refreshing.
	USES	Muscle fatigue, colds, poor circulation, aches and pains, mental fatigue.
Peppermint	ACTIONS	Digestive, refreshing.
	USES	Bad breath, muscle fatigue, toothache, bronchitis, indigestion, travel sickness, sinus congestion.
Lemon	ACTIONS	Refreshing, antiseptic, stimulating.
	USES	Cold sores, cuts, depression, acne, indigestion.
Clary sage	ACTIONS	Warming, soothing.
	USES	Menstrual problems, depression, anxiety, high blood pressure.

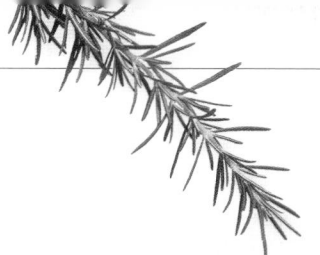

Herbalism

For most purposes keep either the dried herbs or their tinctures. Tinctures will keep, in dark-glass bottles in a cool place, for two or three years. Keep dried herbs in clean screw-top jars and replace them every year. Be sure to label all bottles and jars with the date and contents. Pills can be substituted where available and appropriate. They are especially useful for traveling and for unpleasant-tasting medicines. The creams and lotions can be bought or made at home. See the appropriate entry in the remedies section for methods of use (pages 112–139).

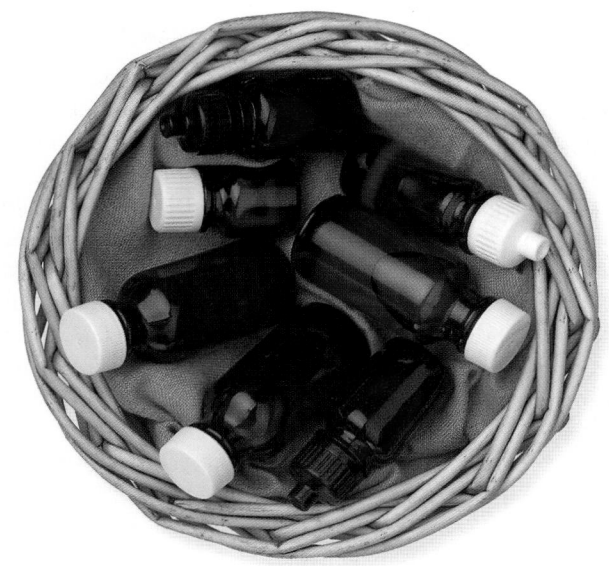

ABOVE *Herbal tinctures must be kept in dark glass bottles to preserve their medicinal actions.*

Angelica   USES   *Coughs, rheumatic pain, travel sickness, fever, pleurisy, nervousness.*

Basil   USES   *Insect bites, vomiting, constipation, nervous complaints.*

Bay   USES   *Rheumatism, fever, bruises, sprains.*

Calendula   USES   *Cuts, bruises, grazes, minor skin problems.*

Chamomile   USES   *Fever, nervous conditions, swelling, sores, fatigue, digestive complaints.*

Comfrey   USES   *Diarrhea, stomach ulcers, bleeding gums, menstrual problems, bruises, bites, sores, lung problems, whooping cough, broken bones.*

Echinacea   USES   *Fighting infection and warding off colds, flu and sore throats; boosts the immune system while acting as a natural antibiotic.*

Elder   USES   *Measles, bronchial problems, scarlet fever, colds, skin complaints.*

Garlic   USES   *Coughs and colds, thrush, wounds, bites, stings, infections, catarrh, cholesterol, high blood pressure.*

Ginger   USES   *Indigestion and wind, circulatory disorders, arthritis, morning sickness, travel sickness.*

Lavender   USES   *Relieves stress and promotes relaxation; treats stress and related disorders, insomnia, headaches, infection.*

BELOW *Chamomile is very versatile: antiseptic, nervine, sedative, and anti-inflammatory.*

Limeflowers   USES   *Tension headaches and the effects of stress, including insomnia.*

Marjoram   USES   *Diarrhea, flatulence, coughs, cramps, colic, sprains, rheumatism, inflammation, sore throats, bruises.*

Meadowsweet   USES   *Pain relief, acid indigestion.*

Mint   USES   *Headaches, insomnia, nervousness, coughs, migraine, flatulence, abdominal aches.*

Parsley   USES   *Rheumatism, cystitis, insect bites, asthma, stings, urinary ailments, coughs.*

Peppermint   USES   *Indigestion, flatulence, headaches, colds.*

Rosemary   USES   *Circulatory disorders, stomach ache, bruises, headaches, migraine, exhaustion.*

Sage   USES   *Gastritis, diarrhea, throat problems, nervousness.*

Thyme   USES   *Coughs and colds, sore throat, catarrh, headaches, whooping cough, diarrhea, rheumatism, bruises.*

Valerian   USES   *Flatulence, nervous headache, insomnia, stress, tension.*

RIGHT *Calendula is a very useful first aid remedy.*

Homeopathy

Although it is better to receive treatment from a qualified homeopath, homeopathy can be very useful in treating minor injuries at home. Bites, stings, bruises, cuts, travel sickness, and so on can be alleviated with the right remedy. But if you are in any doubt, seek professional help. For acute first aid problems in adults, children, and babies, use 30c. For less acute conditions, use 6c. Take every 2 hours up to 6 doses, then three times a day. Do not take more than 30c during pregnancy. Keep remedies in the original bottles. Keep away from essential oils. Replace before the "sell by" date. Homeopathic remedies work best when they fit the full symptom picture. Try to find the remedies that especially suit the individual.

Arnica	USES	Cuts, grazes, broken skin, bruising, burns, scalds, nosebleeds, stings, sprains, dislocated joints, fractures, eye injuries, and shock.
Apis	USES	Stings, hives, water retention, cystitis, bites, puncture wounds allergies affecting the throat, mouth, and eyes.
Bryonia	USES	Fractures, sprains, strains, mastitis, swollen joints, heat exhaustion, colds, flu, bursting headache with nausea.
Calendula	USES	Burns, cuts, grazes (more often used as a cream or tincture).
Cantharis	USES	Blisters, burns, scalds, burning diarrhea, cystitis, any stinging or burning sensation.
Euphrasia	USES	Conjunctivitis, bruising of the eye, sore eyes, eyestrain, constipation, bursting headaches.
Hypericum	USES	Cuts, grazes, bruising, crushed parts such as fingers, lacerations, puncture wounds, cut lip, diarrhea, and indigestion.
Ledum	USES	Cuts, bruises, insect stings, black eye, sore eye, bites, sprains and strains, particularly when they feel numb.
Nux vomica	USES	Travel sickness, digestive problems, hangovers, morning sickness, cystitis, nausea with headache.
Phosphorus	USES	Electrical burns or shock, nosebleeds.
Rhus tox.	USES	Red, swollen, itchy blisters, diaper rash, torn muscles, swollen joints, dislocated joints, cramp, muscle stiffness, arthritic or rheumatic pain which is helped by movement.
Silicea	USES	Splinters, recurrent colds and infection, migraine, spots.

Flower Essences

Rescue Remedy	USES	Shock, trauma, injury, panic, anxiety.
Star of Bethlehem	USES	Shocks of all kind, accidents, bad news, sudden startling noise, trauma.
Walnut	USES	Change of any sort, including menopause, adolescence, divorce, a new school.
Olive	USES	Exhaustion and fatigue on all levels.
Rock Rose	USES	Helplessness, terror, panic.

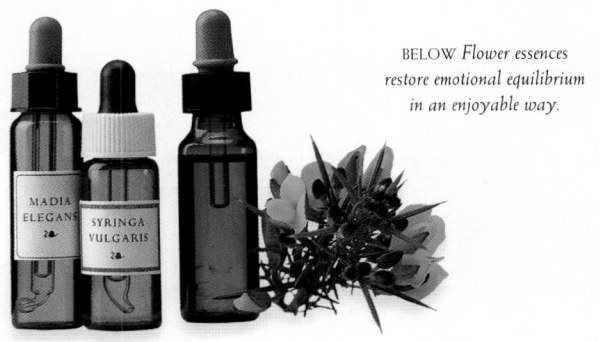

BELOW Flower essences restore emotional equilibrium in an enjoyable way.

Vitamins and Minerals

Royal jelly	USES	Tonic, infections, allergies, stress.
Ginseng	USES	Stress, infections, colds, coughs, fatigue, circulatory problems.
Vitamin C	USES	Colds, infections (bacterial and viral), skin problems, circulatory problems, wounds, gum problems.
Zinc	USES	Colds, arthritis, fatigue, wounds.
Chromium	USES	Blood sugar swings, infections.
Co-enzyme Q10	USES	Colds, infection, heart problems, nervous problems, poor memory.
Calcium	USES	Insomnia, palpitations, arthritis, leg cramps, weak bones and teeth.
Acidophilus	USES	After antibiotics, constipation, diarrhea, infections, digestive problems, respiratory problems.
Charcoal	USES	Digestive problems, flatulence, indigestion.

RIGHT Charcoal has a long tradition of use for flatulence and indigestion.

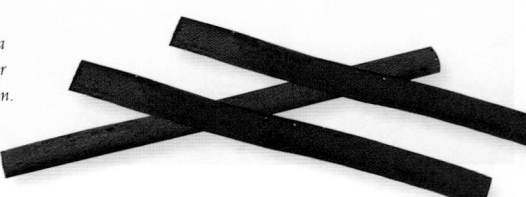

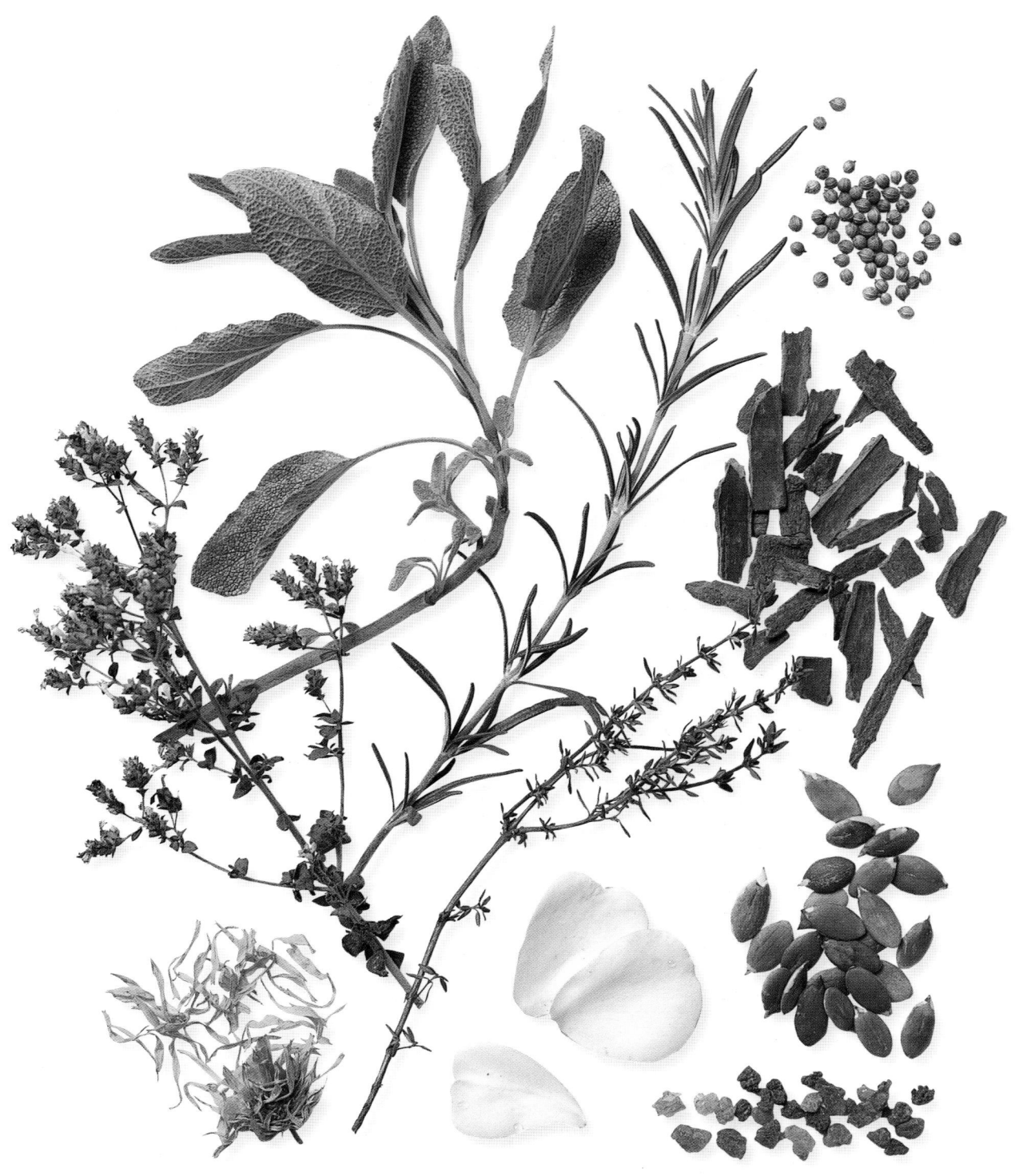

ABOVE *For regular and recurring health problems in the household, it is helpful to make up specific herb combinations. With time you will figure out particular mixtures that are beneficial to you and your family.*

3

REFERENCE
SECTION

GLOSSARY

A

abortifacient
an agent that causes the early expulsion of a fetus

abscess
a self-contained pocket of pus that results from a bacterial infection, and causes inflammation of the local area

absolute
a highly concentrated viscous, semi-solid, or solid perfume, usually obtained by alcohol extraction from the concrete

acute
of sudden onset and brief duration

adaptogen
an agent that modulates hormones

adaptogenic
an agent that adapts itself to respond to the body's needs; for example, lavender is adaptogenic and will relax you if you need to be relaxed, or invigorate you if you are tired

adenoids
lymphatic tissue at the back of the nose

adrenal
the adrenal glands are a pair of endocrine glands, each located on the top of one of the kidneys, which secrete hormones that regulate the functions of other organs and systems into the bloodstream

adrenaline
a substance secreted by part of the adrenal gland that increases the heart rate in response to stress

aerophagia
excessive swallowing of air, which may be a response to stress or a consequence of eating too quickly

aggravation
the exacerbation of symptoms that can occur when taking some natural remedies, particularly in the case of chronic ailments

agni
meaning "fire," or the forces which break down substances consumed; in Indian medicine, considered to be metabolism

agoraphobia
fear of open or crowded places

alcohols
a group of chemical compounds with antiseptic, antiviral, and uplifting properties

aldehydes
chemicals that have a sedative and sometimes anti-inflammatory effect

aldosterone
the steroid hormone which helps the body to control water balance

-algia (suffix)
meaning "pain in"; for example, arthralgia, pain in the joints

allergen
a substance that causes an allergic reaction

allergy
an abnormal response by the body to a food or foreign substance

allopathic
Western medicinal treatment, based on treating symptoms rather than the underlying condition

alopecia
hereditary hair loss

alterative
corrects disordered body functions; works according to the needs of the body. Often used in the same way as "adaptogenic"

ama
in Ayurveda, a toxic substance believed to gather in the weak parts of the body and cause disease. Ama occurs when the metabolism is impaired due to an imbalance of agni

amenorrhea
absence of menses (menstrual periods)

analgesic
pain-relieving

anaphrodisiac
reduces sexual desire

anaphylaxis
an extreme allergic reaction to a foreign substance. Subsequent exposure can produce an overwhelming body reaction called anaphylactic shock

anemia
deficiency in either quality or quantity of red corpuscles in the blood

anodyne
painkilling

anorexia nervosa
psychological problem causing extreme loss of appetite, drastic weight loss, and, sometimes, death

anosmia
loss of the sense of smell. It can be either temporary or permanent

antacid
a remedy or medicine that reduces stomach acidity

anthelmintic
a vermifuge, destroying or expelling intestinal worms

anthraquinone
a powerful laxative which can cause diarrhea and intestinal cramps

antiallergic
an agent that reduces allergic reactions

antiarthritic
an agent that combats arthritis

antibacterial
acts against bacteria; an agent that prevents bacteria forming, e.g. penicillin

antibilious
an agent that helps remove excess bile from the body

antibiotic
an agent that prevents the growth of, or destroys, bacteria

antibody
a chemical produced by the body's immune system to attack what it considers to be an invader, e.g. a bacterium, virus, or allergen

anticarcinogenic
an agent that acts to prevent or treat the development or spread of cancer

anticatarrhal
an agent that helps remove excess catarrh from the body

anticonvulsant
an agent that helps arrest or prevent convulsions

antidepressant
an agent that relieves depression

antidiarrheal
an agent that prevents or treats diarrhea

antidote
the term used to describe other remedies or substances that cancel or nullify the effect of a prescribed remedy

anti-emetic
an agent that reduces the incidence and severity of nausea or vomiting

antifungal
an agent that works to prevent the spread and incidence of fungal conditions

antihistamine
an agent that prevents or treats a histamine reaction (*see Allergy, page 412*)

472

antihypertensive
an agent that works to lower blood pressure

anti-infective
any agent that works to prevent or halt the spread of infection

anti-inflammatory
reducing inflammation

antimicrobial
acts against infection, particularly bacterial infection

antioxidant
a substance that prevents cell degeneration and decay

antiseborrheic
helps to control the production of sebum from sweat glands

antiseptic
helps to counter infection, by fighting bacteria

antispasmodic
prevents contractions of the muscles, or alleviates spasms and cramp

antiviral
inhibits the spread of viruses

aperitif
a stimulant to the appetite

aphrodisiac
increases or stimulates sexual desire; sexual stimulant, increases vitality and builds organs

aromatherapy
the therapeutic use of essential oils

aromatic
a substance with a strong aroma or smell

arteriosclerosis
hardening of the arteries

articulation
range of movement of the joints

asthma
spasm of the bronchi in the lungs, narrowing the airways

astringent
constricts the blood vessels or membranes in order to reduce irritation, inflammation, and swelling; has a binding and contracting effect, usually on the mucous membrane, to give it a protective coating against irritants or infective organisms; also one of the six tastes in Ayurveda; found in potatoes, beans, and witch hazel

athma
in Indian medicine, the unique, individual spirit which occupies the body and which is transferred to another body after death

atopic
persons with allergies are often called atopic. The common atopies include hay fever; asthma; infantile eczema, which is an itchy skin lesion; contact dermatitis, which is a skin inflammation caused by poison ivy or a variety of chemicals that may contact the skin; and perhaps some food or drug allergies

aura
every person, animal, and plant is said to have a visible aura, or magnetic field. These are said to indicate the state of health, emotions, mind, and spirit

autogenic discharge
sensations or muscle movements that accompany the release of stored tensions

autoimmune disorder
occurs when the body creates antibodies against itself and attacks healthy cells

B

bactericidal
an agent that destroys bacteria (a type of microbe or organism)

balsam
a resinous semi-solid mass or viscous liquid exuded from a plant, which can be either a pathological or a physiological product. A "true" balsam is characterized by its high content of benzoic acid, benzoates, cinnamic acid, or cinnamates

balsamic
a soothing medicine or application having the qualities of a balsam

benign
of a tumor, not cancerous or dangerous

bile
thick, oily fluid excreted by the liver; bile helps the body digest fats

biliousness
disorder of bile production (to excess)

bioflavonoids
also called vitamin P, bioflavonoids are widely found in food plants, where they impart color to flowers, leaves, and stems. There are at least 500 naturally occurring varieties, and they are said to strengthen or preserve the integrity of the veins, among other things

biopsy
removal of fluid or tissue from the body for examination

bitter
a tonic component that stimulates the appetite and promotes the secretion of saliva and gastric juices by exciting the taste buds; one of the six Ayurvedic tastes; found in barks, tannins, and resins

blepharospasm
a twitch or tic in which there is spasmodic closure of one or both eyes

Blood
in Chinese medicine, "Blood" has a specialized meaning

bronchio-dilator
a substance which dilates the bronchi, the tubes of the lungs

bursa
a small fluid-filled sac

C

calmative
a sedative agent

calcul
a kidney stone

Candida
Candida albicans, a fungus affecting the mucous membranes and skin; causes thrush

carbuncle
a bacterial infection of the skin, an interconnected group of boils that have many perforations, through which pus drains

carcinogenic
an agent that can cause cancer; cancer-causing

carcinoma
a cancerous tumor

cardiac
pertaining to the heart

cardioactive
an agent that stimulates heart activity

cardiotonic
having a stimulating effect on the heart

carminative
settles the digestive system and relieves flatulence

cathartic
an agent that purges the body, usually the intestine, and cleanses the system

cautery
burning tissue in the body

centesimal scale (c)
in homeopathy, the scale that measures the potency of remedies in hundredths. One drop of mother tincture is mixed with 99 drops of water or alcohol to make a remedy of 1c potency. This remedy is then diluted with a further 99 drops of water or alcohol to make a remedy of 2c potency. The sequence is repeated: 200c is usually the highest dose. The more the remedy is diluted, the more powerful it becomes

cephalic
remedy for problems relating to the head

cerebrovascular accident (CVA)
another term for stroke

chakras
in Eastern medicine, circles which are thought to be found along the mid-line of the body, in line with the spinal column

channels
invisible pathways in which qi (or chi) travels; also called meridians. They appear in and on the body

chelated
of mineral supplements, means that the mineral is combined with amino acids to make assimilation more efficient

chi (or qi)
the life force of the body, which circulates through its meridians or channels

chlamydia
a sexually transmitted disease caused by parasitic bacteria

cholagogue
an agent that stimulates the secretion and flow of bile into the duodenum

cholesterol
a steroid alcohol found in nervous tissue, red blood cells, animal fat, and bile. Excess can lead to gallstones

chronic
persisting for a long time; a state showing no change or very slow change

cicatrizant
an agent that promotes healing by the formation of scar tissue

coagulate
an agent that acts to clot or thicken the blood

complementary
the term used to describe alternative forms of medical treatment – emphasizing the fact that they support rather than replace orthodox medicine

compress
a lint or pad that is soaked in hot or cold substances and applied to the body for relief of swelling and pain, or to produce localized pressure

concomitant
in homeopathy, a symptom coming at the same time, but not directly related to, the main complaint

concrete
a concentrated, waxy, solid, or semi-solid perfume material prepared from previously live plant matter, usually a hydrocarbon type of solvent

congestion
abnormal accumulation of blood

constitutional
homeopathic term relating to the physical and mental constitution of a person, including hereditary factors and underlying health issues

contraindication
any factor in a patient's condition that indicates that treatment would involve a greater than normal risk and is therefore not recommended

cordial
a stimulant and tonic

corticosteroids
adrenal cortico hormones. There are two classes of corticosteroids. The glucocorticoids such as cortisone primarily affect carbohydrate and protein metabolism. They have limited use in the treatment of many immunologic and allergic diseases, such as arthritis. The mineralocorticoids such as aldosterone principally regulate salt and water balance. Synthetic steroids include anti-inflammatory drugs, oral contraceptives, and a synthetic adrenal steroid used to treat Addison's disease

cortisol
the steroid hormone which helps the body to react to stress

coryza
profuse discharge from the mucous membranes of the nose – "common cold"

counter-irritant
an application to the skin that relieves deep-seated pain, usually applied in the form of heat; see also rubefacient

dan tien
energy centers in the body. In Chinese medicine there are considered to be three: an upper (between the eyebrows); a middle (in the centre of the trunk); and a lower (the lower abdomen). Qi is stored here

decimal scale (x)
in homeopathy, the scale that measures the potency of remedies in tenths. One drop of mother tincture is mixed with nine drops of water or alcohol to make a remedy of 1x potency. This remedy is then diluted with a further nine drops of water or alcohol to make a remedy of 2x potency. The sequence is repeated. The more the remedy is diluted, the more powerful it becomes

decoction
a herbal preparation, where the plant material (usually hard or woody) is boiled in water and reduced to make a concentrated extract

decongestant
an agent for the relief or reduction of congestion, e.g. of the mucous membranes

decongestive
relieves or reduces mucus congestion

deficient
condition in Chinese medicine; any disorder that is caused by the body's inability to maintain balance, through improper function of the zangfu

degenerative
a condition in which there is irreversible and progressive decomposition

demulcent
an agent that protects mucous membranes and allays irritation

depurgative
cleanses the blood

detoxificant/detoxifier
an agent that acts to detoxify, or remove toxins from the body

detoxification
external and internal cleaning of the body; the removal of toxins from the body

dhatus
in Indian medicine, seven essential tissues which make up the body

dialogue
discussion on how habitual ideas and emotions can affect your mind, body, and spirit

diaphoretic
an agent that causes sweating

digestive
an agent that promotes or aids the digestion of food

digoxin
a glycoside isolated from the dried leaves of the foxglove plant. It is prescribed to millions of patients suffering from cardiac problems such as rapid atrial fibrillation or heart failure

dina chariya
a daily program recommended by Ayurveda for healthy living

discharge
an excretion or substance evacuated from the body

diuretic
an agent that aids production of urine, promotes urination, or increases flow, reducing the fluid level of the body

DNA
deoxyribonucleic acid, a chemical which makes up our chromosomes

doshas
the three basic constitutional types in Indian medicine – vátha, pitta, and kapha – which are known as the "tri-doshas"

douche
a substance used internally to cleanse or treat the vagina

drawing
draws poisons out from boils and abscesses etc.

dysfunction
abnormal functioning of a system or organ within the body

dysmenorrhea
severe pains accompanying the menstrual period

dyspepsia
difficulty with digestion associated with pain, flatulence, heartburn, and nausea

dyspnea
labored or difficult breathing

ectomorph
one of three basic body types, characterized by thinness and weakness

ectopic
a pregnancy that occurs at a site other than inside the uterus, such as in the Fallopian tube, on the ovary, or at sites outside the abdomen, is termed ectopic

edema
a painless swelling caused by fluid retention beneath the skin's surface

EFAs
essential fatty acids

effleurage
slow, rhythmic massage

eight principal patterns
in Chinese medicine, the system of organizing diagnostic information according to the principles of yin, yang, interior, exterior, cold, hot, excess, and deficiency

emetic
an agent that induces vomiting

emmenagogue
an agent that induces or assists menstruation

emollient
an agent that softens and soothes the skin

Empty Heat
Internal Heat in the body resulting from a yin deficiency

endocrine
the endocrine system consists of specialized glands located in different parts of the body. These glands secrete chemical substances called hormones, which transfer information from one set of cells to another

endometriosis
a common disease in women of reproductive age. It involves tissues of the endometrium, the inner lining of the uterus. During the menstrual cycle, built-up endometrial tissues normally are shed if pregnancy does not occur. In many women some endometrial cells escape from the womb into the pelvic cavity, where they attach themselves and continue their hormone-stimulated growth cycle. They may also migrate to remote parts of the body

endomorph
one of the three basic body types, characterized by roundness, fatness, and heaviness

endorphins
a group of chemicals manufactured in the brain that influence the body's response to pain

engorgement
congestion of a part of the tissues, or fullness (as in the breasts)

enuresis
bed-wetting

enzyme
complex proteins that are produced by the living cells and catalyze specific biochemical reactions

epidural
epidural anesthesia involves depositing anesthetic into the epidural space of the vertebral canal

epigastric
above the navel

epigastrium
the area above the navel

episiotomy
an incision made in the perineum (the area between the anus and the vagina) to prevent tearing while delivering a baby

esophagitis
inflammation of the lining of the esophagus

essence
the pure energy extracted from food that is transformed into qi by the body. Also the integral part of a plant, its life force, as used in flower remedies, herbalism, and aromatherapy

essential oil
a volatile and aromatic liquid (sometimes semi-solid) which generally constitutes the odorous principles of a plant. It is obtained by a process of expression or distillation from a single botanical form or species. A pure, concentrated essence taken from the plant; said to be its life force

esters
chemical compounds that are fungicidal and sedative

estrogen
a hormone produced by the ovary and necessary for the development of female secondary sexual characteristics

etiology
the science of the cause of illness and disease

excess condition
a condition in which qi, blood, or body fluids are imbalanced, accumulating in parts of the body

expectorant
promotes the removal of mucus from the respiratory system

expectoration
coughing up

external
in Chinese medicine, any factors influencing the body from the outside

exudative
a substance or agent that causes something to exude; for example, a warm compress would cause infection or pus to exude from a boil or wound

 F

fast
abstention from all or most foods for a given period

febrifuge
an agent that combats fever

febrile
feverish

feces
excrement, stools

fever
elevation of body temperature above normal (36.8°C/98.4°F)

five elements
the system in Chinese medicine based on observations of the natural world. Built around the elements of fire, water, wood, metal, and earth

fixative
a material that slows down the rate of evaporation of the more volatile components in the composition of a perfume

fixed oil
the name given to a vegetable oil obtained from plants that, in contradistinction to essential oils, is fatty, dense, and nonvolatile, such as olive or sweet almond oil

flavonoids
antioxidants which act on the immune system

fomentation
a hot compress

four levels
the system of diagnosis in Chinese medicine

friction
small circular movements used in massage

fu
hollow yang organs in the body

fungicidal
an agent that prevents and combats fungal infection

fungicide
attacks fungal infestations

 G

galactagogue
an agent that increases the secretion of milk

gan
sweet, used to assign taste to Chinese herbs

ganglion
swelling within a tendon or joint; also a group of nerves

gas exchange
the exchange of water carbon dioxide in the blood for fresh oxygen; it takes place in the alveoli of the lungs

generals
in homeopathy, symptoms relating to the whole person that can be expressed "I am . . ."; compare particulars

germicidal
destroys germs or micro-organisms such as bacteria

ghee
milk or butter fat, clarified by boiling and used in Indian cooking

giardiasis
an infectious parasite that attacks the gastrointestinal tract

giennial
a plant that completes its life-cycle in two years, without flowering in the first year

gliadin
a protein from wheat and rye cereals

gluten
a protein from wheat and other cereals

gum
"true" gum is little used in perfumery, being virtually odorless. However, the term "gum" is often applied to "resins," especially with relation to turpentines, as in the Australian "gum tree." Strictly speaking, gums are natural or synthetic water-soluble materials, such as gum arabic

gunas
in Indian medicine, characteristics which can be attributed to all matter, organic and inorganic, and to thoughts and ideas

 H

halitosis
bad breath

hallucinogenic
causes visions or delusions

harmonize
to balance, or encourage something, such as the body, to work in harmony, with all systems at optimum level

hematoma
a collection of blood

hemorrhage
loss of blood

hemorrhoids
piles, anal varicose veins

hemostatic
stops the flow of blood; a type of astringent that stops internal bleeding or hemorrhaging

hepatic
relating to the liver; an agent that tones the liver and aids its function

herniate
to rupture, or burst out; a slipped disk herniates

holistic
aiming to treat the individual as an entity, incorporating body, mind, and spirit, from the Greek word holos, meaning whole

homeopathy
medical therapy devised by the 19th-century German doctor Samuel Hahnemann, based on the premise that like cures like; sick people are given minute doses of a remedy that will cause the symptoms of their disease, which helps the body to cure itself

homeostasis
the tendency of the internal environment of the body to remain constant in spite of varying external conditions

hormone
a product of living cells that produces a specific effect on the activity cells remote from its point of origin

humors
the four body fluids (blood, phlegm, choler, and melancholy) which are believed to determine emotional and physical disposition, in Chinese medicine

hybrid
a plant originating by fertilization of one species or subspecies by another

hypercalcemia
calcium deposits in the kidneys

hyperglycemia
a condition characterized by an abnormally high level of glucose (sugar) in the bloodstream

hyperhidrosis
excessive sweating caused by overactive sweat glands

hypermetropia
long-sightedness

hyperparathyroidism
secretion of parathyroid hormone resulting from a tumor, enlargement, or cancer of the thyroid glands

hypertension
raised blood pressure

hypertensive
raises blood pressure

hypnotic
causing sleep

hypoglycemia
a condition characterized by an abnormally low level of glucose (sugar) in the bloodstream

hypotension
low blood pressure, or a fall in blood pressure below the normal range

hypotensive
lowers blood pressure

I

immunodeficiency
a deficiency of immune activity

immuno-stimulant
an agent that stimulates immune activity, and the immune system

immunosuppressive
an agent or condition that suppresses the immune system, and normal or excessive immune activity

incontinence
partial or complete loss of control of urination

infection
multiplication of pathogenic (disease-producing) micro-organisms within the body

inflammation
protective tissue response to injury or destruction of body cells characterized by heat, swelling, redness, and usually pain

infusion
immersion of herbs in boiling water; also the liquid obtained from steeping a herb in hot or cold water

inhalant
a remedy or drug that is breathed in through the nose or mouth

insecticidal
an agent that repels or kills insects

insomnia
inability to sleep

internal
refers to aspects of disharmonies that arise within the body, in Chinese medicine

-itis
(*suffix*) "inflammation of"; for example, arthritis, inflammation of the joints

J

jin ye
body fluids – jin refers to the lighter fluids, and ye refers to the denser ones

Jing
the essence of all life in the body – the energy that governs our development

jingluo
Chinese term for the channels, or meridians, which run invisibly through the body, carrying the qi, or life force

K

kapha
the moon force, which is a basic life force or element in Ayurvedic medicine

ketogenic diet
a diet which is high in fat and very low in carbohydrates

ketones
chemical compounds that ease congestion and aid the flow of mucus

ku
bitter; a term used to describe the taste of Chinese herbs

kundalini
an energy which is believed to travel upwards through the chakras, promoting spiritual knowledge

L

lactagogue
a substance which encourages the production of milk in the breasts

laxative
a substance that provokes evacuation of the bowels

legume
a fruit or vegetable consisting of one carpel, opening on one side, such as a pea. Also called a "pulse"

lesion
a term used to describe an abnormality in or damage to the body

leucocyte
white blood cells responsible for fighting disease

leukorrhea
vaginal discharge

liniment
a warming rub, often made by mixing tinctures with herbal infused oils

lithotrophic
dispels stones

liverishness
a term used to describe inadequate liver function

lymph
a colorless fluid which contains mainly white blood cells, which are collected from the tissues of the body and transported through the lymphatic system

lymphatic
pertaining to the lymphatic system. A lymphatic remedy would encourage the flow of lymph

M

macerate
soak or pound until soft

mahabbutas
a Sanskrit term for the elements

malas
in Indian medicine, waste products of the body, including feces, urine, and sweat

malignant
cancerous and possibly life-threatening

MAOI
a type of antidepressant drug known as monoamine oxidase inhibitors

mammograph
an X-ray technique used to aid in the diagnosis of breast cancer in women

mantra
a syllable, word, or phrase which may be spoken aloud and repeated as an aid to meditation

marma puncture
in Indian medicine, the technique of inserting a needle into the marma points for certain treatments

marmas
in Indian medicine, energy points in the body where two or more important functions meet

marrow
in Chinese medicine, the substance that makes up the brain and spinal column

materia medica
a branch of science dealing with the origins and properties of remedies; a complete description of remedies suggested in therapies such as homeopathy and herbalism

medicated oil
2produced by steeping herbs or flowers for one or more months, then straining

meditation
exercising the mind in contemplation

meninges
the membranes that cover the brain and spinal cord

menopause
the normal cessation of menstruation, a life change for women

menorrhagia
an excess loss of blood occurring during menstruation

mentals
in homeopathy, symptoms relating to the mental state, mood, and ideas

meridians
channels that run through the body, beneath the skin, in which the life force, or qi, is carried. There are 14 main meridians running to and from the hands and feet to the body and head

mesomorph
one of the three basic body types, characterized by a muscular and prominent bone structure

metabolism
the complex process that is the fundamental chemical expression of life itself, and the means by which food is converted to energy to maintain the body

metrorrhagia
bleeding that occurs in the middle of the menstrual cycle

microbe
a minute living organism, especially pathogenic bacteria, viruses, etc.

micronutrients
vitamins, minerals, and other health-giving components of our food, such as amino acids, fiber, enzymes, and lipids

micturation
involuntary leakage of urine during coughing, laughing, or muscular effort

modality
in homeopathy, the factor that makes symptoms better or worse

mother tincture
in homeopathy or flower remedies, the source remedy, which is diluted to make the therapeutic dosages prescribed by practitioners

moxa
dried mugwort, which is burned on the end of needles or rolled into a stick, and then heated in moxabustion. It is said to warm the qi in the body in order to increase its flow

moxabustion
see moxa

moxides
a group of chemical compounds with expectorant properties

mucilage
a substance containing gelatinous constituents that are demulcent

mucilaginous
a substance that encourages the body to create more mucus

mucolytic
a substance that thins mucus

mucous membranes
surface linings of the body, which secrete mucus

musculoskeletal
anything pertaining to the muscles and bones (skeletal system) of the body

myopia
short-sightedness

 N

narcotic
an agent that induces sleep; intoxicating or poisonous in large doses

nasya
in Ayurveda, inhalation of oils

naturopathy
treatment based on using natural agents and forces to bring about a cure. The naturopath tends to rely on natural products such as herbs and vitamins, rather than on synthetic drugs and surgery, and may also employ manipulation (such as osteopathy) and electrical treatments

nervine
strengthening and toning to the nerves and nervous system

noradrenaline
a hormone secreted by the adrenal gland

nosode
in homeopathy, a remedy made from a diseased source; for example, tuberculinum, made from tissue infected with tuberculosis

nutritive
a substance that promotes nutrition

nystagmus
abnormal, jerky movements of the eyes

 O

oja
in Indian medicine, the ultimate vital energy that runs through the system

oleo gum resin
a natural exudation from trees and plants that consists mainly of essential oil, gum, and resin

oleoresin
a natural resinous exudation from plants, or an aromatic liquid preparation extracted from botanical matter using solvents. It consists almost entirely of a mixture of essential oil and resin

onycholysis
detachment of the nail from its bed

oophorectomy
removal of the ovaries

opacification
becoming opaque

orchitis
inflammation of the testes

orthodox
a term used to describe conventional medicine

overbreathing
breathing too quickly and too shallowly

P

palindromic
something which can be read the same when taken in reverse order

palpation
examination with the hands

panacea
a cure-all

panchakarma
in Ayurveda, internal cleansing, which consists of five forms of therapy, including vomiting, purging, two types of enema, and nasal inhalation. It is said to prevent disease and to rebalance vitality

parainfluenza
a type of cold virus

parasiticide
prevents and destroys parasites; a parasite killer

paronychia
an infection of the soft tissue around the nail, usually as a result of repeated minor injury, causing pain, swelling and inflammation. Pus may sometimes appear at the edge of the nail

particulars
in homeopathy, symptoms relating to a part of the person that can be expressed "My…"; compare generals

parturient
encouraging the onset of labor

pasteurized
heat treated to destroy harmful microorganisms

pathogenic
referring to any disease-causing agent

peculiars
in homeopathy, strange, rare, and peculiar symptoms which relate to the individual and are not common in illness

peptic
a term applied to gastric secretions and areas affected by them

percussion
vigorous drumming massage

pericarditis
inflammation of the pericardium of the heart

perineal
pertaining to the perineum, the area between the anus and the genital organs

periodontitis
loosening of a tooth, often caused by gingivitis

peristalsis
rhythmic movement of the gut to push food along the intestinal tract

pessary
a treatment that is inserted into the vagina or anus

petrissage
kneading massage movement

pharmacopeia
an official publication of drugs in common use in a given country

phenols
a group of chemical compounds with bactericidal and stimulating properties; they can be irritants

Phlegm
in Chinese medicine a disharmony of the body fluids produces either external (or visible) phlegm or internal (or invisible) phlegm; thick, shiny mucus produced in the respiratory passage

photosensitivity
a sensitivity to light

phototoxic
a substance that becomes poisonous on exposure to light

phthalides
chemicals which have a sedative effect and can ease insomnia

phytotherapy
the treatment of disease by plants; herbal medicine

pitta
in Ayurvedic medicine, the sun force, or one of the three basic life forces or elements controlling all physical and mental processes

plasma
the clear, yellowish fluid part of blood or lymph in which cells are suspended

polyphenols
antioxidants which have beneficial effects on the circulatory system

postnatal
following delivery of a baby; after pregnancy

potencized
diluted to homeopathic prescription

potency
the dilution of a homeopathic remedy; the higher the number, the higher the strength, and the greater the dilution

potentiate
in homeopathy, to shake a remedy to increase its potency

poultice
the therapeutic application of a soft moist mass (such as fresh herbs) to the skin to encourage local circulation and to relieve pain

prakruti
in Indian medicine, a person's individual constitution, determined by their "dosha" type

prana
the vital energy that runs through our bodies; in Indian medicine, also known as our life force

pranayama
the breathing exercises associated with yoga

priapism
prolonged penile erection, usually without sexually desire

progesterone
a female sex hormone that prepares the uterus for the fertilized ovum and maintains pregnancy

prolapse
the sinking or falling-down of an organ – usually refers to the vagina or uterus

prophylactic
preventive of disease or infection

prostaglandins
hormone-like substances that occur in tissues and organs of the human body. They affect several body systems, including the central nervous, cardiovascular, gastrointestinal, urinary, and endocrine systems

prostatitis
inflammation of the prostate gland

proving
the process used in homeopathy for testing a remedy; it can occur when the wrong remedy is prescribed and taken over a period of time, and the symptoms of the condition it is aimed at manifest themselves

psychogenic
symptoms or conditions of mental rather than physical origin

psychosomatic illness
the manifestation of physical symptoms resulting from a mental state

purgative
an agent stimulating evacuation of the bowels

purines
nitrogenous compounds in nucleic acids found in many foods including caffeine, anchovies, sardines, fish roe, sweetbreads and other organ meats. Some people who have difficulty metabolizing purines may be prone to gout

purulent
containing pus

purvakarma
in Ayurveda, a cleansing process involving oil and steam bath therapy

pustular
referring to elevated area of skin containing pus

pyorrhea
any condition characterized by discharge of pus

qi (chi)
the essential energy of the universe which is fundamental to all elements of life. It runs through the whole body in channels or meridians

Qi Ni
rebellious qi, which moves in the wrong direction

Qi Xian
sinking qi, which is too deficient to perform its holding function

Qi Zhi
stagnant qi that is sluggish and not moving efficiently

rajasic
in Ayurveda, energy-producing

rasayana
the branch of Ayurveda which involves rejuvenation

RDA
recommended daily allowance

RDI
recommended daily intake

rectification
the process of redistillation applied to essential oils to rid them of certain constituents

referred pain
pain that is felt in a different part of the body from the area that is actually affected

regulator
an agent that helps balance and regulates the functions of the body

rejuvenative
to invigorate, bring back to life or to the optimum level of functioning; to give new youth or restore vitality

relaxant
a substance that promotes relaxation (either muscular or psychological)

remedy picture
in homeopathy, the collection of symptoms that characterize a remedy

remission
a period in which the symptoms of a disease abate or lessen

Ren
the Chinese meridian that runs down the front of the body, from the lower lip to behind the genitalia

resin
a natural or prepared product, either solid or semi-solid in nature. Natural resins are exudations from trees, such as mastic; prepared resins are oleoresins from which essential oil has been removed

resolvent
an agent that disperses swelling or effects absorption of a new growth

restorative
an agent that helps strengthen and revive the body systems; strengthens and promotes well-being after illness

rhinitis
inflammation (often chronic) of the mucous membranes lining the nasal passage

rhizome
an underground plant stem lasting more than one season

Rishis
wise and holy men of ancient India who meditated and acquired the knowledge that was codified as Ayurveda

RNA
ribonucleic acid, or RNA, is needed in all organisms in order for protein synthesis to occur. It is also the genetic material of some viruses, which are referred to as RNA viruses

rubefacient
a mild irritant which causes redness of the skin

salpingitis
infection of the Fallopian tubes

salty
one of the six Ayurvedic tastes; found in rock salt, seaweed, sea salt, and vegetables

salve
a mixture of beeswax with vegetable oil used to preserve herbs and spices

samagni
in Indian medicine, a balanced appetite, when digestion, absorption, and metabolism function efficiently

san jiao
the triple warmer/heat/burner which is a process organ in the Chinese zangfu system

Sanskrit
ancient Indian language, sacred to Hinduism. Ayurveda was written in Sanskrit

saponins
chemicals which may affect red blood cells

sclerosis
hardening of tissue due to inflammation

seborrheic
involving the sebaceous glands, which secrete sebum into the hair follicles and on to most of the body surface

sebum
an oily, lubricating and protective substance

sedative
an agent that reduces functional activity; calming

self-limiting
a condition that lasts a set length of time and usually clears of its own accord

septic
putrefying due to the presence of pathogenic (disease-producing) bacteria

serotonin
a neurotransmitter in the brain which regulates and induces sleep, and is also said to reduce sensitivity to pain

shad rasa
the six basic food tastes identified by Ayurveda – sweet, acidic, salty, pungent, bitter, and astringent

shen
in Chinese medicine, an important aspect of mind or spirit; the spirit of the person

shiatsu
a type of massage that works on pressure points of the body

shock
sudden and disturbing mental or physical impression; also a state of collapse characterized by pale, cold, sweaty skin, rapid, weak, thready pulse, faintness, dizziness, and nausea

sialogogue
an agent that stimulates the secretion of saliva

six stage patterns
a Chinese diagnostic system

soft tissues
tissues of the body, including muscles, tendons, ligaments, and organs

soporific
an agent that induces sleep; sleep-inducing

sour
one of the six Ayurvedic tastes; found in fats, amino acids, fermented products, fruits, and vegetables

spasm
sudden, violent, involuntary muscular contraction

specific
remedy effective for a particular ailment

spermatorrhea
leaking of sperm

spermicidal
an agent or substance which acts to kill sperm

splenomegaly
abnormal enlargement of the spleen

spondylosis
progressive disease of the spine

sputum
spit

stagnant
when the flow of chi, or qi, is blocked in the meridians

STD
sexually transmitted disease

steroids
fat-soluble organic compounds that occur naturally throughout the plant and animal kingdoms and play many important functional roles

stimulant
increases activity in specific organs or systems of the body, warms and increases energy

stomachic
an agent that stimulates the functioning of the stomach

stroma
connective tissue that forms the foundation of the breast

sty
an infection of the follicle of an eyelash or of a sebaceous gland of an eyelid

styptic
an astringent agent that stops or reduces external bleeding

suan
sour; a description of taste for Chinese herbs

subclinical symptoms
symptoms which are not gross enough to be considered precursors to or evidence of clinically diagnosed disease

subfertility
below-normal fertility

succussion
the shaking method used in preparing homeopathic remedies

sweet
one of the six Ayurvedic tastes, found in sugar, carbohydrates, and dairy products

symptom picture
homeopathic term for the overall pattern of symptoms characterizing each individual patient

symptomatology
the study and interpretation of symptoms

symptoms
perceived changes in, or impaired function of, body or mind indicating the presence of disease or injury

synovial
referring to the fluid that bathes the joints

synthesization
to become synthesized, or amalgamated

T

tachycardia
an unduly rapid heartbeat

TCM
Traditional Chinese Medicine

tenesmus
a spasm of the rectum where one feels the need to defecate without being able to

terpenes
chemical constituents with anti-inflammatory and bactericidal properties

tincture
a herbal remedy prepared in an alcohol base

tisane
a type of herbal infusion, usually drunk as a tea

tissue salt
an inorganic compound essential to the growth and function of the body's cells

tonic
restores tone to the systems, balances, nourishes, and promotes well-being; strengthens and enlivens the whole or specific parts of the body

tonification
a process in Chinese medicine that involves strengthening and supporting the Blood and qi

tonify
to tone or balance; in Chinese medicine, to strengthen and support

topical
local application of cream, ointment, tincture, or other medicine

topical irritant
a substance that irritates the skin

torticollis
wry neck

toxin
a substance that is poisonous to the body

trauma
a physical injury or wound; also an unpleasant and disturbing experience causing psychological upset

trigeminal nerve
a nerve that divides into three and supplies the mandibular (jaw), maxillary (cheek), ophthalmic (eye), and forehead areas

tuber
a swollen part of an underground plant stem of one year's duration, capable of new growth

type
a term used by Bach and other flower remedy therapists to describe a person's general personality and approach to life. Also used by homeopaths to refer to a constitutional picture which relates to a particular remedy

U

ulcer
slow-healing sore occurring internally or externally

ureteric
referring to the ureter, the tube that carries urine from the kidneys to the bladder

urethral
referring to the urethra, the canal that carries urine from the bladder out of the body

uterine tonic
a substance that has a toning effect on the whole reproductive system, in particular the uterus

vátha
the wind force in Ayurvedic medicine – one of the three basic life forces or elements that must be in balance for physical and mental processes to be balanced

V

vaginitis
inflammation or infection of the vagina

vasoconstrictor
an agent that causes narrowing of the blood vessels

vasodilator
an agent that dilates the blood vessels and so improves circulation

Vedic
relating to the Vedas, the ancient, sacred literature of Hinduism

vermifuge
an anthelmintic remedy that kills worms and intestinal parasites

verruca
a plantar wart

vesicant
causing blistering to the skin; a counter-irritant

vibrational medicine
any medicine which treats the body on a vibrational or "energy" level, such as homeopathy and flower essence therapy, based on the theory that we are all dense bodies of energy, and by taking substances that adjust that energy, or the rate at which our energy fields vibrate, we can effect a cure

virulent
extremely infective, or with a violent effect

volatile
unstable, evaporates easily, as in "volatile oil"; see essential oil

vulnerary
an agent that helps heal wounds and sores by external application; assists in the healing of wounds by protecting against infection and stimulating cell growth

vulval
relating to the vulva

W

warming
any agent or substance which warms the body, usually by increasing circulation or the flow of qi

Wei Qi
defensive qi, which protects the body from invasion by external pathogenic factors. It flows just beneath the skin

X

xian
salty; a description of taste for Chinese herbs

xin
acrid; a description of taste for Chinese herbs

xu
deficiency; a common disharmony in Chinese medicine

Y

yang
one aspect of the complementary aspects in Chinese philosophy; reflects the active, moving, and warmer aspects

yin
one aspect of the complementary aspects in Chinese philosophy; reflects the passive, still, reflective aspects

yin/yang
Chinese philosophy that explains the interdependence of all elements of nature. These contrasting aspects of the body and mind must be balanced before health and well-being can be achieved. Yin is the female force, and yang is the male

Ying Qi
nutritive aspects of qi that nourish the body

Yuan Qi
original or source qi; this aspect of qi is passed on from our parents

Z

Zanfu Zhi Qi
qi of the organs; the qi that nourishes the organs of the body

zangfu
the complete yin and yang organs of the body; in Chinese medicine, the term for internal organs (different from those of Western medical science)

Zheng Qi
normal or upright qi; qi that circulates through the channels and the organs of the body

Zong Qi
gathering qi; the qi that gathers in the chest area through the coming together of Gu Qi and Kong Qi

FURTHER READING

Ayurveda

Ayurveda • Scott Gerson
ELEMENT BOOKS, 1993

The Complete Illustrated Guide to Ayurveda
• Gopi Warrier and Dr. Deepika Gunawant
ELEMENT BOOKS, 1997

The Handbook of Ayurveda
• Dr. Shantha Godagama
KYLE CATHIE, 1997

Quantum Healing
• Dr. Deepak Chopra
BANTAM BOOKS, 1989

Return of the Rishi
• Dr. Deepak Chopra
HOUGHTON MIFFLIN CO., 1988

The Seven Pillars of Ancient Wisdom
• Dr. Douglas Baker
DOUGLAS BAKER PUBLISHING, 1982

Chinese Herbalism

Chinese Herbal Medicine
• Richard Craze and Stephen Tang
PIATKUS, 1995

Chinese Herbal Medicine, Ancient Art and Modern Science
• Richard Hyatt
WILDWOOD HOUSE LIMITED, 1978

Chinese Herbal Patent Remedies: A Practical Guide • Jake Fratkin
INSTITUTE FOR TRADITIONAL MEDICINE, 1986

In a Nutshell: Chinese Herbalism
• Eve Rogans
ELEMENT BOOKS, 1997

Chinese Medicine • Tom Williams
ELEMENT BOOKS, 1995

The Chinese Way to Health
• Dr. Stephen Gascoigne
HODDER HEADLINE, 1997

The Complete Family Guide to Chinese Medicine
• Tom Williams
ELEMENT BOOKS, 1997

The Web That Has No Weaver
• Ted J. Kaptchuk
CONGDON & WEED, 1983

Traditional Home and Folk Remedies

In a Nutshell: Aromatherapy
• Sheila Lavery
ELEMENT BOOKS, 1997

The Complete Family Guide to Natural Home Remedies • Karen Sullivan
ELEMENT BOOKS, 1996

The Encyclopedia of Herbs and Herbalism • Malcolm Stuart
ORBIS PUBLISHING, 1979

The Golden Age of Herbs and Herbalists
• Rosetta E. Clarkson
DOVER PUBLICATIONS, 1972

Healing Nutrients • Patrick Quillen
PENGUIN, 1989

Herbal Medicine • Anne McIntyre
OPTIMA, 1987

The Holistic Herbal • David Hoffman
FINDHORN, 1983

In a Nutshell: Natural Home Remedies
• Karen Hurrell
ELEMENT BOOKS, 1996

Neal's Yard Natural Remedies
• Susan Curtis, Romy Frasher, and Irene Kohler
ARKANA, 1988

The Power of Plants • Brendan Lehane
JOHN MURRAY, 1977

Traditional Home and Herbal Remedies
• Jan De Vries
MAINSTREAM PUBLISHING, 1986

The Doctors Book of Home Remedies
• The Editors of *Prevention* Magazine Health Books
RODALE BOOKS, 1990

The Doctors Book of Home Remedies for Children • The Editors of *Prevention* Magazine Health Books
RODALE BOOKS, 1994

The Doctors Book of Home Remedies for Women • The Editors of *Prevention* Magazine Health Books
RODALE BOOKS, 1997

Herbalism

The Complete Illustrated Holistic Herbal
• David Hoffman
ELEMENT BOOKS, 1996

The New Holistic Herbal
• David Hoffman
ELEMENT BOOKS, 1983

The Complete New Herbal
• edited by Richard Mabey
PENGUIN BOOKS, 1991

The Family Medical Herbal
• Kitty Campion
DORLING KINDERSLEY, 1988

The Herb Society's
Complete Medicinal Herbal
• Penelope Ody
DORLING KINDERSLEY, 1993

The Herbal for Mother and Child,
• Anne McIntyre
ELEMENT BOOKS, 1992

Herbal Medicine: The Use of Herbs for
Health and Healing
• Vicki Pitman
ELEMENT BOOKS, 1994

Herbal Remedies: A Practical Beginner's
Guide to Making Effective Remedies in
the Kitchen
• Christopher Hedley and Non Shaw
PARAGON, 1996

In a Nutshell: Herbalism • Non Shaw
ELEMENT BOOKS, 1998

Herbs for Common Ailments,
• Anne McIntyre
GAIA BOOKS, 1992

The Home Herbal • Barbara Griggs
PAN BOOKS, 1995

Natural Medicine for Women
• Julian and Susan Scott
GAIA BOOKS, 1991

Aromatherapy

The Complete Illustrated Guide to
Aromatherapy • Julia Lawless
ELEMENT BOOKS, 1997

Aromatherapy • Christine Wildwood
ELEMENT BOOKS, 1991

Aromatherapy: An A–Z
• Patricia Davis
C. W. DANIEL, 1988

Aromatherapy Blends and Remedies,
• Franzesca Watson
THORSONS, 1996

The Aromatherapy Book
• Jeanne Rose
NORTH ATLANTIC BOOKS, 1994

Aromatherapy for Pregnancy and
Childbirth • Margaret Fawcett
ELEMENT BOOKS, 1993

In a Nutshell: Aromatherapy
• Sheila Lavery
ELEMENT BOOKS, 1997

Aromatherapy: Massage with Essential
Oils • Christine Wildwood
ELEMENT BOOKS, 1991

The Illustrated Encyclopedia of Essential
Oils • Julia Lawless
ELEMENT BOOKS, 1992

The Fragrant Mind
• Valerie Anne Worwood
DOUBLEDAY, 1996

The Fragrant Pharmacy
• Valerie Anne Worwood
BANTAM BOOKS, 1995

Homeopathy

The Challenge of Homeopathy
• Margery Blackie
UNWIN HYMAN, 1981

The Complete Family Guide to
Homeopathy
• Dr. Christopher Hammond
ELEMENT BOOKS, 1996

The Complete Homeopathy Handbook
• Miranda Castro
PAN BOOKS, 1990

Emotional Healing with Homeopathy:
A Self-help Manual • Peter Chappell
ELEMENT BOOKS, 1994

The Family Guide to Homeopathy
• Andrew Lockie
HAMISH HAMILTON, 1990

Homeopathic Drug Pictures
• Margaret Tyler
HEALTH SCIENCE PRESS, 1970

Homeopathy for Mother and Baby
• Miranda Castro
PAN BOOKS, 1995

In a Nutshell: Homeopathy
• Cassandra Marks
ELEMENT, 1997

Homeopathy: Medicine of the New Man
• George Vithoulkas
THORSONS, 1985

The New Concise Guide to Homeopathy
• Nigel and Susan Garion-Hutchings
ELEMENT BOOKS, 1993

The Woman's Guide to Homeopathy
• Andrew Lockie and Nicola Geddes
HAMISH HAMILTON, 1992

Homeopathy for Children
- Henrietta Wells
ELEMENT BOOKS, 1993

Flower Remedies

In a Nutshell: Bach Flower Remedies
- Non Shaw
ELEMENT BOOKS, 1998

The Bach Flower Remedies: Illustrations and Preparations
- Victor Bullen and Nora Weeks
C. W. DANIEL, 1964

The Collected Writings of Edward Bach
- edited by Julian Barnard
FLOWER REMEDY PROGRAM, 1987

Flower Remedies: Natural Healing with Flower Essences • Christine Wildwood
ELEMENT BOOKS, 1991

A Guide to Bach Flower Remedies
- Julian Barnard
C. W. DANIEL, 1987

Heal Thyself • Dr. Edward Bach
C. W. DANIEL, 1931

The Original Writings of Edward Bach
- edited by Judy Howard and John Ramsell
C. W. DANIEL, 1990

The Twelve Healers and Other Remedies
- Dr. Edward Bach
C. W. DANIEL, 1936

Vitamins and Minerals

The Amino Revolution
- Robert Erdmann and Meirion Jones
CENTURY, 1987

The Complete Book of Minerals for Health • J. I. Rodale
RODALE BOOKS, 1976

The Complete Home Guide to All the Vitamins • Ruth Adams
LARCHMONT BOOKS, 1972

Doctor's Book of Vitamin Therapy: Megavitamins for Health
- Harold Rosenberg and A. N. Feldzaman
PUTNAM'S, 1974

The Doctors' Vitamin and Mineral Encyclopedia
- Sheldon Saul Hendler, M.D., Ph.D.
SIMON & SCHUSTER, 1995

Food and Health
- Elizabeth Morse, John Rivers, and Anne Heughan
BARRIE & JENKINS, 1990

Food: Your Miracle Medicine
- Jean Carper
SIMON & SCHUSTER, 1993

Nutritional Medicine
- Stephen Davis and Alan Stewart
PAN BOOKS, 1987

Raw Energy
- Leslie and Susannah Kenton
ARROW BOOKS, 1991

Superfoods • Michael Van Straten and Barbara Griggs
DORLING KINDERSLEY, 1992

Thorsons Complete Guide to Vitamins and Minerals • Leonard Mervyn
THORSONS, 1995

The Vitamin Bible • Earl Mindell
ARROW, 1993

Health Essentials: Vitamins Guide
- Hasnain Walji
ELEMENT BOOKS, 1992

In a Nutshell: Vitamins and Minerals
- Karen Sullivan
ELEMENT BOOKS, 1997

Which Vitamins Do You Need?
- Martin Ebon
BANTAM BOOKS, 1974

The Zinc Solution
- Derek Bryce-Smith and Liz Hodgkinson
ARROW BOOKS, 1987

USEFUL ADDRESSES

Ayurveda

AFRICA

Maharishi Ayurveda Health Centre
P.O. Box 5155
Halfway House
1685 South Africa

South African Ayurvedic Medicine
Association
85 Harvey Road
Morningside
Durban
4001 South Africa

AUSTRALASIA

Maharishi Ayurveda Health Centres
P.O. Box 81
Bundoora, Victoria 3083
Australia

EUROPE

Ayurvedic Company of Great Britain
50 Penywern Road
London SW5 9XS
U.K.

Ayurvedic Living
P.O. Box 188
Exeter EX4 5AB
U.K.

Ayurvedic Medical Association U.K.
The Hale Clinic
7 Park Crescent
London W1N 3HE
U.K.

Eastern Clinic
1079 Garrat Lane
Tooting, London SW17 0LN
U.K.

NORTH AMERICA

The Ayurveda Institute
P.O. Box 282
Fairfield, Iowa 52556
U.S.A.

The Ayurveda Institute
11311 Menaul N.E., Suite A
Albuquerque, New Mexico 87112
U.S.A.

Mapi, Inc.
Garden of the Gods Business Park
1115 Elkton Drive, Suite 401
Colorado Springs, Colorado 80907
U.S.A.

Chinese Herbalism

AFRICA

The Herb Society of South Africa
P.O. Box 37721
Overport
South Africa

Western Cape Su Jok Acupuncture
Institute
3 Periwinkle Close
Kommetjie
7975 South Africa

AUSTRALASIA

Australian College of
Alternative Medicine
11 Howard Avenue
Mount Waverley, Victoria 3149
Australia

Australian College of
Oriental Medicine
24 Price Road
Lalorama, Victoria 3766
Australia

Chinese and Herbal Centre
1st Floor, 2392–2394 Sussex Street
Sydney, New South Wales 2000
Australia

Holistic Health Centre
C.P.O. Box 2273
Auckland
New Zealand

EUROPE

British Acupuncture Council (BAC)
Park House, 206–208 Latimer Road
London W10 6RE
U.K.

British Herbal Medicine Association
P.O. Box 304
Bournemouth BH7 6JZ
U.K.

London School of Acupuncture
and Traditional Chinese Medicine
60 Bunhill Row
London EC1Y 8QD
U.K.

Register of Chinese Herbal Medicine
21 Warbreck Road
London W10 8NS
U.K.

Register of Chinese Herbal Medicine
(RCHM)
P.O. Box 400
Wembley
Middlesex HA9 9NZ
U.K.

NORTH AMERICA

**American Association of
Acupuncture and Oriental Medicine**
1424 16th Street N.W., Suite 501
Washington, DC 20036
U.S.A.

American Herb Association
P.O. Box 1673
Nevada City, California 95959
U.S.A.

American Holistic Nurses Association
P.O. Box 2130
2133 E Lakin Drive, Suite 2
Flagstaff
Arizona 86003–2130
U.S.A.

**American Holistic
Medical Association**
6728 Old McLean Village Drive
McLean, Virginia 22101
U.S.A.

Acupuncture Foundation of Canada
7321 Victoria Park Avenue, Unit 18
Markham, Ontario
Canada L3R 2ZB

**Canadian Holistic
Medical Association**
42 Redpath Avenue
Toronto, Ontario
Canada M4S 2J6

Ontario Herbalists Association
1565 Carling Avenue, Suite 400
Ottawa, Ontario
Canada K1Z 8R1

Herbalism

AFRICA

**South African Naturopaths
and Herbalists Association**
P.O. Box 18663
Wynberg
7824 South Africa

AUSTRALASIA

**National Herbalists
Association of Australia**
Suite 305, BST House
3 Smail Street
Broadway, New South Wales 2007
Australia

EUROPE

**The General Council and
Register of Consultant Herbalists**
18 Sussex Square
Brighton
East Sussex BN2 5AA
U.K.

The Herb Society
77 Great Peter Street
London SW1
U.K.

**National Institute of
Medical Herbalists**
56 Longbrooke Street
Exeter EX4 8HA
U.K.

**School of Herbal
Medicine/Phytotherapy**
Bucksteep Manor
Bodle Street Green
Near Hailsham
Sussex BN27 4RJ
U.K.

NORTH AMERICA

American Herbalists Guild
P.O. Box 1683
Sequel, California 95073
U.S.A.

Canadian Natural Health Association
439 Wellington Street
Toronto, Ontario
Canada M5V 2H7

Aromatherapy

AFRICA

**Association of Aromatherapists
South Africa**
P.O. Box 23924
Claremont
7735 South Africa

EUROPE

Aromatherapy Organisations Council
3 Latymer Close
Braybrooke
Market Harborough
Leicester LE16 8LN
U.K.

**International Federation
of Aromatherapists**
Stamford House
2–4 Chiswick High Road
London W4 1TH
U.K.

**International Society of
Professional Aromatherapists**
Hinckley and District
Hospital and Health Centre
The Annexe
Mount Road
Hinckley
Leicestershire LE10 1AG
U.K.

NORTH AMERICA

**The Aromatherapy
Institute and Research**
P.O. Box 1222
Fair Oaks, California 95628
U.S.A.

American Alliance of Aroma Therapy
P.O. Box 750428
Petaluma, California 94975–0428
U.S.A.

American Aromatherapy Association
P.O. Box 3679
South Pasadena, California 91031
U.S.A.

Nature's Apothecary
6350 Gunpark Drive 500
Boulder, Colorado 80301
U.S.A.

**National Association of Holistic
Aromatherapy**
P.O. Box 17622
Boulder, Colorado 80308–0622
U.S.A.

The Pacific Institute of Aromatherapy
P.O. Box 6842
San Raphael, California 94903
U.S.A.

Homeopathy

AUSTRALASIA

Australian Federation of Homeopaths
238 Ballarat Road
Footscray, Victoria 3011
Australia

Australian Institute of Homeopathy
7 Hampden Road
Artermon
Sydney, New South Wales 2064
Australia

Institute of Classical Homeopathy
24 West Haven Drive
Tawa
Wellington
New Zealand

New Zealand Homeopathic Society
BOX 2929
Auckland
New Zealand

EUROPE

The British Homeopathic Association
27A Devonshire Street
London WC1N 1RJ
U.K.

The Faculty of Homeopathy
The Royal London Homeopathic
Hospital
Great Ormond Street
London WC1N 3HR
U.K.

The Hahnemann Society
Humane Education Centre
Avenue Lodge
Bounds Green Road
London N22 4EU
U.K.

**Homeopathic
Development Foundation**
19A Cavendish Square
London W1M 9AD
U.K.

Society of Homeopaths
2 Artizan Road
Northampton NN1 4HU
U.K.

NORTH AMERICA

**American Foundation
for Homeopathy**
1508 Glencoe Street, Suite 44
Denver, Colorado 80220–1338
U.S.A.

Homeopathic Educational Services
2124 Kitteridge Street
Berkeley, California 94704
U.S.A.

**International Foundation
for Homeopathy**
2366 East Lake Avenue, East Suite 301
Seattle, Washington
U.S.A.

National Center for Homeopathy
801 North Fairfax Street
Alexandria, Virginia 22314
U.S.A.

Canadian Society of Homeopathy
87 Meadowlands Drive West
Nepean, Ontario
Canada K2G 2R9

Flower Essences

AUSTRALASIA

**Martin and Pleasance
Wholesale Pty. Ltd.**
P.O. Box 4
Collingwood
Victoria, New South Wales 3066
Australia

EUROPE

Bach Flower Remedies
The Bach Centre
Mount Vernon
Sotwell
Wallingford
Oxfordshire OX10 9PZ
U.K.

Flower Essence Fellowship
Laura Farm Clinic
17 Carlincott
Peasedown St. John
Bath BA2 8AN
U.K.

Healing Herbs
P.O. Box 65
Hereford HR2 OUW
U.K.

NORTH AMERICA

Dr. Edward Bach Healing Society
644 Merrick Road
Lynbrook, New York 11563
U.S.A.

Ellon (Bach U.S.A.), Inc.
P.O. Box 32
Woodmere, New York 11598
U.S.A.

Vitamins and Minerals

AUSTRALASIA

**Australian College of Nutritional and
Environmental Medicine**
13 Hilton Road
Beamaris, Victoria 3193
Australia

EUROPE

**The Council for Nutrition
Education of Therapy (CNEAT)**
1 The Close
Halton
Aylesbury
Buckinghamshire HP22 5NJ
U.K.

Health Education Authority
Hamilton House
Mabledon Place
London WC1H 9TX
U.K.

Institute of Optimum Nutrition
5 Jerdan Place
London SW6 1BE
U.K.

**Society for the
Promotion of Nutritional Therapy**
P.O. Box 47
Heathfield
East Sussex TN21 8ZX
U.K.

NORTH AMERICA

**American College of Advancement in
Medicine**
P.O. Box 3427
Laguna Hills, California 92654
U.S.A.

**Canadian College of
Naturopathic Medicine**
60 Berl Avenue
Etobicoke, Ontario
Canada M8Y 3C7

National Institute of Nutrition
2565 Carling Avenue, Suite 400
Ottawa, Ontario
Canada K1Z 8RI

INDEX

CONTRIBUTORS

KAREN SULLIVAN

is the author of numerous books on alternative health and nutrition including In a Nutshell: Vitamins and Minerals (Element, 1996). She has also acted as general editor on The Complete Illustrated Guide to Natural Home Remedies (Element, 1996), and is health editor of a woman's magazine. She lectures widely on women's health and general health issues. Canadian by birth, she now lives in London with her two sons.

MARY CLARK

has been a practitioner of healing and esoteric arts for over 20 years. She has studied Ayurveda, nutrition, herbalism, aromatherapy and stress management. Her skills also lie in the area of astrology and consulting the I Ching with a focus on medical diagnosis. She provides a unique combination of approaches in her work for various corporations in the U.S., including Forbes, Sony, Barnes and Noble, and the Hebrew Hospital System in New York.

EVE ROGANS

began studying Traditional Chinese Medicine in 1981, starting with acupuncture and moving onto herbalism. She has undergone clinical training in China on two occasions. As well as working in a private practice, where she specializes in pediatric acupuncture, she is currently working in the field of drug abuse. Eve Rogans is the author of In a Nutshell: Chinese Medicine (Element, 1997). She lives in London and is married with three children.

NON SHAW

is a professional herbalist working from a private practice in North London. Trained in the Western herbal tradition, she also has a wide knowledge of other traditions and natural therapies. She teaches herbalism, massage, and Bach Flower Remedies, and her written work has included the herbalism and Bach Flower Remedy sections of a range of Element's health reference books. She writes for a number of health and women's magazines and is co-founder of a publication for independent herb users.

SHEILA LAVERY

writes widely on healthcare for several prestigious magazines and newspapers in the U.K. Her work, which often focuses on children's health issues, has also been included in various encyclopedias of alternative health. Along with herbalism, aromatherapy is one of her specialties and she is the author of In a Nutshell: Aromatherapy (Element, 1996).

PIPPA DUNCAN

is former editor of one of the U.K.'s leading health magazines and now works from home for a variety of monthly publications, including a number devoted to children's health. She has contributed to several reference books on family healthcare including The Complete Family Guide to Alternative Medicine published by Element. She lives in London with her husband and two children.

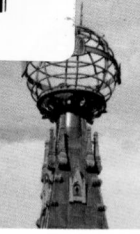

Wesoła, Kleparz and Biskupie

WESOŁA, KLEPARZ
AND BISKUPIE

QUARTER

0 metres   400
0 yards   400

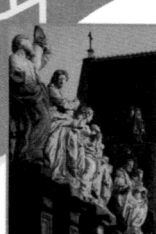

KÓŁ
RADOM
QUARTERS

**Okół and Stradom
Quarters**

KAZIMIERZ
QUARTER

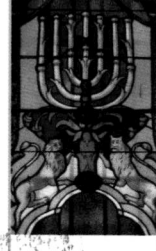

Kazimierz Quarter

KRAKOW

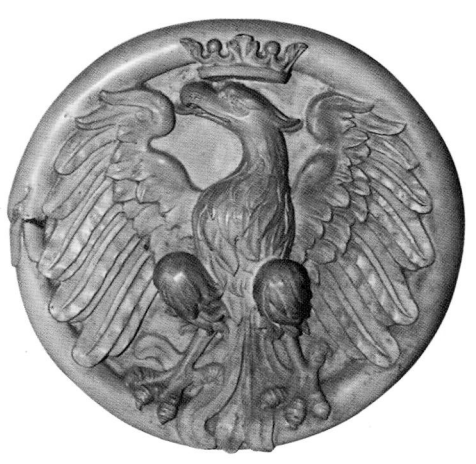

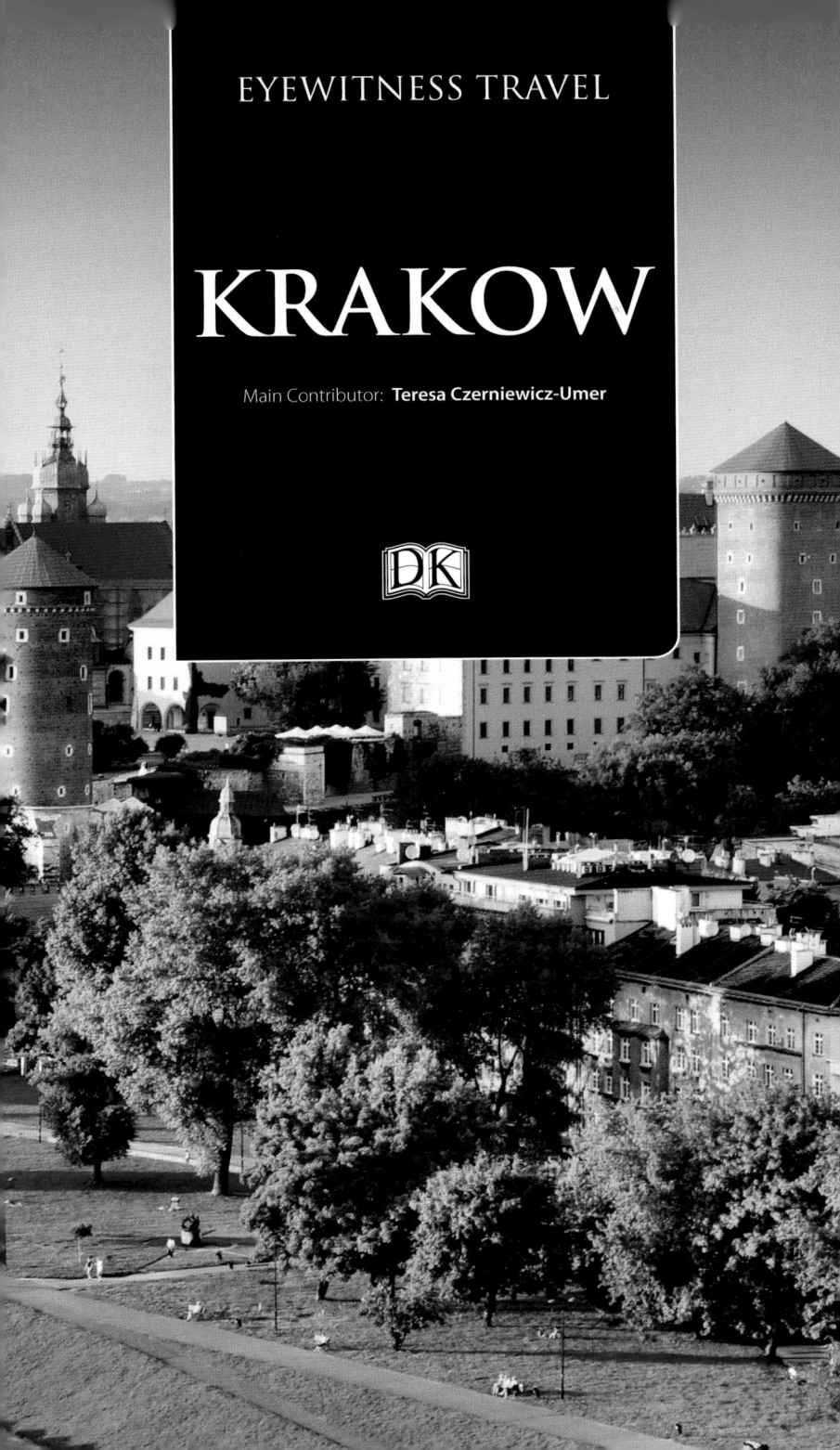

EYEWITNESS TRAVEL

KRAKOW

Main Contributor: **Teresa Czerniewicz-Umer**

DK

LONDON, NEW YORK,
MELBOURNE, MUNICH AND DELHI
www.dk.com

Produced by Wydawnictwo Wiedza i Życie, Warsaw

Managing Editor Ewa Szwagrzyk

Series Editor Joanna Egert

DTP Designer Paweł Pasternak

Consultant Jan Ostrowski

Production Anna Kożurno-Królikowska

Contributors

Teresa Czerniewicz-Umer, Andrzej Betlej, Piotr Krasny,
Robert Makłowicz, Craig Turp

Photographers

Andrzej Chęć, Wojciech Czerniewicz, Piotr Jamski,
Dorota and Mariusz Jarymowicz

Illustrators

Andrzej Wielgosz, Piotr Zybrzycki, Paweł Mistewicz

Printed and bound in China

First published in the UK in 2000 by
Dorling Kindersley Limited
80 Strand, London WC2R 0RL, UK

15 16 17 18 10 9 8 7 6 5 4 3 2 1

Reprinted with revisions 2003, 2007, 2010, 2013, 2015

Copyright 2000, 2015 © Dorling Kindersley Limited, London

A Penguin Random House Company

ISBN 978-1-40937-020-8

MIX
Paper from
responsible sources
FSC™ C018179

Front cover main image: Krakow Cathedral on Wawel Hill

◀ View of the Wawel Royal Castle from across the Vistula River

Contents

How to Use this Guide **6**

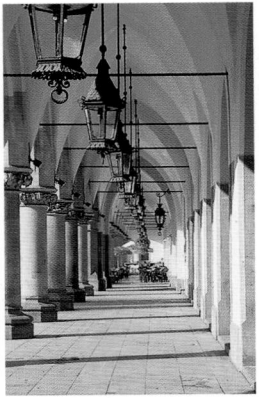

The side arcade of Cloth Hall *(see pp104–5)*

Introducing Krakow

Great Days
in Krakow **10**

Putting Krakow
on the Map **14**

The History of Krakow **20**

Krakow at a Glance **40**

Krakow through
the Year **54**

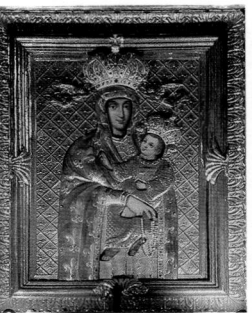

Icon of the Virgin of the Rosary
in the Dominican Church *(see pp118–19)*

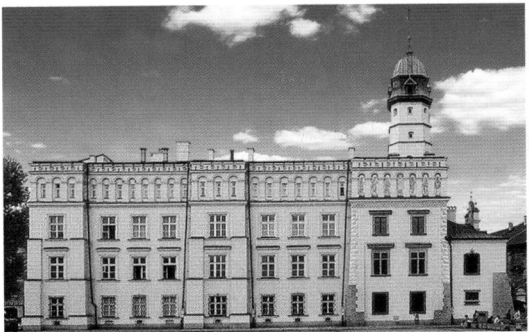
Town Hall in Kazimierz, housing the Ethnographical Museum *(see p125)*

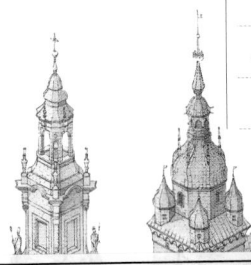
Musicians wearing regional Krakow costumes

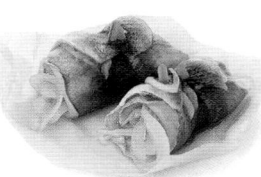
Pickled herrings

on Wawel Hill
(see pp66–7)

HOW TO USE THIS GUIDE

This Eyewitness Travel Guide is intended to help you make the most of your stay in Krakow. It provides detailed practical information and expert recommendations. *Introducing Krakow* tells you about the geographical location of the city, establishes Krakow in its historical context and guides you through the succession of cultural events. The section on *Krakow at a Glance* takes you through the tourist attractions in the city. *Krakow Area by Area* describes the most important sights with photographs, maps and illustrations. It recommends short excursions out of Krakow and offers three walks around the city. Information about hotels, restaurants, shops and markets as well as cafés, bars, entertainment and sport can be found in the section called *Travellers' Needs*. The section headed *Survival Guide* has advice on everything from posting a letter to using public transport to getting medical assistance.

How to Use the Key Indicators

Each of the six quarters has been colour coded for your convenience. Each section gives an introduction to the area, its history and character. The *Street by Street* map shows the most interesting parts of the quarter. Finding your way round is made easy by the numbering system. This reflects the order in which the descriptions are presented.

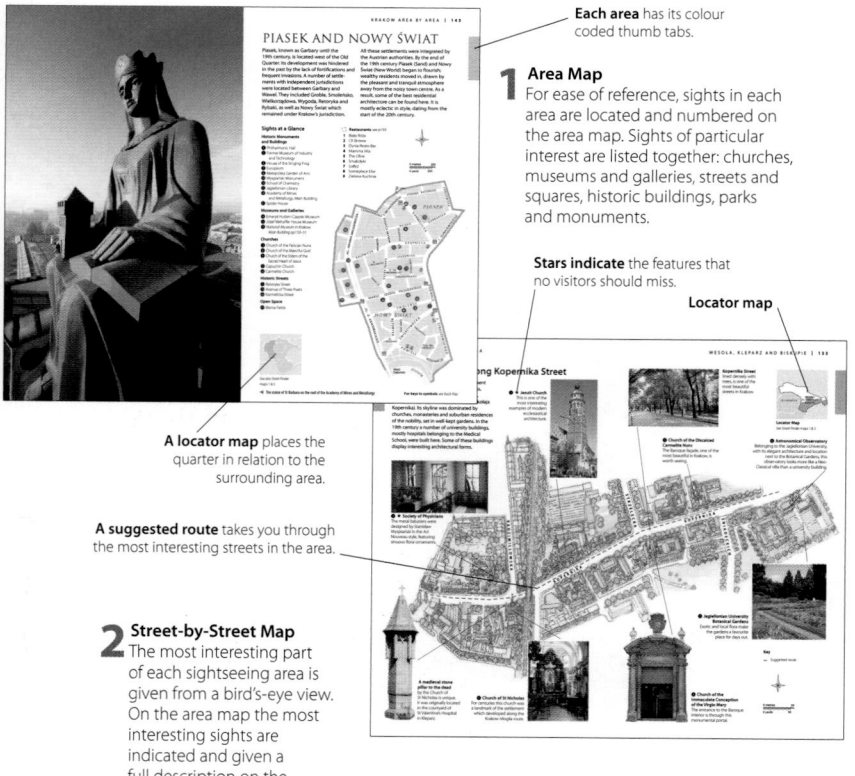

Each area has its colour coded thumb tabs.

1 Area Map
For ease of reference, sights in each area are located and numbered on the area map. Sights of particular interest are listed together: churches, museums and galleries, streets and squares, historic buildings, parks and monuments.

Stars indicate the features that no visitors should miss.

Locator map

A **locator map** places the quarter in relation to the surrounding area.

A **suggested route** takes you through the most interesting streets in the area.

2 Street-by-Street Map
The most interesting part of each sightseeing area is given from a bird's-eye view. On the area map the most interesting sights are indicated and given a full description on the following pages.

Krakow Area Map

This colour-coded map
(see pages 18–19) indicates
the six main sightseeing
quarters described in this
guide. Each of these quarters
is more fully covered in the
Area by Area section (pages 58–
153). In Krakow at a Glance this
same colour coding allows you
to locate the most interesting
places. You will also be able
to orientate yourself during
the three suggested walks
(page 166).

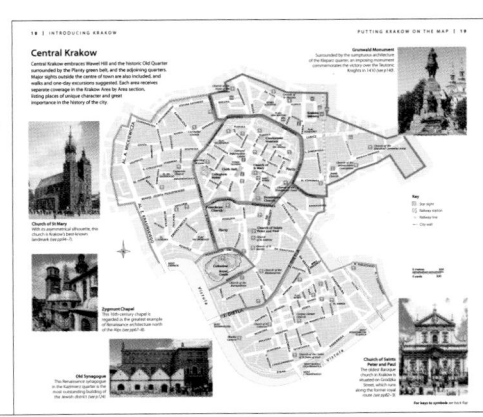

Numbered circles locate the listed
sights on the area map and within
the descriptive section.

Practical information provides everything you need to know to
visit each sight. Map references pinpoint the sight's location on
the Street Finder map (see pp228–37).

3 Detailed Information

Each of the most interesting sights
is described in depth. You will find
them listed in order following the
numbering on the area map.
Practical information, including
map references, opening hours and
telephone numbers is also provided.

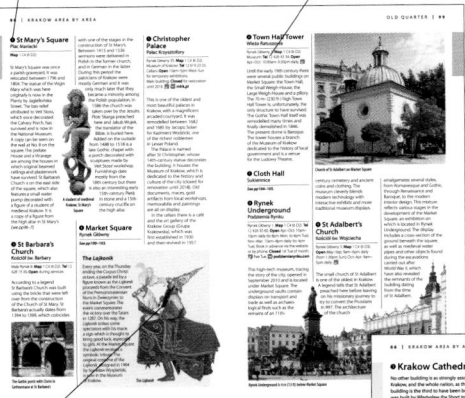

The visitors' checklist
provides useful information you
may need to plan your visit.

The boxes contain detailed information
on a particular subject related to the sight.

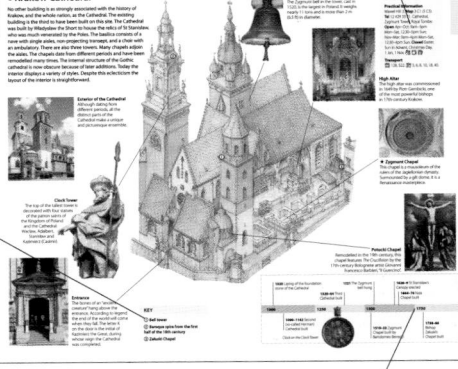

Numbered circles point out key
features of the sight listed in a key.

4 Krakow's Main Sights

Historic buildings are dissected to
reveal their interiors. Museums and
galleries have colour-coded floor
plans enabling you to find
important exhibits.

A timeline indicates important dates in the
history of the building.

The Prussian Homage (1882) by Jan Matejko ▶

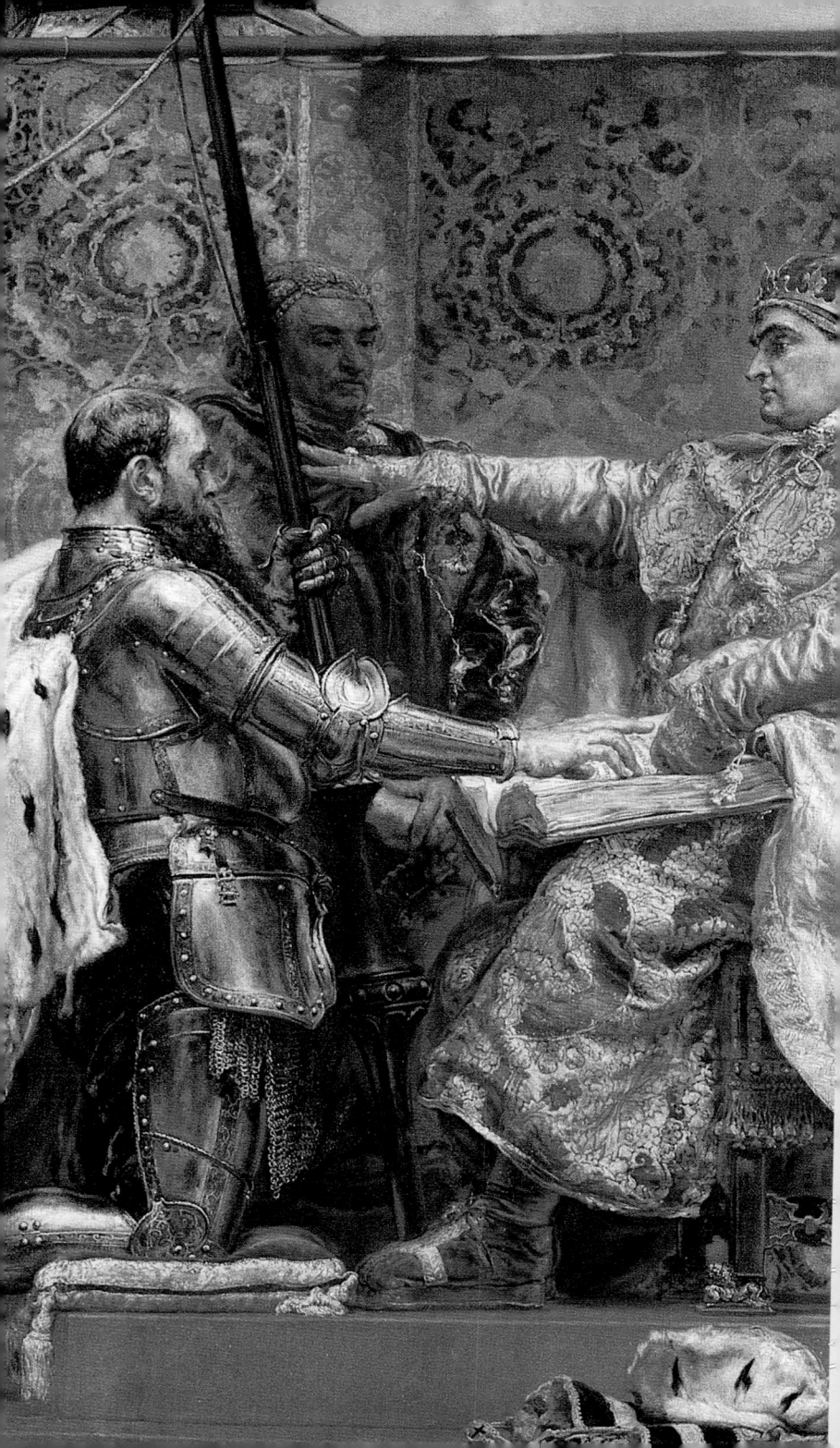

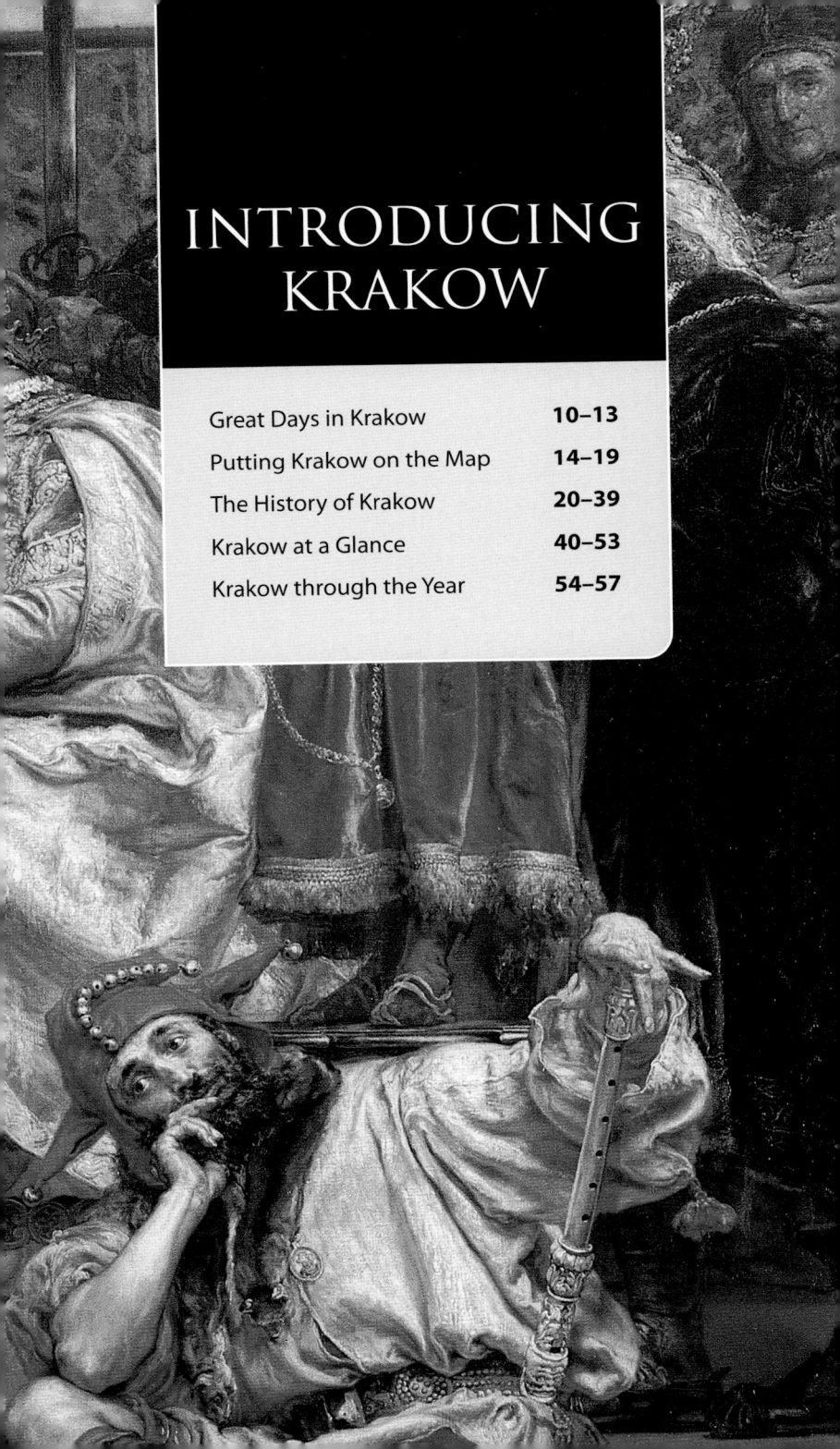

INTRODUCING KRAKOW

GREAT DAYS IN KRAKOW

There are three themes that define the most visited city in Poland – its royal past, Judaism and culture. Some of Krakow's most important sights are along the Royal Route to the Wawel Castle, while the Kazimierz district, home to the city's Jews since the 14th century, is seeing a welcome revival after the tragedy of the Holocaust. As Poland's cultural capital, many museums here house artistic treasures. Krakow is also a surprisingly green city, full of grottoes and parks particularly suited to children. The four days on pages 10–11 are designed to uncover the city from these different viewpoints; the price guides include travel, food and admission fees. The itineraries on pages 12–13 show visitors how to make the most of their time based on length of stay.

Walking the Royal Route

Two Adults allow at least 340zł

- **Explore Krakow's Old Quarter**
- **Great views from the Town Hall Tower**
- **Authentic Polish cuisine**
- **Impressive churches and a cathedral**

Morning

Starting early to avoid the crowds, especially in summer, there is no better way to enter Krakow's Old Quarter than through the 700-year-old **St Florian's Gate** *(see p113)*, one of the few remnants of the city's original defences. Stroll along **Floriańska Street** *(see p116)*, once Krakow's main commercial thoroughfare and still very much a thriving bazaar where artisans and hawkers sell all sorts of souvenirs – look out for watercolours depicting the best of the Old Quarter. Krakow's **Market Square**

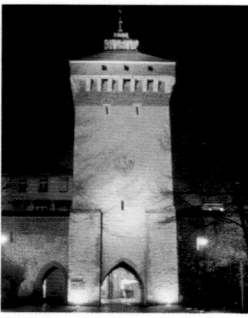
St Florian's Gate

(see pp100–103) is both the geographical and spiritual heart of the city, and is surrounded on all sides by historic treasures; **St Mary's** *(see pp94–7)* and **St Aldabert's** *(see p99)* churches are worth a look. Climb the **Town Hall Tower** *(see p99)* for superb panoramic views and wander around the market inside the 14th-century **Cloth Hall** *(see pp104–5)*. For lunch, enjoy some classic Polish dishes at Krakow's oldest restaurant, **Wierzynek** *(see p192)*.

Afternoon

One of Krakow's oldest streets, **Grodzka** *(see p80)* is a cobbled route of different, but harmonious, architectural styles. Admire the **Royal Arsenal** *(see p81)* and the modest but charming **Church of St Giles** opposite *(see p81)*. A little further down, don't miss the **Church of St Martin** *(see p81)*, set slightly back from the street, or the impressively preserved Romanesque **Church of St Andrew** *(see p80)*. Take a look inside the **Church of Saints Peter and Paul** *(see pp82–3)*, an early Baroque masterpiece. At the end of the Royal Route is **Wawel Hill** *(see pp62–3)*, and late in the afternoon, after the majority of visitors have gone, you can stroll the hill at leisure. Be sure to visit the wonderful **Krakow Cathedral** *(see pp66–71)*, and to wander around the Renaissance-style inner courtyard of the **Wawel Royal Castle** *(see pp72–3)*.

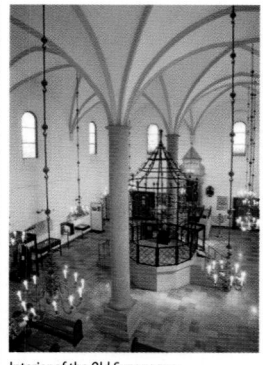
Interior of the Old Synagogue

Jewish Krakow

Two Adults allow at least 180zł

- **The history of Krakow's Jewish population**
- **Great kosher food**
- **World War II Jewish ghetto**
- **The famous Schindler factory**

Morning

Start your day at the **Old Synagogue** *(see p124)*, damaged during World War II, but now restored to its original 16th-century design. The exhibition inside serves as a good introduction to the history of Jews in Krakow. Nearby are two cemeteries: the **New Jewish Cemetery** *(see p125)*, created in the 19th century as a resting place for the city's wealthiest Jews, and **Remu'h Cemetery** *(see pp124–5)* in the courtyard of the Remu'h synagogue. For a kosher lunch head to **Klezmer Hois** *(see p192)*.

Afternoon

Stroll over the Kładka Ojca Bernatka footbridge to the Podgórze district. The Nazis moved the Jews here from Kazimierz in 1941, squeezing them into a ghetto in the area around Bohaterów Getta and Rynek Podgórski. One Polish man, Tadeusz Pankiewicz, owner of the Pharmacy Under the Eagle at Bohaterów Getta 18, stayed on in an attempt to help the city's Jews. Here today, an exhibition portrays life in the ghetto. At Lipowa 4 is the former **Schindler's Factory** (see p158), featured in the film *Schindler's List*. An exhibition details stories from Krakow's Polish and Jewish inhabitants during World War II.

City of Culture

Two Adults allow at least 230zł

- **Admire the only Leonardo da Vinci painting in Poland**
- **Visit the former home of Pope John Paul II**
- **Explore the Collegium Maius**
- **Beautiful Secessionist architecture**

Morning

The **Czartoryski Museum** (see pp114–15) is currently undergoing renovations. During this time, its most famous work of art, Leonardo da Vinci's *Lady with an Ermine*, can be admired at the **Wawel Royal Castle** (see pp72–3). Next, head over to the **Szołayski House** (see p112) to admire the talents of

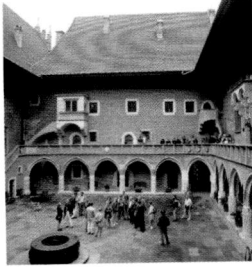
Jagiellonian University

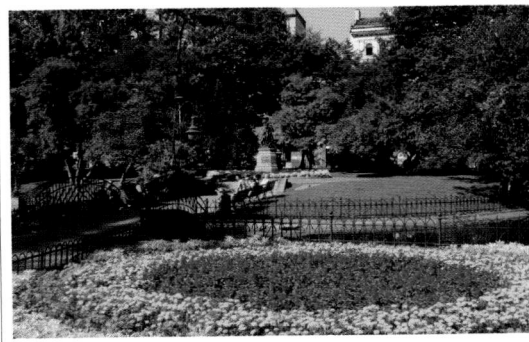
Flowers in bloom in Planty Park

Stanislav Wyspiański, Poland's leading Secessionist painter. Jump on the No. 124 bus for the short ride to the **Archdiocesan Museum** (see p84), home of Poland's finest collection of ecclesiastical art. Today the building is also popular with pilgrims interested in the life of Pope John Paul II; he lived in the building in the 1950s. For lunch, head to **Smak Ukraiński** (see p190) for outstanding Ukrainian food.

Afternoon

A walk through the southern part of **Planty Park** (see pp168–9), past the statue of Copernicus, to the Jagiellonian University and Museum in the **Collegium Maius** (see pp108–9) is the perfect post-lunch stroll. Enjoy the glorious courtyard and take the 30-minute guided tour of the building, then take a quick peek inside the **Church of St Anne** (see pp110–11). If you have an appetite for more art, head to the **"Bunker of Art"** (see p107), home to cutting-edge exhibitions. Next pay a visit to the **Słowacki Theatre** (see p117). It is officially closed unless there is a performance on, but the doorman may just let you in to admire the lovely Secessionist interior. Round off this cultural day with dinner at **Jazz Club U Muniaka** (see p206), Krakow's best jazz café.

Owl statue in Planty Park

A Family Day

Family of Four allow 545zł

- **The magical and mysterious Dragon's Lair**
- **Picnic lunch in the park**
- **Shopping in the Cloth Hall**
- **Cycle round the city**

Morning

Few children will fail to be intrigued by the **Dragon's Lair** (see p65) on Wawel Hill, a warren of tunnels, nooks and crannies. They can then shop for chocolate at **Wawel** (see p201) before you head next door to the deli to buy bread, sausage and cheese for a picnic lunch. Then visit the **Cloth Hall** (pp104–105), which sells excellent wooden toys.

Afternoon

Tram 20 will take you out to the family-friendly Jordan Park, where you can enjoy your lunch while the kids take a paddle-boat on the lake. If you still have some energy, take a bike tour around the sights of the city with Krakow Bike Tour (www.krakowbiketour.com). The tour starts from ul. Grodzka 2 at 3pm. After such an active afternoon, you might want an early dinner; try **U Babci Maliny** (see p191), a cosy basement restaurant serving traditional Polish fare.

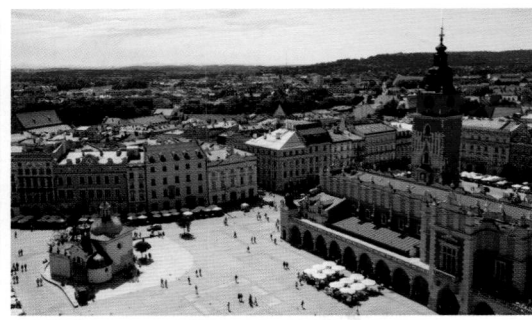

2 Days in Krakow

- Stroll around the buzzing main Market Square
- Admire the tombs of Poland's kings in the Krakow Cathedral
- Explore the mixed Jewish-Christian heritage of the Kazimierz Quarter

Day 1

Morning Start with a circuit of the **Market Square** (pp92–3) before exploring the covered stalls of the Renaissance **Cloth Hall** (pp104–105). Join the crowds milling around at the foot of the **Mickiewicz Statue** (p93), then head for the sumptuously decorated **Church of St Mary** (pp94–7). Try to arrive by 11:50am to observe the ritual unveiling of Veit Stoss's **High Altar** (pp96–7).

Afternoon Walk south through the Okół district along **Grodzka Street** (p80) to **Wawel Hill** (pp60–75), site of the **Krakow Cathedral** (pp66–71) and **Wawel Royal Castle** (pp72–3). Admire the stunning views from the ramparts before taking the spiral steps down to the **Dragon's Lair** cave (p65). Finish the day with a stroll on the Vistula riverbank just below.

Day 2

Morning Explore the multi-cultural past of the **Kazimierz Quarter** (pp120–29) with a stroll around its atmospheric streets and piazzas, notably the former market square of **Szeroka Street** (pp122–3). Visit the **Old Synagogue** (p124) and the **Remu'h Synagogue** (p124) for an evocative taste of Jewish Krakow, then stop at one of the area's many restaurants for lunch.

Afternoon Cross the footbridge at the end of Mostowa Street to reach **Schindler's Factory** (p158), now a moving museum recalling the fate of many Krakovians during World War II. Head back northwards via the western half of Kazimierz,

Krakow's Market Square, with St Adalbert's Church to the left

with its churches of **Corpus Christi** (p125) and **St Catherine** (p128). In the evening, stay in Kazimierz to enjoy the numerous cafés and bars of this bohemian quarter.

3 Days in Krakow

- Step back into Krakow's Middle Ages with a visit to the Rynek Underground
- Tour the former royal apartments of Wawel Royal Castle
- Spend a day at the Auschwitz-Birkenau memorial museum

Day 1

Morning Soak in the sights of the **Market Square** (pp92–3), including the subterranean history museum **Rynek Underground** (p99). Enjoy the rich interior of the **Church of St Mary** (pp94–7) before

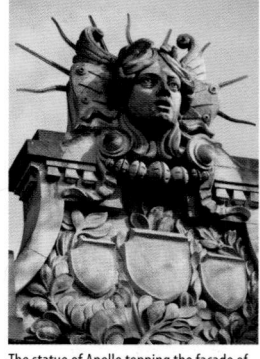

The statue of Apollo topping the façade of the Palace of Art

strolling up **Floriańska Street** (pp116–17) towards the **Barbican** (p116), pausing to admire the 19th-century paintings and furnishings at the **Matejko House** (p116). From here, walk west through **Planty Park** (pp168–9) towards Szczepański Square.

Afternoon Delve into Krakow's Art Nouveau heritage with a visit to the ornate **Palace of Art** (p107) and the inspirational **Szołayski House** (p112). Walk south through the atmospheric University quarter to the **Collegium Maius** (pp108–109) and the Baroque splendour of the **Church of St Anne** (pp110–11). Finish at the **Franciscan Church** (pp88–9), famous for its beautiful Art Nouveau frescoes by Stanisław Wyspiański.

Day 2

Morning Devote a few hours to **Wawel Hill** (pp60–75). Explore the royal tombs in the **Krakow Cathedral** (pp66–71) before choosing to see at least one of the many museum collections located in **Wawel Royal Castle** (pp72–3).

Afternoon Take a stroll around the former Jewish quarter of **Kazimierz** (pp120–29), calling in at renovated synagogues such as the **Tempel** (p124), the **Isaak's** (p124) and the **Remu'h** (p124). Walk through the **Remu'h Cemetery** (pp124–5) and the **New Jewish Cemetery** (p125), filled with reminders of Kazimierz's rich Jewish past. If time allows, cross the river and visit **Schindler's Factory** (p158).

Day 3

Morning Take the bus to Oświęcim for a guided tour of the former **Auschwitz** concentration camp *(pp162–3)*.

Afternoon Visit the nearby killing fields of **Birkenau** *(pp164–5)* before returning to Krakow by bus.

5 Days in Krakow

- Immerse yourself in Krakow's monument-packed Old Town
- Descend into the amazing underground world of the Wieliczka Salt Mines
- Enjoy woodland walks in Las Wolski forest

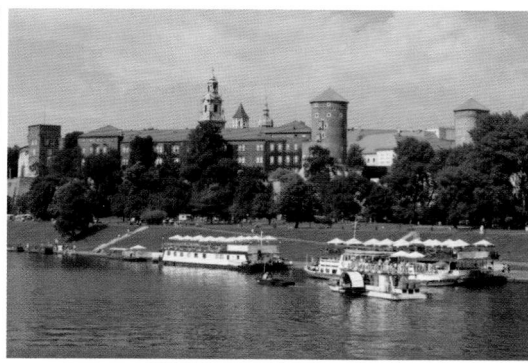

Royal Wawel Castle at Wawel Hill seen from across the Vistula River

Day 1

Morning Explore the **Market Square** *(pp92–3)*, touring the Gallery of Polish Art on the top floor of the **Cloth Hall** *(pp104–105)* before climbing the **Town Hall Tower** *(p99)* for views of the Old Town skyline. Admire the altars of the **Church of St Mary** *(pp94–7)*, then take a peek at **St Barbara's Church** *(p98)* just behind it. Stand beneath the towers of the Church of St Mary on the hour to hear a trumpeter playing the *hejnał* bugle-call *(p94)*.

Afternoon Walk south along **Grodzka Street** *(p80)*, pausing to examine the churches of **St Andrew** *(pp80–81)* and **Saints Peter and Paul** *(pp82–3)*.

Detour into pretty **Kanonicza Street** *(p81)*, where you can visit the medieval art collections of the **Archdiocesan Museum** *(p84)* and the **Palace of Bishop Erazm Ciołek** *(p84)*. Afterwards, spend a leisurely hour or two walking the complete circuit of leafy **Planty Park** *(pp168–9)*.

Day 2

Morning Devote the morning to as many museum collections within **Wawel Royal Castle** *(pp72–3)* as you have time for. If time is at a premium, prioritize the State Rooms and the Private Royal Apartments. Try to arrive early, since there may be queues for tickets.

Afternoon Head for **Kazimierz** *(pp120–29)* and visit the area around **Szeroka Street** *(pp122–3)*, site of the original Jewish quarter. Afterwards, visit the western part of the Kazimierz district, with the **Church of**

St Catherine and the **Paulite Church "On the Rock"** *(p128)*.

Day 3

Morning and afternoon Reserve the whole day for a bus trip to the **Auschwitz-Birkenau** memorial museum *(pp162–5)*, taking time to walk through the extensive Birkenau site.

Day 4

Morning Catch a swift suburban train to **Wieliczka** to take a guided tour of the spectacular man-made caverns of the **Salt Mines** *(p158)*.

Afternoon Return to Krakow by train and take the tram to **Nowa Huta** *(p156)*. You can then stroll from the centre of this 1950s-era suburb to the medieval **Mogiła Monastery** *(p156)* nearby. Again taking the tram, call at the **Polish Aviation Museum** *(p156)* on your way back to the city centre.

Day 5

Morning Explore the extensive art and history collections of the **National Museum in Krakow** *(pp150–51)*. Be sure to leave enough time for the modern paintings on the top floor.

Afternoon Walk, cycle or catch a bus to the Zwierzyniec district in order to scale the **Kościuszko Mound** *(p171)*. Follow this up with a stroll or mountain-bike ride around the **Las Wolski** forest *(pp172–3)*, pausing to visit either **Krakow Zoo** *(p173)* or the **Camaldolese Monastery** *(p172)*.

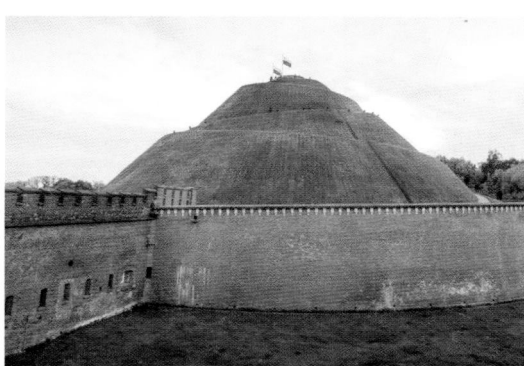

Kościuszko Mound and the fortification surrounding it

Putting Krakow on the Map

The old part of Krakow (Kraków), with the Royal Castle on Wawel Hill, is regarded as a fascinating historic town rich in heritage. The historic quarters constitute only a small part of present-day Krakow, the largest urban development in the Lesser Poland (Małopolska) region. The geographical position makes Krakow an ideal base for excursions to the Polish mountains, Auschwitz or the picturesque Krakow-Częstochowa Valley. The town is also well positioned for international connections to Prague, Brno, Bratislava, Vienna and L'viv.

Baltic Sea

Władysławowo

Gdynia

Słupsk

Gdańsk
Lech Wałęsa

Gdańsk

Koszalin

Bytów

Tczew

POMORSKIE

Starogard
Gdański

Bobolice

Biały Bór

Czersk

Czluchów

Grudziądz

Europe

NORWAY

SWEDEN

ESTONIA

North Sea

DENMARK

LATVIA

LITHUANIA

UNITED
KINGDOM

NETHERLANDS

BELARUS

POLAND

GERMANY

Krakow

BELGIUM

CZECH
REPUBLIC

UKRAINE

SLOVAKIA

AUSTRIA

HUNGARY

FRANCE

SWITZ.

SLOV.

CROATIA

ROMANIA

Atlantic
Ocean

BOSNIA
HERZ.

SERBIA

ITALY

MONTEN.

KOS.

BULGARIA

ALBANIA

MAC.

SPAIN

GREECE

TURKEY

ZACHODNIO-
POMORSKIE

Złotów

Piła

Czlopa

Bydgoszcz

Bydgoszcz

Toruń

Dobiegniew

Rogoêno

KUJAWSKO-
POMORSKIE

Inowrocław

Warta

Oborniki

Gniezno

Poznań-Ławica

Poznań

Wolsztyn

WIELKOPOLSKIE

Konin

LUBUSKIE

Leszno

Jarocin

Kalisz

Głogów

Ostrów
Wielkopolski

Lubin

Wieruszów

Odra

Legnica

Oleśnica

Leipzig

Gorlitz

Wrocław-Copernicus

Wrocław

Kluczbork

Dresden

Jelenia Góra

DOLNOŚLĄSKIE

OPOLSKIE

GERMANY

Liberec

Wałbrzych

Opole

Lubliniec

Teplice

Mlada
Boleslav

Kędzierzyn-
Koźle

Elbe

Carlsbad

Prague

Hradec
Králové

Rybnik

Pardubice

Ostrava

Key

Svitávy

CZECH
REPUBLIC

=== Motorway
or dual carriageway

= = Motorway under construction

— Major road

— Railway line

— National border

--- Provincial border

Humpolec

Olomouc

Brno

Piestany

0 kilometres   100

0 miles   50

For keys to symbols *see back flap*

RUSSIAN FEDERATION
(KALININGRAD)

Gulf of
Danzig

Kaliningrad

Krakow and Environs

Miechów

Olkusz

94

Słomniki

7

Proszowice

Trzebinia

79

79

Wisła

Elbląg

522

Lidzbark
Warmiński

51

A4

See next page

75

Pasłęk

Alwernia

Kraków

KRAKOW

Niepołomice

WARMIŃSKO-
MAZURSKIE

7

Olsztyn

16

Wisła

94

A4

Kwidzyn

Ostróda

Szczytno

44

Skawina

Wieliczka

75

Bochnia

16

Nidzica

53

Skawa

Wadowice

Raba

Dobczyce

52

Brodnica

Mława

7

Ostrołęka

Łomża

28

52

Myślenice

7

MAZOWIECKIE

Ciechanów

Zambrów

Białystok

PODLASKIE

Lipno

10

60

Narew

Ostrów
Mazowiecka

8

Bielsk
Podlaski

Pružany

Włocławek

Płońsk

Wyszków

Bug

19

Płock

61

58

63

BELARUS

Warsaw Modlin

Wisła

Warsaw

Siedlce

Biała
Podlaska

Brest

Kobryn

2

Kutno

Pruszków

Warsaw Chopin

63

Międzyrzec
Podlaski

A2

A1

Łęczyca

A2

Garwolin

17

19

A2

Kock

Włodawa

Łódź

Łódź

58

S7

Kovel'

ŁÓDZKIE

Tomaszów
Mazowiecki

Puławy

12

Radom

12

Wisła

Lublin

Lublin

82

Bełchatów

Piotrków
Trybunalski

7

Iłża

Chełm

74

Skarżysko-
Kamienna

9

LUBELSKIE

Volodymyr-
Volynsky

Ostrowiec

74

Kraśnik

Kielce

Opatów

Zamość

74

Częstochowa

ŚWIĘTOKRZYSKIE

17

ŚLĄSKIE

78

Jędrzejów

Tarnobrzeg

Nisko

19

Zawiercie

7

73

9

Zhovkva

A1

Mielec

77

Katowice

*See map
above*

Rzeszów–Jasionka

Lviv

Katowice

Rzeszów

Radymno

Kraków

KRAKOW

A4

Tarnów

PODKARPACKIE

1

Przemyśl

UKRAINE

51

Bielsko-
Biała

MAŁOPOLSKIE

98

Krosno

98

Rabka

19

Sanok

Sambir

Cadca

Trstená

Nowy Sącz

98

87

Stryi

Žilina

Zakopane

Svidník

Ivano-Frankivsk

D1

Ruzomberok

Poprad

Presov

SLOVAKIA

Košice

Mukacheve

Krakow and its Environs

Until the early 20th century the conurbation of Krakow occupied a relatively small area on the banks of the Vistula (Wisła) River and was made up of several small towns (Kleparz, Kazimierz, Garbary and Podgórze). Greater Krakow was established in 1910 after the incorporation of the extensive lands of Rakowice, Prądnik, Czarna Wieś, Krowodrza, Bielany, Dębnik, Płaszów and Prokocim. A new industrial district of Nowa Huta was constructed outside Krakow after World War II. Long walks in Krakow are always interesting as all the historic quarters have their own unique character.

Kielce

Garlica

Bibice

Zielonki

Węgrzce

Dąbrowa Górnicza

Witkowice

Prądnik Biały

Górka Narodów

Bronowice Małe

Wielkie Pola

Krowodrza

Olsza

Balice

Rząska

Łobzów

Rakowice

Katowice

Mydniki

Nowa Wieś

Warszawskie

John Paul II International Airport

Olszanica

Główny

Balice

Wola Justowska

Błonia

Krakow

Grzegórzki

Piłsudski Mound

Zoo Las Wolski

Kościuszko Mound

Dębniki

Kryspinów

Bielany

Vistula

Podgórze

Płaszów

Bodzów

Krakus Mound

Kostrze

Pychowice

Heltmana

Piekary

Zakrzówek

Bonarka

Wola Duchacka

Tyniec

Cegielniana

Skotniki

Kobierzyn

Borek Fałęcki

Kurdwanów

Kliny Zacisze

Jugowice

Sidzina

Swoszowice

Opatkowice

Wilga

Skawina

Wróblowice

Korabniki

Libertów

Lusina

Oświęcim (Auschwitz)

Gołkowice

Wrząsowice

Ochojno

Zakopane

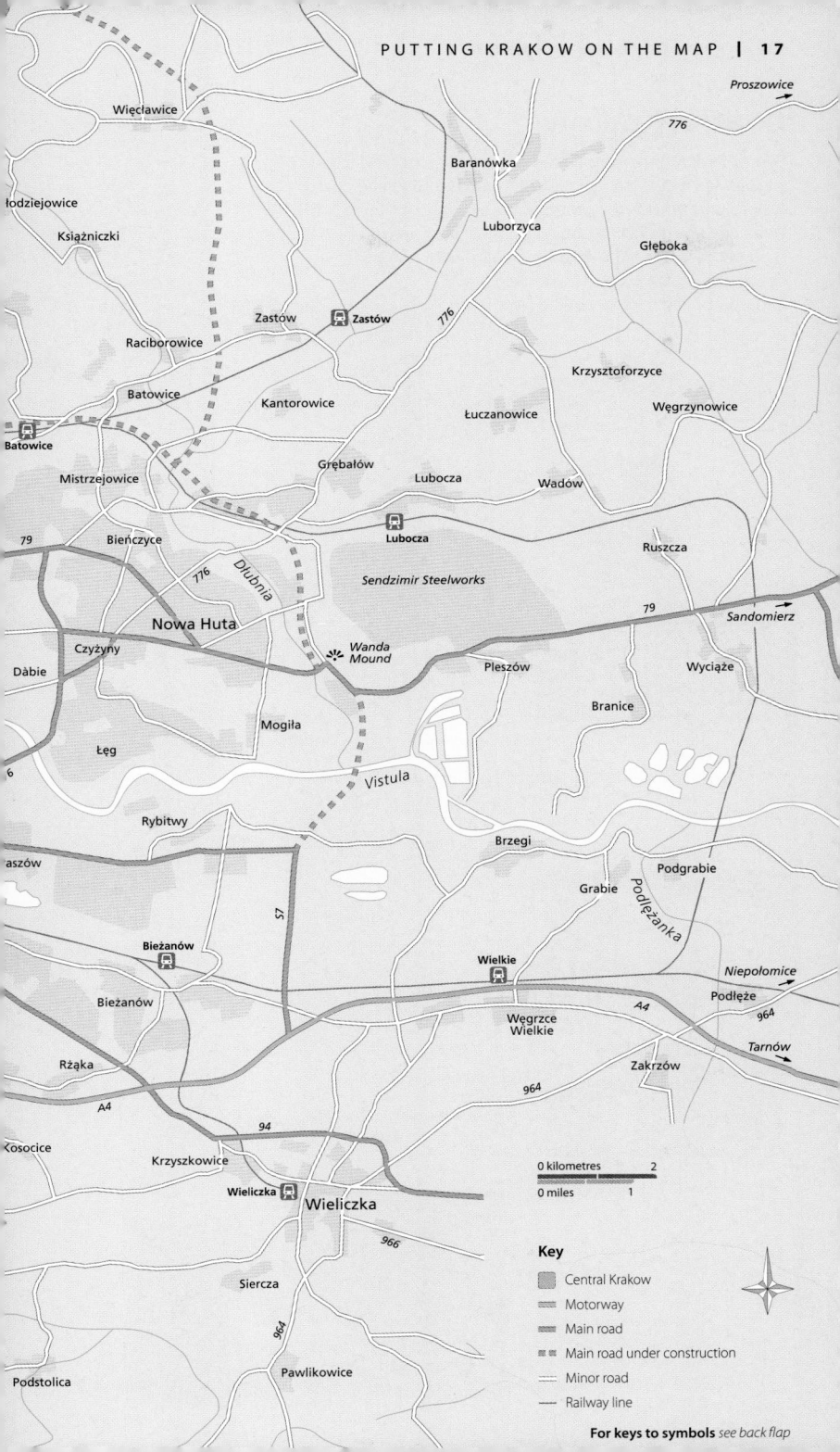

Proszowice

Więcławice

776

Baranówka

Łodziejowice

Luborzyca

Książniczki

Głęboka

Zastów

Zastów

776

Raciborowice

Krzysztoforzyce

Batowice

Kantorowice

Łuczanowice

Węgrzynowice

Batowice

Grębałów

Lubocza

Wadów

Mistrzejowice

79

Bieńczyce

Lubocza

Ruszcza

776

Dłubnia

Sendzimir Steelworks

79

Nowa Huta

Sandomierz

Czyżyny

Wanda
Mound

Wyciąże

Dàbie

Pleszów

Mogiła

Branice

6

Łęg

Rybitwy

Vistula

Brzegi

aszów

Podgrabie

Grabie

Podłężanka

57

Bieżanów

Wielkie

Niepołomice

Bieżanów

Podłęże

Węgrzce
Wielkie

964

Rżąka

A4

Tarnów

A4

Zakrzów

Kosocice

964

94

Krzyszkowice

0 kilometres   2

Wieliczka   Wieliczka

0 miles   1

966

Key

Central Krakow

Siercza

Motorway

Main road

Main road under construction

964

Minor road

Podstolica

Pawlikowice

Railway line

For keys to symbols *see back flap*

Central Krakow

Central Krakow embraces Wawel Hill and the historic Old Quarter surrounded by the Planty green belt, and the adjoining quarters. Major sights outside the centre of town are also included, and walks and one-day excursions suggested. Each area receives separate coverage in the Krakow Area by Area section, listing places of unique character and great importance in the history of the city.

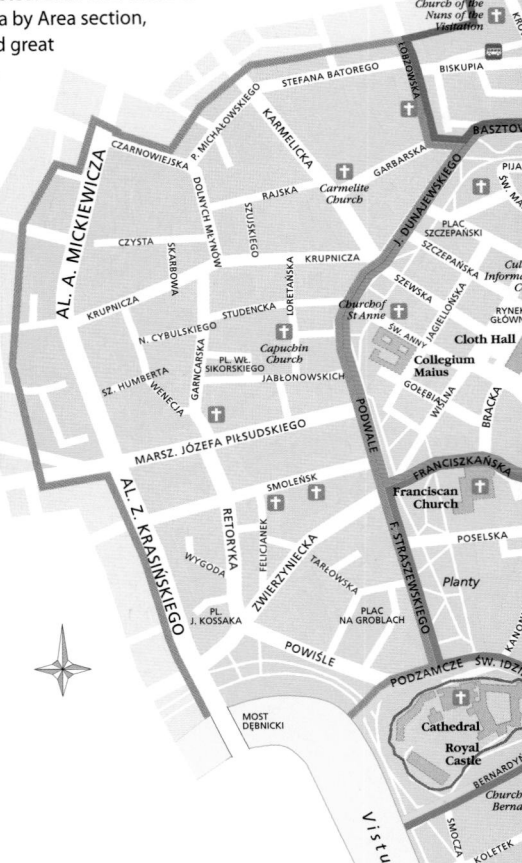

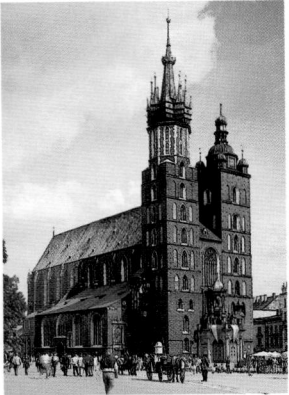

Church of St Mary
With its asymmetrical silhouette, this church is Krakow's best-known landmark *(see pp94–7)*.

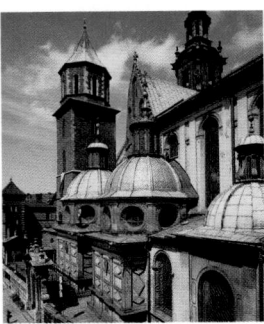

Zygmunt Chapel
This 16th-century chapel is regarded as the greatest example of Renaissance architecture north of the Alps *(see pp67–8)*.

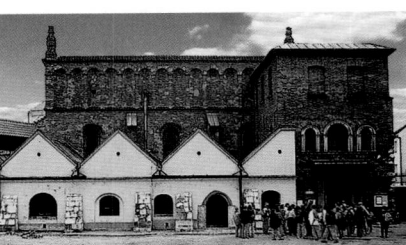

Old Synagogue
This Renaissance synagogue in the Kazimierz quarter is the most outstanding building of the Jewish district *(see p124)*.

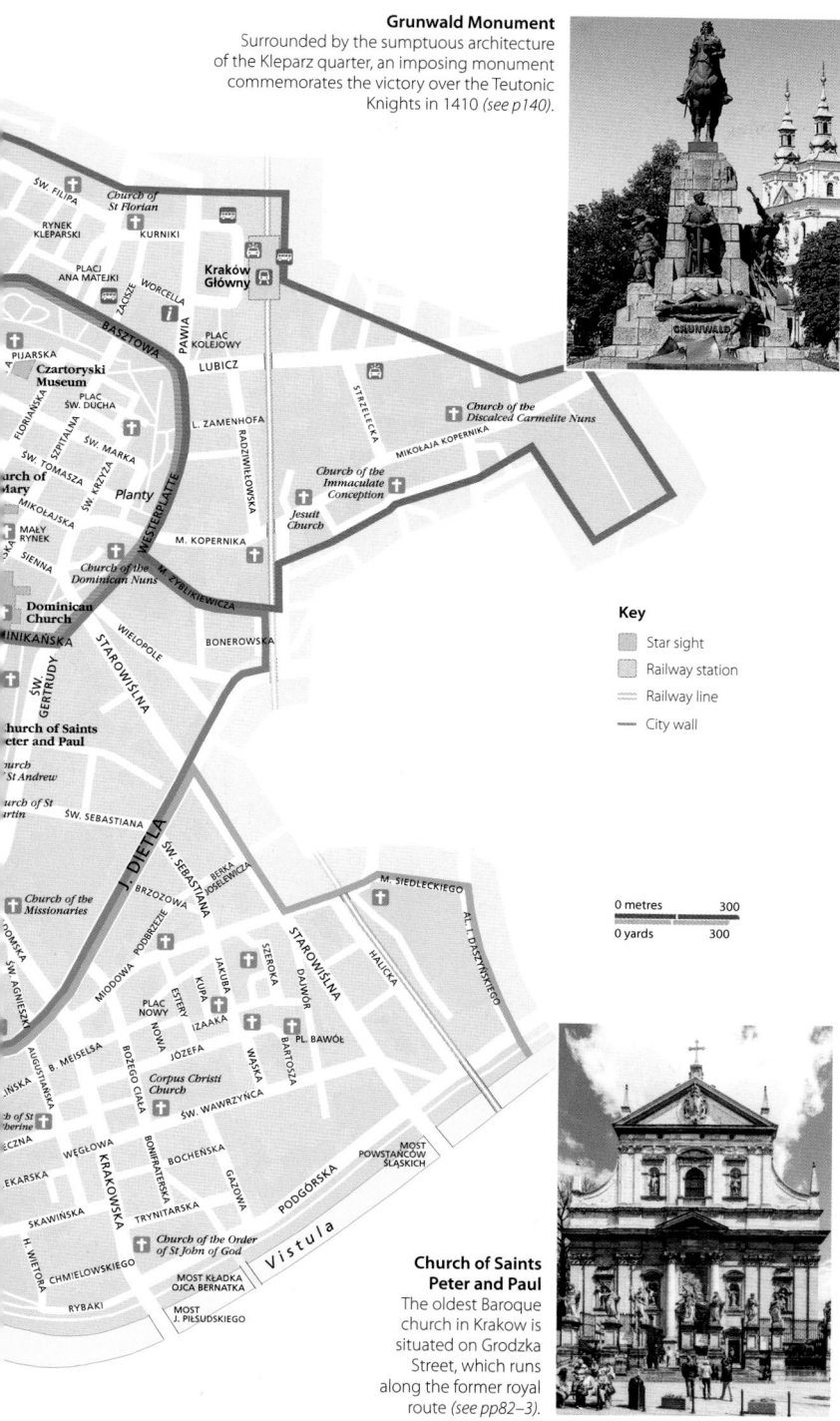

Grunwald Monument
Surrounded by the sumptuous architecture of the Kleparz quarter, an imposing monument commemorates the victory over the Teutonic Knights in 1410 *(see p140).*

ŚW. FILIPA
Church of St Florian
RYNEK KLEPARSKI
KURNIKI
PLACJ ANA MATEJKI
ZACŁKE WORCELLA
PAWIA
Kraków Główny
BASZTOWA
PIJARSKA
Czartoryski Museum
PLAC ŚW. DUCHA
PLAC KOLEJOWY
LUBICZ
FLORIAŃSKA
ŚW. SZPITALNA
ŚW. TOMASZA
ŚW. MARKA
ŚW. KRZYZA
L. ZAMENHOFA
RADZIWIŁŁOWSKA
STRZELECKA
MIKOŁAJA KOPERNIKA
Church of the Discalced Carmelite Nuns
urch of Mary
MIKOŁAJSKA
Planty
WESTERPLATTE
MAŁY RYNEK
SIENNA
Church of the Dominican Nuns
M. KOPERNIKA
Church of the Immaculate Conception
Jesuit Church
M. ŻYBLIKIEWICZA
Dominican Church
INIKAŃSKA
WIELOPOLE
BONEROWSKA
ŚW. GERTRUDY
STAROWIŚLNA
hurch of Saints eter and Paul
urch St Andrew
urch of St artin
ŚW. SEBASTIANA
J. DIETLA
ŚW. SEBASTIANA
BERKA JOSELEWICZA
BRZOZOWA
M. SIEDLECKIEGO
Church of the Missionaries
PODBRZEZIE
STAROWIŚLNA
AL. I. DASZYŃSKIEGO
HALICKA
 MIODOWA
ŚW. AGNIESZKI
ESTERY
KUPA
JAKUBA
SZEROKA
DAJWÓR
NOWA
IZAAKA
PLAC NOWY
PL. BAWÓŁ
BARTOSZA
B. MEISELSA
BOŻEGO CIAŁA
JÓZEFA
WĄSKA
IŃSKA
b of St herine
ECZNA
Corpus Christi Church
ŚW. WAWRZYŃCA
AUGUSTIAŃSKA
WĘGLOWA
BONIFRATERSKA
BOCHEŃSKA
GAZOWA
MOST POWSTAŃCÓW ŚLĄSKICH
EKARSKA
KRAKOWSKA
PODGÓRSKA
SKAWIŃSKA
TRYNITARSKA
Vistula
H. WIETORA
CHMIELOWSKIEGO
Church of the Order of St John of God
MOST KŁADKA OJCA BERNATKA
RYBAKI
MOST J. PIŁSUDSKIEGO

Key

⬜ Star sight
⬜ Railway station
= Railway line
— City wall

0 metres 300
0 yards 300

Church of Saints Peter and Paul
The oldest Baroque church in Krakow is situated on Grodzka Street, which runs along the former royal route *(see pp82–3).*

For keys to symbols *see back flap*

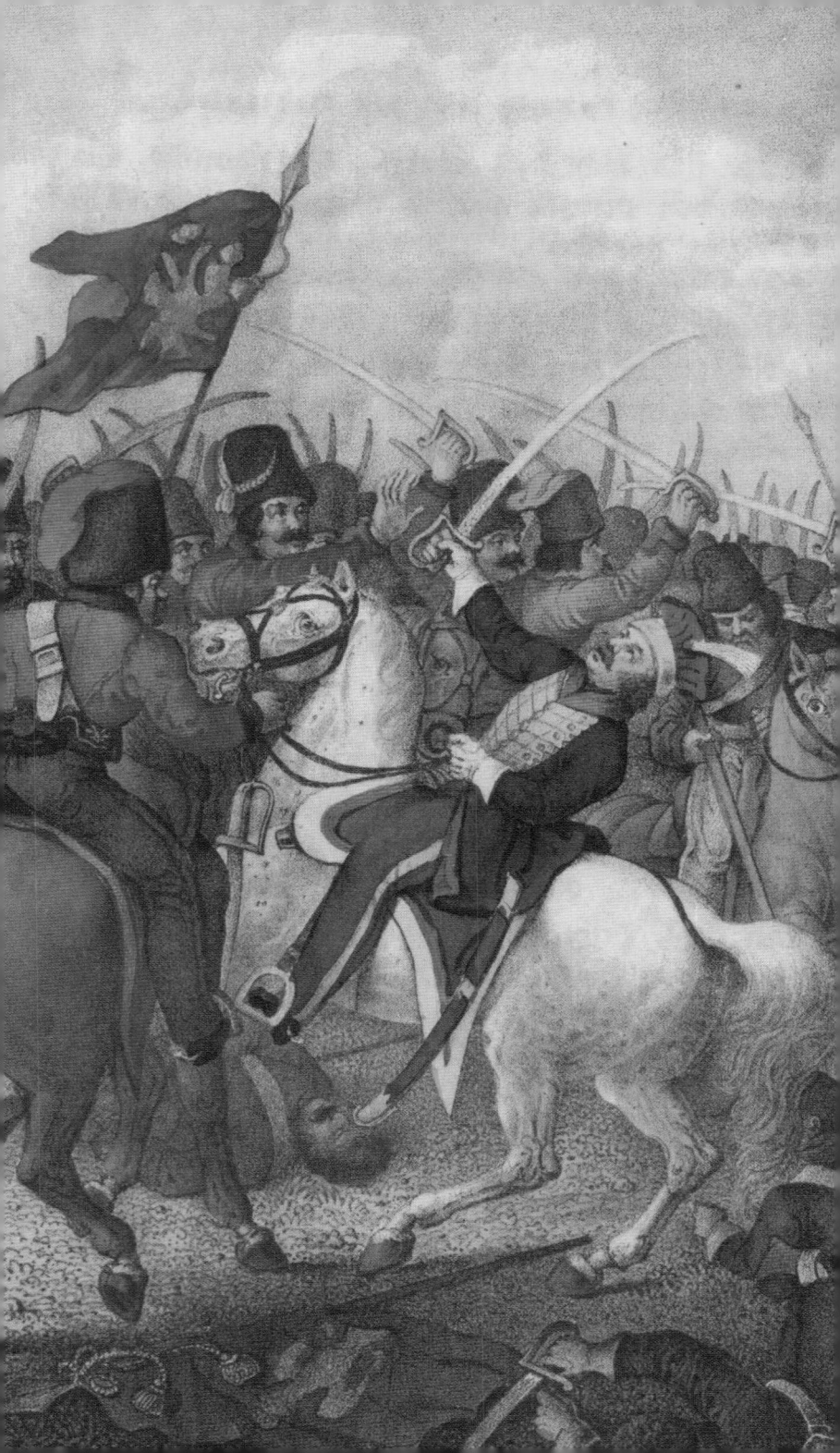

THE HISTORY OF KRAKOW

For many centuries Krakow was the capital of Poland and the country's largest city. Polish rulers resided at Wawel Castle. The royal court moved to Warsaw in 1609, after parliamentary sessions and the election of kings began to take place there. Until the collapse of the First Republic, however, Krakow continued to be regarded as the official capital. Deprived of its former status Krakow suffered a deep crisis in the 18th and 19th centuries.

Despite all the past upheavals, Krakow has retained its magnificence. It is more than 400 years since Krakow ceased to be the seat of national government, and yet the city maintains its leading role in preserving Polish national identity. Wawel, the seat of Polish kings, the Cathedral that bore witness to their coronations and houses their tombs, as well as the Paulite Church "On the Rock" in whose crypt prominent Poles are buried, belong to the most treasured national heritage. The 600-year-old Jagiellonian University, formerly known as the Academy of Krakow, is the oldest and one of the most important universities in the

country and a pillar of Polish culture. Bearing in mind the small population of Krakow (approximately 760,000), visitors may be surprised by the great number of theatres, cabarets, concert halls and art galleries, which are always popular with regular audiences.

Polish historic cities suffered badly during World War II. Luckily, Krakow's losses were minimal. For those interested in old Polish art, Krakow, with its rich heritage, is certainly the place to go. For many years Krakow's architectural treasures were in a state of neglect, hidden beneath peeling plaster, cracking paint and layers of dirt caused by pollution, although many buildings have now been renovated and returned to their former splendour.

Krakow is different from some other large European towns in which historic inner cities have been transformed into open-air museums. The medieval Market Square remains at the heart of today's city. It is the venue for some of the most important events and the traditional meeting place for locals and visitors alike, all of whom enjoy Krakow's unique atmosphere and heritage.

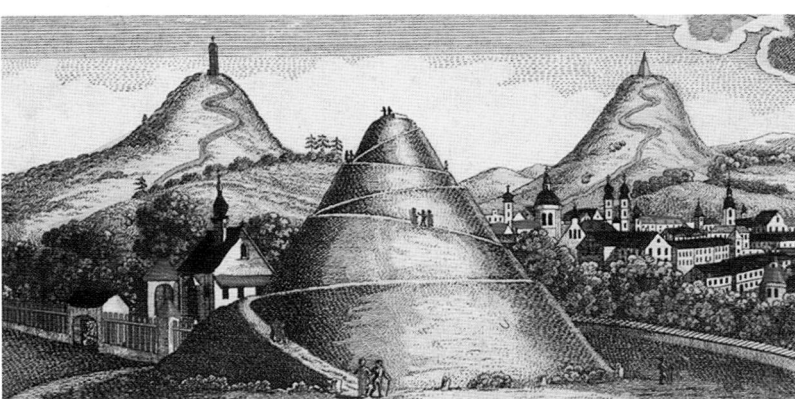

View of Krakow with the Kościuszko Mound (in the foreground), a 19th-century lithograph, Museum of Krakow

◀ *Kościuszko's Defeat against the Russian-Prussian Force at Maciejowice in October 1794* by R. Weibezahl

Krakow's Origins

Krakow is one of the oldest cities in Poland. The archaeological findings provide evidence of a Palaeolithic settlement, as well as those from the Neolithic period, and the Bronze and Iron Ages. The Celtic people and invaders from the east, namely the Scythians and Huns, also left important artifacts. In the early centuries AD Krakow and Lesser Poland bordered and traded with the Roman Empire. Written accounts date only from the 9th century and pertain to the Vistulan settlers who, by the end of the same century, came under the rule of the Great Moravian Empire. The Polish rulers from the House of Piast regained power only at the end of the rule of Mieszko I (around 992).

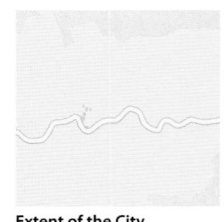

Extent of the City
▨ AD 1000   ▢ Today

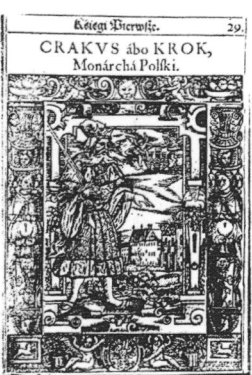

An imaginary view of Wawel Castle

The cave in Wawel Hill

King Krak
The legendary founder of Krakow is believed to have lived in the early 8th century.

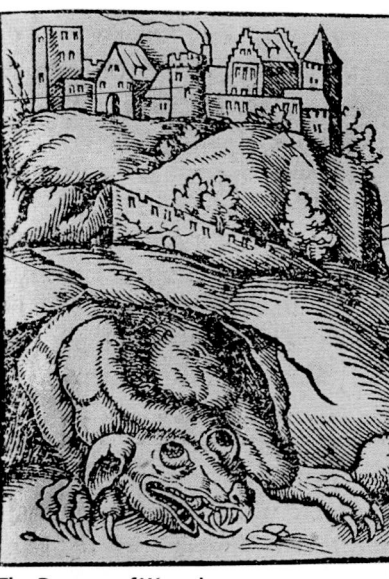

The Dragon of Wawel
This woodcut comes from Sebastian Münster's Cosmographia universalis *of 1544 and shows the legendary dragon and his slayer, the cobbler Skuba, below Wawel Castle.*

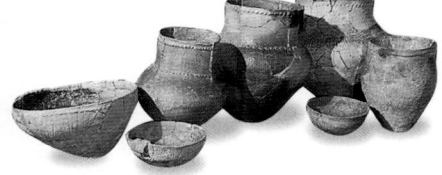

Earthenware with String Ornaments
These earthenware containers were among the 1st-century artifacts excavated at Nowa Huta while constructing the new town.

c. 200,000 BC Earliest evidence of settlements in the Krakow area

c. 1300 BC Lusatian culture flourishes in Lesser Poland

Palaeolithic stone tool

200, 000 BC	20000	0	AD 200

c. 50,000 BC Evidence of a settlement on Wawel Hill

1st – 4th century AD Krakow settlers trade with the Roman Empire

Saints Cyril and Methodius
Methodius and his brother Cyril are two of the three Patrons of Europe. The former failed in his attempt to convert the prince of the Vistulans from paganism to Christianity. Soon after, their land was conquered by the Great Moravian Empire.

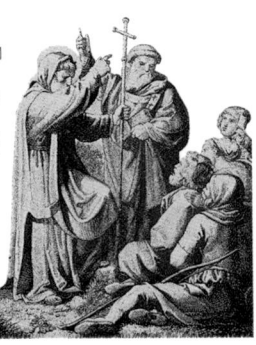

Wawel means a hill surrounded by marshes

Where to See Prehistoric Krakow

Very little has survived from prehistoric times in Krakow. There are, however, two mounds worth a visit: the Krak Mound dominating the southern quarters, and the Wanda Mound near Mogiła village. The Archaeological Museum *(see p85)* houses many interesting artifacts from southern Poland, and the Krakow region in particular. The figure of the four-faced pagan idol Światowid is of special interest.

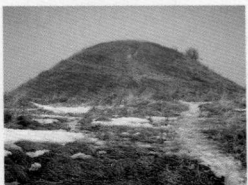

The Krak Mound contains, according to legend, a tomb of Krak, the ancient ruler of Krakow. In reality it was more likely to have been used as a religious site of the Celts.

Iron Treasures
Iron objects in the form of elongated axes found at Wawel Hill were used as a form of payment in the 11th century.

Światowid
This statue represents a four-faced idol holding a cornucopia. Evidence of ancient pagan cults has been found at the Wawel and other sites.

600–1000 Vistulans establish their state, possibly with Krakow as the capital

965 Ibrahim Ibn Yaqub, an Arab traveller, comments on Krakow as a Czech city

| 400 | 600 | 800 | 1000 |

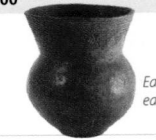

Early medieval earthenware vase

before 885 The Vistulans' state loses its independence. Krakow becomes part of the Great Moravian Empire

before 992 Mieszko I adds the former state of the Vistulans to his other territories

Krakow in the Early Middle Ages

Following the establishment of the bishopric in 1000 and the construction of the cathedral, Krakow became one of the most important centres of the Polish state. After the destruction of other centres in Lesser Poland (Małopolska) by the Czechs in the first half of the 11th century, Kazimierz the Restorer and his successors made Krakow their main seat. Following the death of Bolesław the Wrymouthed Poland was divided into duchies, and the Dukes of Krakow gained suzerain position. From 1138 to 1320 the dukes aimed to unite the remaining provinces. Despite the Tatar invasion in 1241, this period saw Krakow flourish.

Extent of the City
1253   Today

Bishop Stanisław in prayer

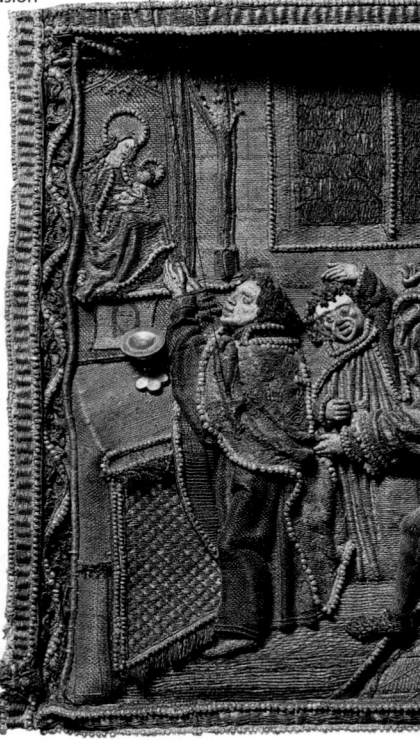

Szczerbiec
According to legend this is the sword of Bolesław the Brave with which he struck the Golden Gate of Kiev on entering the city in 1018. The sword was actually made in the 13th century. Today it is housed in the Crown Treasury as one of the most treasured regalia.

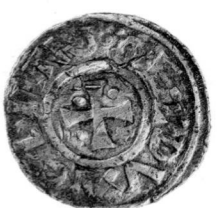

Denarius of Bolesław the Brave
Following the establishment of Krakow's bishopric in 1000, Bolesław made this city one of his seats.

c. 1038 Kazimierz the Restorer makes Krakow the capital of Poland

1000 Bishopric of Krakow established

1079–98 Construction of St Andrew's Church

c. 1044 Benedictine Abbey at Tyniec is established

1090–1142 Construction of second Cathedral at Wawel

| 1000 | 1025 | 1050 | 1075 | 1100 | 1125 |

1020 Construction of first Cathedral in Krakow begins

1079 Martyrdom of St Stanisław

Coat of arms of the Chapter of Krakow

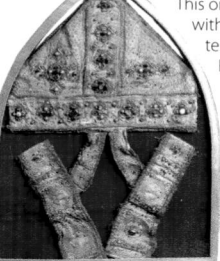

The Supposed Mitre of St Stanisław
This ornate 13th-century mitre decorated with pearls, sapphires and rubies testifies to the riches of metropolitan Krakow, one of the most important bishoprics in medieval Poland.

King Bolesław the Bold

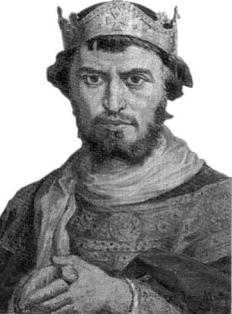

Kazimierz the Restorer
after Jan Matejko
It can be said that Krakow owes its capital status to this ruler, who settled here around 1038 and established a central administration.

Where to See Romanesque Krakow

Krakow is rich in Romanesque architecture. Most buildings have survived in their original form, though they have often been enlarged and refurbished. The Church of St Andrew *(see pp80–81)* dates from this period, as does St Adalbert's *(see p99)* and the remains of the earliest buildings at Wawel, including the Rotunda of the Virgin Mary *(see p65)* and the little Church of the Holy Redeemer *(see p170)*.

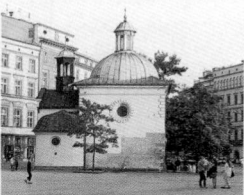

The Church of St Adalbert was, according to legend, consecrated by Adalbert before his missionary journey to Prussia in 997.

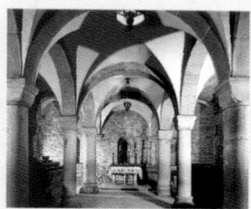

The Crypt of St Leonard is a remnant of Krakow's second cathedral. It was built by Władysław Herman between 1090 and 1142.

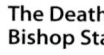

The Death of Bishop Stanisław

The conflict between Bishop Stanisław of Szczepanów (later canonized) and Bolesław the Bold ended with the murder of the bishop in 1079 and the exile of the king. Both events contributed to the weakening of Poland. The cult of St Stanisław began in the 15th century. This scene decorates a 16th-century chasuble (priest's vestment) commissioned by Piotr Kmita.

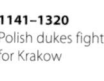

1138 Bolesław the Wrymouthed grants Krakow the status of a capital of the suzerain province

1173 Bolesław the Curly is the first Piast to be buried at Wawel

1241 Tatars led by Batuhan destroy Krakow

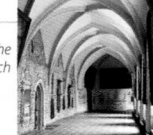

Cloister at the Dominican Church

1150	1175	1200	1225	1250

1141–1320
Polish dukes fight for Krakow

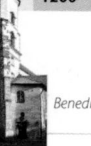

Benedictine Abbey at Tyniec

1250 Consecration of the Dominican Church

Gothic Krakow

The Charter granted to Krakow in 1257 facilitated urban development and allowed for a new and more structured plan. A Gothic defence wall surrounded the city, and Krakow began to flourish anew following the coronation of Władyslaw the Short in 1320. The new satellite towns of Kazimierz and Kleparz both received municipal charters. The architectural panorama of Krakow was substantially transformed by the building of many new churches and the Cathedral in the 14th and 15th centuries. The foundation of the Krakow Academy, and its subsequent renewal, contributed greatly to the development of culture and intellectual activities. The ideas of Italian humanism were known in Krakow early on.

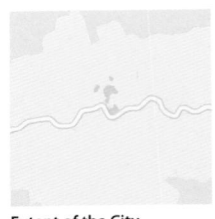

Extent of the City
1370   Today

The coat of arms of the Piasts

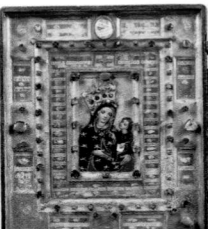 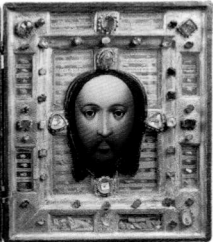

The Diptych Reliquary
A double leaf Gothic reliquary containing the relics of saints is decorated with the image of the Virgin Mary and that of Christ.

Saints Stanisław and Wacław shown standing on the battlement walls are patron saints of Krakow's Cathedral and the Kingdom of Poland.

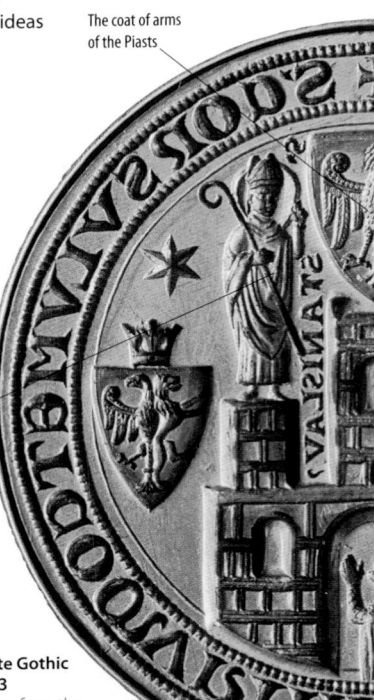

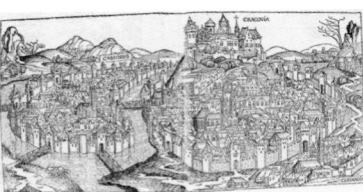

A View of Late Gothic Krakow, 1493
This townscape from the 15th-century *World Chronicle* by Hartmann Schedel is the earliest known view of Krakow.

1285 Construction of Krakow's defence walls begins

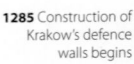

Coat of arms of Kazimierz

1312 Revolt of German burghers, led by Albert

1364 Krakow Academy founded by Kazimierz the Great

1340 Construction of Corpus Christi Church begins

1250	1275	1300	1325	1350

1257 Duke Bolesław the Chaste grants Krakow her Charter on 5 June

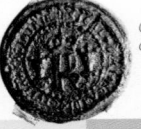

Crown of Kazimierz the Great (replica)

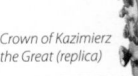

1335 Kazimierz the Great grants Kazimierz its Charter

1366 Kleparz (Florencja) receives its Charter

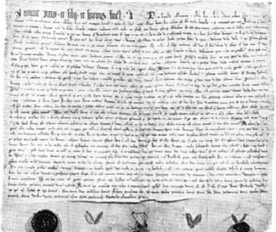

Krakow's Charter
The municipal status granted to Krakow was modelled on the Magdeburg law and contributed to uniform urban development.

Where to See Gothic Krakow

Some of the biggest attractions in Krakow are the Gothic buildings, such as the Barbican (see p116), St Florian's Gate (see p113), the Collegium Maius (see pp108–9), and large churches such as St Mary's (see pp94–5), the Dominican Church (see pp118–19), St Catherine's (see p128) and Corpus Christi (see p125). Some smaller churches, such as the Holy Cross (see p117), are equally interesting. The works by Veit Stoss are gems of Gothic art.

The coats of arms shown on both sides of the gate are those of Bolesław the Chaste who granted Krakow her Charter.

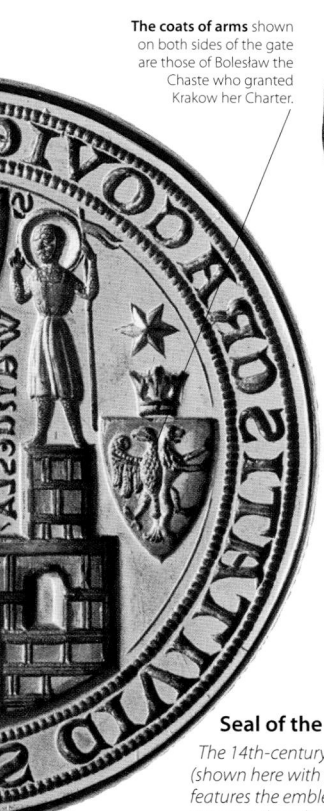

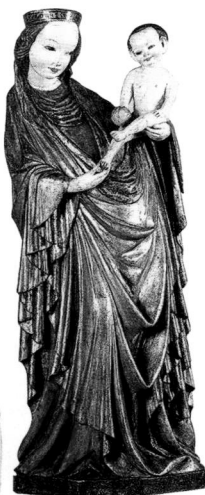

Krużlowa Madonna
This beautiful Madonna with Child is an interesting example of the influence of International Gothic on wood sculpture of Lesser Poland in the 15th century.

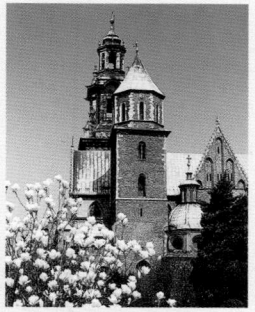

The Cathedral (see pp66–71) is the burial place of kings and the seat of the local archbishop.

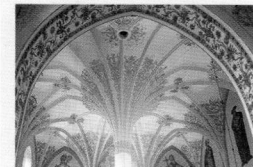

The Church of the Holy Cross has a single nave whose interior is covered with palm vaulting.

Seal of the Royal City of Krakow
The 14th-century Great Seal of Krakow (shown here with the image reversed) features the emblem of Poland, thus stressing the role of Krakow as its capital.

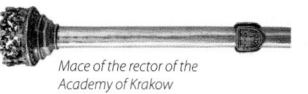

1386 Grand Duke Jogaila of Lithuania becomes King Władysław II Jagiełło of Poland

Mace of the rector of the Academy of Krakow

1473 First Polish printing house of Łukasz Straube issues a calendar

1400	1425	1450	1475	1500

efore 1400 Collegium Maius is established

1400 Władysław Jagiełło reestablishes the Krakow Academy

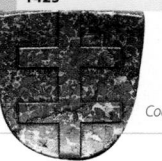

1477–89 Veit Stoss works on the high altar at St Mary's

Coat of arms of the Jagiellonians

1492 Kazimierz Jagiellończyk dies

Renaissance Krakow

Krakow, the capital city, rapidly developed economically and began to change in appearance. The Cloth Hall, the city landmark, was remodelled in the Renaissance style, and the rich merchants of Krakow also began to modernize their houses. The art and culture of the Italian Renaissance was assimilated by the royal courts of King Aleksander and King Zygmunt the Old and his second wife Bona Sforza. Bartolomeo Berrecci, Giovanni Maria Padovano and other outstanding Italian masters established their workshops in Krakow during this time.

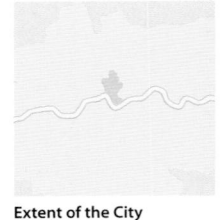

Extent of the City

🟦 1572   ⬜ Today

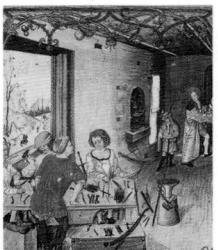

"The Sword Makers" from the Baltazar Behem Codex
This Codex of 1505 contains laws and privileges of the town guilds and is illustrated with 27 illuminations showing craftsmen at work.

Shield with the Polish eagle

Royal sceptre

Royal orb

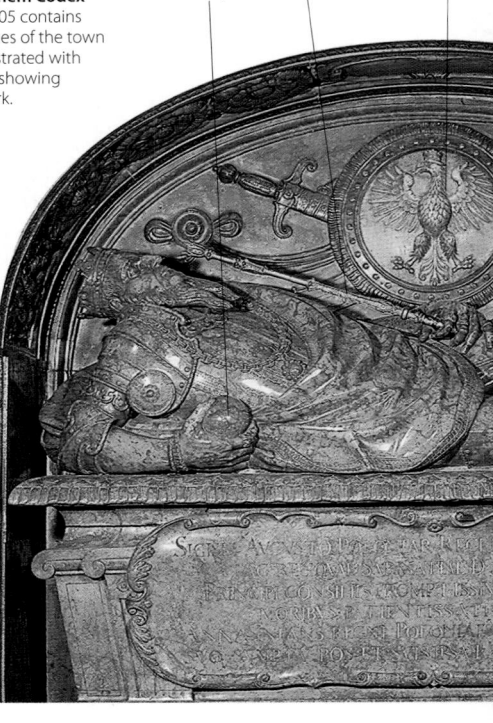

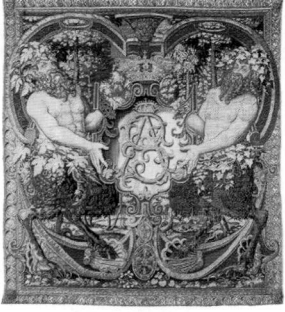

A Tapestry with Satyrs
This is one of 160 tapestries commissioned in the 16th century by Zygmunt August for the Wawel Collection.

1502–5 Erection of King Jan Olbracht's monument, the first work of Renaissance art in Poland

1505 Baltazar Behem Codex made

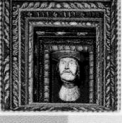
Head in the Hall of Deputies

1525 Homage paid by the Prussians to the Polish King in the Market Square on 10 April

1543 The treatise *De revolutionibus* by Copernicus is published

1500	1510	1520	1530	1540

1504 Rebuilding of the Wawel Castle starts

1513 First Polish book in print from the Ungler House

1521 Zygmunt's Bell is hung

1519 Bartolomeo Berrecci begins work on Zygmunt's Chapel in the Cathedral

NICOLAI CO
PERNICI TORINENSIS
DE REVOLVTIONIBVS ORBI
um cœleſtium, Libri VI.

Detail of the title page from Copernicus's treatise

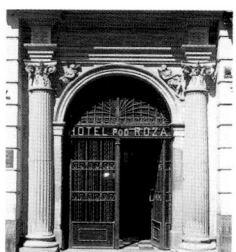

A Renaissance Portal
The first post office in 16th-century Poland, serving the Krakow-Venice route, was situated in the house of Prospero Provana. Today the building houses the Hotel Pod Róża.

Cock of the Marksmen's Brotherhood
This gilt masterpiece, made in 1565, belonged to the members of the Brotherhood whose aim was to support soldiers responsible for the defence of the town.

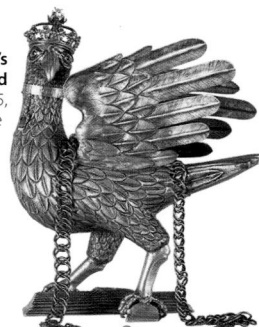

Oval recess
with Renaissance
decoration

Monument of Zygmunt August

King Zygmunt August was a patron of the arts. It was through his commissions that the Royal Castle at Wawel was enriched with an outstanding collection of tapestries. The king's monument was made by Santi Gucci between 1574 and 1575, in Hungarian red marble.

Where to See Renaissance Krakow

Renaissance architecture was introduced by Italian masters during the rebuilding of the Royal Castle at Wawel in the early 16th century. The Zygmunt Chapel (*see pp66–71*), the Montelupis Monument at St Mary's Church (*see pp94–5*) and a number of houses at Kanonicza Street (*see p81*) are among the finest examples of Renaissance art and architecture in the city.

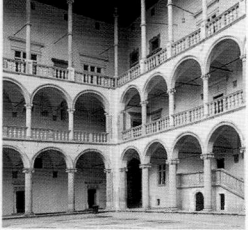

The arcaded courtyard at the Royal Castle at Wawel is one of the most beautiful in Europe (*see pp72–3*).

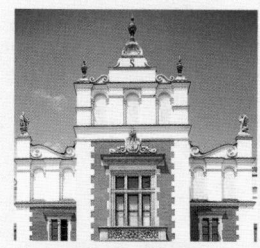

The Renaissance Cloth Hall (*see pp104–5*), topped with a characteristic parapet, displayed the prosperity of Jagiellonian Krakow.

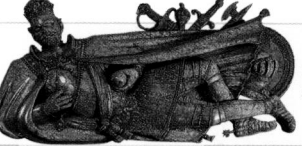

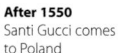

Baroque Krakow

The 17th and 18th centuries saw the decline of Krakow. After the king had moved his residence to Warsaw, he was followed by the noblemen who held high office. Foreign incursions and occupations, wars and the First Partition of Poland in 1772 all added to the city's woes. Despite a number of attempts at reform towards the end of the rule of Stanisław August Poniatowski, Krakow became a provincial, underdeveloped frontier town, though the atmosphere was enlivened by royal coronations and funerals. The failure of the Kościuszko Insurrection of 1794 and the subsequent Third Partition of Poland in 1795 brought an end to Krakow's prominence.

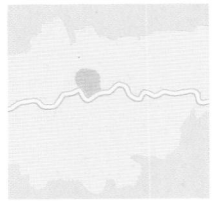

Extent of the City

☐ 1700 ☐ Today

Hood of the 1669 Coronation Cape
The eagle (the emblem of the Commonwealth) on the *cappa magna* of Bishop Tomicki, made for the coronation of Michał Wiśniowiecki, was embroidered with pearls and sapphires.

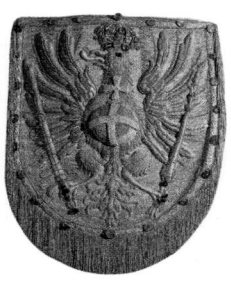

The Evangelists with their symbols: eagle, angel, lion and ox.

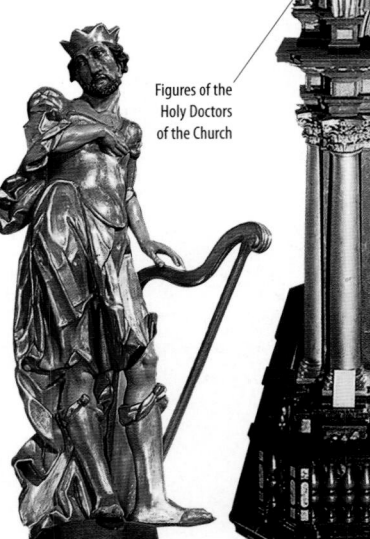

Figures of the Holy Doctors of the Church

Epitaph of King Władysław IV
The monumental and sombre interior of the Vaza Chapel in the Cathedral is decorated with black marble and features splendid memorial plaques of the Vaza dynasty.

King David
This late Baroque dancing figure in the Corpus Christi Church was made by Anton Gegenbaur in the second half of the 18th century.

1626–9 Canopy of St Stanisław is erected in the Cathedral

1619 Church of Saints Peter and Paul is completed

1661 First Polish newspaper "Merkuriusz Polski" published by Jan Alexander Gorczyn's Press

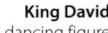

Title page of "Merkuriusz Polski"

1676 University Press is established after the Academy buys Piotrowczyks' Press

1600	1620	1640	1660	1680

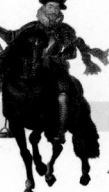

1609 Zygmunt III Vaza finally abandons his Krakow residence in favour of Warsaw on 25 May

Zygmunt III Vaza

1655–7 Swedish, then Transylvanian, armies occupy Krakow

1664–76 Vaza Chapel in the Cathedral is completed

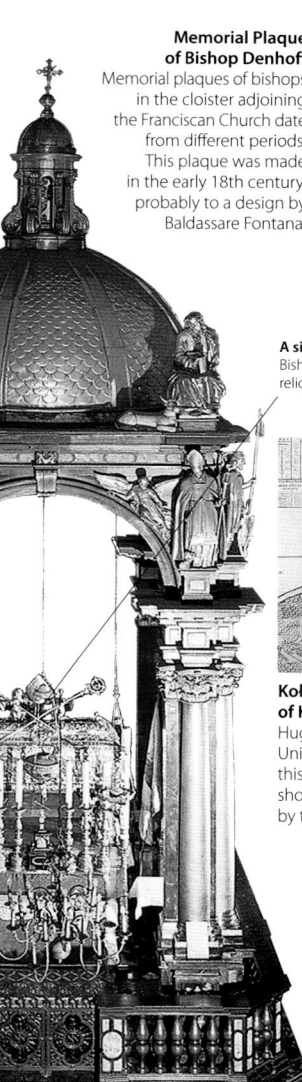

Memorial Plaque of Bishop Denhoff
Memorial plaques of bishops in the cloister adjoining the Franciscan Church date from different periods. This plaque was made in the early 18th century, probably to a design by Baldassare Fontana.

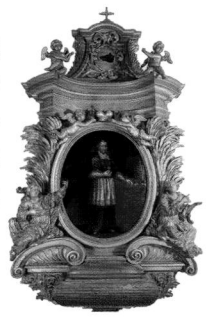

A silver sarcophagus with the Bishop's mitre and crozier is a reliquary of St Stanisław.

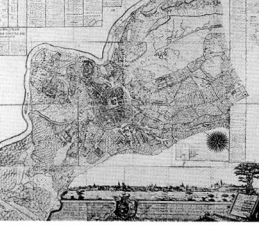

Kołłątaj's Panoramic Map of Krakow
Hugo Kołłątaj led the reform of the University. In 1785 he also created this precise map of Krakow, which shows all the land owned by the city.

Canopy of St Stanisław
This canopy in the Wawel Cathedral was inspired by a number of unexecuted designs for the great baldachin in St Peter's in the Vatican.

Where to See Baroque Krakow

The earliest Baroque church, that was dedicated to Saints Peter and Paul (see pp82–3), as well as much later churches including St Anne's (see pp110–11) and the Church of the Order of St John of God (see p128), represent the best of Baroque architecture from Tylman von Gameren and Kacper Bażanka, among others.

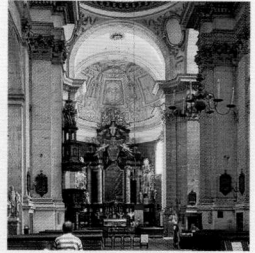

The Church of Saints Peter and Paul is one of the finest early Baroque churches in Central Europe.

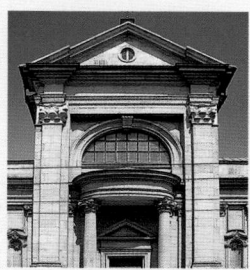

The façade of the Church of the Missionaries (see p87) was inspired by Roman Baroque architecture, in particular by the work of Bernini and Borromini.

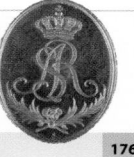

Medal of Virtuti Militari

1734 Coronation of August III Wettin, the last to take place in Krakow, on 17 January

1791 Kazimierz and Kleparz are incorporated into Krakow

1794 Tadeusz Kościuszko takes his oath in the Market Square on 24 March

1768–72 Confederates of Bar fight for Krakow

1700	1720	1740	1760	1780	1800

1705 St Anne's Church is consecrated

1702–05 Krakow is invaded several times by the Swedes

1777–8 Hugo Kołłątaj reforms the Krakow Academy

1788 Astronomical Observatory established

1798 First permanent theatre building established in Krakow

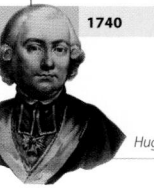

Hugo Kołłątaj

Krakow in Galicia

In 1772 Austria occupied the southern part of Poland, called Galicia. After a period of Austrian occupation, Krakow was briefly incorporated into the Duchy of Warsaw. The Russian occupation followed. In 1815 the Republic of Krakow, which included the area round the city, was established, but by 1846 Krakow was under Austrian rule again. After a period of suppression, Galicia received extensive autonomy from the 1860s onwards. During the 19th century Krakow was the only Polish territory to enjoy relative freedom. It embarked upon a mission of safeguarding traditions and past historic successes, thus becoming the spiritual capital of Poland.

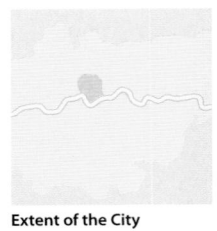

Extent of the City

▨ 1818 ▢ Today

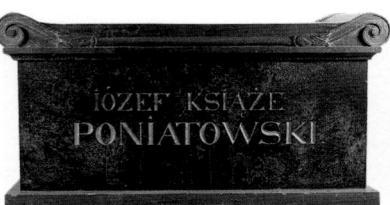

Sarcophagus of Prince Józef Poniatowski
Of all the famous Poles who died abroad, Józef Poniatowski was the first to have his body brought back to receive a solemn funeral, which transformed itself into a patriotic demonstration.

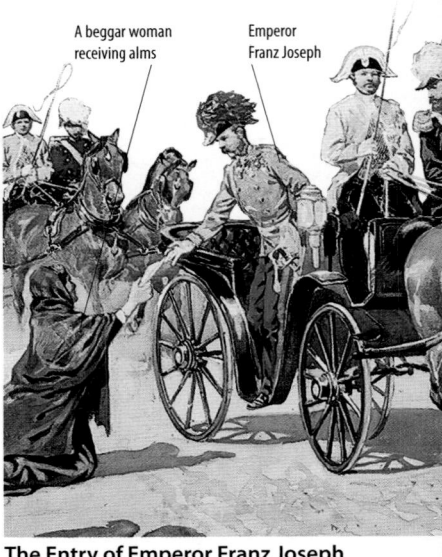

A beggar woman receiving alms

Emperor Franz Joseph

***The Opening of the Sarcophagus of Kazimierz the Great* by Jan Matejko**
An accidental discovery of the remains of the king prompted his second funeral in 1869, which became an event on a national scale, reminiscent of the glorious past.

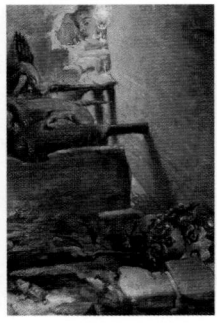

The Entry of Emperor Franz Joseph in 1880

Franz Joseph was a popular ruler with the people of Krakow. He was believed to be behind the development of the city and its autonomy. A series of watercolours by Juliusz Kossak (1824–99), such as this one, depicts his stay in Krakow.

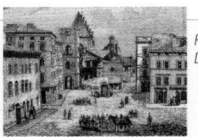

1800 Royal Castle at Wawel made into army barracks

1813–15 Krakow occupied by the Austrians

Ruins of the fire-damaged Dominican Church

1846 Krakow Uprising. Krakow becomes part of Austria

1800	1810	1820	1830	1840

1809 Krakow incorporated into the Duchy of Warsaw

1820–3 Kościuszko Mound constructed

1815 "Free, independent and strictly neutral city of Krakow" and her region established as the Republic of Krakow

1810–14 City walls demolished

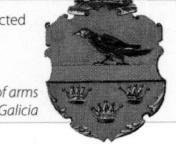

Coat of arms of Galicia

House of Jan Matejko
Jan Matejko, whose particular genre of history painting imprinted in the nation's mind an image of its past, lived in this house *(see p116)*.

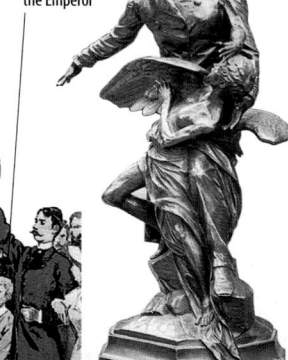

Inhabitants of Krakow greeting the Emperor

Where to See 19th-Century Krakow

The architecture of Krakow in the 19th century was eclectic. The Renaissance Revival style predominated (for example the Academy of Fine Arts, *see p138*), and was often influenced by the monumental architecture of Vienna, the place where many of Krakow's architects trained. The University buildings are a good example of Gothic Revival in which the historic style is blended with vernacular features.

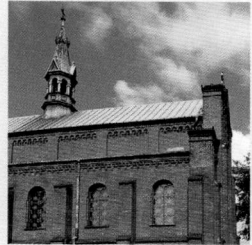

The Church of the Felician Nuns is one of the few buildings in the Romanesque Revival style *(see p146)*.

Design for the Mickiewicz Monument
This model by Antoni Kurzawa was never fully executed. It is held at the National Museum in Krakow.

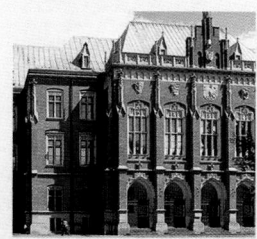

The Collegium Novum is a prestigious Gothic Revival building designed by Feliks Księżarski *(see p106)*.

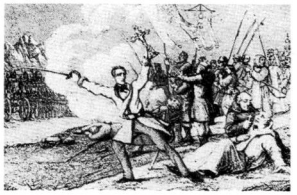

The Krakow Uprising
The uprising of 1846 was intended to spark a revolt in all parts of partitioned Poland, but was suppressed by the Austrians.

1866 Local government established in Krakow with Józef Dietl as Mayor

1872 Academy of Skills established

1876 Czartoryski Collection opens to the public

1854 Society of Friends of Fine Arts established

1883–7 Collegium Novum built

| 1850 | 1860 | 1870 | 1880 | 1890 |

1850 Great fire of Krakow

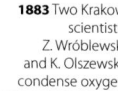

Apparatus for condensing oxygen

1883 Two Krakow scientists, Z. Wróblewski and K. Olszewski, condense oxygen

1893 Słowacki Theatre opens

Modernist Krakow

At the end of the 19th century Greater Krakow was established and became a place of mass excursions from other parts of occupied Poland. People came to see the newly re-established University and the repossessed Wawel, which was then undergoing restoration. It was the period of "art for art's sake", and Krakow became a mecca for Polish artists. Modern life concentrated around artistic cafés, such as the Paon and the Jama Michalika, which were also venues for cabarets. The latter café housed the Zielony Balonik Cabaret. The ambience in Krakow was one of melancholy and decadence but life, permeated by patriotic Neo-Romantic symbolism, was lived here to the full. The outbreak of World War I put an end to this unique bohemian era.

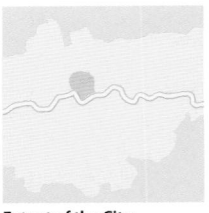

Extent of the City

☐ 1900   ☐ Today

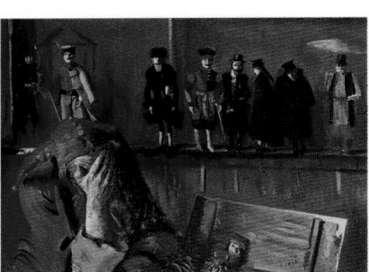

Stańczyk
This painting by Leon Wyczółkowski portrays the court jester, Stańczyk, in pensive mood, playing with marionettes of historic Polish characters.

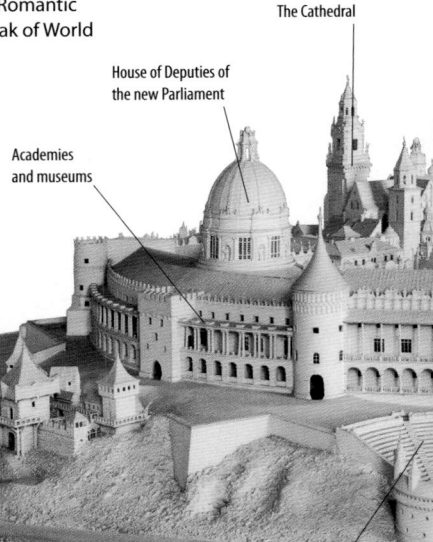

The Cathedral

House of Deputies of the new Parliament

Academies and museums

An amphitheatre modelled on the Barbican in Krakow

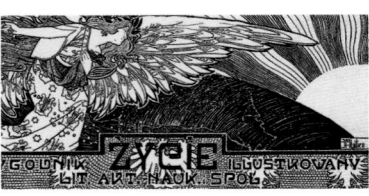

"Życie"
This is the masthead of the magazine of the Polish Modernist movement. The contributors were the leading authors of the time.

1897 "Życie" weekly is established

1898 Stanisław Przybyszewski arrives in Krakow

1901 Palace of Art, the seat of the Society of Friends of the Fine Arts, is built

1903–5 Old Theatre (Teatr Stary) rebuilt in the Art Nouveau style

1895	1897	1899	1901	1903	1905

1895 Adam Mickiewicz's statue is unveiled

1898–1900 Stanisław Wyspiański decorates the Franciscan Church with murals and stained glass

1901 Premiere of *The Wedding* by Stanisław Wyspiański

Wyspiański's Art Nouveau murals in the Franciscan Church

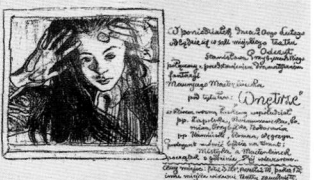

Poster by Stanisław Wyspiański
This poster announces a lecture by S. Przybyszewski followed by a play by M. Maeterlinck.

Where to See Modernist Krakow

Modernist Krakow was, above all, a city of literature and painting. Architecture from this period is scarce. There are, however, some magnificent buildings, such as the spider House "Pod pająkiem" (see p153) and the Palace of Art (see p107). Art Nouveau interiors of exceptional beauty can be found at the Franciscan Church with its stained glass and murals, designed by Wyspiański (see pp88–9), the Society of Physicians building (see p134) and the prestigious former Museum of Industry and Technology (see p145).

Marionettes from the Zielony Balonik Cabaret
This cabaret and New Year's satirical show, staged by Karol Frycz, ridiculed the narrow-mindedness and hypocrisy of the Krakovians.

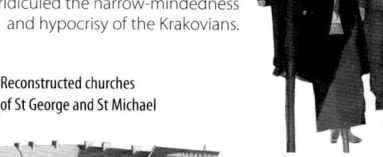

Reconstructed churches of St George and St Michael

Stadium modelled on Roman architecture

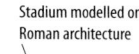

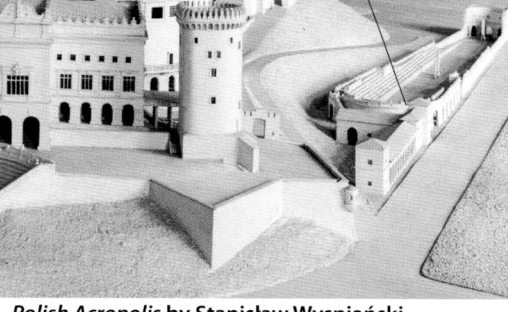

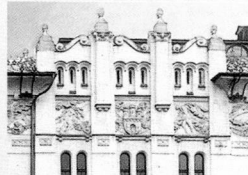

During the rebuilding of the Old Theatre (Teatr Stary) in the Art Nouveau style its façade was decorated with a stucco floral frieze (see p107).

Polish Acropolis **by Stanisław Wyspiański**
The idea behind this design for the rebuilding of the entire Wawel Hill was to transform the Royal Castle into a political, social, academic and cultural centre of the liberated Poland. Its architecture was intended to reflect a synthesis of Polish history.

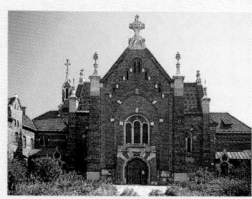

The façade of the Church of the Discalced Carmelite Nuns, with its elaborate decoration, is in sharp contrast to its austere interior.

1906 Krakow sports clubs, Wisła and Cracovia, established

1907 Stanisław Wyspiański dies

1910 Riflemen's Union formed by Józef Piłsudski

1912 First cinema opens in Krakow

A late 19th-century armchair

1907	1909	1911	1913	1915

1906 Building of the Chamber of Commerce and Industry completed

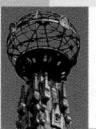

1910 Grunwald Monument unveiled

The sphere at the top of the Chamber of Commerce and Industry Building

1914 First Cadre Brigade of the Polish Legions marches out of Krakow on 6 August

Krakow in the Years 1918–1945

When World War I ended in 1918, Poland regained its independence after 123 years of foreign occupation. In the period between the two World Wars Krakow became a source for political, administrative and army staff for the whole of the Republic of Poland. Above all the city was a cultural and academic centre. The Modernist traditions were still present in the arts but soon gave way to a new generation of artists, such as the Formists, Capists (the Polish variant of Post-Impressionists), the avant-garde Krakow Group and the Cricot Theatre. During World War II the German Governor General had his headquarters in Krakow, and this was reason enough for the city to be spared destruction.

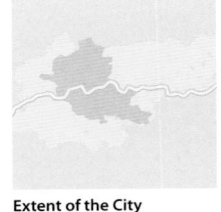

Extent of the City
☐ 1938   ☐ Today

Józef Piłsudski
The Commander by Konrad Krzyżanowski portrays well the personality and character of this uncompromising Polish soldier and politician.

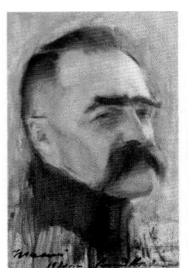

Kościuszko Mound

Marshal Józef Piłsudski

Tribune

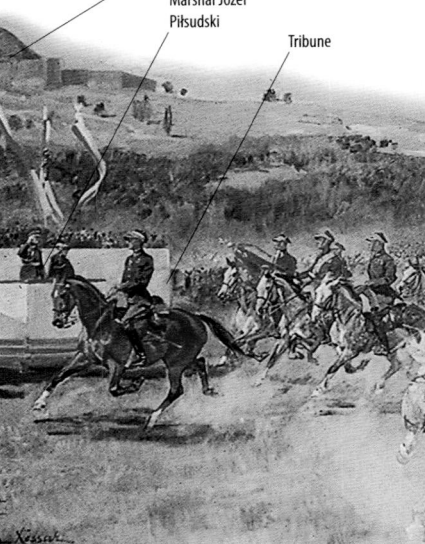

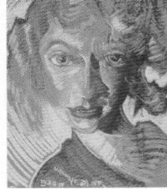

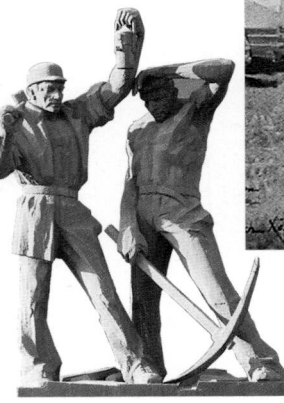

Portrait of Nena Stachurska
This portrait is by S. I. Witkiewicz, who was one of the most unconventional artists of the 20th century. He called for the utopian ideal of "pure art".

Figures decorating the Academy of Mines and Metallurgy Building
The first school of its type in liberated Poland was established to educate specialists for the industry in Silesia.

1918 Austrian Army disarmed in Krakow. Polish Liquidation Commission created on 31 October

1925 Tomb of the Unknown Soldier blessed

1923 Workers' unrest in Krakow

Jagiellonian Library

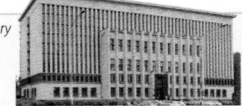

1918	1921	1924	1927	1930

1919 Academy of Mines and Metallurgy established

1921 Jesuit Church at Wesoła consecrated

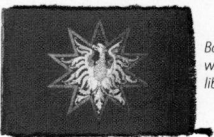

Banner which was raised in liberated Krakow

1927 Juliusz Słowacki's remains brought to Krakow and buried at Wawel

1930–9 Jagiellonian Library completed

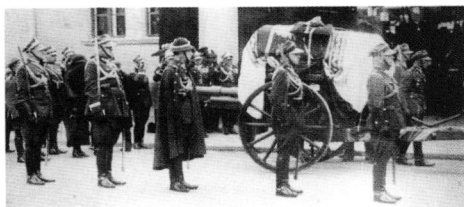

Funeral of Marshal Piłsudski
The funeral of the Commander, who was buried at Wawel in 1935, was the biggest state event in interwar Poland.

Demolition of Mickiewicz's Statue
During the German occupation all monuments of importance were demolished, including those of Mickiewicz, Kościuszko and Grunwald.

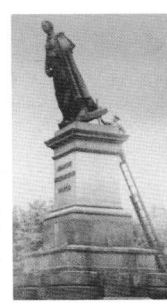

Auschwitz (Oświęcim)

The name Oświęcim may have little meaning for most foreigners but the German name, Auschwitz, raises the spectre of death. During World War II the Nazis established Auschwitz *(see pp162–3)* and the nearby Birkenau (Brzezinka) *(see pp164–5)* concentration camps. Nearly 1.5 million people were put to death in these camps. The Auschwitz camp was set up in 1940 to subject Poles to terror and extermination. Before long the Nazis rounded up and transported people from the whole of Europe, and from 1942 Auschwitz and Birkenau became the largest extermination camps for Jews. A cynical inscription over the gate leading into the Auschwitz camp reads *"Arbeit macht frei"* ("Work makes you free").

It was in the Auschwitz Death Block that Maksymilian Kolbe, a Franciscan priest, gave up his life for another inmate. Kolbe (who was later canonized) was sentenced to death by starvation.

In the old barracks of Auschwitz there is an exhibition telling the history of the camp *(see pp162–3)*. Temporary displays are also organized. In Brzezinka, 3 km (1.8 miles) away, only some of the original 300 barracks remain, along with the loading platform. New prisoners were unloaded from railway wagons and segregated here.

The Cavalry Parade
The parade of the cavalry of the Second Republic took place at Błonie on 6 October 1933. Wojciech Kossak, member of a distinguished Krakow family of artists, painted this grand event.

A military band gallops at the head of the troops.

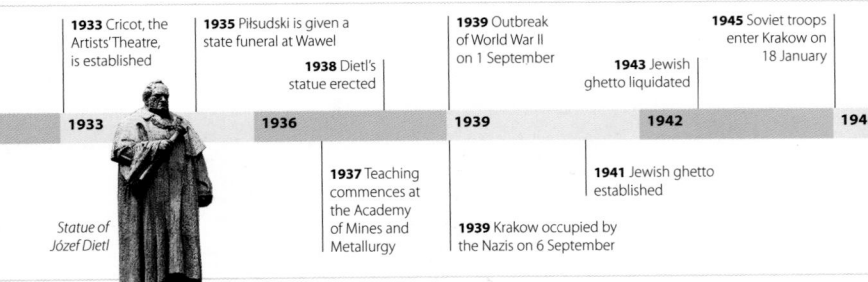

1933 Cricot, the Artists' Theatre, is established

1935 Piłsudski is given a state funeral at Wawel

1938 Dietl's statue erected

1939 Outbreak of World War II on 1 September

1943 Jewish ghetto liquidated

1945 Soviet troops enter Krakow on 18 January

| 1933 | 1936 | 1939 | 1942 | 1945 |

1937 Teaching commences at the Academy of Mines and Metallurgy

1941 Jewish ghetto established

Statue of Józef Dietl

1939 Krakow occupied by the Nazis on 6 September

Krakow after 1945

After World War II ended Krakow did not willingly accept the new Soviet-imposed regime. In 1946 the celebrations of the 3 May Constitution turned into clashes with tragic consequences. Many Krakovians claim that the industrial suburb of Nowa Huta, with its immense steelworks *(see p156)*, was built to "punish" the city for rejecting the 1946 Communist referendum. In fact, the site was chosen because of good rail links, proximity to the river, and Krakow's engineering and scientific heritage. It is also false to claim that pollution from Nowa Huta was meant to damage Krakow's ancient monuments. Krakow's problem with air quality is largely the result of domestic heating furnaces and vehicle fumes.

Tadeusz Sendzimir Steelworks
Formerly known as the Lenin Steelworks, the mills were expected to become a bastion of the Communist proletariat. Paradoxically, they became one of the main centres of opposition.

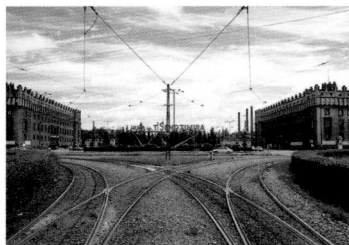

Banner of the Vatican

Papal high altar

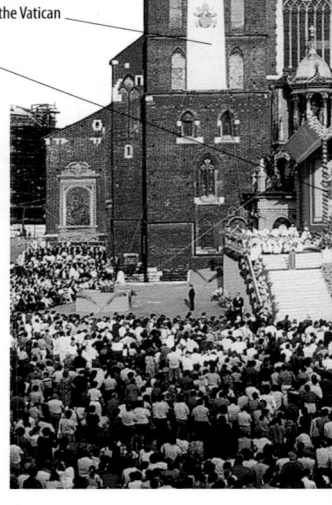

Holy Mass during the Pope's Visit

The political transformation of Poland which took place after 1989 was welcomed in Krakow. The Mass celebrated in 1991 by Pope John Paul II in Market Square attracted unprecedented numbers of worshippers.

Mistrzejowice Church
Built between 1976 and 1983, the church was decorated with sculptures by Gustaw Zemła.

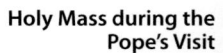

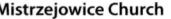

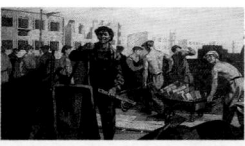

1946 Bloody suppression of 3 May celebrations	*Builders' Brigade by H. Krajewska*		**1967** Construction of the Ark of God Church in Nowa Huta begins	**1978** Krakow included in the UNESCO World Heritage List	**1980** Solidarity established
	1956 Piwnica pod Baranami Cabaret established				

1945	1950	1955	1960	1965	1970	1975	1980

	1950 Nowa Huta becomes a borough of Krakow	**1957** Celebrations of the city of Krakow's 700th anniversary	**1964** 600th anniversary of the Academy of Krakow	**1978** Karol Wojtyła, the Metropolitan of Krakow, elected as Pope John Paul II
1949 Construction of Nowa Huta begins	**1956** Cricot 2 Theatre established		*John Paul II*	

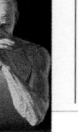

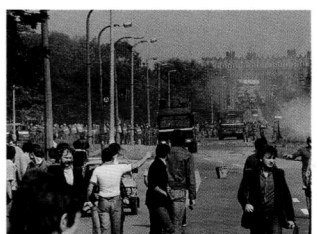

Demonstrations in Nowa Huta
During the period of martial law, street demonstrations in the workers' suburb of Nowa Huta often ended in riots.

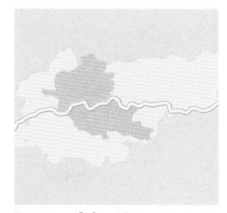

Extent of the City
■ 1945   □ Today

Nobel Prize for Wisława Szymborska
The Krakow poet was awarded the 1996 Nobel Prize for Literature.

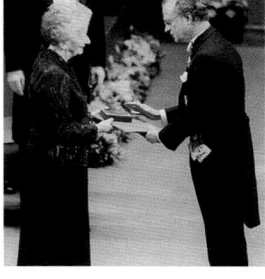

St Mary's Church

Polish banner

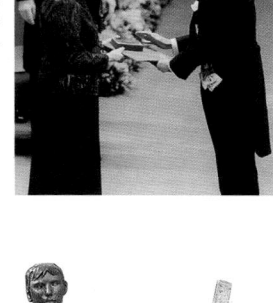

Where to see Modern Krakow

Very few postwar buildings in Krakow deserve notice. However, some examples of ecclesiastical architecture, namely the Abbey of the Fathers of the Resurrection designed by Dariusz Kozłowski, and two churches in Nowa Huta – the Ark of God and Mistrzejowice Church, are exceptional. An extensive programme of building renovation in old Krakow has been undertaken. Completed projects include the Krakow Arena and the Krakow Congress Centre, the latter opposite Wawel Hill.

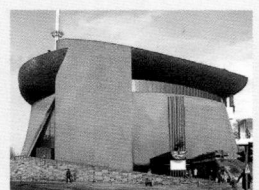

The Ark of God Church in Nowa Huta *(see p156) is an example of modern ecclesiastical architecture, rich in impressive forms and symbolic content.*

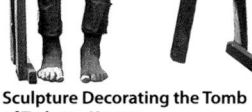

Sculpture Decorating the Tomb of Tadeusz Kantor
The theatre of Tadeusz Kantor (1915–90) had a Polish, as well as a European, dimension. This sculpture on his tomb was originally designed for his play *Wielopole, Wielopole*.

1981 Martial law declared in Poland on 13 December (lifted on 22 July 1983)	**1991** International Cultural Centre established **1992** European Month of Culture celebrations take place in Krakow in June	**1996** Wisława Szymborska is awarded the Nobel Prize for Literature		**2005** Pope John Paul II dies in Rome	**2010** A plane crash kills President Lech Kaczyński and his wife; Bronisław Komorowski elected president of Poland		

1985	1990	1995	2000	2005	2010	2015	2020

1981 Citizens Committee for the Rescue of Krakow established

1993 Czesław Miłosz, the winner of the Nobel Prize for Literature, becomes an honorary citizen of Krakow

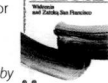

A book by Czesław Miłosz

2004 Poland joins the European Union

2014 Canonization of Pope John Paul II

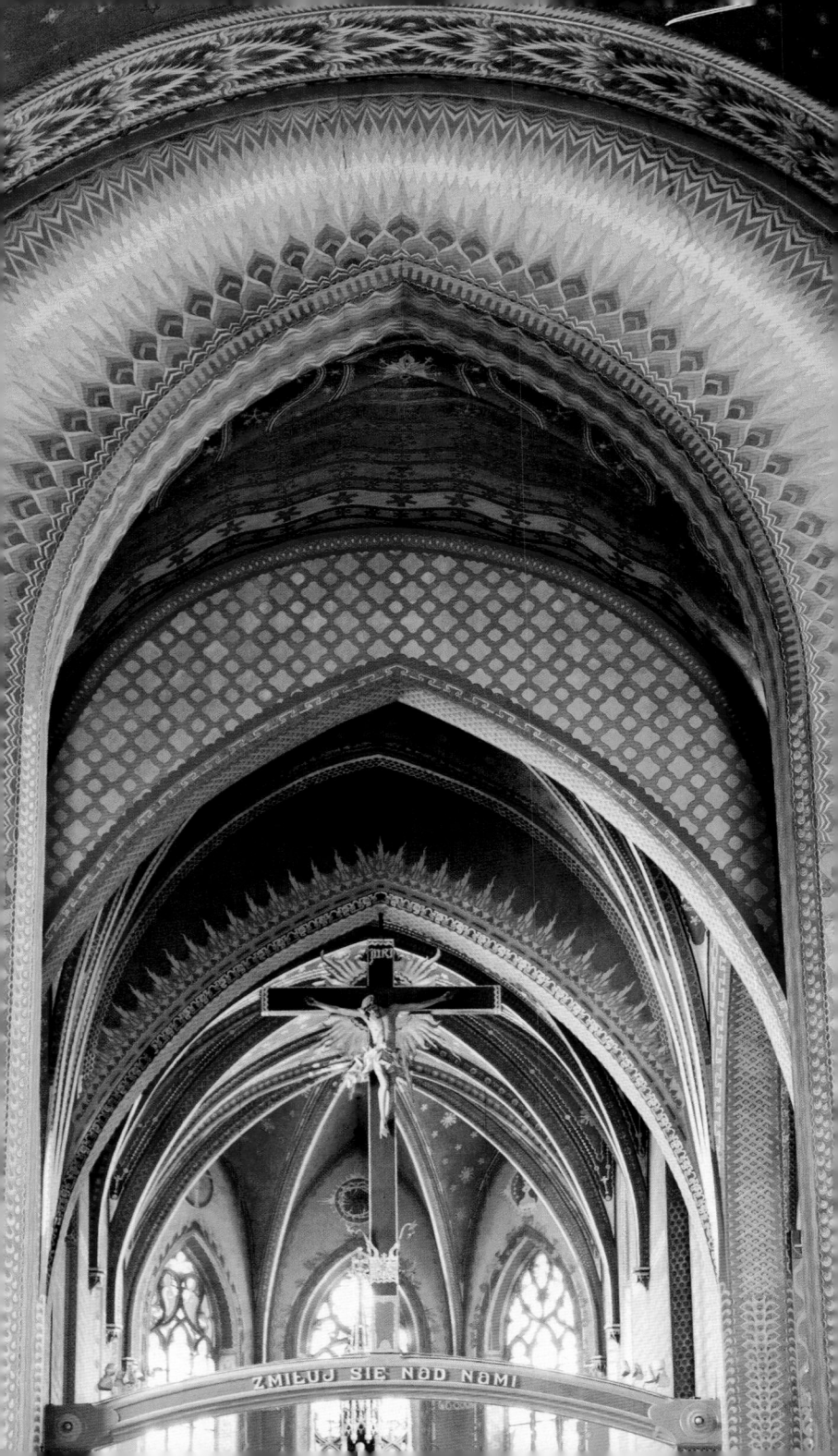

KRAKOW AT A GLANCE

Krakow was one of the few Polish cities to be saved from major destruction during many wars which devastated the country. The city has preserved not only its monuments but also a specific "antiquarian" atmosphere. Already in the 19th century Krakow was a destination for tourists from other countries as well as different parts of Poland. Krakow and Wieliczka were included on the very first UNESCO World Heritage List. The section *Krakow Area by Area* describes many places of interest. To help make the most of your stay, the following 12 pages are a guide to the best Krakow has to offer. Each sight has a cross-reference to its own full entry. Below are the top ten tourist attractions to start you off. Take a journey back in time and enjoy sites of historic interest and beauty.

Krakow's Top Ten Tourist Attractions

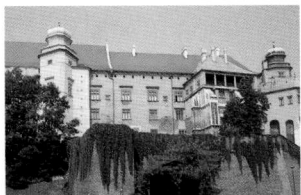

Royal Castle Wawel
See pp72–5.

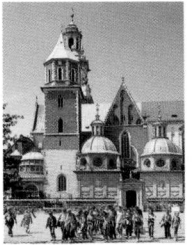

Krakow Cathedral
See pp66–71.

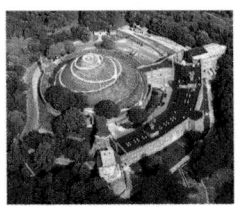

Kościuszko Mound
See p171.

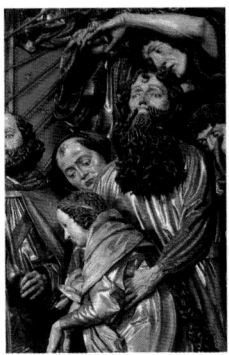

Church of St Mary
See pp94–7.

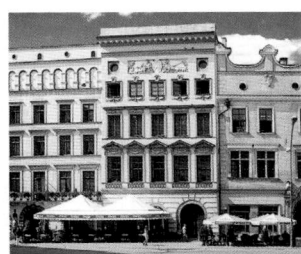

Market Square
See pp100–3.

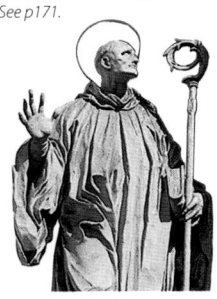

Church of St Anne
See pp110–11.

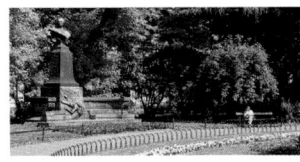

Planty
See pp168–9.

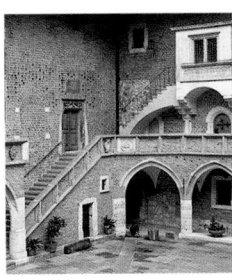

Collegium Maius
See pp108–9.

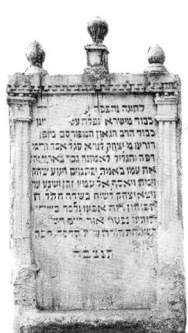

Remu'h Cemetery
See pp124–5.

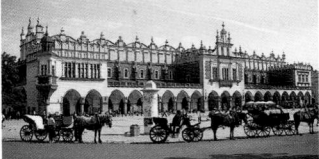

Cloth Hall
See pp104–5.

◀ The splendid Art Nouveau ceiling designed by Stanisław Wyspiański in the Franciscan Church

Krakow's Best: Museums and Galleries

Krakow has dozens of museums, which are very varied in character. The Royal Castle at Wawel is the best known, offering visitors the chance to see collections housed in the royal chambers which date from the time when the Polish kings resided here. The Czartoryski Museum is the best place for Western art. The National Museum has rich collections of Polish art housed in a number of branches in the city centre.

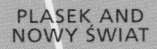

PLASEK AND NOWY ŚWIAT

KARMELICKA

KRUPNICZA

SMOLEŃSK

ZWIERZYNIECKA

F. STRASZEWSKIEGO

Vistula

WAWEL HILL

National Museum in Krakow, Main Building
One of the best collections of 20th-century Polish art is housed here. The collection of Modernist art is particularly rich, and includes excellent sculptures by Konstanty Laszczka.

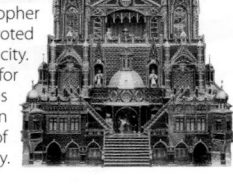

Museum of Krakow
This museum in Christopher Palace is devoted to the history of the city. Krakow is famous for her portable Christmas cribs, and the collection housed here is of great beauty.

Japanese Centre of Art and Technology
This modern building houses a collection of works from the Far East, much of which was donated by Feliks Manggha Jasieński. The *netsuke* (a kind of button) shown takes the form of a tiger.

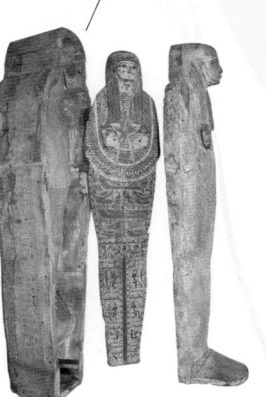

0 metres   500
0 yards   500

Archaeological Museum
Many archaeological finds from the Lesser Poland area, as well as Egyptian mummies, are displayed here.

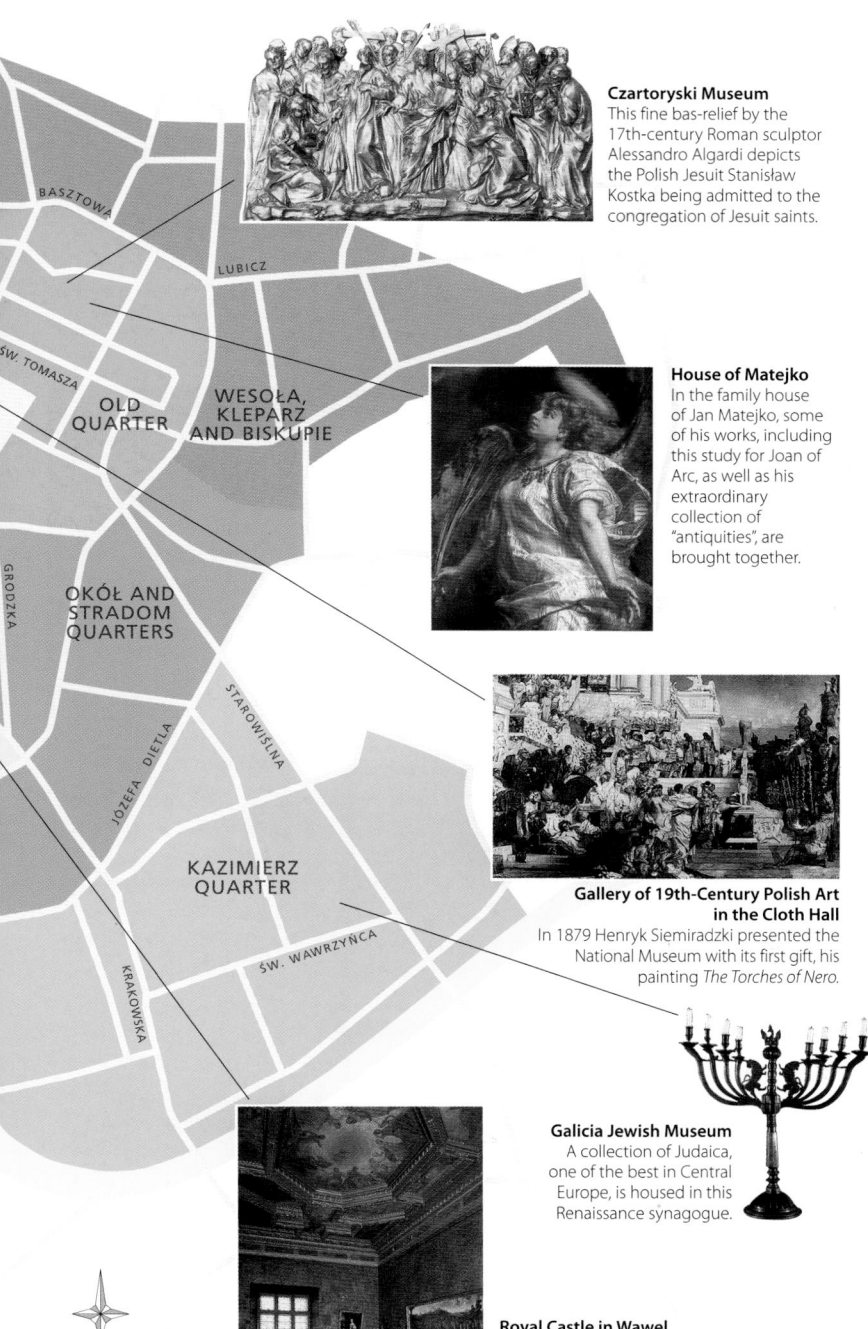

Czartoryski Museum
This fine bas-relief by the 17th-century Roman sculptor Alessandro Algardi depicts the Polish Jesuit Stanisław Kostka being admitted to the congregation of Jesuit saints.

House of Matejko
In the family house of Jan Matejko, some of his works, including this study for Joan of Arc, as well as his extraordinary collection of "antiquities", are brought together.

BASZTOWA

LUBICZ

ŚW. TOMASZA

OLD
QUARTER

WESOŁA,
KLEPARZ
AND BISKUPIE

GRODZKA

OKÓŁ AND
STRADOM
QUARTERS

STAROWIŚLNA

JÓZEFA DIETLA

KAZIMIERZ
QUARTER

**Gallery of 19th-Century Polish Art
in the Cloth Hall**
In 1879 Henryk Siemiradzki presented the National Museum with its first gift, his painting *The Torches of Nero*.

ŚW. WAWRZYŃCA

KRAKOWSKA

Galicia Jewish Museum
A collection of Judaica, one of the best in Central Europe, is housed in this Renaissance synagogue.

Royal Castle in Wawel
This royal residence houses an outstanding art collection which includes paintings, sculptures, gold work, arms and Oriental art. The tapestries are of particular interest.

Exploring Krakow's Museums and Galleries

Krakow's museum collections tell the history of the city and Polish culture in great detail. There are also a few specialized foreign collections. A visit to all the many museums would require several weeks but it is possible to concentrate on just the most important collections and still get to know the city well. For contemporary art, head to the Museum of Contemporary Art in Krakow (MOCAK) and the "Bunker of Art".

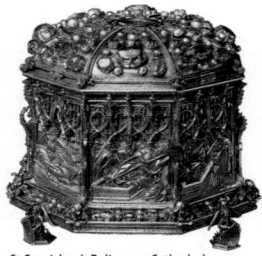

St Stanisław's Reliquary, Cathedral Museum *(see p64)*

The History of Poland and Krakow

The former residence of Polish rulers, the **Royal Castle** at Wawel is the best known of Krakow's museums. Outstanding tapestries and paintings are among the exhibits. The Armoury and Treasury are also open for visits. The latter houses the coronation sword *Szczerbiec*. Worth a visit is the archaeological display "Lost Wawel", which shows the Rotunda of the Virgin Mary (Krakow's first church). A computer-generated model of Wawel gives visitors an overview of the early 10th-century construction. The Gregorian chants sung by the Dominican Friars can be heard while viewing the programme.

The history of the former capital of Poland is told at the **Museum of Krakow**. The collections here include the insignia of municipal governments and those of guilds, seals featuring Krakow's coat of arms and many townscapes showing Krakow in the past.

The Jagiellonian University Museum is housed in the **Collegium Maius**, the oldest of the university's buildings. The museum brings together scientific equipment, of which some items are unique, as well as memorabilia left by former professors. Many rooms have retained their original furnishings.

The borough of Kazimierz was inhabited in the past mostly by Jews. This part of the city became a centre for their culture. The **Galicia Jewish Museum**, with its rich collection of Judaica, including liturgical objects, is dedicated to the Jewish heritage.

The election of the Archbishop of Krakow, Karol Wojtyła, to the pontificate was an important event in the history of the city. A room, recreated in the **Archdiocesan Museum**, commemorates the years spent by Karol Wojtyła in Krakow.

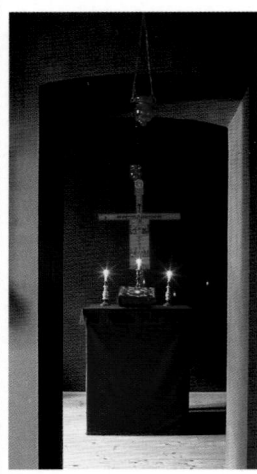

The altar by Jerzy Nowosielski, St Vladimir's Foundation, devoted to the Orthodox Church

Polish Art

In 1879 Henryk Siemiradzki presented Krakow with his painting *The Torches of Nero*. He thus initiated the establishment of the **National Museum in Krakow**. Poland was then still an occupied country and the intention was to raise patriotic awareness and the morale of the Poles. Only Polish art and works relating to the history of Poland were included. As a result, the museum has only a limited selection of Western art. Its collection of historical Polish art, on the other hand, is unparalleled. The museum has a dozen branches throughout the city. A large and outstanding collection of medieval and

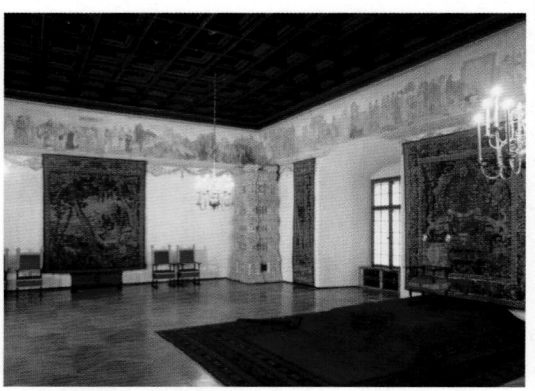

Deputies' Hall in the Royal Castle at Wawel

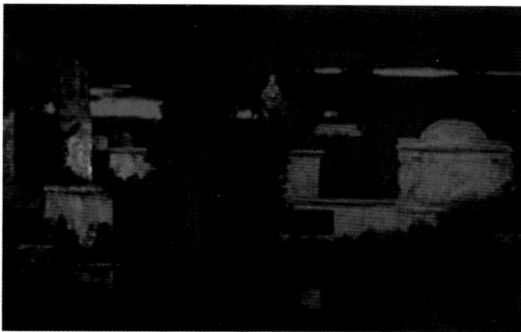
Italian Landscape by Adam Chmielowski, National Museum in Krakow

Renaissance painting and sculpture used to take pride of place in the museum, but it has been moved to the Palace of Bishop Erazm Ciołek *(see p84)* where Polish art up to 1794 is now housed. Nineteenth-century Polish art, housed at the **Cloth Hall Gallery**, is also of great interest. Twentieth-century painting and sculpture can be admired in the Main Building. The museum has a programme of temporary monographic exhibitions concerned with the life and work of great Krakow artists such as Jan Matejko, Stanisław Wyspiański and Józef Mehoffer. The **Europeum** branch houses the museum's collection of Western European art, featuring important works by Brueghel the Younger and Lorenzo Lotto.

The **Cricoteka** displays the works of 20th-century painter and designer Tadeusz Kantor. The museum is housed in a striking modern building on the river bank.

The collection at **St Vladimir's Foundation** is devoted to the culture of the Orthodox Church among whose faithful were the Ruthenians who lived in the eastern borderlands of Poland. The collection features parts of iconostases and single icons from the 16th to 20th centuries.

Contemporary Polish and non-Polish art can be seen at the popular **Museum of Contemporary Art in Krakow (MOCAK)**, as well as at the **"Bunker of Art"**.

The **Archdiocesan Museum** has a magnificent collection of Polish sacred art. The museum also organizes exhibitions of works on loan from leading church treasuries throughout the country as well as other countries.

Foreign Art

Those interested in Western art should visit the **Czartoryski Museum**. There are many fine works here, including *Landscape with the Good Samaritan* by Rembrandt, Romanesque gold work from the Maas region, Italian Renaissance majolica, and Meissen porcelain. The museum is closed for renovation until 2016. During this time, its most celebrated masterpiece, *The Lady with an Ermine* by Leonardo da Vinci, will be on display at Wawel Royal Castle.

The Manggha **Japanese Centre of Art and Technology** covers Japanese art. A bequest of objects from the Far East presented by Feliks Manggha Jasieński constitutes the core of the collection, which also includes works by contemporary artists.

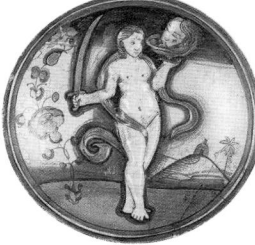
Tin-glazed majolica plate (c. 1545) from the collection of the Czartoryski Museum

Local Culture and Natural History

The **Archaeological Museum** displays important objects found in the 19th century in Galicia *(see p32)*, which was then under Austrian occupation. One of them is the statue of Światowid fished out from the Zbrucz River. Other objects found during the construction of Nowa Huta and renovation works at Kanonicza Street were also added. There is also a notable collection of Egyptian mummies.

The **Ethnographic Museum** houses a large collection of folk art from the Lesser Poland region. Temporary exhibitions, which take place at the Krakowska Street branch, are always of interest.

An extremely well preserved rhinoceros (*coelodonta antiquitatis*) from the Ice Age is a highlight of the **Natural History Museum**.

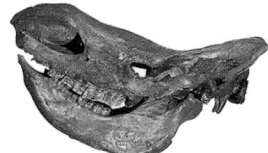
Skull of *coelodonta antiquitatis*, Natural History Museum

Krakow's Best: Churches

The skyline of Krakow is dominated by churches.
There are some 40 churches within the historic
centre alone. There would be even more, however,
as many churches were destroyed or dismantled
in the 19th century. The surviving churches bear
witness to the splendour of Krakow. The interiors
are surprisingly rich in furnishings and house
a variety of works of art in different
artistic styles.

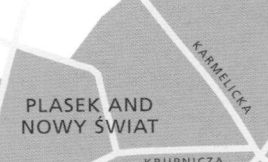

PLASEK AND
NOWY ŚWIAT

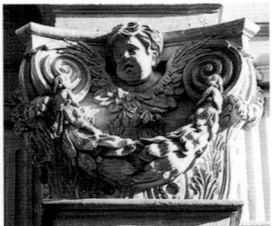

Church of St Anne
This church was created by two
outstanding artists at the end of
the 17th century – the architect
Tylman van Gameren and the
sculptor Baldassare Fontana.

Franciscan Church
Magnificent murals and stained glass
by Stanisław Wyspiański decorate
the Gothic interior of this church.

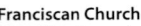

WAWEL
HILL

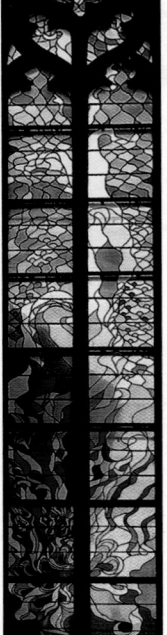

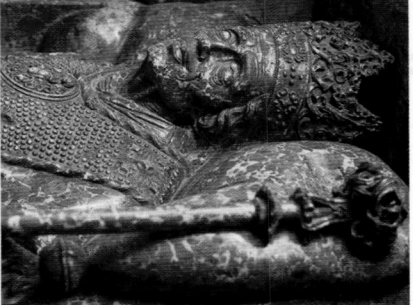

Cathedral
This Cathedral is a place where the
history of the Polish state meets that
of the Church and where national
memorabilia are treasured.

| 0 metres | | 500 |
| 0 yards | | 500 |

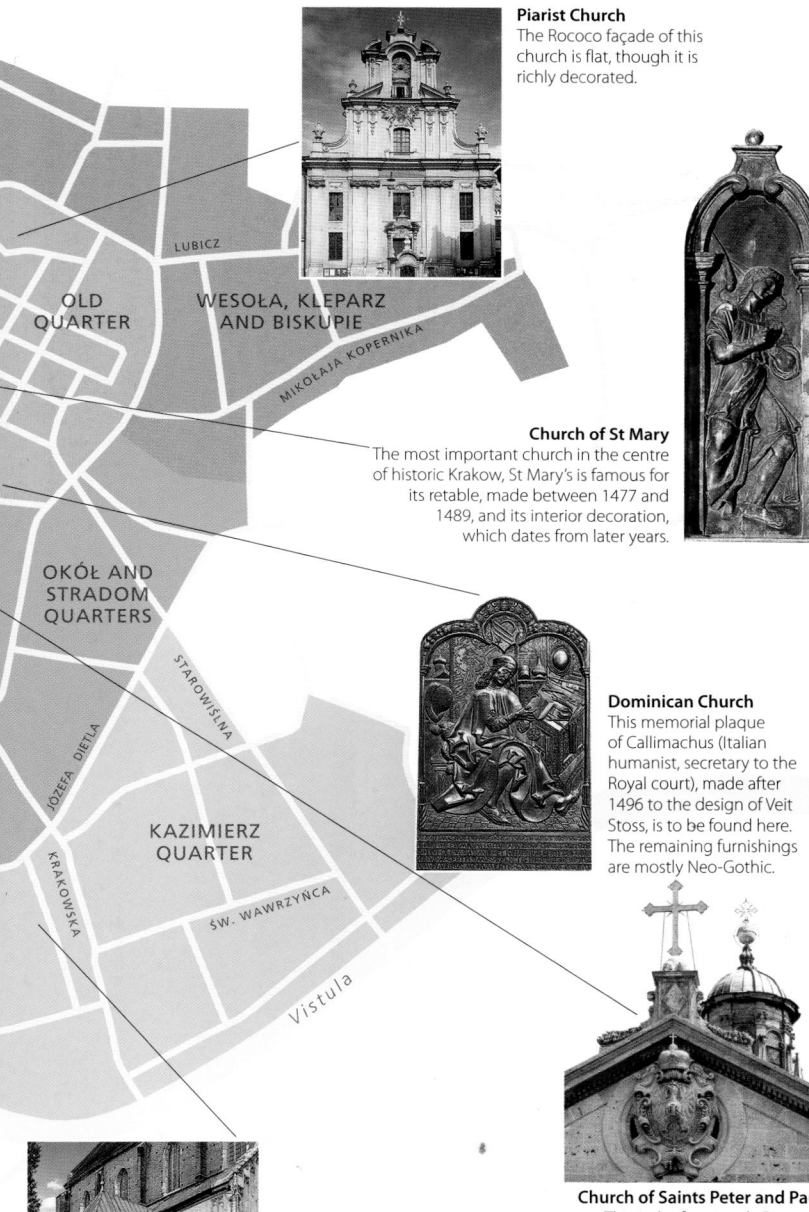

Piarist Church
The Rococo façade of this church is flat, though it is richly decorated.

OLD
QUARTER

WESOŁA, KLEPARZ
AND BISKUPIE

LUBICZ

MIKOŁAJA KOPERNIKA

Church of St Mary
The most important church in the centre of historic Krakow, St Mary's is famous for its retable, made between 1477 and 1489, and its interior decoration, which dates from later years.

OKÓŁ AND
STRADOM
QUARTERS

STAROWIŚLNA

JÓZEFA DIETLA

Dominican Church
This memorial plaque of Callimachus (Italian humanist, secretary to the Royal court), made after 1496 to the design of Veit Stoss, is to be found here. The remaining furnishings are mostly Neo-Gothic.

KRAKOWSKA

KAZIMIERZ
QUARTER

ŚW. WAWRZYŃCA

Vistula

Church of Saints Peter and Paul
This is the finest early Baroque church in Poland from the leading architects of the late 16th century. It is decorated with exquisite carved statues and stuccowork.

St Catherine's Church
While visiting this church one should not miss the south porch decorated with stonework and tracery.

Exploring Krakow's Churches

Krakow's churches represent many different styles, from the Romanesque and Gothic through Baroque and later eclecticism to the modern. Fortunately the majority of churches were saved from wartime destruction and have not been damaged. Today their splendid interiors impress visitors to the city. However, Krakow's churches are not only tourist attractions but also places of pilgrimage. The relics of a number of saints and blessed, as well as many pious figures who enjoy a local cult, are laid to rest in the city's variety of churches.

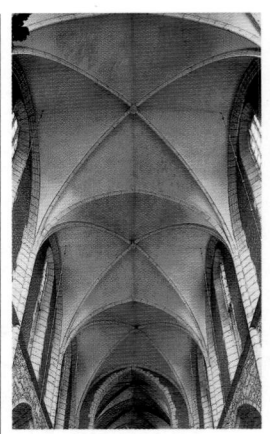

Gothic vault in the nave of the Corpus Christi Church

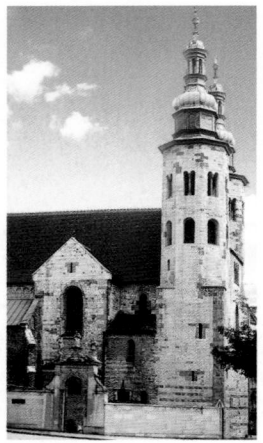

St Andrew's Church

Pre-Romanesque and Romanesque

The earliest stone churches in Krakow date from the second half of the 10th century. They were built on the site of today's **St Adalbert's Church** and at Wawel, where the remnants of a number of rotundas have been found. Today the reconstructed Rotunda of the Virgin Mary *(see p65)*, originally from the late 10th century, can be visited. Built around 1079, **St Andrew's** is exceptional among the Romanesque churches. The **Church of the Holy Redeemer** dates from around the same period. The Crypt of St Leonard beneath the Cathedral is a remnant of the second cathedral built between 1090 and 1142. The remnants of the Church of St Gereon and the Chapel of St Mary of Egypt are also at Wawel.

Gothic

Slender silhouettes of Gothic churches enhance the city. Some buildings were, however, demolished in the 19th century during the programme of "tidying up" the old architecture. The **Franciscan Church** is the oldest to have survived. Its irregular plan of a Greek cross with an asymmetric nave is unusual. The **Church of the Holy Cross**, begun around 1300, is worth visiting for its palm vaulting supported by a single pillar. **Krakow Cathedral** is certainly a major attraction. This three-aisled basilica with a transept and ambulatory, surrounded by chapels, was constructed between 1320 and 1364. The Monastery, **Church of St Catherine** and the **Corpus Christi** were both founded by Kazimierz the Great, while the **Dominican Church** was rebuilt during his reign. All three churches share the same structural and stylistic characteristics and were probably constructed by the same stonemasons, who moved from one site to another. **St Mary's** the city's main civic church, is also Gothic. It was under construction from the end of the 13th century until the late 15th century.

Towers, Domes and Spires in Krakow

The outlines of many church domes and spires dominate the skyline of old Krakow. They also bear witness to the historic and artistic changes that the city has undergone. The Gothic spires of St Mary's and Corpus Christi are among the tallest and most picturesque. Baroque styles are more common and include the Church of Saints Peter and Paul, St Anne's and the Cathedral Clock Tower.

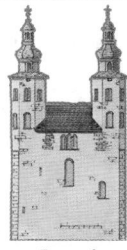

Towers of the Church of St Andrew

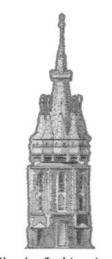

Slender Gothic spire of St Mary's Church

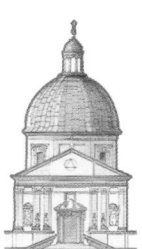

Baroque dome of St Anne's Church

Renaissance and Mannerist

There is no complete church in Krakow in either the pure Renaissance or Mannerist styles, but the Zygmunt Chapel, built from 1519 to 1533, is regarded as the greatest example of Italian Renaissance north of the Alps. The chapel, with its spatial design and decoration, provided a model which was followed faithfully throughout Poland for many years.

Renaissance monuments by Jan Michałowicz of Urzędów and Giovanni Maria Mosca ("Il Padovano") can be seen in a number of churches. The career of the Italian Mannerist Santi Gucci, an equally fine artist, spans the last decades of the 16th century.

Baroque

Although in the 17th century Polish kings no longer resided in Krakow, many new ecclesiastical foundations were undertaken. The Jesuit **Church of Saints Peter and Paul** was the most magnificent. The church was completed by the royal architect

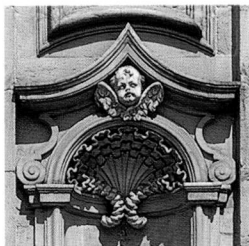

Baroque façade detail of the Church of the Missionaries

Giovanni Battista Trevano in 1609–19. The imposing Zbaraski Chapel in the **Dominican Church**, built between 1629 and 1631, is another fine example of early Baroque. The Canopy of St Stanisław and the Vaza Chapel, both in the Wawel **Cathedral**, exemplify the best of the High Baroque style. In the first half of the 17th century the interiors of a number of Gothic churches, such as St Mark's (see p112) were remodelled in the Baroque style. The century that followed brought about further architectural masterpieces, including **St Anne's Church**. A mention must also be made of the **Church of the Missionaries** whose exterior and interior were both modelled on Roman architecture, the **Piarist Church** with its airy façade, and the **Church of the Order of St John of God** whose façade displays dynamic articulation.

Neo-Classical and Eclectic

The late 18th-century choir and the high altar in the Church of the Norbertine Nuns are the only examples of ecclesiastical Neo-Classicism in Krakow. No building activity was undertaken until Galicia became autonomous, and new churches were only constructed in the second half of the 19th and first half of the 20th centuries. The **Church of the Felician Nuns** was built between 1882 and 1884 to designs by Feliks Księżarski, and the **St Joseph's Church** (1905–09) was designed by Jan Sas Zubrzycki. The **Jesuit Church** designed by Franciszek

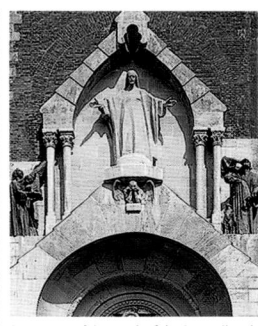

Decoration of the porch of the Jesuit Church

Mączyński and decorated with sculptures by Xawery Dunikowski and Karol Hukan, is an outstanding example of 20th-century architecture.

Modern

A variety of designs were applied to modern churches of the second half of the 20th century. Amongst the most interesting are the **Ark of God** in Nowa Huta (architect Wojciech Pietrzyk, 1967–77), the Church of St Maksymilian Kolbe in Mistrzejowice (architect Józef Dutkiewicz, 1976–83) and the Church of St Jan Kanty at Bronowice Nowe.

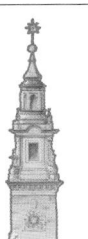

Late Baroque Clock Tower of the Cathedral

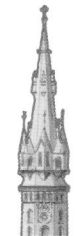

Neo-Gothic spire of St Joseph's Church at Podgórze

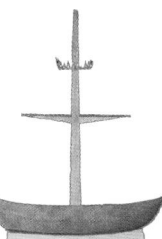

Modern spire of the Ark of God Church in Nowa Huta

Exploring Krakow's Cemeteries

All over Europe the cult of commemorating the dead resulted in the establishment of many large cemeteries, with beautiful sculptures often decorating the tombs. Krakow is no different in this respect. Numerous cemeteries and mausolea in church crypts have been established here over the years. They were already regarded as tourist attractions in the 19th century and continue to be visited by tourists to the city.

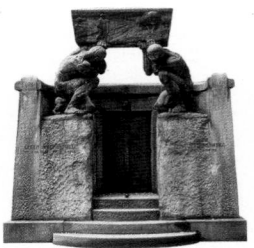
The Jerzmanowski Mausoleum, Rakowicki Cemetery

Christian Cemeteries

At the end of the 18th century a Krakovian noted that "Every time one looks through the window one cannot but see graves and crosses in the centre of the city". At that time cemeteries used to be located near churches. The one at St Mary's was the largest. It was relocated at the end of the 18th century and the original burial site transformed into Mariacki Square. Many tombstones and epitaphs, often medieval, which commemorate those who died centuries ago, have survived on the exterior walls of the churches of St Mary and St Barbara. A number of mausolea, built as chapels by the patrician families of Krakow, also survive on the former site of St Mary's Cemetery.

The **Rakowicki Cemetery** was established outside the city in 1803 and is the oldest cemetery in use. It occupies a vast plot and its layout is transparent. Many old trees give the place a park-like appearance. Some tombstones, especially those made around 1900 by the best Polish sculptors of the time, are true works of art.

In 1920 a **Military Cemetery** was set up by the Rakowicki Cemetery (they have since merged). Polish soldiers who fell in the years 1914–20 and in September 1939, as well as British and Commonwealth airmen who lost their lives in World War II, all rest here.

The **Salwator Cemetery** is a far more modest place with no great monuments, but rather smaller tombstones decorated with small-scale but nevertheless interesting bas-reliefs. It is, however, a lovely place, picturesquely situated on a high hill and rich in varied fauna. One of the best times of year to visit Krakow's cemeteries is a few days either side of 1 November, when they glow under candlelight at night.

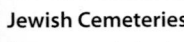

Jewish Cemeteries

For many centuries Jews constituted a substantial part of the population of Kazimierz, the so-called Jewish city. They were interred at the **Remu'h Cemetery**, established in 1533. This small plot, squeezed between buildings, has many layers of tombs which have been

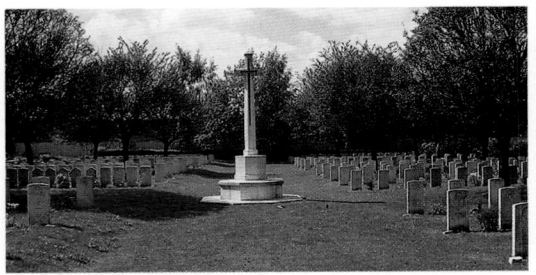
The graves of British airmen, Military Cemetery

Monuments and Tombs

The monuments in Krakow's cemeteries show different ways in which people wished to commemorate the deceased. The medieval monuments show a stiff figure lying on a death bed placed under a canopy. The canopy symbolizes Heaven awaiting the soul. Elements glorifying the deceased were introduced into Baroque monuments. Female figures with attributes personified the virtues. Neo-Classical monuments were influenced by ancient sculpture. Fine sculptures and symbolic content are characteristic of the monuments in the Art Nouveau style.

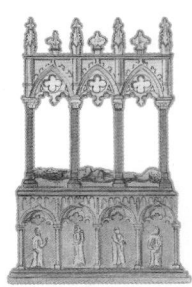
Monument of Kazimierz the Great (died 1370) in the Cathedral

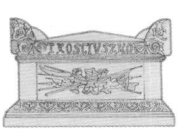
Sarcophagus of Kościuszko in the Cathedral crypt (1818)

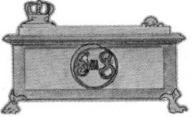
Sarcophagus of Jan III Sobieski in the Cathedral (1760)

placed here over hundreds of years. The tombstones are engraved with Hebrew inscriptions and symbolic images that identify the religion and social rank of the deceased. The dense accumulation of tombstones within a tiny and bare space contributes to the unique character of this Jewish cemetery.

The **New Jewish Cemetery** is different. It was established in the 19th century and given, like other cemeteries, a park-like appearance. Tombstones are scattered randomly and surrounded by luxuriant vegetation. This is one of a few Jewish cemeteries in Poland which is still in use.

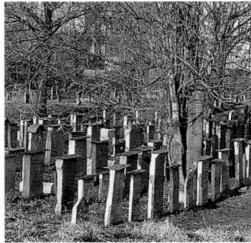

View of Remu'h Cemetery

Crypts with Tombs of Great Poles

During the Partitions period (1795–1918) a number of celebrated Poles received state funerals. These events were intended to raise the patriotic feelings of the Polish people.

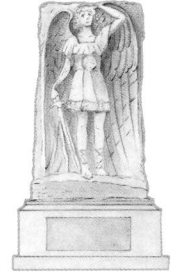

The Angel of Vengeance on the Monument to Victims of the 1848 Bombardment of Krakow (1913)

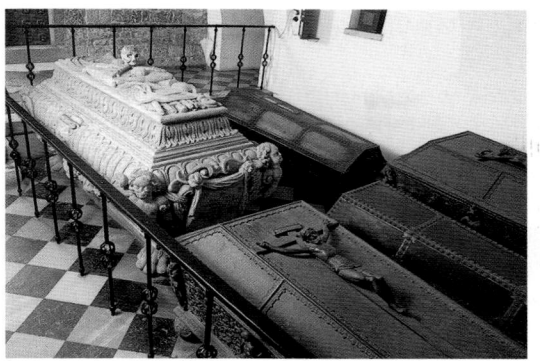

The Vaza Crypt in the Cathedral

Church crypts were open to the public and transformed into pantheons of Poland's greatest citizens. The **Cathedral's Crypt** contains the most solemn royal tombs of all. The crypt is divided into galleries in which Polish rulers, leading poets and national heroes rest. Tadeusz Kościuszko and Prince Józef Poniatowski were interred here during the occupation of Poland; President Lech Kaczyński and his wife, who were killed in a plane crash in 2010, are also buried here.

The **Crypt in the Paulite Church "On the Rock"** is a resting place for those who made great contributions to the arts and sciences. The eminent historian Jan Długosz was buried here in the 15th century.

Monastic Cemeteries

The crypts beneath monastic churches are unique to Krakow. Their character reflects the unusual burial practices of particular religious orders.

The corpses in the **Crypt in the Church of the Reformed Franciscans** have been mummified naturally owing to the crypt's construction and ventilation. One can see here the corpses of poor friars lying on sand with their heads resting on a stone, as well as lay people in rich clothes resting in elaborate coffins. Over 700 laymen and around 250 Franciscan friars were buried here. The **Camaldolese**

Catacombs beneath the church in Bielany are different. Here, the corpses are laid at first in niches cut out in a wall and then bricked up. Some years later the bones are removed and placed in an ossuary with the exception of the skull, which is taken by one of the monks for the purposes of contemplation. The Camaldolese crypt strikingly shows that in the face of death all are equal.

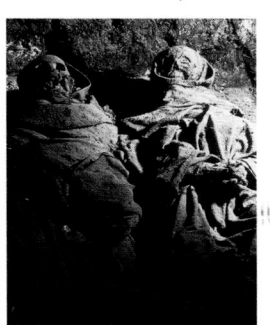

Mummified monks in the Crypt of the Church of the Reformed Franciscans

Finding Krakow's Cemeteries

Krakow's Famous Residents

Many leading personalities of Polish academic, cultural and public life were born in Krakow. Eminent scholars were educated at or drawn to the Jagiellonian University, which was sometimes called "a gem of all knowledge". Famous artists and writers chose to live here, attracted by the unique atmosphere of the city, which was enlivened by old traditions. The cult of such great figures as writer and artist Stanisław Wyspiański, theatre director Tadeusz Kantor and painter Jan Matejko is still alive.

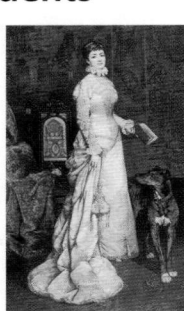

Helena Modrzejewska (1840–1909)
This famous actress began her career at the Old Theatre (Teatr Stary) She is buried in Krakow.

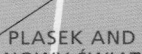

KARMELICKA

KRUPNICZA

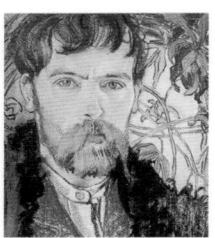

Stanisław Wyspiański (1869–1907)
Best known for his play *The Wedding*, Wyspiański was a dramatist, painter and designer. His great artistic visions are embedded in the Polish perception of national identity. He was born at Krupnicza 26.

PLASEK AND NOWY ŚWIAT

SMOLEŃSK

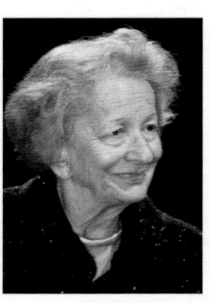

Wisława Szymborska (1923–2012)
This prominent poet was awarded the 1996 Nobel Prize for Literature. Szymborska's links with Krakow span more than 50 years. She lived at Krupnicza 22 in her youth.

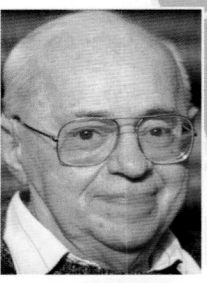

ZWIERZYNIECKA

Stanisław Lem (1921–2006)
One of the most widely read science-fiction authors in the world, Lem was also an essayist and critic. He studied medicine in Krakow.

Vistula

WAW HILL

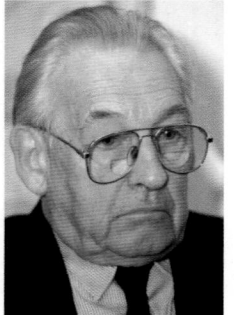

Andrzej Wajda (born 1926)
A leading film and theatre director, Wajda was educated in Krakow. He was the main instigator of the Japanese Centre of Art and Technology, one of the city's best museums. Wajda won an Oscar for Lifetime Achievement in 2000.

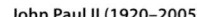

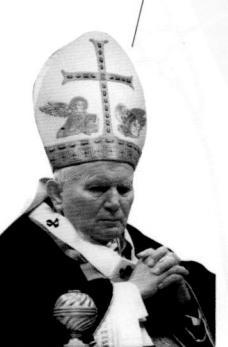

John Paul II (1920–2005)
Before his elevation to the papacy, Karol Wojtyła was Suffragan Bishop, then Archbishop of Krakow from 1963 to 1978. He lived in the Archbishop's Palace on Franciszkańska 3.

Jan Matejko (1838–93)

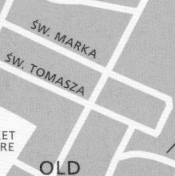

The most renowned Polish painter of the 19th century, Matejko's vision of Polish history has influenced many generations. Krakow's Academy of Fine Arts and the large square next to it are named in his honour.

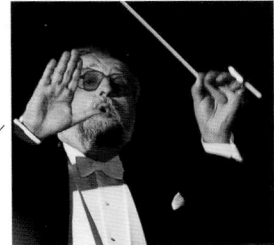

Krzysztof Penderecki (born 1933)

World-renowned composer and conductor, Penderecki was educated in Krakow. He was a Professor and Rector of the Music Academy.

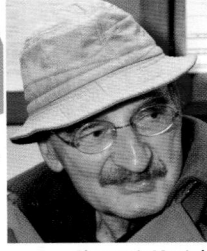

Sławomir Mrożek (1930–2013)

An outstanding playwright and satirist, Mrożek began his career in Krakow as a journalist. After many years abroad, he returned and settled here in 1996. He is buried in the Church of Saints Peter and Paul.

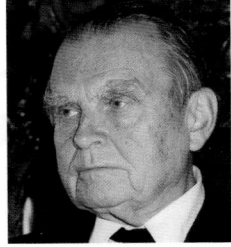

Czesław Miłosz (1911–2004)

A poet, translator, Nobel Prize winner and honorary doctor of the Jagiellonian University, Miłosz was made an honorary citizen of Krakow in 1993. In his final years he lived at W. Bogusławskiego 6.

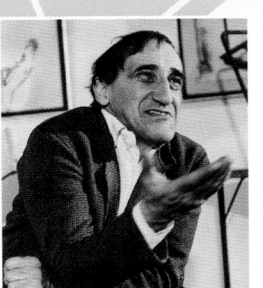

Tadeusz Kantor (1915–90)

A leading European artist and theatre director, Kantor established the world-famous Cricot 2 Theatre. For many years he worked at Kanonicza 5.

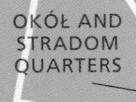
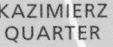

BASZTOWA

LUBICZ

SW. MARKA

SW. TOMASZA

MARKET SQUARE

WESOŁA, KLEPARZ AND BISKUPIE

OLD QUARTER

GRODZKA

OKÓŁ AND STRADOM QUARTERS

STAROWIŚLNA

JÓZEFA DIETLA

KAZIMIERZ QUARTER

KRAKOWSKA

SW. WAWRZYŃCA

0 metres 500
0 yards 500

KRAKOW THROUGH THE YEAR

Beautiful and magical, Krakow is a city where old traditions are maintained. The bugle call that echoes at hourly intervals from the tower of St Mary's Church sets the rhythm of life. And life is lived here slowly, for one should not hurry when surrounded by stones a thousand years old. Embraced by the Planty, which had replaced the medieval walls, the old quarter remains at the heart of the city. It is not an open-air museum that visitors vacate at night. Although no longer the capital of Poland, Krakow is a cultural centre and one of the oldest university cities in Europe. There is something for everyone here. Press listings and other local media, as well as tourist agencies, are good sources of information.

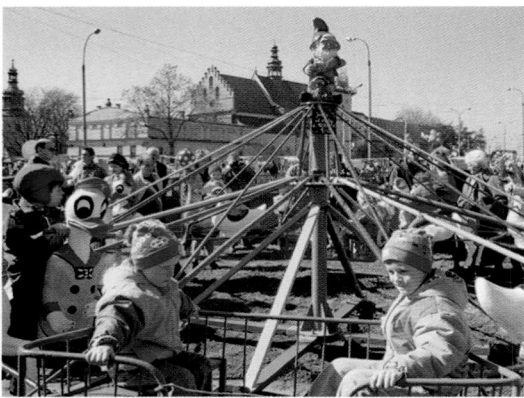

The Emmaus Fair in Zwierzyniec on Easter Monday

Spring

In Podhale, the region at the foothills of the Tatra Mountains, vast fields of crocuses announce the arrival of spring. In Krakow, the opening of street cafés and people spilling onto the pavements heralds the new season.

March

International Festival of Alternative Theatre, Rotunda Club. The oldest event of its kind in which alternative theatres and fans of theatre are brought together.
Jazz Juniors, Rotunda Club. This is an international jazz festival for young musicians.
Festival of Organ Music, various venues. *(Mar–Apr)*.

Easter

Palm Sunday *(Sun before Easter)*. The blessing of palms in churches. A competition for the largest and best decorated palm takes place in Lipnica Murowana village, 41 km (25 miles) east of Krakow.
Holy Saturday is a day when baskets with food are taken to the church for a blessing, and symbolic tombs of Christ are venerated.
Easter Sunday is the most important Catholic feast.
Easter Monday. The Emmaus Fair takes place in Zwierzyniec and people are splashed with water *(Śmigus-dyngus)* throughout the city.

April

Paka Cabaret Festival. Amateur and professional satirical performers, Polish and foreign, all take part.

May

3 May Constitution Day celebrates the first Polish Constitution of 1791 with a Mass said in the Cathedral followed by the laying of wreaths at the Tomb of the Unknown Soldier. Afterwards, there are fairs and picnics.
Procession from Wawel to the Paulite Church "On the Rock" *(first Sun after 8 May, Feast of St Stanisław)*. The Primate and bishops lead the procession and carry the relics of the patron saints of Poland, joined by the faithful in regional costumes.
Juvenalia. Krakow is ruled by students for a couple of days.
Krakow Film Festival *(May–Jun)*. The oldest film festival in the country.
Krakow Spring Ballet Festival Słowacki Theatre, *(May–Jun)*. Leading ballet companies of the world take part.

Archconfraternity of the Passion

Since 1595 the Good Friday processions of the Archconfraternity of The Passion have taken place in the Franciscan Church. The Brothers wear black habits with hoods covering the face. The ritual has remained unchanged for centuries. The Archconfraternity had the right to pardon those condemned to death.

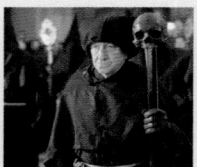

Brothers in Procession

Average Daily Hours of Sunshine

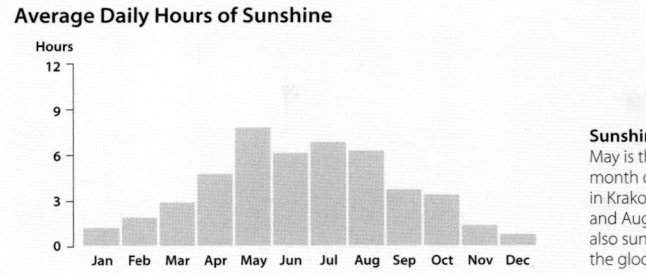

Sunshine Chart
May is the sunniest month of the year in Krakow, but June, July and August are usually also sunny. December is the gloomiest month.

Summer

Summer heat may be difficult to bear in Krakow. This is because of the city's location in a valley and its humid microclimate. Many bars, cafés and restaurants in the Old Quarter are open and busy till the early hours of the morning. Crowds of tourists are attracted not only by the heritage but also the nightlife and cultural events. Organ Recitals at the Benedictine Abbey at Tyniec are among the most famous events.

June

Corpus Christi (Boże Ciało) *(Thu in May or June)*. A great procession proceeds from Wawel to the Market Square. On Thursday a week after Corpus Christi *Lajkonik* canters around the town *(see p98)*.
Enthronement of the "king" Marksman, Market Square. The Marksmen's Brotherhood has existed since the Middle Ages. Its members are burghers who are members of craftsmen guilds. Their leader is the winner of the annual shooting competition. The outgoing leader passes the silver cock to the new "king" during a colourful ceremony.
Midsummer's Eve (Wianki) Sat preceding the eve of St John's Feast *(24 Jun)*. Candle wreaths are set adrift on the Vistula by Wawel and there are fireworks displays.
International Music Festival of Military Bands features gala shows of drill, parades in period uniforms and many concerts.

July

Summer Early Music Festival. Concerts are held in historic houses.
Summer Opera and Operetta Festival. Krakow Jazz Festival (Stary Jazz w Krakowie) *(Jul–Aug)*. A real treat for fans of traditional jazz.
Jewish Culture Festival *(early Jul)*, Kazimierz.

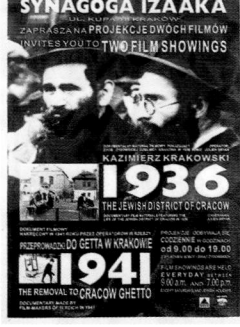

Poster announcing events during the Jewish Culture Festival

Outstanding Jewish performers from all over the world take part in this festival.

August

The Assumption of the Virgin Mary (Święto Wniebowzięcia Matki Boskiej) *(15 Aug)*. A Solemn Mass is said in the Cathedral. This is also the national holiday of the Polish Soldier, marking the 1920 victory over the Bolshevik Army.
International Festival of Music in Old Krakow *(15–31 Aug)*. One of the most prestigious events in Krakow, with recitals and concerts of orchestral and chamber music in the magnificent historic buildings of the Old Quarter.
International Folk Art Fair (Targi Sztuki Ludowj), *(12 days in Aug)*, Market Square. Folk artists and craftsmen from Poland and other countries demonstrate their handicrafts and folklore. One day is dedicated to concerts of folk music by the Polish Highlanders.

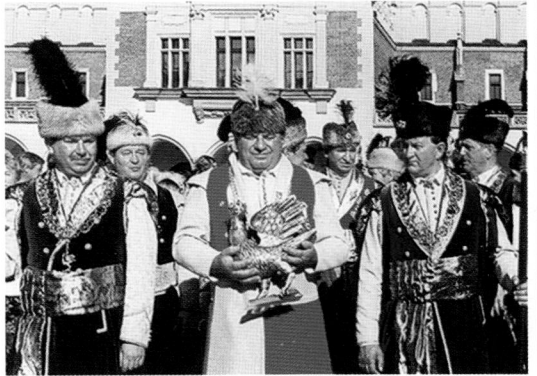

Enthronement of the "king" Marksman in the Market Square

Average Monthly Rainfall

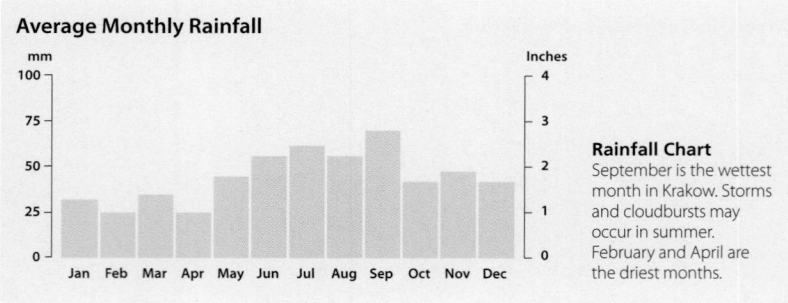

Rainfall Chart
September is the wettest month in Krakow. Storms and cloudbursts may occur in summer. February and April are the driest months.

Autumn

On dry and sunny autumn days Krakow is beautifully shrouded in colours; the Planty chestnut trees turn golden and market stalls display baskets full of wild mushrooms from the woodlands of the mountain foothills.

Students return to Krakow by the end of September to take part in the inaugural celebrations of the new academic year. The hymn *Gaudeamus Igitur* can be heard sung at many colleges, and in particular at the Jagiellonian University, Poland's oldest university, established in 1364.

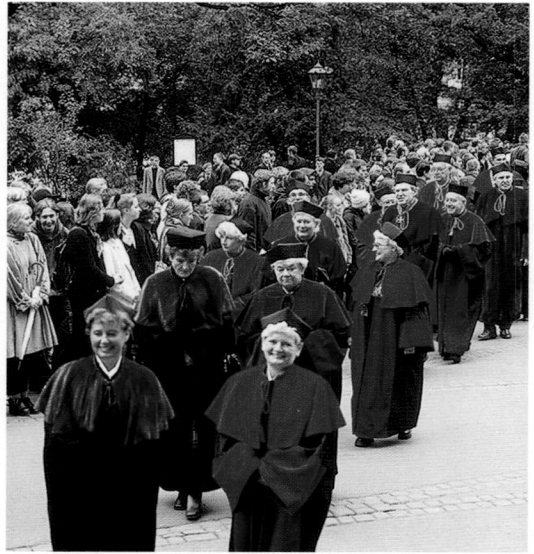
Inauguration of the academic year at the Jagiellonian University

September
Sacrum Profanum Festival
(early to mid-Sep). This annual festival is devoted to 20th-century music of all sorts, whether classical, pop or avant-garde. It has previously included appearances by the likes of Kraftwerk, Aphex Twin and Sigur Rós. Important buildings in the city are adapted and tailored to suit the festival's needs.

October
"Etude" International Film Festival (Międzynarodowy Festiwal Filmowy Etiuda). This festival sees the screening of short films by students from art schools and film schools from all over the world.

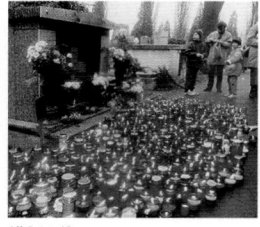
All Saints' Day

Early Music Festival (Festiwal Muzyki Polskiej) *(Oct–Nov)*. Organized simultaneously in a number of cities, the festival presents mainly the music of the Renaissance and Baroque performed on old instruments.

November
All Saints' Day (Dzień Wszystkich Świętych) *(1 Nov)*. Many Krakovians visit cemeteries to lay flowers and light candles on the graves. The views of the old Rakowicki Cemetery or of the beautifully located cemetery on the Hill of the Holy Redeemer (św. Salwator) are unforgettable. It is an old custom of Krakow to be able to buy, on this day only, so-called Turkish honey (caramelized sugar with walnuts or pistachios) at the entrance to cemeteries. Children, especially, look forward to this event.
Independence Day (Święto Niepodległości) *(11 Nov)*. After a Mass at the Wawel Cathedral, wreaths are laid at the Tomb of the Unknown Soldier by the Grunwald Monument in Matejko Square.
All Souls Jazz Festival (Krakowskie Zaduszki Jazzowe). Oldest jazz festival in post-

Average Monthly Temperature

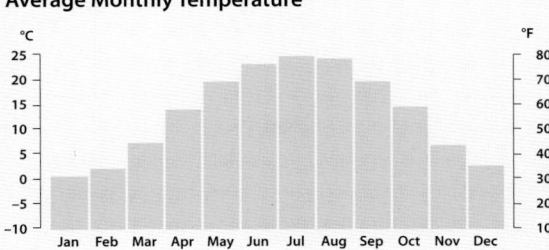

Temperature Chart
Average maximum and minimum temperatures are show here. July and August are the hottest months with the temperature often exceeding 20°C, sometimes even reaching 30°C. Winter is cold and damp. The average temperature in January is -5°C.

communist Europe, with concerts in the Philharmonic hall and jazz clubs.

Winter

Krakow under a blanket of snow is a wonderful sight, but winter also brings misty and bitingly cold days.

Every year on the first Thursday of December a competition for the best Christmas crib *(szopka)* takes place by the Mickiewicz Monument in Market Square. The winning cribs are later displayed at the Museum of Krakow. The tradition of making Christmas cribs, unique to Krakow, goes back to medieval Christmas plays.

Nativity scenes at churches are also worth visiting. The one outside the Franciscan Church, with real people and animals, is best known. It can be seen only on Christmas Eve and Christmas Day.

Stalls selling handmade Christmas decorations and traditional delicacies fill the Market Square during the Christmas Fair.

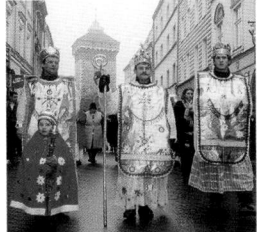

Carol singers in traditional costume in Floriańska Street at Christmas time

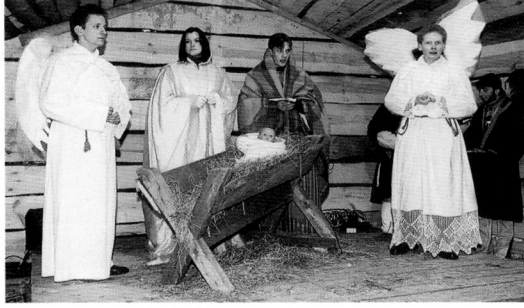

Nativity play being staged at the Franciscan Church

December

Christmas Eve (Wigilia) *(24 Dec)*. The evening begins with a meat-free meal. Midnight Masses are said and the Zygmunt Bell rings at Wawel.
Christmas (Święto Bożego Narodzenia) *(25 and 26 Dec)*. Christmas Day and the day after are public holidays. Masses are celebrated in all churches.
New Year's Eve (Sylwester) *(31 Dec)*. A crowd, several thousand strong, gathers in Market Square to see in the New Year. The Wielopolski Palace, the seat of local government, is the venue for one of the grandest balls in Poland. Distinguished guests arrive from all over the world, and the proceeds go to charity.

Christmas decoration

January

New Year's Day (Nowy Rok) *(1 Jan)*. Public holiday. A month of balls and parties begins on this day.

February

"Fat Thursday" (Tłusty czwartek) *(last Thu before Lent)*. Everybody eats doughnuts. The *Gazeta w Krakowie*, the local supplement to the *Gazeta Wyborcza*, rates the bakeries to help people choose the best doughnuts in Krakow.
Shrovetide (Ostatki), *(last Sat and Tue of the Carnival season, before Ash Wednesday)*. This is a time of parties before Lent.

Public Holidays

New Year's Day (1 Jan)
Epiphany (6 Jan)
Easter Monday (Mar/Apr)
Labour Day (1 May)
Constitution Day (3 May)
Corpus Christi (Thu 8 weeks after Easter)
Assumption (15 Aug)
All Saints' Day (1 Nov)
Independence Day (11 Nov)
Christmas (25 & 26 Dec)

The Gothic cloister at the Collegium Maius ▶

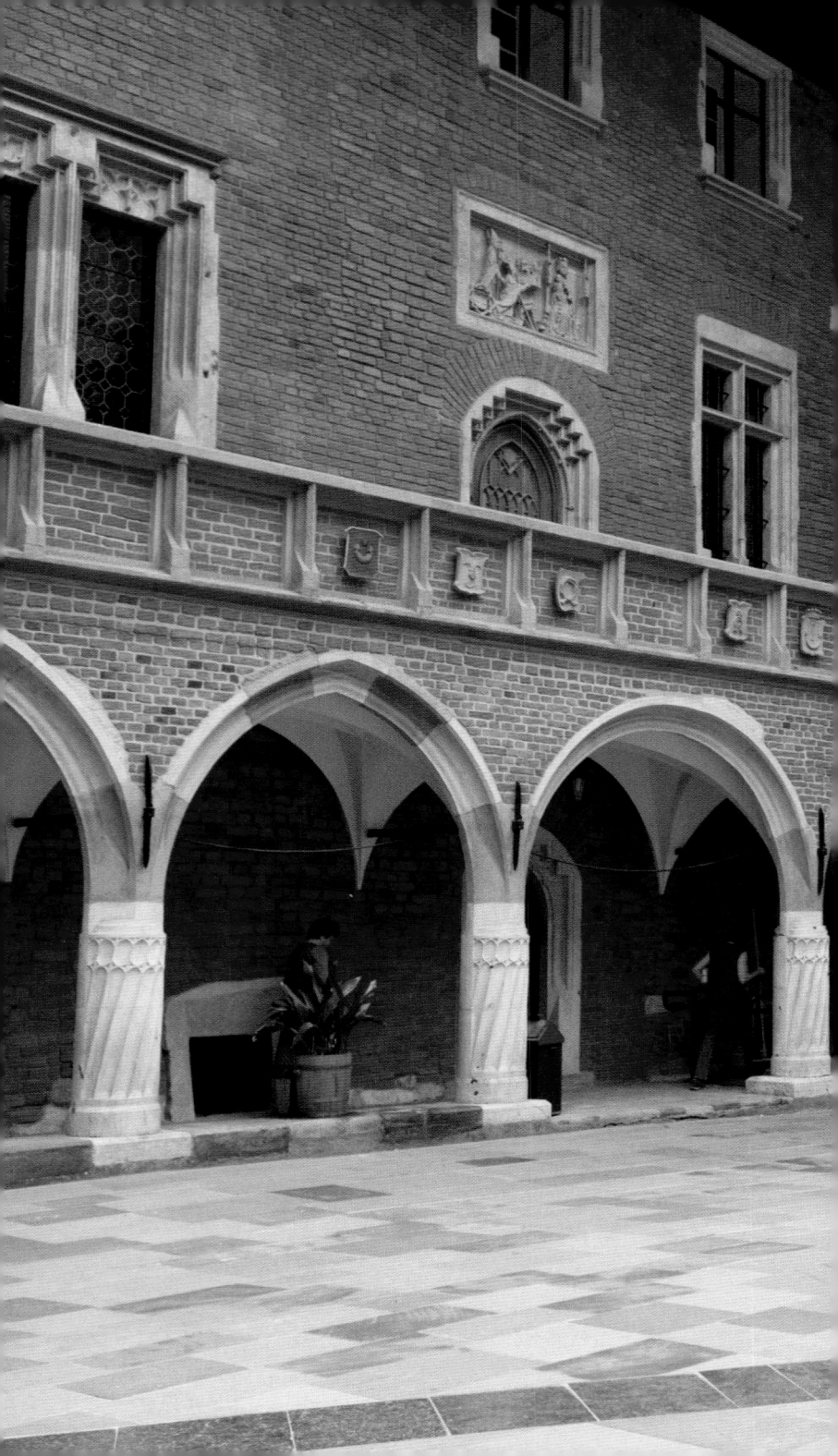

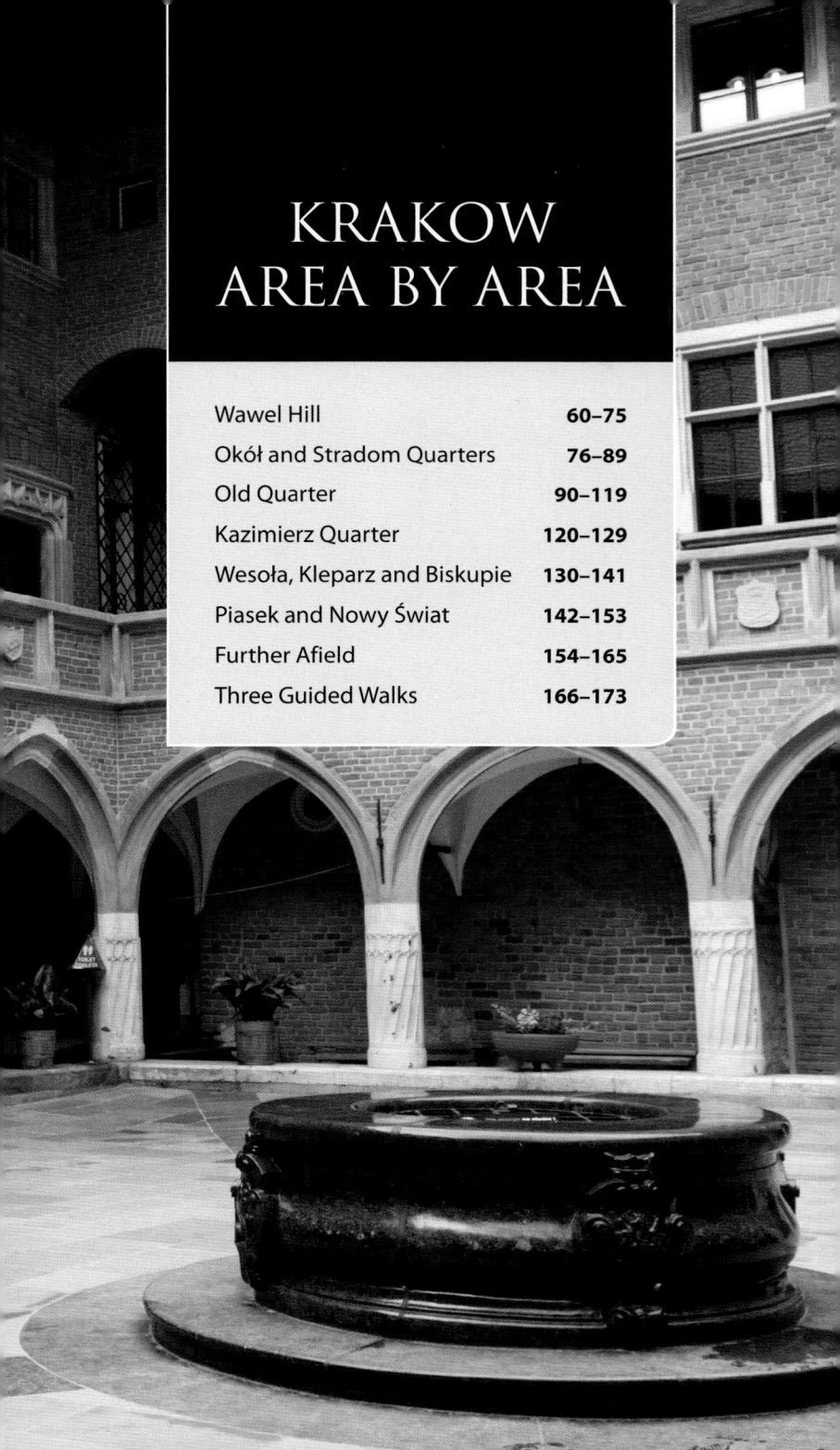

KRAKOW
AREA BY AREA

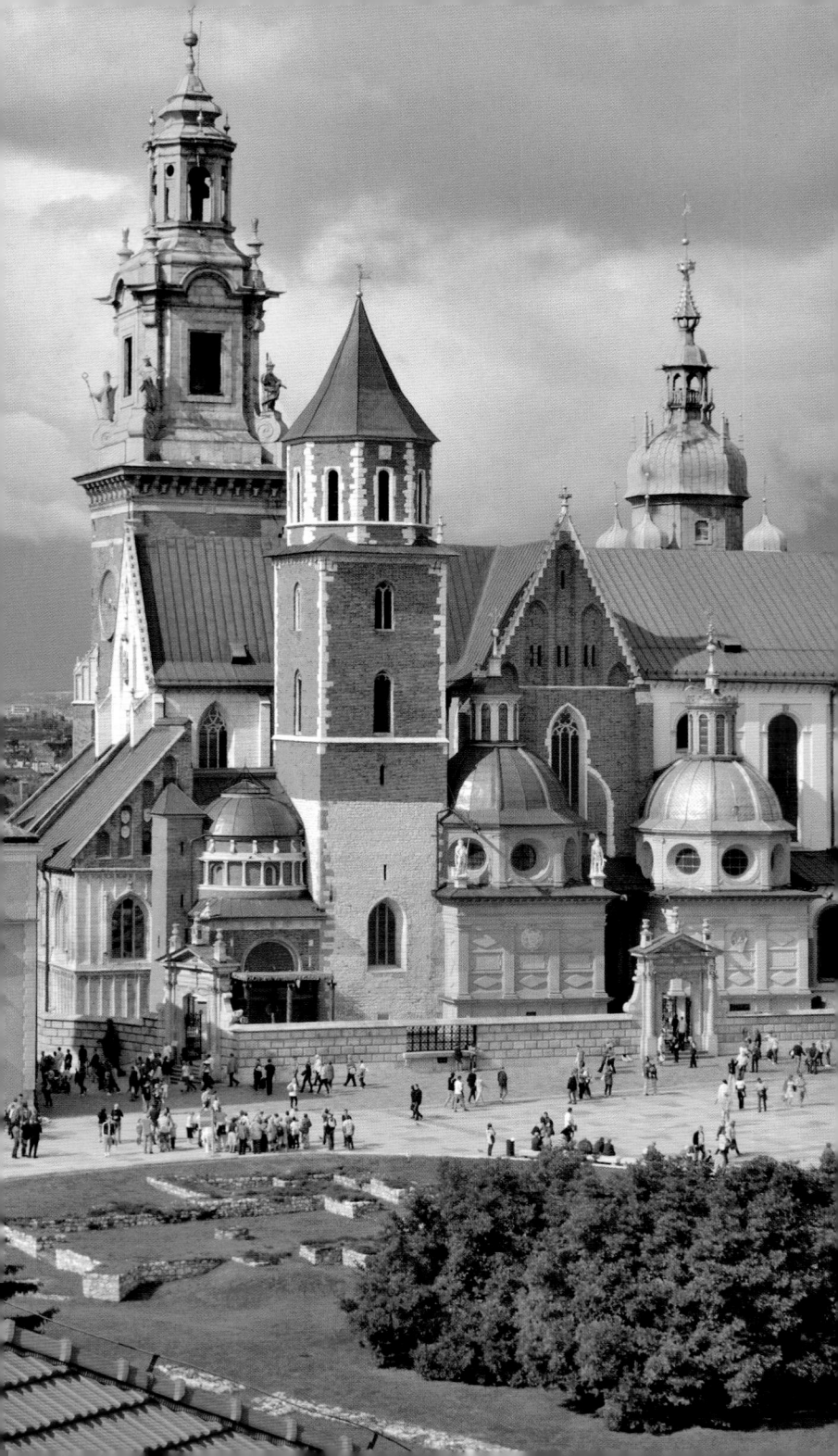

WAWEL HILL

Wawel Hill was inhabited by the Vistulan (Wiślanie) people in ancient times. The settlement came to prominence during the reigns of Bolesław the Brave and Kazimierz the Restorer. The latter made Wawel the seat of his political power. In the late medieval period, from the 14th century onwards, the royal residence and a new cathedral were built. The Cathedral houses the relics of St Stanisław, patron saint of Poland. The last rulers of the Jagiellonian dynasty transformed the Gothic castle into one of the most magnificent Renaissance royal residences in Central Europe. They also endowed the Cathedral with important works of art and architecture. Although the capital of Poland was moved from Krakow to Warsaw at the end of the 16th century, royal coronations and funeral ceremonies continued to take place in Krakow. A series of events in the 17th and 18th centuries led to the dilapidation of the Castle. The Austrian army was garrisoned here from 1795 until the early 20th century. The Castle and Cathedral have both regained their former magnificence through an intensive restoration programme. Fortunately, Wawel was saved from destruction in both World Wars.

Sights at a Glance

Churches
❸ Krakow Cathedral pp66–71

Historic Sights, Buildings and Monuments
❶ Fortifications and Towers
❷ Statue of Tadeusz Kościuszko
❼ Archaeological Site
❽ Dragon's Lair

Museums
❹ Cathedral Museum
❺ Wawel Royal Castle pp72–3
❻ "Lost Wawel" Exhibition

☐ Restaurant see p190
1 Pod Basztą

0 metres   100
0 yards   100

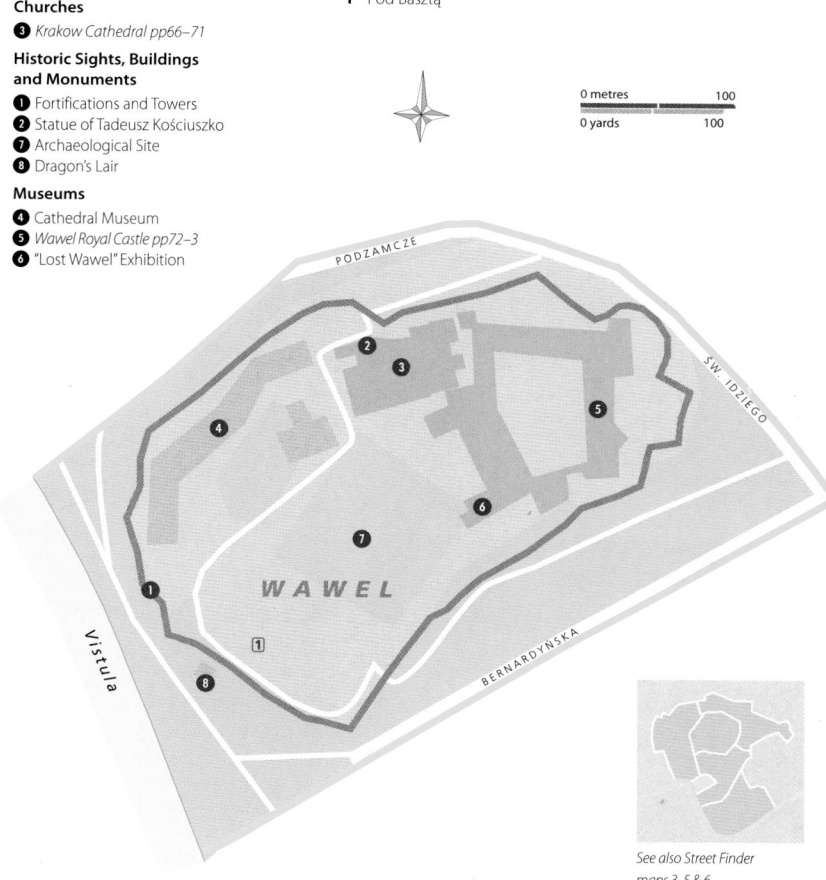

See also Street Finder maps 3, 5 & 6

◀ The grounds of Krakow Cathedral, on Wawel Hill

For keys to symbols see back flap

Street-by-Street: Wawel Hill

The Wawel is exceptional because of its first-class collections and its unique atmosphere. To savour it unhindered by large crowds you should plan an early-morning visit when the Cathedral and Castle courtyard are nearly deserted. Groups of tourists from every corner of the world gather here before noon, thereby enlivening the place. A trip to the Cathedral, where a variety of styles intermingle, as well as to the Royal Castle, is a must for visitors to Krakow.

❷ Statue of Tadeusz Kościuszko
The statue of Kościuszko stands at the entrance to Wawel Castle. Kościuszko was the general who led the Insurrection of 1794 against the Russian army. His ashes rest in the Cathedral crypt.

The Coat of Arms Gate

❹ Cathedral Museum
The museum houses a collection of sacred art, as well as a selection of insignia and memorabilia of the Polish kings, including the coronation robe of Stanisław August Poniatowski.

❽ Dragon's Lair
This cave, consisting of a number of interconnecting chambers, and a sculpture of a fire-belching dragon is a much loved attraction. It is particularly popular with children.

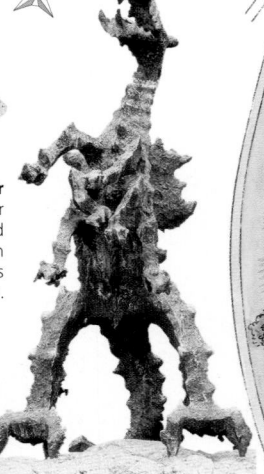

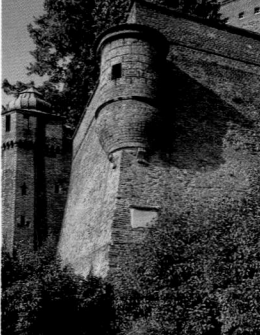

Key

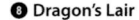 Suggested route

❶ Fortifications and Towers
The compact but varied defence system on Wawel Hill was constructed from the 15th to the 19th centuries.

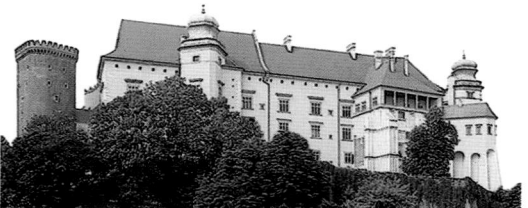

❺ ★ Wawel Royal Castle
A visit to the Castle includes the interior with its display of 16th-century tapestries, regalia, gold treasures and lavish Oriental objects.

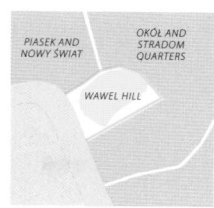

Locator Map
See Street Finder maps 3, 5 & 6

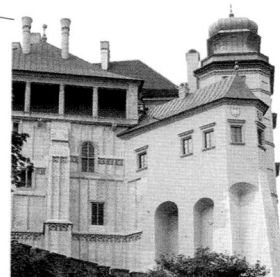

The "Hen's Claw" Wing (Kurza Stopka) is the most prominent remnant of the medieval castle. It was erected during the reign of Jadwiga and Władysław II Jagiełło.

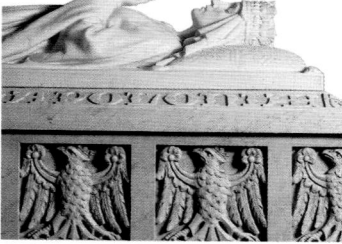

❸ ★ Krakow Cathedral
The 19th-century sarcophagus of St Jadwiga, the Queen of Poland, is among many monuments associated with the history of the Church and Nation.

❻ "Lost Wawel" Exhibition
Arranged in the former royal kitchen in the cellars, this special exhibition includes among its most interesting exhibits a reconstruction of the Rotunda of the Virgin Mary.

0 metres   50
0 yards   50

❼ Archaeological Site
The foundations of medieval buildings are exposed on this site.

❶ Fortifications and Towers

Wawel Hill. **Map** 3 C1 (5 C5). 🚌 304, 522. 🚊 3, 6, 8, 10, 18, 40.

The fortifications surrounding Wawel Hill date from different periods. Three massive towers – the Thief's Tower (Złodziejska), Sandomierz and Senator's Towers (the latter also called Lubranka) are dominant features of the architectural silhouette of the Wawel. They date from the second half of the 15th and early 16th centuries, when the royal residence was rebuilt by the Jagiellonians. New, mainly earth fortifications designed by Jan Pleitner were erected under Władysław IV between 1644 and 1646 on the Castle's northern terrace. The southeast bastion and redan (fortification of two parapets) were constructed in the early 18th century for King August II. Later in the century star-shaped fortifications designed by Bakałowicz and Mehler were built on the side of the Vistula River. The Austrians expanded the system between 1849 and 1852. Two round towers, forming part of the Austrian additions, have survived. The Wawel Castle was thus transformed into a citadel surrounded by a complex defence system.

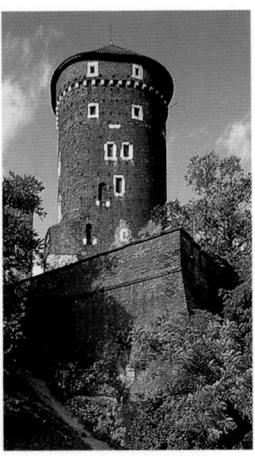

The Sandomierz Tower, one of the three Wawel defence towers

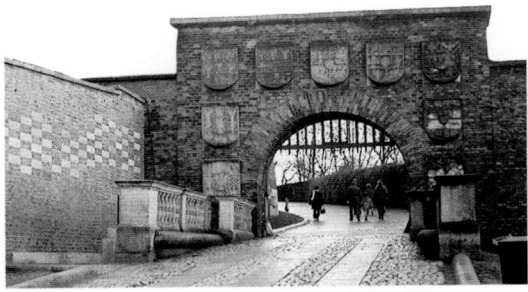

The Coat of Arms Gate and part of the fortifications surrounding Wawel Hill

❷ Statue of Tadeusz Kościuszko

Wawel Hill. **Map** 3 C1 (5 C5). 🚌 304, 522. 🚊 3, 6, 8, 10, 18, 40.

The statue of Tadeusz Kościuszko, general and main leader of the 1794 Uprising in Poland (see p31) and a participant in the American Revolution, was erected in 1921. It was designed by Leonard Marconi and completed by Antoni Popiel. The statue was destroyed by the Germans in 1940. The present reconstruction was donated in 1960. When approaching the Władysław bastion, where the statue stands, you can see a number of plaques mounted in the brick wall. These commemorate the donors who contributed to the restoration works carried out within the Castle during the inter-war years. Also of interest is the Coat of Arms Gate by Adolf Szyszko-Bohusz.

Stirrup that belonged to the Grand Vizier Kara Mustafa, Cathedral Museum

❸ Krakow Cathedral

See pp66–71.

❹ Cathedral Museum

Wawel 3. **Map** 3 C1 (5 C5). **Tel** 12 429 33 21. 🚌 304, 522. 🚊 3, 6, 8, 10, 18, 40. **Open** 9am–5pm Mon–Sat (Nov–Mar: to 4pm). 📷

The Cathedral Museum was established in September 1978 by the then Archbishop Karol Wojtyła, the Metropolitan of Krakow. The display consists of objects from the Cathedral treasury. Among the exhibits are a sword, which was purposely broken in two places at the funeral of the last Jagiellonian king, Zygmunt August; the coronation robe of Stanisław August Poniatowski; the replica of the royal insignia found inside the royal coffins buried beneath the cathedral, and the stirrup of the Grand Vizier Kara Mustafa which was presented to the Cathedral by King Jan III Sobieski following his victory at the Battle of Vienna (1683). The outstanding collection of reliquaries, church vessels and vestments includes objects found in the tomb of Bishop Maur, as well as memorabilia of John Paul II.

❺ Wawel Royal Castle

See pp72–3.

❻ "Lost Wawel" Exhibition

Wawel Hill 5. **Map** 3 C1 (5 D5). **Tel** 12 422 51 55. 🚌 304, 522. 🚊 3, 6, 8, 10, 18, 40. **Open** Apr–Oct: 9:30am–1pm Mon, 9:30am–5pm Tue–Fri, 10am–5pm Sat & Sun; Nov–Mar: 9:30am–4pm Tue–Fri, 10am–4pm Sat & Sun. **Closed** public hols. 📷 Free Mon (Apr–Oct), Sun (Nov–Mar). 🆆 wawel.krakow.pl

This special exhibition, arranged in the basement of the former royal kitchen (now occupied by the administration office), will appeal to those interested in the medieval history of Wawel. There were possibly ten churches on Wawel Hill in the past. The Rotunda of the Virgin Mary (Sts Felix and Adauctus), unearthed in 1917 during excavations carried out by Adolf Szyszko-Bohusz, is of great interest. The excavations also brought to light the remnants of a man's body as well as some articles of jewellery nearby. It is believed that the circular rotunda formed part of the first palatium (the seat of the first ruler of Wawel), and was built sometime in the late 10th or early 11th century. Its plan resembles a quatrefoil, with strong evidence of Czech influences in the design of the structure. The rotunda was almost completety destroyed in the 19th century.

The exhibition also includes a virtual computer model of the Wawel architecture, which enables visitors to travel into the past to the early 10th century. The computer reconstruction of the medieval buildings shows the state of current research into the early history of Wawel. The models of the so-called Rotunda B, the Rotunda of the Virgin Mary and other buildings, including the palatium, the Church of

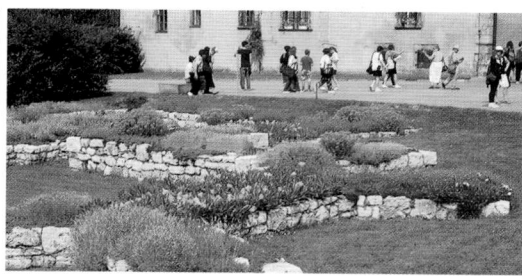

The Archaeological Site

St Gereon and the Cathedral, give a clear picture of the overall layout.

❼ Archaeological Site

Wawel Hill. **Map** 3 C1 (5 C5). 🚌 304, 522. 🚋 3, 6, 8, 10, 18, 40.

The archaeological site is an open area where foundations of medieval buildings can be seen. The buildings were numerous and once formed a small town. A vicarage in the Renaissance style was among them. All the buildings were demolished by the Austrians in 1803–04 and replaced by a drill ground. The lower parts of the walls of St Nicholas, the small Romanesque church rebuilt in the Gothic style during the reign of Kazimierz the Great, are of particular note. This church was an interesting example of

a single nave church, supported on one central column. The plan of the small church of St George is also easy to discern.

❽ Dragon's Lair

Wawel Hill. **Map** 3 C1 (5 C5). **Tel** 12 422 51 55. 🚌 304, 522. 🚋 3, 6, 8, 10, 18, 40. **Open** daily. Apr, Sep & Oct: 10am–5pm; May & Jun: 10am–6pm; Jul & Aug: 10am–7pm.

Within Wawel Hill there are a number of rock caves. The earliest records of these caves date from the 16th century and are thought to be associated with criminality. A pub and a brothel were here in the 18th century. In the 19th century the Austrians sealed the entrance when constructing the fortification walls.

The Lair is open only during the summer months. Some 135 spiral steps lead down into the den, and there are 145 m (476 ft) of tunnels in total, of which only a part can be visited. The bronze statue of the Dragon, designed by Bronisław Chromy, which stands at the exit, was made in 1972.

According to legend, the inhabitants of ancient Krakow were terrorized by a dragon until one day a brave shoemaker, named Skuba, cheated the monster with a sheep stuffed with sulphur. The dragon swallowed the bait. When the sulphur heated its gut, the dragon drank so much water from the Vistula that its body burst. To reward the shoemaker King Krak gave him the hand of his daughter in marriage.

The metal monster belches fire and is seen as a major attraction by younger visitors.

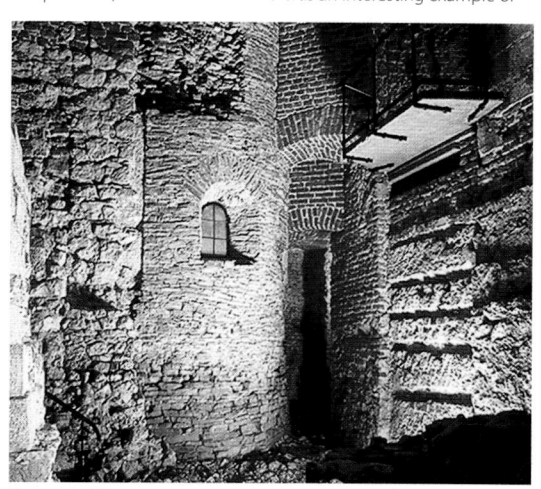

The Rotunda of the Virgin Mary at the "Lost Wawel" Exhibition

❸ Krakow Cathedral

No other building is as strongly associated with the history of Krakow, and the whole nation, as the Cathedral. The existing building is the third to have been built on this site. The Cathedral was built by Władysław the Short to house the relics of St Stanisław, who was much venerated by the Poles. The basilica consists of a nave with single aisles, non-projecting transept, and a choir with an ambulatory. There are also three towers. Many chapels adjoin the aisles. The chapels date from different periods and have been remodelled many times. The internal structure of the Gothic cathedral is now obscure because of later additions. Today the interior displays a variety of styles. Despite this eclecticism the layout of the interior is straightforward.

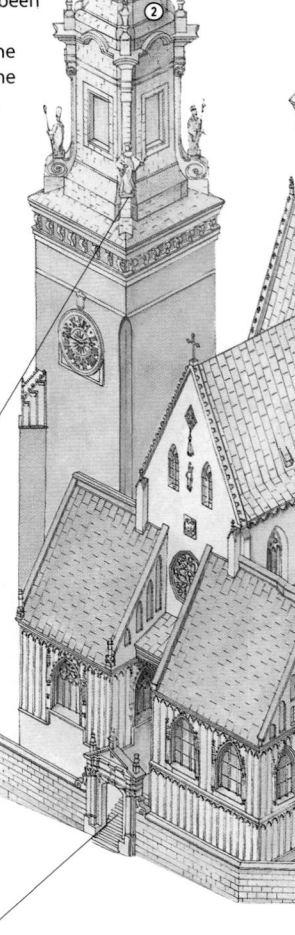

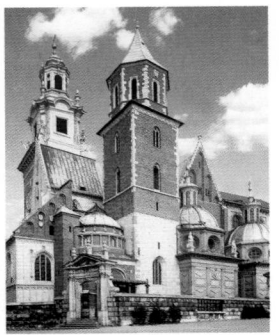

Exterior of the Cathedral
Although dating from different periods, all the distinct parts of the Cathedral make a unique and picturesque ensemble.

Clock Tower
The top of the tallest tower is decorated with four statues of the patron saints of the Kingdom of Poland and the Cathedral: Wacław, Adalbert, Stanisław and Kazimierz (Casimir).

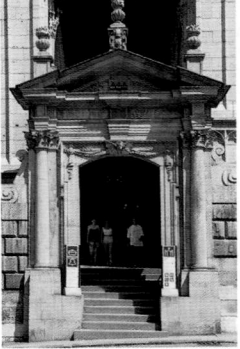

Entrance
The bones of an "ancient creature" hang above the entrance. According to legend the end of the world will come when they fall. The letter K on the door is the initial of Kazimierz the Great, during whose reign the Cathedral was completed.

KEY

① Bell tower

② Baroque spire from the first half of the 18th century

③ Załuski Chapel

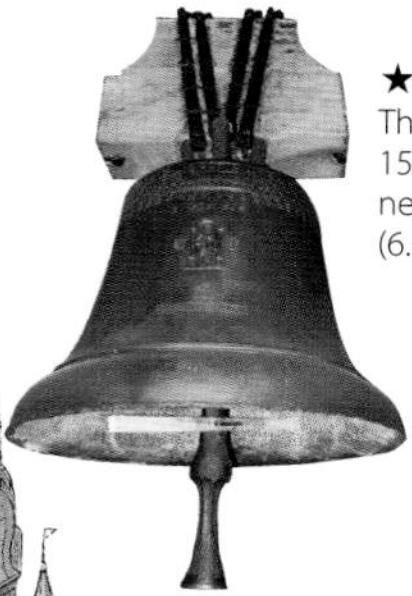

★ Zygmunt Tower
The Zygmunt bell in the tower, cast in 1520, is the largest in Poland. It weighs nearly 11 tons and is more than 2 m (6.5 ft) in diameter.

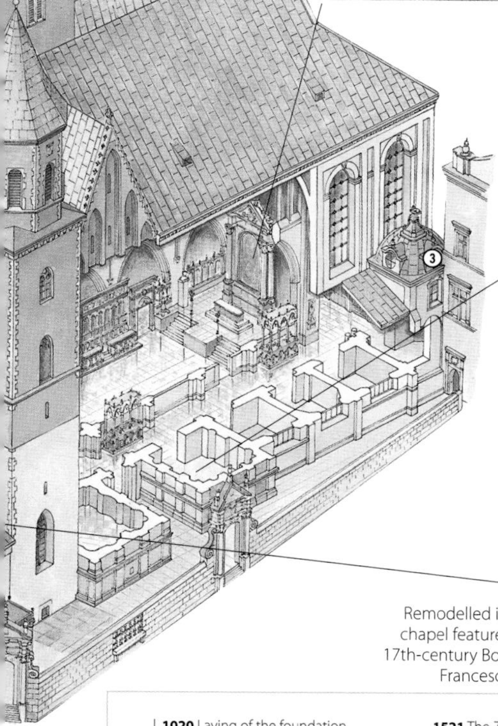

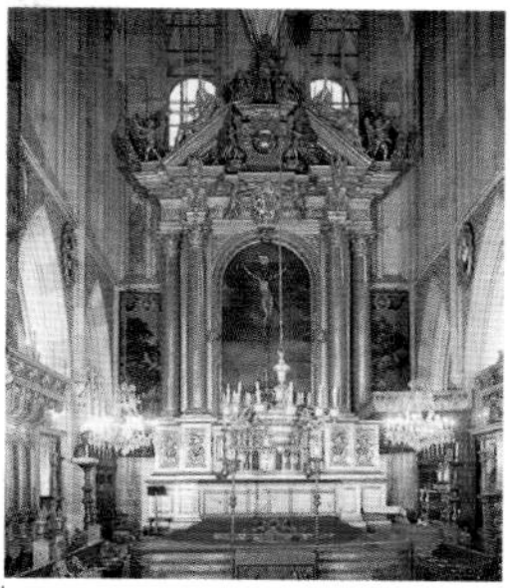

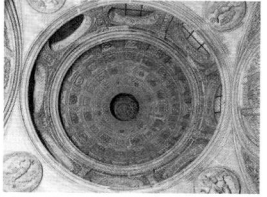

High Altar
The high altar was commissioned in 1649 by Piotr Gembicki, one of the most powerful bishops in 17th-century Krakow.

★ Zygmunt Chapel
This chapel is a mausoleum of the rulers of the Jagiellonian dynasty. Surmounted by a gilt dome, it is a Renaissance masterpiece.

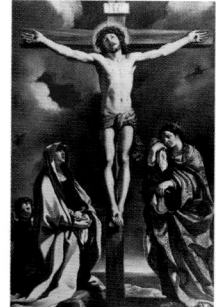

Potocki Chapel
Remodelled in the 19th century, this chapel features *The Crucifixion* by the 17th-century Bolognese artist Giovanni Francesco Barbieri, "Il Guercino".

VISITORS' CHECKLIST

Practical Information
Wawel Hill 3. **Map** 3 C1 (5 C5). **Tel** 12 429 33 21. Cathedral, Zygmunt Tower, Royal Tombs: **Open** Apr–Oct: 9am–5pm Mon–Sat, 12:30–5pm Sun; Nov–Mar: 9am–4pm Mon–Sat, 12:30–4pm Sun. **Closed** Easter, Sun in Advent, Christmas Day, 1 Jan, 1 Nov.

Transport
128, 522. 3, 6, 8, 10, 18, 40.

1020 Laying of the foundation stone of the Cathedral

1090–1142 Second (so-called Herman) Cathedral built

1320–64 Third Cathedral built

1521 The Zygmunt bell hung

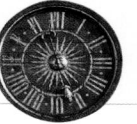

1519–33 Zygmunt Chapel built by Bartolomeo Berrecci

1626–9 St Stanisław's Canopy erected

1664–76 Vaza Chapel built

1758–66 Bishop Załuski's Chapel built

1000 | 1250 | 1500 | 1750

Clock on the Clock Tower

Interior of the Cathedral

The Cathedral of Krakow is exceptional not only for the works of art which are housed here, but also because it has borne witness to many historical events such as coronations, royal weddings and funerals, as well as thanksgiving ceremonies. The Cathedral enjoys not only high sacred status but it also acquired symbolic importance during the occupation of Poland when it became a treasury of objects commemorating national glory. The great Polish playwright Stanisław Wyspiański chose the cathedral as a dramatic setting for his play *Deliverance*. The Cathedral reflects the past but also continues to exert much influence.

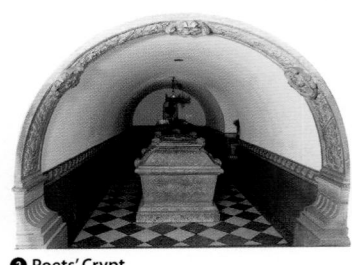

2 Poets' Crypt
Adam Mickiewicz and Juliusz Słowacki, the two foremost Polish poets, are buried here. The remains of Mickiewicz were laid here in 1890 and those of Słowacki in 1929.

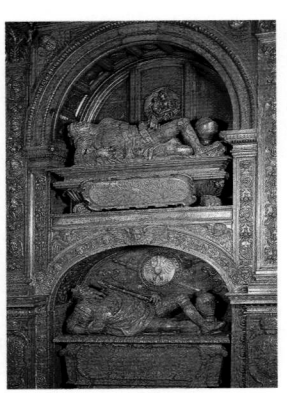

7 Zygmunt Chapel
The splendid double Monument of King Zygmunt the Old (top; by Santi Gucci, 1574–75) and his son, King Zygmunt August (below; by Bartolomeo Berrecci, 1530s) is the outstanding artistic feature of the Cathedral.

Entrance to the Crypt

Czartoryski Chapel

The Cathedral Crypt
houses the tombs of kings and distinguished Poles.

Chapel of the Holy Trinity

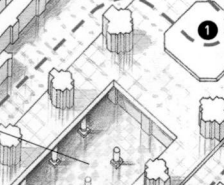

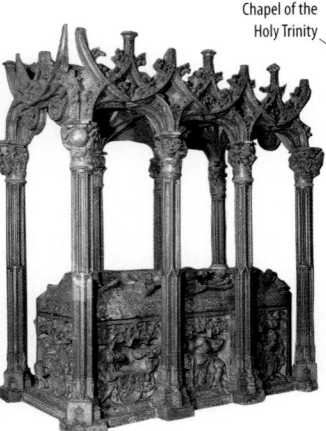

8 Sarcophagus of King Kazimierz Jagiellończyk
One of the most affecting works of Veit Stoss, this was made in 1492, the year of the king's death.

① Canopy of St Stanisław
This altar, the largest in the Cathedral, is dedicated to Poland. It was probably designed by Giovanni Battista Trevano. The silver reliquary in the form of a coffin, containing the relics of St Stanisław, was made by Peter von der Rennen from 1669 to 1671.

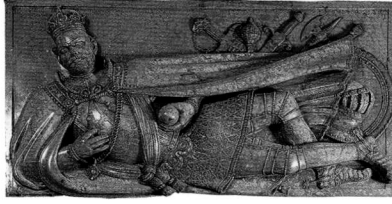

④ Tomb of King Stefan Batory
The work of an outstanding sculptor, Santi Gucci, this tomb was created in 1595. It is a fine example of Mannerist decoration.

Treasury

Sacristy

Chapel of the Virgin
(Batory Chapel)

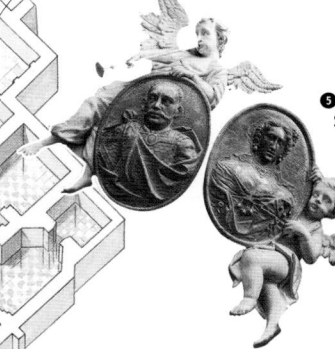

⑤ Tomb of King Jan III Sobieski
Overloaded with Baroque decoration, the tomb of King Jan III (died 1696) and his wife was made in 1760 to the designs of Francesco Placidi.

⑥ Tomb of King Jan Olbracht
Created from 1502 to 1505, the decoration of the recess around the tomb is the earliest example of Renaissance art in Poland. The design is modelled on a Roman triumphal arch. The sarcophagus retains late Gothic forms.

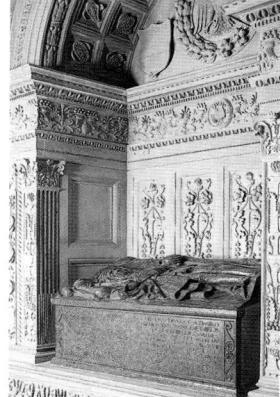

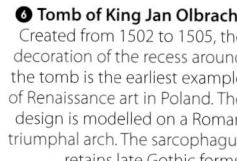

③ Crucifix of Queen Jadwiga
According to legend the Queen prayed in front of this expressive crucifix (c.1380), which has become a place of mass pilgrimage. The relics of the Queen, who became a saint, rest in the altar.

Key

 Suggested route

Exploring Krakow Cathedral

Krakow Cathedral requires more than one visit to do justice to the magnificent building. Its interior with its variety of styles, from medieval to modern, is simply overwhelming. It is worth returning here for a careful visit to all the chapels in the aisles, and to the monuments and tombs of the kings and prominent people in the crypt. It is also possible to look at works in chronological order. The artistic backdrop adds to the spirituality of the Cathedral, which is above all else used for worship. To avoid the crowds, the best time to visit is in the early morning or just before closing time.

Chapels

The chapel of the Holy Cross, erected on the initiative of King Kazimierz Jagiellończyk and his wife Elisabeth von Habsburg, has retained much of its medieval character. The cycle of old Russian wall paintings is one of the largest ensembles to have survived. It is of the Pskov School. Two triptychs of the Holy Trinity and the Virgin Mary of Sorrows both date from the second half of the 15th century. The most interesting furnishing is the tomb of Kazimierz made by Veit Stoss with Huber of Passau. The king is shown in majestic resplendence. It is also a dignified image of death. The stained-glass windows were designed by Józef Mehoffer in the Art Nouveau style.

The Zygmunt Chapel (1519–33), designed by Bartolomeo Berrecci, is of exceptional beauty. The chapel is considered one of the purest examples of the Italian Renaissance outside Italy. It was modelled on the best Italian architectural and decorative works. The silver altar was made between 1531 and 1538 in Nuremberg by Melchior Baier to the designs of Peter Flötner. The royal tombs are equally interesting. The interior is peaceful and majestic and conveys the spirit of 16th-century humanism. Bishop Tomicki's Chapel is also Renaissance in style.

Remodelled by Bartolomeo Berrecci from 1526 to 1535, the chapel played an important role as a model for mausolea for the nobility and gentry. The Chapel of the Virgin Mary (King Stefan Batory's Chapel) houses a 17th-century Baroque tabernacle with the Holy Eucharist. The tomb of Batory and the royal stalls were designed by Santi Gucci. The Vaza Chapel, probably also designed by the same architect, exemplifies a 17th-century interior: monumental,

heavy forms executed in black marble with large epitaphs. It acts as a reminder of the fragility and transience of earthly life.

Among the chapels constructed in the 18th century, two are of particular interest. The Lipski Chapel (1743–7), designed by Francesco Placidi, catches the light and plays with shadows. The decoration of Bishop Załuski's Chapel (1758–66) employs the allegory of the passage through the gate (note the enlarged entrance).

The *Crucifixion* by Guercino and the statue of the Risen Christ by Bertel Thorvaldsen are to be seen in the Chapel of Bishop Filip Padniewski. This Renaissance chapel was remodelled in the 19th century for the Potocki family. The statue of Włodzimierz Potocki in the Holy Trinity Chapel is also by Thorvaldsen.

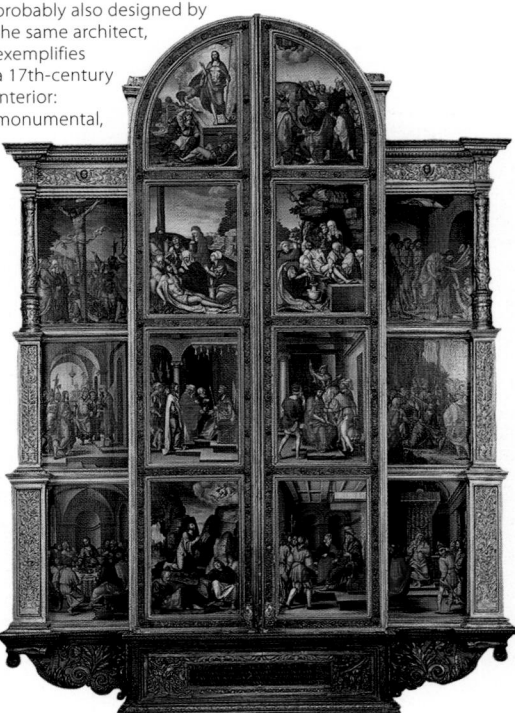

The altar in the Zygmunt Chapel

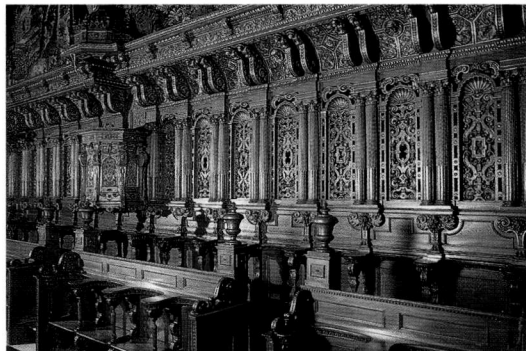

Intricately carved stalls in the choir of the Cathedral

Furnishings

As well as the canopy of St Stanisław, particularly noteworthy are the epitaphs of the bishops of Krakow placed on the pillars, and decorated with busts of the deceased. Marcin Szyszkowski, Piotr Gembicki, Jan Małachowski and Kazimierz Łubieński all rest here, providing eternal company for the relics of St Stanisław. The Baroque stalls in the choir were made around 1620; additions were made in the 19th century. The bas-relief epitaph of Cardinal Fryderyk Jagiellończyk shows superb craftsmanship. It was made after 1503 in the Vischer workshop in Nuremberg. The throne of Bishop Piotr Gembicki has splendid Baroque decoration. The organ loft, made around 1758 to the design of Francesco Placidi, is also of much interest.

Sarcophagi and Tombs

The cathedral is a resting place for Polish rulers, and all its medieval tombs follow a particular model. They show a figure laying in state on a massive sarcophagus, decorated with allegorical figures of the king's subjects lamenting the death of their sovereign. A dog, symbolizing fidelity, is usually placed at the king's feet, and the head of the ruler rests on a lion, the symbol of power. A stone canopy is suspended over the tomb. The tomb of Władysław the Short,

dating from the mid-14th century is the earliest sarcophagus of this type. Kazimierz Jagiellończyk was the last to have such a monument erected.

Two tombs of a much later date were inspired by this early type of sepulchre. The beautiful and majestic tomb of Queen Jadwiga is one of them. It was executed with great delicacy in white Carrara marble by Antoni Madeyski in 1902. The tomb is one of the most visited places of pilgrimage in the Cathedral. The other sarcophagus, also by Madeyski, was erected in 1906. It is a cenotaph (tomb without a corpse) commemorating King Władysław III Warneńczyk, who was killed in 1444 at the Battle of Varna against the Turks. His

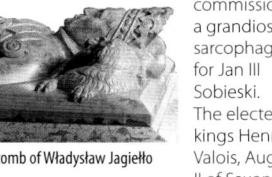

The tomb of Władysław Jagiełło

body was never found, giving rise to stories about his miraculous salvation.

Royal Tombs

The Royal Tombs were placed in the crypt following the construction of the Zygmunt Chapel, which is a mausoleum. Zygmunt the Old and his sons are buried in the crypt under the chapel. Earlier rulers were buried in the Cathedral, except Bolesław the Brave, Bolesław the Bold, Przemysław II, Louis of Anjou, Władysław III Warneńczyk and Aleksander Jagiellończyk. A crypt was also constructed for the Vaza dynasty. Later rulers were buried beneath the Chapel of the Holy Cross and in St Leonard's crypt. In 1783 the last Polish king, Stanisław August Poniatowski, commissioned a grandiose sarcophagus for Jan III Sobieski. The elected kings Henri de Valois, August II of Saxony and Stanisław August Poniatowski do not rest in the Wawel. Two national heroes, Kościuszko and Prince Józef Poniatowski, were laid here during the Partitions of Poland. State funerals of Piłsudski and General Sikorski took place in the Cathedral in the 20th century.

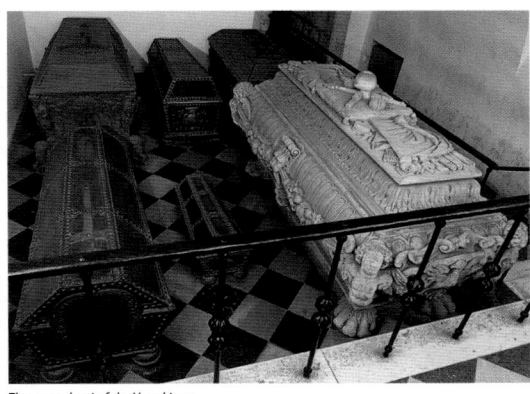

The sarcophagi of the Vaza kings

❺ Wawel Royal Castle

Little is known about the earliest Wawel residence. The Romanesque palatium was probably built by Kazimierz the Restorer; later Władysław the Short started to construct a new building but it was only completed by Kazimierz the Great. The present Renaissance castle was constructed in the first half of the 16th century. At the start of the 17th century the apartments in the north wing were remodelled in the early Baroque style. After the royal court moved from Krakow to Warsaw, the castle fell into ruin. Further devastation was caused by the occupying foreign powers. Early in the 20th century the castle was given back to Krakow, and restoration was begun.

Castle Guide

The Crown Treasury and Armoury, each with a separate entrance, are situated on the ground floor together with a number of state rooms. The remaining state rooms and other apartments are on the first and second floors. After leaving the Senators' Hall a visit to the "Orient in the Wawel Collections" exhibition on the first and second floors in the west wing is recommended.

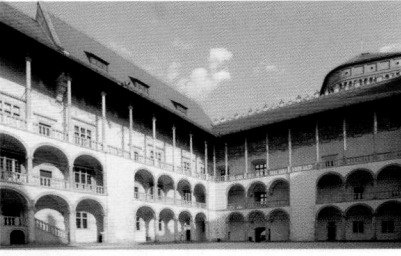

Crown Treasury and Armoury
This 11th-century chalice belonged to the Abbots of Tyniec and is now in the Treasury. Adjacent to the Treasury is the Armoury with its rich collection.

Senators' Hall

Senators' Staircase

First floor

The Castle Courtyard
A mix of architectural styles can be found at the castle. One of the highlights is the beautiful Renaissance-style court-yard, built in the 16th century.

Key

- ▢ Royal Apartments
- ▢ Treasury
- ▢ Armoury
- ▢ "Orient in the Wawel Collections" Exhibition
- ▢ Non-exhibition area

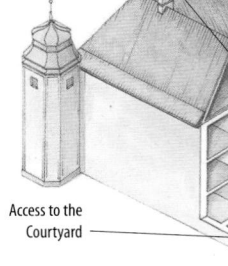

Access to the Courtyard

Entrance to the Crown Treasury and Armoury

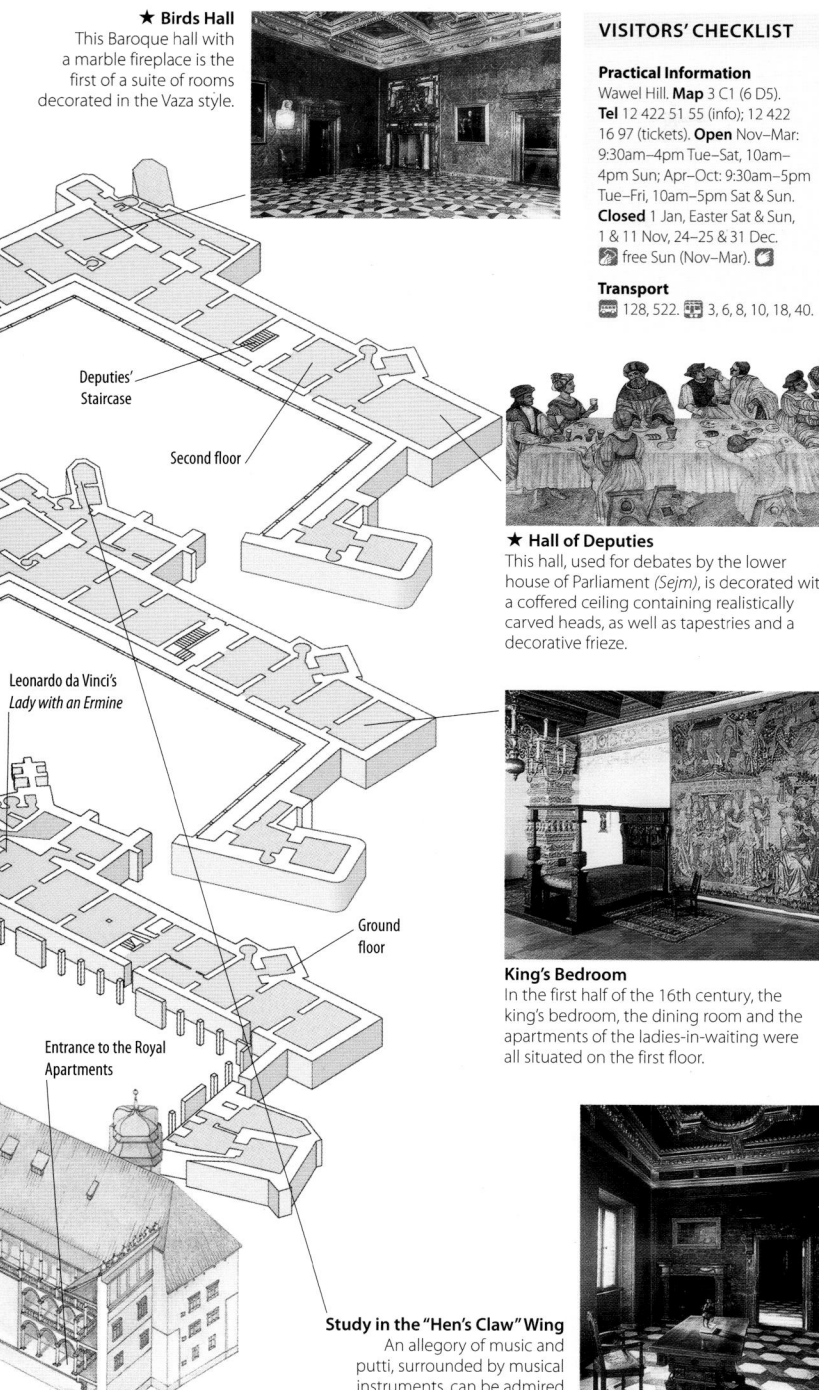

★ Birds Hall
This Baroque hall with a marble fireplace is the first of a suite of rooms decorated in the Vaza style.

Deputies' Staircase

Second floor

Leonardo da Vinci's *Lady with an Ermine*

Ground floor

Entrance to the Royal Apartments

VISITORS' CHECKLIST

Practical Information
Wawel Hill. **Map** 3 C1 (6 D5).
Tel 12 422 51 55 (info); 12 422 16 97 (tickets). **Open** Nov–Mar: 9:30am–4pm Tue–Sat, 10am–4pm Sun; Apr–Oct: 9:30am–5pm Tue–Fri, 10am–5pm Sat & Sun. **Closed** 1 Jan, Easter Sat & Sun, 1 & 11 Nov, 24–25 & 31 Dec. 🎟 free Sun (Nov–Mar). 🛍

Transport
🚌 128, 522. 🚊 3, 6, 8, 10, 18, 40.

★ Hall of Deputies
This hall, used for debates by the lower house of Parliament *(Sejm)*, is decorated with a coffered ceiling containing realistically carved heads, as well as tapestries and a decorative frieze.

King's Bedroom
In the first half of the 16th century, the king's bedroom, the dining room and the apartments of the ladies-in-waiting were all situated on the first floor.

Study in the "Hen's Claw" Wing
An allegory of music and putti, surrounded by musical instruments, can be admired on the ceiling here.

Statues decorating the exterior of Krakow Cathedral, situated on Wawel Hill ▶

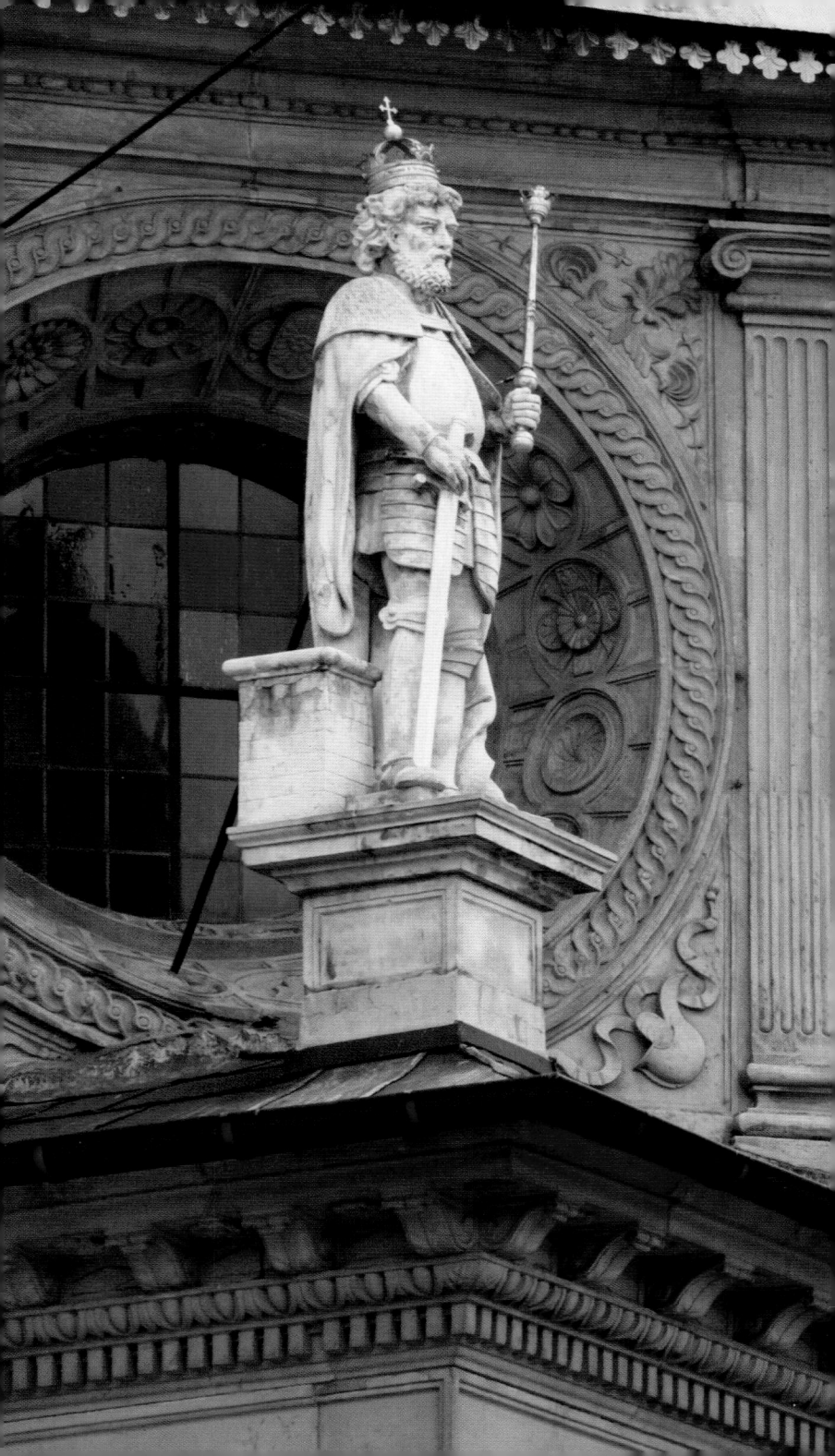

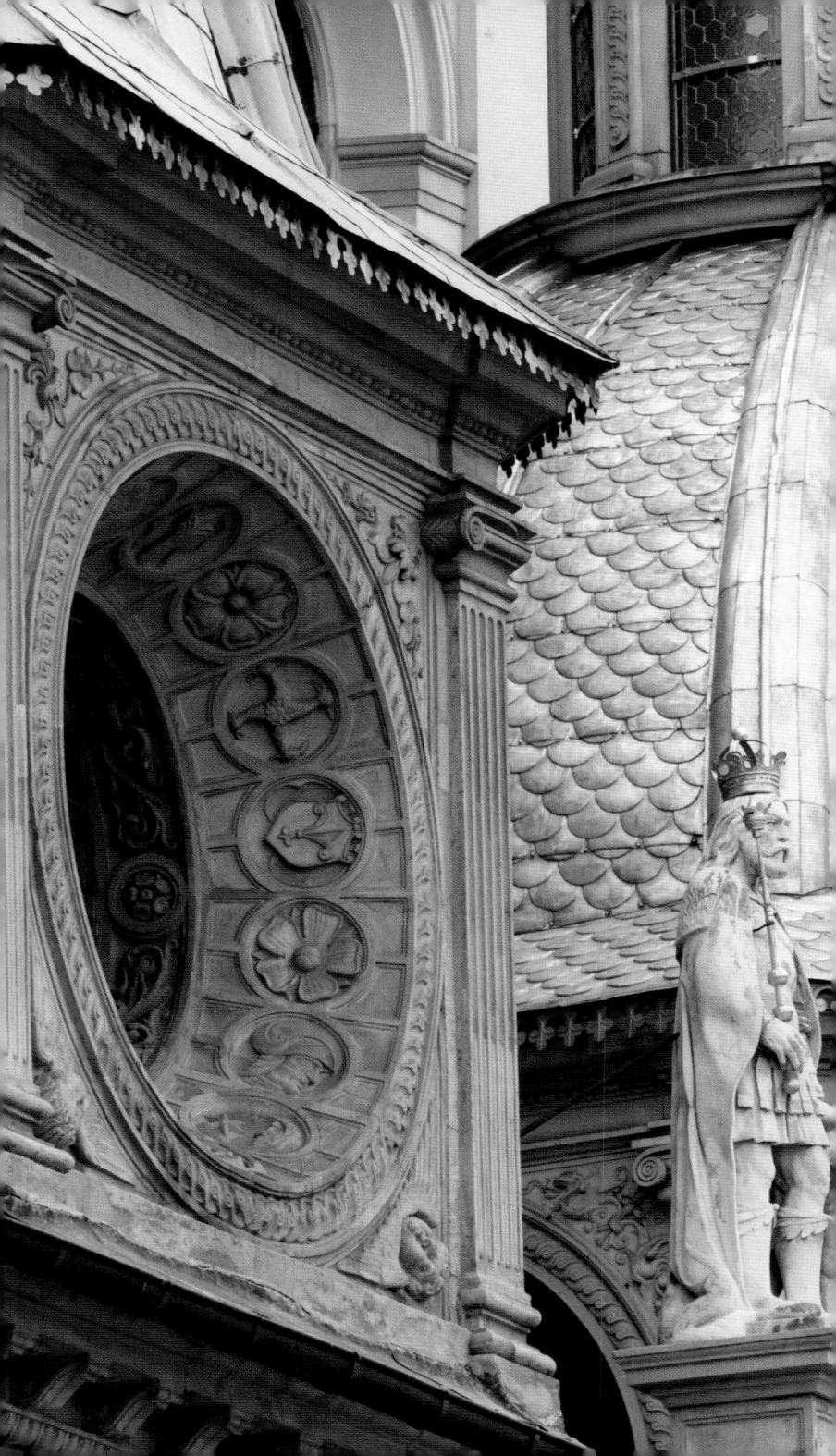

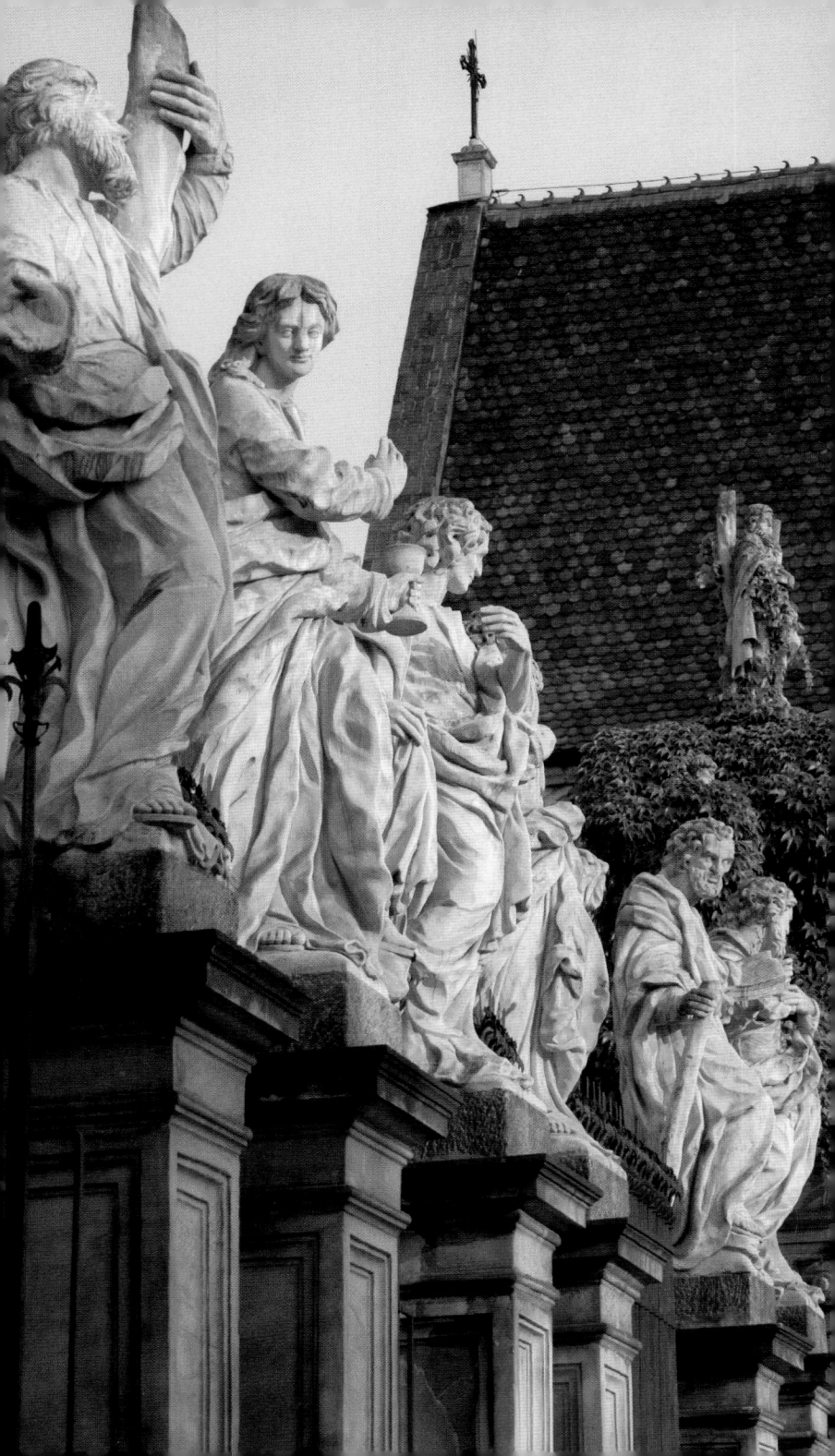

OKÓŁ AND STRADOM QUARTERS

Okół was probably the earliest settlement at the foot of Wawel. Timber-built houses and a palisade enclosure were already here in the 10th century. The settlement developed along the so-called Salt Route which led from Hungary to Greater Poland. The quarter became elitist as a result of its proximity to the Royal Castle and the Cathedral. High-ranking clergy resided here and many churches were built.

The development of Stradom, situated between Okół and Krakow, was hindered by its location on peat marshes and the vicinity of the Wawel fortress. Splendid churches and palaces were constructed here from the mid-17th century. Stradom developed rapidly at the end of the 1800s.

Sights at a Glance

Churches and Monasteries
- ❸ Church of Saints Peter and Paul pp82–3
- ❹ Church of St Andrew
- ❺ Church of St Martin
- ❼ Church of St Giles
- ⓲ Franciscan Church pp88–9
- ⓲ Church of the Bernardine Nuns
- ⓲ Bernardine Church
- ㉑ Church of the Missionaries

Museums and Galleries
- ❿ Archdiocesan Museum
- ⓫ Palace of Bishop Erazm Ciołek
- ⓬ St Vladimir's Foundation
- ⓭ Cricoteka
- ⓮ Archaeological Museum
- ㉒ Natural History Museum

Historic Parks
- ㉓ Dietl Plantations

Historic Monuments and Buildings
- ❷ Collegium Iuridicum
- ❻ Royal Arsenal
- ❾ Deanery
- ⓰ Wielopolski Palace
- ⓱ Statue of Józef Dietl
- ⓴ Częstochowa Seminary

Historic Streets
- ❶ Grodzka Street
- ❽ Kanonicza Street

Restaurants see p190
1. Balaton
2. Il Calzone
3. Copernicus
4. Miód Malina
5. Pod Aniołami
6. Pod Baranem
7. Sakana Sushi Bar
8. Smak Ukrainski
9. Trattoria La Campana

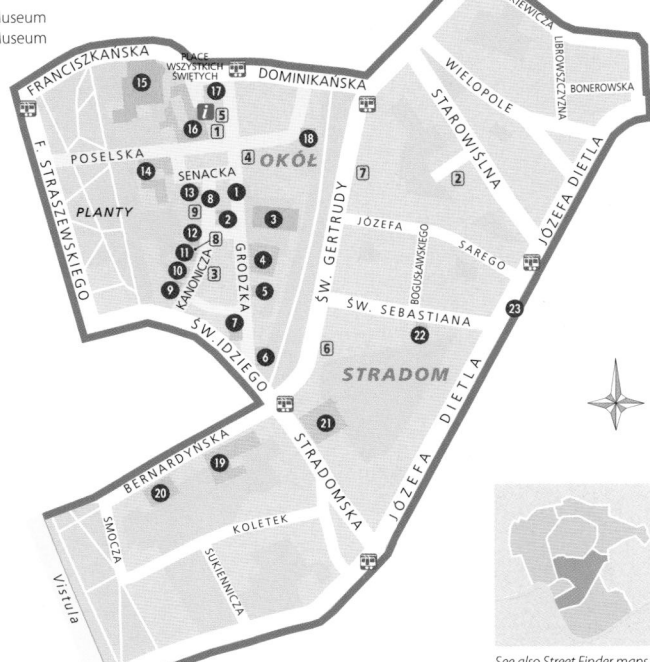

0 metres 200
0 yards 200

See also Street Finder maps 1, 3 & 6

◀ Statues of the Apostles at the entrance to the Church of Saints Peter and Paul

For keys to symbols see back flap

Street-By-Street: Okół

The historic Okół district is more or less in line with the southern part of the medieval centre of Krakow. It is a picturesque area. Those who want a change from the regular plan of the Old Quarter will enjoy Okół's curving streets and dead-end mews, lined with some outstanding buildings. Fortunately the great fire of Krakow in 1850 did not damage the buildings in Okół, and much of the original architecture can still be seen here.

② Collegium Iuridicum
This sculpture, *Luca di Nara*, in the courtyard is by Polish-born Igor Mitoraj. It was presented to the Jagiellonian University by the artist, who now lives in Italy.

⑭ Archaeological Museum
The collections here tell the prehistory of the Polish lands.

⑬ Cricoteka
The Cricot 2 Theatre and Museum are located in this Gothic house.

⑫ St Vladimir's Foundation
This building houses artifacts explaining the life of the Ruthenas in the Polish-Lithuanian Commonwealth.

⑪ Palace of Bishop Erazm Ciołek
This beautiful building is now home to the National Museum's collection of Polish art from the Middle Ages to the beginning of the 19th century.

⑩ Archdiocesan Museum
The collection consists of objects from churches in the Krakow Archdiocese that are no longer used in the liturgy.

SENACKA

KANONICZA

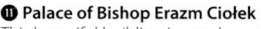

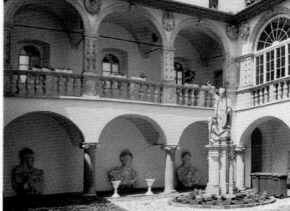

⑨ Deanery
The arcaded courtyard of this small house, formerly a canonry, gives the impression of a magnificent Renaissance residence.

⑧ Kanonicza Street
This quiet street has retained much of the old royal character of Krakow.

❸ ★ Church of Saints Peter and Paul
This early Baroque Jesuit church is a masterpiece of 17th-century Polish architecture. The façade, with its rich sculptural decoration, is remarkable.

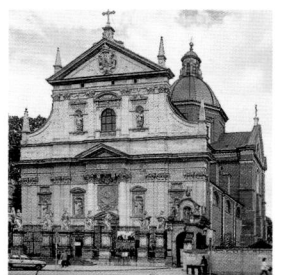

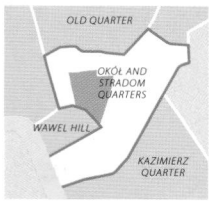

Locator Map
See Street Finder maps 1, 3 & 6

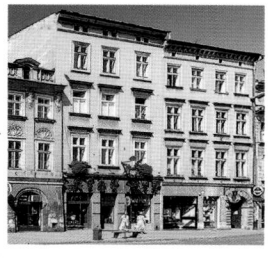

❶ Grodzka Street
The town houses situated along one of the oldest streets in Krakow were once palaces.

❹ ★ Church of St Andrew
This is the best preserved example of Romanesque architecture in Krakow.

❺ Church of St Martin
This small early Baroque church was transformed into the Augsburg Protestant Church in the early 19th century.

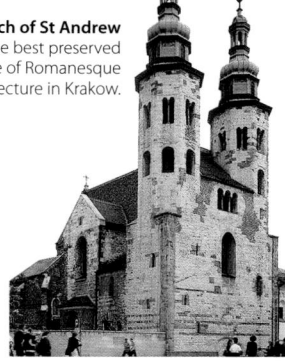

❻ Royal Arsenal
This entrance to the Arsenal is one of the most beautiful 17th-century doorways in Krakow.

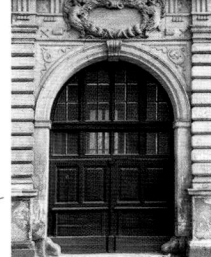

0 metres   50
0 yards   50

Key

— Suggested route

❼ Church of St Giles
This is a rather modest Gothic church dating from the first half of the 14th century.

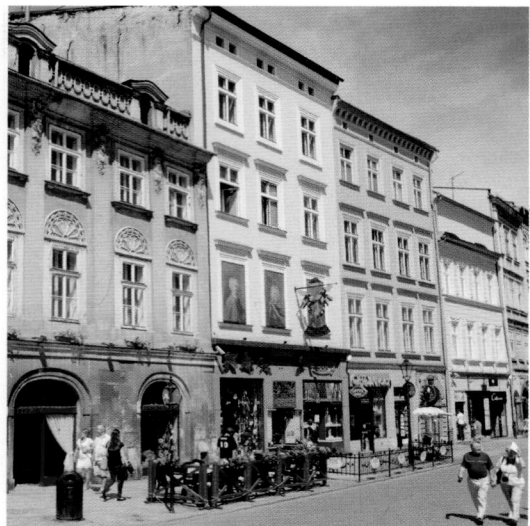

Historic Grodzka Street, lined with picturesque buildings

❶ Grodzka Street
Ulica Grodzka

Map 1 C5 (6 D4). 🚊 1, 3, 6, 8, 18, 40.

Grodzka is one of the oldest streets in Krakow. In the past it formed part of the important Salt Route from Hungary to Greater Poland. As part of the Royal Route it bore witness to coronation and funeral processions of Polish kings.

Grodzka Street was once lined with many palaces and a few churches. These palaces were rebuilt and converted into town houses. Grodzka is a lovely street full of character, owing to its irregular plan, varying width and diverse architecture.

❷ Collegium Iuridicum
ul. Grodzka 53. **Map** 1 C5 (6 D4).
Tel 12 633 63 77. 🚊 1, 3, 6, 8, 18, 40.
Open 10am–1pm Tue & Thu,
11am–2pm Sun.

The Collegium Iuridicum of the Academy of Krakow was founded early in the 15th century through the bequest of Queen Jadwiga. The excavation work carried out at the site has confirmed that the building had replaced a large trade hall, probably built in

the 14th century on the orders of Władysław the Short. The remnants of the hall have survived in the basement. The Collegium Iuridicum was rebuilt several times. The works were funded by Bishop Jan Rzeszowski, among others. The elaborate doorway decorated with the University's emblem was made around 1680. The College was entirely rebuilt after a fire in 1719 and the two-tier arcaded courtyard

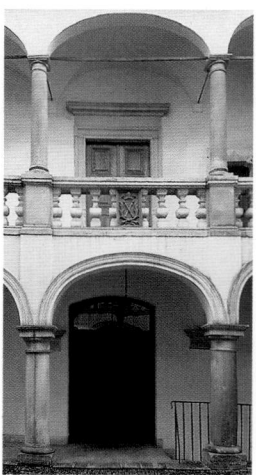

Two-tier arcaded courtyard of the Collegium Iuridicum

added. The Institute of the History of Art is housed here, as was, until recently, the Zoological Museum of the Jagiellonian University. The museum is due to reopen in 2016 in a campus on the outskirts of the city.

In the summer months concerts and theatrical performances take place in courtyard, which features a sculpture by Igor Mitoraj.

❸ Church of Saints Peter and Paul
Kościół św. św. Piotra i Pawła

See pp82–3.

❹ Church of St Andrew
Kościół św. Andrzeja

ul. Grodzka 56. **Map** 1 C5 (6 D4).
Tel 12 422 16 12. 🚊 1, 3, 6, 8, 18, 40.
Open 7:30am–5pm daily and during services.

The Church of St Andrew in Okół is regarded as one of the finest examples of Romanesque architecture in Poland. It was built between 1079 and 1098 as a foundation of Sieciech, the powerful Palatine to Duke Władysław Herman. It was rebuilt around 1200. The towers and aisles were extended and a transept added. According to the chronicler Jan Długosz this was the only church in Krakow to resist the Tatar invasion of 1241. Around 1702 it was remodelled in the Baroque style to the designs of Baldassare Fontana, who also covered the internal walls and vaulting with stuccowork. Mural paintings by Karl Dankwart complete the decoration. Among furnishings worth noting are the pulpit, in the form of a boat, and the high altar with an imposing ebony tabernacle decorated with silver ornaments.

The treasury in the convent adjoining the church houses some priceless objects, such as a portable mosaic depicting the Virgin Mary from the end of the 12th century, 14th-century

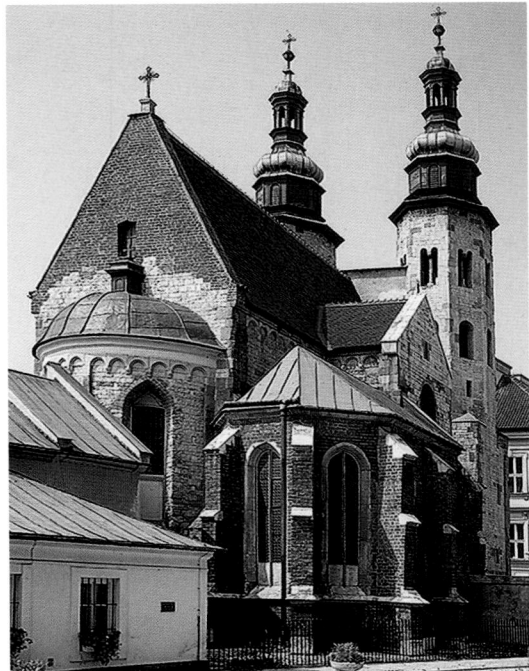

Church of St Andrew with its two spires

marionettes used in Christmas nativity plays, and early medieval reliquaries.

❺ Church of St Martin
Kościół św. Marcina

ul. Grodzka 58a. **Map** 6 D4. **Tel** 12 446 64 30. 8, 10, 18. **Open** 10am–1pm Mon–Sat and during services.

The first church was probably built on this site in the 12th century. In 1612 the Discalced Carmelite Nuns were brought here. The old church was demolished and in 1637–40 the nuns commisioned a new, rather small church in the early Baroque style. After the convent was closed down, the church was taken over by the Protestant community. The interior was converted according to the needs of the Lutheran liturgy. The high altar features a 14th-century crucifix and *Christ Calming the Storm,* painted by Henryk Siemiradzki in 1882.

❻ Royal Arsenal
Arsenał Królewski

ul. Grodzka 64. **Map** 6 D5. 8, 10, 18. **Closed** to the public.

In the first half of the 16th century Zygmunt the Old built an arsenal and a cannon foundry next to the city wall. They formed part of Krakow's fortifications. The present building was remodelled in 1927 by the architect Stanisław Filipkiewicz, who juxtaposed the Baroque structure of the arsenal with an austere extension thus achieving an interesting effect.

❼ Church of St Giles
Kościół św. Idziego

ul. Św. Idziego 1. **Map** 6 D5. 8, 10, 18. **Open** 10am–1pm Tue–Fri.

According to historic evidence made popular by a song by Ewa Demarczyk (of the Piwnica pod Baranami Cabaret), this church was "built in 1082 by Władysław Herman and his wife Judith, after they bore a child through the intervention of St Giles". The present church was built in the early 14th century. In 1595 the Dominicans took over and soon remodelled it.

Among the furnishings, the stone stalls are particularly interesting. They were made in 1629 by reusing fragments of the Renaissance tomb of St Jacek (otherwise known as St Hyacinth) from the Dominican Church.

❽ Kanonicza Street
Ulica Kanonicza

Map 1 C5 (6 D4). 3, 6, 8, 10, 18, 40.

Kanonicza Street formed the last stretch of the Royal Route leading towards Wawel. From the 14th century onwards it was lined with the houses of Krakow's canons, who were given the use of these houses for life when they took up office in the Chapter of Krakow. Each successive inhabitant tended to modernize their house. As a result, Gothic houses acquired arcaded Renaissance courtyards, Baroque doorways or Neo-Classical façades. The canons could afford to spend lavishly owing to their elite status within the church.

The great diversity of architectural styles which can be found within the narrow and winding little Kanonicza Street gives it a picturesque character.

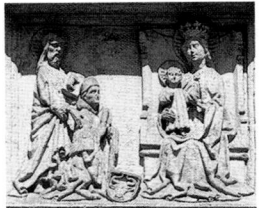

Decorative bas-relief plaque of 1480 on the Długosz House, Kanonicza Street

❸ Church of Saints Peter and Paul

This church, modelled on the Jesuit Church of Il Gesù in Rome, is considered to be one of the most magnificent early Baroque churches in Central Europe. The history of its construction and the name of the architects involved are the subjects of an ongoing debate among architectural historians. The foundation stone was laid in 1596. The leading Jesuit architect, Giovanni de Rosis, contributed the design, and works were carried out by Giuseppe Brizio and Giovanni Maria Bernardoni. In 1605 the church neared its completion but, due to some structural problems, a number of walls had to be dismantled and rebuilt to an altered design. The court architect Giovanni Battista Trevano was put in charge of the second stage.

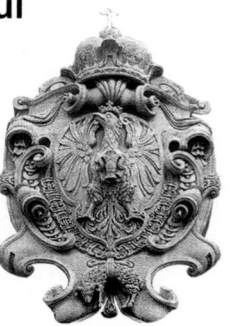

Cartouche with an Eagle
This exquisitely carved coat of arms belonged to the main founder of the church, King Zygmunt III Vaza.

Organ Gallery
The late Baroque organ gallery with a curved balustrade, designed by Kacper Bażanka, is in contrast with the austere and monumental architecture of the church. It is located inside, just above the main entrance.

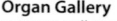

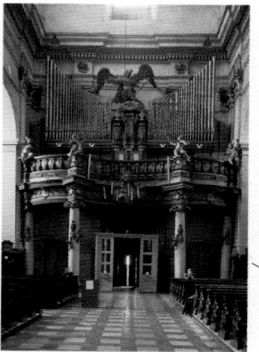

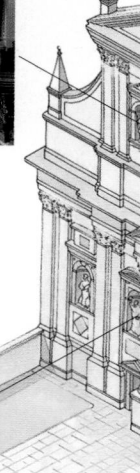

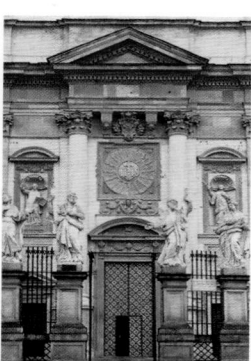

Statues of the Apostles
This railing was designed by Kacper Bażanka and is decorated with copies of statues originally carved by David Heel from 1715 to 1722.

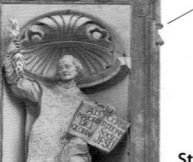

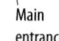

Main entrance

Statue of St Ignatius Loyola
The founder of the Society of Jesus is depicted in this late Baroque sculpture by David Heel. The adjoining statues are of Stanisław Kostka, Francis Xavier and Aloysius Gonzaga.

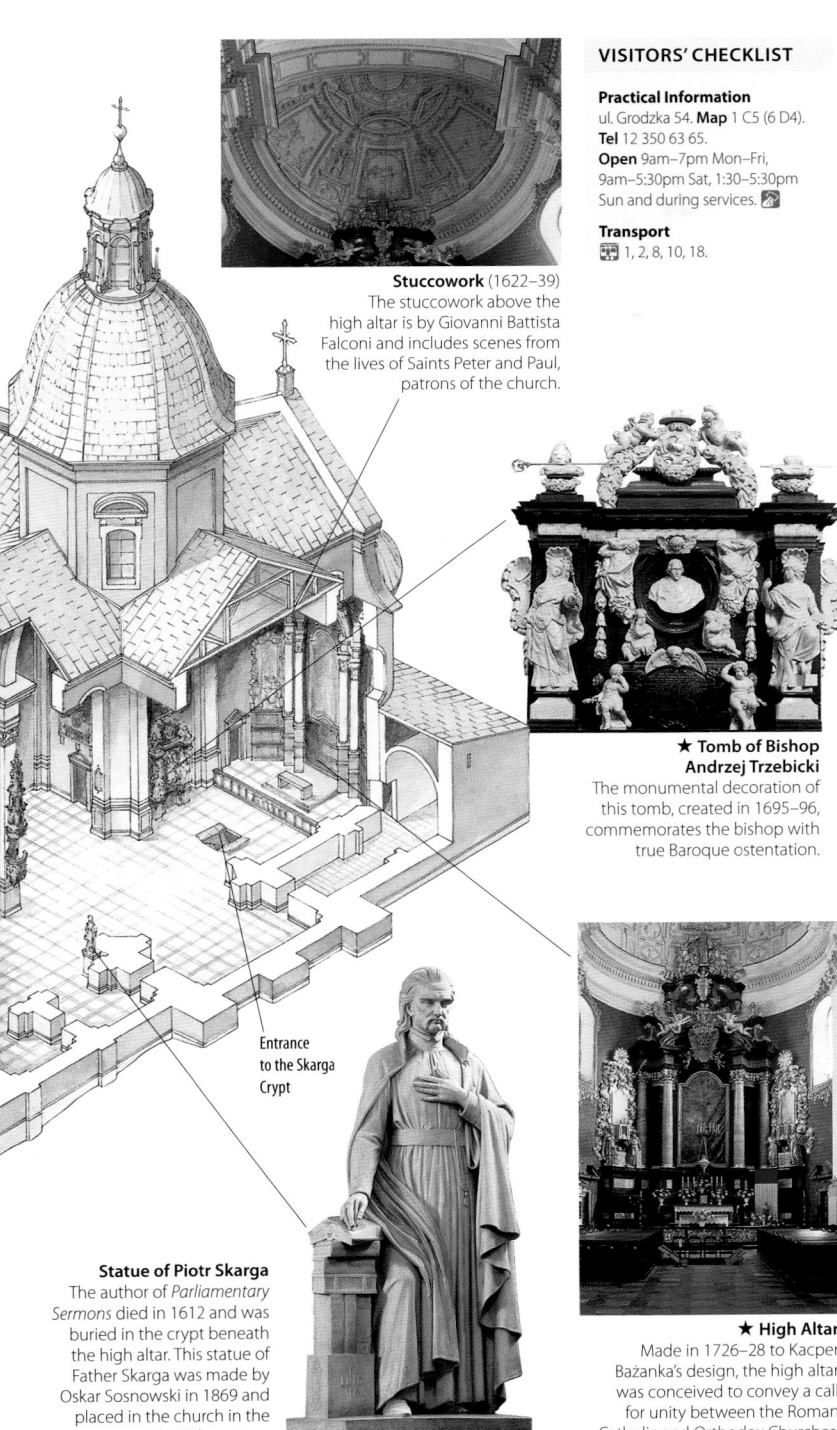

Stuccowork (1622–39)
The stuccowork above the high altar is by Giovanni Battista Falconi and includes scenes from the lives of Saints Peter and Paul, patrons of the church.

VISITORS' CHECKLIST

Practical Information
ul. Grodzka 54. **Map** 1 C5 (6 D4).
Tel 12 350 63 65.
Open 9am–7pm Mon–Fri,
9am–5:30pm Sat, 1:30–5:30pm
Sun and during services.

Transport
1, 2, 8, 10, 18.

★ Tomb of Bishop Andrzej Trzebicki
The monumental decoration of this tomb, created in 1695–96, commemorates the bishop with true Baroque ostentation.

Entrance to the Skarga Crypt

Statue of Piotr Skarga
The author of *Parliamentary Sermons* died in 1612 and was buried in the crypt beneath the high altar. This statue of Father Skarga was made by Oskar Sosnowski in 1869 and placed in the church in the early 20th century.

★ High Altar
Made in 1726–28 to Kacper Bażanka's design, the high altar was conceived to convey a call for unity between the Roman Catholic and Orthodox Churches.

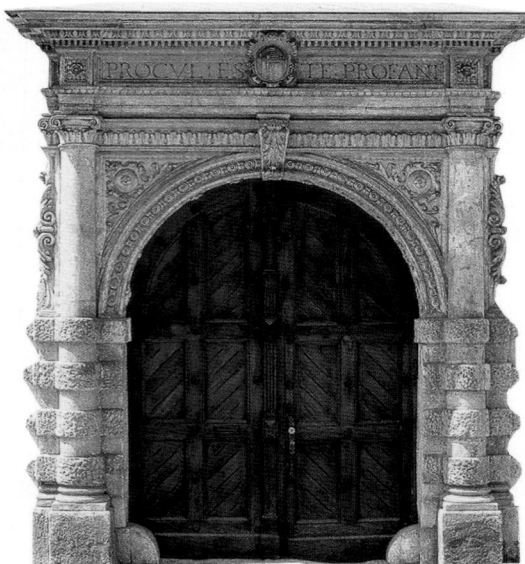
Massive portal of the medieval Deanery

● Deanery
Dom Dziekański

ul. Kanonicza 21. **Map** 1 C5 (6 D4).
🚌 1, 3, 6, 8, 10, 18, 40.

This house is considered to be the most beautiful of all the canons' houses in Krakow. The medieval house was completely rebuilt in the 1580s, probably by the architect and sculptor Santi Gucci. The arcaded courtyard with its magnificent decoration, carved in stone, the impressive portal and the *sgraffiti* on the façade all date from this period. The statue of St Stanisław in the courtyard was added in the 18th century. In the 1960s this was home to the future Pope and then Suffragan Bishop of Krakow, Karol Wojtyła.

● Archdiocesan Museum
Muzeum Archidiecezjalne

ul. Kanonicza 19. **Map** 1 C5 (6 D4).
Tel 12 421 89 63. 🚌 1, 3, 6, 8, 18, 40.
Open 10am–4pm Tue–Fri, 10am–3pm Sat & Sun. 🏛 📷

This house is traditionally associated with the residence of St Stanisław while he was a canon in Krakow, hence the name, St Stanisław's House.

It was actually built in the 14th century but entirely remodelled in the late 18th century. The Archdiocesan Museum is now housed here. It runs a programme of temporary exhibitions of sacred art based on loans from church treasuries in the Krakow Archdiocese. Interesting goldwork displays have taken place here.

Part of the Archdiocesan Museum is given over to the room of Karol Wojtyła, who became Pope John Paul II. The room has been faithfully reconstructed here as it stood originally in the adjoining Deanery, where he lived.

● Palace of Bishop Erazm Ciołek
Pałac biskupa Erazma Ciołka

ul. Kanonicza 17. **Map** 1 C5 (6 D4).
Tel 12 433 59 20. 🚌 6, 8, 10, 18, 40.
Open 10am–4pm Tue–Sun. 🏛 free on Sun (permanent collection).

This museum was once home to the great diplomat and patron of the arts Bishop Erazm Ciołek (1474–1522). A magnificently distinguished residence, it has been extensively renovated and now houses the National Museum's large and notable collection of Polish Art. The house was built in a mix of Gothic and Renaissance styles, while the collection within ranges from the 12th to the 18th centuries. The latter includes such gems as large 15th-century tryptichs from Krakow guilds, exquisite Orthodox icons and encolpions, which reveal the ever-increasing influence and power of Western Europe in the 17th and 18th centuries.

● St Vladimir's Foundation
Fundacja św. Włodzimierza

ul. Kanonicza 15. **Map** 1 C5 (6 D4).
Tel 12 421 92 94. 🚌 1, 3, 6, 8, 10, 18, 40. **Open** call in advance. 🏛

St Vladimir's Foundation is based in a 14th-century house which displays fine Renaissance decoration. Icons from disused Orthodox churches in the Beskidy, Bieszczady and Tomaszów

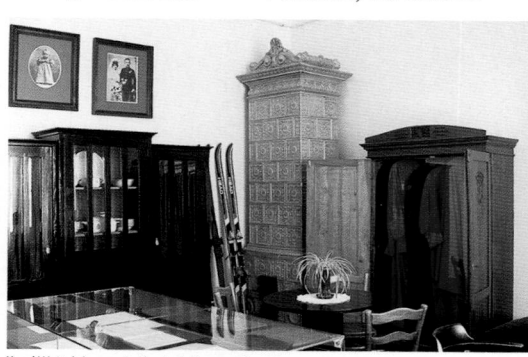
Karol Wojtyła's room in the Archdiocesan Museum

Lubelski regions, dating mainly from the 17th and 18th centuries, are kept here.

The Greek Catholic Chapel is dedicated to the martyr saints Boris and Gleb and is decorated with paintings by Jerzy Nowosielski. This contemporary Krakow artist is influenced by Byzantine art but uses modern forms of expression.

The sanctuary features the miraculous icon of the Korczmin Madonna.

⓭ Cricoteka

ul. Kanonicza 5. **Map** 1 C5 (6 D4). **Tel** 12 422 83 32. 🚋 1, 6, 8, 18. **Open** 10am–2pm Mon & Wed–Fri; 2–6pm Tue. 📷

The former canon's house at 5 Kanonicza Street has retained much of its Gothic form. In 1980 it became the home of the renowned avant-garde theatre Cricot 2. This theatre was founded in 1956 on the initiative of Tadeusz Kantor, the outstanding painter and stage designer. It became famous for performances which were permeated by a symbolic representation of man's existence. Performances relied on traditional theatrical forms while also borrowing from the "happenings" fashionable at the time. The most unusual sets added a surreal flavour. *The Dead Class*, *Wielopole, Wielopole* and *Let Artists Drop Dead* were among Cricot 2's most successful productions. After the death of Kantor in 1990 his actors continued his work.

The house in Kanonicza Street is too small to have a stage, so performances take place in other venues. The Cricoteka housed here is a small museum and archive documenting the work of the theatre since its inception. Costumes, stage designs and props, photographs of the performances, as well as drawings and paintings by Kantor, are all here.

⓮ Archaeological Museum
Muzeum Archeologiczne

ul. Poselska 3. **Map** 1 C5 (6 D4). **Tel** 12 422 71 00. 🚌 304, 522. 🚋 1, 3, 6, 8, 10, 18. **Open** 9am–3pm Mon, Wed & Fri; 9am–6pm Tue & Thu; 11am–4pm Sun (Jul & Aug: 11am–6pm Mon-Fri, 10am–3pm Sun). 📷 free on Sun.

The museum is housed in the former Friary of the Discalced Carmelites, founded in 1606. At the end of the 18th century the Austrian authorities took the building over and converted it into a prison. Mostly political prisoners were held here. In 1945 a group of imprisoned soldiers was rescued following heroic action by the Home Army (AK). After the prison closed down a museum was established here.

The Archeological Museum has its beginings in 1850, it was initially called the Museum of Antiquities.

The collection includes artifacts that tell the earliest history of the Lesser Poland region, but also Egyptian mummies. The statue of the idol Światowid, salvaged from the Zbrucz River, jewellery found in the tomb of a Scythian princess in Ryżanówka, gold objects from the tomb of a Hun from Jakuszowice and iron objects used as a form of payment *(see p23)* are the highlights of the collection.

⓯ Franciscan Church
Kościół Franciszkanów

See pp88–9.

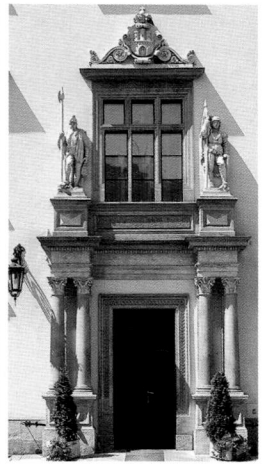

Elaborate porch at the entrance to the Wielopolski Palace

⓰ Wielopolski Palace
Pałac Wielopolskich

Plac Wszystkich Świętych. **Map** 1 C5 (6 D3). **Tel** 12 616 12 07. 🚋 1, 3, 6, 8, 18. **Open** by prior telephone arrangement only.

This palace was sold in the second half of the 19th century and transformed into a seat of municipal administration. Following remodelling work carried out in 1907–12 by architect Jan Rzymkowski, the building acquired a simplified modern form. A porch supported by pseudo-Romanesque columns was added to the wall facing Poselska Street. An Art Nouveau frieze with coats of arms of various cities can also be seen here. Inside the palace, the Debate Room and Portrait Hall are worth visiting.

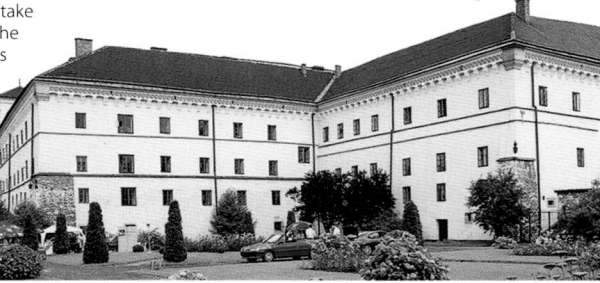

Archaeological Museum and garden

⓱ Statue of Józef Dietl
Pomnik Józefa Dietla

Pl. Wszystkich Świętych.
Map 1 C5 (6 D3). 🚋 1, 3, 6, 8, 18.

Józef Dietl (1804–78) was a medical professor who advocated treating the sick in spas. He was Rector of the Jagiellonian University, and became the first President (Mayor) of Krakow to be elected, in 1866, in the autonomous Galicia. He reformed the education system in Krakow, set up a project for the renovation of the city's heritage and was responsible for the restoration of the Cloth Hall.

The statue of Dietl was made between 1936 and 1938 by Xawery Dunikowski. The artist not only created the monumental figure but also took a great deal of trouble to find it a prominent location. Using a model, he travelled all over Krakow and tried it out in various places before deciding on the present location in All Saints Square. The result is stunning. The Statue of Dietl is regarded as one of the grandest and best located monuments in Poland.

⓲ Church of the Bernardine Nuns
Kościół Bernardynek

ul. Poselska 21. **Map** 1 C5 (6 D4).
Tel 12 422 22 46. 🚋 1, 3, 6, 8, 18.
Open 9am–6:30pm daily and during services.

A small convent of the Bernardine Nuns was established in Poselska Street in 1646. The Church of St Joseph was built here between 1694 and 1703 for the nuns. Though small and modest the church interior displays splendid furnishings which include altars and a pulpit from the workshop of Jerzy Hankis. The miraculous image of St Joseph and Child in the high altar was a gift from Jakub Zadzik, Bishop of Krakow, who possibly received it from Pope Urban VIII.

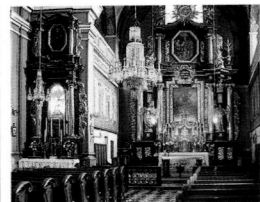
Interior of the small Church of the Bernardine Nuns

A small 17th-century statue of the child Jesus in the side altar is much venerated. It originally came from the Church of the Nuns of St Colette in Stradom and is therefore called the Koletański Christ.

⓳ Bernardine Church
Kościół Bernardynów

ul. Bernardyńska 2. **Map** 3 C1 (6 D5).
Tel 12 422 16 50. 🚋 3, 6, 8, 10, 18.
Open during services only.

Giovanni da Capistrano, the reformer of the Franciscan Order, later canonized, arrived in Krakow in 1453. For the next year he preached repentance and the renouncement of wealth and the immoral way of life. He also incited the people against the Jews. Influenced by his sermons, a few Krakovians took up the habit of the Reformed Franciscans, then called the Observants but known as the Bernardines in Poland. In 1453 Cardinal Zbigniew Oleśnicki built in Stradom a small timber church for this new monastic community, and soon after began building a large brick church. It was completed by Jan Długosz after Oleśnicki's death.

In 1655, while preparing to defend Krakow against the Swedes, Stefan Czarniecki gave orders to set fire to the Bernardine Church, which was located at the foot of Wawel Hill, so that the invaders could not use the church for their own protection. The beautiful statue of the Virgin and Child with St Anne, from Veit Stoss's workshop, and remnants of Mannerist tombs (now on the porch wall) are the only furnishings to have survived.

The new Baroque Church of the Bernardines was built between 1659 and 1680. Krzysztof Mieroszewski is believed to have been the architect. The marble shrine of Blessed Simon of Lipnica was erected in 1662 and the high altar between 1758 and 1766.

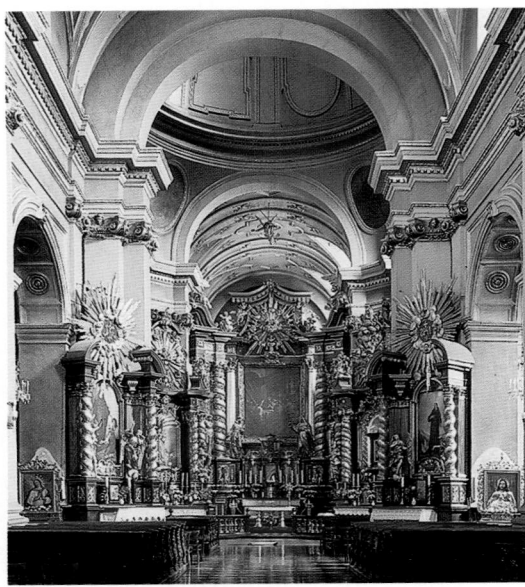
The 17th-century Baroque Bernardine Church

⑳ Częstochowa Seminary
Seminarium Częstochowskie

ul. Bernardyńska 3. **Map** 3 C1 (6 D5).
🚊 3, 6, 8, 10, 18.

In 1925 the Bishop of Częstochowa, Teodor Kubina, founded a seminary affiliated with the Faculty of Theology at the Jagiellonian University, for seminarists from his diocese. The monumental Modernist building was constructed between 1928 and 1930 to the designs of Zygmunt Gawlik and Franciszek Mączyński. The seminary is no longer in operation.

The façade is decorated with sculptures which were carved under the supervision of Xawery Dunikowski, one of the foremost Polish sculptors of the 20th century. The bas-relief at the top is particularly interesting. It shows Christ blessing the allegorical figure of Poland and the representatives of all social ranks, as well as the Virgin Mary accompanied by clergymen. The scene depicting a seminarist tempted by the devil, also on the façade, is worth noting.

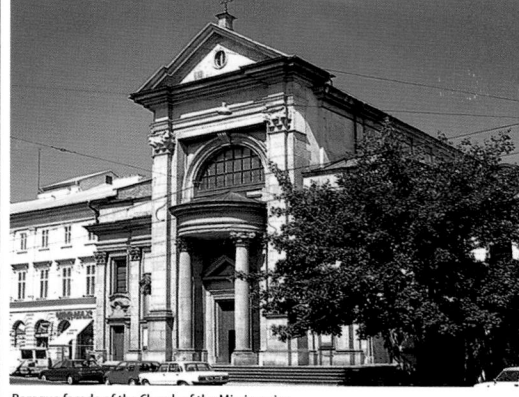

Baroque façade of the Church of the Missionaries

Relief of a seminarist tempted by the devil, Częstochowa Seminary

㉑ Church of the Missionaries
Kościół Misjonarzy

ul. Stradomska 4. **Map** 3 C1 (6 E5).
Tel 12 422 88 77. 🚌 103, 124.
🚊 3, 6, 8, 10, 18. **Open** 2–7pm daily and during services.

The Missionaries were brought to Stradom in 1682 but built the Church of the Conversion of St Paul only in the years 1719 to 1728. The architect, Kacper Bażanka, was influenced in his design by two outstanding examples of Roman Baroque architecture. The interior of the Krakow church resembles that of Francesco Borromini's Church of the Magi at the Collegio di Propaganda Fide, and the exterior is close to Sant'Andrea al Quirinale designed by Gianlorenzo Bernini. Some of the methods applied by Bażanka, such as the use of mirrors in the nave to direct reflected light onto the chapels, are characteristic of High Baroque. The church is regarded as one of the finest examples of 18th-century Baroque Polish architecture.

The same applies to the interior. Most altarpieces were painted by Tadeusz Kuntze and decorated with sculptures by Antoni Frączkiewicz.

㉒ Natural History Museum
Muzeum Przyrodnicze

ul. Św. Sebastiana 9/11. **Map** 3 D1 (6 E5). **Tel** 12 429 10 49. 🚊 3, 6, 8, 10, 18. **Open** 9am–3pm Mon–Fri, 11am–7pm Sat & Sun. 🚻

The core of the Natural History Museum was the collection of the Physiographic Commission of Krakow's Learned Society, established in 1865. It consisted mainly of stuffed birds and invertebrates. Today, the museum keeps live fish, reptiles and mammals; it also boasts a tropical rainforest display. A rhinoceros dating from the Pleistocene era, found in 1920 in Starunia, is a highlight of the collection.

㉓ Dietl Plantations
Planty Dietlowskie

Map 4 D1 (6 E5, F4). 🚌 128, 184.
🚊 12, 22.

The old river bed of the Vistula, from Stradom to Kazimierz, was filled in during the years 1878 to 1880 and transformed into a modern thoroughfare designed by Bolesław Malecki. It was a dual carriageway 1 km (0.6 mile) in length and 100 m (328 ft) wide, with a garden in the middle. The new scheme was named Planty Dietlowskie after Józef Dietl *(see p87)*. This President of Krakow was the first to advocate the filling in of the old Vistula bed which hindered the integration of Krakow with Kazimierz. Both sides of the avenue are lined with high tenement blocks and elegant public buildings, one of which is the PKO Bank built between 1922 and 1924.

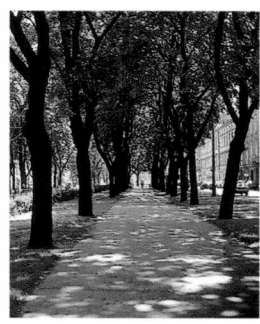

Tree-lined avenue separating Dietl's dual carriageway

⑮ Franciscan Church

The Franciscans arrived in Krakow in 1237. The construction of the church was undertaken in 1255 as a foundation of Duke Bolesław the Chaste and his wife the Blessed Salomea. After the Swedish invasion, which caused much damage, the church was rebuilt in the Baroque style. The great fire of Krakow in 1850 damaged the church again. It was rebuilt partly in the Neo-Romanesque and partly in the Neo-Gothic style. The work of Stanisław Wyspiański on the interior decoration is of prime importance. Around 1900 this artist executed the Art Nouveau murals and designed a series of unusual stained-glass windows in expressive colours.

A 13th-century wall of the first church

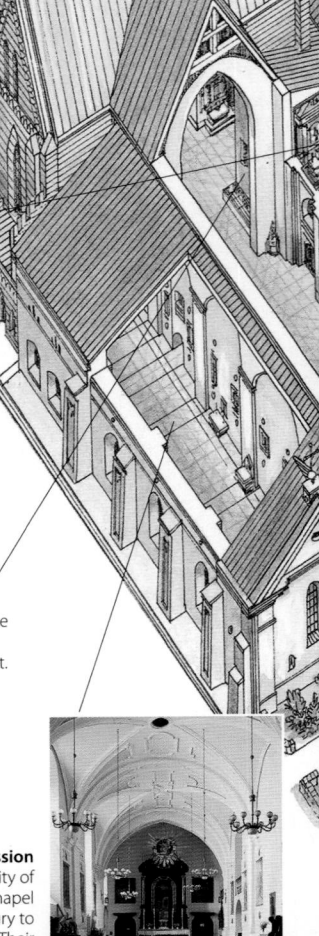

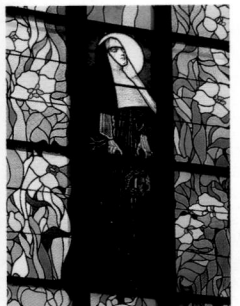

Blessed Salomea
Stanisław Wyspiański's stained glass in the north window of the choir shows the foundress of the church who rejected the ducal coronet before taking the habit of a Poor Clare nun.

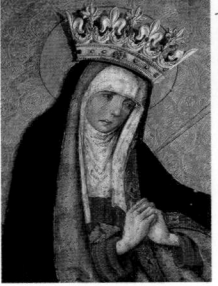

★ **Mater Dolorosa**
This late Gothic image by Master Jerzy, of Mary surrounded by angels holding instruments of Christ's Passion, is much venerated.

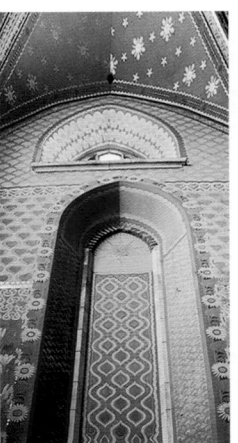

★ **Murals**
The polychrome decoration features flowers and conveys the Franciscan love of nature. This work illustrates the novel means of artistic expression employed by Wyspiański in sacred art.

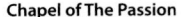

Chapel of The Passion
The brothers of the Confraternity of The Passion have met in this chapel since the end of the 16th century to conduct their rituals (see p54). Their liturgy is theatrical and evokes the spirit of Baroque devotion.

Cloister
Portraits of Krakow's bishops were hung in the cloister of the Franciscan Friary from the 15th to the mid-20th centuries.

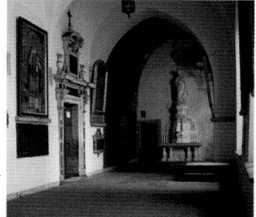

Portrait of Bishop Piotr Tomicki
This beautiful Renaissance portrait of Bishop Tomicki, painted before 1535 by Stanisław Samostrzelnik, is worth seeing in the cloister gallery.

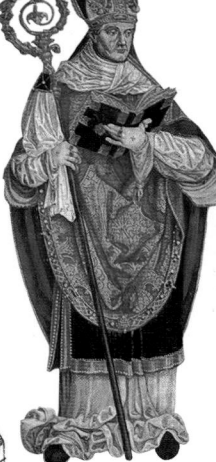

Tomb of Giovanni Gemma (died 1608)
The monument to the Venetian physician to King Zygmunt III Vaza is one of the most interesting sepulchral sculptures of late Mannerism in Poland.

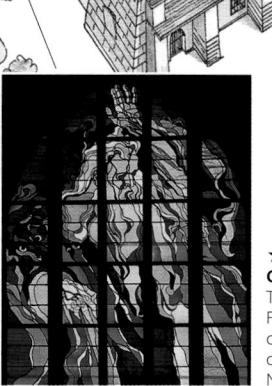

★ Wyspiański's Stained-Glass *Let It Be*
This expressive image of God the Father emerging from the cosmic chaos was rendered using bold colours and sinuous, flowing Art Nouveau forms.

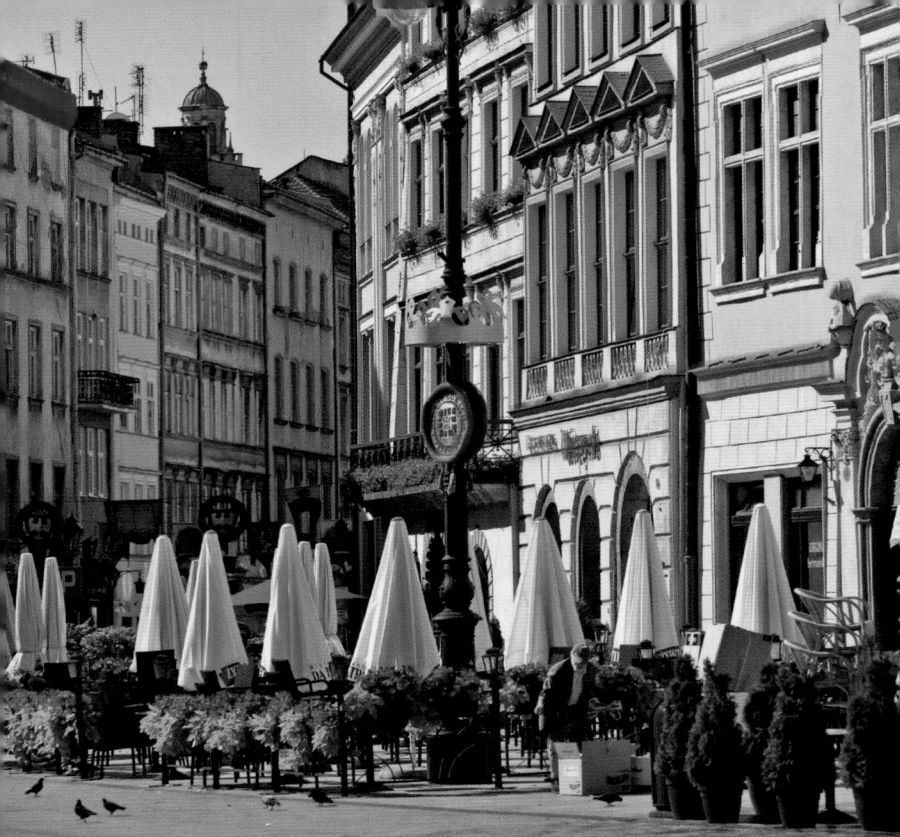

Restaurants lining colourful Market Square

Sights at a Glance

OLD QUARTER

In 1257 Duke Bolesław the Chaste gave Krakow her charter. This law was of key importance to the city as it determined local government and trade privileges, thus stimulating the city's future development. The charter stipulated strict rules for this development: a large, centrally located square surrounded by a regular grid of streets was to become the city centre. The size of each plot determined the size of the houses. Although the architecture became ever more opulent, this urban scheme has survived almost intact. To this day the Old Quarter remains the heart of modern, fast-developing Krakow. It is an area with a great concentration of important historic sights for visitors to enjoy.

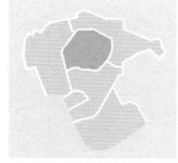

See also Street Finder maps 1, 5 & 6

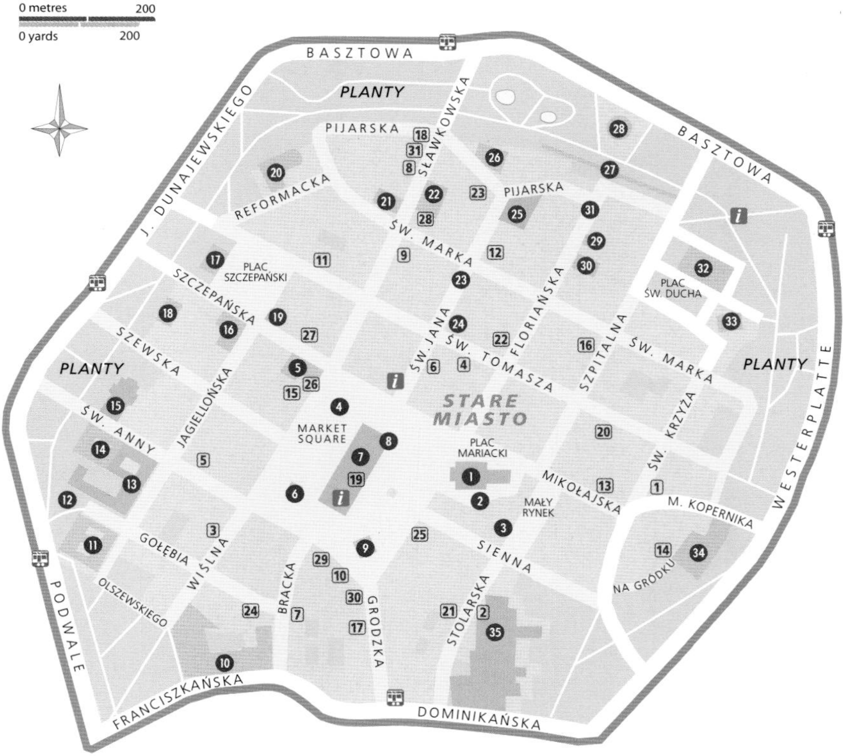

STARE MIASTO

Street-by-Street: Market Square

The Market Square (Rynek Główny) is located in the centre of Krakow's Old Quarter. Public, cultural and commercial activities have always concentrated around the Market Square. Museums and galleries of both old and modern art can be found here. Antiquarian shops selling works of art, bookshops and the best restaurants, cafés and bars are located in the houses around the square. Each summer nearly 30 street cafés open until the early hours. Flower stalls, street musicians, artists selling their works by the Cloth Hall and the general hustle and bustle made by the vendors of souvenirs and their clients all contribute to the lively atmosphere of this area.

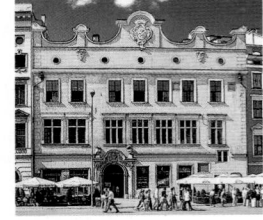

❹ Market Square
This is the largest town square anywhere in Europe. The life of medieval Krakow was centred around the square.

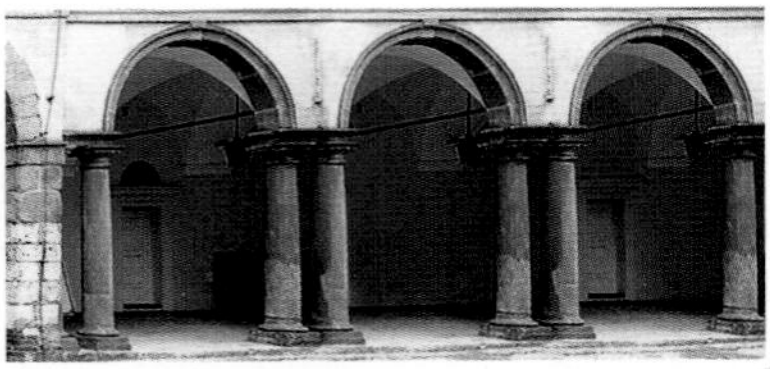

❺ ★ Christopher Palace
A branch of the Historical Museum of the City of Krakow is housed in this palace.

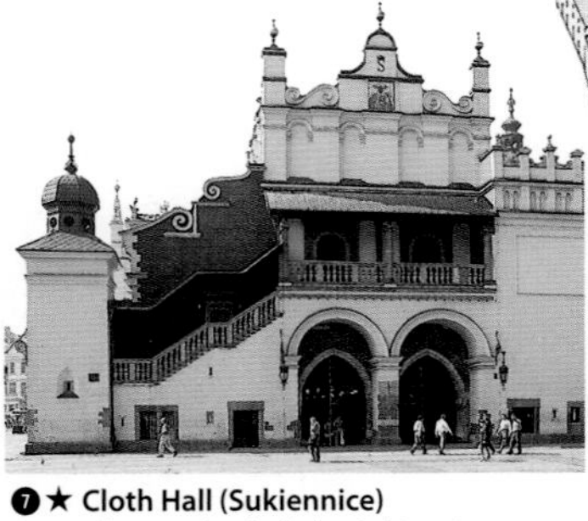

❼ ★ Cloth Hall (Sukiennice)
Originally a market hall, the Sukiennice houses shops, cafés and a renowned gallery of 19th-century Polish art.

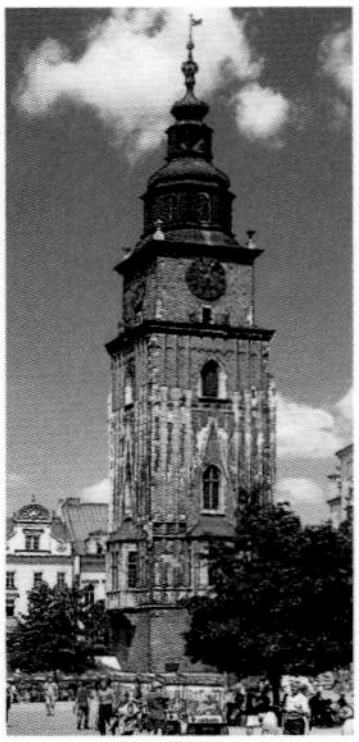

❻ Town Hall Tower
The only remaining fragment of the Old Town Hall, the tower was remodelled after World War II.

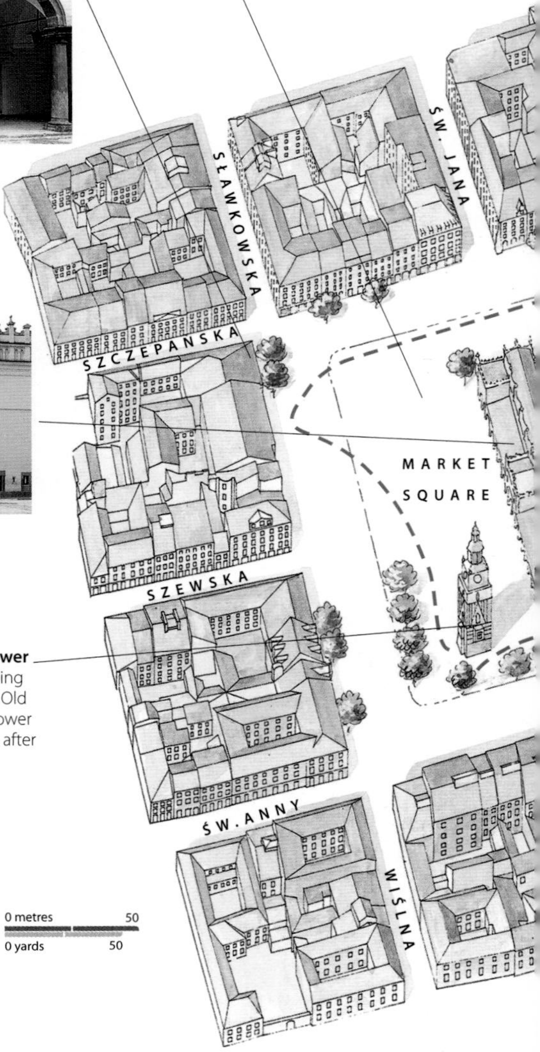

SŁAWKOWSKA

ŚW. JANA

SZCZEPAŃSKA

MARKET SQUARE

SZEWSKA

ŚW. ANNY

WIŚLNA

0 metres   50
0 yards   50

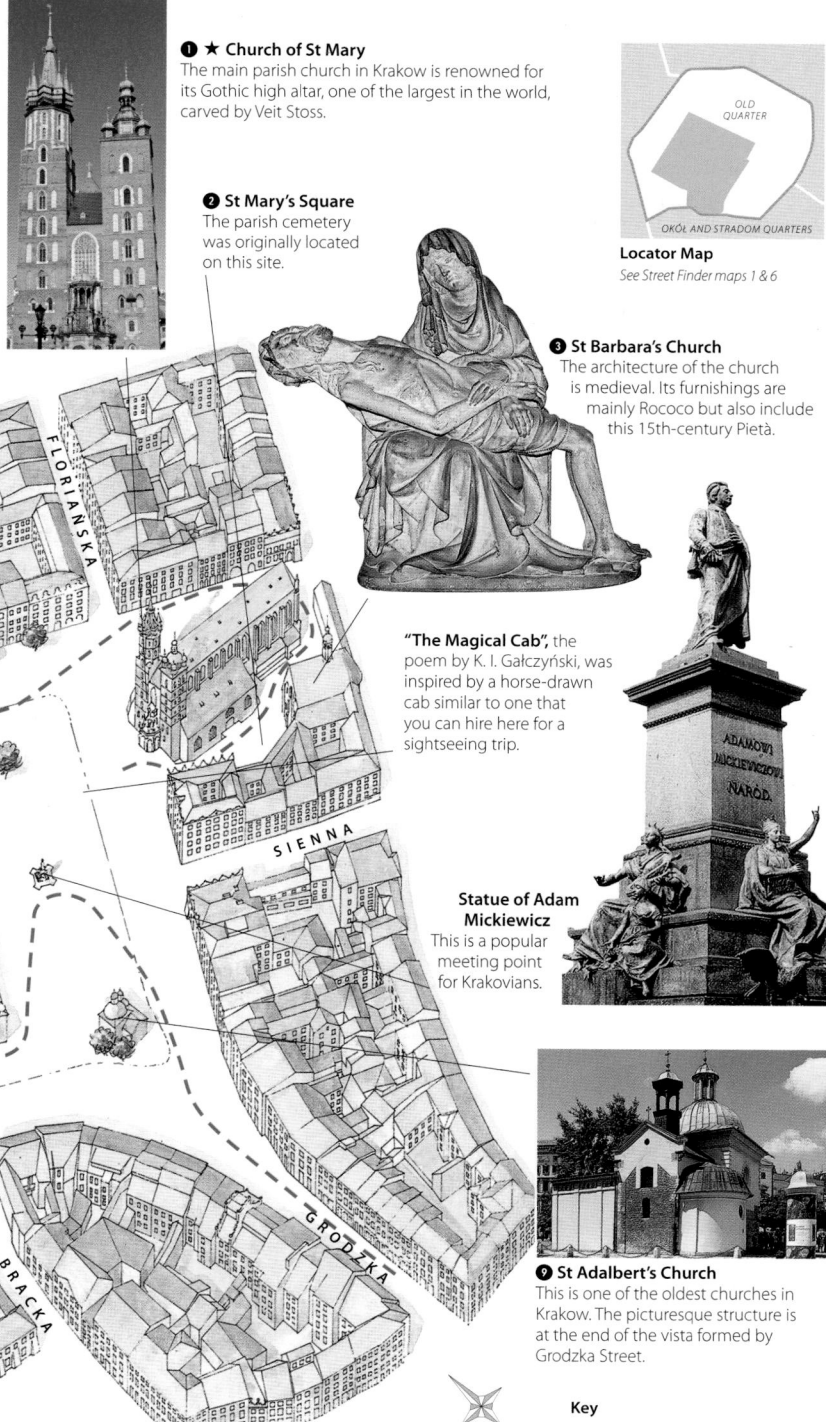

① ★ Church of St Mary
The main parish church in Krakow is renowned for its Gothic high altar, one of the largest in the world, carved by Veit Stoss.

② St Mary's Square
The parish cemetery was originally located on this site.

Locator Map
See Street Finder maps 1 & 6

③ St Barbara's Church
The architecture of the church is medieval. Its furnishings are mainly Rococo but also include this 15th-century Pietà.

"The Magical Cab", the poem by K. I. Gałczyński, was inspired by a horse-drawn cab similar to one that you can hire here for a sightseeing trip.

Statue of Adam Mickiewicz
This is a popular meeting point for Krakovians.

⑨ St Adalbert's Church
This is one of the oldest churches in Krakow. The picturesque structure is at the end of the vista formed by Grodzka Street.

Key

— Suggested route

❶ Church of St Mary
Kościół Mariacki

St Mary's, or the Church of the Assumption of the Virgin, was the main parish church of Krakow's burghers. It is a Gothic basilica composed of nave, aisles and side chapels. There are two towers. The north tower was extended in the early 15th century and in 1478 topped with a spire by Matthias Heringk. It was the city's watch-tower. Inside the church there are many outstanding works of art, among which the magnificent high altar by Veit Stoss *(see pp96–7)* should be mentioned. Other furnishings include the Baroque pulpit, marble altars decorated with paintings by the Italian artist Giovanni Battista Pittoni, and Renaissance tombs in the chapels.

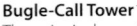

Bugle-Call Tower
The spire is decorated with turrets and topped by a gilt crown. The famous bugle-call *(hejnał)* is played here at hourly intervals and broadcast at noon by the Polish radio.

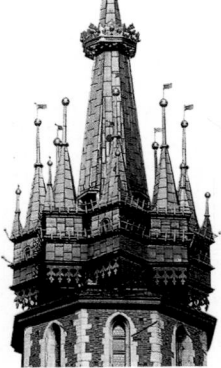

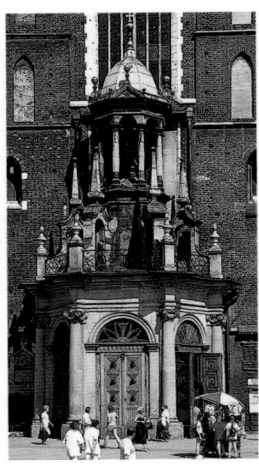

The Porch (1750–52)
The late-Baroque porch was designed by Francesco Placidi. Carved busts of the Apostles and saints by Karol Hukan were added to the door panels in 1929.

Main entrance

1221–2 Building of the Romanesque church

1392–7 Nave and aisles built

1477–89 High altar completed

1585 Choir stalls completed

1200	1300	1400	1500	1600

End of the 13th century Construction of the Gothic church begins

1355–65 New choir built

1478 North tower receives a spire

Detail of the main door

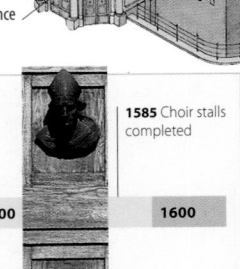

Choir Stalls
The stalls were made in 1585 but the biblical scenes in low relief which decorate the backs of the seats date from 1635.

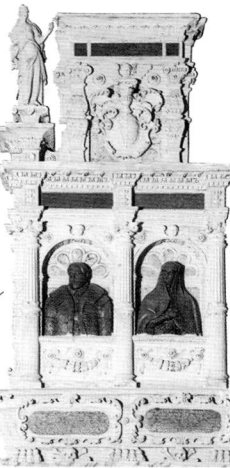

The Montelupi Tomb
This Mannerist tomb of one of the richest Krakow families was made around 1600 in the workshop of Santi Gucci.

Visitors' entrance

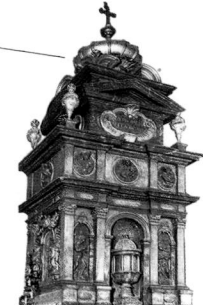

★ **The Ciborium**
This Renaissance ciborium (receptacle for containing the Eucharist) at the entrance to the choir was made around 1552 to the design by Giovanni Maria Mosca.

KEY

① **The tracery of the Great West Window** was designed by Jan Matejko and the stained glass is by Józef Mehoffer and Stanisław Wyspiański.

② **South Bell Tower**

③ **High Altar** (see pp96–7)

④ **The murals** on the walls and vault were designed and executed by Jan Matejko between 1890 and 1892.

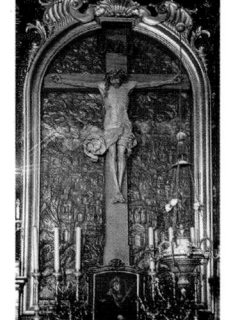

★ **The Slacker Crucifix** (1496)
The figure of the suffering Christ, carved in stone by Veit Stoss, is the most expressive sculpture ever made by the artist.

Exploring St Mary's: The High Altar

The high altar by Veit Stoss was made between 1477 and 1489. It is dedicated, like the church itself, to the Assumption of the Virgin Mary. The altar is a polyptych, some 11 m (36 ft) long and 12 m (39 ft) high. It was even higher originally. The iconography determined its composition. The shutters were closed throughout the liturgical year but opened during important church feasts. The treatment of the human figure is naturalistic, dynamic and dramatically expressive. The low reliefs and figures of saints are masterpieces of late-Gothic art.

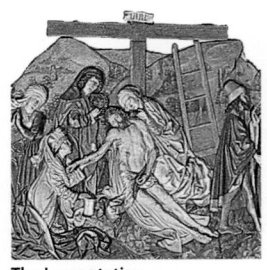

The Lamentation
The design of this particular panel was influenced by Netherlandish painting.

The Meeting of
St Anne and
St Joachim

The middle shutters
are opened every day
at 11:50am.

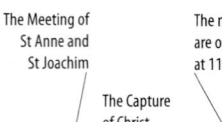

The Capture
of Christ

The Crucifixion

The Three Maries
at the Sepulchre

The Birth of
the Virgin

The Descent into Hell

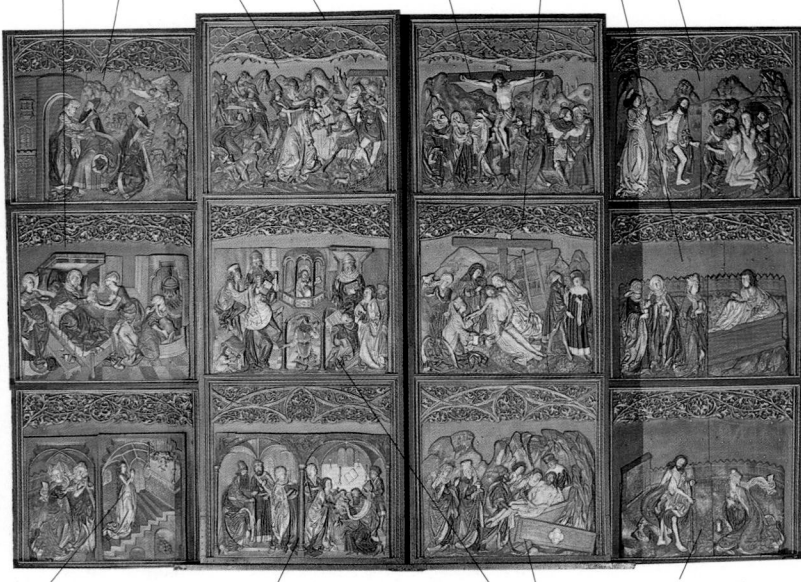

The Presentation of the
Virgin in the Temple

The Entombment

The Risen Christ
appearing to Mary
Magdalene

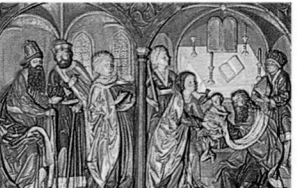

**The Presentation of
Christ in the Temple**
In this scene the artist tries
to recreate the interior
of the temple.

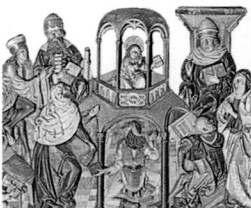

Christ among the Doctors
This scene testifies to Stoss'
masterly depiction of the
diverse physiognomies.

Veit Stoss (Wit Stwosz)

Veit Stoss (1447–1533), one of the greatest wood-carvers of the late Gothic age, was born in Horb am Neckar in Germany. He lived in Krakow from 1477 to 1496, where he was exempted from paying taxes by the City Council. He created a number of sculptural works here.

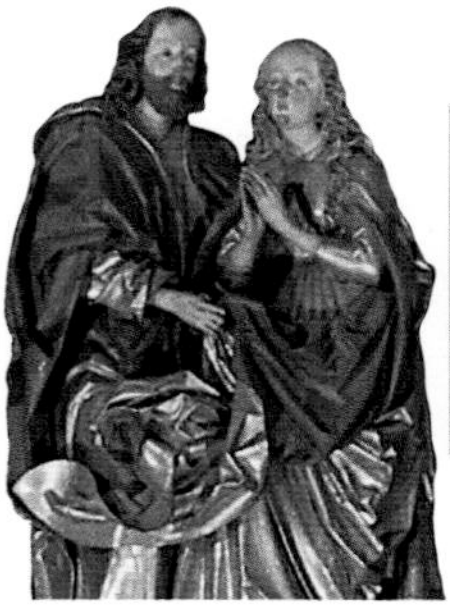

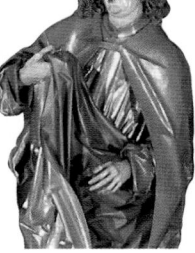

The Assumption
Mary and Christ are raised to Heaven by eight angels.

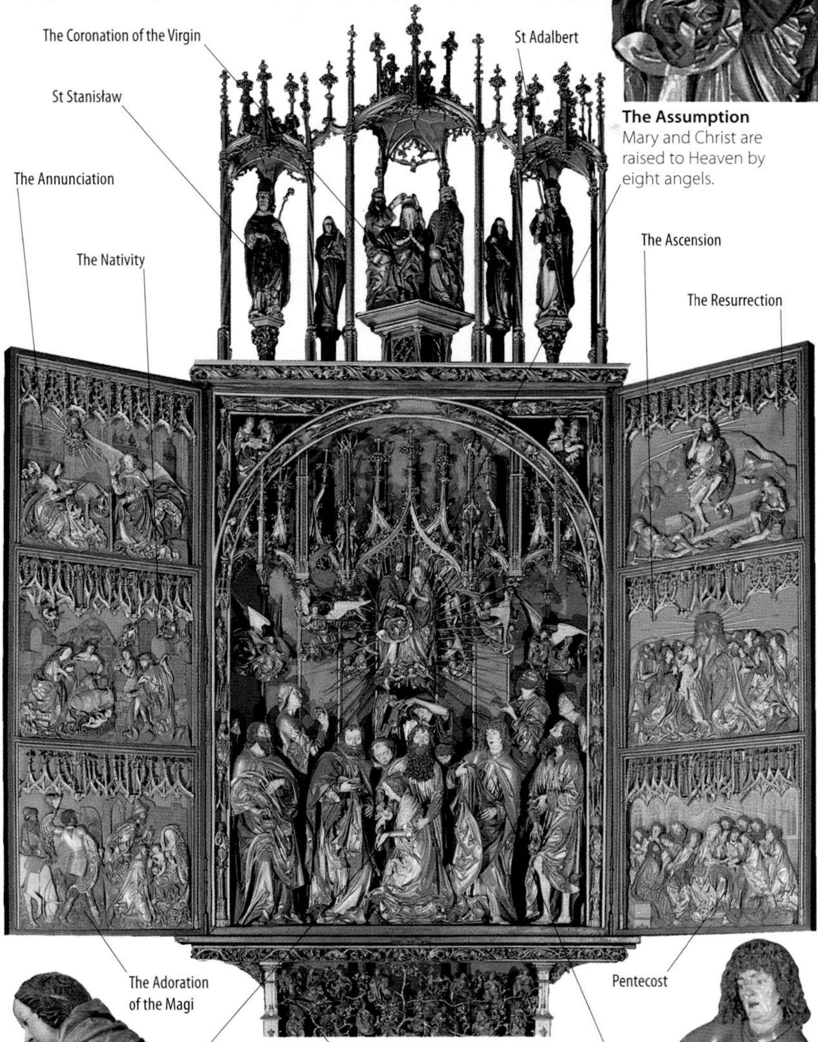

The Coronation of the Virgin

St Adalbert

St Stanisław

The Annunciation

The Nativity

The Ascension

The Resurrection

The Adoration of the Magi

Pentecost

Predella with the Tree of Jesse

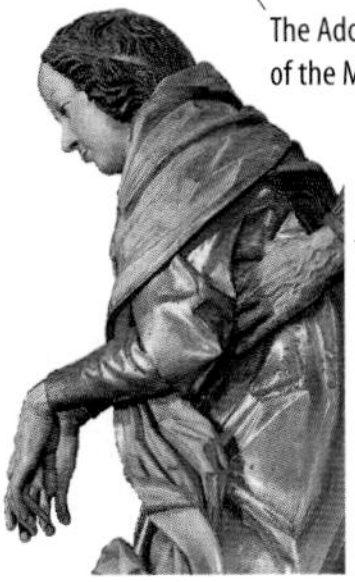

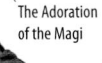

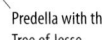

The Death of the Virgin
The figure of the youthful Mary is one of the greatest sculptures ever made in Poland.

St John
Slightly hesitant, the saint is about to put a cape on the fainting Mary.

❷ St Mary's Square
Plac Mariacki

Map 1 C4 (6 D2).

St Mary's Square was once a parish graveyard. It was relocated between 1796 and 1804. The statue of the Virgin Mary which was here originally is now in the Planty by Jagiellońska Street. The bas-relief attributed to Veit Stoss, which once decorated the Calvary Porch, has survived and is now in the National Museum. A copy can be seen on the wall at No. 8 on the square. The prelate House and a Vicarage are among the houses in which original beamed ceilings and plasterwork have survived. St Barbara's Church is on the east side of the square, which also features a small water pump decorated with a figure of a student of medieval Krakow. It is a copy of a figure from the high altar in St Mary's (*see pp96–7*).

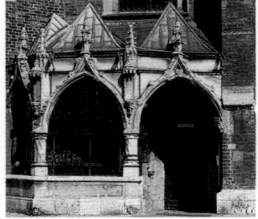

A student of medieval Krakow, St Mary's Square

❸ St Barbara's Church
Kościół św. Barbary

Mały Rynek 8. **Map** 1 C4 (6 D2). **Tel** 12 428 15 00. **Open** during services.

According to a legend St Barbara's Church was built using the bricks that were left over from the construction of the Church of St Mary. St Barbara's actually dates from 1394 to 1399, which coincides

The Gothic porch with Christ in Gethsemane at St Barbara's

with one of the stages in the construction of St Mary's. Between 1415 and 1536 sermons were delivered in Polish in the former church, and in German in the latter. During this period the patricians of Krakow were mostly German and it was only much later that they became a minority among the Polish population. In 1586 the church was taken over by the Jesuits. Piotr Skarga preached here and Jakub Wujek, the translator of the Bible, is buried here. Added on the outside from 1488 to 1518 is a late Gothic chapel with a porch decorated with sculptures made by Veit Stoss' workshop. Furnishings date mostly from the 18th century but there is also an interesting early 15th-century Pietà in stone and a 15th-century crucifix on the high altar.

❹ Market Square
Rynek Główny

See pp100–103.

The *Lajkonik*

Every year, on the Thursday ending the Corpus Christi octave, a parade led by a figure known as the *Lajkonik* proceeds from the Convent of the Premonstratensian Nuns in Zwierzyniec to the Market Square. The event commemorates the victory over the Tatars in 1287. On his way, the *Lajkonik* strikes some spectators with his mace, a sign which is thought to bring good luck, especially to girls. At the Market Square the *Lajkonik* receives a symbolic tribute. The original costume of the *Lajkonik*, designed in 1904 by Stanisław Wyspiański, is now in the Museum of Krakow.

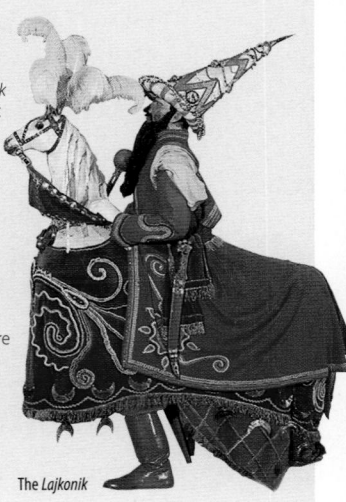

The *Lajkonik*

❺ Christopher Palace
Pałac Krzysztofory

Rynek Główny 35. **Map** 1 C4 (6 D2). Museum of Krakow: **Tel** 12 619 23 03. Cellars: **Open** 10am–5pm Wed–Sun for temporary exhibitions. Main building: **Closed** for restoration until 2018. ♿ **W** mhk.pl

This is one of the oldest and most beautiful palaces in Krakow, with a magnificent arcaded courtyard. It was remodelled between 1682 and 1685 by Jacopo Solari for Kazimierz Wodzicki, one of the richest noblemen in Lesser Poland.

The Palace is named after St Christopher, whose 14th-century statue decorates the building. It houses the Museum of Krakow, which is dedicated to the history and culture of the city (closed for renovation until 2018). Old documents, maces, gold artifacts from local workshops, memorabilia and paintings are all on display.

In the cellars there is a café and the art gallery of the Krakow Group (Grupa Krakowska), which was first established in 1930 and then revived in 1957.

❻ Town Hall Tower
Wieża Ratuszowa

Rynek Główny 1. **Map** 1 C4 (6 D2).
Museum: **Tel** 12 426 43 34. **Open**
Apr–Oct: 10:30am–5:30pm daily.

Until the early 19th century there were several public buildings on Market Square: the Town Hall, the Small Weigh-House, the Large Weigh-House and a pillory. The 70 m- (230 ft-) high Town Hall Tower is, unfortunately, the only structure to have survived. The Gothic Town Hall itself was remodelled many times and finally demolished in 1846. The present dome is Baroque. The tower houses a branch of the Museum of Krakow dedicated to the history of local government and is a venue for the Ludowy Theatre.

❼ Cloth Hall
Sukiennice

See pp104–105.

❽ Rynek Underground
Podziemia Rynku

Rynek Główny 1. **Map** 1 C4 (6 D2). **Tel** 12 426 50 60. **Open** Apr–Oct: 10am–10pm daily (to 8pm Mon, to 4pm Tue); Nov–Mar: 10am–8pm daily (to 4pm Tue). Book in advance via the website or by phone. **Closed** 1st Tue of month. free Tue. **w** podziemiarynku.com

This high-tech museum, tracing the story of the city, opened in September 2010 and is located under Market Square. The underground vaults contain displays on transport and trade as well as archaeological finds such as the remains of an 11th-

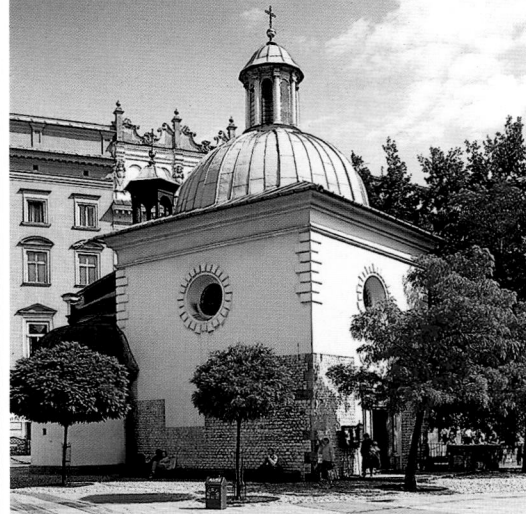

Church of St Adalbert on Market Square

century cemetery and ancient coins and clothing. The museum cleverly blends modern technology with interactive exhibits and more traditional museum displays.

❾ St Adalbert's Church
Kościół św. Wojciecha

Rynek Główny 3. **Map** 1 C4 (6 D3). **Open** May–Sep: 9am–6pm daily (from 1:30pm Sun); Oct–Apr: 9am–5pm daily.

The small church of St Adalbert is one of the oldest in Krakow. A legend tells that St Adalbert preached here before leaving on his missionary journey to try to convert the Prussians in 997. The architecture of the church

amalgamates several styles, from Romanesque and Gothic, through Renaissance and Baroque, to the modern interior design. This mixture reflects various stages in the development of the Market Square, an exhibition on which is located in Rynek Underground. The display includes a cross-section of the ground beneath the square, as well as medieval water pipes and other objects found during the excavations carried out after World War II, which have also revealed the remnants of the building dating from the time of St Adalbert.

Rynek Underground is 4 m (13 ft) below Market Square

❹ Market Square: North and West Sides

The charter given to Krakow in 1257 determined the plan of the city. The square located in the middle of the medieval city has remained the centre of Krakow ever since. This square, some 200 m (656 ft) by 200 m (656 ft), is surrounded by a regular grid of streets, with three streets on each side. Only the off-the-grid location of the Church of St Mary, which pre-dates the charter, and Grodzka Street, with its funnel-like shape, vary the rigidity of the urban planning in this area. There were formerly many buildings in the square, but of those the Cloth Hall and the Town Hall Tower are the only ones to have survived. The square was a venue for many important events, including coronation ceremonies.

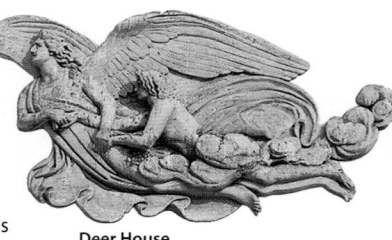

Deer House
This was once an inn. Johann Wolfgang von Goethe and Tsar Nicholas I both stayed here.

North Side

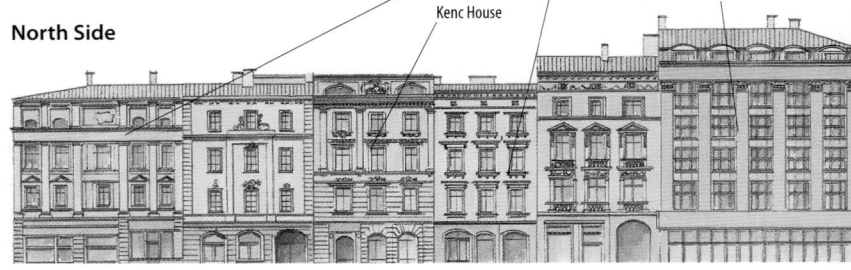

Kenc House

Horse House

Phoenix House

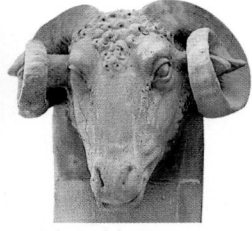

**Palace of the Rams
(Pałac Pod Baranami)**
One of the most magnificent palaces owned by the Potocki family now houses a famous cabaret.

"Piwnica Pod Baranami" Cabaret

The cabaret which is housed in the Palace of the Rams was established in 1956. Although it was originally intended to exist no longer than "five years, possibly even less", the cabaret has been active for more than 50 years and is one of Krakow's top attractions. Piotr Skrzynecki (1930–97) was the founder and heart and soul of the cabaret. Wiesław Dymny, Ewa Demarczyk, Marek Grechuta, Krystyna Zachwatowicz, Zygmunt Konieczny, Leszek Wójtowicz, Anna Szałapak, Grzegorz Turnau and Zbigniew Preisner were among the best-known contributors and performers. The cabaret is a lively place full of poetry and music, joy and laughter.

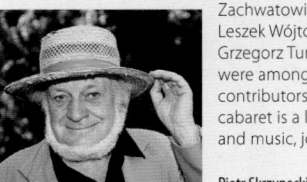

Piotr Skrzynecki

West Side

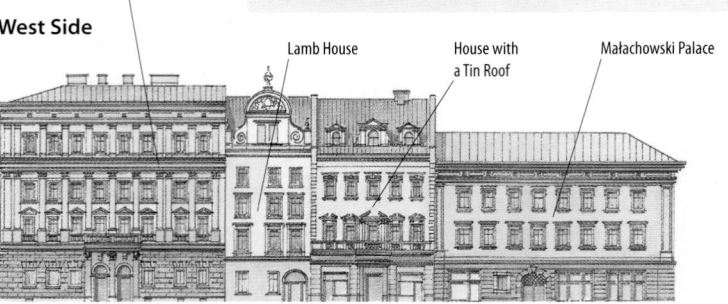

Lamb House

House with a Tin Roof

Małachowski Palace

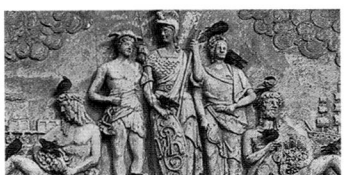

Betman House
This is also known as "Under the Beheaded" after a bas-relief which depicts the martyrdom of St John the Baptist.

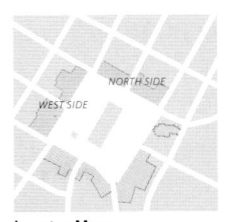

Locator Map

Market Square: North and West sides

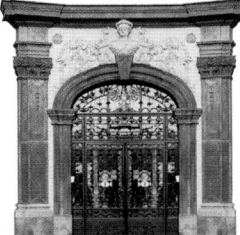

42 Market Square
belonged to the Boner family and in the 19th century to the renowned collector Feliks Manggha Jasieński.

Margrave's House
A former mint and presently a bank, the façade of this house features a splendid Rococo portal.

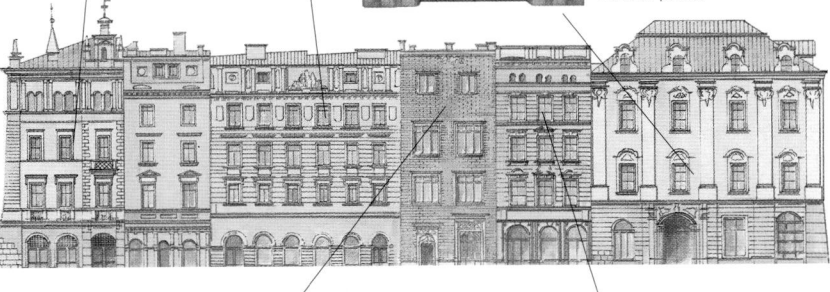

Red House

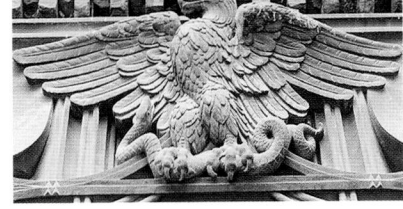

Eagle House (Dom Pod Orłem)
The basement of this fine Renaissance house formerly contained the Starmach Gallery of contemporary art.

House under Three Stars

Christopher Palace (Pałac Krzysztofory)
This palace *(see p98)* houses the Museum of Krakow, among whose highlights is a gilded plaque, made in 1609, depicting St Eligius.

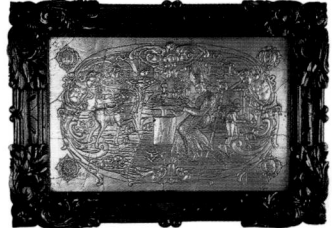

Spiš Palace (Pałac Spiski)
is home to the exclusive Hawełka Restaurant *(see p191)*.

❹ Market Square: South and East Sides

There are many stories about the Market Square. According to one of the legends Krakow's pigeons are the enchanted knights of Duke Henryk Probus, who agreed to their metamorphosis in exchange for gold that he needed to secure papal acceptance for his coronation. The knights were supposed to regain their human form after the coronation. But the duke lost the gold and his knights are still awaiting the promised transformation. The legend about the two brothers who built the St Mary's towers is more popular. When the older mason completed the taller tower he stabbed his younger brother to death in order to prevent him from surpassing his work but then, remorseful, killed himself.

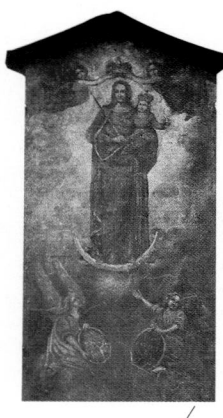

Madonna House (Dom Pod Obrazem)
Formerly the palace of a wealthy burgher family called Cellari, its façade is decorated with the Madonna painted in 1718.

South Side

Wierzynek Restaurant

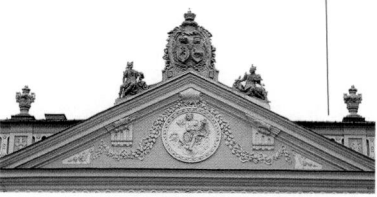

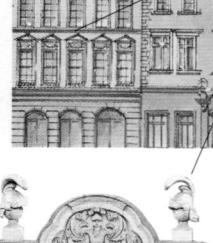

Hetman's House (Kamienica Hetmańska)
The Baroque portal leads to shops on the ground floor, in which Gothic vaults with carved keystones have survived.

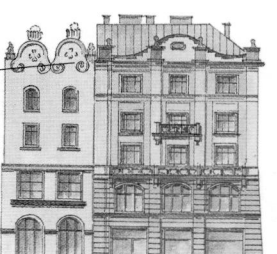

Potocki Palace (Pałac Potockich)
Behind the Neo-Classical façade the original interiors and a small arcaded courtyard have survived.

East Side

Grey House (Kamienica Szara)

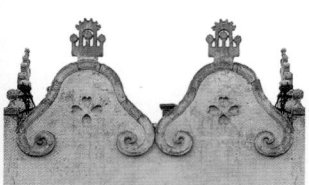

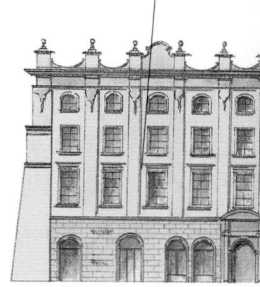

4 Market Square
This is one of a few houses with Art Nouveau decoration. It was added during the remodelling carried out in 1907–8 by Ludwik Wojtyczka.

Prince's House (Kamienica Książęca)
The famous sorcerer Master Twardowski is reputed to have lived here in the 16th century. The house is decorated with a statue of St Giovanni da Capistrano.

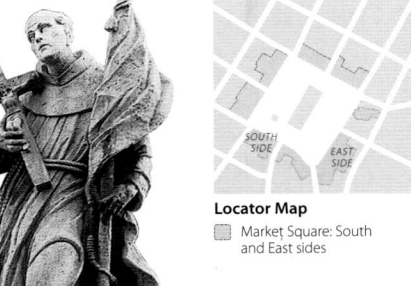

Lanckoroński House, also known as "Under the Evangelists," features the remnants of an 18th-century chapel on the first floor.

Locator Map
Market Square: South and East sides

The pharmacy "Under the Gold Crown" was once housed here. Its emblem has survived above the entrance.

The Raven House (Kamienica Pod Krukiem) is a seat of the International Centre of Culture and Krakow's Cultural Club.

Kromer House (Kamienica Kromerowska)

Canary House (Kamienica Pod Kanarkiem)

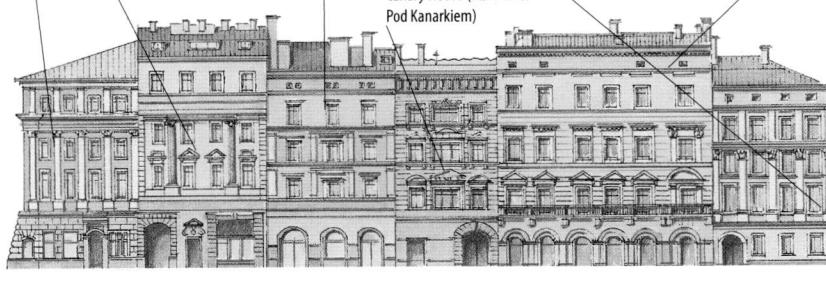

Lizards House (Kamienica Pod Jaszczurami)
Gothic vaults have survived in this house, in which a student club is located.

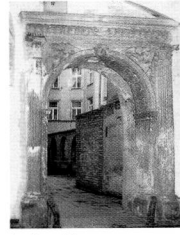

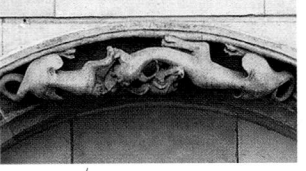

Italian House (Dom Włoski)
The first Polish post office was housed here and coaches passed through this arch.

Boner House (Kamienica Bonerowska)
This is topped by a beautiful Mannerist parapet decorated with herms.

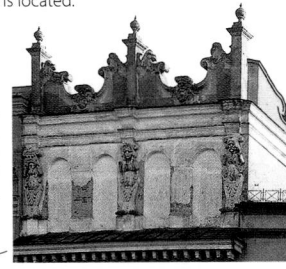

❼ The Cloth Hall (Sukiennice)

The Cloth Hall originated from a covered market. A stone structure protecting the stalls, with an internal passage, was probably here at the time of Kazimierz the Great. It was rebuilt to the design of Giovanni Maria Mosca following a fire in 1555, and remodelled entirely in 1875 by Tomasz Pryliński. The Gallery of 19th-century Polish Art is housed here. The stalls sell a variety of souvenirs. The Noworolski Café, one of the best in Krakow, is a good place to relax after seeing the paintings.

Folly (1894) by Władysław Podkowiński
This Modernist painting aroused much controversy. It began a Symbolist phase in Podkowiński's career.

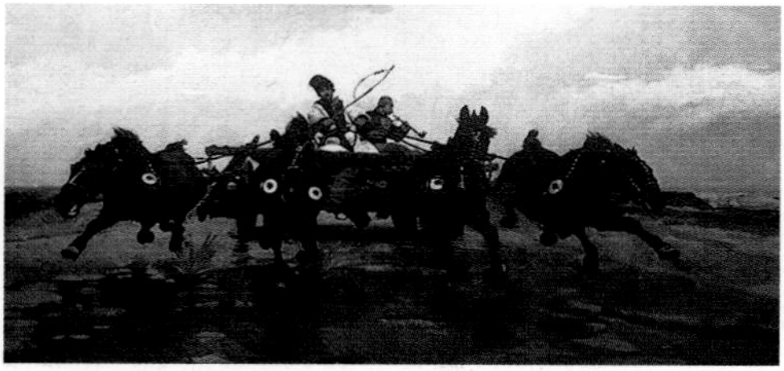

Four-in-hand (1881) by Józef Chełmoński
Paintings by Symbolists as well as Realists are exhibited alongside the _Four-in-hand_.

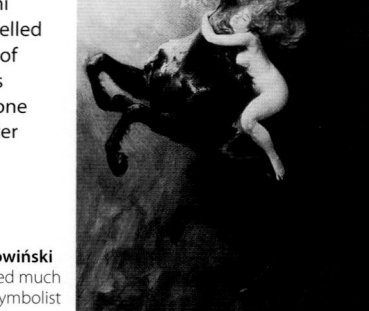

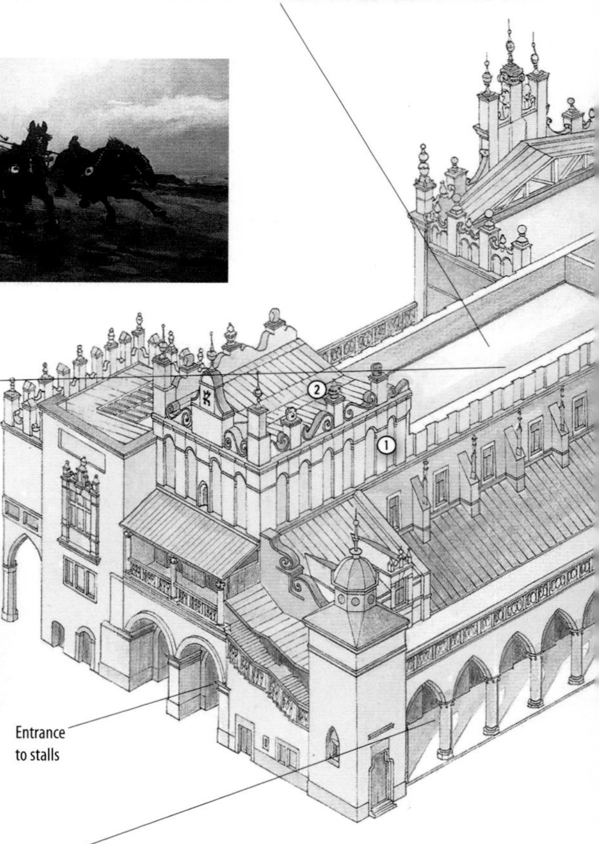

Entrance to stalls

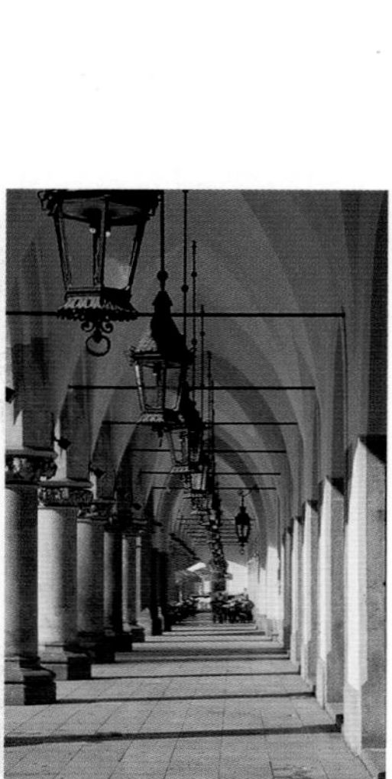

Arcades
The side arcades and oriels were added during the rebuilding in 1875. The arcades echo the medieval architecture of Venice.

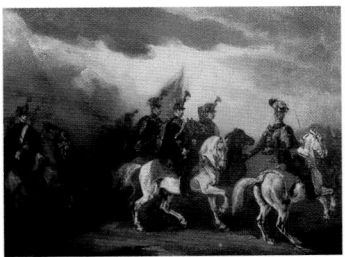

★ Blue Hussars by Piotr Michałowski
A separate room is dedicated to the work of Michałowski, the foremost Polish Romantic artist who lived between 1800 and 1855.

VISITORS' CHECKLIST

Practical Information
Market Square 1/3. **Map** 1 C4 (6 D2). **Tel** 12 433 54 42. **Open** 10am–6pm Tue–Sun. 🖼 free Sun (permanent exhibition only).
📷 🖥 muzeum.krakow.pl

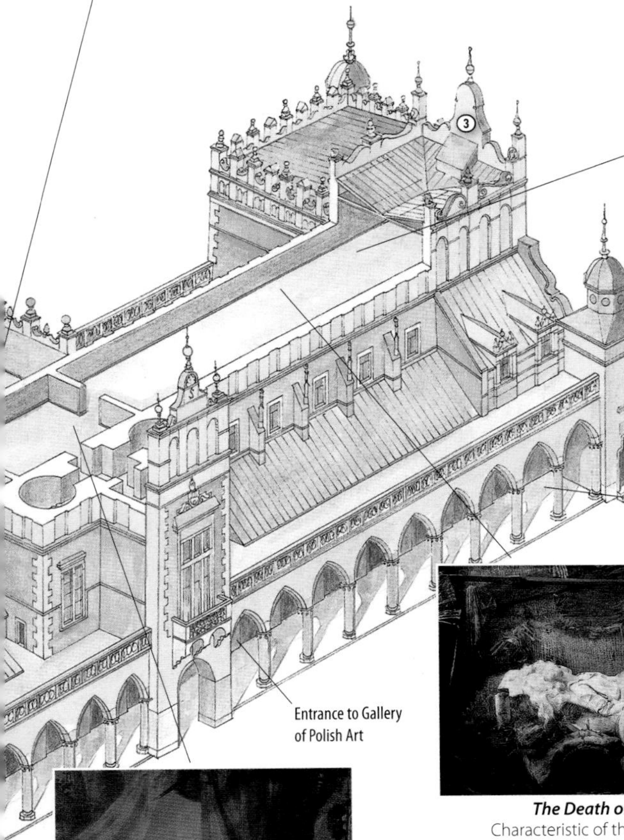

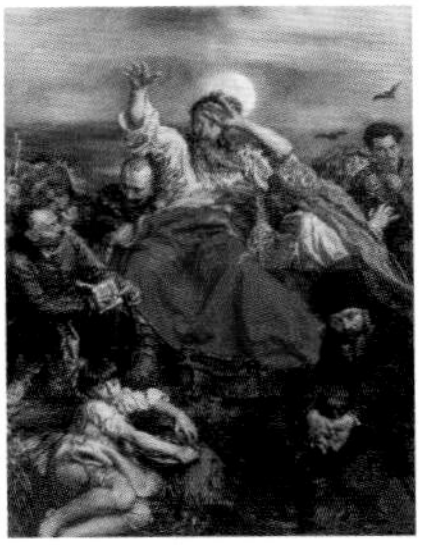

★ Wernyhora by Jan Matejko
Jan Matejko and Henryk Siemiradzki were both exponents of 19th-century history painting which is displayed in the room dominated by Matejko's *Prussian Homage*.

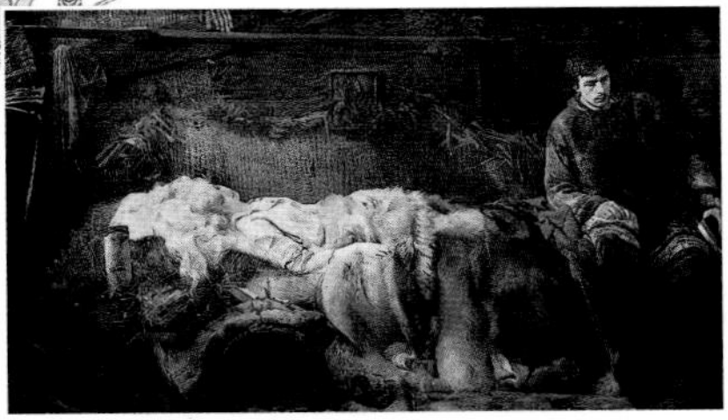

Entrance to Rynek Underground Museum

Entrance to Gallery of Polish Art

The Death of Ellenai by Jacek Malczewski
Characteristic of the artist's early work, which was permeated by the memories of people who had been imprisoned in Siberia, this painting was inspired by a poem by Juliusz Słowacki.

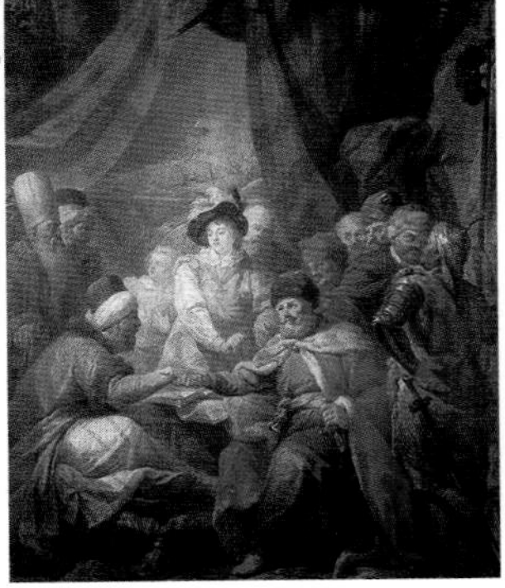

The Chocim Treaty by Marcello Bacciarelli
Late 18th- and early 19th-century Neo-Classical paintings are displayed in the same room.

KEY

① **The Renaissance parapet** is not only decorative but also offers protection from fire.

② **Roof with sunken rafters**

③ **Renaissance parapet**

John Paul II

Karol Wojtyła was born in 1920 in Wadowice *(see p160)*, but lived in Krakow for many years. He arrived here in 1938 to read Polish philology at the Jagiellonian University. The outbreak of World War II put a stop to his studies. During the war he worked for the Solvay Chemical Plant and was active in the underground Rhapsody Theatre. In 1942 he entered the underground theological Seminary. As a devout priest and artists' friend, he became very popular. Despite his election to the Apostolic See in 1978 his

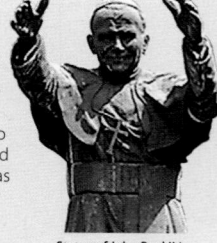

Statue of John Paul II in the courtyard of the Episcopal Palace

links with Krakow remained as close as ever. He continued to return here with his apostolic missions on many different occasions, until his death in 2005.

❿ Episcopal Palace
Pałac Biskupi

ul. Franciszkańska 3. **Map** 1 C5 (5 C3). **Tel** 12 429 74 14. 🚊 1, 3, 6, 8, 18. **Closed** to the public.

First recorded in the 13th century, this is one of the oldest buildings in Krakow. It was damaged by fire and remodelled several times. Giovanni Maria Mosca contributed to the decoration. The present palace dates from the times of Bishop Piotr Tomicki (16th century) and Bishop Piotr Gembicki (17th century). A fire in 1850 caused extensive damage but the splendid furnishings have partly survived.

John Paul II lived here between 1964 and 1978. He was then the Archbishop of Krakow. A statue of him, made in 1980 by Ione Sensi Croci, is in the courtyard.

⓫ Collegium Novum

ul. Gołębia 24. **Map** 1 B4 (5 C3). **Tel** 12 422 10 33. 🚊 1, 8, 15, 18.

The Collegium Novum replaced the Jerusalem College after it was destroyed by fire in the 19th century. The ruins were demolished between 1883 and 1887 and the new building constructed. Its official opening turned into a patriotic demonstration

attended symbolically by delegations from all three parts of the partitioned Poland. According to the contemporary records the architect of the new building, Feliks Księłarski, intended to emulate the vernacular architecture, especially the crystal vaults and decoration of the Collegium Maius, but in fact he imitated German and Austrian models. The magnificent staircase is similar to the one in the Town Hall in Vienna. The College is the seat of the Rector of the Jagiellonian University. It also houses departmental offices, the bursary and the Great Hall where inauguration and graduation ceremonies take place. The Hall has a beamed and coffered ceiling and is decorated with portraits by Jan Matejko.

⓬ Statue of Copernicus
Pomnik Mikołaja Kopernika

ul. Gołębia. **Map** 1 B4 (5 C3). 🚊 1, 2, 8, 15, 18.

The statue of Nicolaus Copernicus was made in 1900 by Cyprian Godebski. The astronomer is represented as a young scholar holding an astrolabe. The statue was originally in the courtyard of the Collegium Maius, but was moved to the present location in front of the Witkowski College in 1953. The statue was intended to function as a fountain.

⓭ Collegium Maius
See pp108–109.

⓮ Collegium Nowodvorianum

ul. Św. Anny 12. **Map** 1 B4 (5 C2). **Tel** 12 422 04 11. 🚊 4, 8, 14, 15, 18. 🚌 124, 152, 502.

The Collegium Nowodvorianum was founded by Bartłomiej Nowodworski, a Knight Hospitaller of St John, Secretary to the King and a warrior in the Battle of Lepanto. This foundation was a result of his bequest of 1617 to the Classes, one of the university colleges and the first secular secondary school in Krakow, established in 1586. The Collegium was built between 1636 and 1643 by

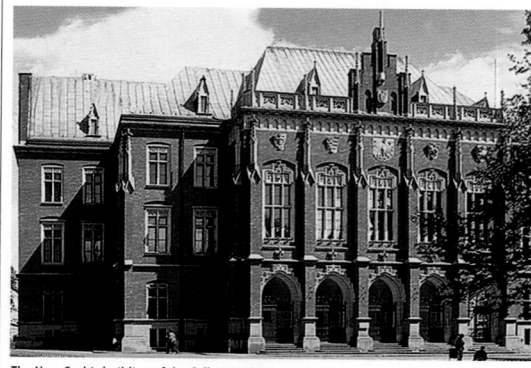

The Neo-Gothic building of the Collegium Novum

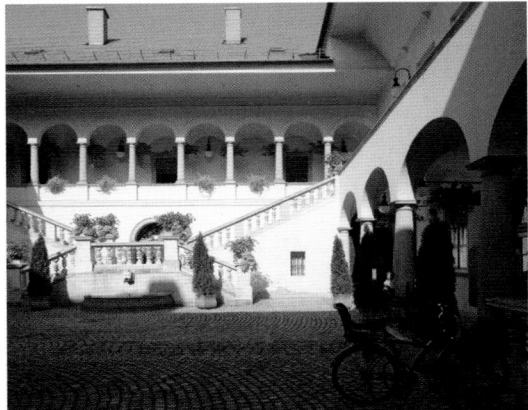
Arcaded courtyard of the Collegium Nowodvorianum

Jan Leitner. A beautiful courtyard with arcades and a grand stairway is one of the best preserved Baroque buildings in Krakow. The offices of the Collegium Medicum are housed here.

⓯ Church of St Anne
Kościół św. Anny

See pp110–11.

⓰ Old Theatre
Teatr Stary

ul. Jagiellońska 1. **Map** 1 C4 (5 C2). **Tel** 12 422 80 20. 2, 4, 8, 13, 14, 15. 124, 152, 502. Museum: **Open** 11am–1pm Tue–Sat and one hour prior to performances.

The Old, or Modrzejewska Theatre is named after the great actress Helena Modrze-jewska. The oldest theatre building in Poland, it has been in use continuously since 1798. It was remodelled in the Neo-Renaissance style between 1830 and 1843 by Tomasz Majewski and Karol Kremer. The next major rebuilding was undertaken from 1903 to 1905 by Franciszek Mączyński and Tadeusz Stryjeński. The reinforced concrete construc-tion applied to the interior, and the exterior Art Nouveau decoration, both date from this time. The stucco frieze was made in 1906 by Józef Gardecki. The plaques on the Jagiellońska Street side commemorate the composer Władysław Żeleński, the director Konrad Swinarski and the actor Wiktor Sadecki.

The Old Theatre is regarded as one of the best in Poland. Many outstanding directors have worked here, including Zygmunt Hübner, Konrad Swinarski and Andrzej Wajda. There is a small theatre museum on the ground floor.

⓱ Palace of Art
Pałac Sztuki

Plac Szczepański 4. **Map** 1 C4 (5 C1). **Tel** 12 422 66 16. 2, 4, 8, 13, 14, 15. 124, 152, 502. **Open** 8:15am–6pm Mon–Fri, 10am–6pm Sat & Sun.

In 1854 the Friends of the Fine Arts Society was established in Krakow for the encouragement of Polish art. The Society embarked upon the organization of exhibitions by living artists, the acquisition of paintings and sculptures and the setting up of a comprehensive records office gathering documents of the history of Polish art in the 19th and early 20th centuries. The Art Nouveau building was designed by Franciszek Màczyński and modelled on the famous Secession Pavilion in Vienna. The finest Krakow artists worked on the decoration. Jacek Malczewski designed the frieze depicting the vicissitudes of fortune and the struggle of artistic genius. The sculptors Antoni Madeyski, Konstanty Laszczka and Teodor Rygier contributed busts of great Polish artists. A portico attached to the façade is topped with a statue of Apollo crowned with a sun halo. Exhibitions of 19th-century and contemporary art are held here.

⓲ "Bunker of Art"
"Bunkier Sztuki"

Plac Szczepański 3a. **Map** 1 C4 (5 C2). **Tel** 12 422 10 52. 2, 4, 8, 13, 14, 15. 124, 152, 502. **Open** noon–8pm Tue–Sun.

This gloomy building in the Socialist Realist style of the 1960s is regarded as one of the ugliest in the city centre. However, it is the venue for some of the most interesting exhibitions of contemporary art, by both Polish and foreign artists. The "Bunker of Art" also features one of Krakow's most popular cafés.

Sculptural decoration on the Palace of Art

⑬ Collegium Maius

The Collegium Maius is the oldest building within the Academy of Krakow (now the Jagiellonian University). It was constructed in the 15th century by amalgamating a number of town houses. Lecture rooms and accommodation for professors were originally located here. In the 19th century the building housed the Jagiellonian Library. Between 1840 and 1870 the architects Karol Kremer, Feliks Księżarski and Hermann Bergman rebuilt the college in the Neo-Gothic style. After World War II the University Museum, established in 1867, was moved here.

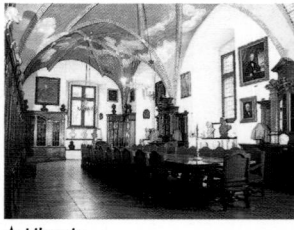

★ Libraria
The Libraria was built in the 16th century as the College Library. Today it is a meeting place of the Senate and is decorated with portraits of rectors and professors of the University.

Oriel
This oriel window projecting from the Stuba Communis enlivens the austere exterior wall.

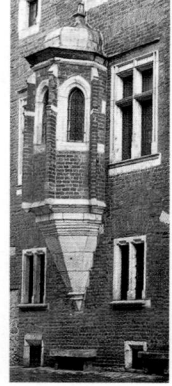

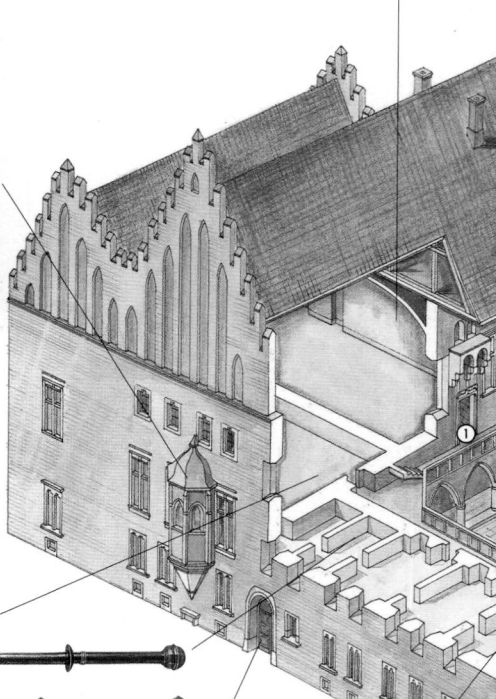

★ Stuba Communis
The Stuba Communis, or Common Room, served as the professors' refectory. The hall features a 14th-century statue of Kazimierz the Great and a 17th-century staircase made in Danzig.

Entrance

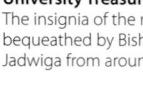

University Treasury
The insignia of the rector, including a late 15th-century mace bequeathed by Bishop Zbigniew Oleśnicki and that of Queen Jadwiga from around 1405, are among the treasures.

Copernicus Room
The Room is dedicated to the great astronomer, who studied here between 1491 and 1495, thus rendering the Academy famous. The display features the so-called Jagiellonian armillary sphere made in 1510.

Cloister
The Gothic cloister, whose columns have a cut crystal-like decoration, is reminiscent of those in medieval Italian universities.

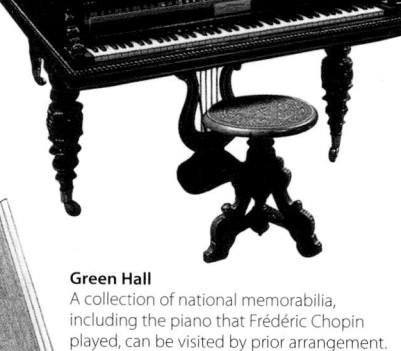

Green Hall
A collection of national memorabilia, including the piano that Frédéric Chopin played, can be visited by prior arrangement.

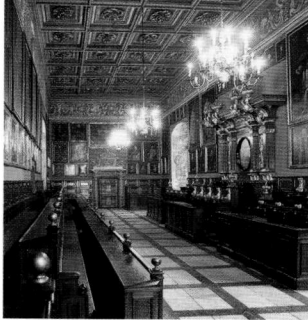

★ Great Hall
The Great Hall features stalls used by the Senate during the ceremonies at which honorary degrees are conferred.

Chapel
The former apartment of John of Kęty, the professor of theology who became the patron saint of the Jagiellonian University, has been converted into a chapel, which is on the ground floor.

KEY

① **Porta Aurea (Golden Gate)**

② **A lavishly inlaid door** was originally in the Senior Room of the old Town Hall.

③ **Rector's Stairs**

⓮ Church of St Anne

A professor of the Krakow Academy, John of Kęty (Jan Kanty) was already considered a saint at the time of his death in 1473, when he was buried in the Gothic Church of St Anne. Following his beatification, the Senate of the Academy commissioned Tylman van Gameren to build a new church. The construction began in 1689 under the supervision of Father Sebastian Piskorski. The Italian architect and sculptor Baldassare Fontana contributed the decoration and most of the furnishings, including the altars, between 1695 and 1703. He was assisted by the painters Carlo and Innocente Monti and Karl Dankwart. St Anne's, with its sumptuous interior, is considered to be a leading example of Baroque ecclesiastical architecture in Poland.

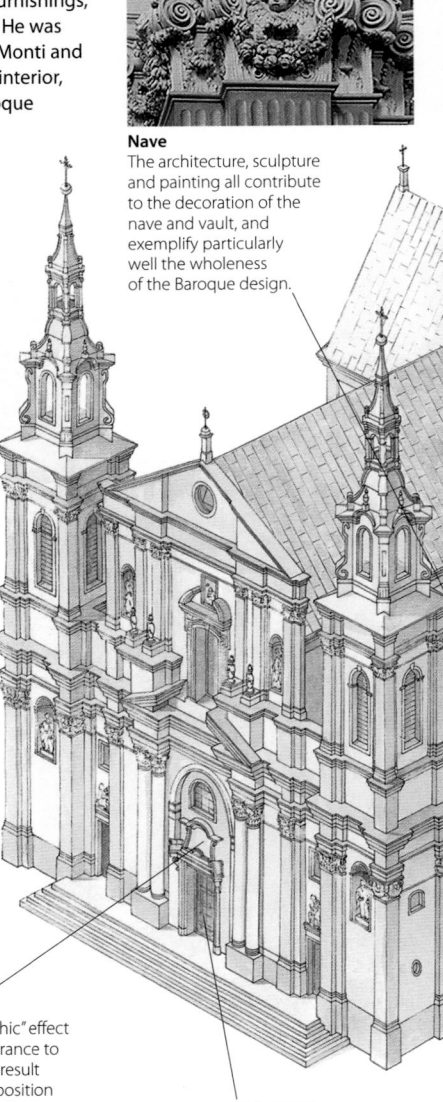

Nave
The architecture, sculpture and painting all contribute to the decoration of the nave and vault, and exemplify particularly well the wholeness of the Baroque design.

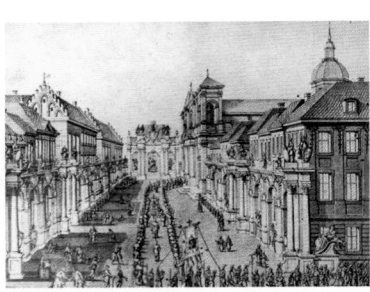

Procession Commemorating St John of Kęty, 1767
To mark the canonization of John of Kęty, a procession with his holy relics was held in Krakow. The saint's relics were carried into the Church of St Anne with great pomp and ceremony.

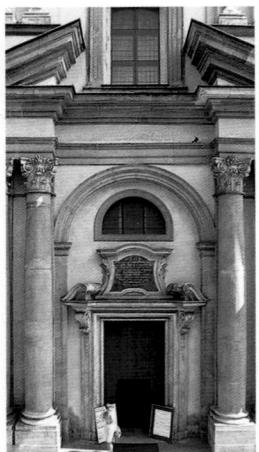

West Portal
The "scenographic" effect of the main entrance to the Church is a result of the superimposition of three portals, one within another.

Main entrance

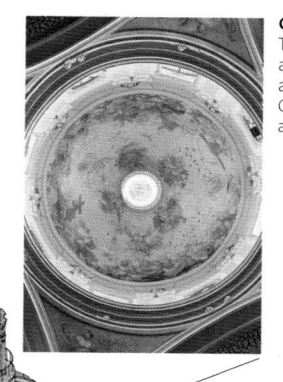

Gloria Domini
The dome fresco by Carlo and Innocente Monti is an allegory of triumphant Catholicism, represented as the true Christian faith.

VISITORS' CHECKLIST

Practical Information
ul. Św. Anny 11. **Map** 1 C4 (5 C2)
Tel 12 422 53 18. **Open** during services only.

Transport
124, 152, 502.
2, 4, 8, 14, 15, 18.

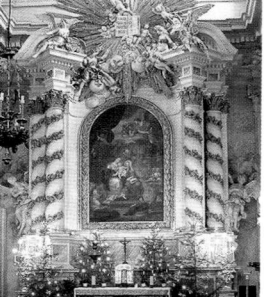

★ High Altar
The high altar is decorated with sculptures by Baldassare Fontana. The altarpiece, depicting the Virgin and Child with Anne, is by Jerzy Eleuter Siemiginowski, painter to Jan III Sobieski.

Pulpit
The angel supporting the pulpit was carved in 1727 by the Krakow artist Antoni Frączkiewicz, who was influenced by the art of Baldassare Fontana.

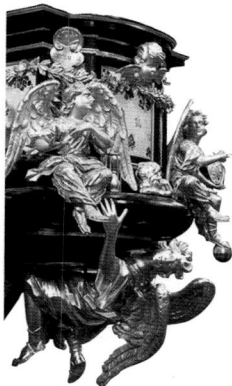

★ Shrine of St John of Kęty
The relics of the saint rest in a sarcophagus supported by four figures personifying the faculties of the Academy of Krakow: Theology, Philosophy, Law and Medicine.

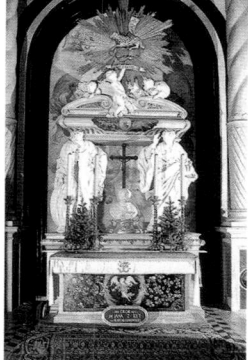

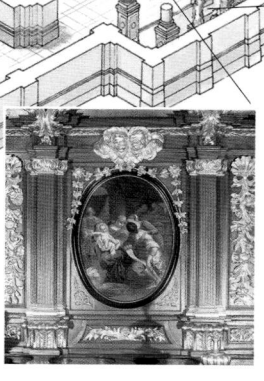

Choir Stalls
The stalls are decorated with paintings by Szymon Czechowicz, a leading Polish painter of the 18th century.

⓭ Szołayski House
Kamienica Szołayskich

Plac Szczepański 9. **Map** 1 C4 (5 D2). **Tel** 12 433 54 50. 🚌 124, 152, 304, 424, 502. 🚊 2, 4, 8, 13, 14, 18, 20, 24. **Open** 10am–6pm Tue–Sat, 10am–4pm Sun. 🎫 free Sun. **W** muzeum.krakow.pl

The oldest parts of this building, which house a branch of the National Museum in Krakow, date from the 15th century. Since then, Szołayski House has served as a private residence, part of a monastery and a newspaper office. Since 1934, it has been an exhibition space, except for a period during World War II when it was occupied by the Nazis. In 2003, it was dedicated to the life and works of Stanisław Wyspiański (1869–1907), Krakow's foremost Art Nouveau artist. Its role has now been expanded to display the works of other Polish artists of the same period, as well as temporary exhibitions on other notable Polish figures.

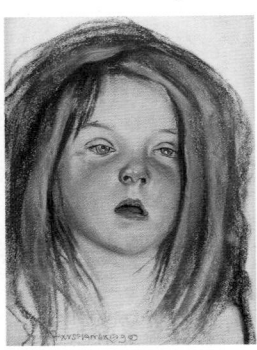

Helenka by Stanisław Wyspiański

⓮ Church of the Reformed Franciscans
Kościół Reformatów

ul. Reformacka 4. **Map** 1 C4 (6 D1). **Tel** 12 422 06 23. 🚌 124, 152, 502. 🚊 2, 3, 4, 8, 13, 14, 15, 20. **Open** during services only.

The Church of the Reformed Franciscans was built between 1666 and 1672. The architecture and modest furnishings conform to the strict rule of the order. The altarpiece

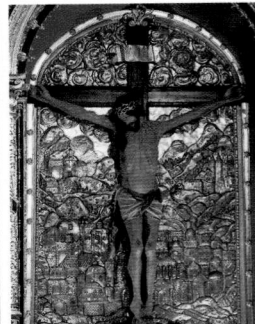

Crucifix on the altar in the Church of St Mark

on the left that depicts St Kazimierz (Casimir) is an outstanding example of 17th-century work.

The specific microclimate within the crypt beneath the church causes the reposing corpses to undergo mummification. Those visitors seeking a shocking experience may request access to the crypt.

⓯ Church of St Mark
Kościół św. Marka

ul. Św. Marka 10. **Map** 1 C4 (6 D1). **Tel** 12 422 21 78. 🚌 124, 152, 502. 🚊 3, 4, 5, 13, 15, 20. **Open** during services only.

The early Gothic church of the Monks of St Mark was founded in 1263 by Duke Bolesław the Chaste. It has been remodelled a number of times throughout its history and the interior acquired an early Baroque appearance in the first half of the 17th century. The high altar, with its lavish Mannerist ornamentation, was made in 1618 in the workshop of Baltazar Kuncz. On the left is the 17th-century tomb of Blessed Michał Giedroyć (died 1485).

⓰ Polish Academy of Skills
Gmach Polskiej Akademii Umiejętności

ul. Sławkowska 17. **Map** 1 C4 (6 D1). **Tel** 12 424 02 00. 🚌 124, 152, 502. 🚊 3, 4, 5, 15, 20. **Open** 9am–4pm Mon–Fri. **W** pau.krakow.pl

The building was constructed between 1857 and 1866 as the seat of the Academic Society of Krakow, which in 1872 became the Academy of Skills, the first academic body to bring together scholars from all three parts of partitioned Poland. It was designed by Filip Pokutyński in the Neo-Renaissance style. The exterior is decorated with portrait medallions of people in low relief who made important contributions to Polish academic and cultural life. Inside, a small meeting room features an impressive coffered ceiling. The rich print collection includes works by Albrecht Dürer and Rembrandt.

⓱ St John Street
Ulica św. Jana

Map 1 C4 (6 D2). 🚌 124, 152, 502. 🚊 3, 4, 5, 13, 15, 20.

This quiet street leading away from the Market Square, and closed off at its

Portal to the House of the Cistercian Abbots of Jędrzejów, 20 St John Street north end by the façade of the Piarist Church, is lined with a selection of fine secular and ecclesiastic Baroque and Neo-Classical buildings.

The House of the Cistercian Abbots of Jędrzejów at No.20 is of particular interest. Remodelled in 1744 by Francesco Placidi, the house is decorated with a magnificent late Baroque portal featuring atlantes.

The Wodzicki Palace at No.11 was given a Neo-Classical façade by Ferdinand Nax after 1781. Around 1818 the Bernardine Friary was converted after a great deal of rebuilding.

❷❹ Church of St John
Kościół św. Jana

ul. Św. Jana 7. **Map** 1 C4 (6 D2). **Tel** 12 422 65 00. 🚌 124, 152, 502. 🚊 3, 4, 5, 15, 20. **Open** during services only.

The chronicler Jan Długosz records that this church was founded in the 12th century. The Romanesque architecture has been lost through much remodelling. The Gothic buttresses still project from the exterior side walls, but the façade and the interior are Baroque. The high altar of 1730 is decorated with sculptures by Antoni Frączkiewicz and the 16th-century miraculous Madonna, the Refuge of Prisoners.

❷❺ Czartoryski Museum
Muzeum Czartoryskich

See pp114–15.

❷❻ Piarist Church
Kościół Pijarów

ul. Pijarska 2. **Map** 1 C4 (6 D1). **Tel** 12 422 17 24. 🚌 124, 152, 502. 🚊 3, 4, 5, 13, 15, 20. **Open** during services only.

This Baroque church was built between 1718 and 1728 probably to designs by Kacper Bażanka. The Rococo façade designed by Francesco Placidi was added in 1759 to 1761. Inside, the church is decorated with frescoes by a master of

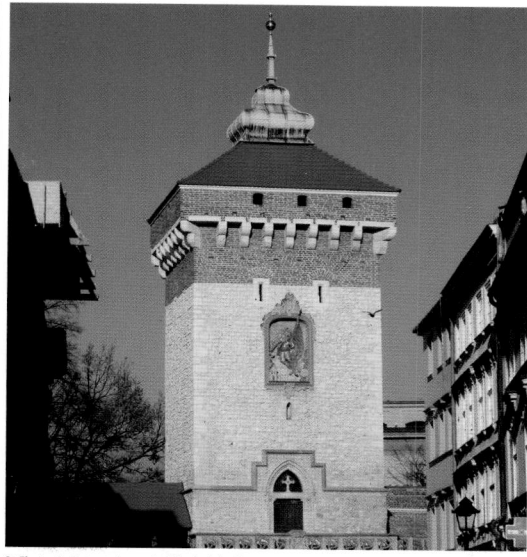
St Florian's Gate at the end of Floriańska Street

illusion, Franz Eckstein. The high altar painted on the wall is by the same artist, as is the fresco in the nave vault that glorifies the name of the Virgin Mary. The altars in the aisles feature .18th-century paintings by Szymon Czechowicz.

The crypt under the church is renowned for the decoration of Christ's Tomb, which usually alludes symbolically to patriotic themes, and is set up here every year during Holy Week. The crypt is also a venue for theatre performances and various exhibitions.

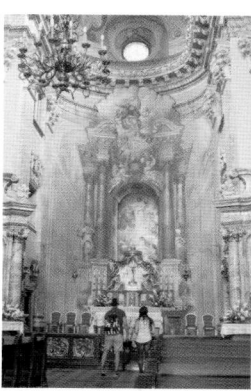
The Rococo interior of the 18th-century Piarist Church

❷❼ St Florian's Gate and the City Wall Remnants
Brama Floriańska i Resztki Murów Miejskich

Map 2 D4 (6 E1). 🚌 124, 152, 502. 🚊 3, 4, 5, 13, 15, 19.

In 1285 Duke Leszek the Black gave Krakow the right to have the city surrounded by walls. These fortifications developed during the following centuries, finally consisting of inner and outer moated walls and 47 towers. Eight fortified gates lead into the city. With the introduction of artillery, the defence system became redundant. Disused, it fell into disrepair by the end of the 18th century. The walls were dismantled early in the 19th century and later replaced by the Planty gardens *(see pp168–9)*. St Florian's Gate, dating possibly from the end of the 13th century, and a small stretch of the adjoining walls have been saved, largely through the efforts of Professor Feliks Radwański. East of St Florian's Gate is the Haberdashers'Tower, and the towers of the Joiners and Carpenters are to the west.

⓲ Czartoryski Museum

At the core of the Czartoryski Museum is the collection assembled late in the 18th century by Princess Izabella Czartoryska. It was initially at Puławy, but partly moved to Paris following the 1830 November Uprising. In 1876 the collection was brought to Krakow, thanks to the efforts of Prince Władysław Czartoryski. It is located in three houses and the adjoining City Arsenal at St John Street, where works are displayed in period interiors but may be subject to changes of location during extensive renovation work.

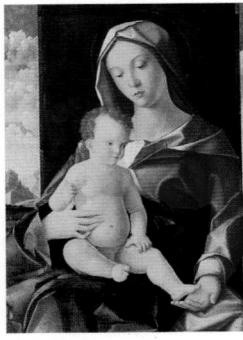

Madonna and Child
By the Venetian Vincenzo Catena, this painting is a highlight of the Czartoryski's Italian collection.

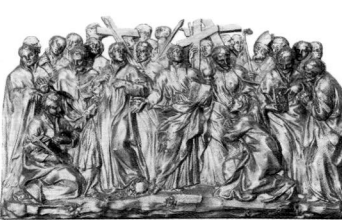

Jesuit Saints
This fine bas-relief by the 17th-century Roman sculptor, Alessandro Algardi, depicts the Polish Jesuit, Stanisław Kostka, being admitted to the congregation of Jesuit saints.

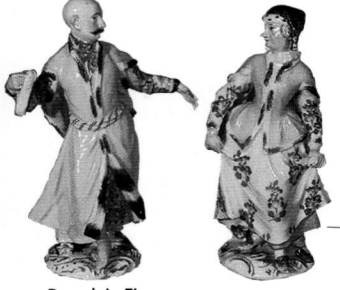

Gallery Guide
There is no gallery space on the ground floor. The first-floor display is dedicated to Polish history of the 14th–18th centuries as well as Western European decorative arts. The picture gallery is on the second floor.

Porcelain Figures
These two figures of a Polish nobleman and noblewoman were made in Meissen.

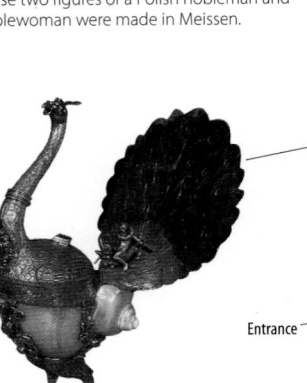

Entrance

Nautilus Cup
The museum collection is rich in decorative arts and includes this 17th-century drinking vessel made in Danzig (now Gdańsk) from a large shell.

★ **Lady with an Ermine by Leonardo da Vinci**
During renovations, this late 15th-century portrait is on display at Wawel Royal Castle *(see pp72–3)*.

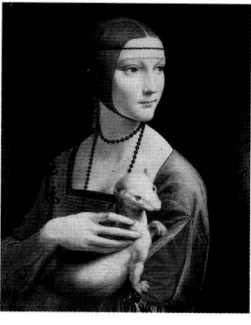

VISITORS' CHECKLIST

Practical Information
ul. Św. Jana 19. **Map** 1 C4 (6 E1).
Tel 12 422 55 66. **Closed** for renovations until June 2016.
🅿 🚻 🌐 **muzeum-czartoryskich.krakow.pl**

Transport
🚋 2, 3, 4, 5, 12, 13, 14, 15, 24.
🚌 124, 152, 424, 502, 512.

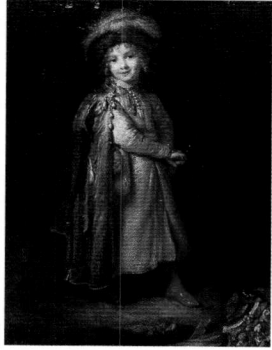

***Portrait of a Boy* by Caspar Netscher**
This sweet little portrait is one of several paintings in the collection by lesser Dutch artists of the 17th century.

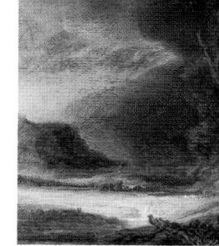

★ ***Landscape with the Good Samaritan* by Rembrandt**
A masterpiece in the collection of Western painting, this treatment of the natural world is breathtaking.

***Landscape* by Alessandro Magnasco**
This dramatic landscape is characteristic of Italian painting of the 18th century.

Second floor

First floor

Ground floor

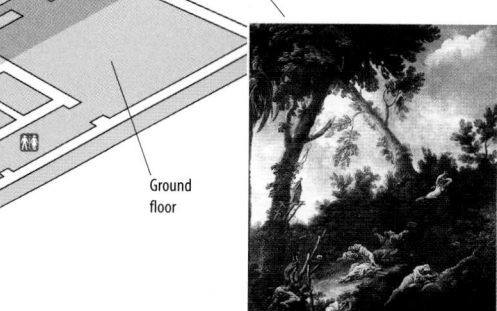

Key

🔲 Non-exhibition space

🔲 History of Poland 1300–1900

🔲 Decorative Arts of Western Europe

🔲 Picture Gallery

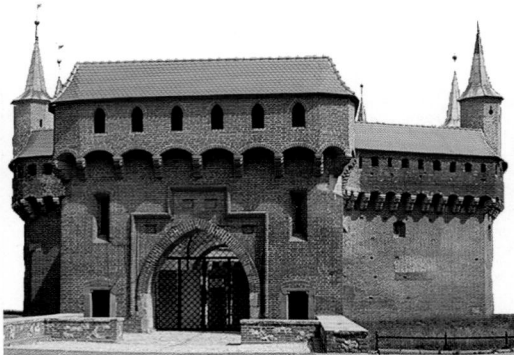

The impressive exterior of the Barbican

㉘ Barbican
Barbakan

ul. Basztowa. **Map** 2 D3 (6 E1). 3, 4, 5, 13, 15. 124, 152, 502.

The Barbican, a round bastion, was constructed in 1498–99 after King Jan Olbracht was defeated by the Turks in Bukowina, and further Turkish incursions were feared. It shows the changes that had been introduced to military architecture as a result of the rapid development of artillery. This relatively low structure projecting from the city walls with a considerable overhang enabled the defenders to fire with precision at the enemy from the loop-holes, positioned at different levels. The Barbican was originally surrounded by a moat and linked to St Florian's Gate by a corridor. It is the best preserved barbican in Europe.

㉙ Jama Michalika Café
Jama Michalika

ul. Floriańska 45. **Map** 2 D4 (6 E1). **Tel** 12 422 15 61. 3, 4, 5, 13, 15. 124, 152, 502. **Open** noon–midnight daily.

In 1895 Jan Michalik opened a patisserie near the Market Square. It became very popular with students of the Fine Arts School who called the place *jama* (grotto) for its lack of windows. Poets, writers and artists soon joined them and in 1905 established the cabaret Zielony Balonik (The Green Balloon) here. The performances, based on texts by Tadeusz Boy-Żeleński, soon attracted a large audience. Satirical Christmas puppet shows, with marionettes by Ludwik Puget and Jan Szczepkowski, became particularly popular.

In 1910 Michalik extended and redecorated the premises to designs by Franciszek Mączyński. The main room received a glass ceiling. Karol Frycz designed the interior decoration, furniture and most of the stained glass in the Art Nouveau style.

The café is still an inviting place where customers can go back in time and enjoy the atmosphere of the fin de siècle, as well as see enduring folk shows.

㉚ Matejko House
Dom Matejki

ul. Floriańska 41. **Map** 2 D4 (6 E1). **Tel** 12 433 59 60. 3, 4, 5, 13, 15. 124, 152, 502. **Open** 10am–6pm Tue–Sat, 10am–4pm Sun. free on Sun.

The artist Jan Matejko was born here in 1838, and in 1873 returned to live with his family. He rebuilt the house and added a new façade designed by Tomasz Pryliński in the Neo-Baroque style. After Matejko died in 1893 the house was transformed into a museum and opened to the public five years later. The statue of a hussar on horseback, on the ground floor, was part of Leon Wyczółkowski's design for the Matejko Monument. The private rooms on the first floor have remained unchanged, while the second floor is used for a display of the artist's works, which include cartoons for the murals that are in the Church of St Mary. His studio on the third floor is full of the props and curiosities he collected. Pieces of old armour and instruments of torture excavated on the site of the old Town Hall are of particular interest.

㉛ Floriańska Street
Ulica Floriańska

Map 1 C4, 2 D4 (6 D2–E1, 2). 3, 5, 13, 15, 20. 124, 152, 502.

This street, leading from St Florian's Gate to the Market Square, formed part of the Royal Route which became fully established after the court moved from Krakow to Warsaw.

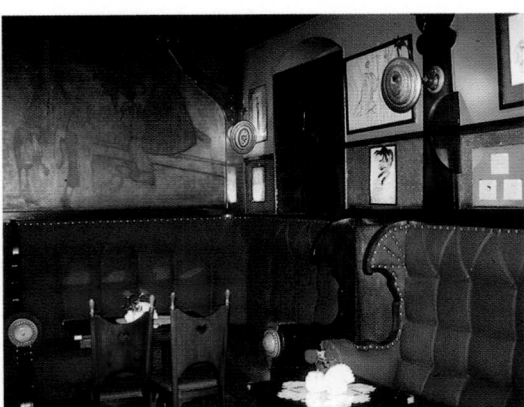

The interior of the Jama Michalika Café

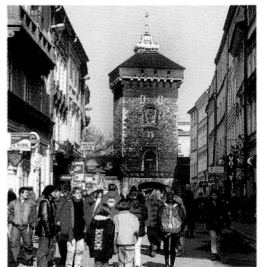

Visitors in front of St Florian's Gate on Floriańska Street

The Royal Route was often used by a sovereign arriving for a coronation, and again when his body was taken in procession for the funeral at Wawel. In the 19th century Floriańska was the busiest street in Krakow, with trams introduced in 1881. Medieval walls have survived in most houses, but the original architecture has been lost through later remodelling. More storeys and new eclectic façades were added to most buildings early in the 20th century, when Floriańska gained its present appearance.

❸❷ Słowacki Theatre
Teatr im. Juliusza Słowackiego

Pl. Świętego Ducha 1. **Map** 2 D4 (6 E2). **Tel** 12 424 45 00. 🚋 2, 4, 5, 8, 13, 15, 20. 🚌 124, 152, 502.

The proposal for a new theatre in Krakow, one which would replace the small and dilapidated Old Theatre, was put forward in 1872. Jan Zawiejski submitted the design and was put in charge of the works which were to be financed entirely through donations. The foundation stone was laid in 1891, and the theatre opened in 1893. Zawiejski designed an opulent building in which vernacular elements, such as the parapet inspired by the Cloth Hall, and foreign influences were blended into an eclectic whole. Allegorical sculptures decorate the exterior of the theatre.

The opulent interior features a grand staircase decorated with stuccowork by Alfred Putz. The four-tiered auditorium can seat up to 900 people. The stage curtain, one of the major attractions, was painted by Henryk Siemiradzki. It depicts Apollo striking an accord between Beauty and Love, surrounded by muses as well as other allegorical figures which represent Art drawing inspiration from man's fate.

❸❸ Church of the Holy Cross
Kościół św. Krzyża

ul. Świętego Krzyża 23. **Map** 2 D4 (6 E3). **Tel** 12 429 20 56. 🚋 2, 4, 5, 8, 15. 🚌 124, 152, 502. **Open** during services only.

The Gothic church of the Order of the Holy Cross was built in two stages. The construction of the choir began immediately after 1300. The main nave and tower date from the first half of the 14th century. The interior is extremely well preserved and the nave impresses with its intricate pattern of vaulting ribs, supported on a single, round pillar. Among its furnishings, the Gothic font made in 1423 by Jan Freudenthal and the late Renaissance triptych in the Węgrzyn Chapel (next to the porch) are of particular interest. There are also various Baroque altars and stalls, as well as a number of memorial plaques of famous sculptors, active at the end of the 19th century, which are worth seeing.

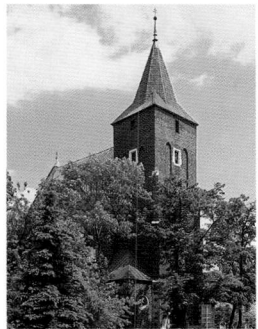

The Church of the Holy Cross

❸❹ Church of the Dominican Nuns
Kościół Dominikanek

ul. Mikołajska 21. **Map** 2 D4 (6 E3). **Tel** 12 422 79 25. 🚋 2, 3, 8, 10, 13, 20. **Open** during services only.

The church, dedicated to the Virgin Mary, Queen of Snow, was founded in 1632–34 by Anna Lubomirska. Prior to the church, a fortified manor of Albert, Krakow's *wójt* (chief officer), was on this site in the 14th century. As a result of Albert's revolt against King Władysław the Short, a new building for the local government was erected. The latter was converted in the 1620s into a convent for the Dominican nuns. The church contains a miraculous 17th-century icon of the Virgin.

❸❺ Dominican Church
Kościół Dominikanów

See pp118–19.

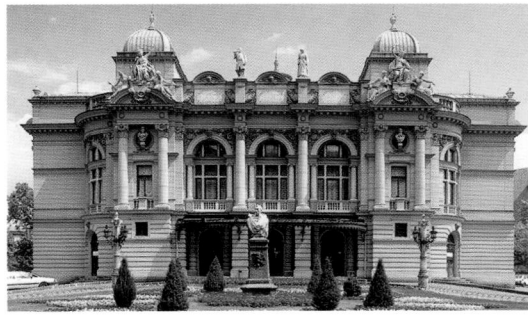

The eclectic façade of the Słowacki Theatre

35 Dominican Church

The Dominicans began the construction of a new church in 1250. It contained the shrine of St Jacek, a place of mass pilgrimage. Opulent mausolea, modelled on the Zygmunt Chapel at Wawel, were added in the 17th century by noble families, and in the 18th century the church was furnished with late Baroque altars. The fire of Krakow in 1850 destroyed the church almost completely. It was rebuilt by 1872 and today is an important evangelical centre which attracts masses of the faithful.

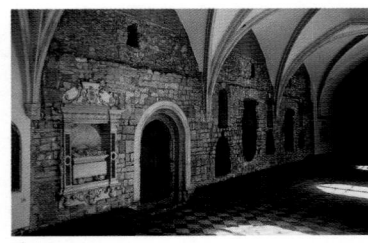

Cloister
The Gothic cloister was a burial place of burghers whose memorial plaques and tombs can still be seen here.

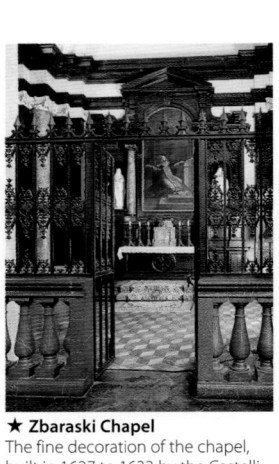

★ Zbaraski Chapel
The fine decoration of the chapel, built in 1627 to 1633 by the Castelli artists, is in sharp contrast with the monumental forms of the altar and tombs in black marble.

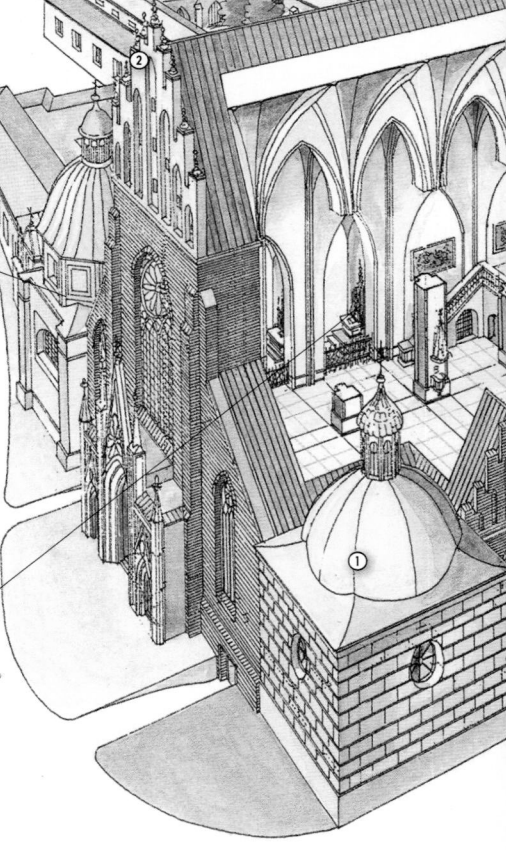

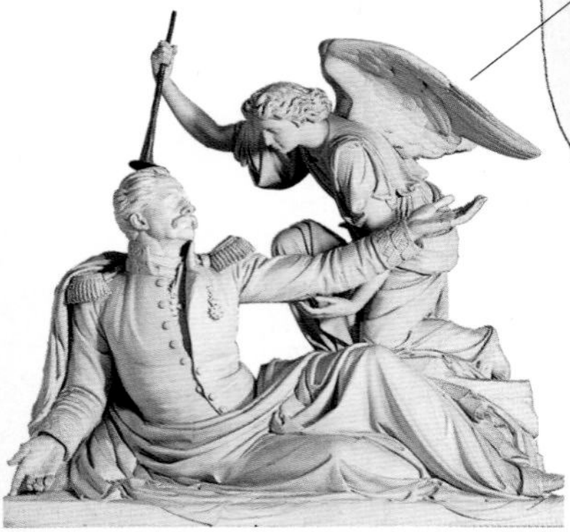

Tomb of General Jan Skrzynecki (died 1860)
This beautiful monument carved by Władysław Oleszczyński commemorates the hero of the November Uprising of 1830.

★ Shrine of St Jacek
The Renaissance Chapel of St Jacek was rebuilt around 1700 by Baldassare Fontana, who also designed this magnificent monument. The chapel is decorated with paintings by Tommaso Dolabella.

VISITORS' CHECKLIST

Practical Information
ul. Stolarska 12. **Map** 1 C5 (6 D3).
Tel 12 423 16 13.
Open 6:30am–8pm daily
🆆 krakow.dominikanie.pl

Transport
🚋 1, 3, 6, 8, 18.

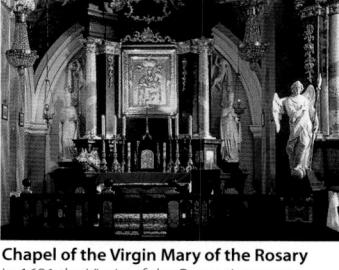

Chapel of the Virgin Mary of the Rosary
In 1621 the Virgin of the Rosary icon was carried in a procession to secure, through prayers, victory over the Turks at Chocim.

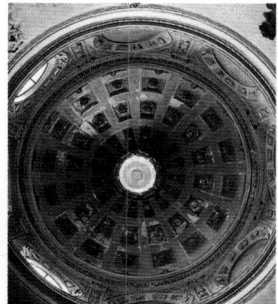

The Myszkowski Chapel
This was built between 1603 and 1614 by masters from Santi Gucci's circle, using marble from the Świętokrzyskie (Holy Cross) Mountains. Portrait busts of the Myszkowskis form part of the splendid decoration of the dome.

KEY

① **The Lubomirski Chapel** displays lovely paintings and sculptures.

② **Crowstep gable**

③ **The memorial plaque of Filippo Buonacorsi (Callimachus)** (died 1496) honours the great humanist at the Polish royal court (see p47).

④ **Choir stalls**, pulpit and confessionals, all in the Neo-Gothic style, date from the second half of the 19th century.

Tomb of Prospero Provano
The monument of this salt magnate (died 1584) is one of the finest Polish sculptural works of circa 1600. It is located next to the Myszkowski Chapel.

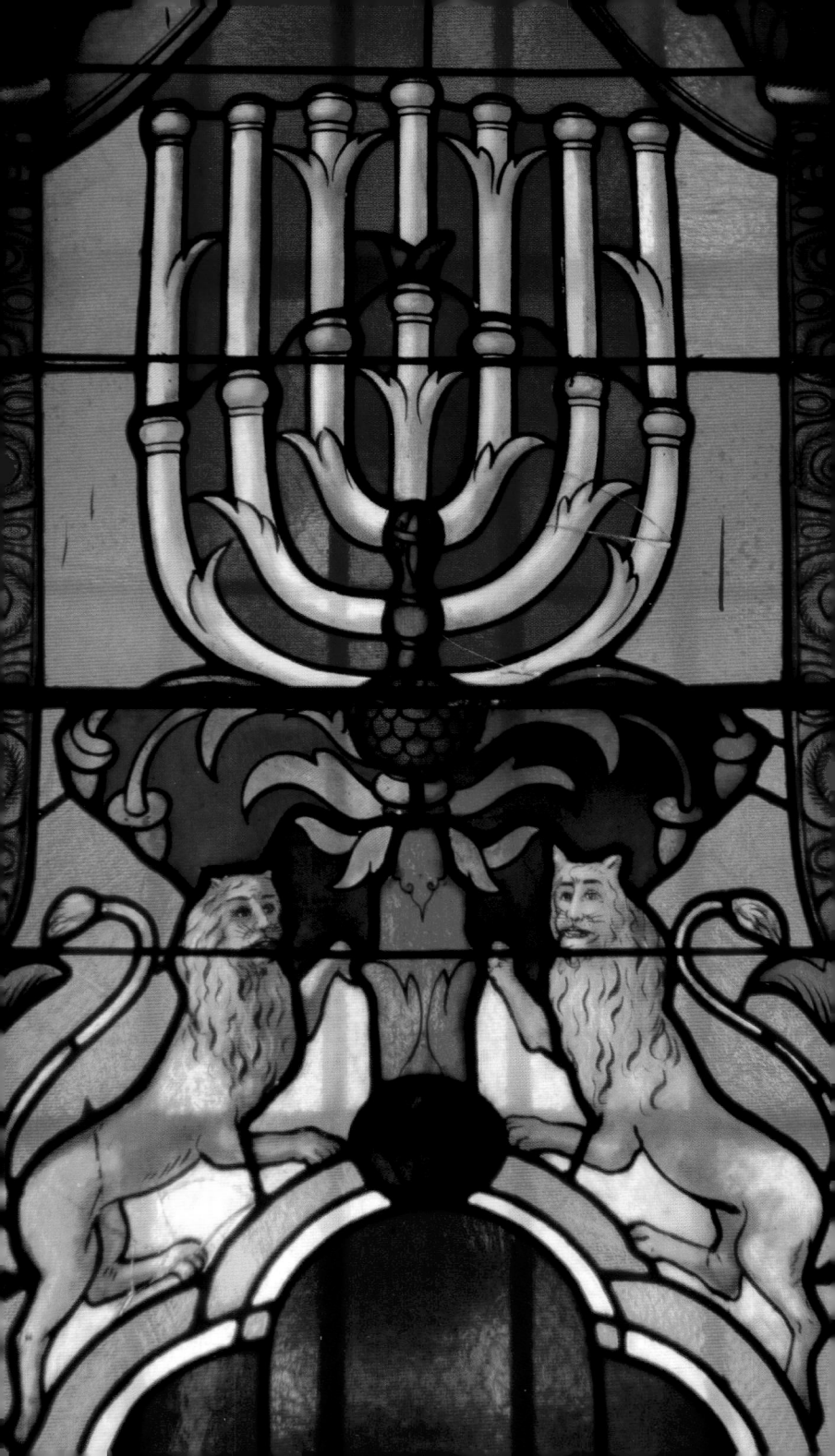

KAZIMIERZ QUARTER

The town of Kazimierz near Krakow was founded in 1335 by Kazimierz (Casimir) the Great. With its own Town Hall and a defence wall, Kazimierz competed with the capital in position and wealth. The king built two large churches, St Catherine's and Corpus Christi, and planned to establish a university here. After King Jan Olbracht had moved the Jewish population here from Krakow in the late 15th century, the separate nature of Kazimierz became more pronounced. The town was soon to become a leading centre of Jewish culture. Although Kazimierz was integrated administratively into Krakow in 1791, the distinctive character of this quarter is still evident. With narrow streets lined with low buildings, it seems to belong to a different world. It bears witness to centuries of the peaceful co-existence of two peoples: Jewish and Polish. Magnificent sacred architecture of both religions can be seen as further confirmation of this symbiosis.

Sights at a Glance

Churches
8 Corpus Christi Church
11 Church of the Order of St John of God
12 Church of St Catherine
13 Paulite Church "On the Rock"

Historic Buildings
9 Kazimierz Town Hall
10 Hospital of the Order of St John of God

Historic Cemeteries
6 Remu'h Cemetery
7 New Jewish Cemetery

Synagogues
1 Tempel Synagogue
2 Isaak's Synagogue
3 High Synagogue
4 Old Synagogue
5 Remu'h Synagogue

Restaurants see pp192–3
1 Dawno temu na Kazimierzu
2 Fabryka Pizzy
3 Genji Sushi Premium
4 Horai
5 Klezmer Hois
6 Manzana
7 Pierogi Mr Vincent
8 Polakowski
9 Studio Qulinarne
10 Trezo
11 Zazie Bistro

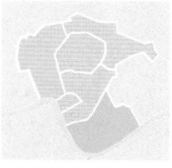

See also Street Finder maps 3 & 4

◀ Stained-glass window in the Tempel Synagogue

For keys to symbols see back flap

Street-by-Street: Szeroka Street Area

The Jewish quarter was located in the east part of Kazimierz and concentrated first around Szeroka Street, then Libusza Square, which was later known as New Square. As well as the Jews displaced here in the late 15th century from Krakow, Czech and German refugees also came to live in Kazimierz. The Jewish community had its own jurisdiction and culture, and was never totally assimilated with the Poles. Many synagogues, baths, schools and cemeteries were established in Kazimierz, which became an active centre of Judaic culture and learning. The Nazis annihilated this unique world. However, a number of art galleries and restaurants have been opened here which evoke the past.

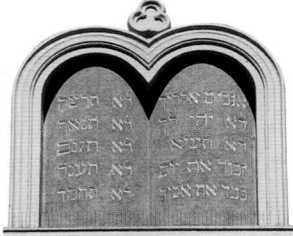

❶ Tempel Synagogue
The decoration of this synagogue, built in the Neo-Renaissance style, was influenced by Moorish art.

Jewish Tombs

The signs carved on tombs convey symbolic meanings. The grave of a rabbi is indicated by hands joined in prayer. Basins and jugs for the ritual ablution of hands can be found on graves of the Levites. Three interlaced snakes feature on the grave of a physician, and a crown of knowledge on that of a learned man. A lion or a six-pointed star of David signifies a descendant of Judah.

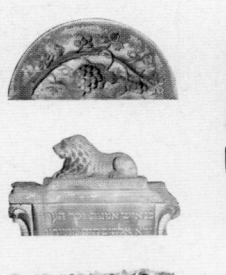

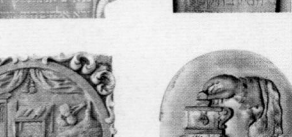

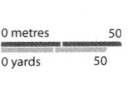

0 metres 50
0 yards 50

Key

— Suggested route

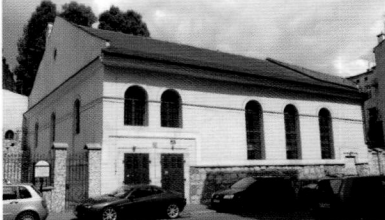

The Kupa Synagogue
This was built in the 17th century and financed by the Kahal of Kazimierz. It was remodelled many times and was also used for non-religious purposes.

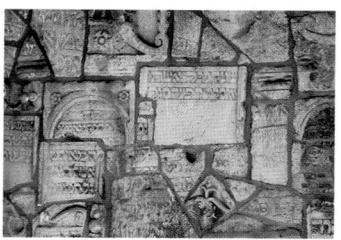

❻ ★ Remu'h Cemetery
The Wailing Wall commemorates the tragic fate of the Jews from Krakow during World War II.

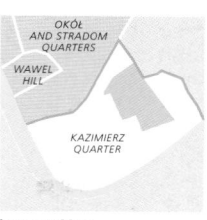

Locator Map
See Street Finder maps 4

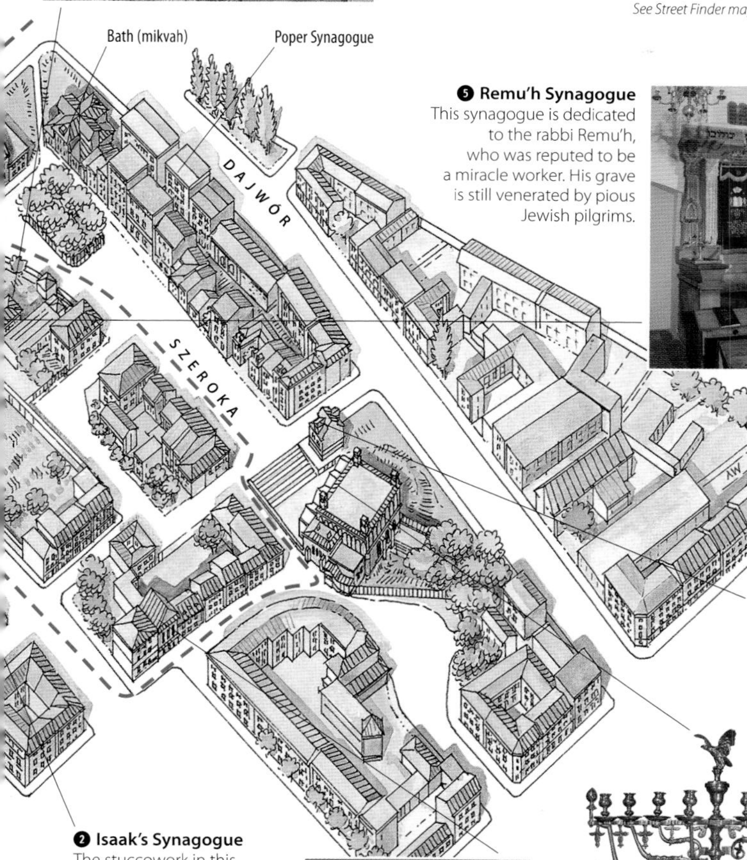

Bath (mikvah)   Poper Synagogue

❺ Remu'h Synagogue
This synagogue is dedicated to the rabbi Remu'h, who was reputed to be a miracle worker. His grave is still venerated by pious Jewish pilgrims.

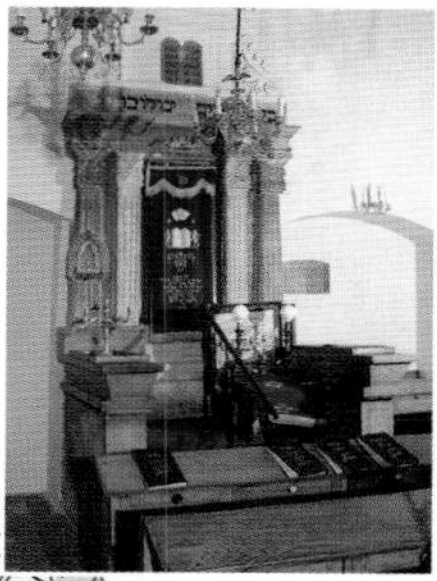

DAJWÓR

SZEROKA

Synagogue on the Hill

❷ Isaak's Synagogue
The stuccowork in this Baroque synagogue is of great interest.

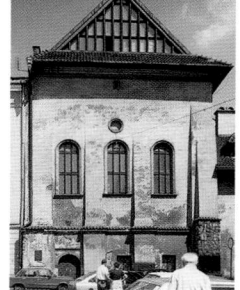

❸ High Synagogue
With its late Gothic architecture and Renaissance decoration, this is one of Krakow's most picturesque synagogues.

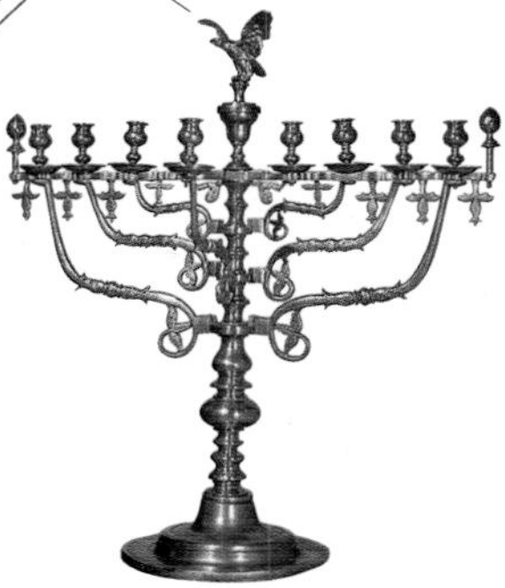

❹ ★ Old Synagogue
This menorah is among the treasures in Poland's oldest synagogue. The building was destroyed by the Nazis, and later restored.

❶ Tempel Synagogue
Synagoga Tempel

ul. Miodowa 24. **Map** 4 D1 (6 F5).
🚊 1, 3, 6, 8, 9, 10, 11, 13, 18, 19, 22.
🚌 128, 184. **Open** Mon–Fri.

The most recent of the synagogues in Kazimierz, the Tempel, was built in the Neo-Renaissance style between 1860 and 1862. It is used by non-Orthodox Jews. Inside note the stained glass and period decoration.

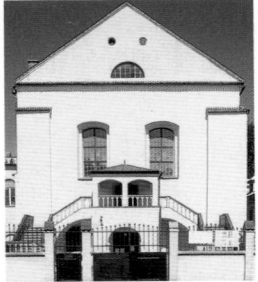

Façade of Isaak's Synagogue

❷ Isaak's Synagogue
Bożnica Izaaka

ul. Kupa 18. **Map** 4 D1. **Tel** 12 430 55 77. 🚊 3, 8, 9, 11, 13. 🚌 128, 184. **Open** 9am–7pm Sun–Fri. **Closed** public hols.

This synagogue was built between 1638 and 1644 as a foundation of Izaak Jakubowicz, an elder of the Jewish community. Inside, the plaster work by Giovanni Battista Falconi has survived in a large nave with a barrel vault. The Jewish Education Centre is housed here.

❸ High Synagogue
Bożnica Wysoka

ul. Józefa 38. **Map** 4 D1.
🚊 3, 8, 9, 10, 11, 13.

This synagogue dates from 1556 to 1563. It is a picturesque structure supported by buttresses. A Renaissance portal is worth noting. Only a few furnishings have survived, including a money box and the remains of an altar. The Studio for the Restoration of Monuments is located here.

❹ Old Synagogue
Synagoga Stara

ul. Szeroka 24. **Map** 4 D1. 🚊 3, 9, 11, 13. Galicia Jewish Museum: **Tel** 12 422 09 62. **Open** Apr–Oct: 9am–5pm Tue–Sun, 10am–2pm Mon; Nov–Mar: 10am–2pm Mon, 9am–4pm Tue–Thu, Sat & Sun, 10am–5pm Fri. **Closed** first Sat & Sun of each month. 🏛 free Mon. 📷

The Old Synagogue was used in the past as a temple and was also a seat of the Kahal and other offices of the Jewish community. Religious and social life was concentrated here. The synagogue houses the Galicia Jewish Museum, which is dedicated to the history and culture of Krakow's Jews.

The brick building dates back to the mid-15th or beginning of the 16th century. Its present appearance is the result of a remodelling in 1557–70. The parapet, and Gothic interior with ribbed vaulting supported by slender columns, all date from then.

The hall used for prayer is almost bare, in accordance with the rule of the Jewish religion. The *bimah*, an elevated platform with an iron balustrade used for readings from the Torah, is the only piece of furnishing.

The east wall features the *aron hakodesh*, an ornamental shrine for the Torah Scrolls.

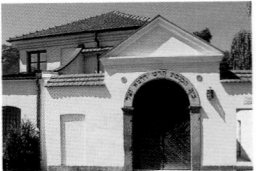

Entrance to the Remu'h Synagogue and Cemetery

❺ Remu'h Synagogue
Bożnica Remuh

ul. Szeroka 40. **Map** 4 D1. **Tel** 12 421 29 87. 🚊 3, 9, 11, 13. **Open** 9am–4pm Sun–Fri (May–Sep: to 6pm). **Closed** during services. 📷 ✉

One of the two still active synagogues, the Remu'h temple is used by Orthodox Jews. It was founded by Israel Isserles Auerbach around 1553 and named after his son, the great author and philosopher Rabbi Moses Remu'h.

Inside, the *bimah* and an ornamental *aron hakodesh* are worth noting.

❻ Remu'h Cemetery
Cmentarz Remuh

ul. Szeroka 40. **Map** 4 D1. 🚊 3, 9, 11, 13, 24. **Open** 9am–4pm Sun–Fri.

The Remu'h Cemetery, established in 1533, is one of the very few Jewish cemeteries

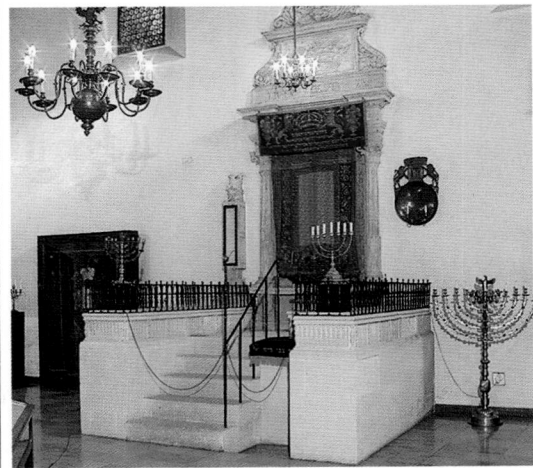

Hall of Prayers in the Old Synagogue

in the whole of Europe with so many tombs, both gravestones *(matzeva)* and sarcophagi. Their rich floral and animal decoration is of particular interest.

The cemetery was almost entirely destroyed during World War II. However, the tomb of Remu'h, which still attracts pilgrims from all over the world, was spared from Nazi destruction. Over 700 tombs have been excavated since World War II. They were probably buried during the Swedish invasion in the early 18th century. The Wailing Wall by the entrance was made using fragments of tombstones destroyed during the war.

❼ New Jewish Cemetery
Nowy Cmentarz Żydowski

ul. Miodowa 55. **Map** 4 E1. 🚋 3, 9, 11, 13, 24. **Open** 9am–5pm Sun–Fri.

Established in the early 19th century, this cemetery is a burial place of the great Jews of Krakow of the 19th and 20th centuries. All Kazimierz's rabbis and many of the great benefactors of Krakow rest here. They include Józef Oettinger and Józef Rosenblatt (professors of the Jagiellonian University), Józef Sare (the city President), and Maurycy Gotlieb (one of the foremost Polish artists of the 19th century).

❽ Corpus Christi Church
Kościół Bożego Ciała

ul. Bożego Ciała 26. **Map** 4 D2. 🚌 128, 184. 🚋 3, 6, 8, 10, 18, 20, 22. **Open** 9am–noon and 1:30–7pm Mon–Sat and during services.

Corpus Christi Church was built on marshland where, according to legend, a monstrance (religious container) with the Eucharist stolen from the Collegiate Church of All Saints had been found. A mysterious light shining in the darkness indicated the site where the profaned monstrance had been abandoned. The construction of

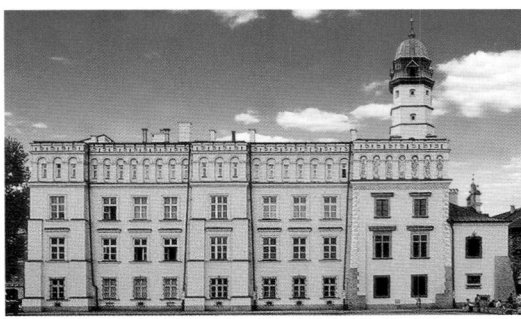

Town Hall in Kazimierz, housing the Ethnographical Museum

the church, founded by King Kazimierz the Great, began in 1340 and was completed in the early 15th century. As a parish church it was bestowed by local burghers with sumptuous furnishings, most of which have survived.

In 1634 to 1637 the high altar was decorated with a painting of *The Nativity* by Tommaso Dolabella, court artist to Zygmunt III Vaza. The large stalls for monks, matching the altar, were made in 1632. An opulent 17th-century stone altarpiece with the relics of Blessed Stanisław Kazimierczyk is located in the north aisle.

The altar of Christ the Redeemer, decorated with sculptures by Anton Gegenbaur, is also worth noting. A slab in the north aisle indicates the burial place of the architect Bartolomeo Berecci, who was assassinated in 1537.

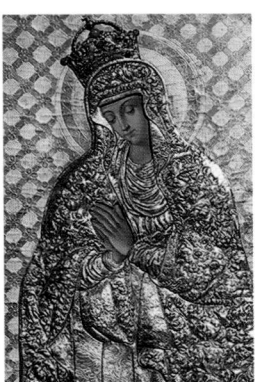

Image of the Madonna in the Church of Corpus Christi

❾ Kazimierz Town Hall
Ratusz kazimierski

Pl. Wolnica 1. **Map** 4 D2. **Tel** 12 430 55 75. 🚌 128, 184, 502. 🚋 3, 8, 10, 40. Ethnographical Museum: **Open** 11am–7pm Tue, Wed, Fri, Sat; 11am–9pm Thu; 11am–3pm Sun. **Closed** public hols. 🚫 📷

The Town Hall was the seat of local government until 1791. The oldest parts of the building date back to 1414, the year of its foundation. After much remodelling, the north section of the Town Hall was finally completed in 1620. The south section was added in 1875 to 1877 by Filip Pokutyński.

The Ethnographic Museum was established here in 1947. Its rich collection includes costumes from Lesser Poland and Silesia, traditional Krakovian Christmas cribs, folk art and musical instruments.

❿ Hospital of the Order of St John of God
Szpital Bonifratrów

ul. Trynitarska 11. **Map** 4 D6. **Tel** 12 379 71 00. 🚌 128, 184, 522. 🚋 8, 10, 12, 18, 22, 40.

This monumental building was constructed between 1897 and 1906 to commemorate the 50th anniversary of Emperor Franz Joseph's reign. Designed by Teodor Talowski in the late Modernist style, the façade, with its central bay projection, is of particular interest.

Krakow's Jewish Community

Before it was all but annihilated in the Holocaust, Krakow had one of the most vibrant, wealthy and prominent Jewish communities in Europe. An important trading post between Prussia, Prague and Vienna, Jews have lived here since the 14th century. In 1938 the Jewish population was over 60,000, one quarter of the total population. However, anti-semitic protests date back to 1369 and in 1495 Jews were expelled from Krakow to Kazimierz *(see p121)*. In 1948, the post-Holocaust Jewish population was 5,900 and by 1978, a mere 600. Today the Jewish population is less than 1,000.

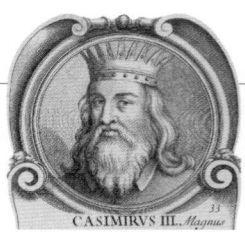

King Kazimierz the Great founded the city that took his name in 1335. Originally a separate town, it became a leading centre of Jewish culture.

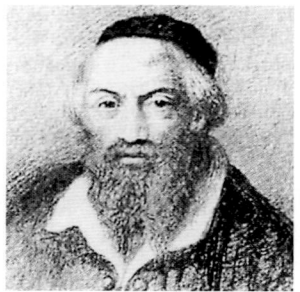

Rabbi Moses ben Isserles (1525–1572) was one of the greatest rabbis of the 16th century, and lived and taught in Kazimierz. He is revered by Jews for his learned additions to the Shulkhan Arukh (the code for everyday life). He was also a keen historian, astronomer, geometrician and philosopher.

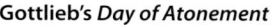

Gottlieb's *Day of Atonement*

This famous painting by Maurycy Gottlieb, a Polish Jew, was executed in 1878. It portrays the artist (the figure in the middle resting on his arm) attending synagogue on the holiest day of the Jewish year, Yom Kippur (the Day of Atonement). Beset with woes, the painter's pose reflects the conflict that faced Polish Jewry as a whole in the late 19th-century: whether they were in the first place Jews or Poles.

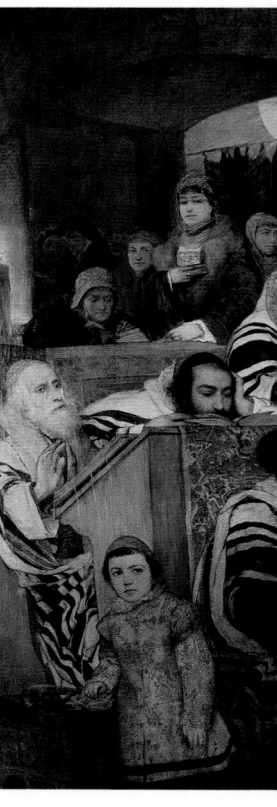

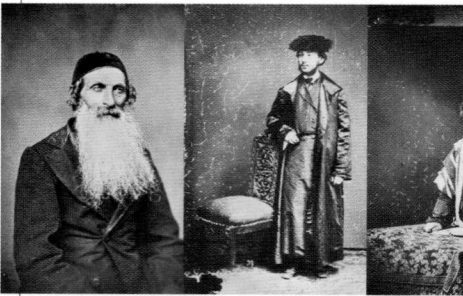

Jewish diversity in Krakow is shown in these three professional portraits from the late 1870s: on the left is an Orthodox Jew and the two on the right are Hassidic Jews. Krakow was long considered to be one of the primary centres of Jewish debate, as all parts of the religious and political spectrum were represented in the city's wide-ranging Jewish population.

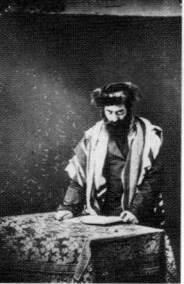

Jewish theatre was a crucial part of Jewish life in Krakow until the late 1930s. Besides entertainment, it also provided one of the last bastions of the Yiddish language.

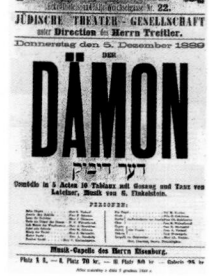

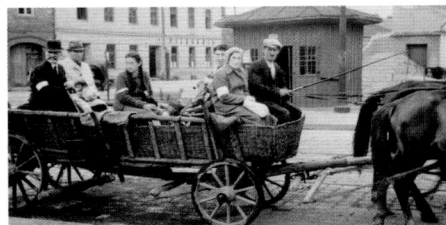

The Nazis ordered large numbers of Jews to move from Kazimierz and enter the Ghetto; often, homes were swapped with Polish families going the other way. The Krakow Jewish Ghetto was centred on Bohaterow Getta Square on the south side of the river.

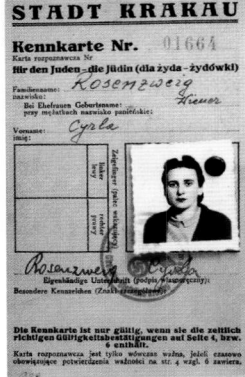

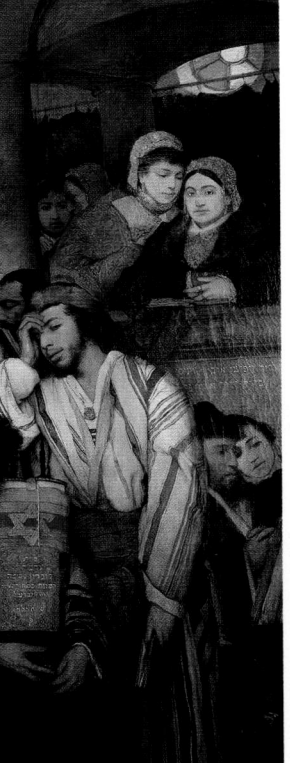

Identity documents were issued even before the creation of the Krakow Ghetto in 1941. All Poles had to carry a card that clearly stated their ethnic provenance in order to limit the civil rights and entitlements of the holder. The card shown here belonged to Cyrla Rosenzweig, a Polish Jew who was rescued from the Holocaust by Oskar Schindler.

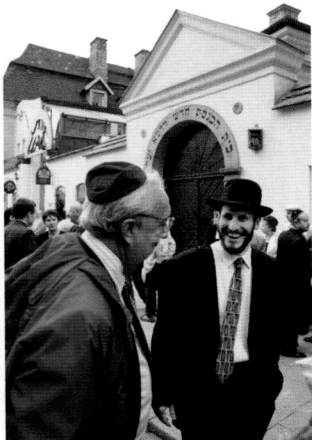

Modern-day Jewish Krakow has become a thriving centre of Jewish tradition and culture since the reintroduction of democracy to Poland in 1989. The growing population is estimated to be well over 5,000. While some are former residents who have returned to their birthplace, many are young descendants of those who later died in the Ghetto and at Auschwitz. Many have found success as entrepreneurs, opening hotels and kosher restaurants.

Schindler's Krakow

Oskar Schindler (1908–78), immortalized in Steven Spielberg film *Schindler's List*, was a German businessman who saved over 1,000 Jews from the gas chambers during World War II, by employing them at his factories. The original Schindler factory at ul. Lipowa 4 has now been transformed into a museum (*see p158*). Schindler lived at ul. Straszewskiego 7, in the upstairs flat.

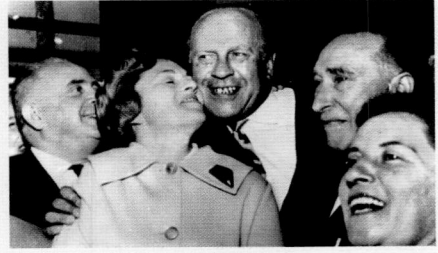

Oskar Schindler with Holocaust survivors in Tel-Aviv

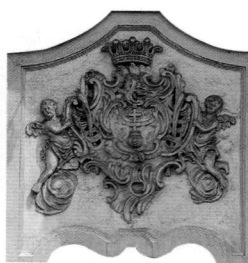

Church of the Order of St John of God, detail of the façade

⑪ Church of the Order of St John of God
Kościół Bonifratrów

ul. Krakowska 48. **Map** 4 D2. **Tel** 12 430 61 22. 📧 128, 184, 522. 🚊 8, 10, 19, 22, 40. **Open** during services only.

This interesting Baroque church was built between 1741 and 1758 to designs by Francesco Placidi. A rather small structure is hidden behind a monumental, wavy façade inspired by the best designs of the leading Roman Baroque architect, Francesco Borromini. The façade, intended to be viewed at an angle, closes the vista formed by Krakowska Street. Inside, the excellent *trompe-l'oeil* painting of the vault was made by Josef Piltz of Moravia in 1757–58. It depicts St John of Matha buying slaves from the heathens. The side altars, with their architectural forms painted directly on the walls, are unusual. They are decorated with Rococo paintings, among which the effigy of St Cajetan is worth noting.

⑫ Church of St Catherine
Kościół św. Katarzyny

ul. Augustiańska 7. **Map** 4 D2. **Tel** 12 430 62 42. 📧 128, 184, 522. 🚊 8, 10, 18, 19, 22. **Open** during services only.

According to the chronicler Jan Długosz, the Church of St Catherine was built by King Kazimierz the Great as a penance for murdering Father Marcin Baryczka in 1349. Baryczka delivered a document issued by bishops excommunicating the king. The king repaid the messenger with the order to have Baryczka drowned in the Vistula. However, the construction of the church possibly began in 1343 and continued until the early 16th century. Regarded as one of the most beautiful Gothic churches in Krakow, its furnishings were lost in the 19th century when it was briefly transformed into a warehouse. The Baroque high altar, decorated with the *Mystical Marriage of St Catherine* by Andrea Venesta, 1634, has survived. Worth visiting is the Gothic cloister which dates from the time of Kazimierz the Great. It features late Gothic murals and large 17th-century paintings. Two chapels adjoin the cloister: one houses the miraculous *Madonna of Consolation* and the other the relics of Blessed Isaiah Boner.

Fresco in the cloister in the Church of St Catherine

⑬ Paulite Church "On the Rock"
Kościół Paulinów Na Skałce

ul. Skałeczna 15. **Map** 3 C2. **Tel** 12 423 09 48. 📧 128, 184, 522. 🚊 8, 10, 18, 19, 22. **Open** 9am–4pm Mon–Sat and during services. The Crypt: **Open** Apr–Oct: 9am–5pm daily; Nov–Mar: on request. 🅿

A small church of St Michael "On the Rock" was recorded already in the 11th century. This was the site where Bishop Stanisław of Szczepanów, later canonized, was murdered (*see pp24–5*).

In the 14th century this small Romanesque church was replaced by a large Gothic church founded by Kazimierz the Great. Four hundred years later it was in danger of collapsing. It was rebuilt in the late Baroque style, between 1733 and 1742. The design by Anton Gerhard Müntzer was modified by Antonio Solari. The uniform furnishings all date from the 1740s. A small font by the church is decorated with a statue of St Stanisław, made in 1731. The tormentors of the saint, who are said to have quartered his body, threw his cut-off finger into the font. The water is reputed to have had healing properties ever since.

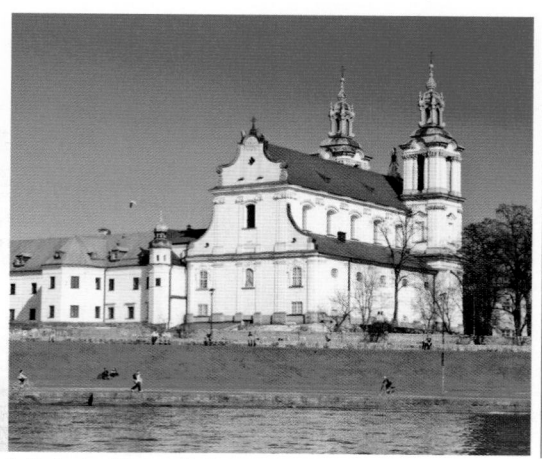

Paulite Church and Monastery "On the Rock"

The Crypt in the Church "On the Rock"

Jan Długosz, the great Polish historian of the Middle Ages, was buried in the crypt beneath the Church "On the Rock" in 1480. In 1876 it was decided to transform the crypt into a national pantheon for the burial of those who had made important contributions to Polish culture. The architect Teofil Żebrawski remodelled the crypt, transforming it into a gallery with a separate chapel housing the altar. Recesses were designed to house the sarcophagi. The stained-glass window above the altar depicts the Madonna of Częstochowa, the Queen of Poland. Coats of arms of provinces of the Polish-Lithuanian Commonwealth were painted on the vault.

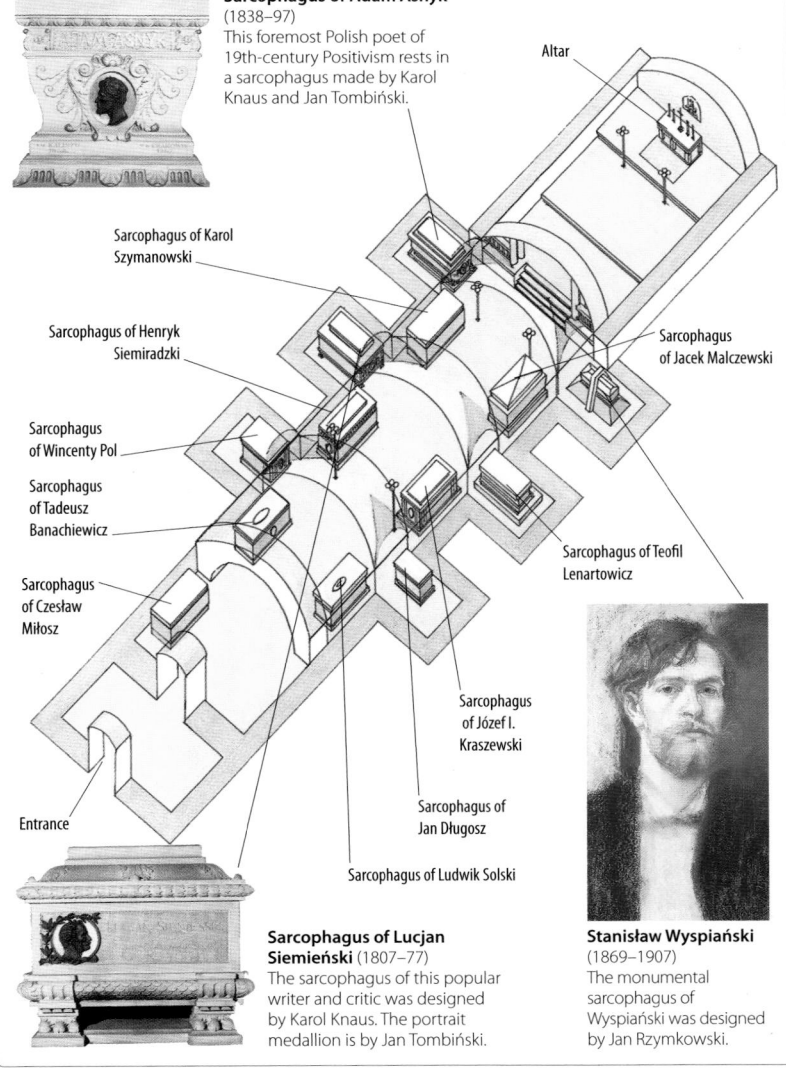

Sarcophagus of Adam Asnyk (1838–97)
This foremost Polish poet of 19th-century Positivism rests in a sarcophagus made by Karol Knaus and Jan Tombiński.

Altar

Sarcophagus of Karol Szymanowski

Sarcophagus of Henryk Siemiradzki

Sarcophagus of Jacek Malczewski

Sarcophagus of Wincenty Pol

Sarcophagus of Tadeusz Banachiewicz

Sarcophagus of Czesław Miłosz

Sarcophagus of Teofil Lenartowicz

Entrance

Sarcophagus of Józef I. Kraszewski

Sarcophagus of Jan Długosz

Sarcophagus of Ludwik Solski

Sarcophagus of Lucjan Siemieński (1807–77)
The sarcophagus of this popular writer and critic was designed by Karol Knaus. The portrait medallion is by Jan Tombiński.

Stanisław Wyspiański (1869–1907)
The monumental sarcophagus of Wyspiański was designed by Jan Rzymkowski.

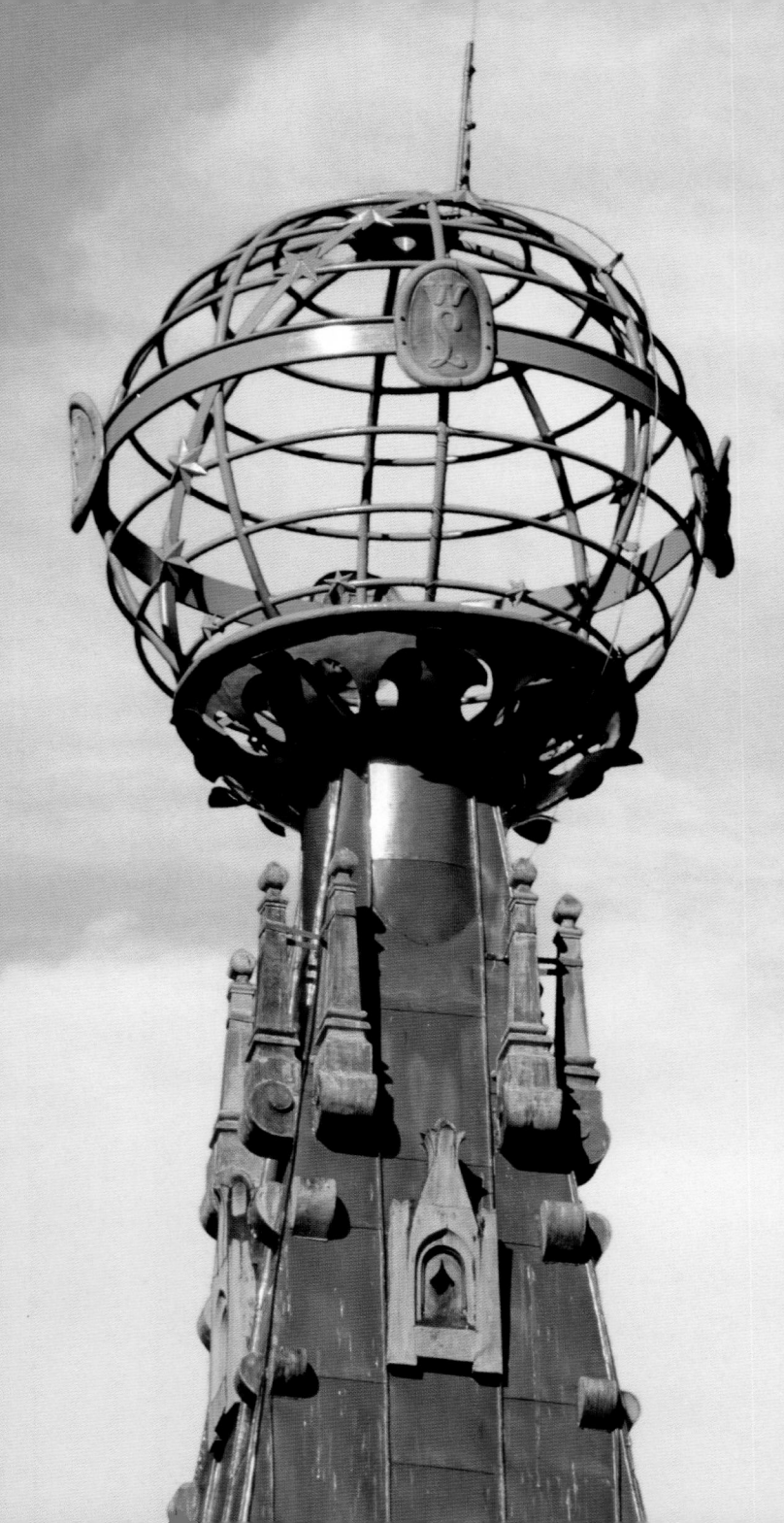

WESOŁA, KLEPARZ AND BISKUPIE

A number of settlements developed around Krakow over the centuries. They were linked culturally and economically with Krakow but were independently administered. As there were no specific boundaries between them and land ownership often changed, the settlements north and east of the city walls developed to constitute a complex urban mosaic, and included Przedmieście Mikołajskie, the royal town of Kleparz, and the privately owned Wesoła, Lubicz and Biskupie. They all looked like small towns. Imposing churches and a few palaces were surrounded by irregularly scattered residential timber buildings. Merchants and craftsmen who were active here avoided paying taxes to the Town Hall, thus contributing to the economic decline of Krakow. As a result, in 1791 the City Council decided to incorporate these quarters into Krakow. This part of the city saw the greatest surge in building activity during the great development of Krakow in the second half of the 19th century.

Sights at a Glance

Historic Monuments and Buildings
2. Society of Physicians
6. Astronomical Observatory
8. Former Main Railway Station
10. Grunwald Monument
11. National Bank of Poland
12. Academy of Fine Arts
13. Polish State Railways Headquarters
15. Globe House

Churches and Monasteries
1. Church of St Nicholas
3. Jesuit Church pp136–7
4. Church of the Immaculate Conception of the Virgin Mary
5. Church of the Discalced Carmelite Nuns
9. St Florian's Church
14. Church of St Vincent de Paul
16. Church of the Nuns of the Visitation

Historic Parks
7. Jagiellonian University Botanical Gardens

▢ **Restaurants** see p193
1. Jarema
2. Trzy kroki w szaleństwo

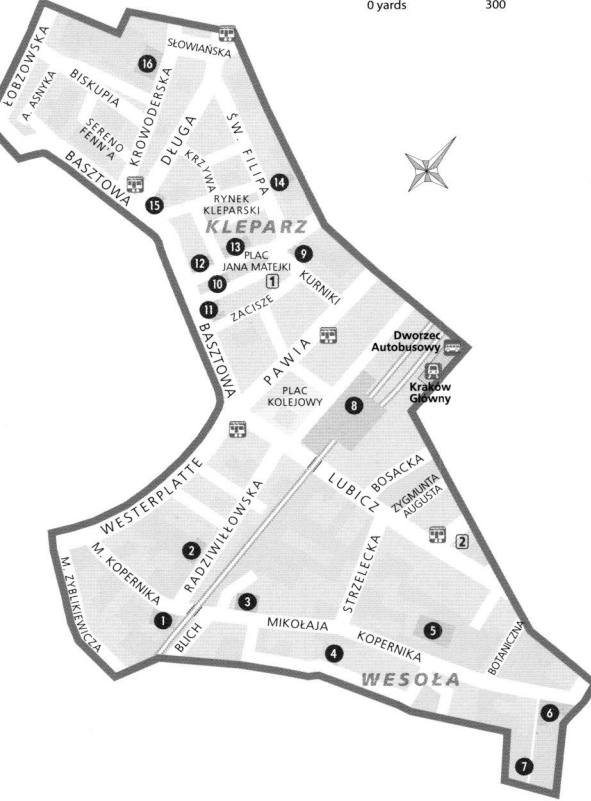

0 metres   300
0 yards   300

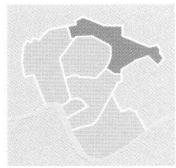

See also Street Finder maps 1, 2 & 3

◀ The metal globe crowning the pyramidal tower of Globe House

For keys to symbols see back flap

Street-by-Street: Along Kopernika Street

Wesoła Quarter, originally a small settlement by the Romanesque Church of St Nicholas, developed along the old route to Mogiła, which is today Kopernika Street (ulica Mikołaja Kopernika). Its skyline was dominated by churches, monasteries and suburban residences of the nobility, set in well-kept gardens. In the 19th century a number of university buildings, mostly hospitals belonging to the Medical School, were built here. Some of these buildings display interesting architectural forms.

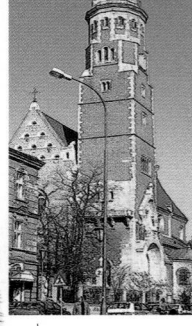

❸ ★ **Jesuit Church**
This is one of the most interesting examples of modern ecclesiastical architecture.

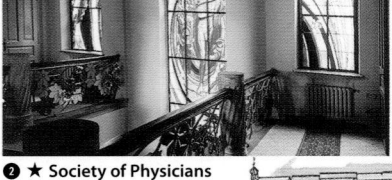

❷ ★ **Society of Physicians**
The metal balusters were designed by Stanisław Wyspiański in the Art Nouveau style, featuring sinuous floral ornaments.

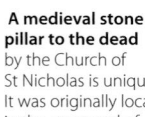

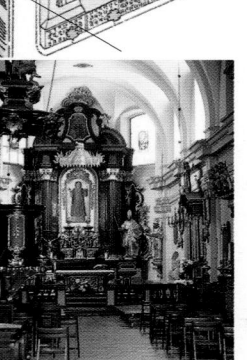

A medieval stone pillar to the dead
by the Church of St Nicholas is unique. It was originally located in the courtyard of St Valentine's Hospital in Kleparz.

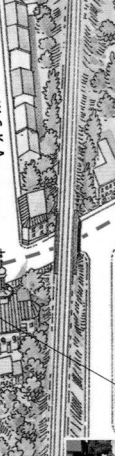

❶ **Church of St Nicholas**
For centuries this church was a landmark of the settlement which developed along the Krakow-Mogiła route.

RADZIWIŁŁOWSKA

KOPERNIKA

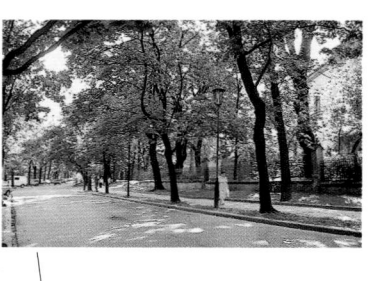

Kopernika Street
lined densely with trees, is one of the most beautiful streets in Krakow.

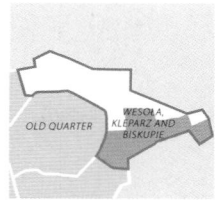

Locator Map
See Street Finder maps 1 & 3

❺ Church of the Discalced Carmelite Nuns
The Baroque façade, one of the most beautiful in Krakow, is worth seeing.

❻ Astronomical Observatory
Belonging to the Jagiellonian University, with its elegant architecture and location next to the Botanical Gardens, this observatory looks more like a Neo-Classical villa than a university building.

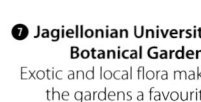
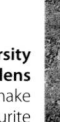

❼ Jagiellonian University Botanical Gardens
Exotic and local flora make the gardens a favourite place for days out.

Key

— Suggested route

❹ Church of the Immaculate Conception of the Virgin Mary
The entrance to the Baroque interior is through this monumental portal.

0 metres   50
0 yards   50

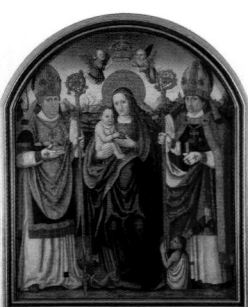

Madonna and Child with Saints Adalbert and Stanisław

❶ Church of St Nicholas

Kościół św. Mikołaja

ul. Kopernika 9. **Map** 2 D4 (6 F3). **Tel** 12 431 22 77. 🚋 1, 10, 11, 13, 14, 15, 19, 22, 40. **Open** during services only.

Recorded in the first half of the 13th century, this is one of the oldest churches in Krakow. The remnants of the Romanesque church and a Gothic portal have survived in the chancel. During Swedish occupation, in 1665, the church was plundered and burned and the present church is the result of a Baroque remodelling undertaken between 1677 and 1682. Furnishings were commissioned by the Academy of Krakow, whose patronage over this collegiate foundation goes back to 1465. A coat of arms of the Academy (a shield with crossed maces) decorates the backs of the stalls. The high altar was probably designed by Francesco Placidi. It features an effigy of St Nicholas and architectural decoration forming coulisses. The church also houses a late Gothic triptych, depicting the Coronation of the Virgin, and a Renaissance Madonna and Child with Saints Adalbert and Stanisław, patron saints of Poland. A bronze font, dating from 1536, is worth noting.
It is also of interest that Feliks Dzierżyński, who was to become the founder of the *Cheka* (Bolshevik secret police) and a Bolshevik revolutionary, was married in this church in 1910.

❷ Society of Physicians

Gmach Towarzystwa Lekarskiego

ul. Radziwiłłowska 4. **Map** 2 D4 (6 F2). **Tel** 12 422 75 47. 🚋 1, 10, 11, 13, 14, 15, 19, 22, 40. **Open** 10am–2pm Tue & Fri, 4–8pm Wed.

This building was constructed in 1904 to designs by the architects Władysław Kaczmarski and Józef Sowiński. A rather modest Neo-Classical exterior is in contrast to the sumptuous interior decoration designed by Stanisław Wyspiański. This multi-talented artist created complex decoration in which, typically for the Art Nouveau movement, the arts and crafts complement each other. Wyspiański chose colour schemes for the walls and designed the exquisite stained glass showing *Apollo, The Solar System*, as well as the metal balusters and furniture.

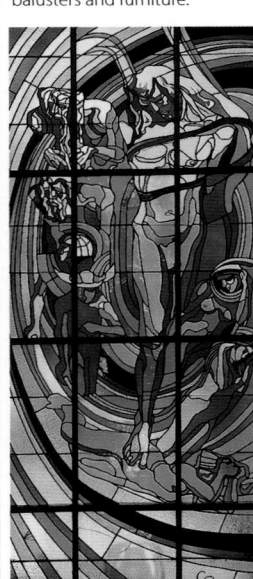

Apollo, The Solar System, a stained-glass window by Stanisław Wyspiański in the Society of Physicians building

❸ Jesuit Church

Kościół Jezuitów

See pp136–7.

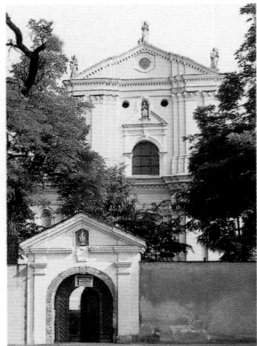

The Baroque Church of the Immaculate Conception

❹ Church of the Immaculate Conception of the Virgin Mary

Kościół Niepokalanego Poczęcia NMP

ul. Kopernika 19. **Map** 2 E4. 🚋 2, 10, 11, 13, 14, 15, 19, 40. **Open** 8am–4pm daily and during services.

This church, also known as the Church of St Lazarus, was used in the past by novices of the order of the Discalced Carmelites. The rigidity of the Baroque architecture of this church, built between 1634 and 1680, reflects the strict building regulations of the Carmelite order. Large and complex, the high altar dominates the small interior. Modelled on the high altar in the Carmelite Church of Santa Maria della Scala in Rome, it was made in 1681 of black marble from the Dębnik quarry, which was owned by the Carmelites.

❺ Church of the Discalced Carmelite Nuns

Kościół Karmelitanek Bosych

ul. Kopernika 44. **Map** 2 E4. **Tel** 12 421 41 18. 🚌 124, 152, 522. 🚋 4, 5, 9, 10, 11, 14, 15, 40. **Open** during services only.

A large convent was built in the neighbourhood of the friary of the same order between 1720 and 1732.

The church is small and has a Greek cross groundplan. The interior with its many columns is impressive. The sumptuous façade has elegant decoration in the late Baroque style.

The architect of the church is unknown. Karol Antoni Bay of Warsaw and Kacper Bażanka are considered likely to have designed it. Due to the strict rule of the order, the church is open to the public only during services. The painting on the high altar depicts Saint Theresa of Avila, to whom the church is dedicated.

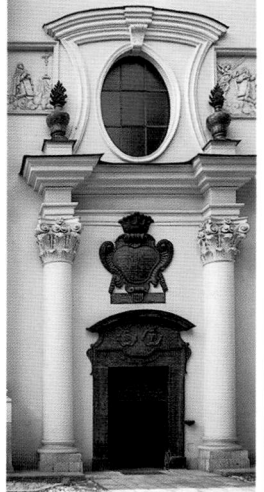

Portal in the Church of the Discalced Carmelite Nuns

❻ Astronomical Observatory
Obserwatorium Astronomiczne UJ

ul. Kopernika 27. **Map** 2 F4. **Tel** 12 425 14 57. 124, 128, 184, 522. 4, 5, 9, 10, 15, 20, 40. **Closed** to the public.

The establishment of the Observatory in Wesoła was directly linked to the reform of the Academy of Krakow carried out in the 1770s by Hugo Kołłątaj, a task he was given by the Commission for National Education. As a result, experimental sciences gained a more prominent role in the curriculum. The suburban Jesuit residence, taken over by the Commission after the abolition of the order, was rebuilt to house the Observatory. Stanisław Zawadzki, the architect to King Stanisław Augustus, redesigned the building in an austere Neo-Classical style. He decorated the façade with astronomical signs.

The building is now occupied by the Jagiellonian Botanical Institute. A modern astronomical observatory is located in the former Skała fortress in Bielany.

❼ Jagiellonian University Botanical Gardens
Ogród botaniczny UJ

ul. Kopernika 27a. **Map** 2 F4. **Tel** 12 421 26 20. 124, 184, 502. 4, 5, 9, 10, 15, 19, 40. **Open** May–Aug: 9am–7pm, Sep–Oct: 9am–5pm. Greenhouses: **Open** 10am–6pm Sat–Thu. Museum of Botanical Gardens: **Open** 10am–2pm Wed & Fri, 11am–3pm Sun.

Next to the Observatory, the Botanical Gardens of the Jagiellonian University are located on the former grounds and lodge of the Czartoryski family. The gardens were established in 1780 by Jan Jaśkiewicz and designed by the Viennese gardener Franz Kaiser. A 500-year-old oak tree in the depths of the garden, as well as exotic and native plants, are particularly worth seeing. Also of interest are late-Gothic pillars, originally from the Collegium Maius, used here as plinths supporting plant pots.

Two of the gardens' palm houses are interesting examples of 19th-century architectural structures. They are

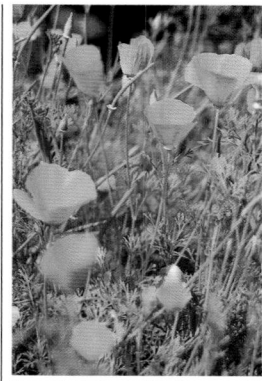

Flowers in the Botanical Gardens

complemented by a third, 20th-century palm house designed by Stanisław Juszczyk and built in 1964 to mark the 6th centenary of the Jagiellonian University. Busts of celebrated botanists decorate the gardens.

❽ Former Main Railway Station
Budynek dawnego dworca głównego

Pl. Kolejowy 1. **Map** 2 D3 (6 F1). most bus and tram routes.

A railway link was established in 1847 between Krakow and Silesia, known as the Northern, or Franz Joseph Railway. Between 1844 and 1847 a new station was built north of the city. Designed by Piotr Rosenbaum, it was considered to be one of the most elegant stations in Europe. It was later rebuilt. In 1898 Teodor Talowski constructed a viaduct next to the station, in the Romanesque Revival style. The building is no longer in use as a station, and ticket offices are now under the platforms nearby.

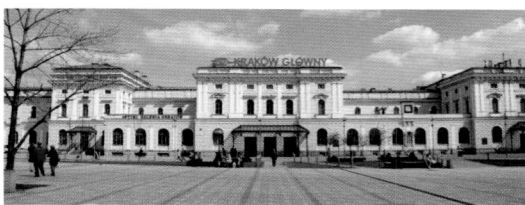

Krakow's Former Main Railway Station

❾ Jesuit Church

This monumental church was built between 1909 and 1921 to designs by the architect Franciszek Mączyński. He applied a number of historic styles which he modified and combined in new ways. What he created is one of the most interesting ecclesiastical buildings of the first quarter of the 20th century in Poland. Leading artists worked on the interior. Karol Hukan carved sculptures for the altars, while Jan Bukowski painted murals of striking beauty and designed unusual confessionals. The mosaic above the high altar is by Piotr Stachiewicz, and the south portal facing Kopernika Street was designed by Xawery Dunikowski. A small statue of Mączyński on the exterior of the east wall is also by Dunikowski.

★ South Portal
The main entrance to the church is through this monumental portal. Note the exquisite ornaments and figures which are both regarded as outstanding examples of Polish sculpture of the early 20th century.

Mosaic in the Porch
Made of mosaic pieces in vivid colours and set against a shiny background, the figures of Mary and Child have an almost unreal, mystical appearance.

Entrance

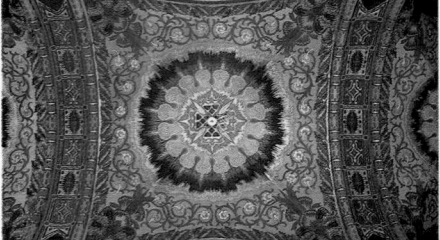

Murals decorating the Nave Vaulting
These murals contribute to the rich and monumental character of the interior. They were painted by Jan Bukowski, who also executed decoration in other churches in Krakow, including St Mary's and the Bernardine Nuns' church, as well as the Loretto Chapel by the Capuchin Church.

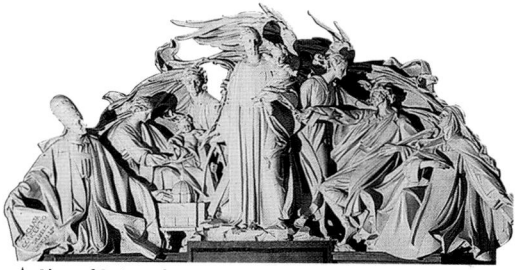

★ Altar of St Joseph
Altars in the aisles were made by the sculptor Karol Hukan. Of particular interest is the altar of St Joseph, made in 1922 to 1923. It features this figurative group, which is rich in dynamic and wavy forms.

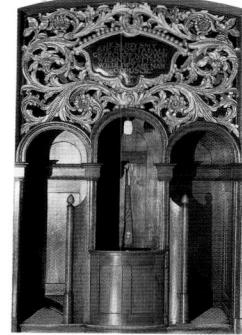

Confessional
The confessionals were designed by Jan Bukowski, Professor of the Industrial School of Art, in the style of the Baroque Revival and are freely decorated with ornaments.

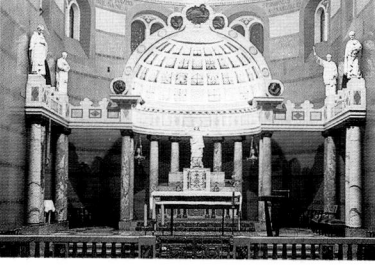

High Altar
The design of the high altar, featuring a half-dome supported by a free-standing colonnade, was influenced by Italian Renaissance architecture. The statues above the altar portray Christ and Jesuit saints.

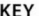

KEY

① **Side porch and tower**

② **Mosaic above the high altar**

Statue of Franciszek Mączyński
The Jesuit Church was Mączyński's most important design. His statue, outside the east wall, is by Xawery Dunikowski.

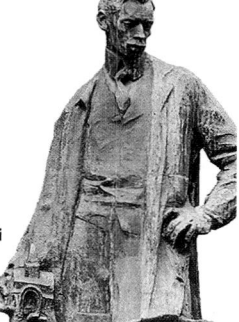

Street-by-Street: Matejko Square

Kleparz, an independent settlement north of Krakow, was granted a municipal charter in 1366. It was incorporated into Krakow in 1791. After the introduction of the railway, Kleparz developed rapidly around the railway station. In the heart of the quarter, the empty space in front of the Barbican was transformed into an elegant square welcoming visitors to Krakow, arriving here by rail or approaching the city from the north, via Warszawska Street.

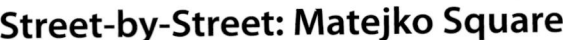

⓾ ★ **Grunwald Monument**
The making of this monument helped to stimulate patriotic feelings in the late 19th century. It is dedicated "to the ancestors' glory and to the brethren with hope".

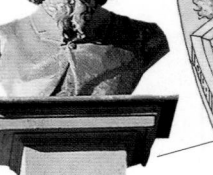

⓬ **Academy of Fine Arts**
The Academy houses a collection of works by its leading professors and students, including a *Self-Portrait* by Jacek Malczewski.

BASZTOWA

A bust of Jan Matejko, carved by Jan Tombiński, can be found above the main entrance to the Academy of Fine Arts. Another monument to the artist is located near the Barbican.

Monument to Jan Matejko

Barbican

Tomb of the Unknown Soldier

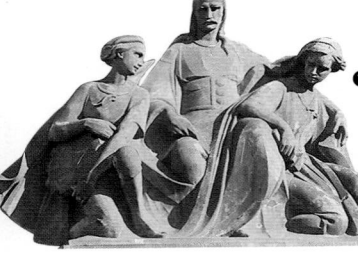

⓫ **National Bank of Poland**
The Allegories of Industry and Agriculture, carved by Karol Hukan, decorate the façade of this bank.

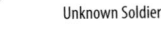

| 0 metres | 50 |
| 0 yards | 50 |

Key

— Suggested route

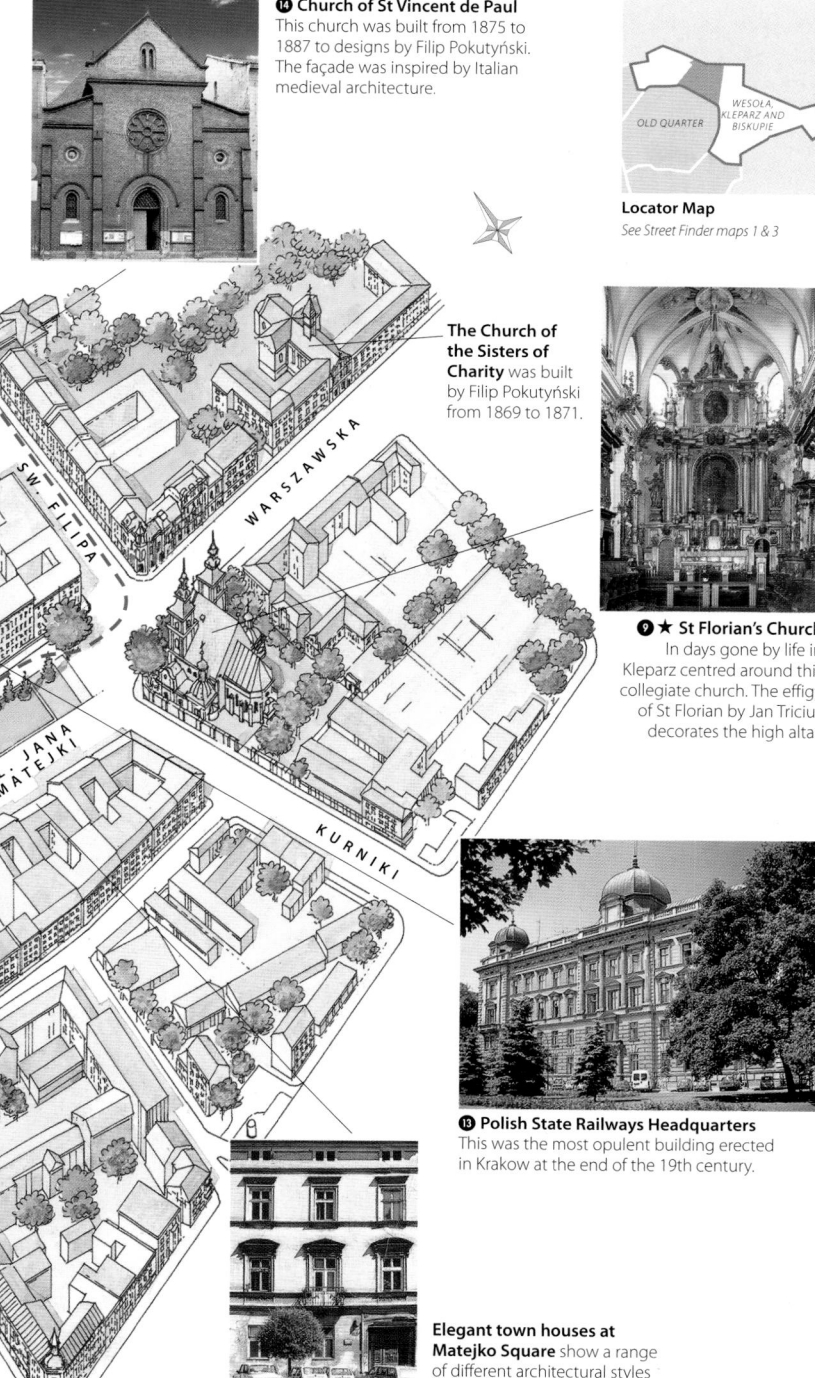

⑭ Church of St Vincent de Paul
This church was built from 1875 to 1887 to designs by Filip Pokutyński. The façade was inspired by Italian medieval architecture.

Locator Map
See Street Finder maps 1 & 3

The Church of the Sisters of Charity was built by Filip Pokutyński from 1869 to 1871.

⑨ ★ St Florian's Church
In days gone by life in Kleparz centred around this collegiate church. The effigy of St Florian by Jan Tricius decorates the high altar.

⑬ Polish State Railways Headquarters
This was the most opulent building erected in Krakow at the end of the 19th century.

Elegant town houses at Matejko Square show a range of different architectural styles of the early 20th century.

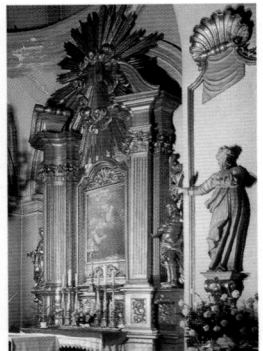

The Baroque altar of St John of Kęty in St Florian's Church

❾ St Florian's Church
Kościół św. Floriana

ul. Warszawska 1B. **Map** 2 D3. **Tel** 12 422 48 42. 124, 152, 154, 192. **Open** during services only.

In 1184 Duke Kazimierz the Just received the relics of St Florian from Pope Lucius III and decided to deposit them in Krakow. The horses which drew the carriage carrying the relics of the martyr stopped suddenly in Kleparz, before reaching the city's gate, and refused to move forward. This was interpreted as a miraculous sign indicating where the relics should be placed. The church was, therefore, built on this spot between 1185 and 1212. After the capital was transferred to Warsaw, the church came to prominence as it was used to receive the deceased royalty brought from Warsaw for burial at Wawel. The funeral processions started here.

The church was damaged by frequent invasions and no trace of the medieval architecture has remained. The present interior and its decoration date from 1677 to 1684. The high altar with an effigy of St Florian, painted by Jan Tricius in the late 17th century, as well as an incomplete late-Gothic altar of St John the Baptist are of interest. The exterior was entirely remodelled by Franciszek Mączyński in the early 20th century.

❿ Grunwald Monument
Pomnik Grunwaldzki

Pl. J Matejki. **Map** 2 D3 (6 E1). 154, 192, 304. 2, 4, 7, 13, 15, 20, 24.

The monument, featuring King Władysław Jagiełło on horseback, was raised to mark the 500th anniversary of the 1410 victory at Grunwald (Tannenberg in German) over the Teutonic Knights. It was commissioned by the states- man, composer and pianist, Ignacy Jan Paderewski, from the sculptor Antoni Wiwulski.

The monument was inspired by grandiose German monu- ments of the second half of the 19th century. It was generally well received but some critics mocked the theatrical treatment of the figures. Some even suggested that the only lifelike figure was that of the dead Grand Master Ulrich von Jungingen. The monument was destroyed by the Nazis in 1939 and only reconstructed in 1975 by the sculptor Marian Konieczny.

⓫ National Bank of Poland

ul. Basztowa 20. **Map** 2 D3 (6 E1). **Tel** 12 618 58 00. 124, 152, 522. 2, 4, 7, 13, 15, 20, 24. **Open** 7am–5pm Mon–Fri.

The bank, built between 1921 and 1925 by the architects Teodor Hoffman and Kazimierz Wyczyński, exemplifies the Neo- Classical style which became popular during the inter-war

years. Neo-Classicism was then applied to important public buildings housing administrative and financial institutions, and was in sharp contrast to the Functionalism favoured in left-wing circles. The exterior sculptural decoration is by Karol Hukan and Stanisław Popławski. Inside, the domed banking hall is worth a visit.

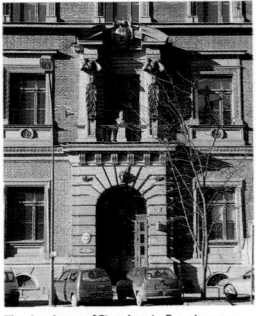

The Academy of Fine Arts in Renaissance Revival style

⓬ Academy of Fine Arts

Pl. J Matejki 13. **Map** 2 D3 (6 E1). **Tel** 12 299 20 14. 154, 192, 304. 4, 7, 13, 15, 20. Museum: by appointment only.

The school of Fine Arts in Krakow gained independent status in 1873 through the efforts of the artist Jan Matejko. Three years later the school was allocated a plot in Kleparz by the city's authorities. The building was constructed in 1879 to 1880 to designs by Maciej Moraczewski. The architect adopted the

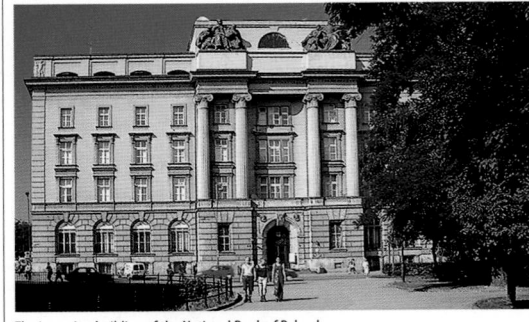

The imposing building of the National Bank of Poland

Renaissance Revival style for this building, in accordance with the spirit of 19th-century Historicism which favoured such forms for school architecture. On the first floor is a studio where Matejko painted his *Kościuszko at Racławice* and *The Vows of King Jan Kazimierz*.

In 1900 the school gained university status, becoming the Academy of Fine Arts. Some of the best Polish artists were among its students. The building in Kleparz is currently the seat of the Academy's governing body and houses the faculties of painting, printmaking and sculpture.

⓭ Polish State Railways Headquarters

Pl. J Matejki 12. **Map** 2 D3 (6 E1).
🚌 154, 192, 304. 🚊 4, 7, 13, 15, 20.
Closed to the public.

This imposing building was constructed in 1888 by an unknown Viennese architect who combined the forms of both Romanesque and Baroque Revival into an eclectic whole. It is possibly the only building in Krakow to have been directly influenced by the 19th-century monumental architecture of its Austrian neighbour, Vienna.

⓮ Church of St Vincent de Paul
Kościół św. Wincentego de Paul

ul. Św. Filipa 19. **Map** 2 D3. **Tel** 12 429 25 33. 🚌 124, 502. 🚊 4, 7, 13, 15, 20.
Open during services only.

The present church was built between 1875 and 1877 and replaced the medieval Church of Saints Philip and James which had been dismantled by the Austrian authorities in 1801. The architect, Filip Pokutyński, was inspired by Italian late-Romanesque architecture. Although modest in design, the church differs from other 19th-century ecclesiastical

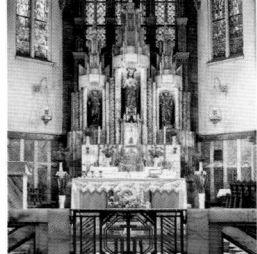

The interior of St Vincent de Paul

architecture in Krakow because of its clear, compact and monumental forms.

The side altar features a miraculous icon depicting Christ Crucified. This much venerated image was brought after World War II from Milatyn near L'viv.

⓯ Globe House
Dom pod Globusem

ul. Długa 1. **Map** 1 C3. 🚌 124, 502.
🚊 4, 7, 12, 13, 15, 20.

This house was built in 1904 to 1906 for the Chamber of Commerce and Industry. It was designed by the architects Franciszek Mączyński and Tadeusz Stryjeński. The building is considered to be one of the best examples of the Art Nouveau style in Polish architecture. It is an interesting asymmetrical structure dominated by a pyramidal tower topped by a globe. The interior decoration, including murals in the great hall, is mainly the work of Józef Mehoffer.

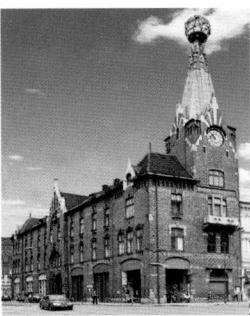

The Globe House, a prime example of Art Nouveau architecture, topped by a pyramidal tower and globe

Stained-glass windows above the stairs depict allegorical subjects such as the progress of mankind through industry and commerce, thus reflecting the function of the building. The several cast-iron decorations are also of interest. Today, the building houses the publishers Wydawnictwo Literackie.

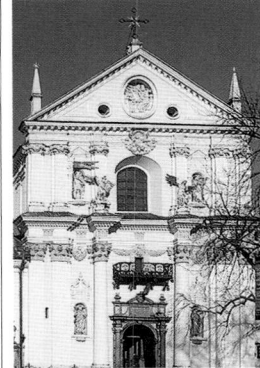

The façade of the Church of the Nuns of the Visitation

⓰ Church of the Nuns of the Visitation
Kościół Wizytek

ul. Krowoderska 16. **Map** 1 C3.
Tel 12 632 16 28. 🚊 3, 5, 19.
Open during services only.

The convent was founded by Bishop Jan Małachowski as a votive offering after he was miraculously saved from drowning in the Vistula. The church is an interesting example of Krakow's Baroque ecclesiastical architecture. It was built from 1686 to 1695 by Giovanni Solari.

The façade is richly decorated with sculptures and ornaments. Some lavish decoration is also characteristic of the interior which, although small, is very elegant. The unusual high altar was made in 1695 by the sculptor Jerzy Golonka. The plasterwork is by Jan Liskowicz. The 18th-century murals decorating the vault have been much altered.

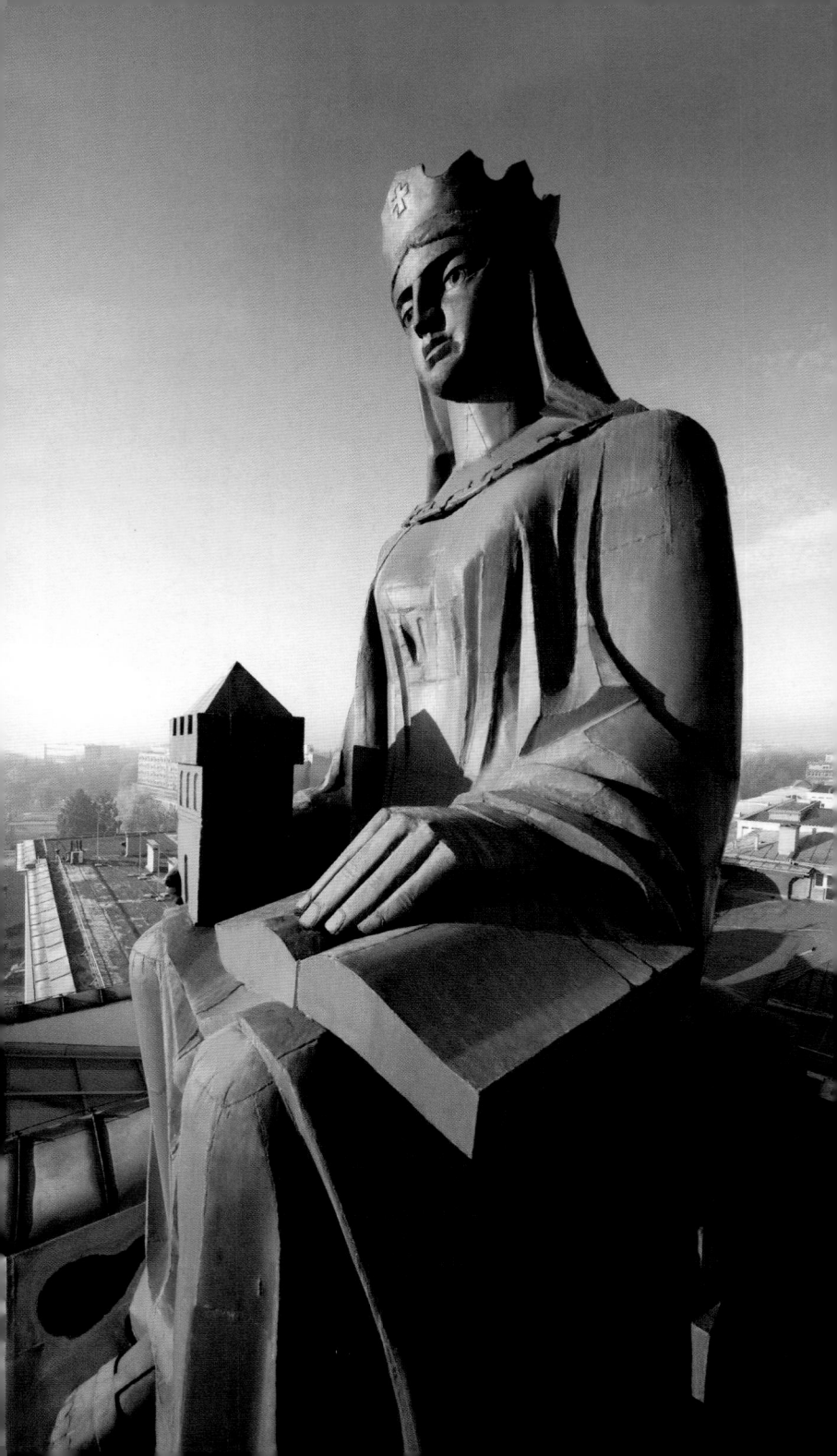

PIASEK AND NOWY ŚWIAT

Piasek, known as Garbary until the 19th century, is located west of the Old Quarter. Its development was hindered in the past by the lack of fortifications and frequent invasions. A number of settlements with independent jurisdictions were located between Garbary and Wawel. They included Groble, Smoleńsko, Wielkorządowa, Wygoda, Retoryka and Rybaki, as well as Nowy Świat which remained under Krakow's jurisdiction.

All these settlements were integrated by the Austrian authorities. By the end of the 19th century Piasek (Sand) and Nowy Świat (New World) began to flourish; wealthy residents moved in, drawn by the pleasant and tranquil atmosphere away from the noisy town centre. As a result, some of the best residential architecture can be found here. It is mostly eclectic in style, dating from the start of the 20th century.

Sights at a Glance

Historic Monuments and Buildings
1 Philharmonic Hall
2 Former Museum of Industry and Technology
6 House of the Singing Frog
7 Europeum
8 Małopolska Garden of Arts
14 Wyspiański Monument
16 School of Chemistry
17 Jagiellonian Library
18 Academy of Mines and Metallurgy, Main Building
21 Spider House

Museums and Galleries
10 Emeryk Hutten-Czapski Museum
12 Józef Mehoffer House Museum
15 National Museum in Krakow, Main Building pp150–51

Churches
3 Church of the Felician Nuns
4 Church of the Merciful God
9 Church of the Sisters of the Sacred Heart of Jesus
11 Capuchin Church
22 Carmelite Church

Historic Streets
5 Retoryka Street
19 Avenue of Three Poets
20 Karmelicka Street

Open Space
13 Błonia Fields

☐ **Restaurants** see p193
1 Biała Róża
2 CK Browar
3 Dynia Resto-Bar
4 Mamma Mia
5 The Olive
6 Smakołyki
7 Solfeż
8 Someplace Else
9 Zielona Kuchnia

0 metres   200
0 yards   200

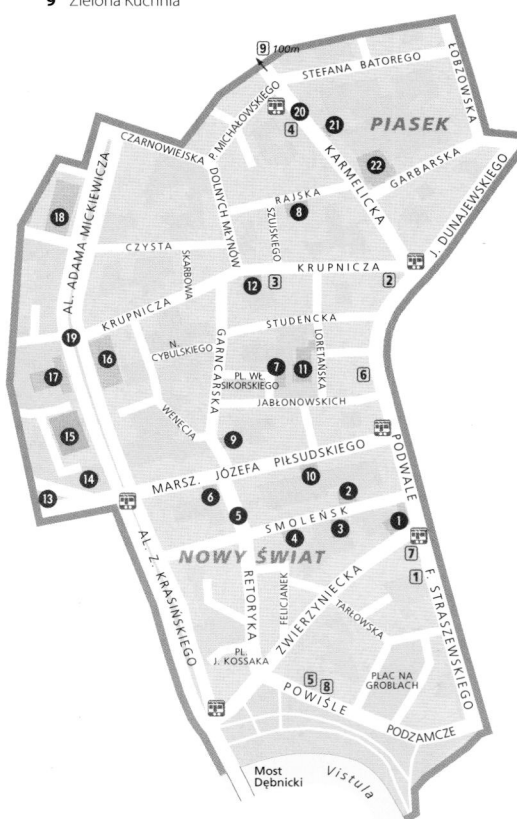

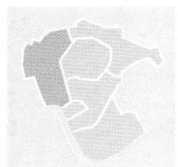

See also Street Finder maps 1 & 5

◀ The statue of St Barbara on the roof of the Academy of Mines and Metallurgy

For keys to symbols see back flap

Street-by-Street: Piłsudski Street

Józefa Piłsudskiego (formerly Wolska) Street formed part of the route connecting Krakow with Wola Justowska. This route was first recorded in the 16th century. After Nowy Świat and the neighbouring jurisdictions were incorporated into Krakow, it became one of the main avenues in this part of town. The vista formed by the street is closed by the vast Błonia Fields with Kościuszko Mound in the distance, behind which Piłsudski Mound can also be seen. Elegant residential and public architecture developed here by the end of the 19th century. Some of the buildings show Polish architecture at its best.

❾ Church of the Sisters of the Sacred Heart of Jesus
The square in front of this church was once a flood plain of the Rudawa river which was filled in prior to the construction of the convent buildings.

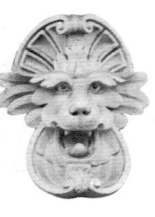

❻ House of the Singing Frog
This house was designed by Teodor Talowski and is decorated with some exquisite, though somewhat overdone, sculptures of fantastic creatures.

0 metres 50
0 yards 50

Key

— Suggested route

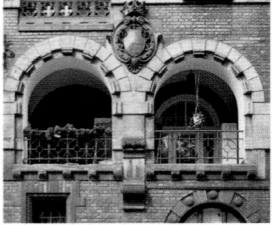

❺ ★ Retoryka Street
The houses designed by Teodor Talowski have a unique "antiquarian" look and contribute to the picturesque character of the street.

⑩ Emeryk Hutten-Czapski Museum
This monster decorates the exhibition pavilion in which Emeryk Hutten-Czapski housed the numismatic collection he brought to Krakow.

Locator Map
See Street Finder maps 1 & 5

❶ Philharmonic Hall
The Hall received a state-of-the-art organ following refurbishment after a fire in 1991.

❷ Former Museum of Industry and Technology
This is one of the most interesting examples of Modernist architecture in Poland.

❸ Church of the Felician Nuns
The church was designed by Feliks Księżarski. Its interior is one of the few examples of Romanesque Revival ecclesiastical architecture in Krakow.

❹ Church of the Merciful God
This memorial plaque of an unknown knight is an exceptional Gothic work surrounded by 19th-century architecture.

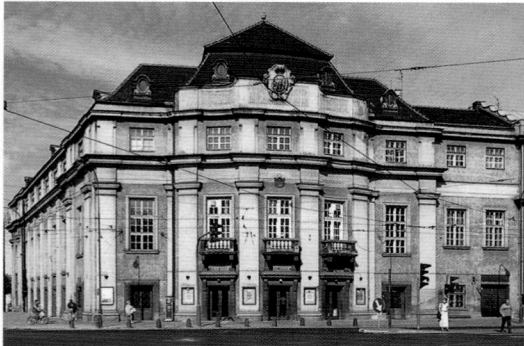

The exterior of the Neo-Classical Philharmonic Hall

❶ Philharmonic Hall
Filharmonia

ul. Zwierzyniecka 1. **Map** 1 B5 (5 C3).
Tel 12 422 94 77. 🚌 124, 152, 502.
🚊 1, 2, 8, 18.

The Society of Friends of Music which was active in Krakow between 1817 and 1884 was regarded as the first philharmonic organization in occupied Poland. The Szymanowski State Philharmonia was established in Krakow in 1945. Walery Bierdiajew, Andrzej Panufnik and Krzysztof Penderecki were among the principal conductors. The orchestra and choir are complemented by the renowned chamber orchestra, Capella Cracoviensis. The Hall is housed in the former Catholic Cultural Institution. It was built between 1928 and 1930 by Pokutyński and Filipkiewicz in the Neo-Classical style which was popular with Polish architects around 1930.

❷ Former Museum of Industry and Technology
Gmach dawnego Muzeum Techniczno - Przemysłowego

ul. Smoleńsk 9. **Map** 1 B5 (5 B3).
🚌 124, 152, 502. 🚊 1, 2, 8, 18.

This museum was established in 1868 by Andrzej Baraniecki who presented the city with his library and large collection of decorative arts. The museum ran courses in fine art, as well as a school of painting for women, and workshops on crafts. Collaboration with other institutions at the forefront of modern design was established. The museum published a number of titles, including journals such as *Przegląd Techniczny* (Technical Revue) and *Architekt* (The Architect). It also played an important role in the development of Polish applied art.

The museum was initially housed in the west wing of the Franciscan friary. The new building was constructed in 1908–14 to designs by Tadeusz Stryjeński. Józef Czajkowski designed the elegant façade, which is rich in geometrical forms. The structure of the building, which uses reinforced concrete, was novel at the time and the layout of the rooms was unusual. It is a leading example of Modernist architecture in Poland. The Museum of Industry and Technology was closed down in 1952. Today the Faculty of Industrial Design of the Academy of Fine Arts is housed here.

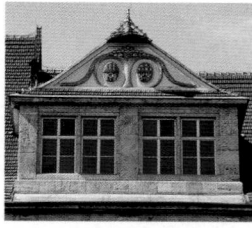

Façade detail, former Museum of Industry and Technology

❸ Church of the Felician Nuns
Kościół Felicjanek

ul. Smoleńsk 4/6. **Map** 1 B5 (5 B3).
Tel 12 422 08 37. 🚌 124, 152, 502.
🚊 2, 5, 8, 18. **Open** 8:30am–6pm daily and during services.

The church of the Felician Nuns is one of the largest churches built in Krakow in the 19th century. This basilica in the Romanesque Revival style was built between 1882 and 1884 to designs by Feliks Księżarski, but modified by Sebastian Jaworzyński. The monumental and austere forms are striking, but softened inside through lavish decoration of the altars. The church houses relics of Blessed Maria Angela Truszkowska, the foundress of the Order, who died in 1899.

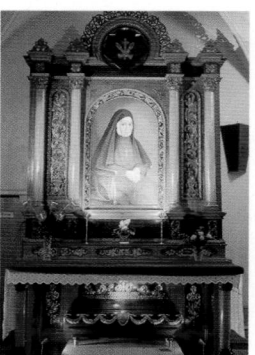

Altar of Blessed Maria Angela, Church of the Felician Nuns

❹ Church of the Merciful God
Kościół Miłosierdzia Bożego

ul. Bożego Miłosierdzia 1. **Map** 1 B5 (5 B3). 🚊 2, 5, 8, 15, 18. **Open** during services only.

In 1555 Jan Żukowski established in Nowy Świat a home for the destitute and a small church. The church was consecrated in 1665. Located outside the city wall, both buildings were badly damaged during a number of invasions. The church has survived. On the outside wall facing Smoleńsk Street, remnants of a Gothic sepulchre, with a kneeling figure of a knight, can be seen.

Among the rather modest Baroque furnishings, the one of most interest is the image of the *Misericordia Domini* (The Suffering Christ and Sorrowful Mary) of 1650, hanging in the chancel.

Adjacent to the church is a presbytery, built in the eclectic style in 1905–6 by Jan Zubrzycki.

❺ Retoryka Street
Ulica Retoryka

Map 1 B5 (5 B3, 4). 🚊 15, 18.

The name of this street comes from the Retoryka jurisdiction, which was established in this area by the Ossolińskis in the first half of the 18th century. In the late 19th century the construction of boulevards began along the Rudawa river, which ran here. They were lined with houses whose architecture was marked by imaginative forms and unusual decoration. In 1910 the river was enclosed in a tunnel beneath street level. The houses designed by Teodor Talowski are most interesting. He used pseudo-antiquarian, intentionally damaged motifs such as mosaics and plaques bearing popular Latin inscriptions for the external decoration. The plaque on his own house reads *festina lente* (hasten slowly) and that on the Ass House, *faber est suae quisque fortunae* (one makes one's own destiny).

The houses in Retoryka Street, designed by Talowski and other leading architects active in Krakow around 1900, are interesting examples of Polish architecture at the dawn of the modern age.

❻ House of the Singing Frog
Dom Pod Śpiewającą Żabą

ul. Retoryka 1. **Map** 1 B5 (5 B3). 🚊 15, 18.

The corner house at No. 1 Retoryka Street is considered

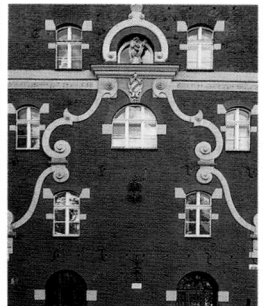

House of the Singing Frog

to be the most interesting of Talowski's designs. It was built in 1889 to 1890. The unusual structure consists of a number of segments varying in height and decoration. It was intended to be viewed at an angle from the adjacent street corner. The name of the house is a joke which refers to both the function and location of the building: it used to house a music school whose singing students were often accompanied by croaking frogs in the nearby Rudawa river.

❼ Europeum

Pl. Sikorskiego 6. **Map** 1 B4 (5 B2). **Tel** 12 433 57 60. 🚌 124, 152, 192. 🚊 15, 18, 20. **Open** 10am–6pm Tue–Sat, 10am–4pm Sun. 🎟️ free on Sun.

The Europeum is home to the most important assemblage of non-Polish European works of art in the National Museum in Krakow collection. Notable exhibits include works by

Lorenzo Lotto, Pieter Brueghel the Younger and Paolo Veneziano.

The gallery is housed in a renovated 17th-century granary set on a quiet, tree-lined square. At the back of the museum is an intriguing collection of masonry fragments from historic buildings all over the city.

❽ Małopolska Garden of Arts
Małopolski Ogród Sztuki

ul. Rajska 12. **Map** 1 B4 (5 B1). **Tel** 12 375 21 50. 🚌 114, 139, 159, 164, 169, 192. 🚊 4, 8, 13, 14. **Open** from 9am; closing times vary. 🌐 mos.art.pl

This multifunctional arts complex features several exhibition spaces, a concert hall, a small cinema and a delightful café, all wrapped up in a strikingly contemporary building that consists of a slatted clay façade, glass frame, industrial beams and a garden courtyard. Opened in 2012, the Małopolska Garden of Arts was built on and around buildings belonging to the Juliusz Słowacki Theatre as a joint project by the theatre and the regional government. The semi-enclosed spaces at the front and side of the building are wonderfully peaceful areas in which to sit and relax, and there are always events or exhibitions taking place inside. Many of Krakow's biggest cultural festivals now use the centre as their main venue.

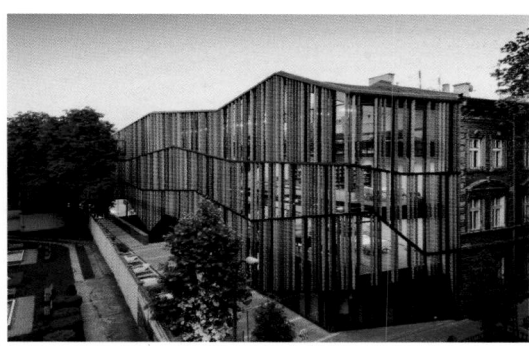

The striking exterior of the Małopolska Garden of Arts

❾ Church of the Sisters of the Sacred Heart of Jesus

Kościół Sercanek

ul. Garncarska 26. **Map** 1 B5 (5 B3). **Tel** 12 422 57 66. 🚊 15, 18. **Open** during services only.

The Convent of the Sisters of the Sacred Heart of Jesus was built between 1895 and 1900 to designs by Władysław Kaczmarski and Sławomir Odrzywolski. The architects designed the building along Garncarska Street so as to close one side of a square located here. They adjusted the façade of the church and the adjoining buildings of the convent to fit the slight bend in the street. This explains the irregularity of the plan.

The church is eclectic in style. The exterior walls show bare brickwork, ornamented in the Romanesque Revival style, as well as with pseudo-Renaissance *sgraffiti* and Neo-Classical sculptures by Jan Tombiński. Furnishings display Neo-Romanesque forms.

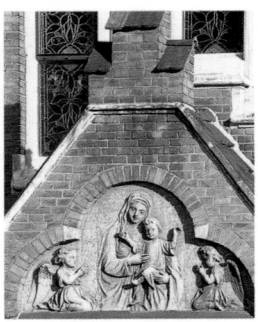

Detail from the Church of the Sisters of the Sacred Heart of Jesus

❿ Emeryk Hutten-Czapski Museum

Muzeum im Emeryka Hutten-Czapskiego

ul. Piłsudskiego 12. **Map** 1 B5 (5 B3). **Tel** 12 422 27 33. 🚊 15, 18. **Open** Access to the collection for professional researchers only.

This small palace in the Renaissance Revival style was built in 1884 by the architect

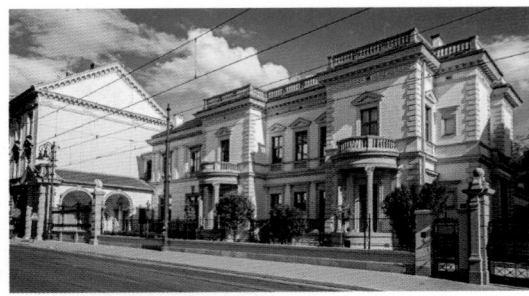

The Emeryk Hutten-Czapski Museum, in the Renaissance Revival style

Antoni Siedek for Hubert Krasiński. A few years later the property was purchased by Emeryk Hutten-Czapski who moved from the Vilnius area, bringing with him an exquisite numismatic collection. A pavilion, purpose-built to house this collection, was added in 1896. It was designed by Tadeusz Stryjeński and Zygmunt Hendel. The inscription decorating the pavilion reads *Monumentis Patriae naufragio ereptis* (To the national heritage salvaged from destruction). In 1903 the Czapskis bequeathed the palace and collection to the city of Krakow.

Today the palace is the seat of the directors of the National Museum and houses the Museum's special holdings. A collection of salvaged architectural fragments can be found outside.

⓫ Capuchin Church

Kościół Kapucynów

ul. Loretańska 11. **Map** 1 B4 (5 B2). **Tel** 12 422 48 03. 🚌 124, 152, 192, 502. 🚊 2, 4, 8, 13, 14, 15, 18. **Open** 9:30am–4:30pm and 5–7pm daily as well as during services.

The Capuchin friars arrived in Krakow in 1695. They began constructing the church and friary a year later. The work was supervised at first by Carlo Ceroni, who was later succeeded by Martino Pellegrini. The architecture and furnishings, the latter dating from 1775, reflect the strict rule of the Order which espouses extreme poverty. Hence the simplicity and functionalism

of the architecture and the modest composition of the altars made of painted timber and lacking decoration. The altars, however, feature good paintings. They include *The Annunciation* by Pietro Dandini, *St Erasmus and St Cajetan*, two 18th-century effigies by Łukasz Orłowski, and *St Francis of Assisi* by Szymon Czechowicz. A number of sepulchres are of interest. A wooden crucifix in front of the church indicates the tomb of the Confederates of Bar who fell in a rebellion against the Russians in 1768.

Between 1712 and 1719 an external Loreto Chapel was built to a design by Kacper Bażanka; this is linked to the church through a cloister. The chapel houses a Neo-Classical altar with a miraculous statue of the Madonna of Loreto and a beautiful tabernacle. The latter was also designed by Bażanka. An animated Christmas crib is erected here every year, featuring historic Polish characters.

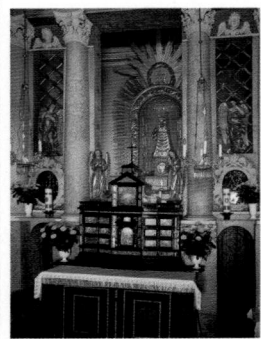

The interior of the Loreto Chapel by the Capuchin Church

⑫ Józef Mehoffer House Museum
Muzeum Józefa Mehoffera

ul. Krupnicza 26. **Map** 1 B4 (5 B2). **Tel** 12 433 58 80. 🚋 124, 152, 173, 179, 502, 512. 🚊 2, 4, 8, 12, 13, 15, 18, 24. **Open** 10am–4pm Wed–Sun. 🏛 free Sun.

Stanisław Wyspiański was born in this house in 1869. In 1930 it was bought by Józef Mehoffer (1869–1946), one of the foremost Modernist artists in Poland. He was also a painter and a stage and interior designer. In 1968 the house was acquired by the National Museum and the Józef Mehoffer House Museum was established. The interiors have been preserved in the tasteful way they were arranged by the artist himself. Many of his works, including paintings, stained glass, cartoons for stained glass and murals, are on display.

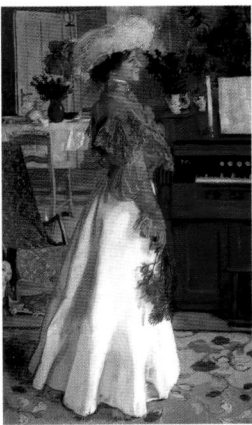
Portrait of Mrs Mehoffer by Józef Mehoffer

⑬ Błonia Fields

Map 1 A5. 🚋 114, 134, 152, 164, 173, 179, 192, 292. 🚊 15, 18.

The Błonia Fields formed part of the grounds owned by the Convent of Premonstratensian (Norbertine) Nuns in Zwierzyniec and were originally used as pastures. In 1366 the nuns made a rather bad deal with the city's authorities and exchanged Błonia for a house in Floriańska Street. The house

proved to be unprofitable and was eventually destroyed by fire. This gave rise to a joke about the nuns who had exchanged pastures for a bonfire. For centuries the nuns tried in vain to regain the land. The Błonia Fields remain the property of the City of Krakow.

Błonia were used in the past as a venue for mass religious and national celebrations. The first football match in Krakow took place here in 1894. Pope John Paul II said a Holy Mass here on four occasions. Today it is a wildlife sanctuary in the centre of Krakow and a popular place for recreation. It should, however, be avoided on days when football matches between Wisła and Cracovia take place.

⑭ Wyspiański Monument
Pomnik S. Wyspiańskiego

Map 1 A5 (5 A3). 🚋 114, 164, 173, 179.

The monument was unveiled in 1982 to mark the 75th anniversary of the death of the great artist and playwright of the so-called Young Poland movement (Polish Modernism). The sculptor, Marian Konieczny, depicted Stanisław Wyspiański surrounded by the characters from two of his plays, *The Wedding* and *November Night*. The monument was badly received and prompted unfavourable

interpretations. Its location, right behind the parking place in front of the National Museum, proved to be particularly unfortunate as the figures seem to emerge from behind parked cars. The agitated gestures of the figures have even been interpreted as an expression of their astonishment at the fast rate of automobile development.

⑮ National Museum in Krakow, Main Building
See pp150–51.

⑯ School of Chemistry
Zespół Szkół Chemicznych

ul. Krupnicza 44. **Map** 1 A4 (5 A2). **Tel** 12 422 32 20. 🚋 114, 164, 169, 173, 179. **Closed** to the public.

In 1834 the Institute of Technology was established in Krakow, funded by the bequest of the architect Szczepan Humbert. It was later transformed into the State School of Industry. In 1912 the school moved to a new building designed by Sławomir Odrzywolski. This irregular brick structure, decorated with Art Nouveau ornaments, now houses the School of Chemistry.

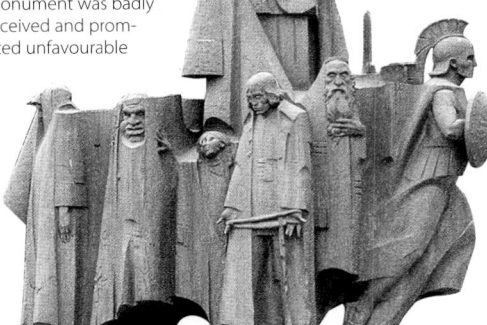
Wyspiański Monument

⓯ National Museum in Krakow, Main Building

The modern building of the National Museum in Krakow was designed by Czesław Boratyński, Edward Kreisler and Bolesław Schmidt in 1934 but the building was not completed until 1989. Permanent galleries display Polish painting and sculpture of the 20th century, decorative arts and arms and other mementos of the Polish Army. Temporary shows are also organized here. The art collection is one of the largest in Poland and includes works by leading Modernist artists, as well as some outstanding works from the period between the two World Wars. Post-1945 art, however, predominates.

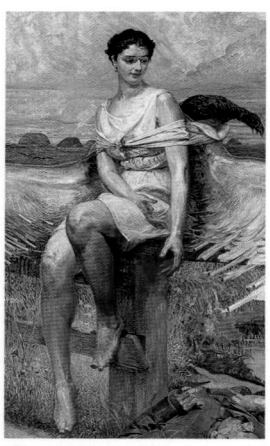

Nike of the Legions
This is one of Jacek Malczewski's symbolic *tours de force*. Nike, the goddess of victory, is sitting by the body of a legionary whose face resembles Józef Piłsudski.

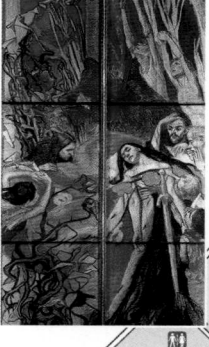

★ *Polonia*, a Cartoon for Stained Glass
Stanisław Wyspiański's cartoons for stained-glass windows in the Cathedral symbolically depict visions of the past but also relate to modern issues.

First floor

The Uniform of Józef Piłsudski
"The uniform of the grey rifleman" reminds one of the tragic but nevertheless victorious history of the Polish Legions between 1914 and 1917.

Audiovisual room

Ground floor

Library and Reading Room

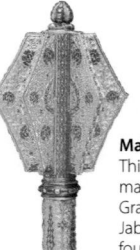

Mace
This gilded "buzdygan" mace belonged to Grand Hetman Stanisław Jabłonowski, who fought in the Battle of Vienna in 1683.

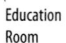

Main entrance

Education Room

VISITORS' CHECKLIST

Practical Information
Al. 3 Maja 1. **Map** 1 A4, 5 (5 A3).
Tel 12 433 55 00. **Open** 10am–
6pm Tue–Sun (to 4pm Sun).
free Sun (permanent exhibition
only). **W** muzeum.krakow.pl

Transport
103, 114, 124, 134, 144, 152,
164, 169, 173, 179, 192, 194.
15, 18.

Second floor

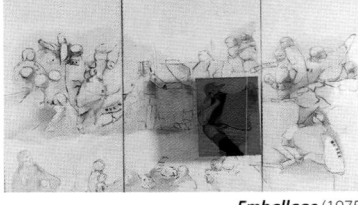

Emballage (1975)
This work by Tadeusz Kantor is an artistic
interpretation of Jan Matejko's great history
piece depicting *The Prussian Homage*.

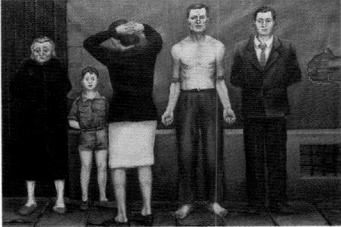

Execution (1949)
The art of Andrzej
Wróblewski, who
died prematurely, is
a personal analysis
of the tragic
war years.

Self-Portrait with Masks
This self-portrait by Wojciech
Weiss (1875–1950) dates from
the early years when the artist
remained under the influence
of Symbolism.

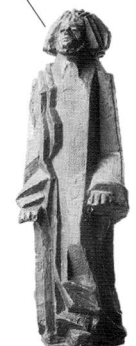

**★ A Design for Mickiewicz's
Statue in Vilnius**
This monumental statue by the
Cubist artist Zbigniew Pronaszko
(1885–1958) was never executed
and exists only as a model.

Key

▨ Temporary exhibitions

▨ Arms and Uniforms in Poland

▨ Gallery of Polish Art of the 20th Century

▨ Gallery of Decorative Arts

▨ Non-exhibition space

Gallery Guide

*Temporary displays and the exhibition "Arms and
Uniforms in Poland" are located on the ground floor.
The display on the first floor is dedicated to decorative
arts and temporary exhibitions. The Gallery of Polish
Art of the 20th Century is housed on the second floor.*

⓱ Jagiellonian Library

Biblioteka Jagiellońska

ul. Oleandry 3. **Map** 1 A4 (5 A2). **Tel** 12 633 09 03. 🚊 15, 18. 🚌 114, 144, 164, 169, 173, 179, 194. **Open** 8:15am–8:50pm Mon–Fri, 9am–4pm Sat.

For many centuries the Library of the Jagiellonian University was housed in the Collegium Maius *(see pp108–9)*. The new building was constructed between 1931 and 1939 to designs by Wacław Krzyżanowski. It has impressive modern forms and a spacious and functional interior. It is not only the success of the design but also the high quality of craftsmanship and the use of luxurious materials that make this building an outstanding example of Krakow's architecture in the interwar years.

During the 1990s work was undertaken on a new wing of the Library, designed by Romuald Loegler. This was completed in 2001, when the University celebrated the 6th centenary of its re-establishment. The additional wing matches the forms of the old building and is one of the most interesting examples of architecture of the 1990s.

The Library's holdings include 25,000 priceless manuscripts and 100,000 rare books and prints.

⓲ Academy of Mines and Metallurgy, Main Building

Al. Mickiewicza 30. **Map** 1 A3, 4 (5 A1). **Tel** 12 617 33 33. 🚌 114, 144, 164, 169, 173, 179, 194. **Open** 7:30am–8pm daily.

The Academy of Mines was established in Krakow in 1919. In 1922 the Faculty of Metallurgy was added. After 1945 the Academy was transformed into a large and well-equipped technological university. It has its own nuclear reactor and modern acoustic laboratory. The enormous main building, with 110,000 sq m (1,183,600 sq ft)

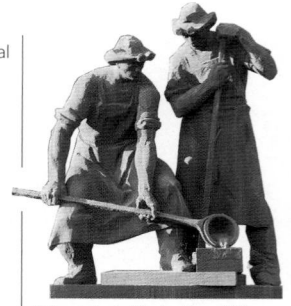

Statues in front of the Academy of Mines and Metallurgy

of floor space, was built between 1923 and 1935. It was designed by Sławomir Odrzywolski and Wacław Krzyżanowski in a Neo-Classical style that is particularly prominent in the façade and portico. The statues of miners and steel workers in front of the building are by Jan Raszka.

In German-occupied Poland the building became the seat of the Governor-General. A museum housed in Building C-1 is dedicated to the history of the Academy.

⓳ Avenue of Three Poets

Aleje Trzech Wieszczów

Map 1 A3, 1 A4, 1 B2, 1 C2. 🚌 114, 129, 139, 144, 164, 173, 179.

In the mid-19th century an earthen embankment was constructed along what is today this avenue, and in 1887 to 1888 a railway line was laid for trains connecting Krakow to Płaszów. East of the embankment, new streets were laid out and new houses constructed in the eclectic and Art Nouveau styles. When in 1910 the borders of Krakow were extended, the railway and the embankment were dismantled. Their site was replaced by a wide avenue comprising a dual carriageway with a belt of greenery in the middle. Each of the sections of the avenue was named after a Romantic poet: Krasiński, Mickiewicz and Słowacki. The intention was to transform the avenue into Krakow's Champs Elysées.

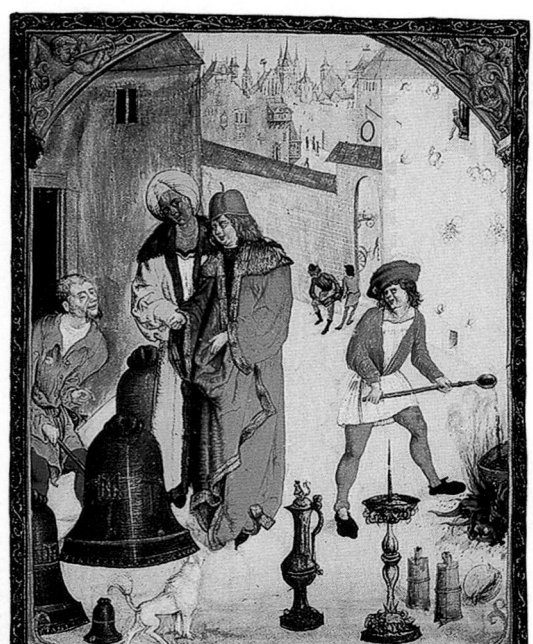

An illuminated page in the Behem Codex, Jagiellonian Library

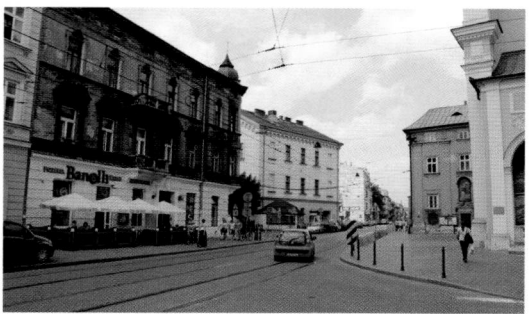

A view looking down Karmelicka Street

⑳ Karmelicka Street
Ulica Karmelicka

Map 1 B3, 5 (B1, C1). 🚌 114, 159, 164, 169, 179. 🚊 4, 8, 13, 14.

Karmelicka Street formed part of the old route connecting Krakow to Czarna Wieś and Łobzów. Formerly known as Czarna, Karmelicka was always the main street in the Garbary quarter. The Carmelite Church and, at No. 12, the Town Hall of Garbary were built here. Initially the street was divided into two parts: the wider part stretched from the Cobblers' Gate to a small bridge, beyond which the street narrowed considerably. This explains why the Carmelite friary building projects into the present-day street.

By the end of the 19th century Karmelicka became one of the most elegant streets in Krakow. Splendid houses were built to designs by Maksymilian Nitsch, Teodor Talowski and Filip Pokutyński. The writers Stanisław Przybyszewski and Tadeusz Boy-Żeleński were among the celebrated residents.

㉑ Spider House
Dom pod Pająkiem

ul. Karmelicka 35. **Map** 1 B3 (5 B1). 🚊 4, 8, 13, 14. **Closed** to the public.

This house was built in 1889 by Teodor Talowski, one of the leading architects in Krakow in the late 19th century. His intention was to give this irregular structure "an ancient appearance" by adding a "Gothic" round corner tower and a high gable in the style of Netherlandish Mannerism. By using different architectural styles of the past he wanted to pretend that the house had been rebuilt many times. He inserted, for example, a parapet modelled on the Renaissance Cloth Hall into the crenellated "Gothic" frieze. The decoration is rich in inventive detail.

㉒ Carmelite Church
Kościół Karmelitów

ul. Karmelicka 19. **Map** 1 B3 (5 C1). **Tel** 12 632 67 52. 🚌 114, 139, 159, 164, 169, 192. 🚊 4, 8, 13, 14. **Open** 9:30am–4:30pm and 5–7pm daily and during services.

According to a legend, Duke Władysław Herman cured his skin disease by rubbing sand on the infected areas. He took the sand from a site miraculously indicated by the Virgin Mary.

This site was therefore named Piasek (sand), and a votive church founded by the duke was built in 1087. Thus was born the legend of the Madonna of the Sand.

The church was actually founded by Queen Jadwiga in 1395. It was almost entirely destroyed during the Swedish invasion in the 17th century and its remnants were incorporated into the new Baroque church which was consecrated in 1679. The magnificent high altar, made in 1698 to 1699, and lavishly decorated with acanthus leaves, is worth noting. The splendid stalls and the balcony with the organ, both by Jan Hankis, are also of interest. An icon of the Madonna of the Sand, painted directly on the wall, is much venerated.

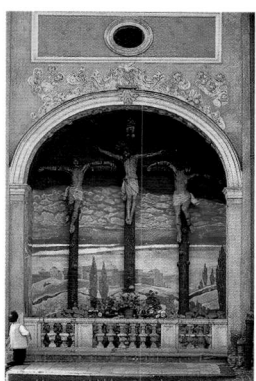

The Calvary Chapel in the side wall of the Carmelite Church

Queen Jadwiga (Hedwig)

Queen Jadwiga (c. 1374–99) was famous for her piety and charity. She contributed to the development of the Academy of Krakow. Venerated since the Middle Ages, she was finally canonized in 1997. A touching legend links Jadwiga to the Carmelite Church. It tells the story of a mason employed at the construction of the church who lamented to Jadwiga about his poverty and lack of money to buy medicine for his wife. The Queen removed a gold brooch from her shoe and offered it to the man. The imprint of her foot can still be seen today.

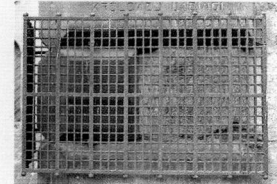

The imprint of Queen Jadwiga's foot

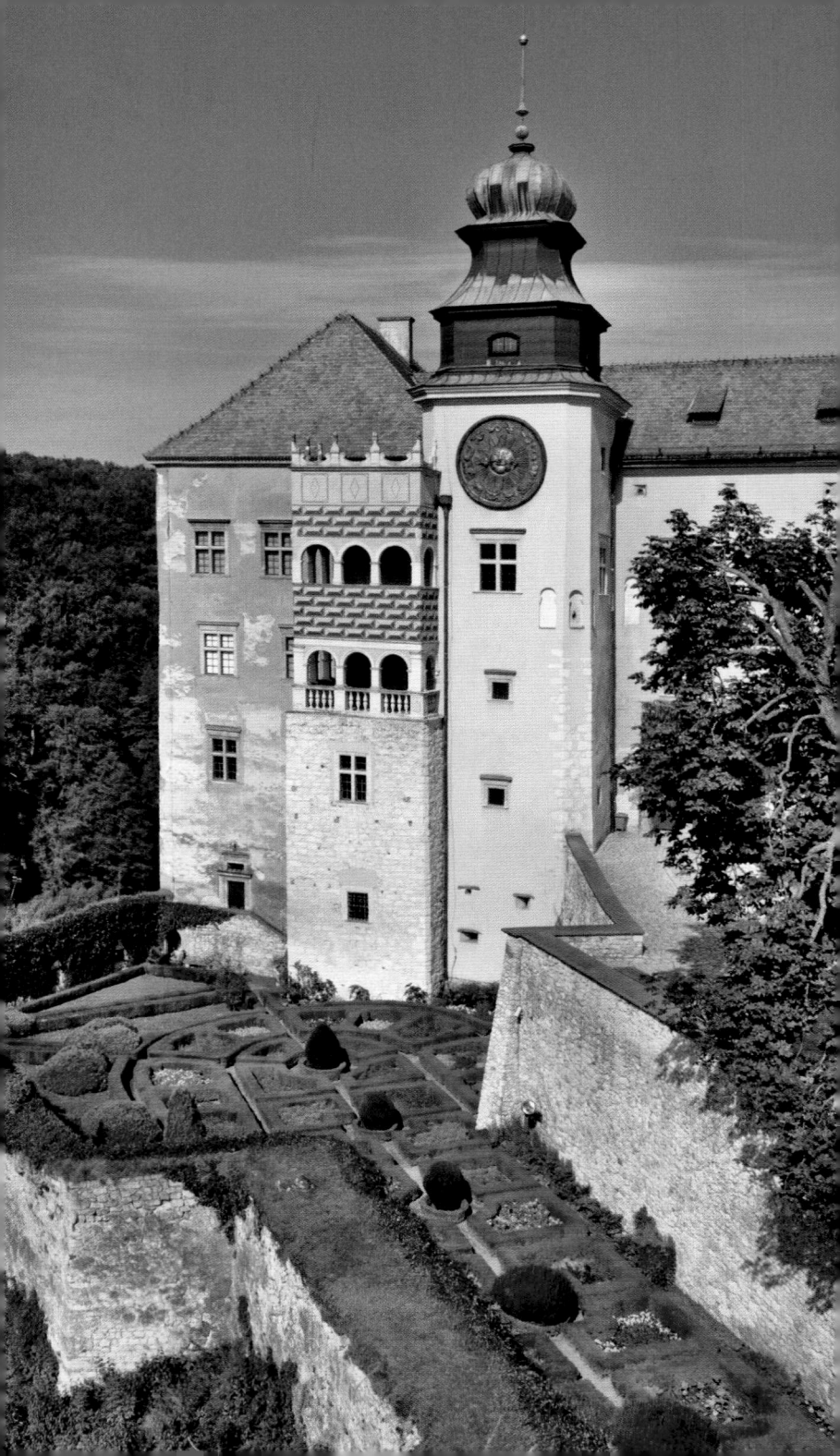

FURTHER AFIELD

Lesser Poland is the most densely populated and richest region of the former Polish-Lithuanian Commonwealth. Until the 17th century the local nobility held the highest offices and played an important political role at the royal court of Krakow, influencing matters of state. The nobles spent their time carrying out official duties in the capital as well as staying in their country estates, where they built castles, churches and monasteries. They introduced the art and culture of Krakow to the rest of Lesser Poland. In the centuries that followed, Krakow continued to dictate the local fashion and was a centre of artists for the whole province. Krakow's strong influence over neighbouring regions contributed to their unique artistic climate, in which the elitist merged with the vernacular, often with surprising effects. To appreciate the long tradition of Krakow's links with the area, visitors should consider excursions out of town. They are ideal for those who are interested in historic or traditional architecture and places of historical interest, as well as those who like to relax in beautiful natural surroundings.

Sights at a Glance

1 Nowa Huta
2 Mogiła
3 Polish Aviation Museum
4 Branice
5 Niepołomice
6 Staniątki
7 Wieliczka
8 Ojców
9 Schindler's Factory
10 Museum of Contemporary Art in Krakow (MOCAK)
11 Grodzisko
12 Pieskowa Skała
13 Tyniec
14 Wadowice
15 *Auschwitz (Oświęcim) (pp162–5)*
16 Kalwaria Zebrzydowska

Key

- ▨ City centre
- ▬ Motorway
- ▬ Major road
- ▭ Minor road
- ── Railway line

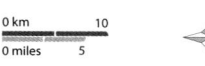

0 km   10
0 miles   5

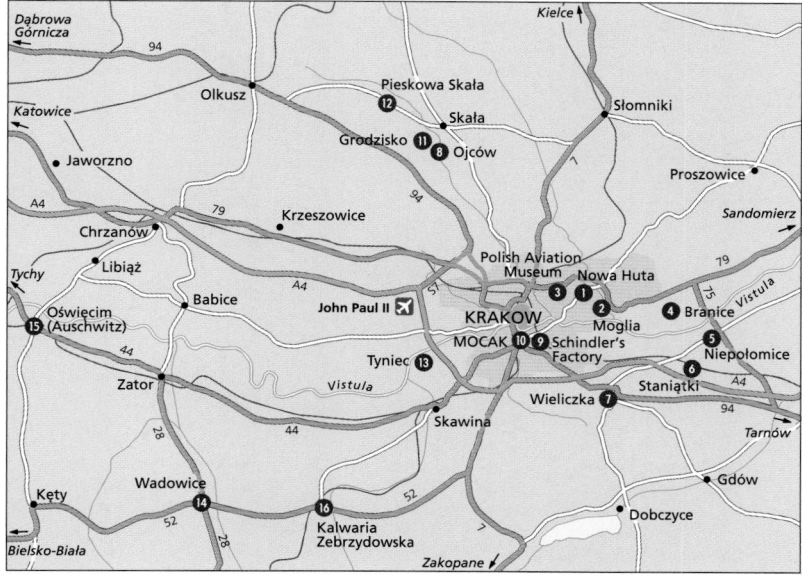

◀ The clock tower at the castle of Pieskowa Skała

For keys to symbols *see back flap*

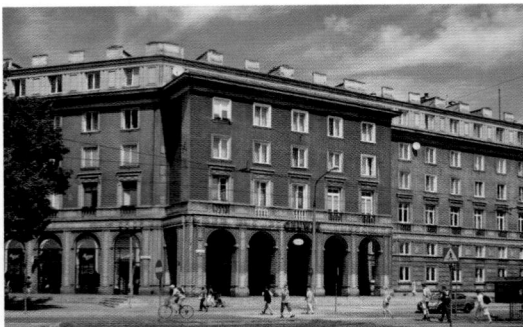

The Socialist Realist architecture of Nowa Huta

❶ Nowa Huta

🚃 117, 132, 138, 139, 142, 148, 149, 163, 174. 🚊 4, 15, 17, 21, 22.

The Communist authorities in Krakow suffered a crushing defeat in the 1946 referendum. This was blamed upon an inappropriate social balance within the class-based society. In order to "rearrange" this balance, they undertook a programme of quick industrialization of the Krakow region to increase the working-class population. In 1948 a contract was signed between Poland and the Soviet Union for a giant steelworks named after Lenin. The construction of a new town named Nowa Huta (New Steelworks) began in 1949. It was designed by Tadeusz Ptaszycki in the Socialist Realist style.

The housing estate, Centre, built between 1949 and 1955, is an interesting example of urban planning. In this "model Communist town" there was no room for churches. However, the people of Nowa Huta demanded one, so despite official intentions, the construction of churches began in the 1970s. Among these, the well-known Ark of God (see p39) is an outstanding piece of modern sacred Polish architecture. During the period of Martial Law (1981–3), the workers residing in Nowa Huta clearly demonstrated that they were not the best allies of the Communists, and the town became notorious for riots.

The Lenin Steelworks have been renamed Sendzimir.

❷ Mogiła

7 km (4 miles) east of Krakow. 🚃 123, 153, 163. 🚊 15. Cistercian Church: Klasztorna 11. **Tel** 12 644 23 31. **Open** 6am–7pm daily.

Mogiła village developed around the Cistercian Abbey. The Cistercians were brought to Poland in 1222, or 1225, by Iwo Odrowąż, the Bishop of Krakow. The new monastery was named Clara Tumba ("Bright Tomb", Jasna Mogiła, in Polish) because of the proximity of the reputed burial place of the legendary princess Wanda.

This Romanesque church followed the strict building regulations of the Cistercian order. The chancel ended with a flat perpendicular wall, and pairs of chapels with a square ground-plan were added to the transept. In 1447 the church was destroyed by fire. Gothic forms were introduced during its rebuilding. Stanisław Samostrzelnik decorated the interior with murals in the first half of the 16th century. These Renaissance paintings are complemented by 18th-century furnishings. The Baroque façade was added by Franz Moser as late as 1779–80. Other wall paintings in the church were made by Jan Bukowski in the early 20th century.

The Gothic cloister built in the time of Kazimierz the Great is the most beautiful part of the Abbey. It leads to the Chapter House, which features murals painted in the 19th century by Michał Stachowicz. These illustrate scenes from the life of Wanda. Not far from the abbey is the Church of St Bartholomew. Built in 1466, it is one of the oldest timber churches in Poland.

❸ Polish Aviation Museum

Al. Jana Pawła II 39. 🚊 5, 9, 10, 15, 40, 73. **Tel** 12 640 99 60. **Open** 9am–7pm Tue–Sun. 🚗 free Tue. 📷 🖳 muzeumlotnictwa.pl

This museum is located on the historic Rakowice-Czyżyny airfield, one of the oldest military airfields in Europe (established in 1912) and the second largest in Poland prior to World War II. The collection consists of more than 200 aircraft, including pre-war Polish fighter planes, Spitfires, German Albatrosses and Soviet Kakaruzniks. Also in the museum are 22 rare aeroplanes that were once part of Hermann Göring's personal collection.

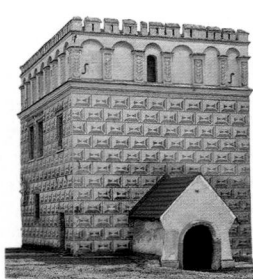

The Renaissance Old Manor in Branice

❹ Branice

12 km (7.5 miles) east from Krakow. Manor: Branice 131.

Branice is situated not far from Niepołomice and is worth visiting for its two manors which exemplify the small-scale residential architecture of the gentry of Lesser Poland. The Old Manor, later converted into a store, was built around 1603 for the Castellan of

Żarnów, Jan Branicki, by an architect from the circle of Santi Gucci. The exterior of the manor is decorated with *sgraffiti* and topped with a parapet. The doors and fireplace inside are lavishly decorated with imaginative Mannerist ornaments carved in stone.

The New Manor was built in the early 19th century in Classical style. Its high hipped roof, and the entrance marked by a small portico supported by columns, make this building characteristic of Polish architecture of this type. Both manors are set in a picturesquely landscaped park, laid out in the 19th century.

Next to Branice is the village of Ruszcza with the Church of St George. The church was built around 1420 by the Royal Master of the Pantry, Wierzbięta of Branice. His Gothic memorial plaque and the Baroque high altar are both of interest.

❺ Niepołomice

24 km (15 miles) southeast of Krakow. 🚌 minibus from Krakow's Main Railway Station. 🚆 from Krakow's Main Railway Station. Church: **Open** 7am–6pm daily. Castle: **Tel** 12 281 30 11. **Open** 10am–5pm daily. 📷

The royal grounds in Niepołomice, situated on the outskirts of a vast woodland, were much favoured by Polish kings. They came here to rest and hunt, and developed magnificent buildings in the town they owned. The Gothic church in Niepołomice was founded by King Kazimierz the Great between 1350 and 1358. Like other sacred buildings founded by this sovereign, this church had two aisles separated by pillars.

It was later rebuilt in the Baroque style. Fragments of the rich stone decoration from the interior of the medieval church have survived and are displayed in the Old Sacristy. Outstanding Gothic paintings made between 1370 and 1375 by an Italian master, commissioned by Princess

Elżbieta (daughter of Władysław the Short), are also in the Old Sacristy.

Next to the church are two mausolea of noble families, both in the form of chapels covered by domes. Built in 1596, the Branicki Chapel is the earlier of the two. It features an ornamental tomb made by the Italian architect and sculptor Santi Gucci in the Mannerist style. In the Chapel of the Lubomirski family, built in 1640, wall paintings depicting scenes from the life of St Carlo Borromeo are of interest. Late-Baroque altars were added in the 18th century.

The hunting lodge in Niepołomice was originally built by Kazimierz the Great. It was transformed by Zygmunt August into a magnificent residence. The new castle was constructed between 1550 and 1571. Its regular plan and the central, square courtyard differ from other royal Renaissance houses in Poland. In 1637 massive stone arcades were added to the courtyard. Part of the castle is used to house the Museum of Hunting.

The dense forest (Puszcza Niepołomicka), a favourite hunting ground of Polish

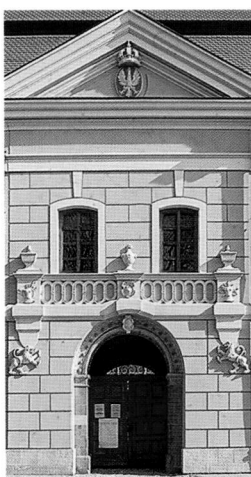

Façade of the palace in Niepołomice, a residence of Polish kings

kings, stretches right behind the town. Brown bears, bison, lynx, wildcat and deer are known to have inhabited it. The forest is not so magnificent as it used to be, though wild areas have been preserved, including the bison sanctuary in the Proszowo forest.

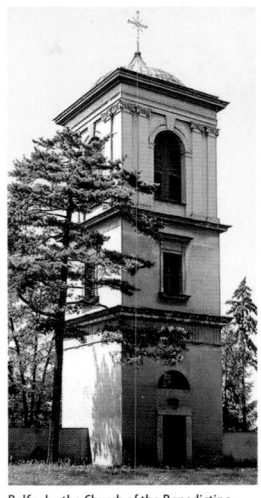

Belfry by the Church of the Benedictine Nuns in Staniątki

❻ Staniątki

24 km (15 miles) southeast of Krakow. 🚆 from Krakow's Main Railway Station and Krakow-Płaszów. Church: **Open** during services only.

The Convent and Church of the Benedictine Nuns in Staniątki is not far from Niepołomice. The convent was founded in 1228 by Klemens of Ruszcza, Castellan of Krakow. The Church of St Mary and St Adalbert, dating from the same period, is Poland's oldest hall-church (a type of church in which the aisles and nave are of the same height).

The church is a brick structure. Its rather modest decoration is carved in stone. The interior was refurbished completely in the 18th century. The lavishly decorated organ gallery, added in 1705, and wall paintings executed in 1760 by the Rococo artist Andrzej Radwański of Krakow, are of great interest.

❼ Wieliczka

12 km (7.5 miles) southeast of Krakow. 🚌 Luxbus coaches from Krakow's Main Railway Station. 🚃 from Krakow's Main Railway Station and Krakow-Płaszów. Salt Mines: ul. Daniłowicza 10. **Tel** 12 278 73 02. 🗎 **Open** Apr–Oct: 7:30am–7:30pm daily; Nov–Mar: 8am–5pm daily. **Closed** 1 Jan, Easter, 1 Nov, 24–25 & 31 Dec. 🌐 kopalnia.pl

Wieliczka developed and was granted a municipal charter in 1290 due to its rich deposits of salt. Salt was probably excavated here as early as the 11th century. The Latin name for Wieliczka was *Magnum Sal* (Great Salt) and indicated the importance of this mine in comparison to a smaller one in nearby Bochnia. According to a legend, the salt in Wieliczka constituted the dowry of St Kinga (Cunegunda) when she marrried Duke Bolesław the Chaste. The salt dowry was supposedly transposed magically from Hungary to Krakow for the wedding.

The salt in Wieliczka was regarded for centuries as a major natural asset of the Kingdom of Poland. A vast network of underground galleries was created here over the centuries. Salt was also used as a building material in the carving of underground chapels and altars in front of which the miners prayed for God's protection against accidents.

The Wieliczka Salt Mine Museum is housed inside the mine. The exhibits on display illustrate the old mining methods and tools. A unique underground sanatorium is also housed here.

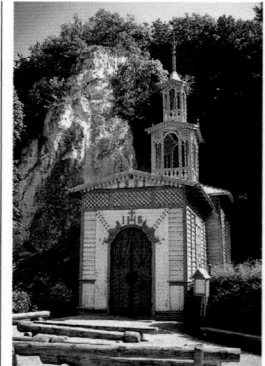

The small chapel overhanging the mountain river in Ojców

❽ Ojców

24 km (15 miles) northwest of Krakow. 🚌 from Krakow's Main Coach Station. Ojców National Park Museum: **Tel** 12 389 20 40. **Open** Apr–Oct: 9am–4:30pm daily; Nov–Mar: 8am–3pm Tue–Fri. Castle Tower: **Open** 13 Apr–11 Nov: from 10am; closing times vary.

The valley of the Prądnik river is the most beautiful part of the local uplands. The river eroded a deep gorge through the limestone. The steep cliffs are overgrown with trees through which stunning rock formations can be seen.

Kazimierz the Great had a number of hill-top castles built in the area to guard the western border of his Kingdom. The one in Ojców was one of the most important fortresses in Poland, but only remnants have survived. In 1956 part of the Prądnik valley was transformed into the Ojców National Park.

After the discovery of the healing properties of the local springs in the mid-1800s, the village at the foot of the castle was transformed into a spa: therapy clinics were set up and luxurious hotels built. The Łokietek Hotel, once the most sumptuous of all the buildings, now houses the museum of the Ojców National Park. During the Partition era, the Tsarist authorities denied planning permission for a church. So only a small timber chapel was built in 1901 to 1902 overhanging the Prądnik river.

❾ Schindler's Factory

ul. Lipowa 4. 🚃 3, 6, 7, 9, 11, 13, 20, 23, 24, 50, 51. **Tel** 12 257 10 17. **Open** Apr–Oct: 10am–8pm daily (to 4pm Mon, to 2pm first Mon of month); Nov–Mar: 10am–6pm daily (to 2pm Mon). 🖼 free Mon. 🗎

Located in the former industrial district of Zabłocie, Schindler's Factory is a symbol of humanitarian courage. In 1943, the factory's German owner, Oskar Schindler *(see p127)*, protected his Jewish workers by claiming that they were essential to the running of his business. The factory, now a branch of the Historical Museum of Krakow, is one of the most visited museums in Poland. The "Krakow during the Nazi Occupation 1939–1945" exhibition illustrates everyday life in the city during World War II using original documents, radio and film recordings, photos and multimedia installations. Visitors follow a trail through time, from the Nazi invasion to the Soviet occupation, delving into specific aspects such as the fate of the city's Jews and the resistance movements.

❿ Museum of Contemporary Art in Krakow (MOCAK)

ul. Lipowa 4. 🚃 3, 6, 7, 9, 11, 13, 20, 23, 24, 50, 51. **Tel** 12 263 40 00. **Open** 11am–7pm Tue–Sun. 🖼 free Tue.

Popularly know as MOCAK, this energetic and constantly evolving institution has carved

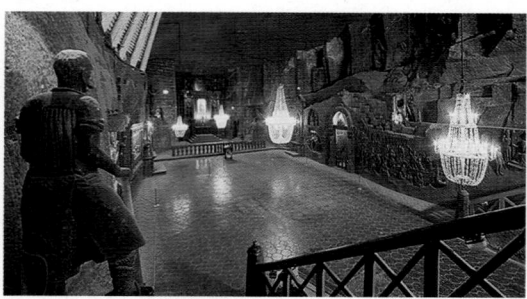

The Chapel of St Kinga in Wieliczka salt mine

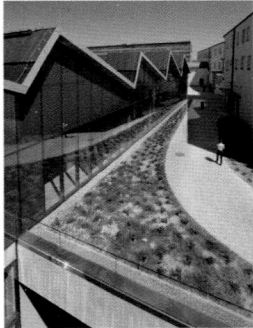

The exterior of MOCAK, housed on the site of the former Schindler's Factory

out an important place for itself in the city's cultural landscape since opening in 2011. The building is the result of a remodelling of parts of Schindler's Factory and features both intimate spaces and open galleries. The MOCAK hosts exhibitions of the most striking contemporary Polish art.

⓫ Grodzisko

28 km (17 miles) northwest of Krakow. 🚉 from Krakow's Main Railway Station. Church: **Open** 9–10am Sun.

Grodzisko is situated on the opposite bank of the Prądnik river from Ojców. The Convent of the Poor Clares was established here in 1262. Blessed Salomea, the sister of Duke Bolesław the Chaste, was the first Mother Superior. The nuns moved to Krakow in 1320 and the convent fell

into ruin. The cult of the Blessed Salomea developed over time, and in 1677 Canon Sebastian Piskorski transformed Grodzisko into a sanctuary devoted to this pious nun. He designed a complex hermitage consisting of a church and a number of chapels enclosed within a wall. There are several charming Baroque touches, like the elephant bearing an obelisk, an idea borrowed from the Italian architect Bernini.

⓬ Pieskowa Skała

35 km (22 miles) northwest of Krakow. 🚌 from Krakow's Main Coach Station. Castle: **Tel** 12 389 60 04. **Closed** for renovation until Apr 2016. 🏛 free Wed.

The castle in Pieskowa Skała was built by King Kazimierz the Great in the 14th century as part of the defence system on the Krakow-Częstochowa Uplands. It became private property in 1377.

Between 1542 and 1544, enlargement of the castle was undertaken by Stanisław Szafraniec and his wife, Anna Dębińska. The commission was probably given to the Italian architect Nicolo da Castiglione.

The castle houses a museum of the history of Polish interiors from medieval times to the "19th century. Some pieces of furniture, tapestries and decorative objects, as well as works of art, are on display.

⓭ Tyniec

10 km (6 miles) west of Krakow. 🚌 112. Benedictine Abbey: Benedyktyńska 37. **Tel** 12 688 54 52. **Open** 10am–6pm daily. 🌐 **tyniec. benedyktyni.pl/en**

The Benedictine Abbey at Tyniec is situated on a rocky escarpment by the Vistula, west of Wawel. The monks were brought to Krakow in 1044, probably by King Kazimierz the Restorer. A Romanesque basilica was built here soon after. Only parts of the walls and a few architectural fragments of this basilica have survived. The new church and monastery were built in the 15th century. The church was remodelled in the early 17th century in the Baroque style, and magnificent stalls were added to the chancel. Large altars in black marble were made in the 18th century.

In the 12th and 13th centuries, during the period when Poland was fragmented into principalities, Tyniec was transformed into a fortress and played an important role during the struggles for the crown of the suzerain province of Krakow. By the end of the 16th century, the fortifications were extended. A number of gates linked through an angled corridor were introduced as part of a defence system modelled on Wawel. Tyniec was a strategic site and as a result often came under attack from the enemy.

Today, the Benedictine Abbey is a picturesque sight.

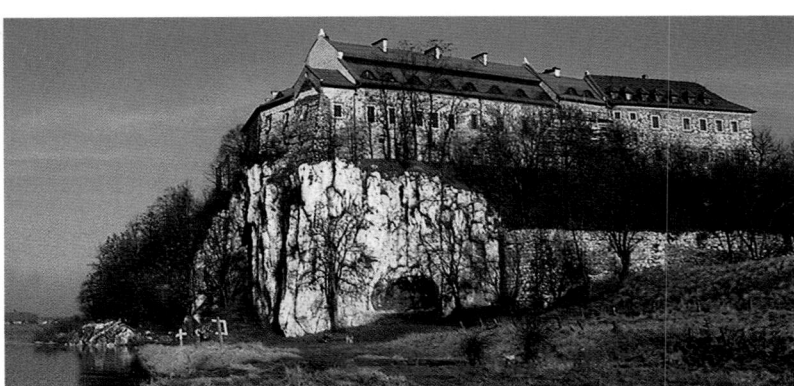

Benedictine Abbey in Tyniec on the Vistula

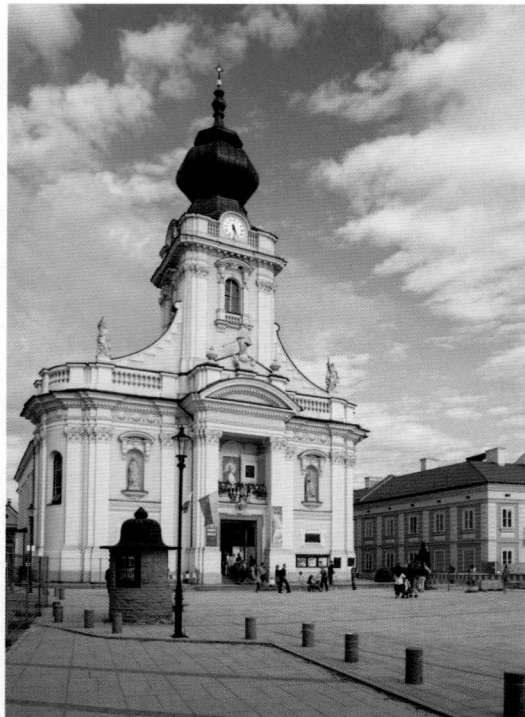

The Church of the Presentation of the Virgin Mary in Wadowice

⑭ Wadowice

40 km (25 miles) southwest of Krakow. 🚌 from Krakow's Main Coach Station. Family House of John Paul II: **Tel** 033 823 2662. **Open** daily. May–Sep: 8:30am–5:30pm, Nov–Mar: 9am–2:30pm, Apr & Oct: 9am–4:30pm.

Wadowice was first recorded in 1327, but the town came to international attention in 1978 when Karol Wojtyła, born here on 18 May 1920, was elected Pope. Almost immediately the town became a place of mass pilgrimage and the local sites associated with the Pope include the Baroque Church of the Presentation of the Virgin Mary in Market Square, where he was baptised, and his family home, which now houses a museum dedicated to the pontiff.

Another site associated with John Paul II is the monumental votive Church of St Peter the Arch-shepherd which was built on the outskirts of Wadowice in

thanksgiving for the Pope's survival of an assassination attempt on 13 May 1981. Designed by Ewa Węcławowicz-Gyurkovich and Jacek Gyurkovich, the walls of its nave seem to give way under the power of light, symbolizing the triumph of good over evil.

The town has had a chequered history, especially in the last century. While under German occupation during World War II, it was renamed Frauenstadt and the entire Jewish population was either executed or sent to nearby Auschwitz *(see below)*. Wadowice has since been growing as a tourist centre, replacing the local industries, which collapsed in the newly democratic economy during the 1990s.

⑮ Auschwitz (Oświęcim)

See pp162–5.

⑯ Kalwaria Zebrzydowska

30 km (19 miles) sw of Krakow. 🚌 from Main Coach Station or Krakow-Dębniki. 🚊 from Krakow's Main Railway Station or Krakow-Płaszów. Bernardine Church: **Open** 6am–7pm daily.

Calavaries, or Ways of the Cross, were introduced in the 16th century and were built throughout Europe to commemorate the Passion and Death of Christ. The landscaping of Calvary grounds had to imitate the topography of Jerusalem. They consisted of structures commemorating the "tragedy of Salvation" and imitations of holy sites connected to the Virgin Mary.

Poland's first Calvary was built by Mikołaj Zebrzydowski from 1600 onwards. He located the chapels representing the Stations of the Cross along Christ's route to Golgotha on the Żary Hill near his residence in Zebrzydowice.

Mystery plays enacting Christ's Passion are staged in Kalwaria during Holy Week. The "funeral of the Virgin" takes place on the feast of the Assumption. Crowds of pilgrims arrive to venerate the miraculous icon of the Mother of God, whose cult in the Bernardine Church goes back to the 17th century. Kalwaria is one of the main religious centres in Lesser Poland.

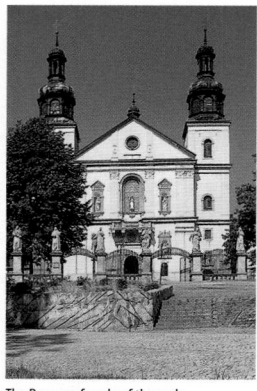

The Baroque façade of the early 17th-century Bernardine Church in Kalwaria Zebrzydowska

Kalwaria Zebrzydowska

The most interesting chapels in the Kalwaria Zebrzydowska are those designed by Paulus Baudarth, a Flemish architect and goldsmith. He was commissioned to design many chapels, and avoiding repetition must have been a difficult task. He applied many different ground-plans, including a Greek cross, a circle and even a triangle. In some chapels he resorted to truly Baroque ideas, and based the plans on the shape of a heart or rose.

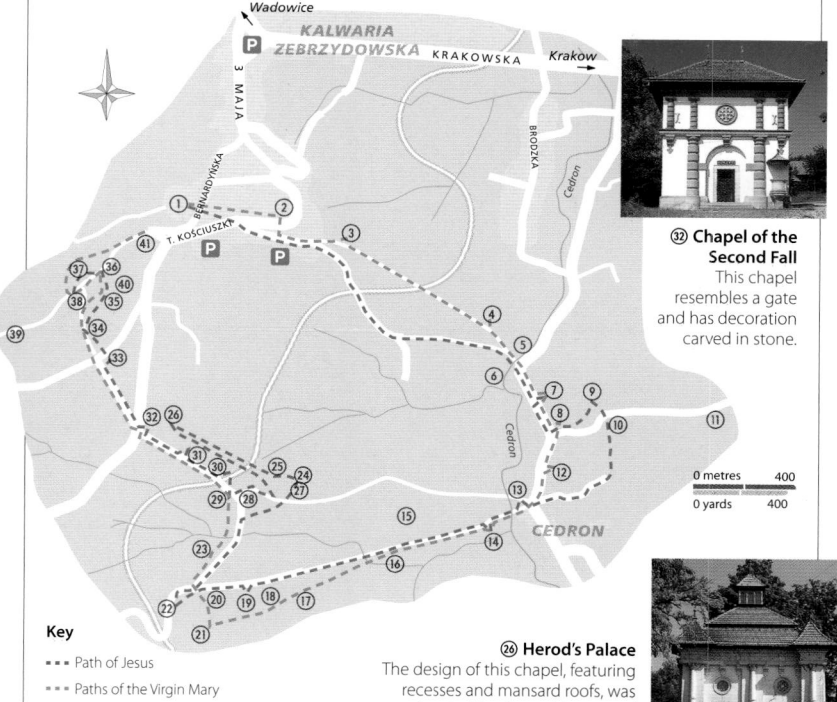

㉜ Chapel of the Second Fall
This chapel resembles a gate and has decoration carved in stone.

㉖ Herod's Palace
The design of this chapel, featuring recesses and mansard roofs, was inspired by the architecture of old Polish manors.

Key

- - - Path of Jesus
- - - Paths of the Virgin Mary

Sights on the Way of the Cross

① St Raphael's Chapel
② Chapel of the Throne
③ Chapel of the Joyful Patriarchs
④ Chapel of the Triumphant Apostles
⑤ Chapel of St John Nepomuk
⑥ Bridge of Angels
⑦ Chapel of Farewell
⑧ Church of the Sepulchre of the Virgin Mary
⑨ Gethsemane
⑩ Chapel of the Arrest of Christ
⑪ Church of the Ascension
⑫ Jewish Chapel
⑬ Bridge over the Cedron
⑭ East Gate
⑮ Bethsaida
⑯ Apostles' Chapel
⑰ Chapel of the Veneration of the Soul of the Virgin
⑱ Angels' Chapel
⑲ House of Annas
⑳ The Cenacle
㉑ House of Mary
㉒ House of Caiaphas
㉓ Chapel of the Fainting Virgin
㉔ Pilate's Town Hall
㉕ The Holy Steps
㉖ Herod's Palace
㉗ Chapel of the Taking up of the Cross
㉘ Chapel of the First Fall
㉙ Chapel of the Heart of Mary
㉚ Chapel of Simon of Cyrene
㉛ St Veronica's Chapel
㉜ Chapel of the Second Fall
㉝ Chapel of the Sorrowful Women
㉞ Chapel of the Third Fall
㉟ Chapel of the Stripping of Christ
㊱ Church of the Crucifixion
㊲ Chapel of the Anointment
㊳ Chapel of the Holy Sepulchre
㊴ Hermitage of St Mary Magdalene
㊵ Hermitage of St Helen
㊶ Chapel of the Madonna of Sorrows

⑮ Auschwitz I

For most people, Auschwitz represents the ultimate horror of the Holocaust. The Nazis began the first mass transportation of European Jews to Auschwitz in 1942 and it soon became the centre of extermination. Over the next three years, at least 1.1 million people, a quarter of those who died in the Holocaust, were killed at Auschwitz and the neighbouring Birkenau camp *(see pp164–5)*, also known as Auschwitz II. Today, the grounds and buildings of both camps are open to visitors, as a museum and a poignant memorial. Auschwitz is now a UNESCO World Heritage site.

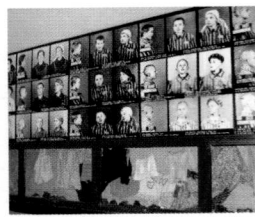

Exhibitions
The daily horrors of life in the camp are today displayed in some of the barracks.

The Camp

Auschwitz I opened in 1940 on the site of former Polish army barracks. Originally built to incarcerate Polish political prisoners, further buildings were added in the spring of 1941 as the number of prisoners dramatically increased. Camp administration was also based at Auschwitz I.

0 metres	100
0 yards	100

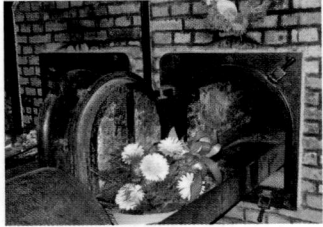

Gas Chambers and Crematoria
The entire Auschwitz complex had seven gas chambers and five crematoria. Six of the gas chambers were in Birkenau but the first was at Auschwitz, operating from 1941.

The Two Camps

Though part of the same camp complex, Auschwitz and Birkenau are in fact 3 km (2 miles) apart. The small Polish town of Oświęcim was commandeered by the Nazis and renamed Auschwitz. Birkenau was opened in March 1942 in the village of Brzezinka, where the residents were evicted to make way for the camp. There were an additional 47 sub-camps in the surrounding area.

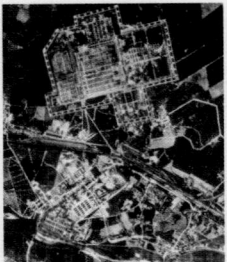

Aerial view of the complex taken by the Allies in 1944. The yellow dotted line marks Birkenau; the blue shows Auschwitz I.

KEY

① **SS Guard house and office of the camp supervisor**

② **"Arbeit Macht Frei" entrance**: the words above the infamous entrance to Auschwitz translate as "Work makes you free". This was certainly not the case for the prisoners transported here, who were often worked to death.

③ **Block 11 was the central jail** that housed prisoners from all over the camp complex.

④ **Store containing the poison, Zyklon B,** first used at Auschwitz to kill prisoners.

⑤ **Camp kitchen**

⑥ **Present-day Information Centre for visitors**

The "Wall of Death"
This is a reconstruction of the wall near Block 11 used for the summary executions by shooting. Usually covered in flowers, it now serves as a place of remembrance.

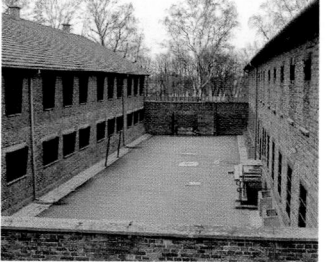

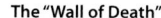

③

④

⑤

⑥

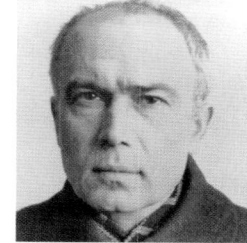

Maksymilian Kolbe
The camp jail, in Block 11, was used for those who broke camp rules. Few emerged alive. Father Kolbe *(see p37)* died here after sacrificing his life for another inmate's.

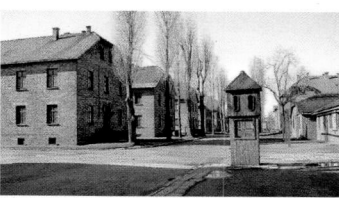

Roll Call Square
Roll call took place up to three times a day and could last for hours. Eventually, due to the increasing numbers of prisoners, roll call was taken in front of individual barracks.

1939 1 Sep, Hitler invades Poland.	1940 First deportation of German Jews into Nazi-occupied Poland.	1941 Hitler reported to have ordered the "Final Solution".		1944 As the Soviet Army closes on Auschwitz, the SS begin destroying all evidence of the camp.	1945 27 Jan, Soviet soldiers liberate the few remaining prisoners at Auschwitz.
			1942 First section of Birkenau camp completed		
1939	**1940**	**1941**	**1942**	**1943** **1944**	**1945**
1940 Oświęcim chosen as the site of the Nazis' new concentration camp.	1941 Himmler makes first visit to Auschwitz and orders its expansion.	1941 First gas chamber goes into operation.	1942 Beginning of mass deportation to Auschwitz.	1943 Four gas chambers built for mass murder. 1945 18 Jan, 56,000 prisoners evacuated on "Death March".	1945 7 May, Germany surrenders to the Allies.

Auschwitz II–Birkenau

Birkenau was primarily a place of execution. Most of Auschwitz's machinery of murder was housed here. In the six gas chambers in use at different stages of the camp's construction, over one million people were killed, 98% of whom were Jewish. Victims included people from over 20 nations. Birkenau was also an enormous concentration camp, housing 90,000 slave labourers by mid-1944 and providing labour for many of the factories and farms of southwestern, Nazi-occupied Poland. The gas chambers were quickly destroyed by the Nazis shortly before the Soviet Army liberated the camp in January 1945.

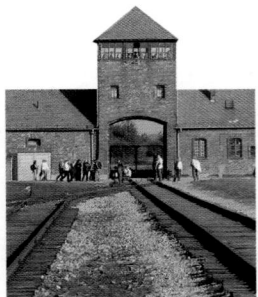

Hell's Gate
In 1944 the numbers arriving began to increase dramatically. A rail line was extended into the camp. The entrance gate through which the trains passed was known as "Hell's Gate".

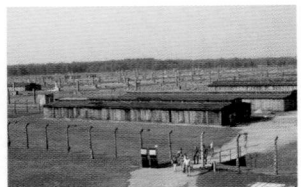

Visiting Birkenau
There is little left of the camp's buildings today; its main purpose is for remembrance. Most visitors come to pay their respects at the Monument to the Victims of the Camp, on the site of the gas chambers.

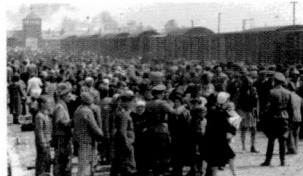

The Unloading Ramp
This was possibly the most terrifying part of the camp. It was here that SS officers separated the men from the women and children, and the SS doctors declared who was fit for work. Those declared unfit (as many as 70 or 80 per cent) were taken immediately to their death.

The Camp

Birkenau was the largest concentration camp in Nazi-occupied Europe. In 1944 the camp had more than 90,000 prisoners, the majority of whom were exterminated. From the unloading ramp to the gas chambers, the crematoria to the ash dumping grounds, the whole process of murder was carried out systematically and on an enormous scale. This reconstruction shows the camp at its peak in 1944, when as many as 5,000 people could be killed every day.

The Liberation of the Camps

With the war all but lost, in mid-January 1945 the Nazi authorities gave the order for all the camps to be destroyed. Such was the speed of the collapse of the German army, however, that only part of Birkenau was destroyed. Between 17–21 January more than 56,000 inmates were evacuated by the Nazis and forced to march west; many died en route. When the Soviet army entered the camps on 27 January 1945, they found just 7,000 survivors.

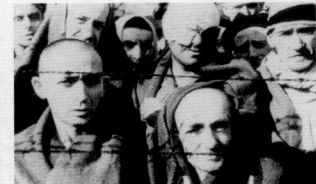

Survivors of Auschwitz II–Birkenau, filmed by Soviet troops

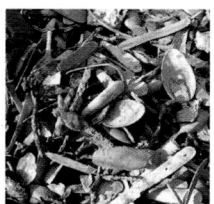

Kanada

"Kanada" was the nickname of the barracks where property stolen from prisoners was stored. It was the preferred place to work at Auschwitz II-Birkenau as it offered opportunities for inmates to pilfer items to barter for food or medicine later.

0 metres	200
0 yards	200

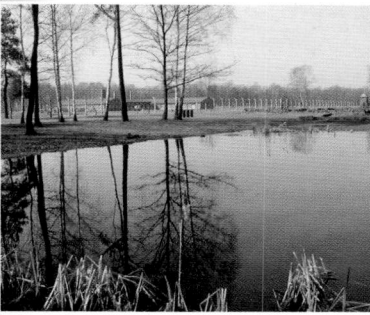

The Sauna

New arrivals selected for work were deloused and disinfected in this building, which became known as the "sauna". Periodic disinfections of existing prisoners were also carried out here.

The Ash Pond

Tons of ash – the remains of hundreds of thousands of Auschwitz victims – were dumped in ponds and troughs dug around the outskirts of the camp.

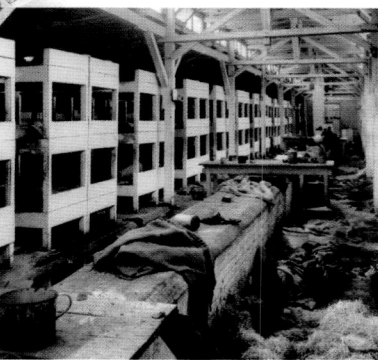

Barracks

The conditions of the living quarters at the camps were terrible. With little or no sanitation, poor nutrition and no medical care, diseases such as typhus spread rapidly. This image shows a typical wooden barracks at Birkenau shortly after liberation.

KEY

① **Towers and barbed wire** isolated the camps from the outside world.

② **Large gas chambers and crematoria (from 1943)**

③ **Area of expansion**, nicknamed "Mexico", never completed.

④ **Wooden barracks**, with 500–600 people living in each.

⑤ **Hell's Gate**

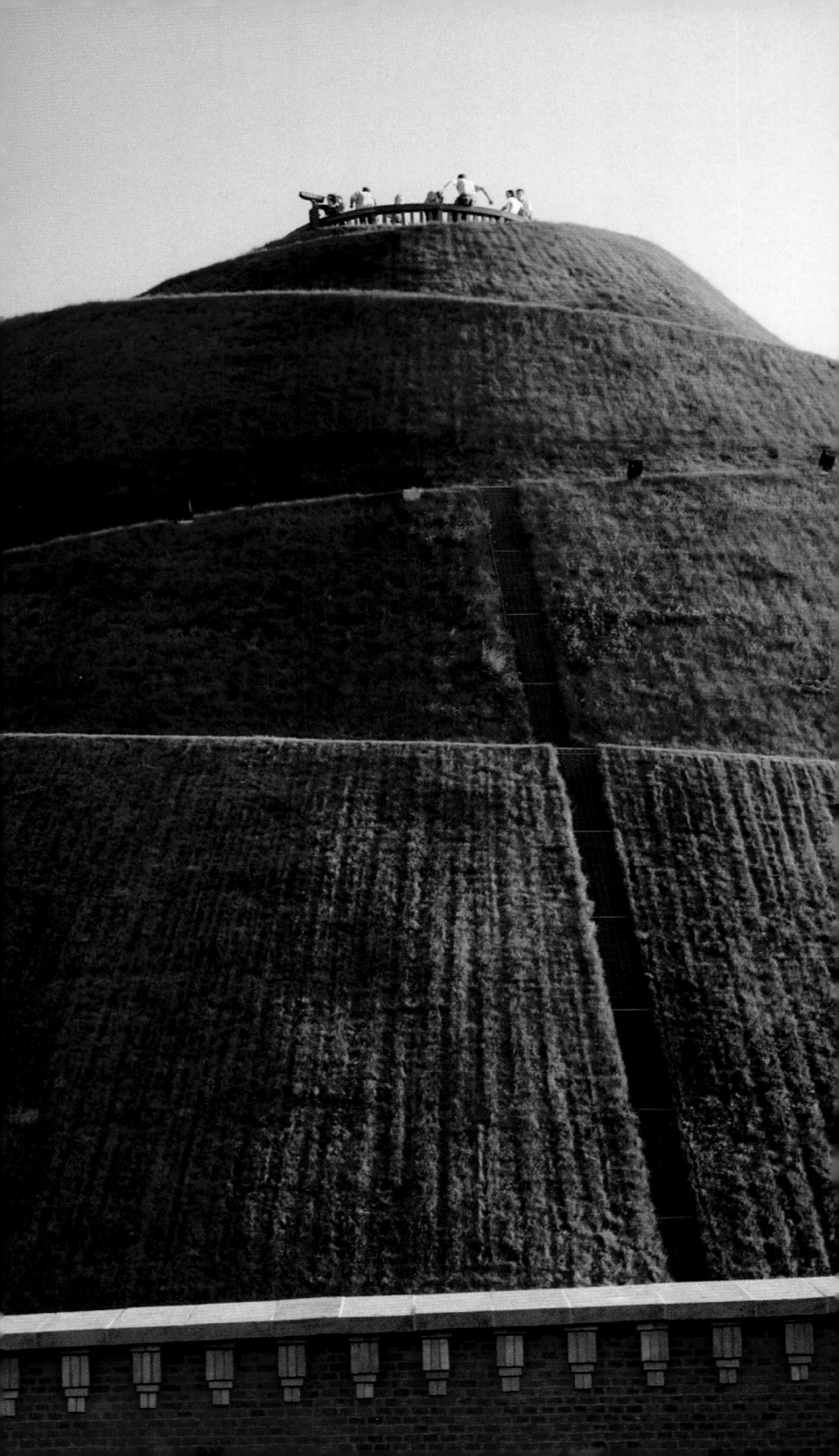

THREE GUIDED WALKS

Krakow is an ideal place for walks. The Old Quarter has become a pedestrian precinct with a large concentration of historic monuments, all within a short walking distance of each other. Suggestions for three walks, each with its own unique character, are included here. The first walk is along the Planty park which was laid out on the site of the medieval wall that surrounded the Old Quarter and Okół. It will give you an idea of the extent of the medieval city and provide an opportunity to enjoy this quiet park in the middle of a densely built city. Many statues decorate this park, commemorating those who had links with Krakow.

The two other walks will lead you away from the busy city centre to suburban Krakow, which has retained much of an idyllic countryside character. Zwierzyniec is rich in heritage and offers beautiful views over Krakow owing to its high location on hills.

Las Wolski (Wolski Wood) is an extensive woodland where you can enjoy nature at her best or visit first-class historic buildings situated on its periphery. Among the finest buildings are the Villa of Decius, famous for its arcaded loggia and today a seat of the European Academy, and the complex of the Camaldolese Monastery. Bear in mind that women are only allowed into the monastery on a few festive days. Children will certainly enjoy a visit to the Zoo in the middle of Wolski Wood.

Greater Krakow is quite large but every district is well served by buses and trams which run from early morning till late at night. An average journey by bus or tram lasts no more than a quarter of an hour. An increasing number of new restaurants, bars and cafés have opened around Krakow. Tourists can visit historic buildings, and enjoy nature and a good meal at the same time.

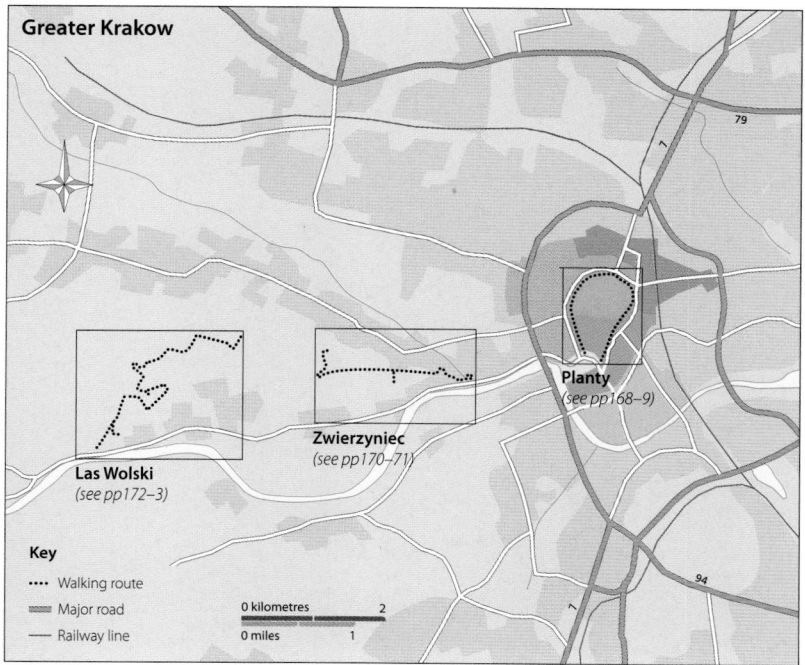

Greater Krakow

Planty
(see pp168–9)

Zwierzyniec
(see pp170–71)

Las Wolski
(see pp172–3)

Key

- •••• Walking route
- ▬▬ Major road
- — Railway line

0 kilometres   2
0 miles   1

◀ Enjoying the views from the top of the Kościuszko Mound

A Two-Hour Walk around Planty

The Planty green belt in Krakow has replaced the city's medieval fortifications, built between the late 13th and 15th centuries. They were demolished early in the 19th century and the small stretch of wall by Floriańska Street is the only fragment to have survived. The gardens of Planty were landscaped to include a network of radiating lanes and beautiful vistas. In the second half of the 19th century the well-kept Planty became a popular venue for socializing. After a period of regeneration the Planty now features period fencing, benches and street lamps.

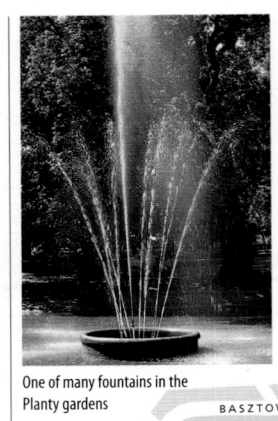

One of many fountains in the Planty gardens

Wawel to the University

The walk begins by the Coat of Arms Gate at Wawel. Walk downhill and cross the street to enter the so-called Wawel gardens. The Gothic Revival Seminary building will be on your right, and a sculpture depicting *Owls* can be seen on your left ①.

Continue down through the park some 40 m (130 ft) towards a little square decorated with a statue of the renowned translator of French literature into Polish, Tadeusz Boy Żeleński, carved by Edward Krzak ②. Turn right and after some 50 m (165 ft) you will reach the wall enclosing the gardens of the Archaeological Museum (*see p85*). Mounted in the wall are small plaques, overrun with greenery, commemorating the contributions made by the honorary Committee for the Renovation of Krakow's Monuments.

Carry straight on and cross Poselska Street. Those interested in archaeology may turn right to visit the museum. On the other side of the street is a plinth indicating the site of one of many medieval towers which formed part of the defence wall. The outline of the wall is marked by sandstones which you can see positioned along the lanes. Take a sharp left turn and walk

down 20 m (65 ft) to a little square where, hidden behind trees, is a statue made in 1884 of Grażyna and Litawor ③, two characters from a poem by Adam Mickiewicz.

From this statue, take a right turn to return to the main lane. You will notice the buildings of the Franciscan Church (*see pp88–9*) and the Episcopal Palace (*see p106*). Go straight ahead and cross Franciszkańska Street to enter the University Gardens. Walk down the main lane along the wall of the Episcopal Palace, passing by the end of Wiślna Street. Some 150 m (492 ft) further down, by Jagiellońska Street, is an 18th-century statue of the Virgin Mary of Grace ④, which originally was in the graveyard of the Church of St Mary. After another 40 m (130 ft), you may choose to rest, looking at the Kościuszko Mound which can be seen through Józefa Piłsudskiego Street in the distance. Then carry on, passing by the façade of the Collegium Novum, the main university building. An oak planted in 1918, known as the Oak of Liberty, can be seen in front of the college. A red-brick paved

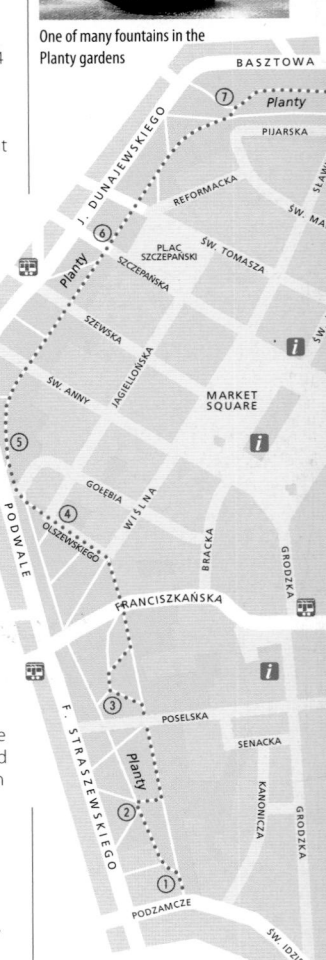

① *Owl* (1964) by Bronisław Chromy

pattern in the square imitates the curves of Copernicus's astrolabe. The statue of the astronomer ⑤ (see p106), surrounded by trees, is to the left of Collegium Novum and in front of the Witkowski College. Further down, you will pass by the Collegium Nowodvorianum (see pp106–7) and after some 50 m (165 ft) cross St Anne's Street. The university Collegiate Church of St Anne (see pp110–11) will be on your right.

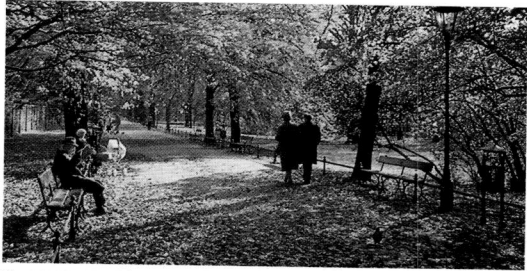

Planty in autumn, with visitors strolling along a path

beautiful statue of Artur Grottger ⑥ made in 1901 by Wacław Szymanowski. Cross St Thomas's Street (ulica św. Tomasza) and after some 300 m (985 ft) turn left. In this "corner" of the Planty is the statue of Lilla Veneda ⑦, the leading character in a play by Juliusz Słowacki. Walk some 200 m (655 ft) down one of the lanes which run alongside Basztowa Street. The next monument you will notice is that of Queen Jadwiga and King Władysław Jagiełło ⑧. It was raised to commemorate the fifth centenary of the union between Poland and Lithuania in 1386. After crossing Sławkowska Street, you will find on your left a large pond where in summer swans can be seen. You can cross a little bridge over the pond and this will lead you to a statue of the Harpist ⑨. Continue down the main lane. Pass by the remains of the defence wall with St Florian's Gate (see p113) to finally reach the Barbican (see p116).

Krakow's Main Railway Station to Stradom

Walk some 300 m (985 ft) through the so-called Station Gardens. The major attractions here are the Słowacki Theatre (see p117) and the Church of the Holy Cross (see p117).

⑦ Statue of Lilla Veneda by Alfred Daun

Continue to the subway entrance by which the Straszewski Obelisk ⑩ is located. Florian Straszewski was the man who laid out Planty. Behind the Church of the Holy Cross is a statue of the playwright Michał Bałucki ⑪. Walk another 300 m (985 ft) cross Mikołajska Street to enter the "Na gródku" Gardens. The Church of the Dominican Nuns (see p117) will be on your right. Continue down the lane and cross Sienna Street. The Dominican Church (see pp118–19) will be on your right. You will pass by an unusual statue of Colonel Narcyz Wiatr-Zawojny ⑫, who was shot dead in 1946 by the secret police (UB). The statue was made in 1992 by Bronisław Chromy. Stroll another 500 m (0.3 mile) downhill to enter the so-called Stradom Gardens and the end of the walk.

Tips for Walkers

Starting point: At the foot of Wawel, by Kanonicza Street.
Length: approx. 5 km (3 miles).
Getting there: Bus Nos. 128, 304, 522; the nearest stop is by Straszewskiego Street.
Stopping-off points: Café at the "Bunker of Art" near the Collegium Novum. There are benches near the Barbican and throughout the park.

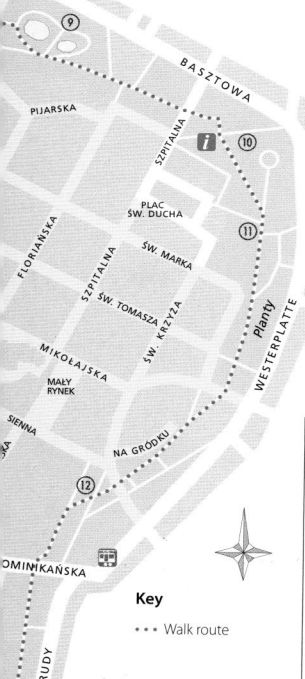

Key

• • • Walk route

Palace of Art to the Barbican

Continue some 100 m (330 ft) and cross Szewska Street. The "Bunker of Art" (see p107) will be on your right. A little further down, some 20 m (65 ft) after crossing Szczepańska Street, continue to walk down the Planty's main lane. You will pass a little square where you will see the Palace of Art (see p107) on the right, while on your left will be a most

For keys to symbols see back flap

A One-Hour Walk around Zwierzyniec

In the 12th century Zwierzyniec was a small village, founded as the endowment to the Premonstratensian nuns, whose convent was located by the Rudawa river, a tributary of the Vistula. Polish sovereigns used to take a rest in the royal gardens located in this village. Henri de Valois is reputed to have organized orgies here to the outrage of his subjects. The richest Krakovians followed in the kings' footsteps by establishing their country residences in Zwierzyniec. Despite being incorporated into Krakow in the early 20th century, Zwierzyniec has managed to retain its original village character.

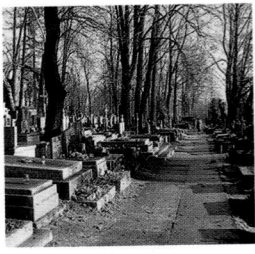

⑤ Salwator Cemetery

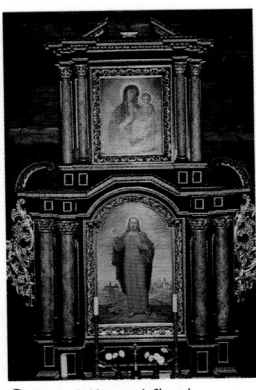

② Altar in St Margaret's Chapel

Salwator

After arriving at the tram depot, walk to the Church of the Premonstratensian Nuns ①. The church was founded in the second half of the 12th century but its appearance today is a result of a remodelling undertaken between 1595 and 1638. The Neo-Classical decoration of the choir is most interesting. It was created between 1775 and 1779 to designs by Sebastian Sierakowski. The convent building next to the church is one of the largest in Poland. It is worth visiting for its courtyard. After leaving the church, go up

the steep Św. Bronisławy Street. The Chapel of St Margaret ②, built in 1690, will be on your left. Those who died of the plague were buried by

the chapel. The Church of the Holy Redeemer ③ is further uphill. According to Polish chroniclers, it was built immediately after

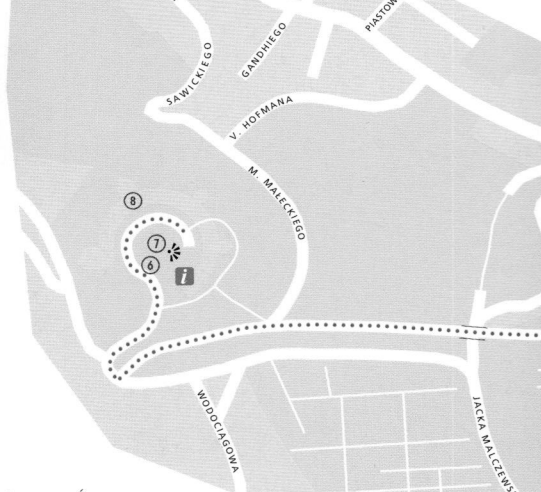

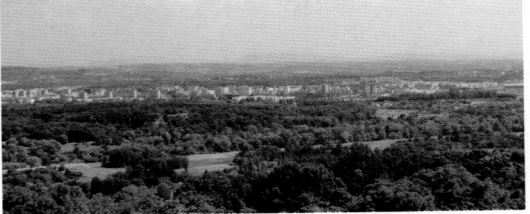

The Kościuszko Mound and Zwierzyniec seen from Wawel

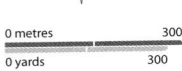

0 metres   300
0 yards   300

Key

••• Walk route

Poland had accepted Christianity in 966, by Duke Mieszko I. The duke presented the church with a miraculous crucifix. Evidence shows, however, that the church was actually constructed later and consecrated in 1148. Despite extensive remodelling, the church has retained much of its Romanesque character. An interesting painting of 1605 by Kasper Kurch depicts a most unusual scene of the crucified Christ shaking off his shoe in order to pass it to a poor fiddler playing under the Cross. A 17th-century pulpit has also survived by the church, as well as a number of interesting tombs from the first half of the 19th century.

A residential estate ④ established in the early 20th century is located near the church. Its Art Nouveau architecture is worth seeing.

Salwator Cemetery

Walk down Anczyca Street and turn right into Aleja Jerzego Waszyngtona

(Washington Avenue). The small Salwator Cemetery ⑤ consecrated in 1865 is located on the outskirts of the Salwator estate. A chapel, built in 1888 to 1889 in the Neo-Gothic style to a design by architect Sebastian Jaworzyńsk can be seen in the middle of the cemetery. A great number of tombs of those who made important contributions to Polish culture can be found here.

Kościuszko Mound

The tree-lined Aleja Jerzego Waszyngtona will lead you to the Kościuszko Mound on Sikornik Hill. At its foot, the Chapel of St Bronisława ⑥ marks the site of the hermitage of the eponymous nun. The chapel was built between 1856 and 1861 by Feliks Księżarski in the Neo-Gothic style. The Kościuszko Mound ⑦ was

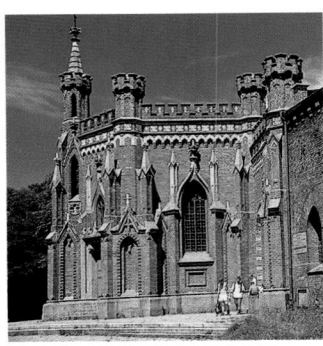

⑥ Chapel of the St Bronisława at the foot of the Kościuszko Mound

erected between 1820 and 1823 to commemorate the leader of the insurrection of 1794. This monument to the hero in the struggle for Polish independence was inspired by the mounds of two mythical Polish rulers, Krak and Wanda, which are located in the environs of Krakow. The construction of the mound became a patriotic endeavour and the monument itself a destination for national pilgrimages arriving in Krakow. Fortifications ⑧ at the foot of the Kościuszko Mound were constructed after 1850 by the Austrians as part of a project which aimed to transform Krakow into a massive fortress. The fortress is currently used as a hotel and houses the popular RMF FM radio station. A bus stop, which serves the city centre, is situated by the entrance to the hotel.

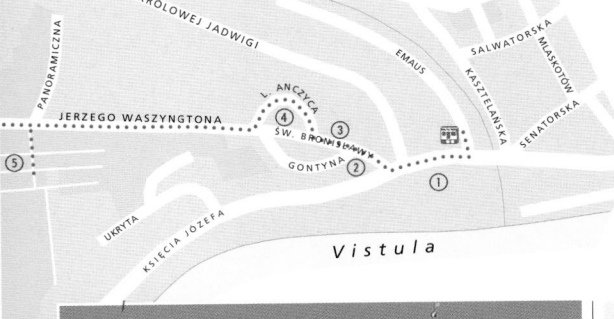

Tips for Walkers

Starting point: The Salwator tram depot.
Length: 2.5 km (1.6 miles).
Getting there: The walk starts from the tram depot in Salwator. You can get there by tram Nos. 1, 2 and 6. Return by bus No. 100 which stops at the foot of the Kościuszko Mound.
Stopping-off points: Benches to relax can be found on Aleja Jerzego Waszyngtona. There is a café and restaurant in the Hotel "Pod Kopcem" on the same street.

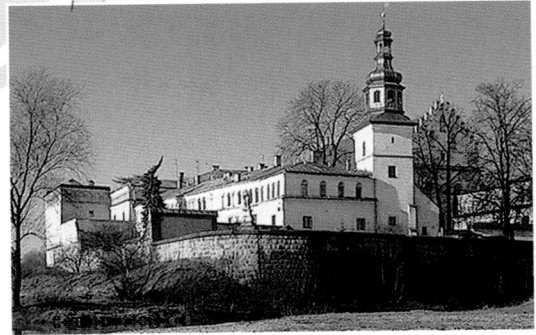

① Church and Convent of the Premonstratensian Nuns at Salwator

For keys to symbols *see back flap*

A Walk in Las Wolski

Las Wolski (the Wolski Wood) is the largest green area in Krakow. It has partly retained its original character as a forest, while the remaining ground is maintained as a park. Paths and lanes wind up and down this hilly terrain, leading to many wild spots of surprising beauty created either artificially or naturally. The lovely architecture of the Camaldolese Monastery and Decius Villa, both on the outskirts of the park, are worth exploring. The walk route described below includes sights in the Wolski Wood and the surrounding neighbourhood.

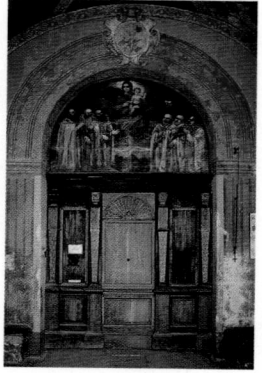

① Entrance to the Camaldolese Monastery

Srebrna Góra (Silver Mount)
The walk begins at the bus stop at the intersection of Aleja Wędrowników (Wędrowników Avenue) and Księcia Józefa Street. Walk some 500 m (0.3 mile) down Aleja Wędrowników then turn right into Aleja Konarowa (Konarowa Avenue).

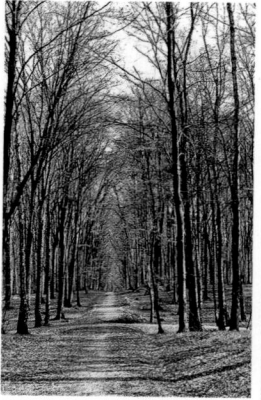

② The Wolski Wood, a favourite place for walks

Climb up the Silver Mount to visit the Camaldolese Monastery ①. The monastery of this strict Reformed Benedictine order was built between 1605 and 1642 by two outstanding architects, Valentin of Säbisch and Andrea Spezza, among others. The stone-clad façade of the church is particularly impressive. The austerity of the interior is in striking contrast with the lavishness of the decoration of the chapels, which feature stuccowork by Giovanni Falconi. The so-called Royal Chapel, dating from 1633 to 1636, is very beautiful. The stairs on either side of the high altar lead down to the crypt which houses a catacomb. This subterranean gallery has recesses excavated in the sides for tombs of the deceased monks. Next to the catacomb is the *ossuarium*, a common grave containing bones removed from the recesses in the catacomb. The hermitages are closed to visitors but can be seen from the ossuary chapel.

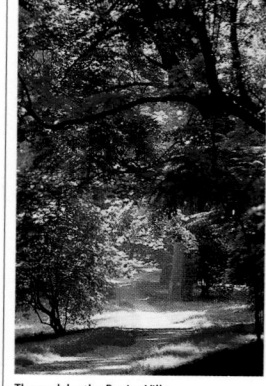

The park by the Decius Villa

Women are allowed into the church on a few festive days only.

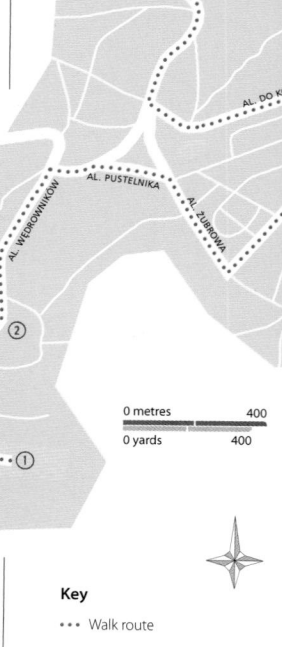

Key

••• Walk route

Wolski Wood (Las Wolski)

Leave the monastery by Aleja Konarowa (Konarowa Avenue), the same route by which you arrived, then turn right into Wędrowników Avenue which is the main lane of Wolski Wood ②. This wood was transformed into a public park in 1917 through the efforts of Juliusz Leo, the President of the City of Krakow. Turn right again into a path which leads to Aleja Żubrowa (Bison Avenue). After a few minutes' walk the entrance to the Zoo ③ will be in front of you. The Zoo was established in 1929. It differs from

constructed between 1934 and 1936 as a monument commemorating the Poles who fell during the long struggle for independence from the three powers that partitioned Poland between 1772 and 1918. The mound is called "a Tomb of Tombs" and contains ashes from many battlefields. Walk down the mound and continue along Aleja Panieńskich Skał (Virgin Rocks Avenue) toward the Sanctuary of the Virgin Rocks ⑤ where you will find picturesque limestone formations. According

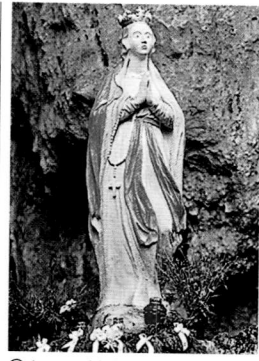
⑤ A statue of the Virgin in Panieńskich Skał

other zoological gardens owing to its location in the middle of a forest. Leave the Zoo via Al Do Kopca (Towards the Mound Avenue) which will take you to the Marshal Piłsudski Mound ④ on top of Sowiniec Mount. The mound was

to a legend, this was the place where the Premonstratensian nuns of Zwierzyniec took refuge and hid from the Tatars. A 16th-century timber church ⑥ at the end of the avenue was moved here from Komorowice.

Wola Justowska

Continue walking along Aleja Panieńskich Skał and turn right at the T-junction into Aleja Kasztanowa (Chestnut Avenue).

Wola Justowska, a fashionable district of Krakow, begins here. Carry on until you see the Decius Villa (Willa Decjusza) ⑦ ahead. Justus Decius was Secretary to King Zygmunt the Old. In 1530 he transformed a late-Gothic manor, dating from the 15th century, into a Renaissance residence. The villa was extended in the first half of the 17th century and a loggia added, offering a view over the area. The Villa houses the European Academy, which is dedicated to the study of European cultural heritage. A nearby bus stop serves the city centre.

Tips for Walkers

Starting point: The bus stop at the intersection of Księcia Józefa Street with Wędrowników Street.
Getting there: Bus routes 109, 209, 229, 239 and 269 will take you to Srebrna Góra. Take bus 134 by the entrance to the Zoo or bus routes 102, 134, 152 and 192 from Wola Justowska to return to the city centre.
Stopping-off points: There are benches to relax on throughout the Wolski Wood. Restaurants are at the foot of Srebrna Góra and near the Zoo and there is a café in the Villa of Decius.
Note: Women are only permitted into the Camaldolese Church on 7 Feb, 25 Mar, Easter Sun, Whit Sun; Whit Mon, Corpus Christi; 19 Jun, Sun after 19 Jun, 15 Aug, 8 Sep, 8 Dec and 25 Dec.

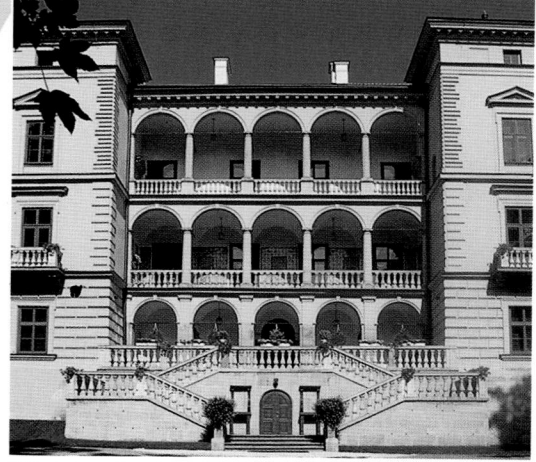
⑦ A suburban residence known as the Villa of Decius

For keys to symbols *see back flap*

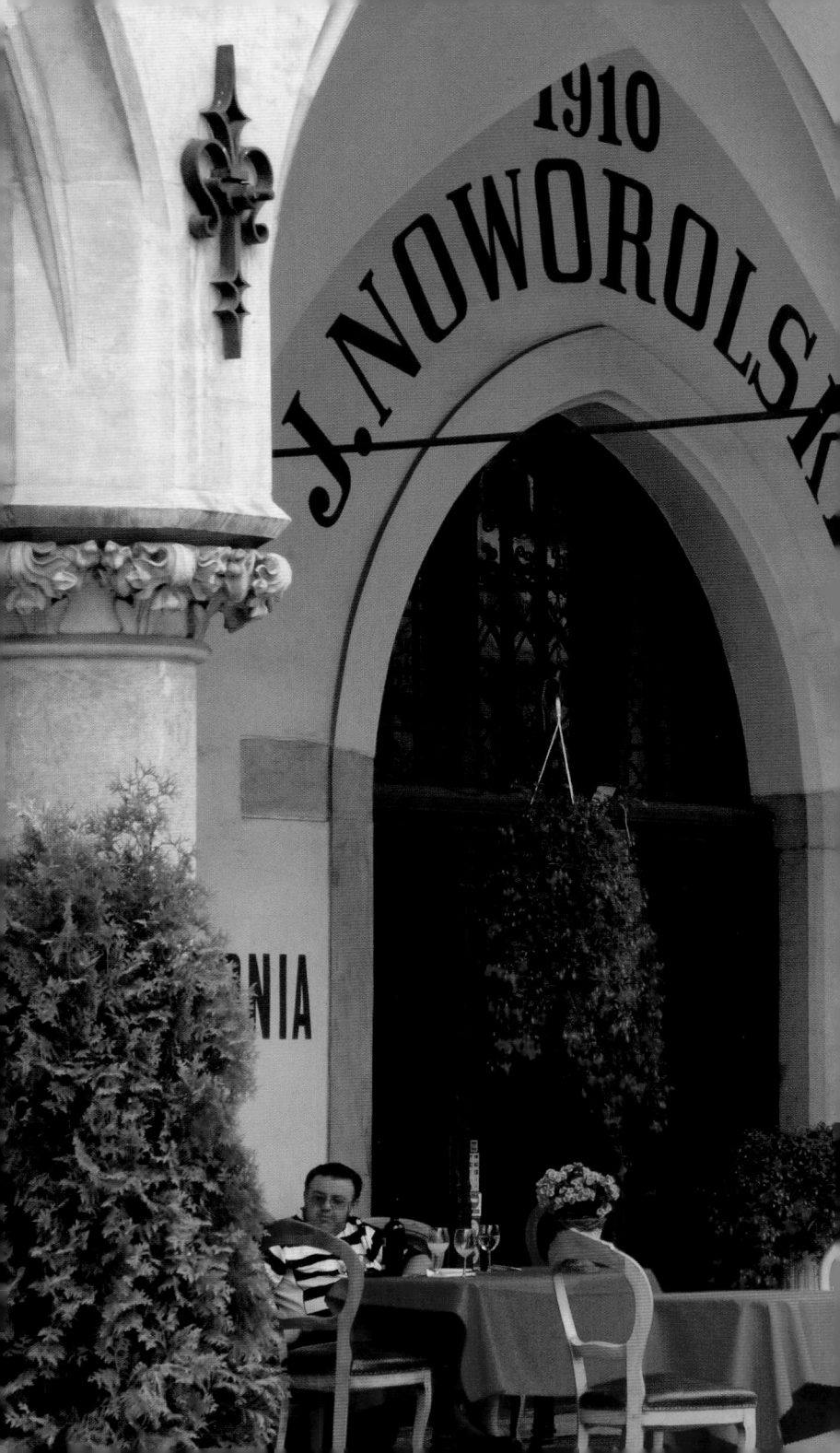

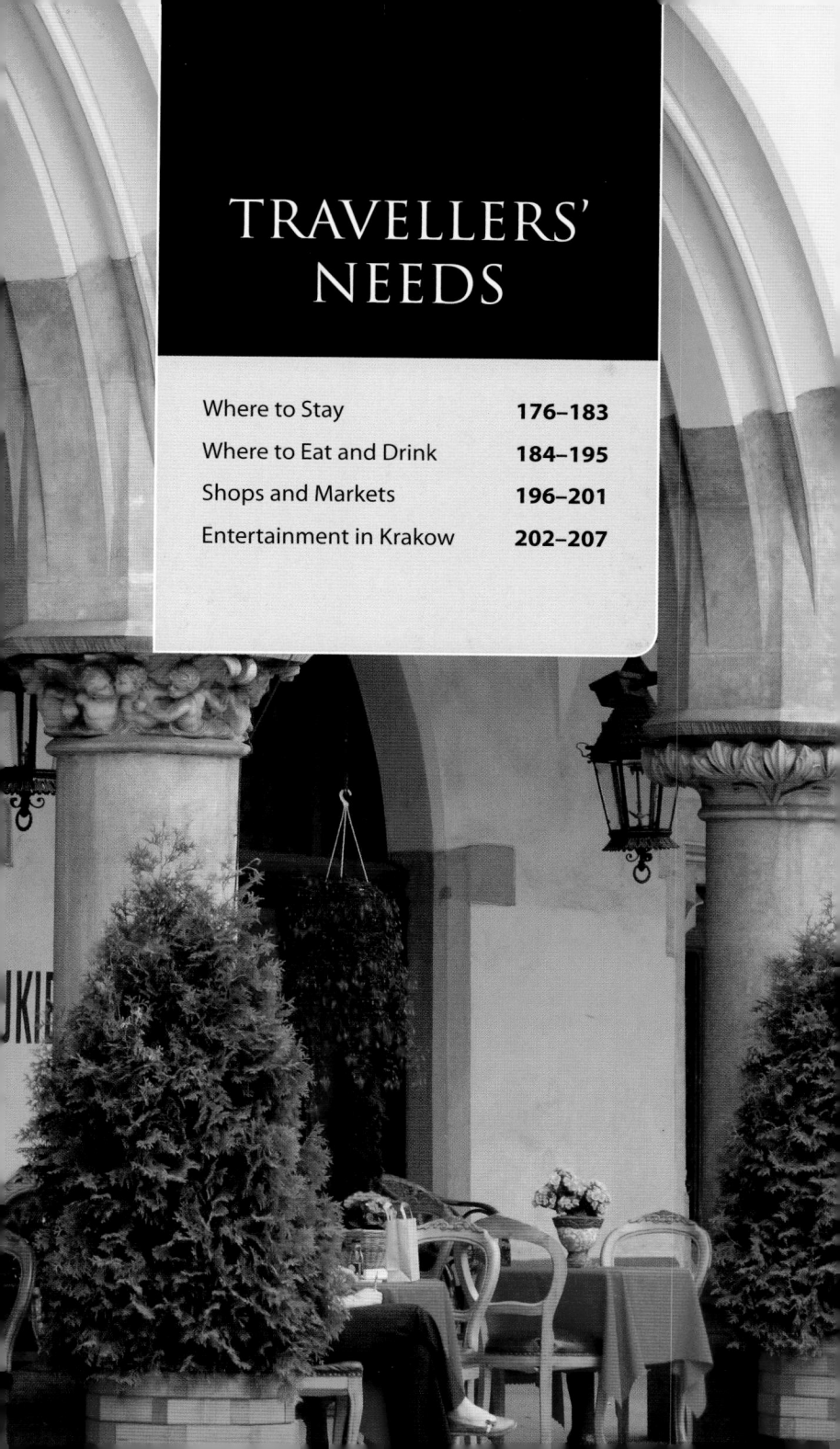

TRAVELLERS' NEEDS

WHERE TO STAY

Krakow is home to some of Poland's best hotels. Besides the big international names, such as Radisson Blu and Sheraton, visitors will also find many independent hotels famed for their architecture, for traditions extending back to the 19th century, and for their *fin-de-siècle* atmosphere. The best of these have managed to recapture the magnificence that was lost during the period of Communist rule. Many of the hotels in the older parts of the city have been renovated, and new establishments have sprung up on the city's fringes and around the river. The number of backpacker hostels has also mushroomed, ensuring that there is a broad choice of accommodation for all budgets. Visitors can still expect to pay a premium for an Old Quarter location, but the competition helps keep prices in check. From all the hotels in Krakow, this section highlights some of the best; they have been listed according to theme, location and price on pages 180–83.

Where to Look

Most of Krakow's hotels are located in the Old Quarter, near the main Market Square; in the former Jewish district of Kazimierz; and in the city-centre districts that surround these two areas. All of these districts are within walking distance of each other, and finding accommodation that is close to the action is never too difficult. Accommodation located outside these central areas is usually linked to the centre by reasonably swift bus or tram services; there are no parts of Krakow where visitors will feel isolated or cut off.

Hotels

Krakow is one of the most atmospheric places to stay in the whole of Central Europe. The city boasts an impressive number of historic, mostly 19th-century hotels, especially grand old establishments like Pod Różą, Pollera, Francuski

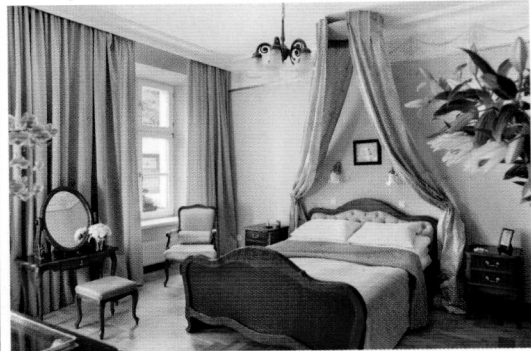

Elegant, flower-filled room at the Polski Hotel Pod Białym Orłem *(see p180)*

and Elektor *(see p180)*, which have preserved the decor and atmosphere of the Belle Époque. There are also many luxury hotels – notably Copernicus *(see p182)*, Stary and Pałac Bonerowski *(see p183)* – that have made good use of old buildings, adapting medieval and Renaissance town houses to the needs of the modern hospitality industry, while leaving much of the original exposed-brick and stone features intact. Modern five-star chains such as Radisson Blu and Sheraton are also present in Krakow, alongside many of the more budget-oriented chains such as Ibis, Best Western, Novotel and Campanile. Recent years have seen the emergence of a breed of boutique and design hotels, such as Pugetów and andel's *(see p182)*, that aim to make best use of the local artistic traditions; and there is also a healthy quantity of B&Bs, offering charming, characterful and informal accommodation in the heart of the city.

Making a Reservation

Most of Krakow's hotels, apartments and hostels are featured on international booking sites such as **Booking**, **Airbnb** and **Hostelworld**.

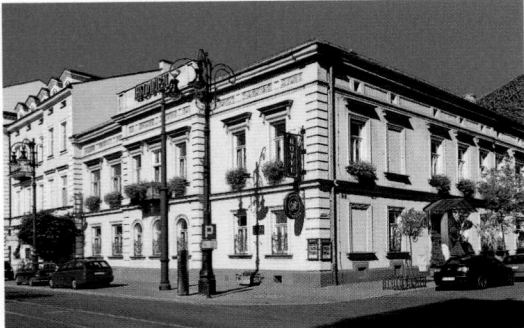

Neo-Classical building housing the Fortuna B&B *(see p181)*

◄ Outdoor dining area at the Noworolski café on Market Square

Reservations can also be made by contacting the establishment directly by phone or email. Early booking is advisable for most of Krakow's hotels, especially during high summer, when finding vacancies may be quite a challenge. Peak times are July and August, the period around the May Day public holiday and New Year's Eve. However, it is worth noting that the tourist season lasts all year round, and only autumn and winter see a decline in the number of tourists. Krakow also sees a constant flow of international conferences, meetings and festivals. Finding a hotel on arrival may prove difficult at any time.

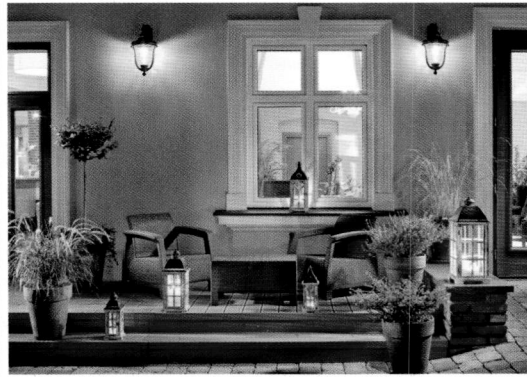

Communal lounge area at the Metropolitan Boutique Hotel *(see p183)*

Facilities

Most hotels offer ensuite rooms with satellite or cable television. The provision of Wi-Fi Internet access is also pretty standard throughout the Polish hotel industry. Even in the better hotels, bathrooms may feature a shower rather than a bathtub, so if you specifically want a bathtub, you should enquire about this when booking. Rooms in the more expensive hotels may have a mini-bar, 24-hour room service and laundry service; some hotels have facilities such as business centres with computers and fax machines. Fitness facilities are increasingly common, but only a handful of hotels in the luxury bracket offer spas or swimming pools. Tourist information is sometimes available at the reception desk, as well as ticket booking facilities for various events.

Check-out time is generally noon, but luggage can usually be left at reception. Hotel personnel frequently speak both English and German.

Discounts

Hotels often advertise rate cuts and budget specials on Internet booking sites. In general, prices tend to fluctuate according to the season, and most hotels in Krakow reduce their prices in autumn and winter. Throughout the year, business and conference hotels, which are often full on weekdays, usually reduce their prices at weekends. There are not many single-bed hotel rooms available for solo travellers, so negotiate a discount when offered a double room for single use.

Wherever you are thinking of staying, it is always worth asking for a discount, and you stand a good chance of getting one if you are planning a longer stay.

Hidden Extras

In accordance with Polish law, the prices quoted or displayed in hotels have to include tax and service. In most places, they also include breakfast, but this is not always the

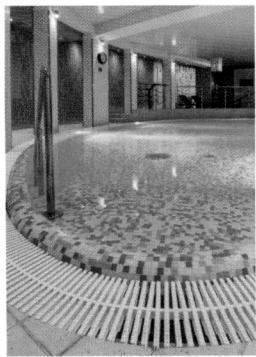

Swimming pool at the contemporary Galaxy hotel *(see p181)*

case, so check in advance. Telephone calls from hotel rooms are never included (even in the best hotels), and they are far more expensive than elsewhere. As an alternative, use one of the numerous card-operated public telephones around town. Phonecards for these are available from newsagents and tobacco kiosks as well as post offices, where you will also find public telephones. Some of the telephone booths situated on the street are specially adapted for wheelchair users.

Although free Wi-Fi Internet access is increasingly standard in the hospitality industry, some hotels (mostly in the business category) may charge for this service; again, it is wise to ask in advance.

Despite these hidden extra costs, Polish hospitality almost always extends to providing guests with a free supply of mineral water. Regardless of the standard of hotel, a fresh bottle of sparkling water is usually left in your room every day. As a rule, if it is not in the mini-bar, it is free.

Tips are not offered to hotel staff, except at the most exclusive hotels where it is customary to offer 10 per cent. You may, however, choose to give less depending on the service you have received. Be aware that saying "thank you" when paying a bill is automatically taken to mean "keep the change".

Travelling with Children

Children are welcome everywhere in Poland. Most hotels offer additional beds for children, and usually no extra charge is made for this as long as the child is under the age of seven or eight. Check when making your reservation. In hotel restaurants there should be no problem in ordering children's portions, and most places also have high chairs. Only the very best hotels offer baby-sitting facilities as part of their service.

Disabled Travellers

Since Poland is a member of the European Union (EU), all hotels must fall in line with EU legislation. This means that any new hotels must include a certain number of rooms for disabled travellers, while all existing hotels must adapt their rooms and common areas to the needs of disabled guests within a strict timeline. The latter part of this legislation has not been strictly enforced, however, and many hotels in Krakow, especially those in the Old Quarter, which have no space for lifts, remain devoid of any facilities for the disabled. As a rule, the newer the hotel (or the more recently it has been renovated), the more likely you are to find suitable access. It is advisable to contact the hotel beforehand to check which facilities for the disabled they have.

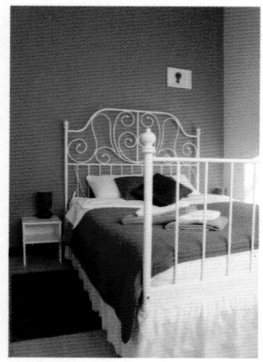

Brightly coloured room at the Secret Garden Hostel *(see p183)*

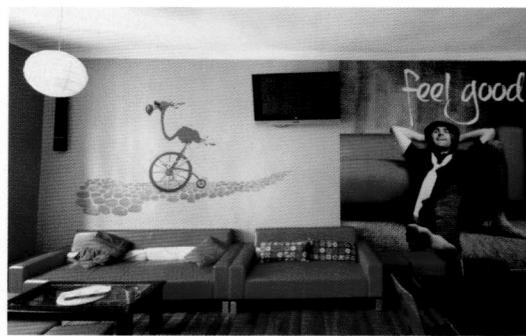

Cheerful decor in the communal lounge at the Flamingo Hostel *(see p183)*

Rooms and Apartments to Let

Many rooms and apartments in Krakow are rented out to tourists for short- or long-term stays. Accommodation of this type can be found in all areas of the city. Apartments in the Old Quarter are often located in beautifully renovated old buildings and are usually more expensive than those further out. Apartments tend to have a fully equipped kitchenette and a TV; many also have Wi-Fi access. Some of the more expensive apartments are cleaned daily or every few days.

Rooms and apartments are often rented out directly by the owner via accommodation websites such as Booking or Airbnb. A number of agents, such as **Krakow Apartments**, **Old City Apartments** and **Sodispar**, rent out holiday apartments in central locations.

B&Bs

There is a small but growing number of bed-and-breakfasts in Krakow, catering for travellers who want something a bit more informal than the average hotel, with the added benefit of friendly and helpful hosts. Krakow's B&Bs tend to have a bit more character than contemporary hotels, frequently featuring homely decor that is in keeping with the often very old buildings in which they are situated. Some of the more characterful B&Bs in Krakow include La Fontaine, Tango House, Wielopole, Klezmer-Hois

and Kolory *(see p181)*. Be aware that rooms might be on the small side. While most B&Bs offer rooms with ensuite bathrooms, some will offer a mixture of ensuite rooms and rooms with shared facilities. Some B&Bs will have someone at reception 24 hours a day, while others may be staffed only at specific daytime hours. Always confirm your arrival time by email or phone to make sure somebody will be there to meet you.

Hostels

There is a huge number of backpacker hostels in Krakow, most of which offer cheap, simple dorm accommodation in fun, informal surroundings. Beds in hostels can be booked via the hostels' own websites or on specialist websites such as Hostelworld. Many hostels offer doubles, triples and quads as well as dorms, and they are increasingly popular with couples and families who enjoy the social aspects of backpacker culture but who want a private room.

Hostels in Krakow vary a great deal in terms of character: some have a bar on site and encourage late-night socializing, while others offer a bit more peace and quiet. The type of atmosphere favoured will be clear from the description on each hostel's website. Many hostels have invested a lot of money in contemporary design and comforts, and are similar in style to small boutique hotels.

Breakfast is available at some Krakow hostels, but not all – this can be checked when making your booking. Due to their popularity, it is advisable to book hostels at least two or three days in advance.

Camping

There is a modest handful of suburban campsites in Krakow, and although they are a fair way from the centre, all are well served by public transport. **Krakowianka** (open from May to September) is a tranquil suburban site next to the wooded Solvay Park, just off the Zakopane road, 6 km (4 miles) south of town. During the summer months there is an open-air swimming pool for the use of the campers, and the Solvay shopping mall is a short walk away; however, there's nothing else of sightseeing or recreational interest in this part of town. **Smok** (open all year) is a privately run site 4 km (2.5 miles) west of town, on the main Oświęcim road, in a pleasant suburban setting with plenty of greenery around.

Recommended Hotels

The places to stay listed on pages 180–83 are the best from a range of accommodation

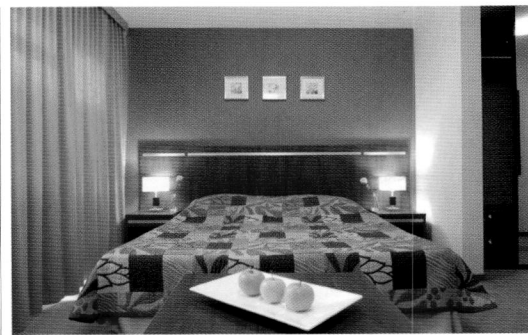

A room in the moden Wyspiański hotel *(see p182)*

types, from charming B&Bs and backpacker hostels to luxury establishments, chains, boutique hotels and the grand, historic hotels for which Krakow is renowned. They are listed by price within each area, be that the narrow alleys of the Old Quarter, bohemian Kazimierz or the pleasant leafy streets just outside the city centre. These lodgings have been featured for their excellent service, wide-ranging facilities or unique character.

Throughout the listings certain hotels have been highlighted as DK Choice. These offer a particularly special experience, such as a beautiful location, spectacular views, a historical setting, outstanding service, a

romantic atmosphere or a combination of these qualities. Whatever the reasons, the DK Choice label is a guarantee of an especially memorable stay. Many of these establishments are popular so it is advisable to book well in advance.

DIRECTORY

Internet Booking Sites

Airbnb
w airbnb.com

Booking
w booking.com

Hostelworld
w hostelworld.com

Rooms and Apartments

Krakow Apartments
Tel 502 501 812.
w krakow-apartments.com

Old City Apartments
Tel 606 941 483.
w oldcityapartments.eu

Sodispar
Tel 12 423 42 44.
w sodispar.pl

Campsites

Krakowianka
ul. Żywiecka Boczna 2.
Tel 12 268 11 33.
w krakowianka.com.pl

Smok
ul. Kamedulska 18.
Tel 12 429 72 66.
w smok.krakow.pl

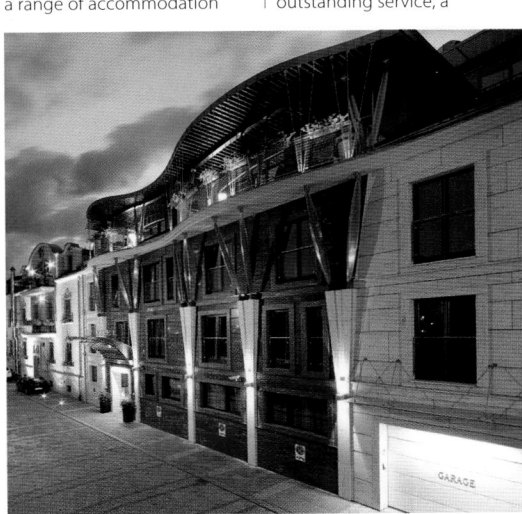

Sleek exterior of the Art Hotel Niebieski, located by the river *(see p183)*

Where to Stay

Historical

Okół and Stradom Quarters

Rezydent zł zł
ul. Grodzka 9
Tel *12 429 54 10* **Map** 6 D3
W rezydent.krakow.pl
Behind its medieval façade, the Rezydent's rooms and suites offer good value for a three-star hotel.

Royal zł zł
ul. Św. Gertrudy
Tel *12 421 35 00* **Map** 6 D5
W hotelewam.pl
Stay in comfortable rooms at the foot of the Wawel Royal Castle in this hotel housed in a 19th-century Art Nouveau building.

Wawel zł zł zł
ul. Poselska 22
Tel *12 424 13 00* **Map** 6 D3
W hotelwawel.pl
In a 16th-century building, the Wawel mixes the old with the new. The large, well-appointed rooms have Art Nouveau-style decor. There is a wellness centre.

Old Quarter

Amadeus zł zł
ul. Mikołajska 20
Tel *12 429 60 70* **Map** 6 E2
W hotel-amadeus.pl
This four-star hotel in a lovely mansion has plush, antique furnishings and a retro feel.

DK Choice

Elektor zł zł
ul. Szpitalna 28
Tel *12 423 23 17* **Map** 6 E2
W hotelelektor.pl
One of the grand old ladies of the Krakow hotel scene, the Elektor preserves an old-world charm. The staff will fall over themselves to help guests, royalty or otherwise: illustrious patrons have included Prince and Princess Takamodo of Japan, King Harald V of Norway and Princess Maha Chakri Sirindhorm of Thailand.

Francuski zł zł
ul. Pijarska 13
Tel *666 195 831* **Map** 6 D1
W hotel-francuski.com
This hotel retains an air of pre-World War I opulence and features retro furnishings and a fine restaurant.

Pod Różą zł zł
ul. Floriańska 14
Tel *12 424 33 00* **Map** 6 E2
W podroza.hotel.com.pl
Balzac and Liszt have stayed in the elegant, high-ceilinged rooms at this hotel, Krakow's oldest.

Pollera zł zł
ul. Szpitalna 32
Tel *12 422 10 44* **Map** 6 E2
W pollera.com.pl
An Art Nouveau classic in the heart of the Old Quarter.

Polski Hotel Pod Białym Orłem zł zł
ul. Pijarska 17
Tel *12 422 11 44* **Map** 6 E1
W podorlem.com.pl
Located next to St Florian's Gate, this comfortable hotel provides traditional accommodation.

Saski zł zł zł
ul. Sławkowska 3
Tel *12 421 42 22* **Map** 6 D2
W hotelsaski.com.pl
A traditional hotel in a 16th-century house, with elegant, retro furnishings and old-school service.

Wit Stwosz zł zł zł
ul. Mikołajska 28
Tel *12 429 60 26* **Map** 6 E2
W hotelws.pl
Housed in an old townhouse just off the main Market Square, this plush hotel has attentive service.

Kazimierz Quarter

Regent zł zł
ul. Bozega Ciala 19
Tel *12 430 62 34* **Map** 4 D2
W rhotels.com.pl
A stylish hotel in a 19th-century building with spacious rooms.

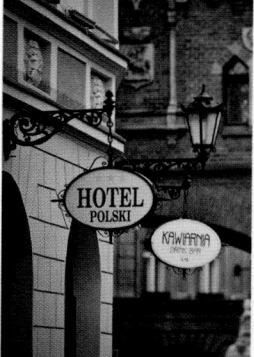
Wrought-iron sign outside the Polski Hotel Pod Białym Orłem

Wesoła, Kleparz and Biskupie

Europejski zł
ul. Lubicz 5
Tel *12 423 25 12* **Map** 6 F1
W he.pl
Founded in the 19th century, this friendly family-run hotel is near the railway station.

Polonia zł zł
ul. Basztowa 25
Tel *12 422 12 33* **Map** 6 F1
W hotel-polonia.com.pl
An Art Nouveau gem dating to World War I, the Polonia is a grand place to stay.

Red Brick Apartments zł zł
ul. Kurniki 3
Tel *12 628 66 00* **Map** 2 D3
W redbrick.pl
These self-catering units in a restored 19th-century building sleep two to six people. Perfect for families or groups.

Piasek and Nowy Świat

Maltanski zł zł zł
ul. Straszewskiego 14
Tel *12 431 00 10* **Map** 5 C4
W donimirski.com
A boutique hotel with luxurious but understated rooms in a restored Neo-Classical building.

Further Afield

Dwór w Tomaszowicach zł zł zł
ul. Krakowska 68, Tomaszowice
Tel *12 419 20 00*
W dwor.pl
In a Neo-Classical manor house, this hotel blends luxury with a rural atmosphere.

B&B

Okół and Stradom Quarters

Globus zł zł
ul. Dietla 91
Tel *12 350 62 65* **Map** 6 F4
W globuskrk.pl
In a converted town house, Globus offers rooms and apartments with elegant decor.

Wielopole   zł zł
ul. Wielopole 3
Tel *12 422 14 75*   **Map** 6 E3
w wielopole.pl
A small, friendly B&B in a 19th-century building.

Old Quarter

Dom Polonii   zł
Rynek Główny 14
Tel *12 422 61 58*   **Map** 6 D2
w wspolnota-polska.krakow.pl
In a classic town house, this guesthouse has three large rooms and friendly staff.

La Fontaine   zł
ul. Sławkowska 1
Tel *12 422 65 64*   **Map** 6 D2
w bblafontaine.com
La Fontaine offers cosy rooms and family-sized apartments.

Tango House   zł
ul. Szpitalna 4
Tel *12 429 31 14*   **Map** 6 E2
w tangohouse.pl
Choose from eight double rooms and two self-catering studios.

Kazimierz Quarter

Abel   zł
ul. Jozefa 30
Tel *12 411 87 36*   **Map** 4 D1
w abelkrakow.pl
The characterful, individually furnished rooms here all have en-suite bathrooms.

Alef   zł
ul. Św. Agnieszki 5
Tel *12 424 31 31*   **Map** 3 C1
w alef.pl
Wooden antique beds, retro furnishings and a hearty breakfast feature at this popular B&B.

Klezmer-Hois   zł
ul. Szeroka 6
Tel *12 411 12 45*   **Map** 4 E1
w klezmer.pl
This characterful guesthouse is full of 19th-century artifacts.

DK Choice

Kolory   zł
ul. Estery 10
Tel *12 421 04 65*   **Map** 4 D1
w kolory.com.pl
The bright, homely rooms at Kolory are decorated with Polish folk art. It is in the centre of the nightlife zone, so ask for a room at the back of the building to minimize street noise. Breakfast is served in Les Couleurs café on the ground floor, whose croissants and coffee rank among the best in Krakow .

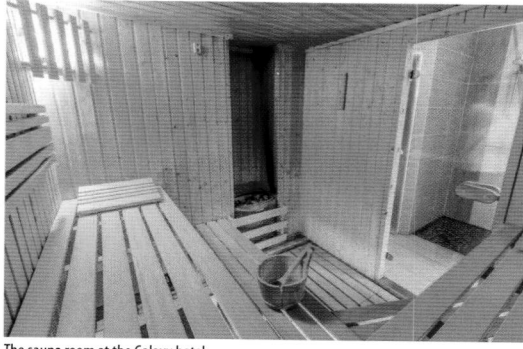
The sauna room at the Galaxy hotel

Tournet   zł
ul. Miodowa 7
Tel *12 292 00 88*   **Map** 4 D1
w nocleg.krakow.pl
Tournet offers simply furnished, well-maintained rooms on one of Kazimierz's quieter streets.

Eden   zł zł
ul. Ciemna 15
Tel *12 430 65 65*   **Map** 4 D1
w hoteleden.pl
Offering large but simple rooms, Eden also has a kosher restaurant and a healing salt grotto.

Wesoła, Kleparz and Biskupie

Jordan   zł
ul. Długa 9
Tel *12 430 02 92*   **Map** 1 C3
w nocleg.jordan.pl
Above a travel agent, Jordan offers simple, pleasant rooms on a lively shopping street near colourful markets.

Piasek and Nowy Świat

Fortuna   zł zł
ul. Czapskch 5
Tel *12 422 31 43*   **Map** 5 B3
w hotel-fortuna.com.pl
In a charming building, Fortuna has decent-sized rooms and large bathrooms. Friendly service.

Modern

Okół and Stradom Quarters

Best Western Krakow Old Town   zł zł
ul. Św. Gertrudy
Tel *12 422 76 66*   **Map** 6 E4
w bwkrakow.pl
This four-star hotel is well placed for visiting the Old Quarter.

Old Quarter

Floryan   zł zł
ul. Floriańska 38
Tel *12 431 14 18*   **Map** 6 E2
w http://floryan.com.pl
At the top of a historic town house, this highly individual hotel has contemporary design and an intimate vibe.

Unicus Hotel   zł zł
ul. Św. Marka 20
Tel *12 433 71 11*   **Map** 6 E2
w hotelunicus.pl
In a historic building, Unicus is contemporary on the inside, with a grey and brown colour scheme.

Kazimierz Quarter

Columbus   zł zł
ul. Starowiślna 57
Tel *12 252 75 50*   **Map** 4 E1
w hotelcolumbus.pl
The Columbus has rooms decked out in warm colours, attentive staff and a good buffet breakfast.

Galaxy   zł zł
ul. Gęsia 22a
Tel *12 342 81 00*   **Map** 4 F1
w http://galaxyhotel.com
A hotel with designer rooms in bright colours, Galaxy also has a pool and a spa centre.

Karmel   zł zł
ul. Kupa 15
Tel *12 430 67 00*   **Map** 4 D1
w karmel.com.pl
A welcoming guesthouse with high-ceilinged rooms, the Karmel features an antique-meets-modern decor.

Kazimierz   zł zł
ul. Miodowa 16
Tel *12 421 66 29*   **Map** 4 D1
w hk.com.pl
The comfortable modern rooms in this contemporary building feature stained-glass windows with scenes from local history.

For more information on types of hotels *see pages 176–9*

Secesja zł zł
ul. Paulinska 24
Tel *12 430 74 64* **Map** 3 C2
🅦 hotelsecesja.pl
On the quieter side of Kazimierz, this cosy hotel has Art Nouveau-inspired decor in warm colours.

Wesoła, Kleparz and Biskupie

Ibis Budget Stare Miasto zł
ul. Pawia 11
Tel *12 355 29 50* **Map** 2 D3
🅦 ibisbudget.com
Next to the main railway station, this no-frills hotel has well-equipped but functional rooms.

Atrium zł zł
ul. Krzywa 7
Tel *12 430 02 03* **Map** 1 C3
🅦 hotelatrium.com.pl
A good option near the railway station, Atrium offers 50 rooms and two suites with kitchenettes.

Batory zł zł
ul. Soltyka 19
Tel *12 294 30 30* **Map** 2 E5
🅦 hotelbatory.pl
This brightly decorated hotel in a quiet location has friendly staff and a cosy atmosphere.

Puro Hotel zł zł
ul. Ogrodowa 10
Tel *12 314 21 00* **Map** 2 D3
🅦 purohotel.pl
Opposite the railway station and the Galeria shopping centre, Puro has sleek, minimalist but well-equipped rooms with large windows.

Wyspiański zł zł
ul. Westerplatte 15
Tel *12 422 95 66* **Map** 6 F2
🅦 hotel-wyspianski.pl
This large, functional hotel is a reliable option, offering three-star comforts close to the Old Town.

DK Choice

andel's zł zł zł
ul. Pawia 3
Tel *12 660 00 10* **Map** 6 F1
🅦 andelskrakow.com
Jutting out into the plaza in front of the main railway station like an ocean liner, andel's offers design-conscious, supremely comfortable rooms in harmonious colours. It is a place for spending quality time in rather than just sleeping, while its location opposite Planty Park and the Old Quarter makes it a perfect sightseeing base.

Piasek and Nowy Świat

Kossak zł zł
Pl. Juliusza Kossaka 1
Tel *12 379 59 00* **Map** 5 B4
🅦 hotelkossak.com
A smart hotel with contemporary design touches. Rooms on the upper floor offer good views of the castle and the river.

Logos zł zł
ul. Szujskiego 5
Tel *12 631 62 00* **Map** 1 B4
🅦 hotel-logos.pl
The stylish Logos offers large rooms with great bathrooms. There are sauna and spa facilities.

Further Afield

Dom Goscinny Przegorzaly zł
ul. Jodlowa 13
Tel *12 429 71 15*
🅦 dg.uj.edu.pl/przegorzaly
This student campus on the fringes of Las Wolski forest offers tourist accommodation over the summer. Rooms are bright and plain; the surroundings, peaceful.

Ruczaj zł
ul. Ruczaj 44
Tel *12 269 10 00*
🅦 ruczajhotel.pl
Rooms have large windows and enormous beds at this charming hotel in a leafy suburb. It has a sauna and solarium.

Teresita zł
ul. Schweitzera 3
Tel *12 657 94 77*
🅦 teresita.pl
Kitsch decor and loud colours make the gypsy-themed Teresita a fun place to stay, with simple but comfortable rooms.

Chopin zł zł
ul. Przy Rondzie 2
Tel *12 299 00 00*
🅦 vi-hotels.com
This functional hotel, a 20-minute walk from the city centre, offers brightly coloured rooms, efficient staff and good facilities.

Ibis Krakow Centrum zł zł
ul. Syrokomli 2
Tel *12 299 33 00*
🅦 accorhotels.com
Just a short tram ride from the city centre, this hotel offers spacious, comfortable rooms.

Novotel Centrum zł zł zł
ul. T. Kościuszki 5
Tel *12 299 29 00* **Map** 5 C5
🅦 accorhotels.com
Bright rooms, great service and a generous buffet breakfast are the main draws here. There is a gym, sauna and swimming pool.

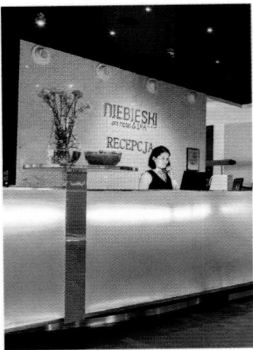

The sleek reception area of the luxurious Art Hotel Niebieski in Zwierzyniec

Luxury

Okół and Stradom Quarters

Copernicus zł zł zł
ul. Kanonicza 16
Tel *12 424 3400* **Map** 6 D4
🅦 copernicus.hotel.com.pl
In a Renaissance town house, this hotel features beautiful historic interiors and spacious rooms.

Pugetów zł zł zł
ul. Starowislna 15a
Tel *12 432 4950* **Map** 6 E4
🅦 donimirski.com/hotel-pugetow
This hotel has original artworks and sumptuous rooms.

Queen Boutique Hotel zł zł zł
ul. Dietla 60
Tel *12 433 3333* **Map** 6 E5
🅦 queenhotel.pl
In a 19th-century town house, this hotel offers plush rooms with contemporary furnishings.

Senacki zł zł zł
ul. Grodzka 51
Tel *12 422 7686* **Map** 6 D4
🅦 hotelsenacki.pl
This hotel with well-equipped rooms is in a historic building.

Old Quarter

Grodek zł zł
ul. na gródku 4
Tel *12 431 9030* **Map** 6 E3
🅦 donimirski.com/hotel-grodek
Adjoining a Dominican convent, the opulent 5-star Grodek offers high-end comfort.

Grand zł zł zł
ul. Slawkowska 5–7
Tel *12 424 0800* **Map** 6 D2
🅦 grand.pl
A historic hotel with antique furnishings and superb amenities.

Pałac Bonerowski zł zł zł
ul. Św. Jana 1
Tel *12 374 13 00* **Map** 6 D2
Ⓦ palacbonerowski.pl
This 16th-century mansion retains
some historic features. The
bathrooms are totally modern.

DK Choice

Stary zł zł zł
ul. Szczepańska 5
Tel *12 384 08 08* **Map** 6 D2
Ⓦ stary.hotel.com.pl
In a 15th-century merchant's
house, Stary retains many
original features, such as
exposed brick and stone, high
ceilings and wall paintings.
Furnishings are contemporary
and bathrooms have the
highest quality marble.
Amenities include a swimming
pool, saunas and a spa centre
that boasts salt inhalation
among its treatments.

Wentzl zł zł zł
Rynek Główny 19
Tel *12 430 26 64* **Map** 6 D3
Ⓦ wentzl.pl
Elegant rooms here have views
over the main Market Square.

Kazimierz Quarter

**Metropolitan
Boutique Hotel** zł zł zł
ul. Berka Joselewicza 19
Tel *12 442 75 00* **Map** 4 D1
Ⓦ hotelmetropolitan.pl
This plush, modern hotel offers
large rooms in soothing colours
and a generous buffet breakfast.

Wesoła, Kleparz and Biskupie

Komorowski zł zł zł
ul. Długa 7
Tel *505 989 371* **Map** 1 C3
Ⓦ hotelkomorowski.com
Ideal for a romantic break, this
boutique guesthouse has rich
colours and lavish furnishings.

Piasek and Nowy Świat

Amber Design zł zł zł
ul. Garbarska 8–10
Tel *12 421 06 06* **Map** 5 C1
Ⓦ hotel-amber.pl
Murals inspired by the Art
Nouveau artist Stanisław
Wyspiański adorn the rooms here.

Sheraton zł zł zł
ul. Powisle 7
Tel *12 662 10 00* **Map** 5 B4
Ⓦ sheraton.pl/krakow
The Sheraton offers high-end
comfort and service by the river.

Further Afield

Art Hotel Niebieski zł zł zł
ul. Flisacka 3
Tel *12 297 40 00*
Ⓦ niebieski.com.pl
Large rooms have all mod cons
at this tranquil hotel by the river.

Qubus zł zł zł
ul. Nadwislańska 6
Tel *12 374 51 00* **Map** 4 E2
Ⓦ qubushotel.com
Large and superbly equipped,
this hotel south of the Vistula is
perfect for exploring Kazimierz.

Sympozjum zł zł zł
ul. Kobierzynska 47
Tel *12 261 86 00*
Ⓦ sympozium.com.pl
A popular conference hotel with
great dining and a lively bar.

Hostel

Okoł and Stradom Quarters

DK Choice

Mundo Hostel zł
ul. J. Sarego 10
Tel *12 422 61 13* **Map** 6 E4
Ⓦ mundohostel.eu
Rooms at this boutique hostel
have a geographic theme and
contain ethnic-influenced *objets
d'art* and textiles. There is a
communal kitchen. A quieter
option than some of the other
backpacker places in town.

Old Quarter

Flamingo Hostel zł
ul. Szewska 4
Tel *12 422 00 00* **Map** 6 D2
Ⓦ flamingo-hostel.com
A firm favourite, this hostel is off
the main square, on a lively street.

Tulip Hostel zł
Pl. Wszystkich Świętych 8
Tel *513 399 690* **Map** 6 D3
Ⓦ tuliphostel.pl
Tulip has two-, three- and four-
bed rooms with wooden floors.
There is a fully equipped kitchen .

Tutti Frutti zł
ul. Floriańska 29
Tel *12 428 00 28* **Map** 6 E2
Ⓦ tuttifruttihostel.com
A mixture of dorms and four-bed
rooms is on offer at this central
but relaxing hostel.

Kazimierz Quarter

Goodbye Lenin zł
ul. Berka Joselewicza 23
Tel *12 421 20 30* **Map** 4 E1
Ⓦ goodbyeleninhostel.com
In a ramshackle old house
adorned with Pop Art murals, this
is an enjoyable, sociable hostel.

Secret Garden Hostel zł
ul. Skawińska 7
Tel *12 430 54 45* **Map** 3 C2
Ⓦ thesecretgarden.com
Hidden away in a quiet corner of
Kazimierz, this hostel offers bright
dorms and double rooms, and a
relaxing vibe. Closed 24–27 Dec.

Wesoła, Kleparz and Biskupie

Greg & Tom Hostel zł
ul. Pawia 12–17
Tel *12 422 41 00* **Map** 6 F1
Ⓦ gregtomhostel.com
This hostel has dorms and double
rooms with neat furnishings and a
fully equipped kitchen .

Mosquito Hostel zł
Rynek Kleparski 4–6
Tel *12 430 14 61* **Map** 1 C3
Ⓦ mosquitohostel.com
Mosquito offers a mixture of
dorms and private rooms.

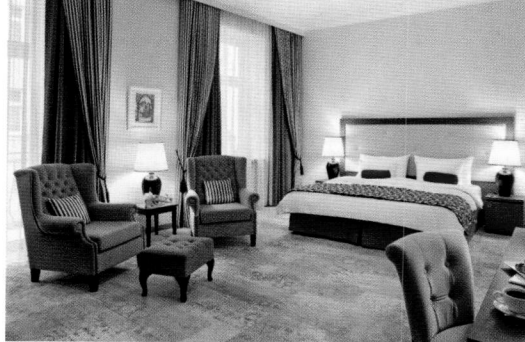

An elegant room at the Metropolitan Boutique Hotel

For more information on types of hotels *see pages 176–9*

WHERE TO EAT AND DRINK

Krakow has always been known as a good place for eating out. Even during the Communist era, when Polish restaurants were notorious for having very little on the menu, Krakow's culinary culture survived unscathed. Now one of the busiest tourist destinations in the country, Krakow boasts hundreds of restaurants, many of the highest quality. Traditional Polish food is at its best here – whether in the budget canteen restaurants where customers queue up to order at the counter, or in the finer restaurants serving traditional specialities like roast duck with apples. There is a growing number of haute cuisine restaurants offering Mediterranean, French and contemporary Polish cooking, often blended with Asian influences. Italian, Asian, Mexican and South American eateries can all be found in Krakow. Some of the best eateries in the city are listed on pages 190–93.

Restaurants

Those who enjoy good food in a pleasant atmosphere will not be disappointed in Krakow. Many of the city's restaurants are housed in historic buildings or medieval cellars, usually painstakingly restored and tastefully furnished. Eateries in the bohemian quarter of Kazimierz frequently opt for a range of retro styles, with candles on the table and antique furniture. Restaurants on the main Market Square and on Szeroka Street in Kazimierz have large areas of outdoor seating, although pavement terraces are a rarity elsewhere. Evenings and weekends tend to be particularly busy, so booking a table in advance is advisable. Wherever you go, restaurants are not too formal, and there is no real dress code.

Canteen Restaurants and Vodka-and-Herring Bars

Much of the best local food can be enjoyed in a *jadłodajnia* (also known as a *bar mleczny* or

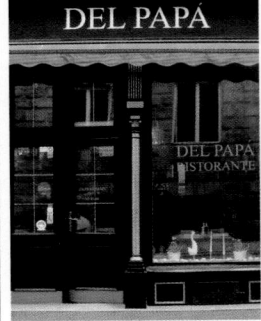

Del Papá, considered by many to be one of Krakow's best Italian restaurants *(see p192)*

"milk bar"), a budget canteen restaurant where customers order at the counter, choosing from a menu of inexpensive soups, *pierogi*, potato pancakes, pork chops and other Polish staples. The decor is often plain in these places, but prices are rock bottom – visitors can enjoy a three-course meal for as little as 20zł. *Jadłodajnias* often close early – usually late afternoon or early evening, or when the food has sold out.

The Krakow dining scene is witnessing a rise in the number of vodka-and-herring bars, some of which are open round the clock. These places sell spirits and traditional bar snacks (marinated herring being one ubiquitous favourite) for very little money.

Street Food

Krakow pretzels, or *obwarzanki*, are sold by street vendors throughout the city and make an excellent snack. Very much a local speciality, they are traditionally coated with salt crystals, poppy seeds or sesame seeds. You will also see street sellers offering delicious hunks of *oscypek*, smoked sheep's cheese from the Tatra Mountains.

Arguably Poland's favourite street snack, the *zapiekanka* is a halved baguette covered in meat, cheese and vegetables, then toasted. *Zapiekanki* are sold from fast-food kiosks all over the city, notably on plac Nowy, the centre of nightlife in Kazimierz.

Another ubiquitous feature of the Krakow street-food scene is the grilled sausage. The best sausages are sold at the outdoor grill on plac Nowy in Kazimierz and at the kiosk near the Market Hall in Grzegórzecka Street, where they are available until 3 o'clock in the morning.

Eating at Night

The majority of restaurants in Krakow close around midnight, but several establishments in

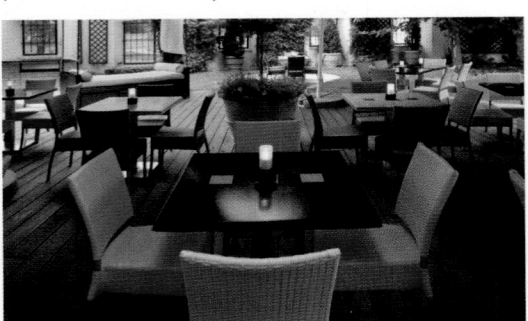

The chic outdoor area at Someplace Else, within the Sheraton Hotel *(see p193)*

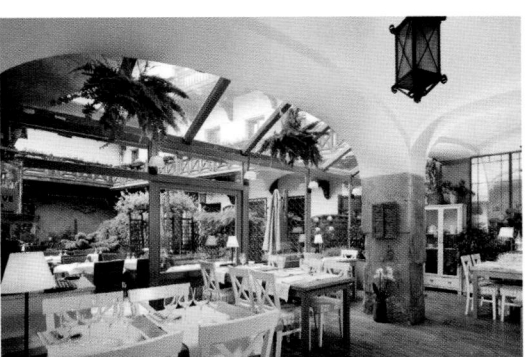

Pimiento Argentino, with decor in the style of an Argentinian hacienda *(see p191)*

Kazimierz are open till 1 or 2am. Several vodka-and-herring bars in the Old Quarter stay open round the clock. Plenty of street-food outlets keep going beyond midnight, and it is usually possible to pick up a pizza slice or a *zapiekanka* in the Old Quarter or in Kazimierz well into the early hours.

Prices and Tips

The price of food in Krakow's restaurants is below the European average. A three-course meal without alcohol will cost about 100zł per person in all but the most expensive places. However, drinking alcohol with your meal will add a substantial amount to your bill.

Credit cards are becoming ever more popular and should be readily accepted by all the larger restaurants and those located on the main tourist trail. Signs on windows or doors indicate which cards are accepted by the establishment.

All over Poland a customary tip amounts to about ten per cent of the bill.

Vegetarian Food

The majority of restaurants in Krakow serve at least a handful of vegetarian dishes. Traditional local specialities, such as *pierogi* (dumplings) filled with wild mushrooms,

cheese, sauerkraut or fruit, are very popular, as are all kinds of savoury pancakes, omelettes and *knedle* (potato dumplings). A choice of many colourful and tasty salads is available in all restaurants. Beetroot, carrots, cabbage, cauliflower, celeriac and leeks are traditional Polish favourites. Broccoli, aubergines, celery, endives and courgettes have also been introduced to Polish cuisine. Vegetarian food is available not only from most ethnic restaurants, but also from salad bars, which are very popular and also serve freshly pressed fruit and vegetable

juices. In some restaurants you can create your own salad from a selection of ingredients.

Recommended Restaurants

The restaurants listed on pages 190–93 have been selected to give a cross-section of the most noteworthy places to eat in Krakow. Whether located in the lively main Market Square, the medieval brick cellars of the Old Quarter and Okół or the former Jewish quarter of Kazimierz, they all have an evocative ambience.

The listings cover a vast variety of eateries and cuisine types, from traditional Polish canteens to pizzerias and ethnic restaurants, from places specializing in fish and seafood to designer bistros, and from characterful cafés to smart, elegant restaurants offering fine dining.

Throughout the listings some establishments have been labelled as DK Choice. These stand out from the crowd and offer something particularly special, such as superb local specialities, excellent value for money, a beautiful location, a historical setting, a romantic atmosphere, particular charm or a combination of these factors.

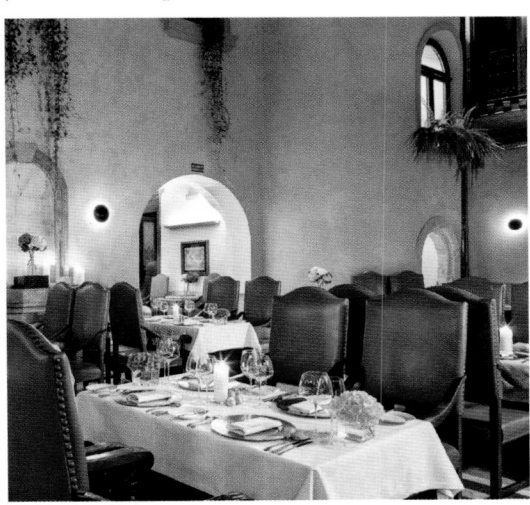

The elegant dining area at Copernicus *(see p190)*

The Flavours of Krakow

Polish cuisine, like that of many central European countries, makes heavy use of meat, especially pork, which is often served quite plainly with potatoes or rice and cabbage. However, because of the long Baltic coastline in the north of the country, fish is also likely to feature on many menus. Carp, trout and herring are particular favourites. Around Krakow, in the south, the local forests yield a bounty of quality game, with duck being very popular. The legacy of former rule by Austria is also evident in the south, especially in some of the sophisticated cakes and pastries.

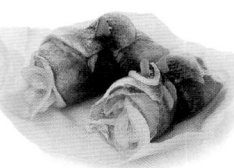

Pickled herring

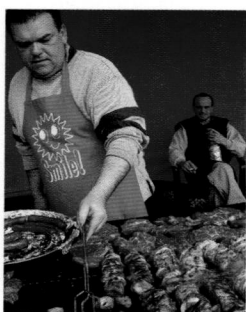

Barbecuing meat at a street celebration on Palm Sunday

Meat

Pork (wieprzowina) is the most popular meat by far in Poland. It usually comes as a steak (kotlet schabowy) or on the bone (golonka wieprzowa) and also appears in soups, sausages and as hams. Polish hams are generally cured and have a rich, sweet flavour. Ham is mainly served cold as an appetizer with cheese and pickles, though it may also be eaten for breakfast. Poland also produces high quality veal (cielęcina), which is often dished up with a rich mushroom sauce (cielęcina po staropolsku) or with cabbage and raisins.

Poultry and Game

Chicken (kurczak) is a staple food in Poland and drumsticks (podudzie) are especially popular. Chicken livers (wątróbka), served with a fruit sauce, are considered a delicacy.

A wide variety of game roams the forests of southern Poland. Pheasant (bażant), duck (kaczka), goose (gęś), venison (comber), rabbit (królik) and hare (zajqc) are found on many local menus. Availability varies with the season; autumn is the best time to enjoy game.

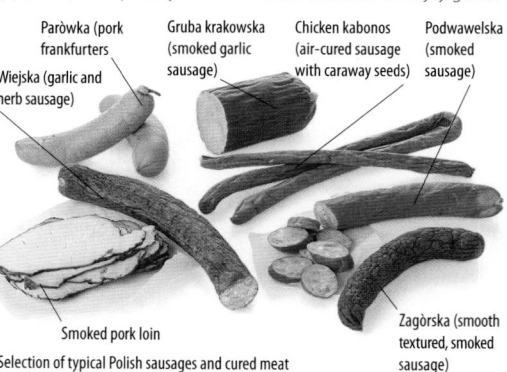

Paròwka (pork frankfurters

Gruba krakowska (smoked garlic sausage)

Chicken kabonos (air-cured sausage with caraway seeds)

Podwawelska (smoked sausage)

Wiejska (garlic and herb sausage)

Smoked pork loin

Zagòrska (smooth textured, smoked sausage)

Selection of typical Polish sausages and cured meat

Local Dishes and Specialities

Many classic Polish dishes are offered at restaurants all over the country, but fish also features prominently on northern menus, while those of the the south offer a range of game. The most varied and cosmopolitan cuisine is found in large cities, such as Warsaw and Krakow, where top chefs run the kitchens of some of the grand hotels. The national dish, bigos, comes from eastern Poland. It is hearty and warming for the long, bleak winters found there, as is another dish from this chilly region, pierogi (pasta dumplings, stuffed with meat, cheese or fruit). Both are influenced by the food of neighbouring Russia. Polish cakes and desserts also tend to be heavy and rich, although most originate in the warmer south, once ruled by Austria.

Green cabbage

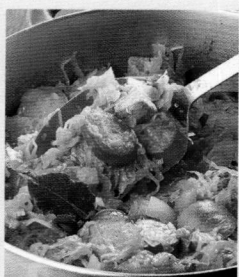

Bigos Chunks of meat and sausage are simmered with sauerkraut, cabbage, onion, potatoes, herbs and spices.

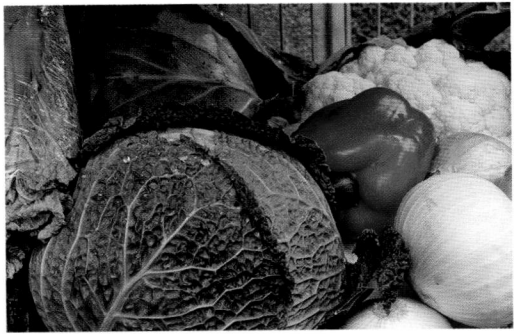

A colourful display of locally grown vegetables at a city market stall

Fish

Fish features strongly on menus in northern Poland, where herring *(śledź)* is a central part of the diet. It comes pickled, in oil, with onions, with soured cream – in fact, with just about everything. *Rolmops po kaszubsku* (marinated herring wrapped around pickled onion, then spiked with cloves and dipped in soured cream) are widely enjoyed. Other popular fish are freshwater trout *(pstrąg)* – served simply grilled with boiled potatoes; carp *(karp)* – often accompanied by horseradish sauce; and salmon *(łosoś)*. A treat in early summer is smoked salmon served with spears of fresh asparagus *(łosoś wędzony ze szparagami)*, which is then in season.

Vegetables

Poland produces many fine quality vegetables. The hardy cabbage *(kapusta)* remains the country's top vegetable. It is used in so many ways, including raw in salads and simply boiled to partner meat or fish. Cabbage soup

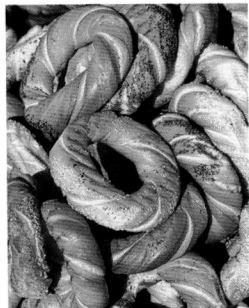

Polish pretzels on sale in a Krakow bread shop

(kapuśniak) and sauerkraut are on every menu. Potatoes are also a staple. They come boiled, baked and mashed, though rarely roasted. Peppers are popular too, often served stuffed with rice and minced meat or pickled in summer salads. Root vegetables such as carrots, parsnips, swede (rutabaga), turnips and beetroot make their way into a range of dishes. Mushrooms grow wild all over Poland and come both cooked and pickled as a tasty addition to many meals.

SNACKS

Sausages A wide range of smoked and unsmoked varieties are on offer at the profusion of street stalls and snack bars that can be found on most city streets.

Precles (pretzels) Another favourite street snack, these are popular, freshly baked, at train and bus stations first thing in the morning.

Zapiekanki Often referred to as Polish-style pizzas, these are tasty, open-top baguettes, spread with cheese and tomato, then toasted and served piping hot. They are also a common item on street-stall menus.

Smalec This snack consists of fried lard, liberally sprinkled with sea salt, and eaten with chunks of crusty bread. It can be found as a bar snack in most pubs and makes a good accompaniment to beer.

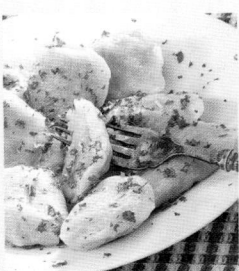

Pierogi These ravioli-style dumplings may be stuffed with meat, sauerkraut, mushrooms, cheese or fruit.

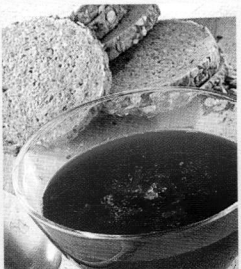

Barszcz This beetroot soup, flavoured with lemon and garlic, may be served clear or with beans or potatoes.

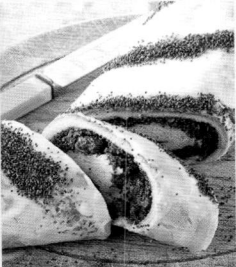

Poppy seed roll A rich yeasted dough is wrapped around a sweet poppy-seed filling and baked until lightly golden.

What to Drink in Krakow

In Krakow, as indeed anywhere in Poland, you may try many different brands of exquisite vodkas, both clear and flavoured. Beer is becoming ever more popular and its production is growing rapidly. There are many bars in Krakow that offer a large selection of beers, especially beers brewed in Poland. Poland does not produce quality wines but shops and restaurants offer a large selection of brands imported from all over the world, especially from throughout Europe and the New World.

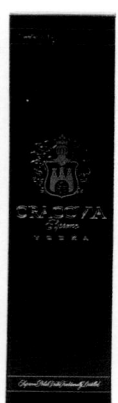
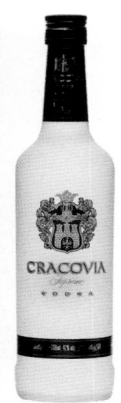

Cracovia, one of the best Polish clear vodkas

Vodka

Vodka distilled from potatoes or grain is a Polish speciality. Such brands as clear *Wódka Wyborowa* and dry but flavoured *Żubrówka* are both world-famous. The variety of vodka brands produced in Poland may be bewildering. Clear *Cracovia*, which has been produced in Krakow for some years, is very popular. *Starka* is definitely the oldest brand among quality vodkas. For centuries *starka* was made from unrectified grain spirit, which was aged for at least six years in reused oak wine-casks. The casks used to be buried for ageing, but this is no longer the case. Krakow *Starka* was once regarded as the "queen" of all *starkas*, but has lost this status.

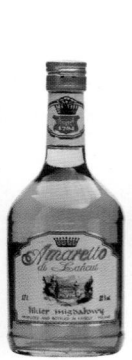

Starka krakowska vodka

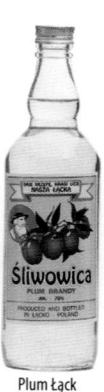

Dzięgielówka, a dry vodka flavoured with angelica root

Polish distilleries have been decentralized, but have retained the recipes imposed during Communist rule. Above all the lack of an *appellation contrôlée* has resulted in the fact that, if you buy a *Starka krakowska* (Krakow starka), be prepared to accept that it may have been produced elsewhere. (Another example is the renowned Goldwasser liqueur which was unique to Gdańsk but is now produced in Poznań.) *Starka bankietowa* is aged for longer and is definitely one of the best. It is sold in crystal-glass bottles and is a luxurious drink difficult to find elsewhere.

Good kosher plum vodka is distilled in Poland. *Śliwowica łącka* is the best and most famous of all plum vodkas. Paradoxically, it is produced illegally owing to the lack of proper regulations. It is home-made in the small village of Łącko in the mountain region, some 70 km (43 miles) south of Krakow. Śliwowica Łącka is not available from off-licences (liquor stores) but is offered in many households in Krakow.

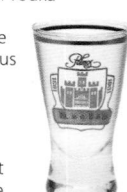

A vodka glass

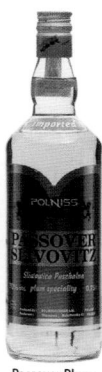

Amaretto liqueur

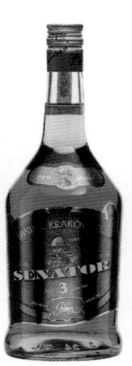

Plum Łąck brandy

Passover Plum vodka

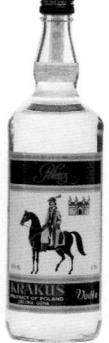

Senator vodka

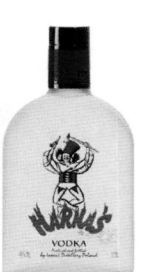

Krakus vodka

Harnaś vodka

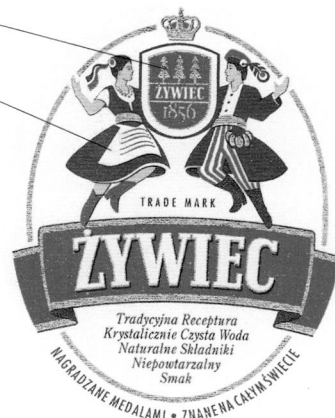

Żywiec logo with the date of establishment

A dancing couple in traditional costumes from the Krakow region

Żywiec Beer Label

Many brands of beer are produced by the Żywiec Brewery, but bottles with the couple dressed in traditional Krakow costumes sell best.

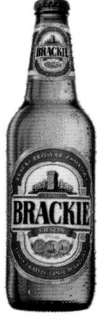

Brackie beer from Żywiec

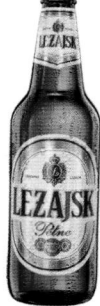

Lezajsk beer from Żywiec

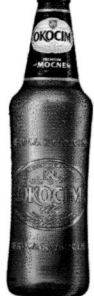

Beer from the Okocim Brewery

Beer

Polish breweries have developed rapidly over the years. The production of quality beer has grown and been modernized. Figures show that Poles are drinking more and more beer and less strong alcohol.

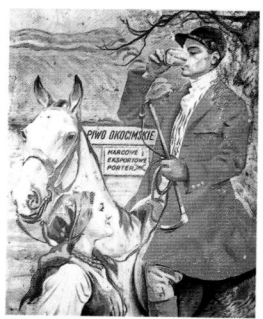

Pre-1939 advertisement of the Okocim Brewery

Beers from Okocim and Żywiec are traditionally the most popular in Krakow. Kracovians are still very aware that both breweries were established in Galicia. The Okocim brewery was founded by the Goetz family who were raised to the rank of hereditary barons by Emperor Franz Joseph. The Żywiec brewery was set up and owned, until World War II, by the Habsburg Archdukes. The grim paradox was that this Żywiec branch of the Habsburgs, who took up Polish citizenship after World War I, had their brewery confiscated by the Nazis after they refused to sign the *Volkslist*. After World War II the Communists nationalized Żywiec as a former German property. Heineken, the Dutch brewer, acquired a majority holding in the enterprise a few years ago, and the brewery is now one of the most technologically advanced in Europe.

Wine

Although vineyards were cultivated in the Krakow area quite successfully, they disappeared in the 15th century. Large quantities of quality wine were produced until World War II in the Zaleszczyki region on the then Romanian border. Today only a few vineyards can be found near Zielona Góra in the far west of the country, which means that Poland's wine production is negligible. Any visitor to Krakow wishing to drink wine will find a large selection of imported wines both in shops and restaurants.

Wine comes from many countries, including France, Italy, Spain and Austria, as well as California, Australia, Chile and New Zealand. Hungarian wine, however, is to be recommended in Krakow. This is not only because of its budget price. For centuries Krakow was a place where Tokay wines were stored for ageing, in barrels housed in large cellars beneath Market Square, before being exported all over the world.

Non-Alcoholic Drinks

Mineral water, sparkling and still, is the most popular non-alcoholic drink. Many brands of mineral water come from the springs in the mountain foothills or highlands not far from Krakow. Fruit juices are also popular. Apple and blackcurrant juices are Polish specialities.

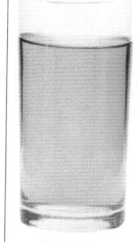

Apple juice

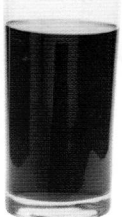

Blackcurrant juice

Where to Eat and Drink

Wawel Hill

Pod Basztą   zł
Traditional Polish   **Map** 3 C1
Zamek Wawel 9
Tel *12 422 75 28*
This stalwart has a well-earned
reputation for good authentic
Polish cooking and reasonable
prices despite its very touristy
Wawel Hill location.

Okół and Stradom Quarters

Balaton   zł
Hungarian   **Map** 1 C5 & 6 D4
ul. Grodzka 37
Tel *12 429 51 41*
A plain-looking restaurant,
Balaton has been around for a
long time and still serves the best
goulash soups and *pörkölts*
(paprika-rich stews) in town.
Savour them with wine from the
excellent Hungarian list.

Smak Ukrainski   zł
Ukrainian   **Map** 1 C5 & 6 D4
ul. Kanonicza 15
Tel *12 421 92 94*
Hearty meat-and-potato dishes
and dumplings from Poland's
eastern neighbour are served by
costumed staff in a lively cellar.
Wash them down with a
selection of Ukrainian beers.

Il Calzone   zł zł
Italian   **Map** 2 D5 & 6 E3
ul. Starowiślna 15a
Tel *12 429 51 41*
This is the restaurant to visit for a
range of high-quality fish and
pasta dishes, plus a long menu
of inexpensive pizzas. There is a
terrace for outdoor dining.

DK Choice

Miód Malina   zł zł
Traditional Polish   **Map** 6 D4
ul. Grodzka 40
Tel *12 430 04 11*
Occupying lovely barrel-vaulted
rooms decorated in raspberry
shades of red, Miód Malina
("Honey Raspberry") is one of
the most welcoming places to
eat in Krakow. Traditional Polish
festive fare is the main focus,
with generous portions of
meat and poultry followed
by delicious desserts.

Pod Baranem   zł zł
Polish   **Map** 2 D5 & 6 E4
ul. Św Gertrudy 21
Tel *12 429 40 22*
There are few better places in
Krakow for Polish cuisine with a
modern European twist, made
with locally sourced ingredients.

Sakana Sushi Bar   zł zł
Asian   **Map** 2 D5 & 6 E4
ul. Św. Gertrudy 7
Tel *12 429 30 86*
Enjoy a range of sushi, tempura
dishes and soba noodles at one
of Krakow's best Asian restaurants.

Trattoria La Campana   zł zł
Italian   **Map** 1 C5 & 6 D4
ul. Kanonicza 7
Tel *12 430 22 32*
This is a great place for a romantic
dinner. Ingredients in the dishes
are imported from Italy.

Copernicus   zł zł zł
Fine dining   **Map** 1 C5 & 6 D4
ul. Kanonicza 16
Tel *12 424 34 21*
This atmospheric hotel restaurant
specializes in superlative modern
Polish cuisine and lots of game.

Pod Aniołami   zł zł zł
Traditional Polish   **Map** 6 D3
ul. Grodzka 35
Tel *12 421 39 99*
Classic Polish recipes, superbly
prepared, are served in
meticulously restored medieval
cellars that were once home to
goldsmiths' workshops.

Old Quarter

DK Choice

Ambasada Śledzia   zł
Polish   **Map** 6 D3
ul. Stolarska 8/10
Tel *662 569 460*
An outstanding example of the
vodka-and-snack bars cropping
up all over Poland, the "Herring
Embassy" serves traditional
Polish bar food, such as
marinated fish and potato pie
meat in aspic at rock-bottom
prices. Drinks are similarly good
value; no wonder the outdoor
terrace is constantly full.

Camelot   zł
Café-patisserie   **Map** 6 D2
ul. Św. Tomasza 17
Tel *12 421 01 23*
This mildly bohemian café with
a cabaret club downstairs is
famous for its good coffee, fine
cakes and delicious apple pie.

Chimera   zł
Polish   **Map** 5 C2
ul. Św. Anny 3
Tel *12 292 12 12*
At this buffet restaurant in a
medieval cellar, you pay
according to the size of your
plate. It is ideal for sampling a
variety of different dishes.
Vegetarian options aplenty.

Green Day   zł
Vegetarian   **Map** 6 E2
ul. Mikołajska 14
Tel *12 431 10 27*
A good-value buffet restaurant,
Green Day serves all kinds of
meat-free fare, including filling
soups, generous salads and tasty
savoury pancakes.

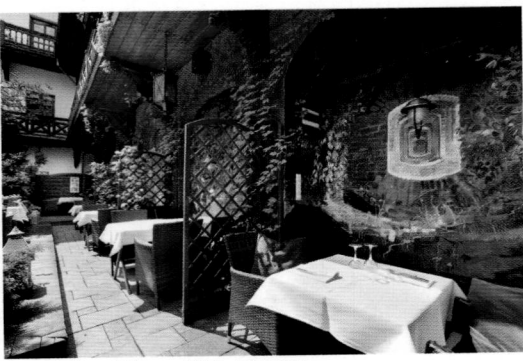
The sunny alfresco dining area at Pimiento Argentino

Noworolski

zł

Cafe-patisserie **Map** 6 D2

Rynek Główny 1/3

Tel *12 422 47 71*

This beautifully preserved Art Nouveau treasure attracts both locals and visitors eager for a cup of coffee and a slice of something sweet. Try the *sernik* (cheesecake).

DK Choice

La Petite France

zł

Cafe-patisserie **Map** 6 E2

ul. Św. Tomasza 25

Tel *12 370 20 74*

A combined delicatessen and café, this ideal lunchtime spot is dominated by the aroma of fresh cheeses and charcuterie. As well as strong coffee, La Petite France serves some of the finest quiches in Poland and delicious gourmet sandwiches. With only eight tables and a few bar stools, it's a cosy, intimate space.

U Babci Maliny

zł

Traditional Polish **Map** 6 D1

ul. Sławkowska 17

Tel *12 422 76 01*

Krakow has no shortage of queue-at-the-counter budget restaurants, and this is one of the best, serving all manner of classic Polish fare in a folksy bench-filled basement.

Zapiecek

zł

Traditional Polish **Map** 6 D1

ul. Sławkowska 32

Tel *12 422 74 95*

This is something of a temple to the humble *pierogi* (stuffed dumplings), which are served with a range of fillings. The savoury, sweet and baked versions are all well represented.

Chłopskie Jadło

zł zł

Traditional Polish **Map** 6 D2

ul. Św. Jana 3

Tel *12 429 51 57*

Polish classics dominate the menu at this characterful, folk-styled restaurant, with plenty of meat dishes in heavy sauces. There is also a long list of typical Polish alcoholic spirits.

CK Dezerter

zł zł

Eastern European **Map** 1 C5

ul. Bracka 6

Tel *12 422 79 31*

Large portions of meaty Polish and Austro-Hungarian classics are served at this charming restaurant. The soups are terrific, and cabbage has never tasted as good as in the sauerkraut here.

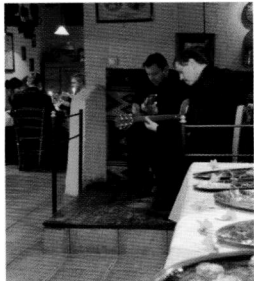

Diners enjoying their meal accompanied by live music at CK Dezerter

Czerwone Korale

zł zł

Traditional Polish **Map** 6 D1

ul. Sławkówska 13–15

Tel *12 430 61 08* **Closed** *lunch Sat & Sun*

Decorated with dolls in Polish costume and pictures of folk-dancing villagers, this is the perfect place to feast on traditional fare. All dishes are reasonably priced.

Farina

zł zł

Seafood **Map** 6 D1

ul. Św. Marka 16

Tel *12 422 18 60*

An informal, Mediterranean-themed restaurant that specializes in fish and seafood. Fine white fish is served grilled, pan-fried or baked.

Hawelka

zł zł

Traditional Polish **Map** 6 D2

Rynek Główny 34

Tel *12 422 06 31*

For fine Polish cuisine in a historic setting, it is difficult to do better than Hawelka, which has been serving roast duck and other classics since 1876 and is somewhat a local institution.

Leonardo

zł zł

Italian **Map** 6 E2

ul. Szpitalna 20-22

Tel *12 429 68 50*

Exquisite cuisine, including superb pasta dishes, is served in this basement dining room decked out to look like a Mediterranean piazza.

Marmolada

zł zł

Tradtional Polish **Map** 6 D3

ul. Grodzka 5

Tel *12 396 49 46*

Classic Polish cuisine and Italian pizzas are on the menu at this smart restaurant. A profusion of candles and cut flowers provide a soothing ambience. There is live classical music on Saturday and Sunday evenings.

Miód i Wino

zł zł

Traditional Polish **Map** 6 D1

ul. Sławkowska 32

Tel *12 422 74 95*

Enjoy classic Polish food in a traditional setting, with waiting staff in folk costumes and wooden-bench seating. This is a good place for meat-heavy feasting washed down with local beer.

Pimiento Argentino

zł zł

Argentinian **Map** 6 D3

ul. Stolarska 13

Tel *12 422 66 72*

Meat-lovers will relish the steaks freshly imported from Argentina at this grill restaurant. The menu includes everything from beef empanadas to ribeye steaks. South American wines complete the picture.

Restauracja we Francuskim

zł zł

Contemporary Polish **Map** 6 D1

ul. Pijarska 13

Tel *666 195 831*

This hotel restaurant with understated decor is famous for reinventing European classics (such as Wiener Schnitzel and beef Stroganoff) with great skill. Waiters dressed in white serve the freshly prepared dishes at your table.

Resto Illuminati

zł zł

International **Map** 6 D3

ul. Gołębia 2

Tel *12 430 73 73* **Closed** *lunch (Jul & Aug)*

Boasting exposed-brick interiors, Iluminati is a good restaurant to sample the best of modern Polish cuisine. Traditional meat and poultry dishes are cooked with a Mediterranean twist. There is often live piano music in the evenings.

Amadeus

zł zł zł

International **Map** 6 E2

ul. Mikołajska 20

Tel *12 423 03 40*

International and Polish dishes take pride of place on the menu of this restaurant in the hotel of the same name. The service is outstanding; the wines exemplary. The decor is themed on Wolfgang Amadeus Mozart.

Aqua e Vino

zł zł zł

Italian **Map** 6 D1

ul. Wiślna 5/10

Tel *12 421 25 67*

The dishes at this outrageously trendy restaurant appear as carefully designed as the interior. Expect imaginative takes on classic recipes made from fresh ingredients, and superb desserts.

For more information on types of restaurants *see pages 184–5*

DK Choice

Cyrano de Bergerac zł zł zł
Fine dining Map 6 D1
ul. Sławkowska 26
Tel *12 411 72 88*
If prices are high, the diners
who book days in advance here
don't seem to mind. This is a
world-class French restaurant,
set in two elegant rooms, with a
quiet patio for the summer. The
food is exquisite (leave room for
the extravagant desserts), and
the service impeccable. Look
out for affordable set-menu
lunches on weekdays.

Da Pietro zł zł zł
Italian Map 6 D2
Rynek Główny 17
Tel *12 422 32 79*
The quality food here is made
with ingredients imported from
Italy. The unrivalled main-square
location is reflected in the prices.

Del Papá zł zł zł
Italian Map 6 D2
ul. Św. Tomasza 6
Tel *12 421 83 43*
This is one of Krakow's best
Italian eateries, with a menu that
features classic meat dishes as
well as Mediterranean seafood.

Grodek zł zł zł
Fine dining Map 6 E3
ul. Na Grodku 4
Tel *12 431 90 30*
Polish and international cuisine
prepared with flair is served in
the brick-lined basement of the
historic Grodek hotel.

Pod Różą zł zł zł
International Map 6 E2
ul. Floriańska 14
Tel *12 424 33 81*
Under a glass-covered atrium
at the Pod Różą hotel, this
restaurant combines tradition
and creativity in its dishes.
Game is a speciality.

Szara zł zł zł
International Map 6 D2
Rynek Główny 6
Tel *12 421 66 69*
An imposing place with vaulted
ceilings, crisp linens and a grand
menu that spans the globe, Szara
has a reputation for quality.

Tetmajerowska zł zł zł
Traditional Polish Map 6 D2
Rynek Główny 34
Tel *12 422 06 31*
From the elegant decor to the
sublime service, everything at this
modern restaurant contributes to
a special experience.

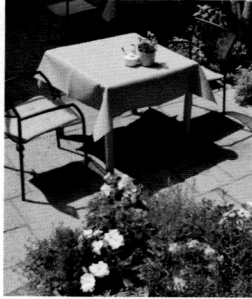

The courtyard at Del Papá, perfect for
alfresco dining in warm weather

Trzy Rybki zł zł zł
Fine dining Map 6 D2
ul. Szczepańska 9
Tel *12 384 08 01*
The cosy flagship restaurant of
the Stary hotel offers a seasonally
changing menu of European fare.

Wentzl zł zł zł
International Map 6 D3
Rynek Główny 19
Tel *12 429 52 99*
Savour Polish and European food
in a historic room with oak floors,
high ceilings and lavish fabrics.

Wierzynek zł zł zł
Traditional Polish Map 6 D3
Rynek Główny 15
Tel *12 424 96 00*
Claiming to be the oldest
restaurant in Krakow, Wierzynek
serves sumptuous Polish fare in
elegant, wooden-beamed rooms.

Kazimierz Quarter

Dawno temu na Kazimierzu zł
Traditional Polish Map 4 E1
ul. Szeroka 1
Tel *12 421 21 17*
Enjoy classic Polish and Jewish
fare in a room full of retro
furnishings and memorabilia.

Fabryka Pizzy zł
Italian Map 4 D2
ul. Jozefa 34
Tel *12 433 80 81*
The "Pizza Factory" serves some
of the tastiest and best-value
thin-crust pizzas in Poland, plus
a good selection of pasta dishes.

Manzana zł
Mexican Map 4 D1
ul. Miodowa 11
Tel *12 422 22 77*
This is the place for tacos, burritos,
fajitas and other Mexican classics.
It also has the biggest selection
of tequila in Krakow.

DK Choice

Pierogi Mr Vincent zł
Polish Map 4 D2
ul. Bożego Ciała 12
Tel *506 806 304*
Pierogi (stuffed pastry pockets)
are among Poland's most
emblematic dishes, yet they
rarely receive the culinary
attention they deserve. This tiny
restaurant offers only *pierogi*
with all kinds of creative fillings,
including exotic spicy versions.

Polakowski zł
Polish Map 4 D1
ul. Miodowa 39
Tel *12 421 21 17*
This popular order-at-the-
counter restaurant offers the best
in Polish cooking, including *bigos*,
pierogi and *żurek* (rye soup), plus
pancakes and Jewish specialities.

Zazie Bistro zł
French Map 4 D2
ul. Józefa 34
Tel *500 410 829*
Everything from onion soup and
bouillabaisse to mussels with fries
is served at this bistro. With
low prices and little space, it's
often busy.

Genji Sushi Premium zł zł
Japanese Map 6 E5
ul. Dietla 55
Tel *12 429 59 59*
This restaurant offers a full range
of Japanese dishes. The decor is
Far Eastern too, with one room
carpeted in dried rushes.

Horai zł zł
Asian Map 4 D2
pl. Wolnica 4
Tel *12 430 03 58*
The menu at Horai spans the
entire Asian continent, with solid
standards across the board. The
Thai curries are especially strong.

Trezo zł zł
Traditional Polish Map 4 D1
ul. Miodowa 33
Tel *12 374 50 00*
Classic meat, poultry and fish
dishes are presented with style in
an interior that mixes modern
minimalism with exposed brick.
Live music at weekends.

Klezmer Hois zł zł zł
Jewish Map 4 E1
ul. Szeroka 6
Tel *12 411 16 22*
Quality Jewish and Central
European fare is served in
this restaurant filled with bric-a-
brac. There is Klezmer
music nightly.

DK Choice

Studio Qulinarne zł zł zł
Contemporary Polish **Map** 4 D2
ul. Gazowa 4
Tel 12 430 69 41
Studio Qulinarne uses traditional Polish ingredients, Mediterranean style and the odd touch of Oriental spice to conjure up an original menu. Game and seafood feature strongly. The bright interior is filled with bookshelves and wine bottles; the garden is one of Krakow's loveliest.

Wesoła, Kleparz and Biskupie

Trzy kroki w szaleństwo zł zł
International **Map** 2 E4
ul. Lubicz 28
Tel 12 430 04 38
An attractive brick-lined cellar is the setting for this contemporary restaurant, offering inventive pasta and fish dishes, steaks and delicious desserts.

Jarema zł zł zł
Eastern European **Map** 2 D3 & 6 E1
pl. Matejki 5
Tel 12 429 36 69
Cuisine from the eastern margins of what used to be the Polish–Lithuanian commonwealth are on the menu here, including plenty of hearty meat dishes sourced from old recipe books.

Piasek and Nowy Świat

Mamma Mia zł
Italian **Map** 5 C1
ul. Karmelicka 14
Tel 12 430 04 92
A classy pizzeria that draws local families in droves, Mamma Mia opts for authenticity rather than experimentation in its traditional pizza toppings. There are also many pasta alternatives.

Smakołyki zł
Traditional Polish **Map** 5 C4
ul. Straszewskiego 28
Tel 12 430 30 99
Located opposite the main university building, this contemporary, bright canteen restaurant is the ideal place to try filling, inexpensive Polish favourites such as potato pancakes, stuffed cabbage leaves and borscht.

CK Browar zł zł
Traditional Polish **Map** 6 D1
ul. Podwale 6–7
Tel 12 429 25 05
This large brewery-restaurant is an excellent place to enjoy local favourites such as sausages and *bigos*, plus the house-brewed ales.

Dynia Resto-Bar zł zł
International **Map** 5 B2
ul. Krupnicza 20
Tel 12 430 08 38
The "Pumpkin" excels in pasta dishes, salads and fresh cakes. It has a wonderful walled garden.

Someplace Else zł zł
Mexican **Map** 3 B1 & 5 B4
ul. Powiśle 7
Tel 12 662 10 00
The bar of the Sheraton offers an affordable menu of Mexican specialities, plus burgers and chicken wings. Sporting events are shown on the big screen.

Zielona Kuchnia zł zł
Organic **Map** 1 B3
ul. Grabowskiego 8/9
Tel 12 634 55 22 **Closed** *Sat, Sun*
The emphasis at this sleek eco-restaurant is on organic produce and naturally reared meats. There are also vegetarian options.

Biała Róża zł zł zł
International **Map** 1 C5 & 5 C4
ul. Straszewskiego 16
Tel 12 421 51 90
This convivial restaurant between the Philharmonic Hall and Wawel Hill serves Polish classics with French and Italian influences.

The Olive zł zł zł
Mediterranean **Map** 3 B1 & 5 B4
ul. Powiśle 7
Tel 12 662 16 60
The Sheraton Hotel's showpiece restaurant offers refined Polish and Mediterranean fare, especially fish and seafood. Good wine list.

Solfeż zł zł zł
International **Map** 1 C5 & 5 C4
ul. Straszewskiego 17
Tel 12 618 88 88
Enjoy inventive European cuisine and attentive service in the elegant Radisson Hotel.

Further Afield

Stylowa zł
Traditional Polish
osiedle Centrum C bl. 3 (Aleja Róża)
Tel 12 644 26 19
One of the few restaurants in Nowa Huta, Stylowa is like a step back in time, with its 1980s decor and old-fashioned (but delicious) meat-and-potatoes menu.

U Ziyada zł zł
International
ul. Jodłowa 13
Tel 12 429 71 05
Perched high on a hill, this café-restaurant on the edge of Las Wolski forest has superb views across the Vistula River and serves quality Polish, European and Kurdish cuisine.

Zakładka zł zł
French **Map** 4 E3
ul. Józefińska 2
Tel 12 442 74 42 **Closed** *Mon lunch*
Just across the river from the Kazimierz Quarter, this bistro offers a creative and seasonally changing menu. You can also pop in simply for a sandwich and a glass of wine.

Villa Decius zł zł zł
Fine dining
ul. 28 Lipca 1943 17a
Tel 12 425 33 90
A luxurious restaurant in a park-fringed Renaissance villa, Decius serves classic Polish and other European cuisines with old-school finesse.

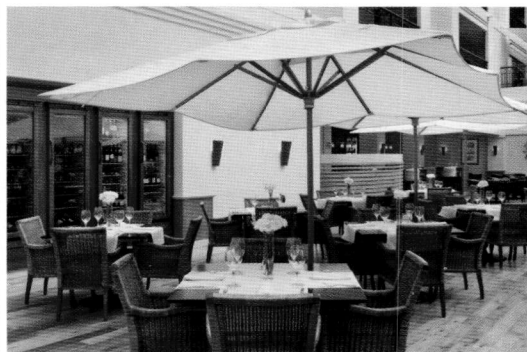
The airy interior of The Olive, located inside the Sheraton Hotel

For more information on types of restaurants *see pages 184–5*

Cafés and Bars

Krakow's cafés are an important part of everyday life and are often institutions in their own right. It would be unthinkable to deny a Krakovian his or her daily 15 minutes or so spent chatting with a friend or reading a newspaper in a café. The majority of cafés have regular customers, who come year in, year out to their chosen place, every day except at weekends.

Cafés

Situated in the heart of the city, **Kawiarnia Noworolski** is one of the longest established cafés. It is housed in the Cloth Hall, with its entrance facing the Mickiewicz Monument. It dates back to the end of the 19th century. The interior, modelled on Viennese cafés, has preserved its original appearance. A visit to the **Jama Michalika** *(see p116)*, renowned for the Zielony Balonik (Green Balloon) Cabaret, is a must. However, the Art Nouveau rooms offer a feast for the eye rather than the palate. They are now often deserted, possibly because of a total ban on smoking (smoke would damage the historic interior).

The **Pożegnanie z Afryką** (Out of Africa) is the best place for lovers of good coffee. The coffee served here will satisfy even the most demanding customer. Situated in St Thomas Street (ul. Św. Tomasza), it is a coffee bar and shop. A variety of brands are available here, which can be prepared in small espresso machines. The smell is so fantastic that it is hard to resist buying or trying a cup. There are many outlets of Pożegnanie z Afryką in other cities throughout Poland but the company started in Krakow and has its headquarters here.

The **Café Zakopianka** occupies meticulously restored 19th-century premises right on the Planty Park and has a distinctly Parisian feel and live music. If you want to travel back in time and see how a patisserie looked in the early 19th century, then **Europejska** in Market Square is the place to visit, to see the original period furnishing.

This café was established by a Swiss man, Lorenzo Paganino Cortesi, in 1823, but the name Redolfi refers to its second owner, also Swiss. Lunch is also served here.

Krakow's very large student population is one of the main reasons the city's cafés continue to thrive and haven't become gentrified curiosities for tourists. Students of all subjects, ranging from art to philosophy and astrophysics, can be found lounging around in the cafés that surround the old university buildings. These include **Nowa Prowincja**, with its legendary hot chocolate, and **Café Gołębia 3**, a down-at-heel hangout where you could meet anyone from a professor of literature to the CEO of one of the city's many hi-tech startups. Apple cake *(szarlotka)* is the usual order, and provides delicious fuel for conversation.

Tasty canapés served on bread from the highlands and tea with home-made raspberry syrup are just two specialities of the **Café Camelot**. The walls here are decorated with pictures by the celebrated Polish naive artist Nikifor. The **Dym** (Smoke) is next door, serving delicious Pischinger cake as well as beer and spirits.

Street Cafés

Most of the eateries in Market Square (Rynek Główny) open street bars and cafés in the spring and summer. The square is thus transformed into a huge open-air café for thousands of customers.

A little away from the square, the corner of ul. Św. Tomasza and ul. Św. Jana is a tiny pavement café paradise.

The street café set up by the **Black Gallery** is very busy at night, sometimes till the early hours. An enormous parachute will protect you from rain, and the house drink Kamikaze, a deceptive mixture of Blue Curacao, vodka and lemon juice, may well help you not notice any change in the weather.

If you decide to eat at one of the outdoor restaurant tables, expect a lunch rather than a full dinner menu. Dishes served outside are less elaborate. Bear in mind that the journey from the kitchen to the table is a long one and makes serving an exotic *flambé* lobster, for example, almost impossible.

All sorts of street buskers roam and play in and around the street cafés. They request gratuities but you are not obliged to give any. It is worth listening to the gypsy band, with a partially paralysed fiddler in a wheelchair, who plays his violin holding it like a double-bass.

Bars

An increasing number of bars have opened in Krakow. They are often called "pubs" as in England. They are housed in cellars and are open till late, and live music is played in many. The **Free Pub** in the Old Quarter and **Singer** in Kazimierz were the first and remain firm favourites. Hot hangouts for the younger crowd include **Pauza**, **Alchemia**, **Kitsch** and **Piękny Pies**.

The **Pod Złotą Pipą** is popular with more conservative customers. The place is nostalgically decorated in the Austro-Hungarian style and features many portraits of His Imperial Majesty Franz Joseph and the Empress Sissi. White sausage with cabbage and peas is served here, and to accompany this you may order authentic Czech Budweiser on draught. The fruits of Poland's rocketing craft-beer revival can be sampled at **Omerta** and the appropriately named **House of Beer**.

DIRECTORY

Afera
ul. Sławkowska 13.
Map 1 C4 (6 D1).
Tel 12 421 17 71.

Albo Tak
ul. Mały Rynek 4.
Map 2 D4 (6 E3).
Tel 12 421 11 05.

Alchemia
ul. Estery 5.
Map 4 D1.
Tel 12 421 22 00.

Antycafe
ul. Sławkowska 12.
Map 1 C4 (6 D2).
Tel 506 48 18 88.

Aperitif
ul. Sienna 9.
Map 1 C4 (6 D3).
Tel 12 432 33 33.

Ariel
ul. Szeroka 18.
Map 4 E1.
Tel 12 421 79 20.

Arlekin
Rynek Główny 24.
Map 1 C4 (6 D2).
Tel 12 430 24 57.

Black Gallery
ul. Mikołajska 24.
Map 2 D4 (6 E2).
Tel 12 423 00 30.

Bomba
Plac Szczepański 2/1.
Map 1 C4 (5 C1).
Tel 782 60 19 99.

Bunkier Café
Plac Szczepański 3A.
Map 1 C4 (5 C1).
Tel 12 431 05 85.

Café Camelot
ul. Św. Tomasza 17.
Map 1 C4 (6 D2).
Tel 12 421 01 23.

Café Czekolada
ul. Bracka 4.
Map 1 C4 (6 D3).
Tel 12 430 24 08.

Café Gołębia 3
ul. Gołębia 3.
Map 1 C4 (5 C3).
Tel 12 430 24 19.

Café Manekin
ul. Św. Tomasza 25.
Map 2 D4 (6 E2).

Café Numero
Rynek Główny 6.
Map 1 C4 (6 D2).
Tel 12 421 13 05.

Café Zakopianka
ul. Św Marka 34a.
Map 1 C4 (6 D1).
Tel 12 421 40 45.

Carpe Diem
ul. Floriańska 33.
Map 2 D4 (6 E2).
Tel 12 431 22 67.

Charlotte
Plac Szczepański 2.
Map 1 C4 (5 C1).
Tel 600 807 880.

Dym
ul. Św. Tomasza 13.
Map 1 C4 (6 D2).
Tel 12 429 66 61.

Dynia Resto Bar
ul. Krupnicza 20.
Map 1 B4 (5 A2).
Tel 12 430 08 38.

Europejska
Rynek Główny 35.
Map 1 C4 (6 D2).
Tel 12 429 34 93.

Free Pub
ul. Sławkowska 4.
Map 1 C4 (6 D2).
Tel 0802 90 82.

Le Fumoir
ul. Sławkowska 26.
Map 1 C4 (6 D2).
Tel 12 429 54 28.

Hamlet
ul. Miodowa 9.
Map 4 D1 (6 F5).
Tel 12 422 12 11.

Hot Chili
ul. Pijarska 9.
Map 1 C4 (6 D1).
Tel 12 422 12 92.

House of Beer
ul. Św. Tomasza 35.
Map 1 C4 (6 D2).
Tel 12 794 222 136.

Jama Michalika
ul. Floriańska 45.
Map 2 D4 (6 E2).
Tel 12 422 15 61.

Jazz Rock Café
ul. Sławkowska 12.
Map 1 C4 (6 C1).
Tel 511 433 506.

Kawiarnia Noworolski
Rynek Główny 1,
Cloth Hall.
Map 1 C4 (6 D2).
Tel 12 422 47 71.

Kitsch
ul. Grodzka 20.
Map 1 C5 (6 D4).
Tel 12 518 879 055.

Krzysztofory
ul. Szczepańska 2.
Map 1 C4 (6 D2).

Lamus
ul. Karmelicka 54.
Map 1 B3.

Manggha
ul. Marii Konopnickiej 26.
Map 2 D5 (6 E3).
Tel 12 267 27 03.

Nowa Prowincja
ul. Bracka 3–5.
Map 1 C5 (6 D3).
Tel 12 430 59 59.

Omerta
ul. Kupa 3.
Map 4 D1.
Tel 12 501 508 227.

Pauza
ul. Floriańska 18.
Map 2 D4 (6 E2).
Tel 12 422 48 66.

Piękny Pies
ul. Bożego Ciała 9.
Map 4 D2.

Pierwszy Lokal
ul. Stolarska 6.
Map 1 C5 (6 D3).
Tel 12 431 24 41.

Pod Białym Orłem
Rynek Główny 45.
Map 1 C4 (6 D2).
Tel 12 421 57 97.

Pod Papugami
ul. Św. Jana 18.
Map 1 C4 (6 D2).
Tel 12 422 82 99.

Pod Złotą Pipą
ul. Floriańska 30.
Map 2 D4 (6 E2).
Tel 12 421 94 66.

Poezja Smaku
ul. Jagiellońska 5.
Map 1 C4 (6 D2).
Tel 12 292 80 20.

Pożegnanie z Afryką
ul. Św. Tomasza 21.
Map 1 C4 (6 E2).
Tel 12 644 47 45.

Ratuszowa
Rynek Główny 1.
Map 1 C4 (6 D2).
Tel 12 421 13 26.

Royal Art Café
ul. Św Gertrudy 29.
Map 2 D5 (6 E4).

Senacka
ul. Grodzka 51.
Map 1 C5 (6 D4).
Tel 12 422 76 86.

Singer
ul. Estery 20.
Map 4 D1.
Tel 12 292 06 22.

Stare Mury
ul. Pijarska 21.
Map 2 D4 (6 E1).
Tel 12 421 38 98.

U Literatów
ul. Kanonicza 7.
Map 1 C5 (6 D4).
Tel 12 421 86 66.

U Louisa
Rynek Główny 13.
Map 1 C4 (6 D3).
Tel 12 617 02 22.

Vis-a-vis
Rynek Główny 29.
Map 1 C4 (6 D2).
Tel 12 422 69 61.

Wiśniowy Sad
ul. Grodzka 33.
Map 1 C5 (6 D3).
Tel 12 430 21 11.

Yummie
Rynek Główny 25.
Map 1 C4 (6 D2).
Tel 12 421 34 44.

SHOPS AND MARKETS

Krakow has always been a favourable place for merchants and recent reforms have stimulated trade. Unlike in other Polish cities, most of the prewar buildings in Krakow have remained in private hands. After 1989 the number of new shops opening surged with house owners either opening shops themselves or letting premises out. A profusion of shop-signs appeared on façades, inner courtyards and basements. Quality soon took over and big Western names also began to appear. Today one can hardly tell the difference between a Krakow shop and its Viennese or Parisian counterpart. The area around Market Square is especially good for shopping. It offers a variety of elegant shops, little traffic and many cafés. Markets and street stalls offer a different kind of shopping and a lively atmosphere. There is something for everyone.

Shopping Hours

In Poland, unlike in many other Western European countries, there is no law regulating the hours of trade. Each shop owner decides for themselves when to open and close their shop, and this is regarded as a necessary part of a free-market economy. Grocers open in Krakow at 6 or 7am and close at 7pm at the earliest. Many remain open until 10pm or longer, and a dozen or so shops are open 24 hours. Other types of shops are generally open between 10am and 7pm on weekdays, but on Saturdays close at 2 or 3pm. All shops within the Planty green belt tend to trade on Sundays for similar periods to those on Saturdays. All shops are customarily open on the Sunday preceding Christmas and Easter Day. Supermarkets are at their busiest on Friday afternoon and evening. The great number of tourist shops in the centre attract customers all

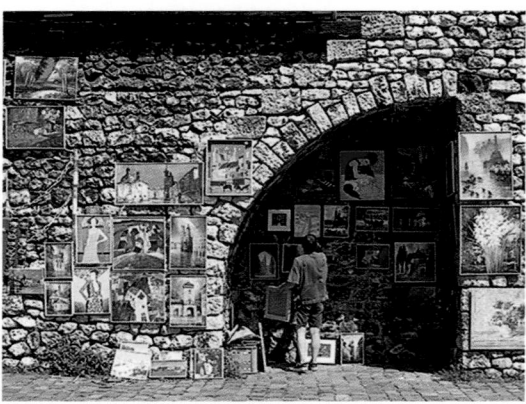

Pictures for sale, displayed on the wall near St Florian's Gate

the time regardless of the day of the week but Saturdays are possibly the busiest.

How to Pay

Cash is the most popular form of payment throughout Poland. The situation is different in major cities, where most of the shops in the city centre do accept major credit cards, as indicated by stickers displayed in their windows. Supermarkets and department stores also accept credit cards as well as cheques, but the latter must be issued by a Polish bank. All the prices displayed are inclusive of VAT.

Department Stores and Shopping Malls

Jubilat, built in the mid-1970s, is the largest department store in Krakow. The food department is on the ground floor, and on the other floors you will find household goods, furniture and electrical appliances, clothes, shoes and cosmetics, as well as toys and books. The large **Galeria Krakowska** shopping mall is located by the main train station, and there is another large mall, **Galeria Kazimierz**, on

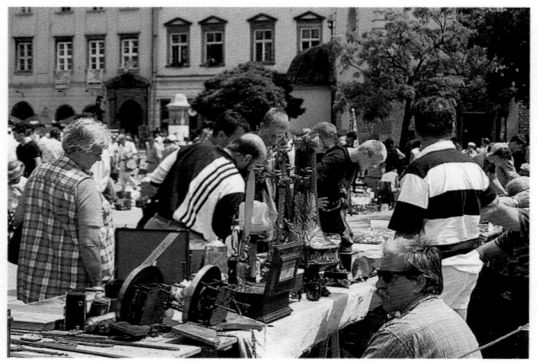

A collectors' fair in Market Square

the opposite side of town. Both contain dozens of stores, including international names, and at least one large supermarket. A little out of town, but served by many bus routes, is a large branch of the **Factory** clothes discount store.

Right on the Market Square (Rynek Główny) is the **Pasaż 13** shopping centre. Converted from a beautiful old townhouse, it has 17 designer and boutique shops, plus a restaurant.

Krakow now has at least eight large shopping malls further out from the centre, with more opening all the time. They include mega supermarkets, DIY stores and all the usual services you would expect elsewhere in Europe.

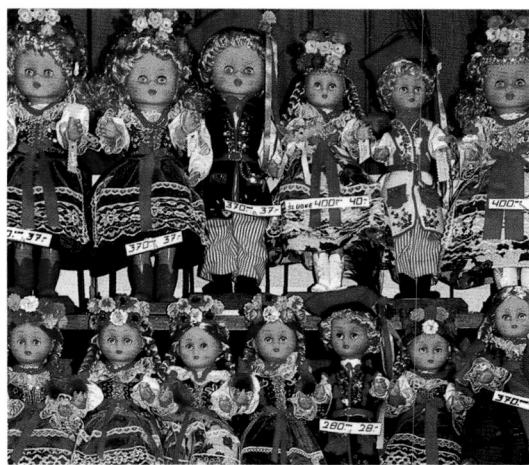

Dolls in regional costumes sold in the Cloth Hall

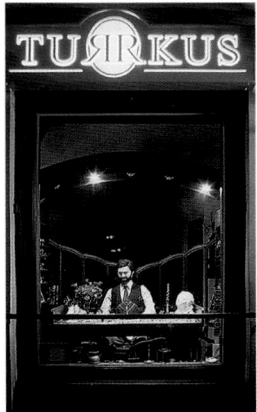

Jewellery shop on Floriańska Street

Markets and Fairs

Krakow's markets are never called bazaars as in other Polish towns. Here the term bazaar has a pejorative connotation. In Krakow locals go to the "square" to buy fruit and vegetables, cheese, meat, fish or other produce from the stallholders.

The Old Kleparz market is the nearest to the city centre. The New Kleparz market sells not only food but also flowers and clothes, while every Tuesday and Friday you will find stalls selling brooms, clay pots and wickerware. The market in Grzegórzecka Street by the Market Hall is the biggest

and full of stalls selling meat, fruit and vegetables. On Sundays you have the added attraction of book and antique stalls.

The unique atmosphere of the New Market in Kazimierz was used to good effect in the filming of *Days and Nights (Noce i dnie)*, a Polish film after a well-known novel by Maria Dąbrowska of the same title. The late 19th-century round butchers stalls, which are centrally located, are still in use. These stalls are surrounded by vegetable and fruit stands. On Sundays this place becomes an extensive flea market, where among other things you can buy famous Harris tweed jackets from Scotland and woollen coats and Tyrolean tunics from Austria. The Tomex Market in

Nowa Huta is dominated by sellers from the former Soviet Union. The so-called Tandeta Market sells mostly clothes. Although *tandeta* means rubbish in Polish, this term is used in Krakow to mean an ordinary clothes market and has no derogatory meaning.

Sales

Seasonal sales are now quite common in a number of larger shops but, in terms of the selection of goods on offer and the prices, they are not as attractive as those in other Western European countries. Goods are no longer reduced because they are imperfect or no longer in fashion, as used to be the case, but because of promotions, end of season sales or the arrival of new collections.

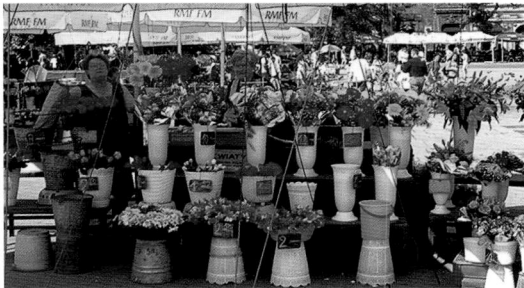

A flower stall in Market Square

Shopping in Krakow

If you are a Western visitor you can expect to be able to find everything in Krakow you can buy at home. It is no longer necessary to bring items for everyday use. On the other hand you should not expect luxury Western merchandise, such as perfumes, alcohol, designer clothes and shoes and other branded items, to be cheaper in Poland. You may, however, find bargains in shops and galleries selling handicrafts, silver jewellery, contemporary paintings and prints, as well as leather goods, bric-à-brac and coffee-table books.

Book and Record Shops

There are many excellent bookshops in Krakow. **Massolit Books** sells second-hand and new books in English. It also features a café that serves teas and superb cakes. It's common to find people pouring over books in here for hours on end. This is typical of Krakow, where the way of life is still heavily influenced by artists, professors and students. Massolit also hosts literary readings, art exhibitions and musical events.

Empik, one of Poland's leading book retailers, has nine branches in Krakow, with the two biggest in the Galeria Krakowska and Kazimierz malls. Galeria Krakowska is also home to **The American Bookstore**, which sells only English-language books.

For visitors with more literary tastes, the prestigious **Znak** bookshop in Kościuszki Street has a large selection of foreign titles. Academic books and fiction can be bought at the **Ossolineum** and Elefant bookshops. The **Księgarnia Muzyczna Kurant** in Market Square specializes in music books, scores and recordings. The shop of the **Polskie Wydawnictwo Muzyczne** (Polish Music Publishers) has a similar assortment with an emphasis on classical music. Among many shops in the centre selling CDs and cassettes, the one in Poselska Street offers a particularly good selection of jazz and classical recordings. It also has a useful sale-or-return section. The music shop found in Mikołajska Street specializes in jazz.

Antiques

Krakow is possibly the best place in Poland for antiques because the city was saved from destruction during World War II and Krakovians did not have to migrate. Foreigners are advised that exporting pre-1945 antiques from Poland is illegal without special permission, which is very difficult to obtain *(see p210)*. As far as valuable works of art are concerned, as well as those which form part of the cultural heritage, such as paintings, furniture, jewellery, old prints, rare books and maps, this law is rigorously observed, but less so in the case of objects of lesser value and bric-à-brac, which are plentiful in Krakow.

Antique dealers are mainly located in the area around the Planty gardens. Occasional antique markets take place in Market Square. Every Sunday, sellers of collectors' items and second-hand books put up their stalls by the Market Hall in Grzegórzecka Street. They are worth visiting.

Folk Art

The annual folk Art Fair in Market Square takes place in September. Dozens of stalls are set up, selling sculpture, earthenware, woven rugs and wood carvings made in various parts of Poland.

The stalls in the **Cloth Hall** offer a large selection of crafts and are a must for the tourist. You will find here colourful, embroidered traditional costumes of the Krakow and Podhale regions, as well as walking sticks from the highlands, cratfted with an axe-like handle; ornate chess sets and jewellery boxes, devotional statues and Jewish objects all carved in wood; paper cut-outs, painted Easter eggs, traditional dolls and much more.

Crafts and Contemporary Art

The stands in the Cloth Hall also sell silver jewellery, amber *objets d'art*, leather items and fabrics for the home. Shopping in this Renaissance hall has the added bonus of sustaining a trading tradition that goes back to the 16th century. The charming **Kramy Dominikańskie** (Dominican Stalls) also specialize in crafts. The **Galeria Osobliwości** (Gallery of Curiosities) in Sławkowska Street sells rare and unusual objects. The **Calik** Gallery is famous for Christmas decorations and attracts customers from all over the world.

Krakow is a good centre for Polish contemporary art, which is enjoying an ever-greater demand. Works by contemporary artists can be found in the **Starmach Gallery**, **Zderzak**, **Space Gallery**, **Galeria Mariana Gołogórskiego**, **Dominik Rostworowski Gallery**, **Kocioł Artystyczny** and many others. The open-air gallery by St Florian's Gate is the place for lovers of images of sunsets and sunrises, galloping horses or large-scale nudes. This kind of painting is displayed on the city wall throughout the year. Fans of satirical drawings by **Andrzej Mleczko** will find a visit to his gallery in St John's Street (Św. Jana) a must.

Clothes and Shoes

Jeans can be found in abundance in almost any clothes shop and those who prefer the well-known brands can go to the shops of **Levi Strauss**, **Diesel**, **Wrangler** or Lee. There are also shops that sell the leading brands of sports shoes: **Reebok** and **Puma**.

Timberland has fashion for the young, while designer menswear is available from **Pierre Cardin**. Polish brands, such as **Vistula**, offer less expensive suits for men, and **Wólczanka** specializes in shirts. **IDEA FIX** is a hothouse of Polish design, mixing fashion, art, music and photography. **Linen Dream** sells unique shawls, tunics and coats made by Polish artisans with organic materials.

Promod offers a good selection of clothes and shoes from both leading foreign brands and designers as well as Polish names.

The **Zebra** chain of shops is best for Italian shoes and the **Nico** store is great for Italian fashion for the whole family – men, women and children.

Food Shops and Off-Licences (Liquor Stores)

The only supermarket in the centre of Krakow is in the **Galeria Krakowska** mall. The Delikatesy general grocery store next to the Hawełka Restaurant is the largest in Market Square. Its selection of alcoholic drinks is particularly good. Apart from a number of small shops close to Market Square there are several self-service ones.

The large supermarkets such as **Real** and **Tesco** are located away from the centre and cater for shoppers who come by car. There are supermarkets on most of the housing estates, catering for local needs.

Most Krakovians purchase their fruit and vegetables from local stalls and markets. The Old Kleparz market is the closest to the city centre just a few minutes' walk away. The selection of coffee brands available from the charming **Pożegnanie z Afryką** (Out of Africa) is hard to beat. Julius Meinl's famous Viennese coffee is only available from the Meinl supermarket in the Azory (Azores) housing estate. The little and delightfully decorated **Pod Aniołami** (Angels) shop sells exquisite cold meats prepared according to old Polish recipes, *bundz* and

oszczypek cheese from the highlands, as well as country-style bread baked in log-fired ovens. Wines are also sold here but the largest selection from around the world can be found in the off-licence (liquor store) **In Vino Veritas**, as well as in the drinks department at the Galeria Krakowska. Those who favour strong spirits may choose the **Polmos** shop, where they can not only buy but also sample drinks at the bar.

Lovers of chocolate will be welcomed in the **Wawel** shop in Market Square, selling goods from the local sweet factory, Zakłady Przemysłu Cukierniczego. Many patisseries throughout Krakow offer a wonderful selection of cakes and pastries. The best doughnuts can be bought at **Michałek** and nougat at **Cichowski**. Look out for *kremówka*, a delicious puff-pastry cake filled with custard and available in the city's main patisseries. Note that what is known as *kremówka* in Krakow, in Warsaw is called *napoleonka*.

Other language differences between Mazovia and Lesser Poland include the names given to fruits of the forest, blueberries are called *borówki* in Krakow and Galicia, and *czarne jagody* in the Warsaw region. All berries, including the non-edible varieties, are called *jagody* in Krakow; *brusznice* is the name given to small red berries, which are called *borówki* in Warsaw, but in both regions *żurawiny* is the name for cranberries.

There are further differences in bread terminology which will probably confuse first-time visitors to the city. A long white loaf of bread called *weka* in Krakow is known as Wrocław bread in Warsaw.

Cosmetics

All chemists (drug stores) and supermarkets sell basic cosmetic goods, but expensive international brands are best purchased from specialist shops where expert advice is also available. **Guerlain** and Yves Rocher have their own outlets and beauty clinics.

Well-known foreign brands of perfumes, such as Gucci, Biagotti, Trussardi, Bulgari, Carolina Herrera and Burberry are available from the large **Marionnaud** shop or from **Sephora**. Another place to find a good selection of brands is in hotel shops.

Pharmacies

The majority of drugs are available from Polish chemists on prescription only. Prescriptions issued by overseas doctors are generally accepted without any problem. Non-prescription drugs and medicines are readily available throughout the city. In the city centre, there are many chemists in the following streets, among others: **Szczepańska, Grodzka** or **Dunajewskiego**. If you need some medication after normal opening hours, then go to one of the chemists that are open 24 hours; their addresses are displayed in all the chemists' shop windows. A 24-hour telephone service (12 94 39) will provide you with general medical information, including the location of the nearest hospital with an accident and emergency unit.

Florists

Krakow would not be Krakow without the flower stalls by the Mickiewicz statue in Market Square. On the day of the great poet's birthday, these street vendors have made it a tradition to lay flowers at the base of the statue in tribute. They also regularly make a gift of flowers to visiting foreign VIPs. On warm summer days you can buy flowers till late into the evening. There are many flower stalls to be found in New Kleparz market. Of the specialist florist shops, **Niezapominajka** (Forget-me-not) is particularly well known. Alternatively, you can buy bunches of flowers in one of the many 24-hour shops and at petrol stations.

DIRECTORY

Department Stores and Shopping Malls

Factory Outlet
ul. Różańskiego 32.
Tel 12 297 35 00.

Galeria Kazimierz
ul. Podgórska 34.
Map 4 F1.
Tel 12 433 01 01.

Galeria Krakowska
ul. Pawia 5.
Map 2 D3 (6 F1).
Tel 12 428 99 00.

Jubilat
al. Krasińskiego 1–3.
Map 1 B5 (5 B4).
Tel 12 619 33 00.

Pasaż 13
Rynek Główny 9.
Map 1 C4 (6 D2).
Tel 12 422 77 13.

Book and Record Shops

American Bookstore
ul. Pawia 5 (Galeria Krakowska).
Map 2 D3 (6 F1).
Tel 12 628 75 73.

Empik
ul. Pawia 5 (Galeria Krakowska).
Map 2 D3 (6 F1).
Tel 12 451 03 85.

Inter Book
ul. Karmelicka 27.
Map 1 B3.
Tel 12 632 10 08.

Księgarnia Muzyczna Kurant
Rynek Główny 36.
Map 1 C4 (6 D2).
Tel 12 422 98 59.

Massolit Books
ul. Felicjanek 4.
Map 1 B5 (5 B4).
Tel 12 432 41 50.

Ossolineum
ul. Św. Marka 12.
Map 2 D4 (6 E2).
Tel 12 422 58 44.

Polskie Wydawnictwo Muzyczne (Polish Music Publishers)
al. Krasińskiego 11a.
Map 1 B5 (5 B4).
Tel 12 422 70 44 ext.121.

Znak
ul. Sławkowska 1.
Map 1 C4 (6 D2).
Tel 12 422 45 48.

Rare and Second-Hand Books

Antykwariat AB
Rynek Główny 43.
Map 1 C4 (6 D2).
Tel 12 421 69 03.

Antykwariat księgarski
ul. Stolarska 8/10.
Map 1 C5 (6 D3).
Tel 12 422 62 88.

Bibliofil
ul. Szpitalna 19.
Map 2 D4
(6 E2). **Tel** 12 422 18 61.

Krakowski Antykwariat Naukowy
ul. Św. Tomasza 8.
Map 1 C4 (6 D2).
Tel 12 421 21 43.

Rara Avis
ul. Szpitalna 11.
Map 2 D4 (6 E2).
Tel 12 422 03 90.

Antiques

Antique
ul. Św. Tomasza 19.
Map 1 C4 (6 D2).
Tel 503 517 171.

Connaisseur
Rynek Główny 11.
Map 1 C4 (6 D2).
Tel 12 503 517 171.

Desa
ul. Floriańska 13.
Map 1 C4 (6 D2).
Tel 12 422 27 06.

ul. Grodzka 8.
Map 1 C5 (6 D4).
Tel 12 421 54 54.

Galeria Kersten
ul. Sławkowska 5/7.
Map 1 C4 (6 D1).
Tel 12 424 08 49.

Sopocki Dom Aukcyjny
Rynek Główny 45.
Map 1 C4 (6 D2).
Tel 12 429 12 17.

Folk Art

Cloth Hall
Rynek Główny 1/3.
Map 1 C4 (6 D2).

Crafts and Contemporary Art

Autorska Galeria Andrzeja Mleczki (Mleczko Gallery)
ul. Św. Jana 14.
Map 1 C4 (6 D2).
Tel 12 421 71 04.

Bunkier Sztuki
Pl. Szczepański 3A.
Map 1 C4 (5 C2).
Tel 12 422 10 52.

Calik
Rynek Główny 7.
Map 1 C4 (6 D2).
Tel 12 421 77 60.

Dominik Rostworowski Gallery
ul. Św. Jana 20.
Map 1 C4 (6 D2).
Tel 12 423 21 51.

Galeria Jana Siuty
ul. Sławkowska 14.
Map 1 C4 (6 D1).

Galeria Mariana Gołogórskiego
ul. Grodzka 29.
Map 1 C5 (6 D4).
Tel 12 421 44 19.

Galeria Osobliwości
ul. Sławkowska 16.
Map 1 C4 (6 D1).
Tel 12 429 19 84.

Galeria Związku Polskich Artystów Plastyków (Gallery of the Association of Polish Artists)
ul. Łobzowska 3.
Map 1 C3 (5 C1).
Tel 12 632 46 22.

Kocioł Artystyczny
ul. Sławkowska 14,
1st floor.
Map 1 C4 (6 D2).
Tel 12 429 17 97.

Kramy Dominikańskie
ul. Stolarska 8/10.
Map 1 C5 (6 D3).
Tel 12 422 19 08.

Mocak
ul. Lipowa 4.
Map 3 F2.
Tel 12 263 40 01.

Pryzmat
ul. Łobzowska 3.
Map 1 C3 (5 C1).
Tel 12 632 46 22.

Space Gallery
ul. Św. Marka 7.
Map 1 C4 (6 D1).
Tel 12 432 29 20.

Starmach Gallery
ul. Węgierska 5.
Map 4 E3.
Tel 12 656 43 17,
12 656 49 15.

Zderzak
ul. Floriańska 3.
Map 1 C4 (6 D2).
Tel 12 429 67 43.

Clothes and Shoes

Diesel
Rynek Główny (Pasaż 13).
Map 1 C4 (6 D2).
Tel 12 617 02 16.

IDEA FIX
ul. Bocheńska 7 .
Map 4 D2.
Tel 12 422 12 46.

Levi Strauss
ul. Floriańska 9.
Map 1 C4 (6 D2).
Tel 12 428 15 73.

Linen Dream
ul. Grodzka 63.
Map 1 C5 (6 D4).
Tel 790 46 61 03.

Nico
ul. Modlnica 214.
Tel 12 637 03 95.

Pierre Cardin
ul. Kamieńskiego 11
(Bonarka City Center).
Map 4 D5.
Tel 506 457 825.

Promod
ul. Floriańska 18.
Map 1 C4 (6 D2).
Tel 694 462 950.

Puma
ul. Pawia 5.
Map 2 D3 (6 F1).
Tel 12 628 76 35.

Reebok
ul. Pawia 5.
Map 2 D3 (6 F1).
Tel 12 628 76 48.

Timberland
ul. Szewska 20.
Map 1 C4 (5 C2).
Tel 12 432 84 40.

Troll
ul. Pawia 5.
Map 2 D3 (6 F1).
Tel 12 628 78 67.

Vistula
ul. Pawia 5 (Galeria
Krakowska).
Map 2 D3 (6 F1).

Wólczanka
Pl. Mariacki 1.
Map 1 C4 (6 D2).
Tel 12 421 83 16.

Wrangler
ul. Pawia 5.
Map 2 D3 (6 F1).
Tel 12 428 99 00.

Zebra
Rynek Główny 7.
Map 1 C4 (6 D2).
Tel 12 421 40 34.

Food Shops

Carrefour
ul. Witosa 7.
Tel 12 639 48 00.

Chichowsky
ul. Starowišina 21.
Tel 12 421 02 27.

Krakowski Kredens
ul. Grodzka 7.
Map 1 C5 (6 D4).
Tel 12 423 81 59.

Michałek
ul. Krupnicza 6.
Map 1 B4 (5 C2).
Tel 12 422 47 05.

Pod Aniołami
ul. Grodzka 35.
Map 1 C5 (6 D4).
Tel 12 421 39 99.

Polo Market
ul. Św. Gertrudy 5.
Map 2 D5 (6 E4).
Tel 518 014 075.

**Pożegnanie z
Afryką**
ul. Św. Tomasza 21.
Map 2 D4 (6 D2).
Tel 12 644 47 45.

Real
ul. Bora Komorowskiego
37. **Tel** 12 617 06 00.

Tesco
ul. Dobrego Pasterza 67.
Tel 12 412 75 34.

ul. Kapelanka 54.
Map 3 A3.
Tel 12 255 25 00.

ul. Włoska 2.
Tel 12 655 76 71.

ul. Wybickiego .10.
Tel 12 633 43 99.

Wawel
Rynek Główny 33.
Map 1 C4 (6 D2).
Tel 12 423 12 47.

Cosmetics

Guerlain
ul. Św. Jana 20.
Map 1 C4 (6 D2).
Tel 12 422 39 45.

Marionnaud
ul. Szpitalna 34.
Map 2 D4 (6 E2).
Tel 12 421 30 55.

Sephora
ul. Floriańska 19.
Map 1 C4 (6 D2).
Tel 12 421 24 24.

Off-Licences (Liquor Stores)

Baryłeczka
ul. Szczepańska 9.
Map 1 C4 (5 C2).
Tel 12 429 62 67.

Dom Wina
ul. Starowiślna 66.
Map 2 D5 (6 E3).
Tel 12 431 03 68.

In Vino Veritas
ul. Łobzowska 26.
Map 1 B2 (5 C1).
Tel 12 606 805 51.

Polmos
ul. Starowiślna 26.
Map 2 D5 (6 E3).
Tel 12 423 11 18.

Regionalne Alkohole
ul. Miodowa 28a.
Map 4 D1 (6 F5).
Tel 533 59 33 35.

Strefa Piwa
ul. Krowoderska 37.
Map 1 B2.

Pharmacies

ul. Dunajewskiego 2.
Map 1 B4 (5 C2).
Tel 12 422 65 04.

ul. Grodzka 34.
Map 1 C5 (6 D4).
Tel 12 421 85 44.

Apteka Bonifratrów
ul. Krakowska 50.
Map 4 D2.
Tel 12 426 80 10.

**Apteka
Niezapominajka**
ul. Starowiślna 1.
Map 2 D5 (6 E3).
Tel 12 421 08 08.

Dbam o Zdrowie
ul. Podwale 6.
Map 1 B4 (5 C2).
Tel 12 429 49 43.

Europa
ul. Karmelicka 42.
Map 1 B3.
Tel 12 632 72 57.

Pod Złotym Lwem
ul. Długa 4.
Map 1 C2
Tel 12 422 62 04.

Pod Złotym Tygrysem
ul. Szczepańska 1.
Map 1 C4 (5 C2).
Tel 12 422 92 93.

Świat. Apteka
ul. Szpitalna 38.
Map 2 D4 (6 E2).
Tel 12 422 65 34.

Ziko
ul. Dunajewskiego 2.
Map 1 C4 (5 C1).
Tel 12 687 57 47.

Florists

BeA
ul. Łobzowska 33/10.
Map 1 B3.
Tel 601 504 436.

Konwalia
ul. Zwierzyniecka 23.
Map 1 B5 (5 B4).
Tel 12 422
93 52.

Margareta
ul. Długa 74.
Map 1 C2.
Tel 12 633 78 63.

Niezapominajka
al. Krasińskiego 1.
Map 1 A5 (5 B4).
Tel 12 619 33 31.

Sofi-Flora
ul. Pawia 5.
Map 2 D3 (6 F1).
Tel 12 628 78 77.

ENTERTAINMENT IN KRAKOW

Krakow is the cultural capital of Poland, and visitors looking for entertainment may find themselves spoiled for choice. Local theatres are among the best in the country and often host leading international companies. The Szymanowski Philharmonic Orchestra and Choir and the Capella Cracoviensis have excellent reputations. There are many concerts and festivals of classical and folk music organized in the magnificent interiors of historic houses and churches. The history of Krakow's cabarets goes back some 100 years, attracting both domestic and foreign audiences. The busy nightlife can be compared to that offered by Italian or Spanish cities. You only have to walk a couple of minutes to find a variety of music clubs, discotheques and bars. They are usually housed in Gothic or Renaissance cellars and are open until very late or even till the early hours of the morning. Theatre, film, music and ballet festivals take place throughout the year.

Useful Information

Full listings of cultural events in Krakow appear in the *Karnet – Krakowskie Aktualności Kulturalne* monthly, published by **InfoKraków** in both Polish and English. For the electronic version of the *Karnet* see their website on: www.karnet. kracow.pl. Current listings and reviews of cinemas, theatres and other events, as well as a guide to restaurants, discos and clubs (live music) are published on Friday in the *Gazeta Wyborcza* supplement entitled *Co jest grane?* (What's on?). Listings also appear in local newpapers on a daily basis. Information in English, German, French and Russian is also available on the website www.krakow.pl, under the heading "Calendar of Events". *Magiczny Kraków* is also a good source of information in English.

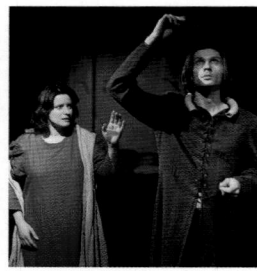
A theatre performance

Booking Tickets

Tickets for all major events can be purchased from the InfoKraków tourist office. This is also the best place to make enquiries about how and where to buy other tickets or to make an advanced booking. Staff at the Centre speak English, French, German and Italian. Booking is also possible through travel agents and hotel receptions.

Seats for the Philharmonic Hall and the theatres are available from their respective box offices, which also take advance bookings. Cinema tickets can be booked over the phone. Bear in mind that some performances require booking months in advance.

Ticket Prices

Ticket prices have increased considerably in recent years, but they are still cheaper than in the West. Theatre seats are more expensive in Krakow compared to anywhere else in Poland, and in greatest demand. Average prices vary from 25 to 40 zł per person. Cinema tickets cost between 13 and 20 zł. Museum tickets are good value; in some museums entrance is free on one day of the week.

Night Transport

Bus and tram day-routes stop around 11pm. Night buses and trams operate according to timetables displayed at stops or online; visit www.mpk.krakow.pl for more information. Tickets can be purchased from ticket machines at some stops and on most trams and buses.

Taxis are a better option. A radio-taxi booked over the phone is cheaper than one at a taxi-rank but you can rely on the taxis waiting at the ranks in the city centre. Most taxi drivers are honest, but it is best to

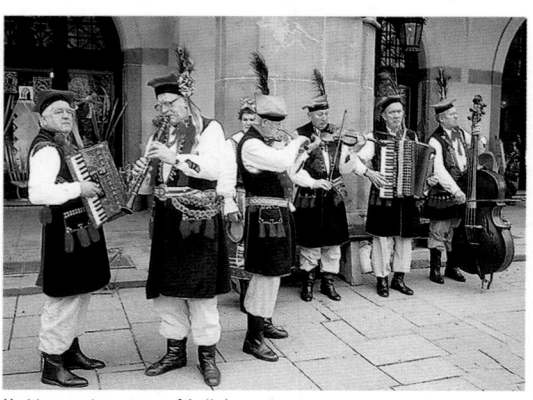
Musicians wearing costumes of the Krakow region

avoid the taxi rank by the main Railway Station. If you require a taxi while in the main Railway Station area, go to the radio-taxi rank situated at roof level above the platforms (use the platform stairway).

Festivals

The city plays host to a multitude of cultural festivals; the only problem is how to choose the most interesting. The International Festival of Alternative Theatre will appeal to theatre fans, the Krakow Film Festival to film lovers, the Krakow Spring Ballet Festival to ballet aficionados, the International Festival of Music in Old Krakow to admirers of classical music, while enthusiasts of brass instruments may enjoy the International Music Festival of Military Bands.

Walks and Open-Air Events

The tradition of open-air fairs in Krakow goes back to at least the early part of the 19th century when folk festivals were organized on the Błonia fields, then located out of town. One of the attractions was to try to climb a pole smeared in soap, a flask of alcohol and sausages attached to the top of the pole awaiting the successful climber. The event has since disappeared but the Błonia is still a venue for public events, of either a traditional or light entertainment nature. Two great cavalry parades in the inter-war years, attended by Marshals Józef Piłsudski and Edward Rydz Śmigły respectively, took place here. The masses celebrated on these fields by Pope John Paul II, and attended by millions of the faithful, are commemorated by a granite block brought here from the Tatra Mountains.

All kinds of concerts, festivals and fairs also take place at the Błonia.

The Jordan Park, situated opposite the Błonia fields, is very popular with mothers with toddlers. Doctor Henryk Jordan, a Krakow physician, introduced the idea of playing fields which are now found throughout the country and are named after this celebrated physician. The Jordan Park in Krakow was the first-ever public playground for small children.

The Wolski Wood (Las Wolski) is not far from Krakow and offers many walking routes (see pp172–3). For Krakovians it is one of the favourite destinations for a day out, though the zoo (see p173) is also popular. At weekends and on public holidays there is no access to the zoo by car, so use bus or taxi services. On weekdays a charge is made to enter the zoo by car.

Summer concerts in the open air are organized in the Wawel Castle courtyard, in the gardens of the Archaeological Museum and in Radio Kraków's amphitheatre as well as in the courtyard of the Collegium Iuridicum and on a temporary stage in Market Square.

A pillar advertising cultural events

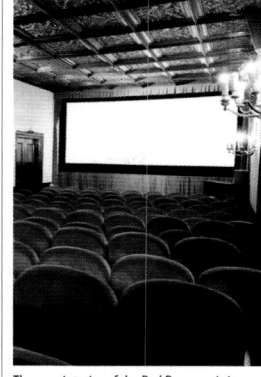
The cosy interior of the Pod Baranami cinema

Out of Town Trips

A number of appealing sights are located within close proximity to Krakow. A trip to the Ojców National Park (see p158), one of the smallest but most beautiful of Polish national parks, is an unforgettable experience. White limestone rocks, such as Hercules's Club, have very unusual shapes.

The Salt Mines at Wieliczka (see p158) have been included by UNESCO on their World Heritage List. The mines and the underground sanatorium housed here are unique. Niepołomice (see p157) has a 14th-century castle and the remnants of an ancient forest where bison are bred. The Benedictine Abbey in Tyniec (see p159) is beautifully located on the Vistula and worth visiting, as is Schindler's Factory (see p158), in the former industrial district of Zabłocie.

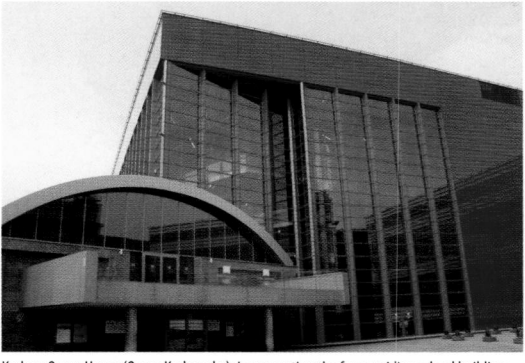
Krakow Opera House (Opera Krakowska), incorporating the former riding school building

Theatre, Music, Nightlife and Sports

Krakow is famous for its cultural traditions. The renowned Stary Theatre gained its fame through productions directed by Konrad Swinarski and counts as one of Europe's leading theatre companies. The city resounds with music of every kind, ranging from classical concerts and opera to hip-hop, techno, rock and jazz in the lively clubs. Cabarets continue the best of traditions that go back to the beginning of the 20th century. As well as myriad cultural events, Krakow also offers good sporting facilites for those who like to keep active.

Foreign-Language Performances

Krakow does not have a theatre company that performs in a foreign language on a permanent basis. The annual Festival of French-speaking Theatre takes place in May and attracts many companies from French-speaking countries. The city occasionally hosts foreign theatre companies from all parts of the world who perform in their own languages.

A number of bodies, such as the **Institut Français**, the **Goethe Institut**, the **Instituto Cervantes de Cracovia**, the **Istituto Italiano di Cultura** and the **Manggha Japanese Centre of Art and Technology**, are all actively involved in artistic patronage. They usually organize events in the language of their country, and information about these events can be obtained from **InfoKraków**.

Theatre

The first professional theatre company was established in Krakow in 1781, and today there are many theatres. The most renowned is **Stary Teatr** (Old Theatre). The best actors, directors and set designers work for the Stary Teatr whose performances are mostly based on Polish and other Eastern European classics and Romantic literature.

The **Teatr im. Juliusza Słowackiego** shares the same traditions and types of plays. The building, modelled on the Opéra Garnier in Paris, opened in 1893. Its splendid Art Nouveau interior features a curtain designed by the painter Henryk Hektor Siemiradzki. As an added bonus, spectators may watch the performance from the box originally used by the Austro-Hungarian Emperor, Franz Joseph and his wife Sissi.

The **Krakowski Teatr Scena Stu** gained fame through unconventional performances, sometimes staged in the open air, and other grand productions. In their main venue in aleja Krasińkiego, their performances are predominantly of the classics. Benefit performances celebrating theatre stars take place here, and are broadcast by television. These have became classics in their own right.

The **Ludowy Theatre** in Nowa Huta has a young cast who perform not only in Nowa Huta but also in two other venues in Krakow – in the cellars beneath the Town Hall and in Kanonicza Street.

The **Bagatela Theatre** specializes in light satirical productions. The **Teatr Lalki i Maski Groteska** generally performs for children but has also staged a number of plays for adults.

The experimental productions of the world-famous Cricot 2 theatre ceased following the death of its radical founder and director, Tadeusz Kantor, in 1990. The **Cricoteka** is a museum that documents the history of this major theatre and the art of Tadeusz Kantor, and includes photographs and set designs.

Opera and Ballet

After many years without a permanent venue, the **Opera Krakowska** moved into its premises on ul. Lubicz in 2008. It continues to stage occasional performances at various venues across the city, including the courtyard of Wawel Castle and underground at the Wieliczka Salt Mines. The productions here include Galician all-time favourites by Kalman, Lehar and the Strausses.

For many years, ballet was rather unpopular in Krakow, but regular performances now take place at the Opera Krakowska building. Two festivals, the annual Krakow Spring Ballet Festival, which takes place in May and June, and the International Ballet Festival have played an important role in increasing the popularity of ballet.

Cabaret

Cabaret artists are much in demand in Krakow and can always rely on good audiences and sell-outs. Opened in 1956, the literary **Piwnica Pod Baranami**, is the longest-running cabaret in Krakow and is famous throughout Poland. Despite the death of its founder Piotr Skrynecki in 1997, the cabaret continues and is very popular.

The **Loch Camelot** is artistically affiliated to the Piwnica and also performs in cellars. Very popular is the **Kabaret Pod Wyrwigroszem**, which puts on shows in various venues across town.

Lovers of the classic, satirical texts of the **Jama Michalika** Cabaret may still attend a performance here. In surroundings which include Art Nouveau objects and caricatures dating from the early 20th century, they may listen to Tadeusz Boy-Żeleński's verses. The original decadent ambience of this place is, however, difficult to recreate today, the menu lacks absinthe and there is a total ban on smoking.

Cinemas

Krakow has many multiplex cinemas, but the largest and best independent cinema is **Kijów.Centrum**. Besides its regular programme, it is also a venue for a number of festivals, including the Krakow Film Festival and one dedicated to commercials. Food and drinks are available on the first floor. A truly Parisian-style multiplex, the **Kino ARS**, is situated at the junction of św. Jana and św. Tomasza. It comprises several auditoria named after historic cinemas, such as Gabinet, Kiniarnia, Salon, Aneks and Reduta. Cafés can be found in all of them.

The small **Pod Baranami** cinema, housed in the Palace of the Rams, is very popular with those seeking independent and art-house films from around the world. Its prime location is an added bonus. After a show, walk a few steps to enjoy a drink in the Piwnica Pod Baranami bar. Among other cinemas worth recommending are the **Kika** and **Mikro**.

Classical Music

The most prestigious concert hall in Krakow is the Szymanowski Philharmonic Hall, home of the **Filharmonia**. Classical music is, however, best enjoyed in the more informal setting of one of the city's many historic houses. Among the many venues are the Wawel Castle, the National Museum in the Cloth Hall and the **Akademia Muzycna** (Music Academy), as well as churches, such as St Mary's (see pp94-7), St Catherine's (see p128) and the Holy Cross (see p117). In summer, concerts are also organized outside in such open-air venues as the arcades of the Wawel Castle, Collegium Maius's courtyard, in the former prison of St Michael (now the Archaeological Museum), and in the Radio Kraków amphitheatre, housed in the former Tarnowski Palace. For those prepared to travel a little, then there are the renowned organ recitals in the Romanesque Benedictine Abbey in Tyniec near Krakow (see p159).

Music Clubs

Any jazz fan visiting Krakow should seek out the **Jazz Club u Muniaka**. Here on Fridays and Saturdays Janusz Muniak, one of Poland's most celebrated jazzmen, plays to the accompaniment of other musicians. Jazz concerts take place at the **Harris Piano Jazz Bar, Mile Stone Jazz Club**, and **Jazz Club Kornet** (traditional jazz) as well as Piwnica pod Baranami. Apart from jazz, **U Louisa** provides blues music and during the break you can surf the Internet using one of several terminals provided.

The **Rotunda-Orlik** and **Pod Jaszczurami** student clubs are also venues for rock groups, blues bands and student cabaret songs. Live music, and rock in particular, can be heard in a number of pubs such as **Alchemia, Klub Piękny Pies** and **Jazz Rock Café**.

Nightclubs and Discos

The best venue for techno music, experimental music and drum and bass is the barrel-vaulted **Krzysztofory**. **Afera Club, Pod Papugami, Społem, Frantic** and **Prozak 2.0** discos are also popular, with a good party atmosphere.

Drukarnia caters for fans of avant-garde hip-hop, grunge and acid jazz music. Lovers of music of the sixties will enjoy the **Bosto** club, which offers a retro atmosphere on its small dance floor. The front end of a Syrena car, mounted in the wall, is a reminder of this unforgettable period.

If you feel exhausted after having a wild time in a disco, **Kitsch, Free Pub** and **Black Gallery** are good places to go to to relax.

Krakow's nightclubs do not have any specific hour at which they close. In summer, especially, a club-goer may simply leave a club and go straight to work.

Sports

As far as sports facilities are concerned, Krakow has much to offer. Two neighbouring sports clubs, **KS Cracovia** and **TS Wisła**, are the oldest and most popular in the city. Both clubs have their own swimming pools, which are open to the public.

The artificial lake in Kryspinów has clean water and is a good place for both beach lovers and windsurfers. A supervised swimming area can be found in the **Nad Zalewem Recreation Centre**. However, here there is a charge for the use of the centre and the lake's beaches. The sports grounds in the Jordan Park (see pp212–13) are a good place for badminton players. Other sports clubs include **Korona, Olsza** and **Zwierzyniecki**.

Tennis courts are available at **Centrum tenisowe, Klub tenisowy "Kosłówek"** and **Hotel Crown Piast**. The courts at the Olsza and Zwierzyniecki sports centres are open all year round.

Horse-riding facilities are available at the University Riding Club, as well as at a number of stables located on the outskirts of the city and further afield.

Increasingly, Krakovians have shown an interest in healthy living. Sauna, sun bed and health and beauty clinics have opened in all parts of the city, as have fitness clubs such as **Relax Body Club** and **Fit-Styl**. The **Korona Club**, which is attached to the hotel of the same name, offers a covered swimming pool (filled with sea water), fitness centre and sauna facilities.

If you want to go for a run during your visit, take advantage of Błonia Fields (see p149), the expansive meadow in the middle of the city.

Billiards can be played in a number of venues throughout Krakow. Billiards and snooker clubs include **Daddy's Bilard, Frame Snooker & Bilard** and **Prominent**.

DIRECTORY

Booking Tickets

InfoKraków
ul. Św. Jana 2.
Map 1 C4 (6 D2).
Tel 12 421 77 87.

Foreign and International Institutes

The British Council
Rynek Główny 6.
Map 1 C4 (6 D3).
Tel 12 428 59 30.

Goethe Institut
Rynek Główny 20.
Map 1 C4 (6 D3).
Tel 12 422 58 29.

Institut Français
ul. Stolarska 15.
Map 1 C5 (6 D3).
Tel 12 424 5350.

Instituto Cervantes de Cracovia
ul. Kanonicza 12.
Map 1 C5 (6 D4).
Tel 12 421 32 55.

International Cultural Centre
Rynek Główny 25.
Map 1 C4 (6 D3).
Tel 12 424 28 11.

Istituto Italiano di Cultura
ul. Grodzka 49.
Map 1 C5 (6 D4).
Tel 12 421 89 46.

Manggha Japanese Centre of Art and Technology
ul. Konopnickiej 26.
Map 3 B1.
Tel 12 267 27 03.

Theatre

Bagatela Theatre
ul. Karmelicka 6.
Map 1 B4 (5 C2).
Tel 12 424 52 12.

Cricoteka
ul. Kanonicza 5.
Map 1 C5 (6 D4).
Tel 12 422 83 32.

Krakowski Teatr Scena Stu
al. Krasińskiego 16–18.
Map 1 A5 (5 A4).
Tel 12 422 27 44.

KTO
ul. Gzymsików 8.
Tel 12 623 73 00.

Ludowy Theatre
Os. Teatralne 34.
Map 1 B4 (5 C2).
Tel 12 680 21 16.

Opera Krakowska
ul. Lubicz 48. **Map** 2 F3.
Tel 12 296 62 60.

Stary Teatr
ul. Jagiellońska 5.
Map 1 C4 (5 C2).
Tel 12 422 90 80.

Stowarzyszenie Teatralne „Łaźnia"
ul. Paulińska 28. **Map** 3 C2. **Tel** 12 680 23 41.

Teatr im. J. Słowackiego
Pl. Świętego Ducha 1.
Map 2 D4 (6 E1).
Tel 12 424 45 26.

Teatr Lalki i Maski Groteska
ul. Skarbowa 2.
Map 1 B4 (5 A2).
Tel 12 632 92 00.

Zależny
ul. Kanonicza 1.
Map 1 C5 (6 D4).
Tel 12 628 24 88.

Cabaret

Jama Michalika
ul. Floriańska 45.
Map 2 D4 (6 E2).
Tel 12 422 15 61.

Kabaret Pod Wyrwigroszem
Tel 609 45 11 05.

Loch Camelot
ul. Św. Tomasza 17.
Map 1 C4 (6 D2).
Tel 501 426 404.

Piwnica Pod Baranami
Rynek Główny 27.
Map 1 C4 (6 D2).
Tel 12 421 25 00.

Cinema

Agrafka
ul. Krowoderska 8.
Map 1 C3.
Tel 12 430 01 79.

Cinema City
ul. Podgórska 34
(Galeria Kazimierz).
Map 4 F1.
Tel 12 254 54 54.

Kijów.Centrum
al. Krasińskiego 34.
Map 1 A5 (5 A3).
Tel 12 433 00 33.

Kika
ul. I. Krasickiego 18.
Map 3 C4.
Tel 12 296 41 52.

Kino 18
ul. Floriańska 18.
Map 2 D4 (6 E2).
Tel 882 041 881.

Kino ARS
ul. Św. Jana 6.
Map 1 C4 (6 D2).
Tel 12 421 41 99.

Mikro
ul. J. Lea 5. **Map** 1 A3.
Tel 12 634 28 97.

Paradox
ul. Krupnicza 38.
Map 1 B4.
Tel 12 430 00 15.

Pod Baranami
Rynek Główny 27.
Map 1 C4 (6 D2).
Tel 12 423 07 68.

Sfinks
Os. Górali 5.
Tel 12 644 27 65.

Świt
Os. Teatralne 10.
Tel 503 021 896.

Wrzos
ul. J. Zamojskiego 50.
Map 4 D3.
Tel 12 656 10 50.

Classical Music

Akademia Muzyczna
ul. Św. Tomasza 43.
Map 2 D4 (6 E2).
Tel 12 422 04 55.

Capella Cracoviensis
ul. Zwierzyniecka 1.
Map 1 B5 (5 C3).
Tel 602 620 698.

Centrum Kultury „Dworek Białoprądnicki"
ul. Papiernicza 2.
Tel 12 420 49 50.

Filharmonia
ul. Zwierzyniecka 1.
Map 1 B5 (5 C3).
Tel 12 619 87 33.

Radio Kraków SA
al. Słówackiego 22.
Map 2 D2.
Tel 12 630 60 00.

Sinfonietta Cracovia
ul. Papiernicza 2.
Tel 12 416 70 75.

Willa Decjusza
ul. 28 lipca 17a.
Tel 12 425 36 44.

Music Clubs

Alchemia
ul. Estery 5.
Map 4 D1.
Tel 12 421 22 00.

Harris Piano Jazz Bar
Rynek Główny 28.
Map 1 C4 (6 D2).
Tel 12 421 57 41.

Jazz Club u Muniaka
ul. Floriańska 3.
Map 1 C4 (6 D2).
Tel 12 423 12 05.

Jazz Klub Kornet
al. Krasińskiego 19.
Map 1 A5 (5 A4).

Jazz Rock Café
ul. Sławkowska 12.
Map 1 C4 (6 D2).
Tel 511 433 506.

Klub Piękny Pies
ul. Bożego Ciała 9.
Map 4 D2.

Mile Stone Jazz Club
ul. Nadwiślańska 6.
Map 4 E2.
Tel 12 374 5100.

Pod Jaszczurami
Rynek Główny 8.
Map 1 C4 (6 D3).
Tel 12 429 45 38.

Rotunda-Orlik
ul. Oleandry 1.
Map 1 A4.
Tel 12 634 34 12.

U Louisa
Rynek Główny 13.
Map 1 C4 (6 D3).
Tel 12 617 02 22.

Nightclubs and Discos

Afera Club
ul. Sławkowska 13/15.
Map 1 C4 (6 D2).
Tel 12 421 17 71.

Black Gallery
ul. Mikołajska 24.
Map 2 D4 (6 E2).
Tel 724 630 154.

Bosto
ul. Floriańska 33.
Map 2 D4 (6 E2).
Tel 12 421 16 93.

Drukarnia
ul. Nadwiślańska 1.
Map 4 E3.
Tel 12 656 65 60.

Frantic
ul. Szewska 5.
Map 5 C2.
Tel 12 423 04 83.

Free Pub
ul. Sławkowska 4.
Map 1 C4 (6 D2).
Tel 080 290 82.

Kitsch
ul. Dajwor 16.
Map 4 E1.
Tel 518 879 055.

Krzysztofory
ul. Szczepańska 2.
Map 1 C4 (6 D2).
Tel 12 421 36 02.

Pod Papugami
ul. Św. Jana 18.
Map 1 C4 (6 D2).
Tel 12 422 82 99.

Prozak 2.0
pl. Dominikański 6.
Map C5 (6 D3).
Tel 733 70 46 50.

Społem
ul. Św. Tomasza 4.
Map 1 C4 (6 D2).
Tel 12 421 79 79.

Sports Clubs

Korona
ul. Kalwaryjska 9/15.
Map 4 D3.
Tel 12 656 13 68.

KS Cracovia
ul. Kałuży 1.
Map 1 A5.
Tel 12 294 66 05.

Olsza
ul. Siedleckiego 7.
Tel 12 421 10 69.

TS Wisła
ul. Reymonta 22.
Tel 12 630 45 52.

Zwierzyniecki
Na Błoniach 1.
Tel 12 425 18 46.

Tennis Courts

Centrum tenisowe
Na Błoniach 1.
Tel 12 425 29 98.

Gołaski Sport
ul. Królowej Jadwigi 220.
Tel 12 425 39 00.

Hotel Crown Piast
ul. Radzikowskiego 109.
Tel 12 683 26 00.

Klub tenisowy „Kozłówek"
ul. Spółdzielców 13.
Tel 12 655 55 54.

KS Wieczysta
ul. Chałupnika 16.
Tel 12 442 42 70.

Nadwiślan
ul. Koletek 20. **Map** 3 C1.
Tel 12 422 21 22.

Olsza
ul. Siedleckiego 7.
Tel 12 421 10 69.

Tenis servis
al. Jana Pawła II 37.

Swimming Pools

Clepardia
ul. Mackiewicza 14.
Tel 12 415 16 74.

Krakowianka
ul. Bulwarowa 1.
Tel 12 644 14 21.

Park Wodny
ul. Dobrego Pasterza 126.
Tel 12 616 31 90.

Polfa
ul. Eisenberga 2.
Tel 12 411 40 88.

Wisła
ul. Reymonta 22. **Map** 1 A4. **Tel** 12 630 45 00.

Billiards and Snooker Clubs

Daddy's Bilard
ul. Krowoderska 28.
Map 1 C3.

Frame Snooker & Bilard
ul. Smolki 11A.
Map 4 D3.
Tel 12 423 57 06.

Prominent
ul. Kamienna 17.
Map 2 D1.
Tel 12 632 10 58.

Horse-Riding

Decjusz
al. Kasztanowa 1.
Tel 12 425 24 21.

Krakowski Klub Jazdy Konnej
ul. Kobierzńyska 175.
Tel 12 262 14 18.

Krakus
ul. Kąpielowa 51.
Tel 12 654 72 10.

Pegaz
ul. Łowińskiego 1.
Tel 12 425 80 88.

Pod Żubrem
Niepołomice,
Targowa 5.
Tel 12 281 19 96.

Stadnina Podskalany
ul. Podskalany 61.
Tel 606 91 50 09.

Stary Młyn
ul. Wilczkowice 50.
Tel 12 411 10 91.

Health, Fitness and Sauna Clubs

Fit-Styl
ul. Miodowa 21.
Map 4 D1.
Tel 12 421 95 34.

Forteca Climbing Centre
ul. Racławicka 60.
Tel 12 632 83 33.

Korona Club
ul. Kalwaryjska 9–15.
Tel 12 656 53 89

Nad Zalevem Recreation Centre
ul. Bronowicka 19.
Tel 12 292 75 53.

Relax Body Club
ul. Mogilska 70.
Map 2 F3.
Tel 12 411 03 60.

Tribal Fitness
ul. Św. Filipa 9a.
Map 2 D3.
Tel 12 632 68 48.

Yoga International
ul. Św. Marka 34
Map 6 E2.
Tel 692 41 41 47.

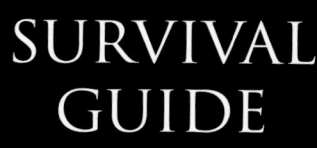

SURVIVAL
GUIDE

PRACTICAL INFORMATION

Krakow attracts more tourists than any other Polish city, and visitor facilities are generally first class. Points of arrival such as the main railway and bus stations have been thoroughly modernized in recent years, and the John Paul II Airport at Balice boasts a speedy rail link to the city centre. Tourist signage makes it easy to find your way around on foot and many of the city's sights are within walking distance from each other. The increased use of bicycles is a sign that Krakow is becoming much more eco-friendly. The communications system is good: postal services are easy to use, and the provision of Wi-Fi access is increasingly widespread. The tourist season lasts all year round in Krakow, but summer is particularly busy thanks to the warm weather.

When to Go

Krakow is a popular destination for visitors throughout the year and tourist facilities are open for business during every season. Spring and summer bring warm, dry weather, when the city is filled with visitors and café tables cover the pavements. Autumn and winter, although cold, can also be a magical time, with Advent markets on the main city squares and an atmosphere of celebration in restaurants and bars.

Hotel prices are at their highest from Easter to August and around Christmas and New Year. It is best to travel outside these times if you want to enjoy an inexpensive holiday without the crowds.

Culture-lovers should take note that most theatres and classical-music venues take an annual break from June to mid-September.

Visas and Passports

Citizens of the European Union, USA, Australia, Canada and New Zealand can enter Poland without a visa, on production of a valid passport for stays of up to 90 days. Citizens of other countries should check the latest visa regulations with their local Polish embassy. Poland is a member of the Schengen group of European Union countries, which means that there are unlikely to be any border controls at immigration when entering Poland from another Schengen-zone country.

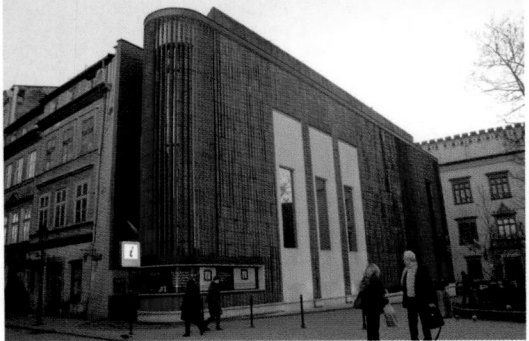
Façade of InfoKraków

Customs Information

If you are travelling to or from another EU country there are few restrictions on items brought in and out of Poland for personal use.

Visitors from outside the EU should check the customs regulations of their home country – there are likely to be limits on the amount of cigarettes, alcoholic beverages, toiletries and gifts that can be taken home. The maximum value of currency that can be brought into or taken out of Poland is €10,000 (or equivalent). Sums in excess of this must be declared to the customs authority. A licence is required to export any item more than 100 years old or any artwork over 50 years old and exceeding more than 16,000zł in value. For more information contact the **Ministry of Culture and National Heritage**. Value Added Tax (VAT) can be claimed on goods totalling 200zł or more and that are taken out of the country within 30 days of purchase.

Tourist Information

Krakow's municipal tourist office operates information centres at several locations around the city centre. Their locations are shown on the Street Finder maps towards the end of this book (see pp232–7). The main office is situated in the **Cloth Hall** on Market Square. There is also a branch at **Planty Park** and at **John Paul II Airport**. All offices offer brochures with museum and gallery opening times, and lists of accommodation.

Electronic displays with information on the availability of hotels can be found at the main railway station and John Paul II Airport. **InfoKraków**, just off the Market Square on ul. Św. Jana, provides information on upcoming concerts and shows. Hotel and hostel reception desks can be useful sources of information, although they sometimes only advertise tourist companies with whom they have a commercial agreement.

Admission Prices

Admission charges to museums and galleries are modest but may be increased substantially for a temporary exhibition. Reduced rates are available for children, students and senior citizens. Overseas students should possess a valid international student card in order to qualify for a discount (see p212).

Opening Hours

The opening hours of the museums and galleries listed in this guide are given individually for each sight. Most state museums and galleries are closed on Mondays and private galleries of contemporary art are generally closed on Sundays. Opening times vary depending on the day of the week, but late openings are normally on Thursdays.

Churches usually remain open from the first to the last service without closing at midday, but there are some variations. Food stores are open 7am–7pm, but there are no strict rules about opening hours, which are at the owner's discretion. Other shops tend to open between 10am and 7pm. For information on opening times of banks and bureaux de change see p216.

Restaurants are open until 11pm although there are many pubs and bars that serve food and stay open until the early hours. Twenty-four-hour bars serving cheap drinks and snacks are popular with the locals and easy to find.

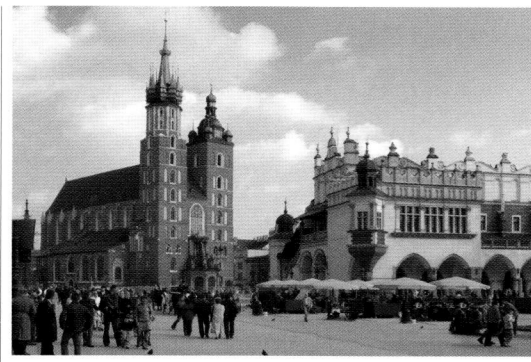
Tourists in Market Square, with the Church of St Mary in the background

Language

Language learning has undergone something of a boom in recent years, and most young Krakovians speak English and maybe one other world language as well. Older-generation Poles are a bit less forthcoming when it comes to foreign languages, although they will make an attempt to communicate with the few words they may have.

Some taxi companies use drivers who speak foreign languages, so you may, for example, request an English-speaking driver. Staff at museums, hotels and restaurants generally speak English, and possibly also one other major European language. In many cases staff in shops, post offices and banks communicate in Polish only, especially outside the city centre. It is worth making an effort to learn a few words and phrases in Polish; the Phrase Book is a useful place to start (see pp255–6).

Etiquette and Smoking

There are nearly 100 Roman Catholic churches in Krakow and masses take place at all times of day throughout the week. Sightseeing is allowed when there are no services taking places but visitors should refrain from making noise and use cameras discreetly. In some churches, signs banning photography are clearly visible on the door. When visiting places of worship, it is polite to dress

modestly: as well as the torso, upper arms and legs should be covered.

Smoking is banned in most public places. Almost all restaurants and cafés are completely smoke-free indoors, although smoking is permitted outside at restaurants and cafés that have a pavement terrace or a garden. Only a handful of bars and clubs have retained a self-contained indoor area where smoking is still allowed.

Accessibility to Public Conveniences

There are free-of-charge public conveniences in big shopping centres such as Galeria Krakowska next to the main railway station, and Galeria Kazimierz on ul. Podgórska near the Kazimierz Quarter. Pay-to-use toilets are scattered throughout the centre and can be found in the Cloth Hall, in Planty Park by Sienna and Reformacka streets, and at the parking area by the Wawel. All restaurants, bars and cafés have facilities. Most of these are free to use if you are a customer, although one or two restaurants do charge.

Taxes and Tipping

It is common to give a tip in cafés and restaurants with waiting staff, although there are no strict rules as to how much this should be. Adding 10 per cent to the bill or rounding it up to a suitable number is considered polite.

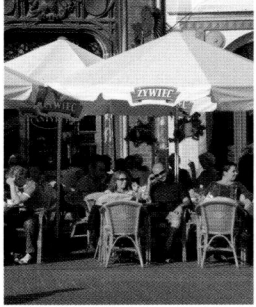
Visitors enjoying street cafés in Market Square

Travellers with Special Needs

Facilities for people with disabilities are still limited in Krakow. Moving around in a wheelchair is not easy due to the lack of contoured pavements and the large number of cars parked in pedestrian areas. Improvements are being made: some pedestrian crossings have low kerbs, and the number which are equipped with an audio message for the blind is on the increase. Wheelchair access and lifts are available at the main railway station.

Good facilities can also be found in a number of museums, including the National Museum in Krakow's Main Building (see pp150–51), most of the National Museum's other branches, and the Japanese Centre for Art and Technology (see p45), as well as in some cinemas and theatres. The Main Post Office also offers easy access. All hotels four stars or above offer at least a couple of rooms for wheelchair users (see p178). An increasing number of trams and buses have low-level entry floors for wheelchair access.

There are several organizations which assist the disabled in Krakow, including the **Polish Association for the Blind** and the **Polish Assocation for the Deaf**. The **Radio Taxi Partner** company operates a fleet of vehicles especially adapted for wheelchair users.

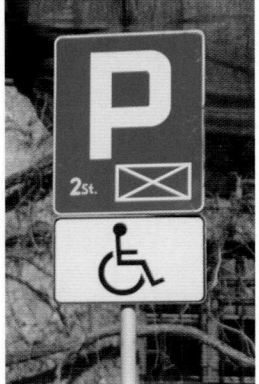
Disabled parking sign in a Krakow street

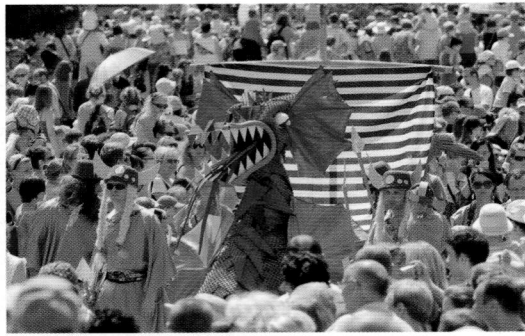
Crowds watching the annual Dragon Parade on Market Square

Travelling with Children

Krakow is an enjoyable and safe environment for children, thanks to the largely pedestrianized city centre and the extensive areas of park in the surrounding areas.

One of the best public playparks is in **Jordan Park**, west of the Old Town. The **Stanisław Lem Garden of Experiments**, east of the centre towards Nowa Huta, is an open-air, hands-on science museum that encourages children to learn about science by playing on large pieces of apparatus.

Groteska Theatre is Krakow's leading children's theatre, whose productions often mix puppets with live action. Groteska also organizes the annual Dragon Parade in June, when puppet monsters descend on Market Square followed by fireworks beside the River Wisła.

Finding child-friendly accommodation in Krakow is usually problem-free (see p178).

Gay and Lesbian Travellers

Although Krakow is more liberal than many other European cities, Poland as a whole is a conservative country and the gay and lesbian scene remains discreet. Krakow has a handful of clubs specifically tailored to gay men and lesbians, and a broader choice of bars, particularly in the Jewish Kazimierz quarter in the west of the city, that encourage a mixture of all customers. The annual

Tolerance March, a gay-pride-style event that takes place in mid-May, attracts many supporters from across the social spectrum – but also draws large numbers of conservative counter-demonstrators.

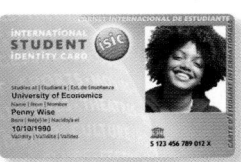
An ISIC card (International Student Identity Card)

Travelling on a Budget

In comparison to other major European cities, Krakow is not that expensive and with some planning it is possible to get around on a low budget.

For young travellers, international youth and student cards such as **ISIC** (International Student Identity Card) and **European Youth Card** are worth obtaining. Both cards entitle holders to reduced rates in museums, tourist attractions, hotels, hostels and on intercity buses. A wide range of other Krakow businesses offer discounts to bearers of both cards, including car-hire firms, cafés, hairdressers, pizzerias, travel agents and theatres. The logos of the cards are displayed in the windows of those businesses offering discounts.

An ISIC card is available to anyone who is either a full-time student or who is under the age of 26. You can obtain one in your home country or through youth-tourism specialists **Almatur** in Krakow, providing you have documentary evidence of your status.

The European Youth Card is available to anyone under the age of 30 and can be bought from numerous outlets throughout Europe, or online via their website.

Time

Poland is in the Central European time zone, which means that Krakow is 1 hour ahead of Greenwich Mean Time, 6 hours ahead of US Eastern Standard Time, and 11 hours behind Australian Eastern Standard Time. From late March until late October clocks are set forward 1 hour.

Electricity

The voltage in Poland is 230 volts. Plugs are of the two-pin type, as is the case in most countries in Europe. Buy a European travel adaptor before you leave home.

Responsible Tourism

Travelling responsibly is largely a matter of common sense. Eating in chain restaurants or fast-food outlets increases the likelihood that you will be consuming cheaply supplied products that have not come from ecological sources. If you eat Polish food in Polish restaurants, it is more likely that food has been locally sourced. When shopping for your own food, aim for outdoor markets rather than the large supermarkets. Stall-holders at the Stary Kleparz market at Rynek Kleparski near Planty are far more likely to sell seasonal produce of local provenance, and will frequently advertise the fact by chalking up signs advertising the Polish origin of their vegetables. Organic food shops include Naturalny sklepik at Krupnicza 8; and Natura at Krupnicza 21. Both sell many Polish specialities. Take a multiple-use bag of your own rather than using plastic bags.

If you have rubbish to dispose of, ask locals to direct you to the recycling bins located on many street corners. There is usually a trio of containers set aside for paper, glass and plastics.

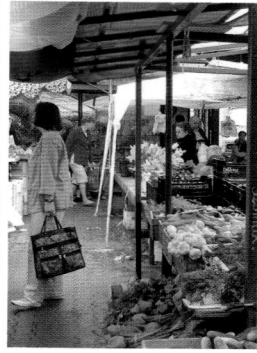

Fresh fruit and vegetables at a Krakow food market

DIRECTORY

Embassies and Consulates

Australia
3rd floor, Nautilus Building, ul. Nowogrodzka 11, Warsaw. **Tel** 22 521 34 44. W australia.pl

Canada
ul. Jana Matejki 1/5, Warsaw.
Tel 22 584 31 00.
W poland.gc.ca

Ireland
ul. Mysia 5, Warsaw.
Tel 22 849 66 33.
W embassyofireland.pl

United Kingdom
ul. Św. Anny 9.
Map 1 B4 (5 C2).
Tel 12 421 70 30.
W http:// ukinpoland. fco.gov.uk

United States of America
ul. Stolarska 9.
Map 1 C5 (6 D3).
Tel 12 424 51 00.
W krakow.usconsulate. gov

Customs Information

Ministry of Culture and National Heritage
W mkidn.gov.pl

Tourist Information

Cloth Hall
Rynek Główny.
Map 1 C4 (6 D2).
Tel 12 433 73 10.

InfoKraków
ul. Św. Jana 2.
Map 1 C4 (6 D2).
Tel 12 421 77 87.
W infokrakow.pl

John Paul II Airport
Tel 12 295 58 00.

Planty Park
ul. Szpitalna 25.
Map 2 D4 (6 E1).
Tel 12 432 01 10.
W infokrakow.pl

Travellers with Special Needs

Polish Association for the Blind
ul. Dr. Józefa Babińskiego 29, blok 23/3.
Tel 12 262 53 59.
W pzn.malopolska.pl

Polish Association for the Deaf
ul. Św. Jana 18.
Map 1 C4 (6 D2).
Tel 12 422 73 45.
W pzg.krakow.pl

Polish Society for the Rehabilitation of the Disabled
al. 29 Listopada 130. **Tel** 12 312 14 00.
W pfron.org.pl

Radio Taxi Partner
Tel 196 33, 196 88.
W taxi-partner. krakow.pl

Travelling with Children

Groteska Theatre
ul. Skarbowa 2.
Map 1 B4 (5 A2).
Tel 12 633 48 22.
W groteska.pl

Jordan Park
al. 3 Maja.

Stanislaw Lem Garden of Experiments
al. pokoju. **Tel** 12 346 12 85. W ogroddos wiadczen.pl

Travelling on a Budget

Almatur
Rynek Główny 27.
Map 1 C4 (6 D2).
Tel 12 422 46 68.
W almatur.pl

European Youth Card
W europeanyouth card.org

ISIC
W isic.org

Personal Security and Health

Krakow is one of the safest cities in Poland. Although the number of reported crimes is generally on the increase, Krakow is a quiet place and visitors can feel safe in most parts of the city. The same safety rules apply here as everywhere, so beware of pickpockets, do not leave any property visible in a car, and use guarded car parks. The local police take a tough line on rowdy, alcohol-influenced behaviour on the streets. Anyone suffering a minor health problem should seek advice at a pharmacy, while hotels can usually arrange a doctor's visit.

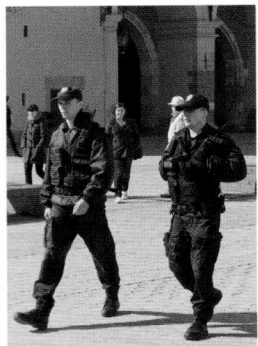

Police officers patrolling Krakow's Market Square

Police

In Krakow the police are assisted by other services, including town wardens and private security guards. Serious crime should be reported to a uniformed officer at a police station. Major police stations are indicated on the Street Finder maps (see pp232–7). Police are often visible, especially on weekend nights when people showing signs of bad behaviour under the influence of alcohol will usually be apprehended. Blue and silver police cars are used for patrolling the streets. Town wardens are unarmed and have no power of arrest. They tend to perform traffic wardens' duties by fining owners of illegally parked vehicles. Private security agencies are generally responsible for security in large shops and public buildings, as well as at public events. They are usually uniformed and should always carry identification badges.

What to Be Aware Of

Krakow is a popular venue for weekend party tourism. Late-night noisy behaviour is a frequent annoyance, but outright public disorder is very rare. Local police are taking an increasingly hard line on drunkenness, and anyone creating a disturbance late at night is likely to be apprehended and fined.

Ulica Szewska in the Old Quarter is at the centre of the weekend party scene. Most of the bars and clubs here are legitimate, although one or two establishments on this strip are notorious for overcharging tourists. Male visitors travelling solo or in small groups should be particularly aware of over-friendly young females suggesting a drink in a nearby bar; a hugely inflated bill will probably be the result.

Anyone found driving under the influence of alcohol will be arrested and must appear in court the following day. Be aware that cyclists riding a bicycle under the influence of alcohol will receive the same treatment as car drivers. The level of alcohol in the blood for both car drivers and cyclists is so low that it is advisable to not drink and drive at all. In the event of a serious road accident you are required by law to call an ambulance, the fire brigade and also the traffic police – see Directory opposite.

Petty thieves and pick-pockets are active in crowded bars, on public transport and at busy markets. Keep a close eye on your bag or rucksack, and carry it securely fastened across your body. Passports, wallets and other valuable items should never be carried in a back pocket or in the external pockets of a rucksack. Pickpockets frequently operate in gangs, and a sudden push or other distraction caused by them will hardly ever be accidental.

Valuables should never be left unattended in a car. Car break-ins are a big problem in Krakow. If you can remove the radio and take it with you, you may save your windows from being smashed. A car alarm offers no protection against professional thieves, so guarded parking may be a good option. A number of guarded car parks are available in the centre.

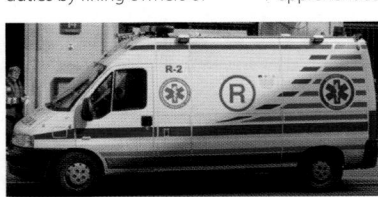

Ambulance

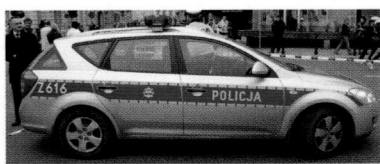

Police car

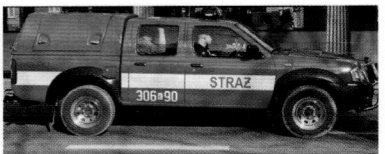

Fire engine

In an Emergency

Call 112 for emergencies requiring medical, police or fire services. An operator will answer (most speak English) and will direct your call. Minor health problems can often be dealt with in a pharmacy, where trained staff can provide advice on remedies. Prominent pharmacies are listed in the directory below. For more serious injury or illness, head for the casualty unit of one of the big city-centre hospitals.

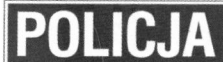

Police sign

Lost and Stolen Property

If you lose something at a venue in Krakow there is a good chance that staff will keep it for a day or two, in the expectation that you will return. It is a good idea to write your mobile phone number inside bags or wallets – in the event of loss, a good citizen or conscientious policeman may call to inform you that it has been found.

There are several lost property offices in Krakow, one for property lost on public transport and one for items misplaced elsewhere in the city. Items left on aeroplanes, intercity trains or buses will be kept at lost property offices at the airport, railway and bus station respectively. Never leave luggage unattended in public, as this can lead to theft or security alerts.

Hospitals and Pharmacies

Both state and private health care are available in Krakow. First aid is provided free of charge. Other treatment may be subject to a fee, which is usually required in advance, along with showing a passport for identification. It is very important to obtain a receipt for any payment made and it is advisable to take out insurance cover before you travel.

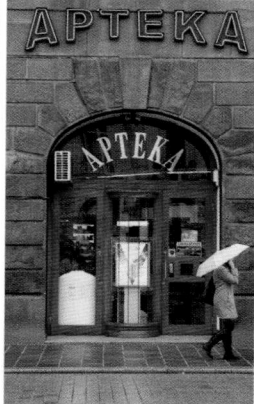

A typical pharmacy window in Krakow

Treatment for minor problems is available at pharmacies located throughout the city. If you require treatment after normal opening hours visit a 24-hour pharmacy. Their addresses are usually displayed in any pharmacy window (see p199). The ambulance service is on call day and night and should be contacted in case of an accident or emergency. There are several hospitals in Krakow including **Szpitzal Wojskowy**, north of the city centre. Hospitals with casualty units are shown on the Street Finder maps (see pp232–7).

Travel and Health Insurance

Travel insurance that includes provision for health care is highly recommended. The longer you stay abroad, the more important it is to ensure that you have substantial cover in case of loss, theft, or medical emergencies that will require repatriation help.

Many airlines and travel agents offer you insurance when you book your ticket. The Australian-based **World Nomads** is a reputable service that offers travel insurance to citizens of 150 countries.

All EU nationals are entitled to state healthcare in Poland on production of a valid **European Health Insurance Card** (EHIC). In the UK, this can be obtained from a post office or online from the EHIC website. It includes a booklet that details what healthcare you are entitled to, and where and how to claim. You may still have to pay in advance to obtain treatment, and then reclaim the money back later. As not all treatments are covered, it is advisable to take out additional insurance.

Make sure you travel with all relevant insurance documents. Keep a copy in your hotel room or with a reliable family member or friend back home, and itemize any valuables you are taking with you.

Banking and Local Currency

Financial transactions are easy in Krakow. ATMs accepting all major cards are located throughout the city. Foreign visitors will find many bureaux de change in the city centre, offering more favourable exchange rates than the banks. Credit and debit cards are accepted by most of Krakow's shops and restaurants. Signs displayed by the entrance to the establishment indicate which cards are accepted.

Banks and Bureaux de Change

Banks can be found throughout the city, both in and around the centre, as well as on the outskirts. They are usually open 9am–5pm Monday–Friday and many are open until 1pm on Saturday. Banks are often busy so expect to queue. Some branches have a ticketing system – take a numbered ticket at the entrance and wait until the number is displayed before approaching the counter.

Most banks have their own exchange service but better rates are offered by the independent bureaux de change (*kantor*), which do not charge commission. In Krakow these include **Dukat, Euro-Kantor, JPJ, Kantor Exchange** and **Pod Arkadami**. Foreign currency can also be changed at hotels, but rates are more expensive.

Large Polish banks with branches in Krakow include **PKO** and **Pekao**. International banks include **ING, HSBC** and **Raiffeisen**.

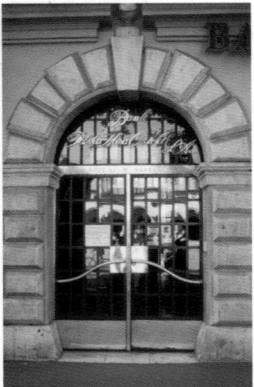

Entrance to the PKO Bank in Market Square

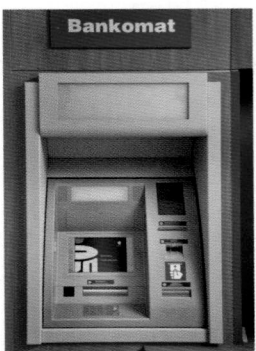

Bankomat automated teller machine (ATM) for dispensing cash

ATMs

ATMs (*bankomat*) are easy to find in Krakow and instructions are usually available in a choice of languages. The types of card accepted will be displayed on the ATM itself. Check these carefully before inserting your card – the vast majority accept Visa, Maestro and MasterCard. ATM withdrawals will be marginally more expensive than changing cash. The exchange rate for the amount withdrawn in złoty is slightly less advanta-geous than the one you will receive in a bank or bureau de change. A small fee will be charged by your bank for each ATM transaction carried out when abroad.

Be aware of your surroundings when using an ATM and always shield the keypad when entering your PIN.

Credit and Debit Cards

Credit and debit cards payments are accepted in most hotels, museums, restaurants, and shops. There may be a minimum expenditure in some restaurants and shops, below which they will not accept credit card payments; ask first. Cards are unlikely to be accepted in markets, suburban railway stations, and in smaller shops and cafés in the suburbs so it is advisable to carry a small amount of Polish cash.

All major credit cards such as American Express, VISA and MasterCard are widely accepted. Establishments normally indicate which cards they accept by displaying appropriate stickers on their windows.

It is a good idea to notify your bank before you travel so that they expect your card to be used in Poland.

DIRECTORY

BANKS

Bank Pekao
Rynek Główny 31.
Map 1 C4 (6 D2).

HSBC
Rynek Główny 13.
Map 1 C5 (6 D3).

ING Bank Śląski
ul. Św. Tomasza 20.
Map 1 C4 (6 E2).

PKO Bank
ul. Wielopole 19.
Map 2 D5 (6 F4).
Rynek Główny 21.
Map 1 C4 (6 D2).

Raiffeisen
ul. Długa 55.
Map 1 C2.

Bureaux de Change

Dukat
ul. Starowiślna 12. **Map** 2 D5 (6 E4). **Tel** 12 421 1203.

Euro-Kantor
ul. Szewska 21. **Map** 1 C4 (5 C2). **Tel** 12 421 55 65.

JPJ
ul. Wielopole 3. **Map** 2 D5 (6 E3). **Tel** 12 421 74 67.

Kantor Exchange
ul. Pawia 5 (Galeria Krakowska shopping mall) **Map** 2 D3 (6 F1). **Tel** 12 430 0761.

Pod Arkadami
ul. Grodzka 40. **Map** 1 C5 (6 D5). **Tel** 12 421 50 21.

Currency

The Polish unit of currency is the złoty, a term that literally means golden and which dates back to the Middle Ages, when gold pieces were used. Złoty is most commonly abbreviated to zł, although you will see the abbreviation PLN in banks and on your credit or debit ard statement. One złoty equals 100 groszy, abbreviated to gr.

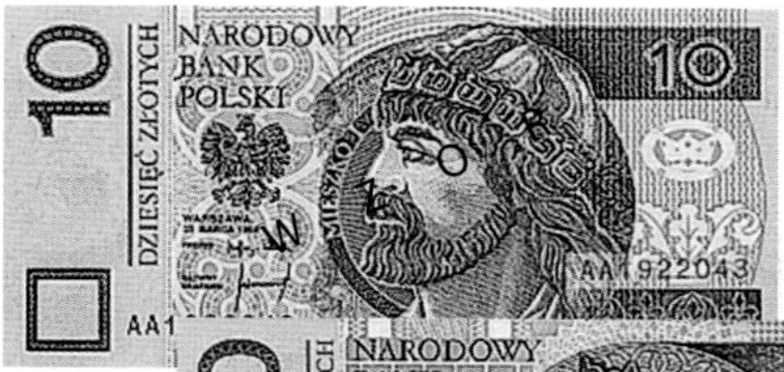

10 złoty

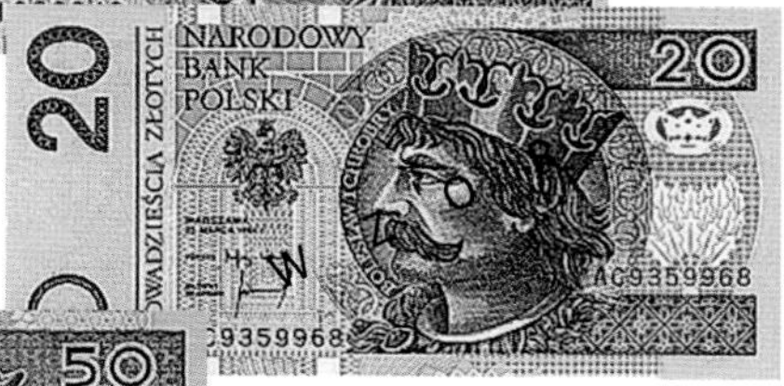

20 złoty

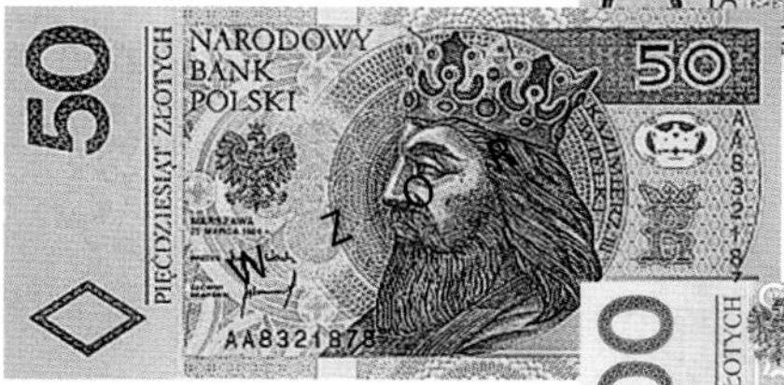

50 złoty

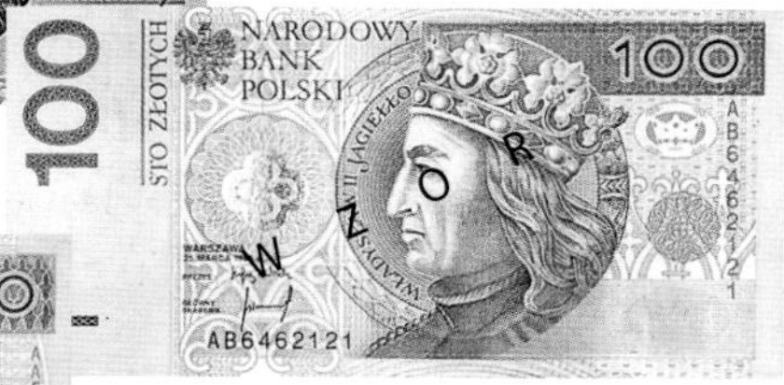

100 złoty

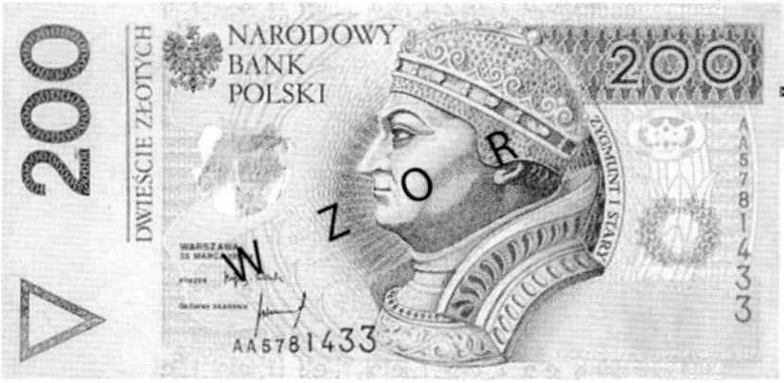

200 złoty

Bank Notes

Bank notes come in denominations of 10, 20, 50, 100 and 200 zł. Each bank note bears the portrait of a Polish king.

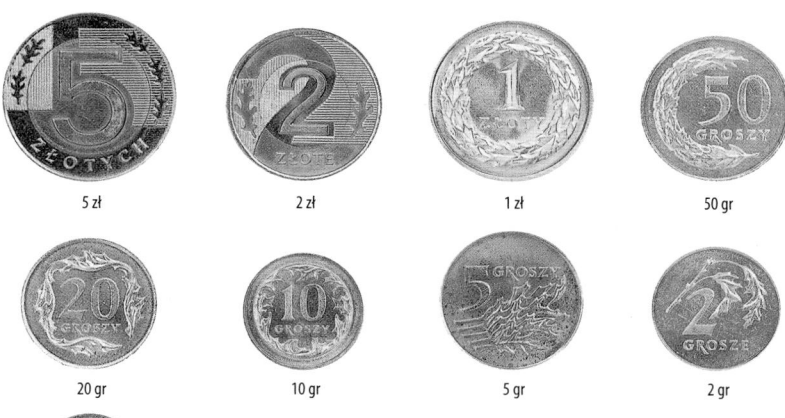

5 zł

2 zł

1 zł

50 gr

20 gr

10 gr

5 gr

2 gr

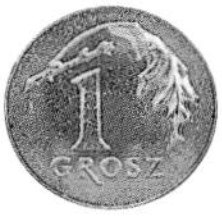

Coins

Polish coins come in denominations of 1, 2, 5, 10, 20, 50 gr and 1, 2, 5 zł. They all feature on one side a crowned eagle, the emblem of Poland.

1 gr

Communications and Media

The main Polish telephone service is provided by Telekomunikacja Polska (TP), although there are numerous mobile phone operators such as Plus, Orange and T-Mobile. There are many public telephones in the centre of Krakow, and these are mainly card-operated. Some phone booths are wheelchair-accessible. Many hotels and cafés offer guests free Wi-Fi access, and international newspapers and magazines are widely available. Offices of the efficient Polish postal service (*Poczta Polska*) are located throughout the city.

International and Local Telephone Calls

To make a telephone call you may choose to use a public telephone or go through the operator service at the post office. Keep in mind that calling from a hotel room is much more expensive, so it is always better to find a public telephone at the hotel or in its vicinity.

The vast majority of public phones are card-operated. Telephone cards (*karty telefoniczne*) can be purchased from newsagents and post offices. These cards are available in units of 15 (9zł), 30 (15zł) and 60 (24zł). A local call will only use up a few units of a phone card, but for long-distance calls it is advisable to use a higher-priced card.

Mobile Phones

Most mobile phones will function perfectly well in Krakow and elsewhere in Poland. However mobile phones supplied by providers in the US may only have limited global coverage. Contact your service provider for clarification.

To use your mobile phone abroad you will need to check with your provider that the roaming facility has been enabled. Remember that you will be charged for the calls you receive as well as the calls you make, and you will have to pay a substantial premium for the international part of the call.

If you are staying in the area for a reasonable amount of time, a popular option is to purchase a local SIM card that uses the local mobile phone networks and can be topped up with credit. You can only do this if your handset is "unlocked", as some operators lock their phones to specific networks. Some of the local/international networks are **Orange**, **T-Mobile** and **Plus**. If you are using a smart phone, beware that charges for data roaming can be high. If you want to make and receive calls while abroad but do not want to be charged for use of the Internet or other data, you can switch this service off and continue using the telephone functions as normal.

Check your insurance policy in case your phone gets stolen and keep your network operator's helpline number handy in case of emergencies.

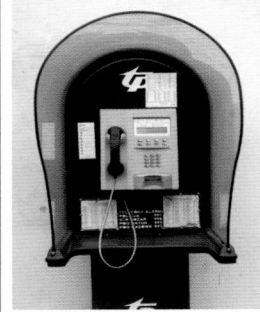

A typical public telephone booth in Krakow

Public Telephones

To make a telephone call, lift the receiver and wait for a continuous dialling tone. Insert a telephone card when the words "włóż kartę" (insert card) are displayed. The display will indicate the amount of credit (*kredyt*) available. Dial the number and await connection. Note that a short, rapidly repeating tone indicates that the number is engaged. When you have finished the call, replace the receiver and remove the ejected card.

Internet Access

If you are travelling with a laptop or a smartphone, there are numerous opportunities to log on to the Internet for little or no cost. A growing number of hotels, cafés and bars provide their guests with Wi-Fi access. In most places it is free but some establishments do charge. Look out for a Wi-Fi sticker in the window. There is also a free public Wi-Fi zone on the main Market Square.

For those travelling without a Wi-Fi-enabled device, most

tp

Telekomunikacja Polska – the biggest Polish telecoms company

Telephone Directories and Dialling Codes

- Local (Krakow) directory enquiries in English can be reached on 118 811.
- National (Polish) directory enquiries dial 118 913.
- International directory enquiries dial 118 912.
- Local calls within Krakow first dial 12, the city's area code. For calls within Poland always include the area code.
- To call overseas dial 0 and wait for the tone, dial 0 again followed by the country code, followed by the area code (omit the initial 0), and then the subscriber's number.
- Country codes: UK 44; Eire 353; Canada and USA 1; Australia 61; South Africa 27; New Zealand 64.

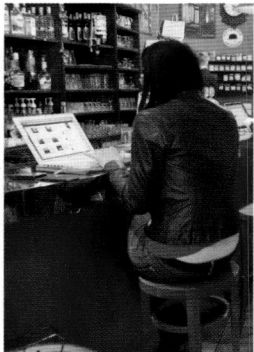

One of many bars in Krakow offering Wi-Fi access

hotels and hostels have at least one computer with Internet access in the lobby for guests to use. There are also several Internet cafés (*Kafejki Internetowe*) scattered throughout the city, including **Garinet**, **Hetmańska** and **Nandu** offering reasonable rates for Internet use – fares rarely exceed 10zł per hour.

Postal Services

Branches of the post office are scattered liberally throughout central Krakow and the suburbs. The main post office, **Poczta Głowna**, is situated at the junction of Westerplatte and Wielopole streets. It is open 8am–8pm Monday–Friday, and 8am–2pm Saturday, and offers a wide range of services. You can send letters, faxes, telegrams and parcels, as well as make international money transfers and operator-initiated calls. Stamp collectors can buy

from the philatelic counter. A *poste restante* (mail-holding) service is also available. The post office branch near the railway station has a 24-hour counter.

Stamps can be purchased at post office counters and from selected newsagents. Inland letters arrive after 2 to 3 days but international mail can take a week or maybe a little longer. Letters or cards sent via the more expensive express service will arrive sooner. Courier service is the fastest postal method, but is very costly. This service is available from larger post office branches, as well as from **DHL** and other similar courier companies.

Newspapers and Magazines

Foreign newspapers and magazines are available from the larger newsagents and bookshops. The widest choice is available at the **Empik** multimedia store in the Galeria Krakowska mall, which sells English-language and other foreign publications.

The most popular quality newspapers in Krakow are the nationals *Gazeta Wyborcza* and *Rzeczpospolita*, and the local *Dziennik Polski* and *Gazeta Krakowska*. Populist tabloid *Fakt* is the biggest-selling daily paper in the country. *Dziennik Polski* and *Gazeta Wyborcza* have the best "what's-on" information. English-language monthly *The Krakow Post* is a good source of local news and views, and can be picked up from many bars and restaurants free of charge.

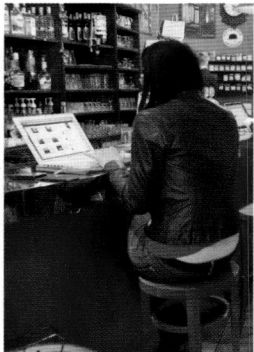

A post office housed in an old palace by the main railway station

TV and Radio

Most hotels have a television in the room offering a handful of Polish-language stations and a choice of German-, English-, Italian- and French-language stations. News channels such as CNN or BBC are more common than entertainment or film channels. Polish TV stations broadcast many English-language films and drama, although the voices are usually dubbed into Polish or read by a single actor.

Popular radio stations include RMF FM (96 FM), Trójka (99.4 FM), Radio Kraków (101.6 FM) and Radio Zet (104.1 FM).

GETTING TO KRAKOW

Krakow has good connections with other Polish and European cities. Direct air routes serve John Paul II airport from Warsaw as well as an ever-increasing number of European and American cities. There are direct trains from Berlin, Prague, Warsaw and other major Polish cities. In addition, Krakow is served by intercity buses from a growing range of European cities and from most cities in Poland itself.

Driving to Krakow is relatively easy and will take you through some wonderful scenery, with plenty of roadside restaurants and petrol stations along the way. Krakow has good, fast road connections if you are approaching from the west. Road routes from the north, south and east however are not in such good condition, and journeys via these routes are generally more time-consuming.

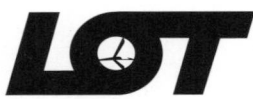

The logo of Polish Airlines

Arriving by Air

Krakow's **John Paul II Airport** at Balice is served by direct flights from a large number of European and Polish cities. Travellers from other continents will find that connections to Krakow – usually involving a change of plane in another European city – are easy to organize.

From the UK there's a choice of **LOT Polish Airlines** flights from London Heathrow; **Ryanair** from East Midlands, Edinburgh, Leeds-Bradford, Liverpool and London Stansted; **easyJet** from Belfast, Bristol, Edinburgh, Liverpool and London Gatwick; and **Jet2** from Newcastle. From Ireland, both **Aer Lingus** and Ryanair fly direct from Dublin.

Travellers from North America will need to make at least one stop en route. LOT airlines fly from Chicago, Toronto and New York to Krakow with a transfer in Warsaw. **Lufthansa** offer flights from various North American cities to Krakow with a change of plane in either Frankfurt or Munich. Visitors from Australasia can choose between one-stop flights via a major European hub such as London, or two-stop flights with connections in Singapore or Bangkok. LOT also operate domestic flights to Krakow from Warsaw; while Eurolot

fly to Krakow from Gdańsk, Poznań and Szczecin.

Krakow also has another international airport, **Katowice**, which is served by the budget airlines Wizz and Ryanair as well as Lufthansa. These airlines fly from numerous European destinations, in particular from Eastern Europe.

John Paul II Airport

Situated 15 km (9 miles) west of the city centre, John Paul II Airport is modern, comfortable and easy to get around. Although it has all the facilities that you would expect from an international airport, including cafés, restaurants, shops, money exchange and ATMs, it is small, and doesn't offer the variety found in larger airports. The international terminal is about 1 km (0.5 miles) away from the domestic terminal. There is a regular shuttle bus that transports passengers between the two; the same bus also goes to the airport's small railway station.

There is a tourist information office in the international arrivals hall, and car rental firms operate from their desks in the nearby concourse area.

Katowice Airport

Katowice international airport is located about 80 km (50 miles) northwest of Krakow in Pyrzowice. The airport has two busy passenger terminals. Facilities include souvenir shops, money exchange, duty-free and a post office. Car rental outlets can be found on the ground floor in Terminal A.

Tickets and Fares

Ticket prices vary enormously according to time of year and how far in advance you book. Peak periods such as Easter, June–August and the festive winter season are expensive times to travel whichever airline you book with. In general, tickets booked direct from the airline's website a month in advance or earlier are cheaper than tickets booked through

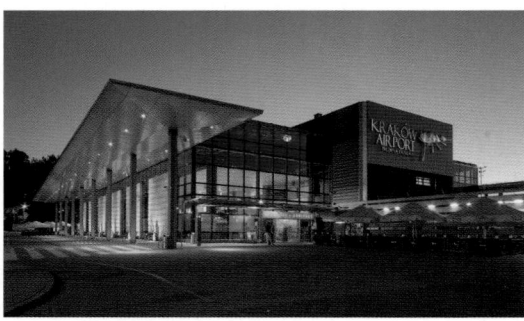

Krakow-John Paul II Airport

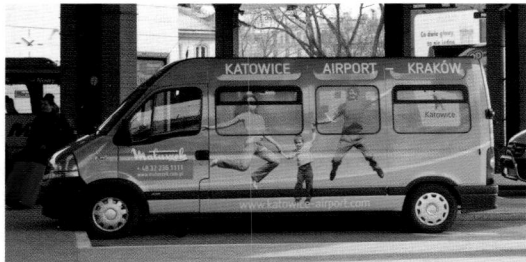

Matusek bus connecting Katowice Airport and Krakow city centre

travel agents or those booked near to your date of travel.

Budget airlines specialize in offering low-cost tickets and should be your first port of call if you are looking for inexpensive deals. Be aware however, that each item of hold baggage is usually charged extra.

Some airlines offer reductions for children under 12 but this is not standard practice across the whole industry. Children under 2 years old usually travel free, providing they occupy the same seat as the accompanying parent.

Getting into Town

John Paul II Airport is connected to Krakow's main railway station, Kraków Główny (see pp222–3), by fast suburban trains. There is a railway station in the departure terminal of the airport. Trains run every half hour (between approximately 6am and 11pm) and take 20 minutes. Tickets (10zł) can be bought from a machine near the central exit of Terminal 1 or from the conductor on board.

There are two regular bus services from the airport to the railway station: bus numbers 208 and 292, which depart from the airport forecourt. The journey time is about 40 minutes depending on traffic, and although slower than the train, the route runs through parts of west Krakow where several hotels are situated. If you are staying in this area and you have clear directions to your accommodation, these buses are very useful. Between 11pm

and 5am, there is also a night bus service, number 902.

Bus tickets (4zł) can be purchased from a newsagent stand inside the airport terminal, from the ticket machine beside the bus stop or from the driver on the bus (coins only) prior to commencing your journey. Large pieces of luggage are subject to an additional charge.

Taxis are located at the terminal's main exit. Here you will find Radio Taxis (see p227). The journey into town takes about 20 minutes but can take longer in rush hour. A Radio Taxi to the centre should cost around 50zł but may cost more at night and weekends. Credit cards are accepted. Expect to pay more if you are travelling to the suburbs, or if you book with an alternative taxi company.

From Katowice Airport, **Matusek** offers a bus service to Krakow central bus station, which takes about two hours. A single ticket costs 44zł if booked in advance or 50zł if bought on board.

DIRECTORY

Arriving by Air

Aer Lingus
w aerlingus.com

easyJet
w easyjet.com

Jet2
w jet2.com

LOT Polish Airlines
w lot.com

Lufthansa
w lufthansa.com

Ryanair
w ryanair.com

Airports

John Paul II Airport
Tel 12 295 58 00 or
801 055 000.
w krakowairport.pl

Katowice Airport
Tel 32 39 27 000.
w katowice-airport.com/en

Getting into Town

Matusek
w matusek.com

Pyrzowice Ekspress
w pyrzowiceekspres.pl

Alternatively, you can hire a private car with a driver through **Pyrzowice Ekspress**. For a standard car, with up to four passengers, the journey to Krakow costs 310zł (price is per trip). Cars must be booked at least five days in advance.

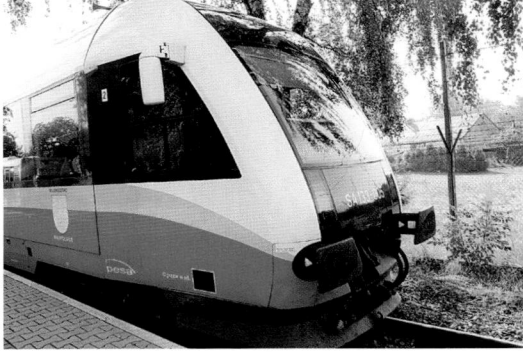

Train operating between John Paul II Airport and the city

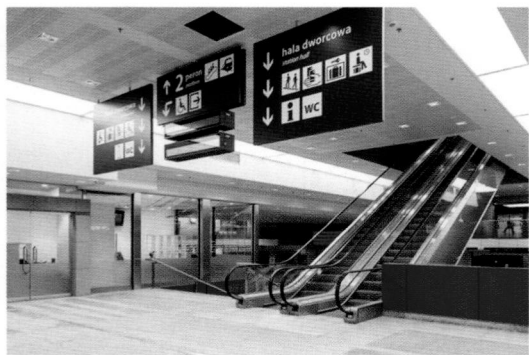

Escalators to the ticket hall in Kraków Główny, Krakow's main railway station

Travelling by Rail

You can get to Krakow by train from almost any Polish city and town, as well as from many other European cities. There are stretches of high-speed track between Warsaw and Krakow, but otherwise journey times are slow and in some cases travel by road may well be faster.

The Polish rail network is operated by various different companies. Most express intercity trains are run by **PKP InterCity** (Polskie Koleje Państwowe), who operate fast and relatively expensive services, as well as the slightly slower and slightly cheaper TLK (Twoje Linie Kolejowe) services. A number of other express trains are operated by **Przewozy Regionalne** (and go under the name of InterRegio). Przewozy Regionalne also operate slower trains that stop at more stations en route.

As a rule, train tickets in Poland are cheaper than in western Europe. Prices vary widely according to class of train, however travelling by express train will be two or three times more expensive than covering the same route on a slower local train.

Tickets for one service will not be valid for travel on another. Buying tickets is relatively straightforward as each of the ticket counters at Krakow's main railway station sell tickets for all of the above companies. Tickets can be bought in advance or on the day of travel from the ticket counters in the main railway station. Queues are common, so

allow at least half an hour to buy your ticket. You can also purchase one from the train conductor, but you must inform him that you require a ticket upon boarding the train. Bear in mind that tickets bought from the conductor are 10–20 per cent more expensive than those bought from counters at the station.

InterCity and Express Trains

Trains operated by PKP InterCity offer the fastest and most comfortable way to travel. First and second class seating is available. Seat reservations are obligatory and are made at the time of purchasing the ticket. Express trains operated by InterRegio are not as fast as PKP InterCity and only offer second-class seating although they are much cheaper and also allow bicycles. A PKP InterCity train from Warsaw to Krakow takes just under 3 hours and costs 120zł one-way (160zł in first class). An InterRegio train from Warsaw to Krakow takes 3 hours 15 minutes and only costs 50zł one-way.

PKP InterCity services offer a complimentary hot drink and a pastry, and also have a buffet car and trolley service offering a limited range of drinks and snacks. Other trains do not always carry a buffet car, so buy refreshments before boarding.

Railway Stations

Krakow's main railway station, Kraków Główny, is located in the heart of the city, a 10-minute walk northeast of Market Square. All international and domestic trains pass through this station, and the Krakow airport train terminates and departs from here. The main ticket hall is located under the train platforms and can be accessed from the Krakow bus station immediately to the east, the Dworzek Głowny tram stop, the Galeria Krakowska shopping mall to the west and via a covered walkway from the square in front of the shopping mall. Parking places and taxi ranks are located on the station roof, accessible by lift directly from the platforms.

Station signage is good, with digital displays notifying passengers of train departures and platform numbers. The main ticket hall contains two rows of counters for domestic departures, an information counter, and two counters (clearly marked in Polish and English) for international tickets. Queues at the international ticket counters can be very long in summer.

If catching a train outside central Krakow, beware that smaller railway stations have

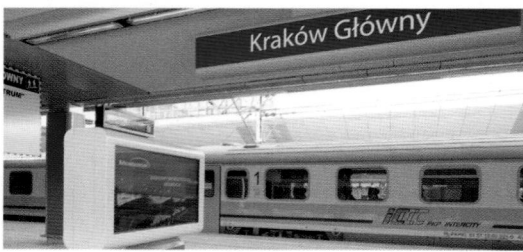

An InterCity train at Krakow's main railway station

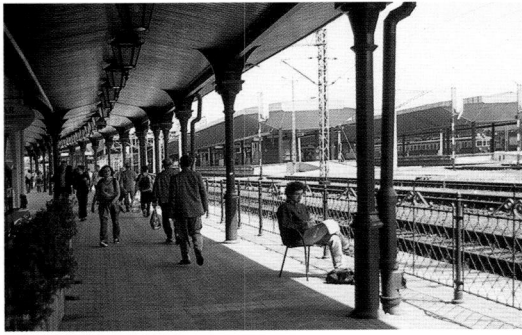

A platform at Kracow's main railway station

DIRECTORY

Travelling by Rail

InterRegio
W interregiorail.eu

PKP InterCity
W rozklad-pkp.pl

Train timetable information
Tel 22 39 19 757.
W rozklad-pkp.pl

Travelling by Coach

Coach timetable information
W rda.krakow.pl

Jordan
W jordan.pl

PolskiBus
W polskibus.com

Sindbad
W sindbad.krakow.pl

Travelling by Car

Polish Automobile Association
Tel 196 37.

---

poor information displays. Always allow plenty of time to buy your ticket and find the right platform.

Travelling by Coach

Regular coach services to Krakow operate from many Polish and European cities. The main coach station, Dworzec Autobusowy, is located in the city centre, immediately east of the main railway station. Local, domestic and most international coach services operate from this station. The coach station is linked to the Old Town, emerging outside the Galeria Krakowska shopping mall, via the underground pedestrian concourses that connect the bus station with the train station platforms.

The coach station has good facilities and clear timetable information, however there are insufficient ticket windows to deal with demand (especially on summer weekends), and long queues soon build up. International coach tickets can be bought from the coach station or from operating agencies **Jordan** or **Sindbad**.

Coach services are operated by various companies. Those offering prime intercity routes often use more modern, comfortable coaches. Services to nearby towns and villages are also operated by mini-buses. Tickets sell out quickly, especially at weekends.
PolskiBus runs services to and from Krakow from Warsaw as well as from other Polish and Central European cities. Tickets are sold online, *see directory*. Pick-up and drop-off points are located in the suburbs of Krakow.

Travelling by Car

Major roads into Krakow are well signposted, but you will need time and patience to find a safe parking space. Prominent car parks in the city are located on the Street Finder maps *(see pp232–237)*.

Driving licences issued in other countries are generally valid in Poland. If you drive in Poland you must carry a valid driving licence and vehicle registration document, as well as a Green Card, which is confirmation of your international insurance cover. If you drive a rental car, a hire certificate is also obligatory. A sticker identifying the country in which the car is registered must be displayed on the vehicle. The wearing of seat belts is compulsory, and children under 12 are not allowed to travel in the front of the car. Headlights must be on, day and night, regardless of the weather.

Road signs at the Polish border indicate strictly observed speed limits (in km). If ignored, foreign drivers are required to pay hefty fines on the spot.

The permitted alcohol content in blood is so low in Poland that drinking and driving should be avoided altogether.

In the event of a break-down, call the **Polish Automobile Association**.

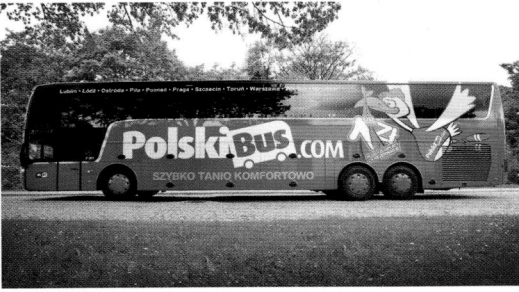

A PolskiBus service operating between Warsaw and Krakow

GETTING AROUND KRAKOW

Central Krakow is small and compact so moving around on foot, by bike or by public transport is best. Children in particular will enjoy a sightseeing ride on one of Krakow's blue trams, and tours in a horse-drawn cab are very popular with visitors too. A small electric "meleks" vehicle can also be hired for group sightseeing, with qualified guides who speak foreign languages. Both meleks vehicles and horse-drawn carriages await passengers in Krakow's historic Market Square. If you are visiting attractions outside the city centre, using the public transport system is more environmentally friendly than hiring a car or using taxis. This guide lists the bus and tram routes which you can use to get to the sights described in the Krakow Area by Area section. Maps of Krakow's tram and bus systems can be found on the inside back cover.

Green Travel

There are a great many private cars in circulation in central Krakow, leading to traffic congestion and a shortage of parking spaces. Foreign visitors should try and refrain from adding to this pressure on the local infrastructure and consider alternative ways of getting around the city.

Krakow's centre is easy to navigate on foot and the city is also bike-friendly – the local authorities are trying to extend the number of cycle lanes in busy areas. Otherwise, the electric-powered meleks vehicles available for hire in the Market Square provide an emissions-free alternative to hiring a taxi within the Old Quarter. When exploring further afield, the public transport network is a perfectly adequate way of reaching suburbs such as Nowa Huta or recreation areas such as Las Wolski forest.

Walking

Krakow is ideal for exploring on foot. Much of the city centre is pedestrianized and distances between the main sightseeing areas are small.

Walking from the Old Town to the Kazimierz quarter takes around 20 minutes and there is much to see on the way. Planty Park runs round three sides of the Old Town, and the tree-shaded paths offer a pleasant walk from one part of the centre to another.

Pedestrians should take care at zebra crossings as drivers do not always stop.

Cycling

Cycling is a wonderful way to see Krakow, and the number of bike-rental outlets is increasing. Beware that marked cycle lanes are not widespread and cycling on main roads can be unnerving. It is permissible to cycle on the pavement, although pedestrians have right of way. The broad avenues of Planty Park are an ideal way of getting around the Old Town by bike.

A stop and give way road sign

There are several rental outlets around town and your hotel or hostel will know where the nearest one is. Prices depend on the type and age of the bike you are hiring, but you should expect to pay 40–70zł per day. A scheme called **KMK Bike** allows you to pick up rental bikes from one of 16 automated bike parks located throughout the city, although registering online is required. If you are hiring a bike for just one day or if you prefer to pay by cash, use **Eccentric Bike Rental** or **Bike Trip**.

Driving

Visitors are advised to walk, cycle or use public transport as access to the historic centre is limited to licenced taxis, delivery vans and local residents. Outside the Old Town traffic is busy and parking places are hard to find.

If you do drive, note that congestion is common during rush hours, especially on Friday afternoons. Main roads into the city have numerous traffic lights and junctions causing frequent tailbacks. A ring road runs around the west and south sides of the city, but is yet to be extended all the way round.

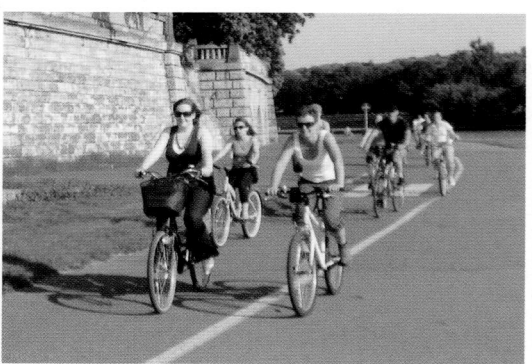

Tourists cycling by the Vistula River

Popular excursion routes in the environs of Krakow are well serviced by public transport, although you will need a car in order to explore the countryside in depth. Car hire in Krakow is problem-free, with several car-hire counters in the international arrivals hall of John Paul II airport, and car-hire deals offered by virtually all of the city's hotels and hostels *(see p223)*. Major car hire companies include **Avis**, **Europcar**, **Hertz** and **Sixt** and the Polish car rental company, **Joka**.

Parking

Parking areas are divided into zones. Most of the Old Town (zones A and B) is a no-parking zone for non-residents, although there is a limited amount of space available for hotel guests – you should enquire about availability when booking your room. Street parking is possible in a belt of territory surrounding the Old Town (zone C), but places are hard to come by. Parking in zone C costs 4zł per hour, payable at roadside parking meters, between 10am and 6pm Monday–Friday, but is free outside that time.

The most convenient car park for the Old Town is at Starowiślna 13 (6–8zł per hour). The largest underground parking garage is near Wawel Castle at Na Groblach (8zł per hour).

Illegally parked vehicles are prone to clamping. Details of where to pay the fine and get the clamp removed will be posted on the windscreen.

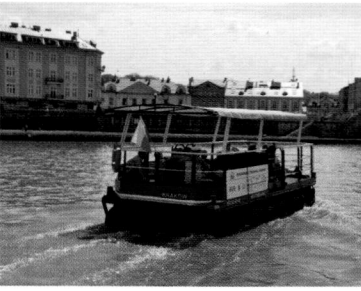
A water tram on the Vistula River

Water Trams

Water trams *(tramwaj wodny)* run during the tourist season from May to October. One service runs between Flisacka (in the suburb of Zwierzyniec) and Kazimierz, passing Wawel Castle on the way. Another less frequent service sails from Flisacka to Tyniec Abbey on the western fringes of Krakow. They function very well as scenic excursions, but are slower than other modes of public transport and should not be used to travel anywhere if you are in a hurry.

Tickets are bought on the boat and cost 8zł one-way on the Flisacka-Kazimierz route and 25zł one-way on the Flisacka-Tyniec route. Buying return tickets works out about 20 per cent cheaper than buying two singles.

Guided Tours

Guided sightseeing tours of Krakow are strongly recommended. The multi-lingual meleks drivers are situated by the Church of St Adalbert in Market Square. Bike-hire and horse-drawn cabs can also be found here.

Top sightseeing spots, such as **Wawel Castle** have their own guides, and many local travel agencies also offer specialist sightseeing tours. **Crazy Guides** focus on the communist past, frequently using old-style Trabant cars as transport. **Krakow City Tours** operate themed tours such as Jewish Krakow and ghost walks, as well as organizing trips to the Auschwitz-Birkenau memorial site. **Discover Krakow** arrange tailor-made city centre and John Paul II tours.

DIRECTORY

Cycling

Bike Trip
ul. Zwierzyniecka 10.
Tel 667 712 054.
ꟼ biketrip.pl

Eccentric Bike Rental
ul. Grodzka 2. **Map** 1 C5
(6 D3). **Tel** 12 430 20 34.
ꟼ krakowbiketour.com

KMK Bike
ꟼ kmkbike.pl

Driving

Avis
ul. Lubicz 23. **Map** 2 E4.
Tel 12 629 61 08.
ꟼ avis.pl

Europcar
ul. Nadwislanska 6.
Map 4 E2.
Tel 12 374 56 96.
ꟼ europcar.pl

Hertz
Al. Focha 1. **Map** 1 A5.
Tel 12 429 62 62.
ꟼ hertz.com.pl

Joka
ul. Zacisze 7.
Map 2 D3 (6 E1).
Tel 12 429 66 30.
ꟼ joka.com.pl

Sixt
John Paul II Airport.
Tel 12 639 32 16.
ꟼ sixt.pl

Water Trams

**Water Tram
(Tramwaj Wodny)**
ꟼ ktw.krakow.pl

Guided Tours

Crakow City Tours
ul. Floriańska 44.
Map 2 D4 (6 E1).
Tel 12 421 13 33.
ꟼ cracowcitytours.com

Crazy Guides
ul. Floriańska 38.
Map 2 D4 (6 E1).
Tel 500 091 200.
ꟼ crazyguides.com

Discover Cracow
Rynek Główny 7–10b.
Map 1 C4 (6 D3).
Tel 12 346 38 99.
ꟼ discovercracow.eu

Wawel Castle Guide Service
Wawel 5.
Map 3 C1 (6 D5).
Tel 12 422 51 55.
ꟼ wawel.krakow.pl

Buses, Trams and Taxis

Krakow is covered by an extensive public transport network. Trams and buses are frequent on weekdays, with rush hours between 7 and 8am and 2 and 5pm, but less so at weekends and on public holidays. A few trams and buses operate at night. Tickets, valid for both buses and trams, are inexpensive, especially if you opt for a 24- or 48-hour travel pass. A number of private firms operate minibus services, which will stop on request within the inner and outer city. Taxi ranks are located around the Old Town, and their prices are reasonable.

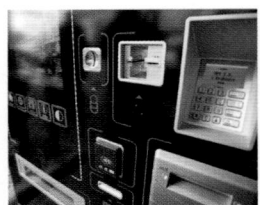
Ticket machine

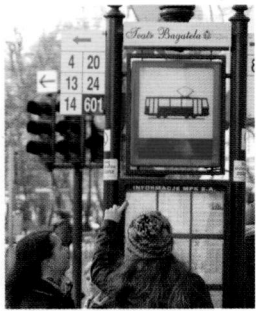
Tourists planning a route at a Krakow tram stop

Tickets and fares

One type of ticket is used for both trams and buses. Tickets can be purchased from kiosks on the street, from ticket machines at some stops and on most buses and trams. There are two zones: zone 1 covers the city of Krakow and includes all tram and bus routes numbered 100 to 194. Zone 2 covers the outer suburbs, outlying villages and John Paul II Airport.

Several types of ticket are available: in zone 1, a ticket for a single journey by tram or bus is 3.80zł, a ticket for two journeys by bus or tram costs 7.20zł. Tickets valid for unlimited travel within a specific time period include the 20-minute ticket, which costs 2.80zł (useful if you're only travelling a few stops), as well as a 40-minute (3.80zł), 60-minute (5zł), 90-minute (6zł), 24-hour (15zł), 48-hour (24zł) and 72-hour (36zł) ticket. A weekly ticket is also available, which costs 48zł. Family tickets, allowing for unlimited travel for two adults and two children at weekends, cost 16zł. A group

ticket for up to 20 people costs 36zł. If you are travelling to zone 2, a single ticket is priced at 4zł and a ticket for two journeys is 7.60zł. Children under 4 and senior citizens over 70 travel for free.

After boarding, passengers must validate each ticket (even those purchased on board) by inserting it in one of the orange machines. Weekly tickets require the holder to carry identification.

Ticket Inspectors

Tickets are subject to regular checks on Krakow's trams and buses. Ticket inspectors operate in plain clothes but carry ID bearing an MPK symbol and a photograph. A passenger without a valid, punched ticket is liable to pay a fine, which is up to 250zł. Fines may be paid on the spot or at a post office with a penalty ticket. Foreign visitors, however, must pay on the spot.

Machines for checking the validity of your ticket are located throughout the city.

Travelling by Bus

Krakow is well served by buses that take passengers to all parts of the city. Bus routes numbered from 100 to 194 operate in the city centre and those numbered 201 to 297 link the city with outer suburbs and villages. Express buses, which do not go to every stop, begin with a 3 or a 5 and are three digits long. The frequency of buses varies from every few minutes to approximately every 20 minutes Monday–Friday, but they are less regular at weekends and on public holidays.

Bus stops are marked by a blue sign with a picture of a bus on it. When boarding the bus remember to validate your ticket. Approaching stops are read out by a pre-recorded voice and – in the newer vehicles – displayed on an electronic sign. To request a stop, push one of the red buttons near the doors. Some of the more modern buses have low floors, which allow easier wheelchair, pram and pushchair access.

Bus routes beginning with a 6 or a 9 are night buses. These

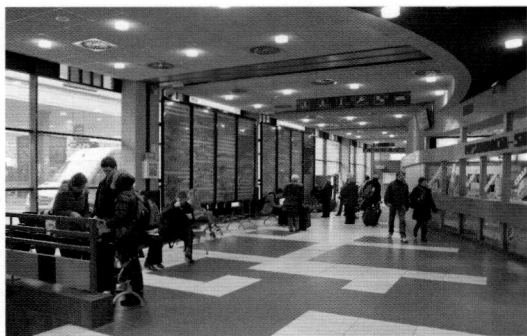
Interior of main bus station in Krakow

buses run about once an hour and cross the city in all directions. The fare is the same as for any other bus journey.

Private minibus services operate on many routes within the city and in the suburbs. You can purchase a ticket directly from the driver which costs approximately twice the fare of the MPK public transport. Most of these minibuses depart from the main railway station or nearby.

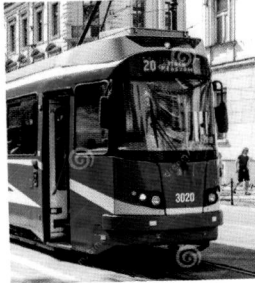

A Krakow tram operating in the city centre

Travelling by Tram

Trams are the main form of public transport in central Krakow, running round either side of the Old Town and fanning out towards outlying suburbs. They are the best means of travelling between the major bus and rail stations, and they are also the quickest way of reaching outlying attractions in the suburbs of Podgórze, 3 km (2 miles) south of the centre and Nowa Huta, 7 km (4 miles) east. Trams run from around 5:15am–11:15pm daily. Most tram routes operate every 10–15 minutes in the middle of the day, and every 20–25 minutes early in the morning and in the evening. Many vehicles have low floors enabling easy wheelchair access,

but it is not always possible to tell when one of these trams is due at your stop.

Taxis

Taxis are easy to locate in central Krakow and rates are reasonably low. Various taxi companies are in operation – vehicles vary in colour and make, and have different signs, depending on which company they belong to. All have an identification number clearly marked on the side of the car, as well as an illuminated "taxi" sign on the roof displaying the name of the company.

Taxis wait in taxi ranks rather than driving round the city looking for custom, so it is highly unlikely that you will be able to hail a taxi on the street. Those ordered by phone are usually cheaper than those picked up at a taxi rank.

Taxi ranks can be found all around the Old Town area. The biggest are on ul. Sienna, a short walk east of the main Market Square, and pl. Wszystkich Świętych, close to the Franciscan and Dominican churches. There are also plenty of taxis on or near pl. Nowy in the Kazimierz quarter. The

taxi rank for the main railway station is located on its roof – take the escalator or lift up from the platform.

There is an initial charge of 7zł, followed by 3zł per kilometre. Rates rise by 50 per cent between 11pm and 5am. Bear in mind large items of luggage will increase the fare.

Radio Taxi-Partner runs a fleet of taxis for disabled passengers. Fares are cheaper than those of regular taxis. These must be booked in advance.

DIRECTORY

Travelling by Bus and Tram

Tram and Bus Information
Tel 191 50.
🆆 mpk.krakow.pl

Taxis

Radio Taxi
Tel 19191.

Radio Taxi Barbakan
Tel 19661.

Radio Taxi-Partner
Tel 19633.

Wawel Taxi
Tel 19666.

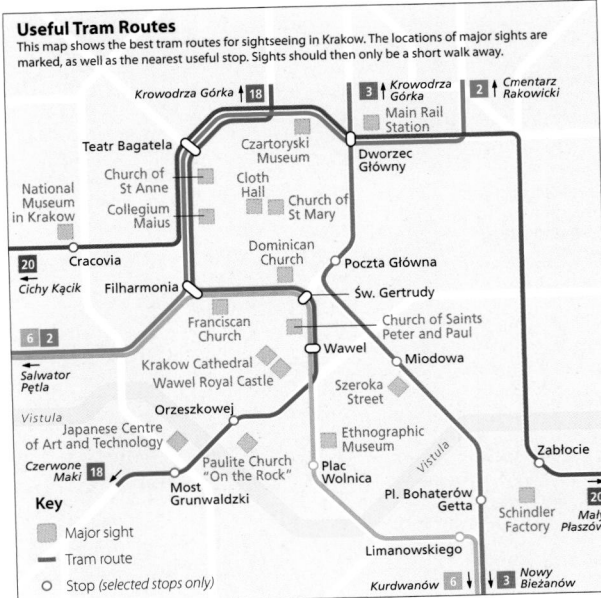

Useful Tram Routes
This map shows the best tram routes for sightseeing in Krakow. The locations of major sights are marked, as well as the nearest useful stop. Sights should then only be a short walk away.

Krowodrza Górka ↑ **18**

3 ↑ Krowodrza Górka

2 ↑ Cmentarz Rakowicki

Teatr Bagatela

Czartoryski Museum

Main Rail Station

Dworzec Główny

National Museum in Krakow

Church of St Anne

Cloth Hall

Collegium Maius

Church of St Mary

20 Cracovia

Dominican Church

Poczta Główna

Cichy Kącik

Filharmonia

Św. Gertrudy

6 2

Franciscan Church

Church of Saints Peter and Paul

Salwator Pętla

Krakow Cathedral
Wawel Royal Castle

Wawel

Miodowa

Vistula

Orzeszkowej

Szeroka Street

Japanese Centre of Art and Technology

Ethnographic Museum

Zabłocie

Czerwone Maki **18**

Paulite Church "On the Rock"

Plac Wolnica

Vistula

Most Grunwaldzki

Pl. Bohaterów Getta

Schindler Factory

20 Mały Płaszów

Key

◼ Major sight

— Tram route

○ Stop (selected stops only)

Limanowskiego

Kurdwanów **6**

3 ↓ Nowy Bieżanów

STREET FINDER

Map references, given for each sight within its individual entry in this guide relate to the map on the following pages only. The same applies to the hotels *(see pp180–83)* and restaurants *(see pp190–93)* listed. The first figure indicates the map number, while the middle letter and the last number refer to the relevant grid. The key map on the right shows Krakow divided into six parts which correspond to the maps that follow. All symbols used are explained in the key. You will find the Street Finder Index on pp230–31. Note that Polish is an inflected language and street names require different name endings (Jan Kowalski but Jana Kowalskiego Street).

Top sights and attractions are indicated on the maps.

Key to Street Finder

- Major sight
- Other sight
- Railway station
- Coach terminal
- Tram stop
- *i* Tourist information
- Hospital
- Police station
- Boat pier
- Church
- Synagogue
- = Railway line
- Pedestrian street
- — City wall

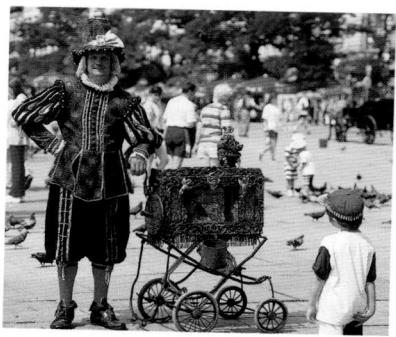
A hurdy-gurdy man in Market Square

Scale of Maps 1–4

0 metres 200
0 yards 200
1:13,000

Scale of Maps 5–6

0 metres 150
0 yards 150
1:8,500

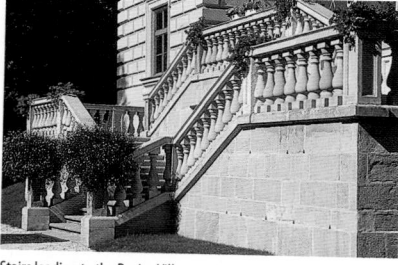
Stairs leading to the Decius Villa

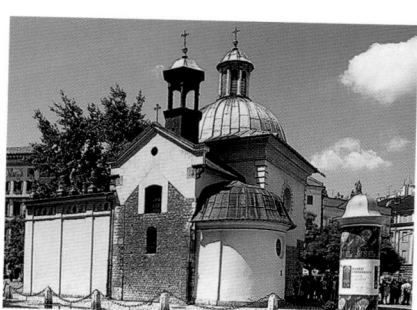
Church of St Adalbert in Market Square

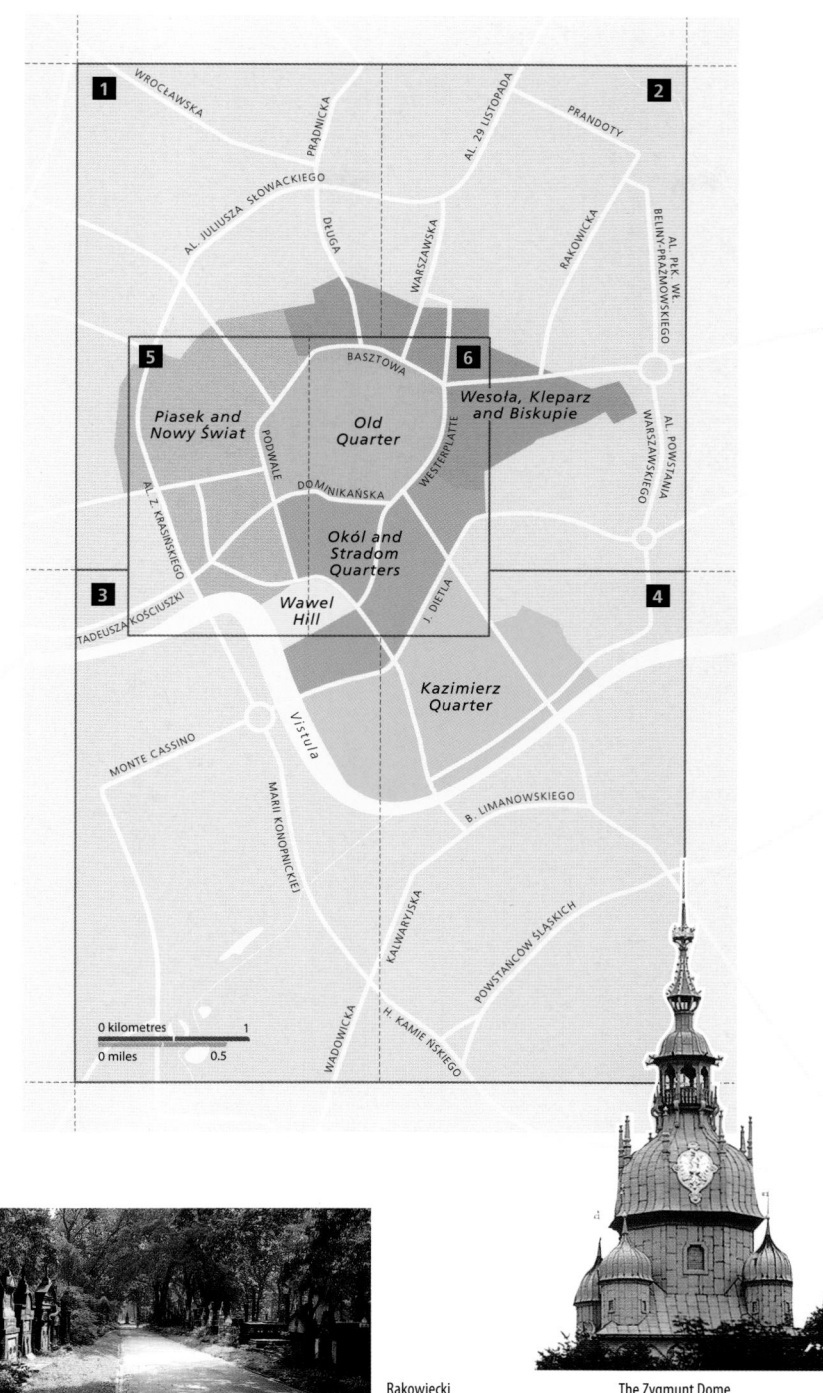

1 WROCŁAWSKA

2 PRANDOTY

PRĄDNICKA

AL. 29 LISTOPADA

AL. JULIUSZA SŁOWACKIEGO

DŁUGA

WARSZAWSKA

RAKOWICKA

AL. PŁK. WŁ. BELINY-PRAŻMOWSKIEGO

5 BASZTOWA **6**

Wesoła, Kleparz and Biskupie

Piasek and Nowy Świat

Old Quarter

PODWALE

WESTERPLATTE

AL. POWSTANIA WARSZAWSKIEGO

AL. Z. KRASIŃSKIEGO

DOMINIKAŃSKA

3 Okół and Stradom Quarters **4**

TADEUSZA KOŚCIUSZKI

Wawel Hill

J. DIETLA

Kazimierz Quarter

Vistula

MONTE CASSINO

B. LIMANOWSKIEGO

MARII KONOPNICKIEJ

KALWARYJSKA

POWSTAŃCÓW ŚLĄSKICH

0 kilometres 1
0 miles 0.5

WADOWICKA

H. KAMIEŃSKIEGO

Rakowiecki Cemetery

The Zygmunt Dome of the Cathedral

Street Finder Index

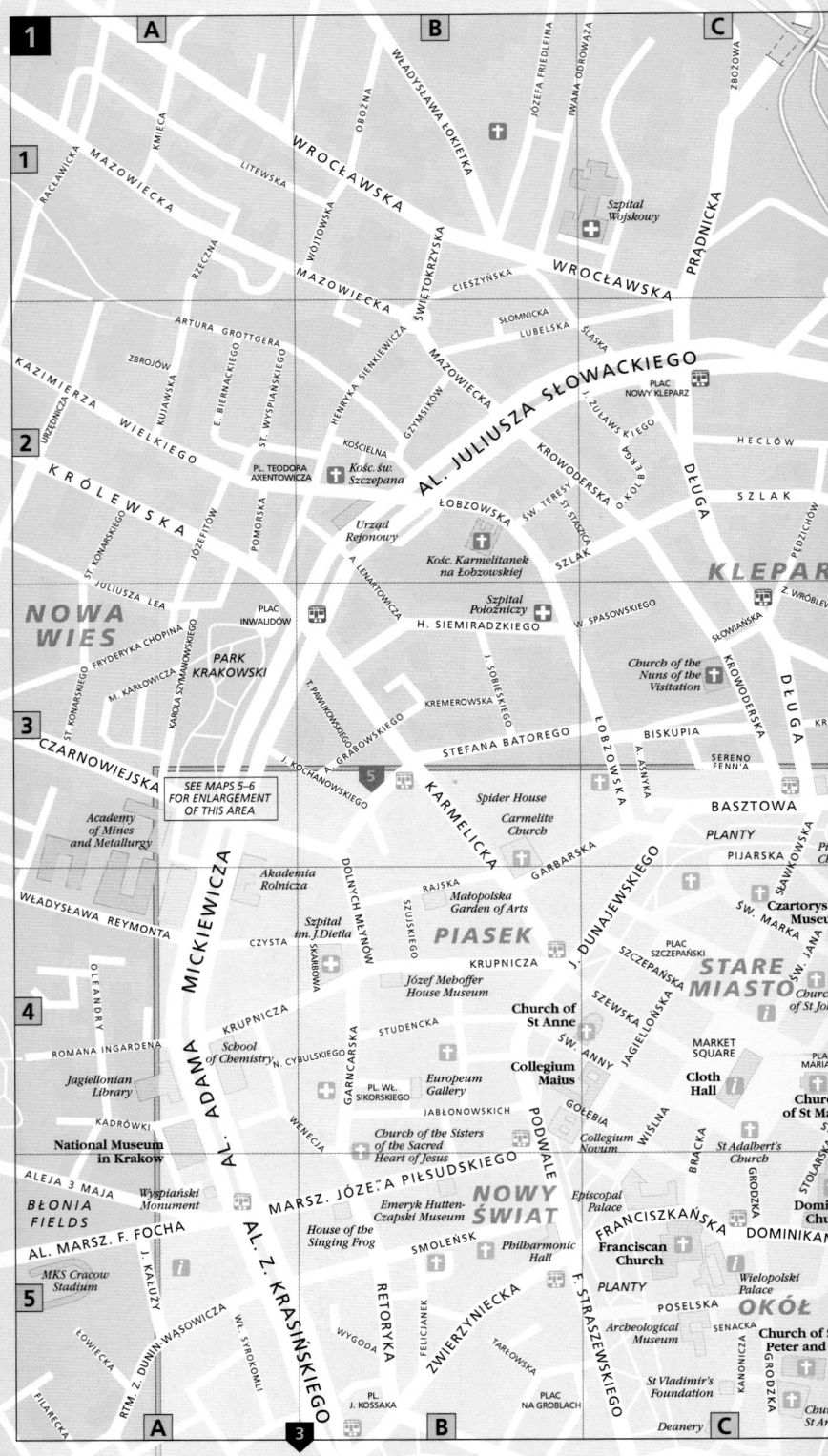

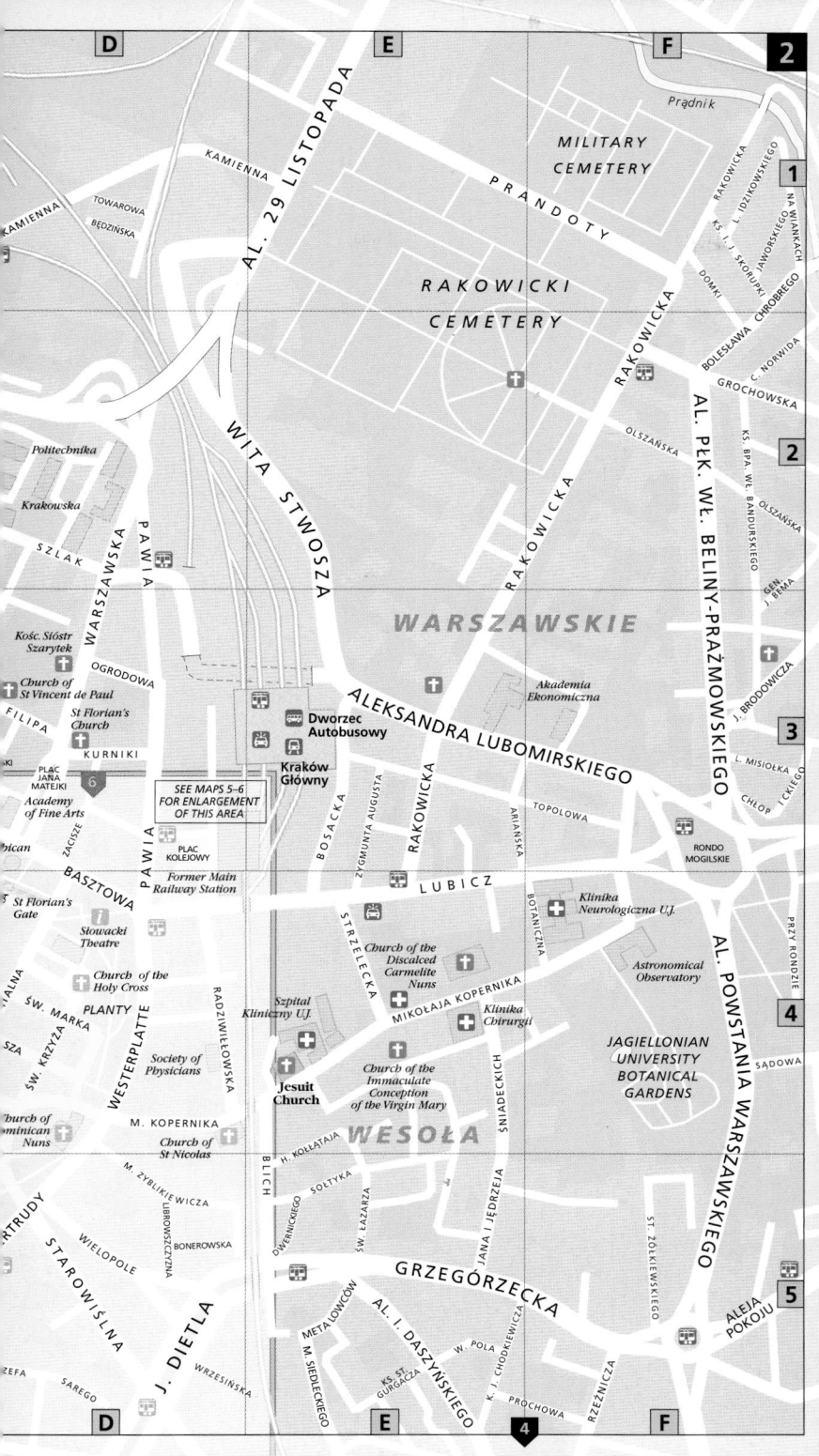

D **E** **F** **2**

1

Prądnik

MILITARY CEMETERY

KAMIENNA

AL. 29 LISTOPADA

PRANDOTY

RAKOWICKI CEMETERY

TOWAROWA

BĘDZIŃSKA

KAMIENNA

RAKOWICKA

RAKOWICKA

KS. J. SKORUPKI

JAWORSKIEGO

KS. I. IDZIKOWSKIEGO

NA WIANKACH

DOMKI

BOLESŁAWA CHROBREGO

C. NORWIDA

GROCHOWSKA

2

Politechnika

Krakowska

WITA STWOSZA

WARSZAWSKA

PAWIA

SZLAK

AL. PŁK. WŁ. BELINY-PRAŻMOWSKIEGO

OLSZAŃSKA

RAKOWICKA

KS. BPA. WŁ. BANDURSKIEGO

OLSZAŃSKA

SEN. J. BEMA

J. BRODOWICZA

3

Kośc. Sióstr Szarytek

Church of St Vincent de Paul

St Florian's Church

OGRODOWA

FILIPA

KURNIKI

WARSZAWSKIE

Dworzec Autobusowy

Kraków Główny

ALEKSANDRA LUBOMIRSKIEGO

Akademia Ekonomiczna

L. MISIOŁKA

CHŁOP ICKIEGO

PLAC JANA MATEJKI **6**

Academy of Fine Arts

BASZTOWA

PAWIA

ZACISZE

SEE MAPS 5–6 FOR ENLARGEMENT OF THIS AREA

PLAC KOLEJOWY

Former Main Railway Station

BOSACKA

ZYGMUNTA AUGUSTA

RAKOWICKA

ARIAŃSKA

TOPOLOWA

RONDO MOGILSKIE

PRZY RONDZIE

4

St Florian's Gate

Słowacki Theatre

Church of the Holy Cross

PLANTY

WESTERPLATTE

ŚW. MARKA

ŚW. KRZYŻA

RADZIWIŁŁOWSKA

STRZELECKA

LUBICZ

Church of the Discalced Carmelite Nuns

MIKOŁAJA KOPERNIKA

BOTANICZNA

Klinika Neurologiczna U.J.

Astronomical Observatory

AL. POWSTANIA WARSZAWSKIEGO

SADOWA

Society of Physicians

Szpital Kliniczny U.J.

Klinika Chirurgii

JAGIELLONIAN UNIVERSITY BOTANICAL GARDENS

Church of Dominican Nuns

M. KOPERNIKA

Church of St Nicolas

Jesuit Church

Church of the Immaculate Conception of the Virgin Mary

ŚNIADECKICH

WESOŁA

H. KOŁŁĄTAJA

BLICH

DWERNICKIEGO

SOŁTYKA

ŚW. ŁAZARZA

JANA I JĘDRZEJA

ŚT. ŻÓŁKIEWSKIEGO

5

TRUDY

STAROWIŚLNA

WIELOPOLE

M. ZYBLIKIEWICZA

LUBOMIRSKIEGO

BONEROWSKA

J. DIETLA

WRZESIŃSKA

GRZEGÓRZECKA

METALOWCÓW

M. SIEDLECKIEGO

AL. I. DASZYŃSKIEGO

KS. ST. GURGACZA

W. POLA

K. J. CHODKIEWICZA

K. J. PRÓCHOWA

RZEŹNICZA

ALEJA POKOJU

ZEFA

SAREGO

D **E** **F**

4

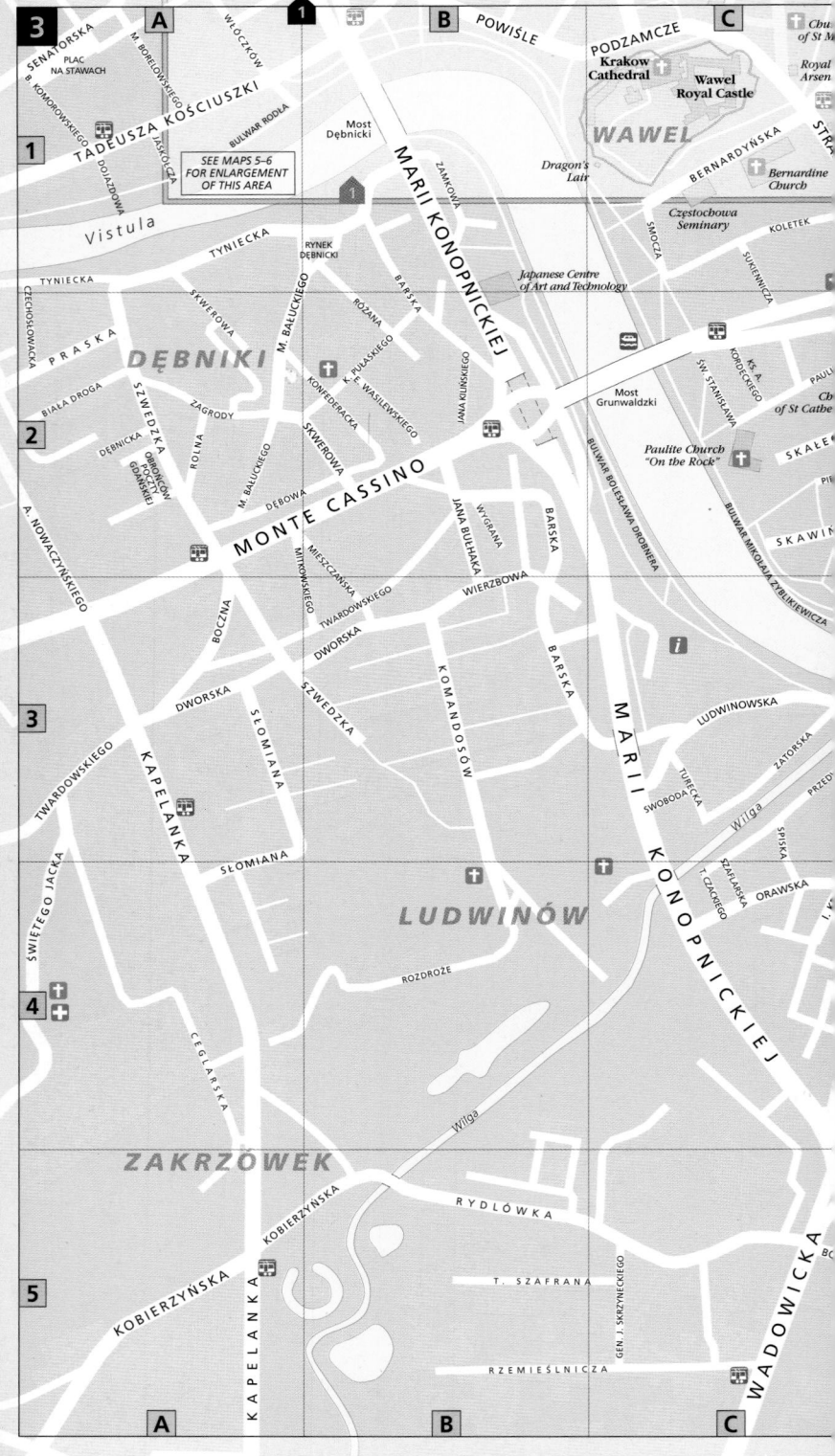

3

A	B	C

1

WŁOCZKÓW

SENATORSKA

M. BOROWSKIEGO

PLAC NA STAWACH

KOMOROWSKIEGO

DOJAZDOWA

BULWAR RODŁA

TADEUSZA KOŚCIUSZKI

JAKÓBA

SEE MAPS 5–6 FOR ENLARGEMENT OF THIS AREA

Most Dębnicki

POWIŚLE

PODZAMCZE

Krakow Cathedral

WAWEL

Wawel Royal Castle

Chu of St M

Royal Arsen

STRA

Vistula

ZAMKOWA

Dragon's Lair

BERNARDYŃSKA

Bernardine Church

TYNIECKA

RYNEK DĘBNICKI

MARII KONOPNICKIEJ

SMOCZA

Częstochowa Seminary

KOLETEK

2

CZECHOSŁOWACKA

TYNIECKA

SKWEROWA

RÓŻANA

BARSKA

Japanese Centre of Art and Technology

SUKIENNICZA

PRASKA

M. BAŁUCKIEGO

RÓŻANA

K.-E. WASILEWSKIEGO

PUŁASKIEGO

KONFEDERACKA

JANA KILIŃSKIEGO

KS. A. KORDECKIEGO

ŚW. STANISŁAWA

Ch of St Cathe

DĘBNIKI

BIAŁA DROGA

SZWEDZKA

ZAGRODY

DĘBNICKA

OBROŃCÓW GDAŃSKA

ROLNA

M. BAŁUCKIEGO

SKWEROWA

DĘBOWA

Most Grunwaldzki

Paulite Church "On the Rock"

SKAŁE

PIE

A. NOWACZYŃSKIEGO

MONTE CASSINO

MIESZCZAŃSKA

MITKOWSKIEGO

JANA BUŁHAKA

WYGRANA

WIERZBOWA

BARSKA

BULWAR BOLESŁAWA DROBNERA

BULWAR MIKOŁAJA ZYBLIKIEWICZA

SKAWIN

3

TWARDOWSKIEGO

BOCZNA

TWARDOWSKIEGO

DWORSKA

SZWEDZKA

KOMANDOSÓW

BARSKA

MARII KONOPNICKIEJ

LUDWINOWSKA

ZATORSKA

KAPELANKA

DWORSKA

SŁOMIANA

SWOBODA

TURECKA

Wilga

PRZED

SPISKA

ŚWIĘTEGO JACKA

SŁOMIANA

T. CZACKIEGO

SZAFLARSKA

ORAWSKA

I. K

4

CEGLARSKA

LUDWINÓW

ROZDROŻE

Wilga

5

ZAKRZÓWEK

KOBIERZYŃSKA

KAPELANKA

KOBIERZYŃSKA

RYDLÓWKA

T. SZAFRANA

GEN. J. SKRZYNECKIEGO

WADOWICKA

BO

RZEMIEŚLNICZA

KOBIERZYŃSKA

A	B	C

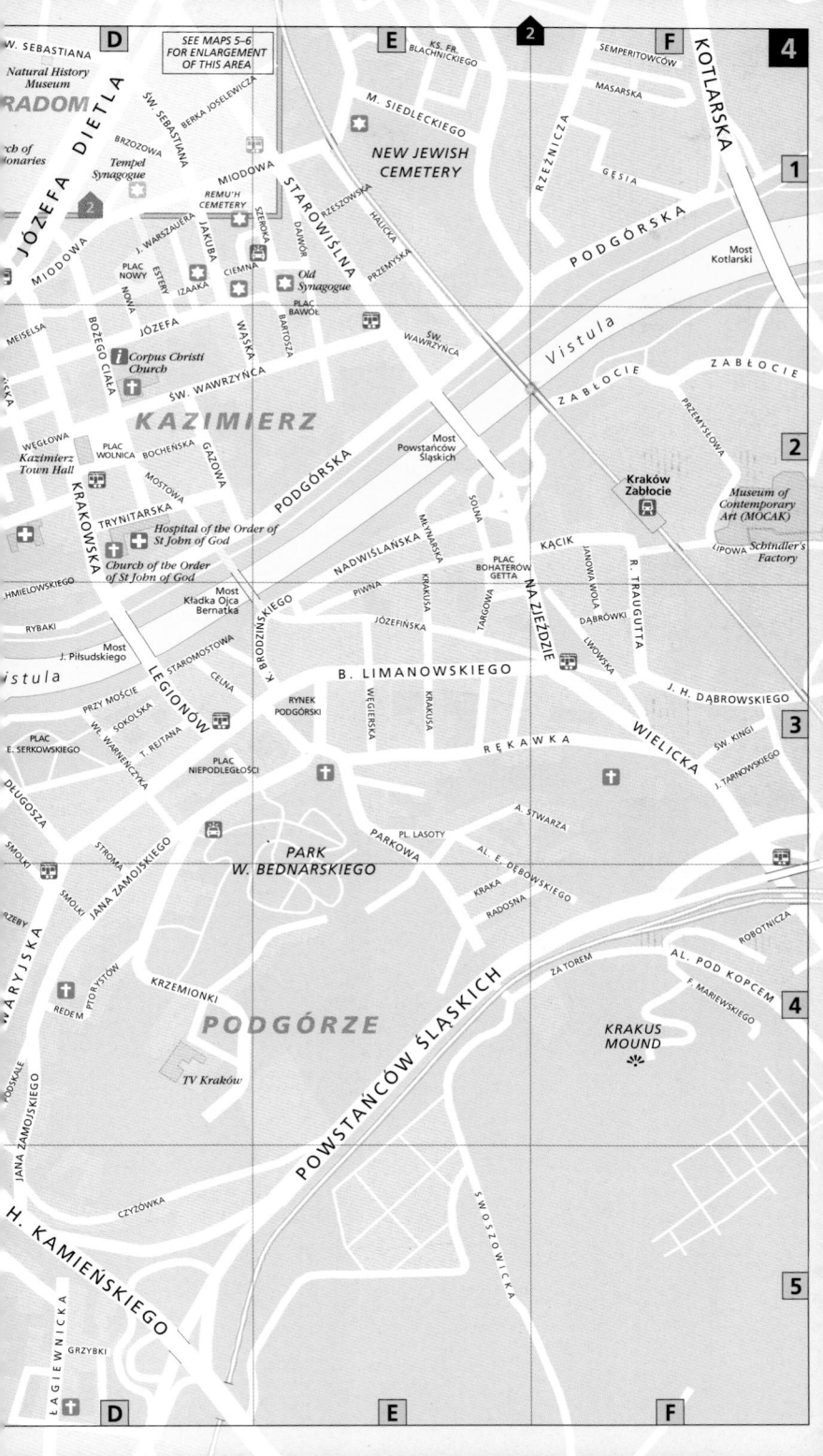

D · **E** · **2** · **F** · **4**

W. SEBASTIANA

Natural History Museum

RADOM

SW. SEBASTIANA

BERKA JOSELEWICZA

KS. FR. BLACHNICKIEGO

SEMPERITOWCÓW

KOTLARSKA

rch of onaries

BRZOZOWA

M. SIEDLECKIEGO

MASARSKA

Tempel Synagogue

2

MIODOWA

STAROWIŚLNA

NEW JEWISH CEMETERY

RZEŹNICZA

GĘSIA

1

REMU'H CEMETERY

J. WARSZAUERA

JAKUBA

SZEROKA

RZESZOWSKA

DAJWÓR

HALICKA

PODGÓRSKA

Most Kotlarski

MIODOWA

PLAC NOWY

ESTERY

IZAAKA

CIEMNA

PRZEMYSKA

MEISELSA

NOWA

JÓZEFA

WĄSKA

Old Synagogue

PLAC BAWÓŁ

Vistula

ZABŁOCIE

ZABŁOCIE

BOŻEGO CIAŁA

PLAC BARTOSZA

SW. WAWRZYŃCA

ZABŁOCIE

PRZEMYSŁOWA

i *Corpus Christi Church*

SW. WAWRZYŃCA

2

KAZIMIERZ

WĘGLOWA

PLAC WOLNICA

BOCHEŃSKA

GAZOWA

PODGÓRSKA

Most Powstańców Śląskich

Kraków Zabłocie

Museum of Contemporary Art (MOCAK)

Kazimierz Town Hall

MOSTOWA

KRAKOWSKA

TRYNITARSKA

Hospital of the Order of St John of God

NADWIŚLAŃSKA

MŁYNARSKA

SOLNA

KĄCIK

JANOWA WOLA

LIPOWA

R. TRAUGUTTA

Schindler's Factory

Church of the Order of St John of God

Most Kładka Ojca Bernatka

PIWNA

KRAKUSA

PLAC BOHATERÓW GETTA

TARGOWA

DĄBRÓWKI

RYBAKI

JÓZEFIŃSKA

NA ZJEŹDZIE

LWOWSKA

Most J. Piłsudskiego

LEGIONÓW

K. BRODZIŃSKIEGO

STAROMOSTOWA

CELNA

B. LIMANOWSKIEGO

J. H. DĄBROWSKIEGO

3

Vistula

PLAC E. SERKOWSKIEGO

PRZY MOŚCIE

WŁ. SOKOLSKA

WL. WARNEŃCZYKA

T. REJTANA

RYNEK PODGÓRSKI

WĘGIERSKA

KRAKUSA

RĘKAWKA

WIELICKA

SW. KINGI

J. TARNOWSKIEGO

DŁUGOSZA

STROMA

SMOLKI

JANA ZAMOYSKIEGO

PLAC NIEPODLEGŁOŚCI

PARKOWA

PL. LASOTY

A. STWARZA

AL. E. DĘBOWSKIEGO

ROBOTNICZA

RZEŹBY

MARYJSKA

SMOLKI

PARK W. BEDNARSKIEGO

KRAKA

RADOSNA

ZA TOREM

AL. POD KOPCEM

F. MARIEWSKIEGO

REDEM

PTORYSTÓW

KRZEMIONKI

PODGÓRZE

KRAKUS MOUND

4

PODSKALE

JANA ZAMOJSKIEGO

TV Kraków

POWSTAŃCÓW ŚLĄSKICH

H. KAMIEŃSKIEGO

CZYŻÓWKA

S W O S Z O W I C K A

5

ŁAGIEWNICKA

GRZYBKI

D · **E** · **F**

SEE MAPS 5–6 FOR ENLARGEMENT OF THIS AREA

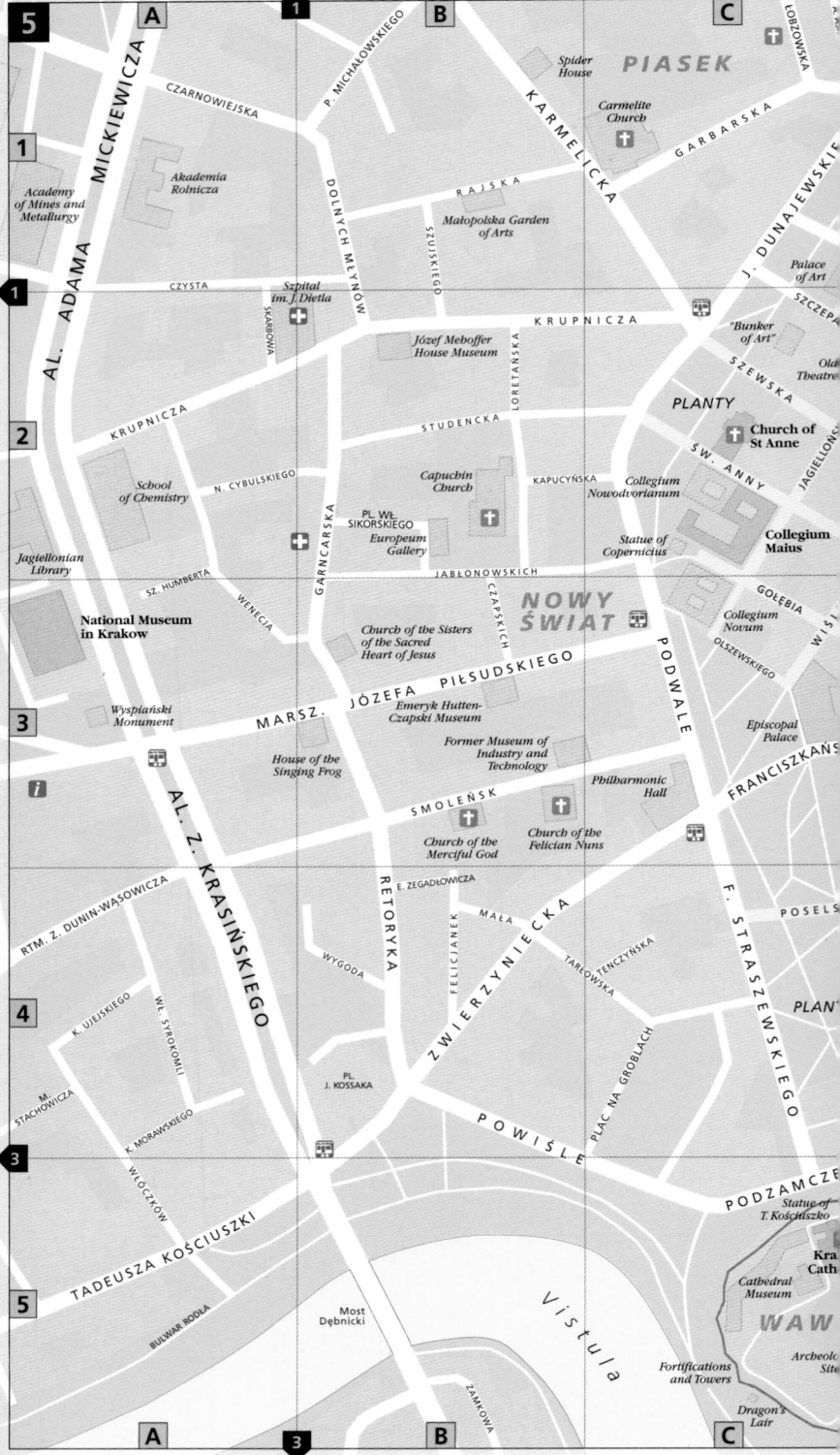

5

A · **1** · B · C

1 Academy of Mines and Metallurgy

CZARNOWIEJSKA

AL. ADAMA MICKIEWICZA

P. MICHAŁOWSKIEGO

Akademia Rolnicza

DOLNYCH MŁYNÓW

SZUJSKIEGO

Spider House

PIASEK

ŁOBZOWSKA

KARMELICKA

Carmelite Church

GARBARSKA

RAJSKA

Małopolska Garden of Arts

J. DUNAJEWSKIE

Palace of Art

SZCZEPA

1 CZYSTA

SKARBOWA

Szpital im. J. Dietla

KRUPNICZA

"Bunker of Art"

SZEWSKA

Old Theatre

Józef Mehoffer House Museum

LORETAŃSKA

PLANTY

2 KRUPNICZA

STUDENCKA

ŚW. ANNY

Church of St Anne

JAGIELLOŃS

N. CYBULSKIEGO

School of Chemistry

Capuchin Church

KAPUCYŃSKA

Collegium Nowodvorianum

GARNCARSKA

PL. WŁ. SIKORSKIEGO

Europeum Gallery

Statue of Copernicus

Collegium Maius

Jagiellonian Library

SZ. HUMBERTA

WENECJA

JABŁONOWSKICH

CZAPSKICH

NOWY ŚWIAT

GOŁĘBIA

Collegium Novum

W. SI

OLSZEWSKIEGO

National Museum in Krakow

Church of the Sisters of the Sacred Heart of Jesus

PODWALE

3 Wyspiański Monument

MARSZ. JÓZEFA PIŁSUDSKIEGO

Emeryk Hutten-Czapski Museum

Episcopal Palace

FRANCISZKAŃS

AL. Z. KRASIŃSKIEGO

House of the Singing Frog

Former Museum of Industry and Technology

Philharmonic Hall

i

SMOLEŃSK

Church of the Merciful God

Church of the Felician Nuns

3

E. ZEGADŁOWICZA

POSELS

RTM. Z. DUNIN-WĄSOWICZA

RETORYKA

FELICJANEK

MAŁA

TENCZYŃSKA

TARŁOWSKA

F. STRASZEWSKIEGO

PLAN

K. UJEJSKIEGO

WŁ. SYROKOMLI

WYGODA

ZWIERZYNIECKA

4 M. STACHOWICZA

K. MORAWSKIEGO

PL. J. KOSSAKA

PLAC NA GROBLACH

POWIŚLE

PODZAMCZE

WŁÓCZKÓW

Statue of T. Kościuszko

3

TADEUSZA KOŚCIUSZKI

Kra Cath

Cathedral Museum

5 BULWAR RODŁA

Most Dębnicki

ZAMKOWA

Vistula

WAW

Archeolo Site

Fortifications and Towers

Dragon's Lair

A · **3** · B · C

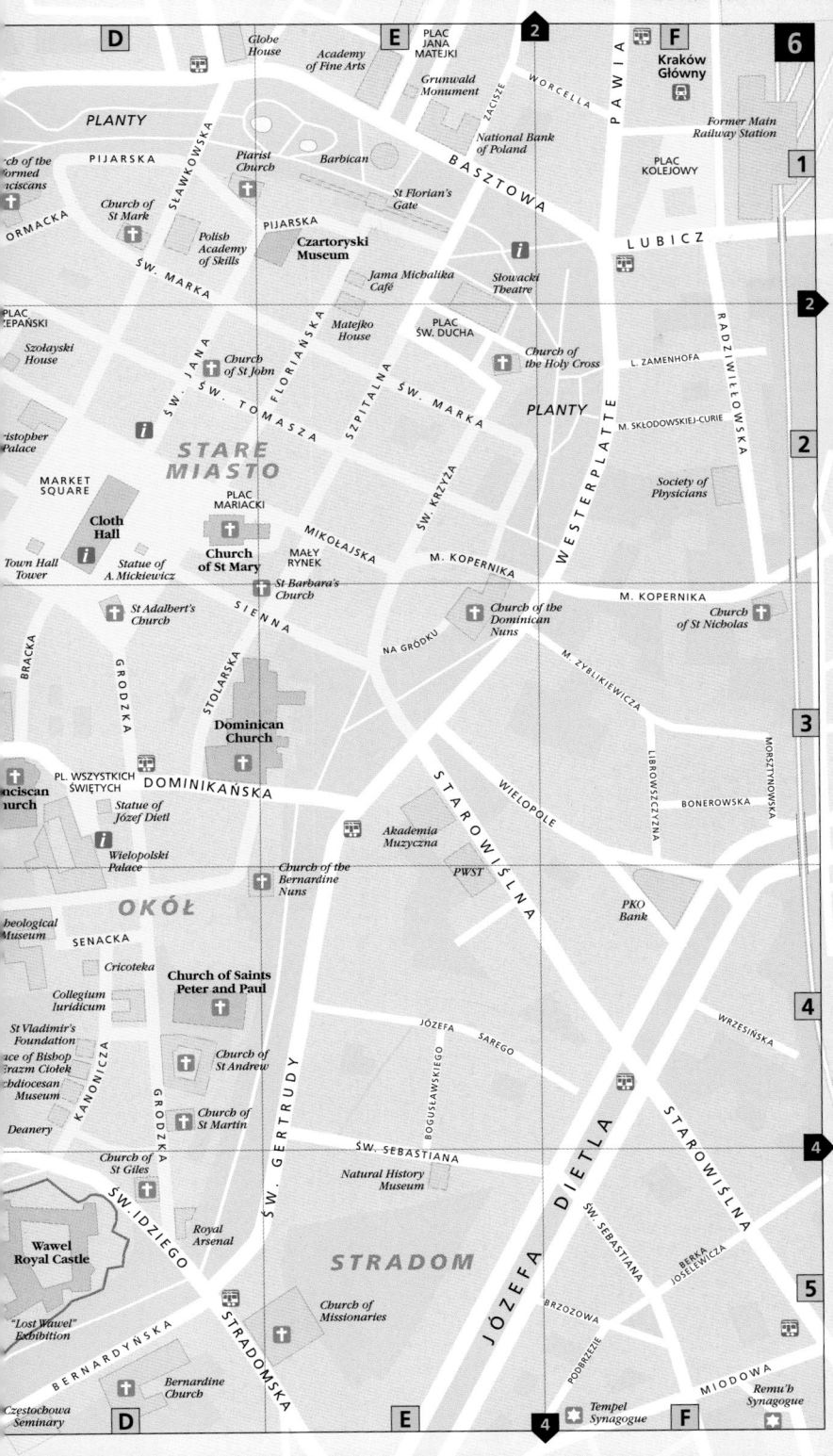

D | **E** | PLAC JANA MATEJKI | **2** | **F** | **6**

Globe House
Academy of Fine Arts
Grunwald Monument
Kraków Główny
PLANTY
PIJARSKA
Piarist Church
Barbican
National Bank of Poland
Former Main Railway Station
ch of the formed nciscans
ORMACKA
Church of St Mark
Polish Academy of Skills
PIJARSKA
St Florian's Gate
BASZTOWA
ZACISZE
WORCELLA
PAWIA
PLAC KOLEJOWY **1**
ŚW. MARKA
Czartoryski Museum
Jama Michalika Café
Słowacki Theatre
LUBICZ
PLAC ĆEPAŃSKI
Szołayski House
SW. JANA
Church of St John
Matejko House
PLAC ŚW. DUCHA
Church of the Holy Cross
L. ZAMENHOFA
i
RADZIWIŁŁOWSKA **2**
ristopher Palace
ŚW. TOMASZA
FLORIAŃSKA
SZPITALNA
ŚW. MARKA
PLANTY
M. SKŁODOWSKIEJ-CURIE
WESTERPLATTE
i
STARE MIASTO
MARKET SQUARE
PLAC MARIACKI
Church of St Mary
MIKOŁAJSKA
ŚW. KRZYŻA
M. KOPERNIKA
Society of Physicians **2**
Cloth Hall
i
Statue of A. Mickiewicz
Town Hall Tower
MAŁY RYNEK
St Barbara's Church
St Adalbert's Church
SIENNA
NA GRÓDKU
Church of the Dominican Nuns
M. KOPERNIKA
Church of St Nicholas
BRACKA
GRODZKA
STOLARSKA
Dominican Church
M. ZYBLIKIEWICZA
LIBROWSZCZYZNA
BONEROWSKA
MORSZTYNOWSKA **3**
PL. WSZYSTKICH ŚWIĘTYCH
nciscan urch
DOMINIKAŃSKA
Statue of Józef Dietl
i
Wielopolski Palace
OKÓŁ
STAROWIŚLNA
WIELOPOLE
Akademia Muzyczna
Church of the Bernardine Nuns
PWST
PKO Bank **4**
beological Museum
SENACKA
Cricoteka
Collegium Iuridicum
St Vladimir's Foundation
ace of Bishop razm Ciołek
chdiocesan Museum
Deanery
Church of Saints Peter and Paul
Church of St Andrew
Church of St Martin
KANONICZA
GRODZKA
ŚW. GERTRUDY
JÓZEFA
SAREGO
BOGUSŁAWSKIEGO
WRZESIŃSKA
Church of St Giles
ŚW. IDZIEGO
Royal Arsenal
ŚW. SEBASTIANA
Natural History Museum
JÓZEFA DIETLA
STAROWIŚLNA **4**
Wawel Royal Castle
"Lost Wawel" Exhibition
STRADOM
ŚW. SEBASTIANA
BERKA JOSELEWICZA
BRZOZOWA **5**
BERNARDYŃSKA
STRADOMSKA
Bernardine Church
Church of Missionaries
Czestochowa Seminary
D
Bernardine Church
E
PODBRZEZIE
Tempel Synagogue
MIODOWA
Remu'h Synagogue
F
4

General Index

Acknowledgments

Dorling Kindersley would like to thank the following people whose assistance has made the preparation of this book possible.

Managing Editor Helen Townsend
Managing Art Editor Kate Poole
Senior Managing Editor Louise B. Lang
Art Director Gillian Allan
Additional Photography Jakub Hałun, Jamie Howard, Krzysztof Kotowski, Piotr Kozłowski, Wojciech Kozłowski, Ian O'Leary, Kamil Szymaczek.
Revisions Team Claire Baranowski, Sonal Bhatt, Hilary Bird, Jonathan Bousfield, Arwen Burnett, Caroline Elliker, Eli Estaugh, Rhiannon Furbear, Lydia Halliday, Victoria Heyworth-Dunne, Elly King, Piotr Kozłowski, Ferdie McDonald, Gordon McLachlan, Casper Morris, Scarlett O'Hara, Catherine Palmi, Susie Peachey, Rada Radojicic, Simon Ryder, Sands Publishing Solutions, Sadie Smith, Jamie Stokes, Leah Tether, Conrad Van Dyk, Vinita Venugopal, Deepika Verma, Stewart J. Wild.

Dorling Kindersley wish to thank the following institutions, picture libraries and individuals for their kind permission to reproduce photographs of objects in their care and for the use of other photographic material:

Magdalena Maros the Director, and Krystyna Litewka at the Public Record State Office, Krzysztof Zamorski, Director of the Jagiellonian Library, Stanisław Waltoś the Director, Lucyna Bełtowska and Robert Springwald at the Collegium Maius, Matejko House, St Vladimir Foundation, Katarzyna Bałus, Princes Czartoryski Foundation, Jama Michalika, Prelate Janusz Bielański, Krakow Cathedral and Cathedral Museum, Church of the Bernardine Nuns, Bernardine Church, Father Mirosław Pilśniak, OP, Dominican Church, Sister Wanda Batko, Church of the Felician Nuns, Brother Bogumił Stachowicz, OFM, Franciscan Church, Father Edward Stoch, SJ, Jesuit Church in Wesoła, Capuchin Church, Father Dr Bronisław Fidelus, Church of St Mary, Father Jan Mazur, Paulite Church "On the Rock", Church of St Anne, Father Henryk Dziadosz, Church of St Barbara, Church of St Florian, Church of St Catherine, Church of the Holy Cross, Church of St Mark, Church of St Peter and St Paul, Church of St Vincent, Wieliczka Salt Mine, Father Dr Józef A. Nowobilski, the Metropolitan Curia and Archdiocesan Museum, Balice Airport, Archaeological Museum, Andrzej Szczygieł, Director of the Museum of Krakow, Anna Studnicka, National Museum, Natural History Museum, Zbigniew Święcicki the Director, and Mirosław Ciunowicz at the Polish Military Museum in Warsaw, PAP Polish Press Agency, Society of Physicians, Pieskowa Skała Castle.

Dorling Kindersley are grateful to the following individuals for their kind permission to reproduce their photographs:
Jacek Bednarczyk, Olaf Beer, Maja Florczykowska, Michał Grychowski, Stanisława Jabłońska, Dorota i Mariusz Jarymowiczowie, Beata i Mariusz Kowalewscy, Grzegorz Kozakiewicz, Wojciech Mędrzak, Stanisław Michta, Hanna i Maciej Musiałowie, Tomasz Robaczyński, Maciej Sochor, Jan Zych.

All the dishes whose photographs feature in this guide were prepared in the restaurant Pod Aniołami. We wish to thank the owner, Jacek Łodziński for his help. We are also grateful to Marcin Duszyński, Madropol for his kind assistance.

Key: a=above; b=below/bottom; c=centre; f=far; l=left; r=right; t=top.

Works of art have been reproduced with the permission of the following copyright holders: © ADAGP, Paris and DACS, London 2011

collegium luridicum by Igor Mitoraj 78tr. **123RF.com:** kaetana 80tl; qumran 153tl.
AKG-Images: 20; 163cr; Ullstein Bild-KPA/HIP/Jewish Chronicle Ltd 127br. **Alamy Images:** AA World Travel Library 170bl; David Crausby 218cr; David Sanger Photography/David Sanger 187tl; Kevin Foy 126tl, 187c; Kevin George 113bc; Karolek 10cr; kpzfoto 135br; lookGaleria 11bl, 127cb; Look Studio 90tl; G Owston (Poland) 222tl; Pegaz 76, 211bl; Magdalena Rehova 166; David Robertson 74-75; Sherab 120; Paul Springett 72clb; Peter Svarc 10bl; Krystyna Szulecka 186cl; Matthew Taylor 174-175; VIEW Pictures Ltd 147br; John Warburton-Lee Photography 40; Jan Włodarczyk 208-209. **Archaeological Museum:** 22clb, 22bc, 23cr, 23cb, 23bl, 42b. **The Art Archive:** Laurie Platt Winfrey 127cra. **Art Hotel Niebieski:** 179bl, 182tr. **Auschwitz-Birkenau Memorial & Museum:** 162tr, 162cl, 162bl, 163tc, 164clb, 165cr, 164br; Ryszard Domasik 162tl, 163crb, 164cla, 165tl, 165tr; Jarek Mensfelt 164tr. **AWL Images:** Katie Garrod 58-59. **Carlsberg polska:** Chris Biggs 189c. **Cathedral Museum:** 24–5c, 26cla, 27cla, 46cl, 62ca, 64c. **Collegium Maius:** 27cb, 33b, 108–9. **Cool Tour Company:** 224bl. **Copernicus Restaurant:** 185br. **Corbis:** Bettmann 127tl; Jon Hicks 74–5; Historical Picture Archive 126tr. **Czartoryski Museum:** 43t, 45b, 114–15. **CK Dezerter:** 190bc. **Del Papa:** 184c, 192tc. **Dreamstime.com:** Artur Bogacki 225tr; Roksana Bashyrova 93tl; Dimaberkut 12tr; Jorg Hackemann 19br; Mbonaparte 128bl; Krzysztof Nahlik 2-3, 154; Neirfy 13tr; Nightman1965 160tl; Puchan 211tr; Tatiana Savvateeva 60; Jacek Sopotnicki 13bl; Simon Thomas 227cla. **FM Dutton, uk:** 213cra. **Edyta Gawron:** 126br. **Encyclopaedia Judaica:** 126cl. **Flamingo Hostel:** 178tr. **Hotel Fortuna:** 176bl. **Hotel Galaxy:** 177bc, 181tr. **Groteska Theatre:** Anna Kaczmarz 212tr. **Jagiellonian Library:** 22–3c, 26clb, 28tl, 28cra, 28b, 32b, 32crb, 30br, 34cb, 152bl. **Dariusz Jedrzejewski:** 11tr. **Kraków Airport:** 220br; 221br. **Krakow Festival Office:** 210cr. **Matejko House:** 25cr. **Metropolitan Hotel Krakow:** 177tr, 183br. **MOCAK The Museum of Contemporary Art in Krakow:** Rafał Sosin 159tl. **Museum of Krakow:** 20, 21b, 29ca, 31cb, 36b, 37ca, 37cr, 42cr, 43cbr, 94tr, 101br; Emeryk Hutten Czapski Museum 148tr. **Muzeum Historyczne Miasta Krakowa:** Ignacy Krieger 126clb, 126cb, 126crb. **National Museum:** 8–9, 24bc, 25tc, 26b, 27cr, 31br, 32bl, 32–3c, 33cr, 34tc, 34–5c, 35t, 35tr, 36cl, 36–7c, 39bl, 42tr, 43tcl, 43c, 45t, 52cl, 53tl, 52cl, 104tr, 104c, 105, 112cl, 149l. **Natural History Museum:** 45c; **Novotel Krakow Centrum:** 177tr. **Pimiento Argentino:** 185tl, 191tr. **PKO Bank Polski:** Wojciech Czerniewicz 216c, 216bl. **Pod Baranemi:** 203tr. **Polskibus.com:** 223br. **Polski Hotel Pod Bialym Orlem:** 176cra, 180bl. **Polskie Koleje Panstwowe S.A.:** PKP InterCity 222br. **Public Record State Office:** 26–7c, 26bl. **Robert Harding Picture Library:** Bennet Dean 12bc, Henryk T. Kaiser 107tl, 130. **Secret Garden Hotel:** 178bl. **Sheraton Krakow Hotel:** 179tl. **The Olive 193br, SomePlace Else 184bl. **STA Travel Group:** 212cr. **SuperStock:** age fotostock / age fotostock 156tl, Henryk T. Kaiser / age fotostock 142. **Tel Aviv Museum of Art:** Jews Praying in the Synagogue on Yom Kippur by Maurycy Gottlieb, oil on canvas, gift of Sydney Lamon, New York 126–7c; **Telekomunikacja Polska:** 218c. **Topfoto.co.uk:** Roger-Viollet 165br. **Urzad Miasta Krakowa:** P. Krawczyk 226tr. **Hotel Wyspianski:** 179tr. s Żywiec group: 189cl; 189fcl.
Front Endpapers: Alamy Images: Look Studio Lclba; Pegaz Rc; Sherab Rcr. **Dreamstime.com:** Tatiana Savvateeva Lcrb. **Robert Harding Picture Library:** Henryk T. Kaiser Rtr. **SuperStock:** Henryk T. Kaiser / age fotostock Lcla.

Sheet Map Cover - Superstock: Travel Library Limited.
Jacket
Front main and spine t – Superstock: Travel Library Limited.

All other images ©Dorling Kindersley.
For further information see: www.dkimages.com

Phrase Book

Summary of Pronunciation in Polish

ą a nasal *"awn"* as in *"sawn"* or *"an"* as in the French *"Anjou"* but barely sounded
c *"ts"* as in *"bats"*
ć, cz *"ch"* as in *"challenge"*
ch *"ch"* as in Scottish *"loch"*
dz *"j"* as in *"jeans"* when followed by **i** or **e** but otherwise *"dz"* as in *"adze"*
dź *"j"* as in *"jeans"*
dż *"d"* as in *"dog"* followed by *"s"* as in *"leisure"*
ę similar to *"en"* in *"end"* only nasal and barely sounded, but if at the end of the word pronounced *"e"* as in *"bed"*
h *"ch"* as in Scottish *"loch"*
i *"ee"* as in *"teeth"*
j *"y"* as in yes
ł *"w"* as in *"window"*
ń similar to the *"ni"* in *"companion"*
ó *"oo"* as in *"soot"*
rz similar to the *"s"* in *"leisure"* or, when it follows **p, t** or **k**, *"sh"* as in *"shut"*
ś, sz *"sh"* as in *"shut"*
w *"v"* as in *"vine"*
y similar to the *"i"* in *"bit"*
ź, ż similar to the *"s"* in *"leisure"*

Emergencies

Help!	**pomocy!**	*pomotsi*
Call a doctor!	**zawołać doktora!**	*zawowach doctora*
Call an ambulance!	**zadzwonić po pogotowie!**	*zadzvoneech po pogotovee*
Police!	**policja!**	*poleetsya*
Call the fire brigade!	**zadzwonić po straż pożarną!**	*zadzvoneech po stras posarnAWN*
Where is the nearest phone?	**Gdzie jest najbliższa budka telefoniczna?**	*gjeh yest nIbleezhsha boodka telefoneechna*
Where is the hospital?	**Gdzie jest szpital?**	*gjeh yest shpeetal*
Where is the police station	**Gdzie jest posterunek policji?**	*gjeh yest posterunek politsyee*

Communication Essentials

Yes	**Tak**	*tak*
No	**Nie**	*n-yeh*
Thank you	**Dziękuję**	*jENkoo-yeh*
No thank you	**Nie, dziękuję**	*n-yej jENkoo-yeh*
Please	**Proszę**	*prosheh*
I don't understand.	**Nie rozumiem.**	*n-yeh rozoom-yem*
Do you speak English? (to a man)	**Czy mówi pan po angielsku?**	*chi moovee pan po ang-yelskoo*
Do you speak English? (to a woman)	**Czy mówi pani po angielsku?**	*chi moovee panee po ang-yelskoo*
Please speak more slowly	**Proszę mówić wolniej.**	*proseh mooveech voln-yay*
Please write it down for me.	**Proszę mi to napisać.**	*prosheh mee to napeesach*
My name is…	**Nazywam się…**	*nazivam sheh*

Useful Words and Phrases

Pleased to meet you (to a man)	**Bardzo mi miło pana poznać**	*bardzo mee meewo pana poznach*
Pleased to meet you (to a woman)	**Bardzo mi miło pania poznać**	*bardzo mee meewo pan-yAWN poznach*
Good morning	**Dzień dobry**	*jen-yuh dobri*
Good afternoon	**Dzień dobry**	*jen-yuh dobri*
Good evening	**Dobry wieczór**	*dobri v-yechoor*

Good night	**Dobranoc**	*dobranots*
Goodbye	**Do widzenia**	*do veedzen-ya*
What time is it…?	**Która jest godzina?**	*ktoora yest gojeena*
Cheers!	**Na zdrowie!**	*na zdrov-yeh*
Excellent!	**Wspaniale**	*wspan-yaleh*

Shopping

Do you have…? (to a man)	**Czy ma pan…?**	*che ma pan*
Do you have…? (to a woman)	**Czy ma pani…?**	*che ma panee*
How much is this?	**Ile to kosztuje?**	*eeleh to koshtoo-yeh*
Where is the… department?	**Gdzie jest dział z…?**	*gjeh yest jawuh z*
Do you take credit cards? (to a man)	**Czy przyjmuje pan karty kredytowe?**	*chi pshi-yuhmoo-yeh pan karti kreditoveh*
Do you take credit cards? (to a woman)	**Czy przyjmuje pani karty kredytowe?**	*chi pshi-yuhmoo-yeh panee karti kreditoveh*
bakery	**piekarnia**	*p-yekarn-ya*
bookshop	**księgarnia**	*kshENgarn-ya*
chemist	**apteka**	*apteka*
department store	**dom towarowy**	*dom tovarovi*
exchange office	**kantor walutowy**	*kantor valootovi*
travel agent	**biuro podróży**	*b-yooro podroozhi*
post office	**poczta,**	*pochta*
	urząd pocztowy	*ooZHAWNd pochtovi*
postcard	**pocztówka**	*pochtoovka*
stamp	**znaczek**	*znachek*
How much is a postcard to…?	**Ile kosztuje pocztówka do…?**	*eeleh koshtoo-yeh pochtoovka do*
airmail	**poczta lotnicza**	*pochta lotneecha*

Staying in a Hotel

Have you any vacancies? (to a man)	**Czy ma pan wolne pokoje?**	*chi ma pan volneh poko-yeh*
Have you any vacancies? (to a woman)	**Czy ma pani wolne pokoje?**	*chi ma panee volneh poko-yeh*
What is the charge per night?	**Ile kosztuje za dobę?**	*eeleh koshtoo-yeh za dobeh*
I'd like a single room.	**Poproszę pokój jednoosobowy.**	*poprosheh pokoo-yuh yedno-osobovi*
I'd like a double room.	**Poproszę pokój dwuosobowy.**	*poprosheh pokoo-yuh dvoo-osobovi*
I'd like a twin room.	**Poproszę pokój z dwoma łóżkami.**	*poprosheh pokoo-yuh z dvoma woozhkamee*
I'd like a room with a bathroom.	**Poproszę pokój z łazienką.**	*poprosheh pokoo-yuh z wazhenkAWN*
bathroom	**łazienka**	*wazhenka*
bed	**łóżko**	*woozhko*
bill	**rachunek**	*raHoonek*
breakfast	**śniadanie**	*shn-yadan-yeh*
dinner	**kolacja**	*kolats-ya*
double room	**pokój dwuosobowy**	*pokoo-yuh dvoo-osobovi*
full board	**pełne utrzymanie**	*pewuhneh ootzhiman-yeh*
guest house	**zajazd**	*za-yazd*
half board	**dwa posiłki dziennie**	*dva posheewuhkee jen-yeh*
key	**klucz**	*klooch*
restaurant	**restauracja**	*restawrats-ya*
shower	**prysznic**	*prishneets*
single room	**pokój jednoosobowy**	*pokoo-yuh yedno-osobovi*
toilet	**toaleta**	*to-aleta*

Eating Out

A table for one, please.	**Stolik dla jednej osoby proszę.**	*stoleek dla yednay osobi prosheh*
A table for two, please.	**Stolik dla dwóch osób proszę.**	*stoleek dla dvooh osoob prosheh*
Can I see the menu?	**Mogę prosić jadłospis?**	*mogeh prosheech yadwospees*

Can I see the wine list?	**Mogę prosić kartę win?**	*mogeh prosheech karteh veen*
I'd like…	**Proszę**	*prosheh*
Can we have the bill, please?	**Proszę rachunek?**	*prosheh raHoonek*
Where is the toilet?	**Gdzie jest toaleta?**	*gjeh yest to-aleta*

Menu Decoder

baranina	mutton, lamb
barszcz czerwony	beetroot soup
bażant	pheasant
befsztyk	beef steak
bigos	hunter's stew *(sweet and sour cabbage with a variety of meats and seasonings)*
bukiet z jarzyn	a variety of raw and pickled vegetables
ciasto	cake, pastry
cielęcina	veal
cukier	sugar
cukierek	sweet, confectionery
dania mięsne	meat dishes
dania rybne	fish dishes
dania z drobiu	poultry dishes
deser	dessert
flaki	tripe
grzybki marynowane	marinated mushrooms
herbata	tea
jarzyny	vegetables
kabanos	dry, smoked pork sausage
kaczka	duck
kapusta	cabbage
kartofle	potatoes
kasza gryczana	buckwheat
kaszanka	black pudding
kawa	coffee
kiełbasa	sausage
klopsiki	minced meat balls
lody	ice cream
łosoś	salmon
łosoś wędzony	smoked salmon
makowiec	poppy seed cake
naleśniki	pancakes
piernik	spiced honeycake
pierogi	ravioli-like dumplings
piwo	beer
prawdziwki	ceps (type of mushroom)
przystawki	entrées
pstrąg	trout
rolmopsy	rollmop herrings
sałatka	salad
sałatka owocowa	fruit salad
sok	juice
sok jabłkowy	apple juice
sok owocowy	fruit juice
sól	salt
śledź	herring
tort	cake, gâteau
wieprzowina	pork
wino	wine
woda	water
ziemniaki	potatoes
zupa	soup

Health

I do not feel well.	**Źle się czuję.**	*zhleh sheh choo-yeh*
I need a prescription for…	**Potrzebuję receptę na…**	*potzheboo-yeh retsepteh na*
cold	**przeziębienie**	*pshef-yENb-yen-yeh*
cough (noun)	**kaszel**	*kashel*
cut	**skaleczenie**	*skalechen-yeh*
flu	**grypa**	*gripa*
hayfever	**katar sienny**	*katar shyienny*
headache pills	**proszki od bólu głowy**	*proshkee od booloo gwovi*
hospital	**szpital**	*shpeetal*
nausea	**mdłości**	*mudwosh-che*
sore throat	**ból gardła**	*bool gardwa*

Travel and Transport

When is the next train to…?	**Kiedy jest następny pociąg do…?**	*k-yedi yest nastENpni pochAWNg do…*
What is the fare to…?	**Ile kosztuje bilet do…?**	*eeleh koshtoo-yeh beelet do*

A single ticket to … please	**Proszę bilet w jedną stronę bilet do…**	*prosheh beelet v yednAWN stroneh beelet do*
A return ticket to … please	**Proszę bilet w obie strony do…**	*prosheh beelet v obye strony do*
Where is the bus station?	**Gdzie jest dworzec autobusowy?**	*gjeh yest dvozhets awtoboosovi*
Where is the bus stop?	**Gdzie jest przystanek autobusowy?**	*gjeh yest pshistanek awtoboosovi*
Where is the tram stop?	**Gdzie jest przystanek tramwajowy?**	*gjeh yest pshistanek tramvi-yovi*
booking office	**kasa biletowa**	*kasa beeletova*
station	**stacja**	*stats-ya*
timetable	**rozkład jazdy**	*rozkwad yazdi*
left luggage	**przechowalnia bagażu**	*psheHovaln-ya bagazhoo*
platform	**peron**	*peron*
first class	**pierwsza klasa**	*p-yervsha klasa*
second class	**druga klasa**	*drooga klasa*
single ticket	**bilet w jedną stronę**	*beelet v jednAWN stroneh*
return ticket	**bilet powrotny**	*beelet povrotni*
airline	**linia lotnicza**	*leen-ya lotna-yeecha*
airport	**lotnisko**	*lotn-yeesko*
arrival	**przylot**	*pshilot*
flight number	**numer lotu**	*noomer lotoo*
gate	**przejście**	*pshaysh-cheh*
coach (bus)	**autokar**	*awtokar*

Numbers

0	**zero**	*zero*
1	**jeden**	*yeden*
2	**dwa**	*dva*
3	**trzy**	*tshi*
4	**cztery**	*chteri*
5	**pięc**	*p-yENch*
6	**sześć**	*shesh-ch*
7	**siedem**	*sh-yedem*
8	**osiem**	*oshem*
9	**dziewięć**	*jev-yENch*
10	**dziesięć**	*jeshEnch*
11	**jedenaście**	*yedenash-cheh*
12	**dwanaście**	*dvanash-cheh*
13	**trzynaście**	*tshinash-cheh*
14	**czternaście**	*chternash-cheh*
15	**piętnaście**	*p-yENtnash-cheh*
16	**szesnaście**	*shesnash-cheh*
17	**siedemnaście**	*shedemnash-cheh*
18	**osiemnaście**	*oshemnash-cheh*
19	**dziewiętnaście**	*jev-yENtnash-cheh*
20	**dwadzieścia**	*dvajesh-cha*
21	**dwadzieścia jeden**	*dvajesh-cha yeden*
22	**dwadzieścia dwa**	*dvajesh-cha dva*
30	**trzydzieści**	*tshijesh-chee*
40	**czterdzieści**	*chterjesh-chee*
50	**pięćdziesiąt**	*p-yENchjeshAWNt*
100	**sto**	*sto*
200	**dwieście**	*dv-yesh-cheh*
500	**pięćset**	*p-yENchset*
1,000	**tysiąc**	*tishAWNts*
1,000,000	**milion**	*meel-yon*

Time

today	**dzisiaj**	*jeeshl*
yesterday	**wczoraj**	*vchorl*
tomorrow	**jutro**	*yootro*
tonight	**dzisiejszej nocy**	*jeeshAYshay notsi*
one minute	**jedna minuta**	*yedna meenoota*
half an hour	**pół godziny**	*poowuh gojeeni*
hour	**godzina**	*gojeena*

Days of the Week

Sunday	**niedziela**	*n-yejela*
Monday	**poniedziałek**	*pon-yejawek*
Tuesday	**wtorek**	*vtorek*
Wednesday	**środa**	*shroda*
Thursday	**czwartek**	*chvartek*
Friday	**piątek**	*p-yAWNtek*
Saturday	**sobota**	*sobota*

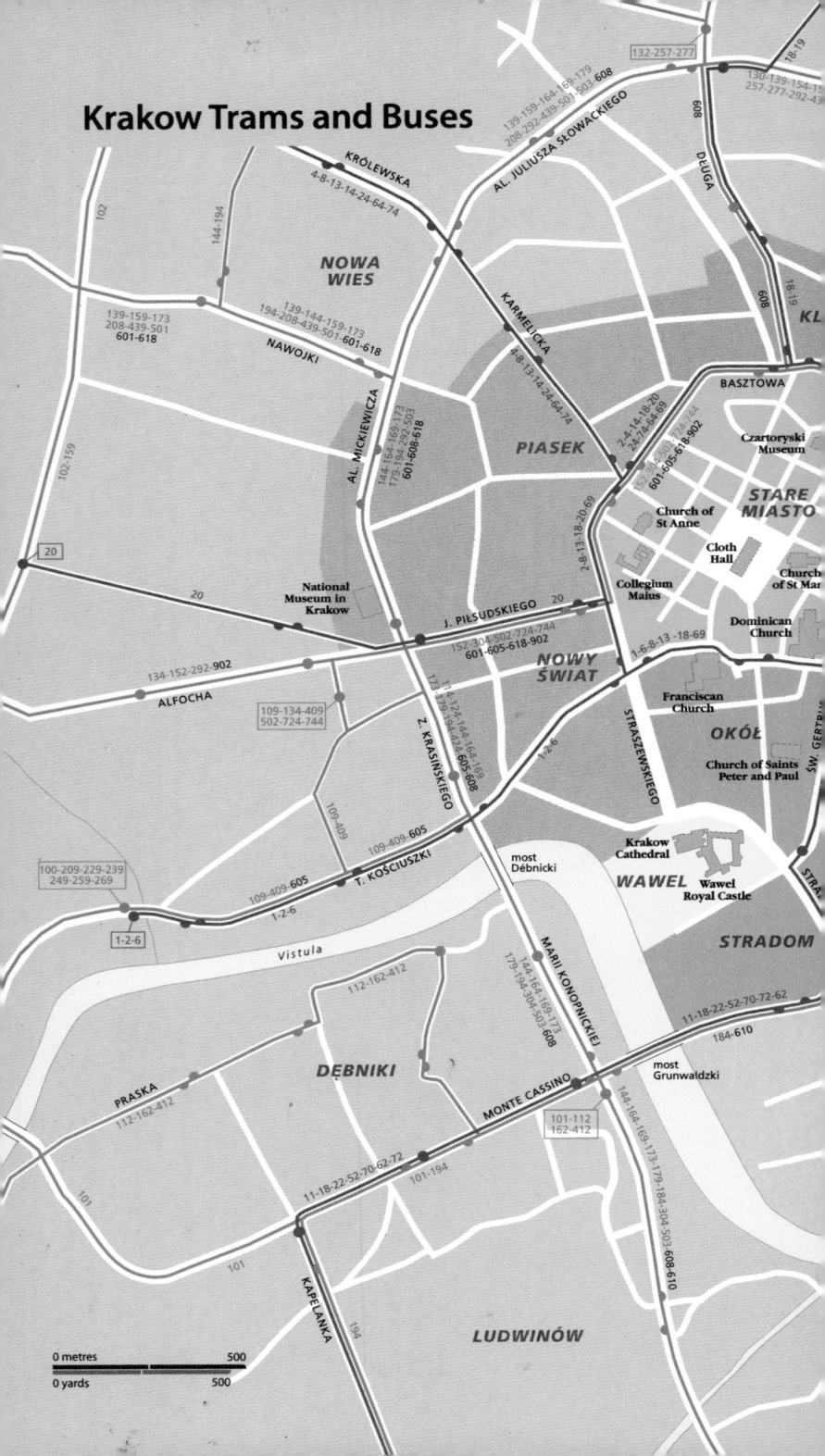

Krakow Trams and Buses

NOWA WIES

KRÓLEWSKA

4-8-13-14-24-64-74

AL. JULIUSZA SŁOWACKIEGO

139-159-164-169-179
208-292-439-501-503-608

132-257-277

130-139-154-173
257-277-292-439

18-19

DŁUGA

608

KL

18-19

102

144-194

144-194

139-159-173
208-439-501
601-618

139-144-159-173
194-208-439-501-601-618

NAWOJKI

KARMELICKA

BASZTOWA

4-8-13-14-24-64-74

AL. MICKIEWICZA

144-164-169-173
179-194-292-503
601-608-618

PIASEK

2-4-14-18-20
24-74-64-69

Czartoryski
Museum

STARE
MIASTO

601-605-618-902

Church of
St Anne

Cloth
Hall

Church
of St Mary

102-159

20

20

National
Museum in
Krakow

J. PIŁSUDSKIEGO

2-8-13-18-70-69

Collegium
Maius

20

152-304-502-724-744
601-605-618-902

Dominican
Church

1-6-8-13-18-69

134-152-292-902

ALFOCHA

109-134-409
502-724-744

173-179-144-164-169
11-124-144-164-169
601-605-608

NOWY
ŚWIAT

Franciscan
Church

STRASZEWSKIEGO

OKÓŁ

SW. GERTRUDY

109-409

Z. KRASIŃSKIEGO

1-2-6

Church of Saints
Peter and Paul

100-209-229-239
249-259-269

109-409-605

T. KOŚCIUSZKI

most
Dębnicki

Krakow
Cathedral

WAWEL

Wawel
Royal Castle

STRA

1-2-6

109-409-605
1-2-6

Vistula

STRADOM

112-162-412

MARII KONOPNICKIEJ

144-164-169-173
179-194-304-503-608

11-18-22-52-70-72-62

184-610

PRASKA

112-162-412

DĘBNIKI

MONTE CASSINO

most
Grunwaldzki

101-112
162-412

144-164-169-173-179-184-304-503-608-610

101

11-18-22-52-70-62-72

101-194

KAPELANKA

194

LUDWINÓW

0 metres   500
0 yards   500